TEXTBOOK OF NEUROPATHOLOGY

TEXTBOOK OF NEUROPATHOLOGY

RICHARD L. DAVIS, M.D.

Professor
Department of Pathology
University of California, San Francisco
San Francisco, California

DAVID M. ROBERTSON, M.D.

Professor and Head
Department of Pathology
Queen's University
Kingston, Ontario

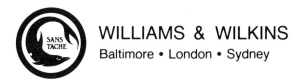

WILLIAMS & WILKINS
Baltimore • London • Sydney

Editor: George Stamathis
Associate Editor: Joseph E. Seitz
Copy Editor: Andrea Clemente
Design: JoAnne Janowiak
Illustration Planning: Wayne Hubbel
Production: Anne G. Seitz

Accurate indications, adverse reactions, and dosage schedules for drugs are provided
in this book, but it is possible that they may change. The reader is urged to review
the package information data of the manufacturers of the medications mentioned.

Made in the United States of America

Library of Congress Cataloging in Publication Data

Main entry under title:

Textbook of neuropathology.

   Includes bibliographies and index.
   1. Nervous system—Diseases. I. Davis, Richard L. II. Robertson, David M.
[DNLM: 1. Nervous System Diseases. WL 100 G326]
RC347.G46 1985   616.8   84-11882
ISBN 0-683-02343-8

Composed and printed at the
Waverly Press, Inc.

Dedicated to
those who taught us Neuropathology

Preface

The decision to write this volume was not lightly taken. The need for an authoritative text in general neuropathology was obvious, but it was recognized from the beginning that producing a text that would be useful to general pathologists, neurosurgeons, neurologists, as well as neuropathologists would not be an easy task. Further, if the volume was to be reasonably up-to-date it must be produced rapidly so that the textual material was not outdated at the time of publication. Exploratory talks were held with numerous colleagues from the North American continent and from overseas, and there was uniform encouragement for the project. At the same time we consulted with a number of possible publishers and one of them, Williams & Wilkins, strongly supported the concept.

Of importance, we believe, was the manner in which we selected contributors for the various chapters. Expertise in neuropathology and in the area of the particular chapter was of great significance, but we felt it equally imperative that the individual be willing and able to write in an interesting and clear manner. To this end we roughed out a table of contents with major areas and subdivisions and then looked for some novel approaches that would make the book more valuable and give greater insight into at least some of the problems of modern neuropathology. We then compiled lists of individuals with particular expertise in these areas and through personal knowledge, a review of some of their written work, or through recommendations of colleagues, or some combination of these determined which individuals would meet the criteria of both expertise and an ability to write interestingly and well. Some of the authors had particular viewpoints relative to their subject; we asked that they present a balanced description and discussion of other possible interpretations while indicating their own preference. Further, although we developed a uniform structure for the chapters, we did not attempt to impose rigorous uniformity on style or content, preferring the refreshing variety of approaches spontaneously used by our authors.

Our next consideration was what to include, and therefore, what would not be covered. It seemed to us and those we consulted that a number of areas of neuropathology had been recently and expertly addressed in quality texts, and that repetition of coverage would be expensive both to produce and to buy. Thus we decided not to include nervous system neoplasms, peripheral nerve pathology, and diseases of skeletal muscle in this text.

With the final decision to go ahead, it seemed that the book would have clear sailing. This early optimism did not take into account, however, the realities of academic life, and in the following months it seemed that almost everyone who had agreed to participate in the project for good reasons suffered delays in scheduling. Cautious persistence has, in the long run, paid off, and we are proud to present to the reader the results of the collaborative efforts of the authors, and, we know, many others. Throughout this effort we were given strong encouragement and support by Williams & Wilkins.

Finally we would like to give tribute to our families and particularly to our patient, tolerant wives who forgave us our absences, tolerated our depressed times, and shared with us our exhilaration as this product moved through its various phases.

Richard L. Davis, M.D.
David M. Robertson, M.D.

Contributors

Laurence E. Becker, M.D., F.R.C.P. (C)
Associate Professor of Pathology, University of Toronto; The Hospital for Sick Children, Toronto, Ontario, Canada

Richard L. Davis, M.D.
Professor of Pathology, Neurology, and Neurological Surgery, University of California, San Francisco, San Francisco, California

Clarisse L. Dolman, B.A., M.D., F.R.C.P.(C), F.R.C.Path.
Clinical Professor of Pathology, University of British Columbia; Vancouver General Hospital, Vancouver, British Columbia, Canada

Michael L. Dyer, M.D.
Fort Sanders Regional Medical Center, Knoxville, Tennessee

Julio H. Garcia, M.D.
Professor of Pathology, University of Alabama in Birmingham, Birmingham, Alabama

Floyd H. Gilles, M.D.
Burton E. Green, Professor of Pediatric Neuropathology, Childrens Hospital of Los Angeles; Professor of Pathology (Neuropathology), Neurosurgery, and Neurology, University of Southern California, Los Angeles, California

Jocelyn B. Gregorios, M.D.
Assistant Professor of Pathology and Neurology, University of Miami, Miami, Florida

John M. Hardman, M.D.
Professor of Pathology, University of Hawaii at Manoa, Honolulu, Hawaii

Asao Hirano, M.D.
Professor of Neuropathology and Neuroscience, Albert Einstein College of Medicine; Montefiore Medical Center, Bronx, New York

Jan E. Leestma, M.D.
Professor of Pathology, Northwestern University; Children's Memorial Hospital, Chicago, Illinois

Samuel K. Ludwin, M.D., B.Ch, F.R.C.P. (C)
Professor of Pathology (Neuropathology), Queen's University, Kingston, Ontario, Canada

J. Gordon McComb, M.D.
Associate Professor of Neurosurgery, University of Southern California; Head, Division of Neurosurgery, Childrens Hospital of Los Angeles, Los Angeles, California

Michael D. Norenberg, M.D.
Professor of Pathology and Neurology, University of Miami, Miami, Florida

Margaret G. Norman, M.D., F.R.C.P. (C)
Associate Professor of Pathology, University of British Columbia; British Columbia Children's Hospital, Vancouver, British Columbia, Canada

Joseph C. Parker, Jr., M.D.
Professor of Pathology and Medical Biology, University of Tennessee, Knoxville, Tennessee

David M. Robertson, M.D., F.R.C.P. (C)
Professor and Head, Department of Pathology, Queen's University, Kingston, Ontario, Canada

Cedric S. Raine, Ph.D., D.Sc.
Professor of Pathology (Neuropathology) and Neuroscience, Albert Einstein College of Medicine, Bronx, New York

Sydney S. Schochet, Jr., M.D.
Professor of Pathology, (Neuropathology), West Virginia University, Morgantown, West Virginia

William C. Schoene, M.D.
Associate Professor of Pathology, Harvard University; Brigham and Women's Hospital, Boston, Massachusetts

Robert D. Terry, M.D.
Professor of Neuroscience and Pathology, University of California, San Diego, La Jolla, California

Allan Yates, M.D., Ph.D., F.R.C.P. (C)
Professor of Neuropathology, Ohio State University, Columbus, Ohio

Contents

CHAPTER 1 ────────────────────────

Neurons, Astrocytes, and Ependyma

ASAO HIRANO, M.D.

NEURONS

The function of the central nervous system is the generation and propagation of electrical impulses among cells. The cells responsible for carrying out this function are the neurons.

In keeping with this function neurons all have a basic architecture consisting of a cell body and, usually, extensive cell processes. This configuration results in relatively large surface areas available for synaptic contact as well as the ability to propagate impulses over long distances.

Perhaps the major distinction between the architecture of the central nervous system and that of other areas of the body resides in the fact that each neuron occupies a unique place in the quasielectrical network of the central nervous system. The origin of the specific placement of each neuron arises from the highly ordered development of the central nervous system.

The neurons and glia of the central nervous system all arise from the single layer of neuroepithelial germinal (138) or matrix (42) cells of the primitive neural tube. These cells enclose the primitive central canal and are joined by small adhesive junctions forming a terminal bar. The cells multiply by mitosis. Eventually, some cells begin to migrate peripherally and form a mantle layer.

In general, in any one area of the developing nervous system, neurons differentiate before glial cells. Furthermore, among the neurons, the larger ones move towards their ultimate domain and differentiate before the smaller ones which are considered to be local circuit neurons (138).

In most regions, such as the cerebral cortex, the cells of the deeper layers form first, and they are followed by those of the more superficial layers (138). Certain exceptions to this rule occur. In the cerebellar cortex, for example, the granular cell layer is formed by the inward migration of cells from the external germinal layer. The guidance for the migrating neurons is thought to be supplied by the so-called radial glia (10, 197). In still other areas such as the thalamus the first cells to take up their position migrate along a lateromedial gradient (138).

During their migration most neurons have an elongated shape but do not achieve their characteristic architecture, including the long cell processes, i.e., the axons and dendrites, until well after they have come to rest. The axon is generally the first cell process to form. It elongates at its leading point, i.e., the growth cone (138, 192). Unlike the mature axon, the growth cone contains substantial numbers of organelles. It is capable of pinocytosis and like the motile cell processes of other cells contains a network of microfilaments. The axon continues its growth until it reaches its target cell, either another neuron or a muscle or gland, etc. At this point the cytological features of the axons assume their final form.

Dendritic development generally follows axonal formation. Finally, synaptic terminals are completed, and glial ensheathment occurs at the surface of the maturing neuron.

1

At maturity the neuron may be conveniently divided into three components. First is the cell body or soma which contains the nucleus and perikaryon (Fig. 1.1). The latter contains virtually all the elements observed in epithelial cells. These include the synthetic machinery of the cell, especially the rough endoplasmic reticulum which is aggregated in large accumulations known as Nissl substance, free ribosomes, and the Golgi apparatus. In addition, lysosomes including residual bodies (lipofuscin), mitochondria, neurofilaments, and microtubules as well as various other inclusions are present in the perikaryal cytoplasm.

The other two major components of the neurons are the dendrites and axons which are processes of the cell bodies. The dendrites, especially in their proximal portions, are substantially similar to the perikaryon. However, the preponderance of synaptic elements on the dendrites clearly indicates that their major function is to act as receptors of synaptic transmissions. The axons

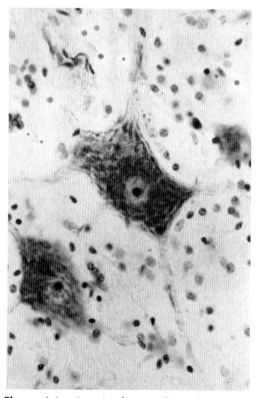

Figure 1.1. Anterior horn cells in the lumbar cord. Nissl stain. (Original magnification ×360.)

have relatively few organelles besides neurofilaments, microtubules, smooth endoplasmic reticulum and mitochondria. Their size and shape clearly reflect their function as propagators of impulses.

Thus, the cytology of the neuron is closely related to the function of the various parts. The cell body is the trophic center of the cell and provides the dendrites and axons with their functional and metabolic needs. This enables the structure of the latter two components to be virtually totally devoted to their highly specific functions.

Within the constraints imposed by its function the final shape and size of the neuron varies remarkably from region to region, and several neuronal types may be found even within the same region. One method of classification is based on the size of the neuron and the extension and form of the axon (186). According to this scheme the Golgi type 1 or macroneuron is large, and its usually myelinated axon extends for long distances into other parts of the nervous system before its terminal arborization. Purkinje cells and the large anterior horn cells are good examples of Golgi type 1 neurons. The smaller microneurons, or Golgi type II neurons, are considerably smaller, and their unmyelinated axons generally arborize locally. These cells are considered to be local circuit neurons. The granule cells of the cerebellum are typical examples of Golgi type II neurons.

Neuronal shape can vary from pyramidal, such as the Betz cells of the motor cortex, to the spherical shape of the ganglion cells in the dorsal roots. Other neurons such as the Purkinje cells have their own distinctive shapes. The distribution of size is very wide. The large anterior horn cells of the cervical and lumbar cord, the Betz cells and the dorsal root ganglia cells may be up to 100 μm in diameter. The tiny granule cells of the cerebellum, however, are only 5 or 6 μm wide.

The overall shape of the neuron is influenced by the number and distribution of the cell processes, especially the dendritic tree. In a typical neuron there is a single axon and a number of branching dendritic trunks arising either from the opposite side of the cell body or from various points on it. One may not easily generalize, however, and the precise distribution of the cell processes varies greatly among the neuronal types.

Despite the prominence of the cell body, the numerous and lengthy cell processes occupy the bulk of the neuronal cytoplasm. In the large dorsal root ganglia or Betz cells, for example, it has been estimated that the axon contains over 100 times the volume of the cell body. On the other hand, the axon of the granule cell apparently accounts for less than twice the volume of the soma (186).

As might be expected from the relative volumes of the soma and axons the latter have a surface area many fold greater than the cell body. Even more significant, however, is the surface area of the dendrites, since these are the predominant sites of synaptic contact. Unlike the axon, the dendrites are characterized by enormous arborization. Those dendrites which show spine formation have another complete level of arborization.

An appreciation of the different types of neurons is important not only for an understanding of the microscopic anatomy of the nervous system. The different shapes and sizes of the various neuronal types are reflections of a fundamental, probably developmental, relationship among the neurons of a specific type. The transmitter substance might be expected to be the same among the neurons in one type and may be different from those of another category of neuron. Furthermore, many disease processes affecting the nervous system are quite selective and involve only certain neuronal types while sparing other neurons, some of which may be in the immediate vicinity. For example, granule cell type cerebellar degeneration results in the loss of cerebellar granular cells, but leave their immediate synaptic mates, the Purkinje cells, intact. Similarly, in amyotrophic lateral sclerosis, the principal target cell is the large anterior horn cell of the spinal cord which is profoundly affected, while the nearby sensory neurons and the cells of the autonomic nervous system are spared.

The bases for the selective nature of these neuropathological processes are unknown. The answer, no doubt, lies in understanding the cell biology of the neurons. In an effort to contribute to this understanding the remainder of this work is devoted to an explication of the morphological features, under both normal and pathological conditions, of the neuron, astrocyte, and ependymal cell.

Nucleus

Neuronal nuclei are essentially similar to those found in other cells. Their sizes are related to their sizes of the cell bodies, but large neurons have a substantially smaller nucleocytoplasmic ratio than smaller neurons (Fig. 1.1). The nuclei are generally found in the center of the soma, but in some cells, such as those in Clarke's column, they are often eccentrically placed. Most neuronal nuclei are considered to be diploid, but some of the larger ones such as Purkinje cells, Betz cells, pyramidal cells of the hippocampus, and some large anterior horn cells are reported to be tetraploid (186).

Most large nuclei contain a prominent single nucleolus (Fig. 1.2), which is a convenient marker distinguishing neurons from nearby astrocytes. In some smaller neurons, however, such as the granule cells of the cerebellum, the nucleoli are not conspicuous due to a dense chromatin material that fills most of the nucleoplasm.

A variety of pathological conditions may affect the neuronal nucleus. Frequently these result in the appearance of eosinophilic intranuclear inclusions. In some instances, such as herpes virus infection (152) or in subacute sclerosing panencephalitis (153, 191) these inclusions do, indeed, consist of viral particles and serve as aids in the diagnosis of viral encephalitis. However, it is important to point out that eosinophilic intranuclear inclusions may be seen in a number of nonviral conditions.

Most often the inclusions simply represent cytoplasmic invagination into an irregularly shaped nucleus. This phenomenon suggests a reactive change of some sort but not necessarily an infection.

Eosinophilic fibrillar lattice-like intranuclear inclusions have also been observed in both normal and in experimentally altered animals. These appear as curved, rod-

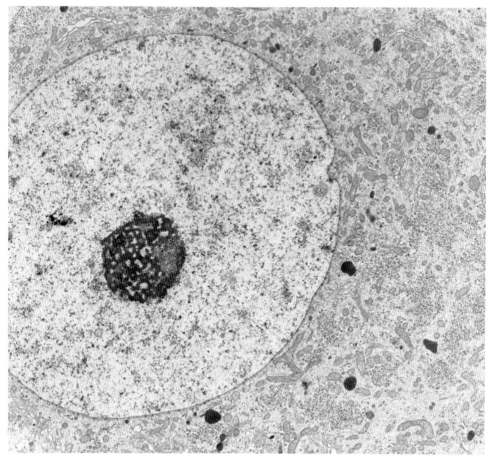

Figure 1.2. The perikaryon of a neuron in the gasserian ganglion of a normal animal. The nucleus with a prominent nucleolus is at the left. The cytoplasm contains scattered groups of rough endoplasmic reticulum, Golgi apparatus, and occasional dense bodies. Filaments, microtubules and mitochondria may be seen between them. (Original magnification ×9,000.) (From N. Malamud and A. Hirano (163).)

like inclusions in the light microscope. They are nonspecific changes and, when studied at the fine structural level, are found to consist of circular or arciform arrays of 5- to 7-nm diameter filaments. The filaments are arranged in interlacing curved lamellae (25, 213). The filaments forming a single lamella are parallel to one another and at a 60° angle to the filaments of adjacent lamellae.

Marinesco bodies are eosinophilic intranuclear inclusions found in pigmented neurons, especially in the substantia nigra, and are unrelated to viral infections (Fig. 1.3). A good review of the subject was published by Schochet in 1972 (206). These bodies

were first described by Marinesco in 1902 in the locus ceruleus and substantia nigra. In 1963 in a study of 160 random autopsies, Yuen and Baxter found them in the majority of individuals over 21 yr of age. They increased in numbers with advancing age. Yuen and Baxter were the first to apply the eponym "Marinesco body." From one to four of these intranuclear inclusions may be present in a single nucleus. They range in size from 2 to 10 μm in diameter, but most are as large as the nucleolus. The size does not change with age.

Marinesco bodies are eosinophilic in contrast to the basophilic nucleoli (Fig. 1.3). They stain pink with Masson's trichrome

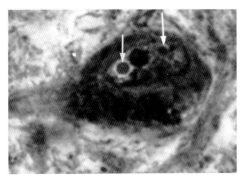

Figure 1.3. Marinesco bodies (*arrows*). H&E. (Original magnification ×1080.)

stain and are negative for both periodic acid-Schiff (PAS) and Feulgen.

The fine structure was first described by Leestma and Andrews (159). Marinesco bodies are devoid of a limiting membrane. They consist of an aggregate of moderately osmiophilic granular material. In some cases they are associated with a lattice-like arrangement of filaments. Similar structures have been described in the substantia nigra in an aged monkey (131).

The significance of the Marinesco body is obscure. It has not been correlated with any disease. Schochet (206) has raised the possibility that they may be a variant of the nuclear bodies seen in astrocytes.

Occasionally, large neurons which apparently contain two nuclei have been seen under certain conditions, such as tuberous sclerosis or ganglioglioma. Since these "binucleated neurons" are seen in section, it is often difficult to rule out the possibility that instead of two separate nuclei these profiles actually represent a section through two lobes of a single deformed or lobulated nucleus.

Nissl Substance and Golgi Apparatus

NORMAL

Prominent Nissl bodies, which stain blue with aniline dyes, are characteristic features of large neurons (Figs. 1.1 and 1.4). They are found in the perikaryon and in the proximal portion of dendrites but are absent in the axon, including the axon hillock.

The electron microscope has revealed that, in fact, the Nissl bodies correspond to the rough endoplasmic reticulum of other cells. They consist of stacks of flattened, membranous, anastomosing cisterna. Numerous ribosomes are attached to the outer surface of the cisterns. Polysomes are found apparently free-floating in the cytoplasmic areas between the cisterns, as well as in other parts of the perikaryal cytoplasm and proximal portions of the neuronal cell processes.

The Nissl substance is considered to be the organelle in which proteins destined for export from the neuron are synthesized, while proteins required for use within the cell are formed on the free ribosomes. This divergence of function is reflected in the fact that free ribosomes predominate in immature neurons.

Clusters of stacks of smooth membranous cisternae and sacs, forming a Golgi apparatus, are found in the perikaryon of large neurons arranged around the nucleus. For the most part they consist of closely packed fenestrated cisternae and numerous associated small vesicles and vacuoles. The interconnected stacks form a reticulum encircling the nucleus. In contrast, in small neurons such as the granule cells of the cerebellum, the Golgi apparatus is restricted to a single area.

PATHOLOGY

Chromatolysis

The loss of Nissl substance and its attendant change in the staining patterns of the neuron is known as chromatolysis, especially as seen in the large motor neurons of the hypoglossal nucleus or in the anterior horn cells (138, 160, 194). Chromatolysis may be found in various diseases but has been most extensively studied after experimental axotomy.

Experimental axotomy results in the well-known Wallerian degeneration which will be discussed below (see p. 44). Chromatolysis also follows axotomy. The closer the injury is to the cell body the sooner chromatolysis occurs.

Chromatolytic neurons are characterized by a swollen perikaryon. During the early phase, so-called "central" chromatolysis is seen in which the nuclei becomes eccentric,

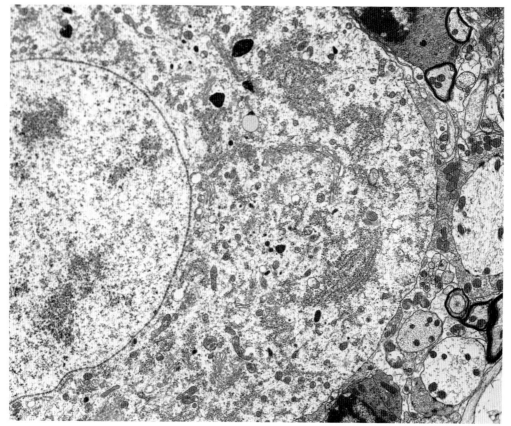

Figure 1.4. A portion of an anterior horn cell surrounded by a neuropil in the spinal cord of a normal animal. (Original magnification ×5,000.)

and the powdery remains of the Nissl substance are confined to the periphery of the cell (Fig. 1.5). Most of the cytoplasm appears homogeneous. Dendritic retraction follows these changes. The Golgi apparatus may be displaced to the periphery of the cell (retispersion).

Fine structural studies reveal that rough endoplasmic reticulum is relatively sparse, and the bulk of the perikaryal cytoplasm is filled with filaments, tubules, smooth endoplasmic reticulum, and mitochondria. Free ribosomes become comparatively more abundant. Lysosomes, too, are increased in number. While these changes are characteristic of chromatolytic neurons, some cells such as Betz cells, for example, do not show all of these changes (5). In these cells Nissl substance is lost, but filament accumulation is reported to be absent.

Chromatolysis is accompanied by an increase in RNA and protein synthesis. Ap-

parently, the chromatolytic reaction to axotomy represents a shift of protein synthesis from that destined for export to protein required for domestic use in regeneration (138).

While the chromatolytic process may be a straightforward reaction to cell injury, the possibility has been raised that it is also a reaction to the loss of contact with target organs. In this way the neurons return to a state more similar to their condition during development, and the accompanying cytological changes are consistent with this alteration. It should be noted that axotomy during development, i.e., during a period in which the bulk of the protein synthesis is devoted to dendritic growth and to synaptogenesis, results in little or no chromatolysis (138).

It is also interesting in this connection that chromatolysis is sometimes accompanied by "satellitosis" in which glial cells

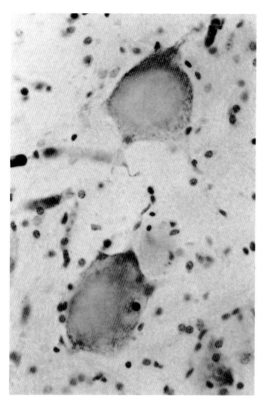

Figure 1.5. Chromatolysis in the lumbar anterior horn cells. Nissl stain. (Original magnification ×360.)

surround the cell body. This is preceded by a lifting of the boutons from the surface of the soma so that the cell body is deprived of its normal synaptic contact. The surrounding glial cell processes are interposed between the separated boutons and the perikaryal surface (9, 138, 145). The contacts are reestablished when the neuron completes its regeneration and recovers its normal cytology.

Chromatolytic changes are often associated with conditions other than axotomy. In cases such as motor neuron disease or pellagra the cell body undergoes cytological changes virtually identical to those seen after axotomy.

Other Alterations of Nissl Substance

Certain other alterations of the Nissl substance are characterized by a change of the membrane configuration rather than a frank loss of the organelle. These have all become apparent after fine structural study

and at times may be quite striking in appearance. It is difficult to assign a role in pathogenesis to these alterations, since they are sometimes seen in apparently normal tissue in certain neurons and in certain species and, indeed, may even be artifactitious in some circumstances. It is, however, important to be familiar with these structures because of their occasional prominence in some cells and in some conditions. The neuropathologist must be cautious before making a judgment concerning pathology based on the presence of these unusual configurations.

The "lamellar body" (Figs. 1.6 and 1.7) consists of short stacks of membranous cisterns packed so closely together that virtually no cytoplasm or ribosomes are found between the individual cisterns (62). Their relationship to rough endoplasmic reticulum is evidenced by the presence of ribosomes on the outermost cisterns. Lamellar bodies are most obvious in Purkinje cells, especially after inadequate preservation. They may be related to anoxic changes or other, unknown, insults. They have been occasionally observed in other neurons under certain experimental conditions.

Closely related to the lamellar bodies are the "annulated lamellae" (Fig. 1.8). These are essentially identical to the lamellar bodies, but in annulated lamellae the membranes of a single cistern are fused at fairly regular intervals. A dense material often accumulates at the cytoplasmic surface of the fused areas. In many ways the fused areas are highly reminiscent of the nuclear pores. Annulated lamellae also differ from lamellar bodies by the fact that they sometimes form concentric whorls rather than short stacks. Annulated lamellae are apparently normal constituents of oocytes and certain developing cells. They have been seen in neurons in the lateral geniculate body and, in some species, of the dorsal root ganglia (74). Under pathological conditions they are reported in certain neoplasms and in degenerating anterior horn cells in experimental animals or in human motor neuron diseases.

A third form of alteration of the Nissl substance is manifested by the formation of "membrane particle complexes" or "glycogen-membrane complexes" (188) (Figs. 1.9 and 1.10). In this configuration the

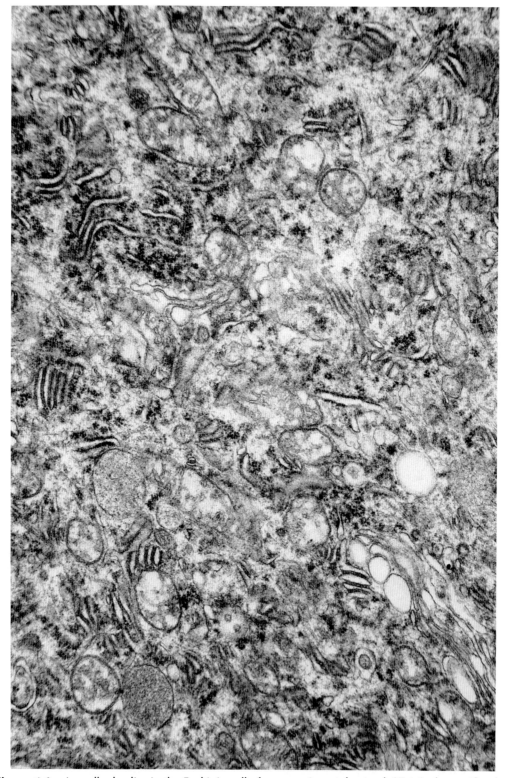

Figure 1.6. Lamellar bodies in the Purkinje cell of an experimental animal. (Original magnification ×36,000.) (From A. Hirano (79).)

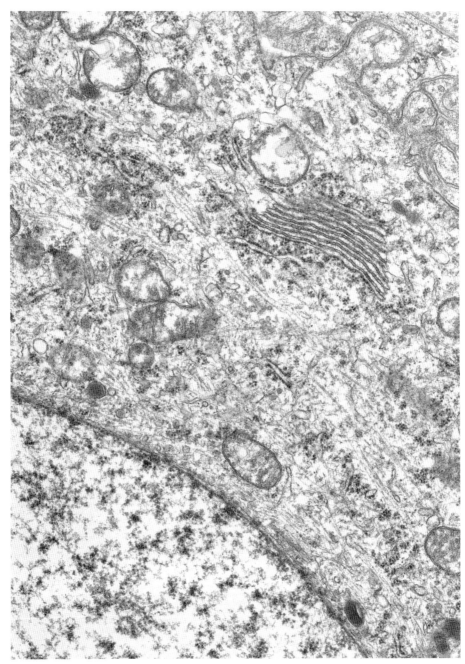

Figure 1.7. A lamellar body in a dorsal root ganglion of a mutant hamster with hindleg paralysis. (Original magnification ×26,000.)

membranes also form stacks or concentric whorls of cisterns, but the space between adjacent cisterns is relatively wide. However, instead of ribosomes on the membrane surfaces 20- to 30-nm particles, considered to be glycogen, occupy the space between the cisterns. Membrane particle complexes have been seen in neurons of the dorsal root ganglia in the normal animal as well as in certain mutants (74).

As suggested above, the significance of the lamella bodies, annulated lamellae, and

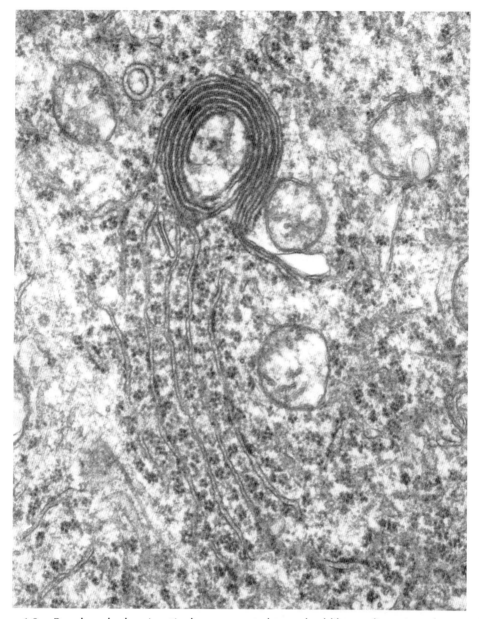

Figure 1.8. Rough endoplasmic reticulum connected to a whorl-like configuration of an annulate lamellae-like structure. (Original magnification ×50,000.) (From A. Hirano (74).)

membrane particle complexes is not clear. On rare occasions single bodies have been observed in which elements of all three alterations are present simultaneously (Fig. 1.11).

A well known neuropathological alteration is the formation of "colloid" inclusions. More will be said of these structures in a later section. At this point, however, we should point out that they actually consist of lake-like distentions of cisternae of the Nissl substance (174).

Other alterations of the Nissl substance are not as striking. Glycogen granules have been reported within distended cisterns of the rough endoplasmic reticulum in neurons of the substantia nigra (6) or cochlear nuclei (141) of the Gunn rat. Microtubule-

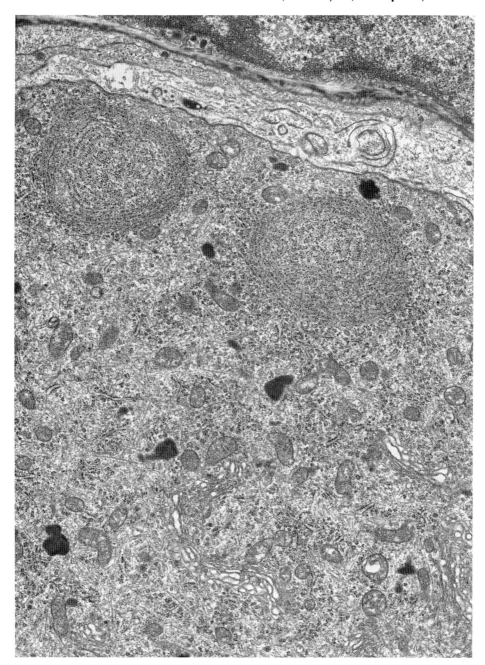

Figure 1.9. Two, dense, lamellated structures are seen in the dorsal root ganglion of a hamster. (Original magnification ×5,000.)

like structures have also been observed in PAS-positive granules in cortical neurons of certain species of aged dogs. The granules actually consist of distended cisterns of the Nissl substances (225). Finally, virus particles have been observed within the cisterns of the rough endoplasmic reticulum in the dorsal root ganglia of certain hamsters (Fig. 1.12). The mere presence of virus particles, however, is not necessarily an indication that they are the etiological agent of the condition being studied. It is difficult, often, to rule out the possibility of contamination.

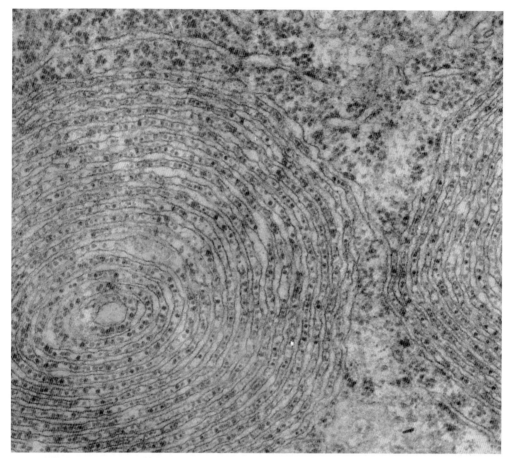

Figure 1.10. Higher magnification of structures similar to those illustrated in Figure 1.9 disclose a membrane-particle complex. (Original magnification ×15,000.)

Lipofuscin and Other Pigments

LIPOFUSCIN

Accumulation of lipofuscin granules in neurons is a common feature of aged brains. In hematoxylin and eosin (H&E) preparations, these granules retain their inherent yellow-brown color; they are metachromatic and stain green with the Nissl stain. In contrast to neuromelanin, they remain unstained with silver impregnation methods, but the margins of the granules become outlined, resulting in a honeycomb-like configuration. Histochemical studies suggest that lipofuscin is a heterogenous substance containing lipids, proteins, and carbohydrates (206). The inclusions have significant quantities of hydrolytic enzymes such as acid phosphatase and are generally considered to be residual bodies derived

from lysosomes (206). At the ultrastructural level, the lipofuscin granule consists of a membrane-bounded particle containing a dense, finely granular substance and/or a lighter, homogeneous hyaline-like material (Fig. 1.13).

Aged brains show a characteristic topographic distribution of lipofuscin granules. While they are fairly widespread throughout much of the nervous system they are especially prominent in the inferior olivary nuclei, dentate nuclei, dorsal root ganglia and anterior horn cells of the spinal cord. Certain neurons such as the Purkinje cells of the cerebellum do not usually show a significant amount of lipofuscin detectable by light microscopy, but the small amount they contain has been observed with the electron microscope.

The effects of lipofuscin accumulation

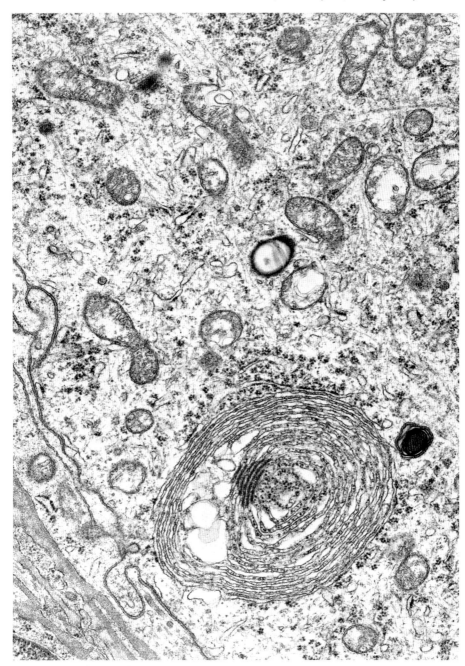

Figure 1.11. A single membranous accumulation which contains three types of alterations of the endoplasmic reticulum: a lamellar body, a membrane-particle complex, and annulate lamellae. (Original magnification ×33,000.) (From A. Hirano (74).)

are not known. It is generally assumed that lipofuscin accumulation is a sign of neuronal degeneration leading to death (pigmentary degeneration). On the other hand, different interpretations have been proposed. Certain neuronal groups such as the inferior olivary nuclei have abundant lipofuscin granules resulting in ballooning of the cell body in normal, elderly people. However, this phenomenon has not been associated with any dysfunction and interestingly, without any appreciable neuronal

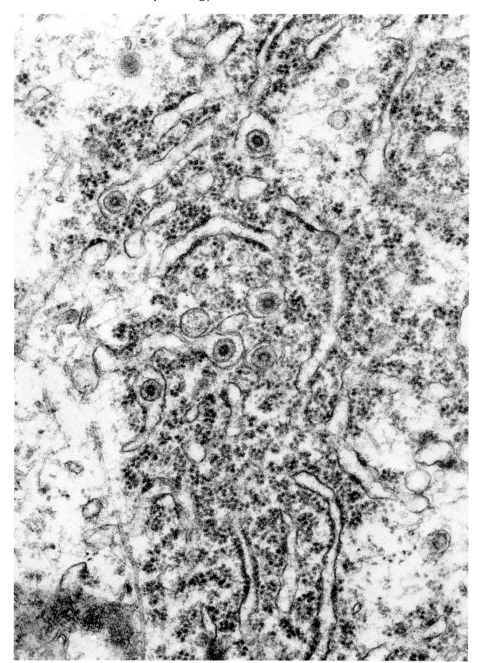

Figure 1.12. Virus particles, referred to as "R" particles (Bernard and Towiner: Am. Inst. Pasteur 107:447, 1964), within the cisterns of the rough endoplasmic reticulum in a neuron of a hamster. (Original magnification ×50,000.) (From A. Hirano (74).)

loss. Apparently, these neurons have been able to survive pigment accumulation (230, 234).

Intraneuronal lipofuscin granules have also been observed in a number of experimental animals (234). It increases in sev-

eral animal species on vitamin E-deficient diets (234).

Accumulations of lipofuscin granules are prominent in certain parts of the central nervous system in senile dementia, Alzheimer's disease, and in amyotrophic lat-

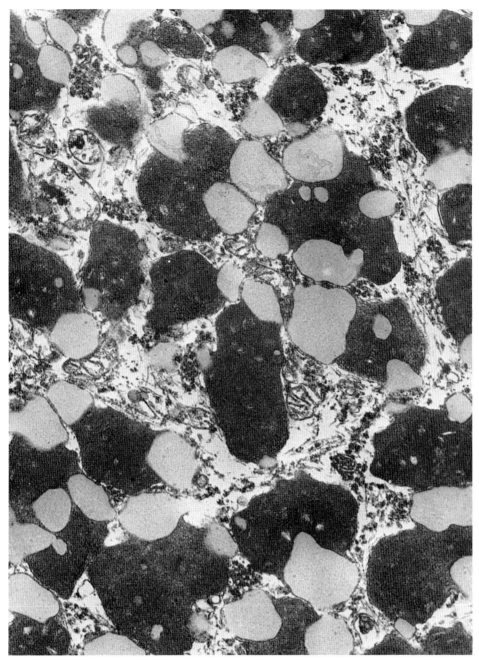

Figure 1.13. Lipofuscin granules in the anterior horn cell of a patient with amyotrophic lateral sclerosis. (Original magnification ×36,000.) (From A. Hirano (79).)

eral sclerosis, etc. In lipofuscinosis, a kind of lipidosis, there is an increase in the number of lipofuscin granules spread over a wider than normal distribution involving a number of neuronal systems (260). In other types of lipofuscinosis abnormal curvilinear bodies (37, 39, 52, 240) and finger print-like inclusions (223) have been seen.

The prominence of lipofuscin granules in aged neurons is presumably related to the fact that neurons do not turn over and so, like cardiac muscle, may accumulate residual bodies. Why certain neurons do so to a greater degree than others is a mystery. Schochet (206) and Tomlinson (234) have published concise reviews of the current literature on lipofuscin and other changes associated with aging.

NEUROMELANIN

Neuromelanin bears certain similarities to lipofuscin but shows distinct differences as well. Both may be present as intraneuronal inclusions, especially in aged brains, and their fine structures are very similar except for the coarser, electron-dense granules found in neuromelanin (126) (Fig. 1.14). They have different staining characteristics as well. Neuromelanin is darker in H&E preparations where it appears very dark brown compared to the yellowish brown of lipofuscin. Furthermore, neuromelanin is strongly argentophilic, while only the periphery of lipofuscin granules takes up the silver stain.

Another difference between lipofuscin and neuromelanin is the distribution of the two pigments. Unlike lipofuscin which may be widely distributed throughout the nervous system, neuromelanin is generally confined to only certain groups of neurons. These include the zona compacta of the substantia nigra and the locus ceruleus where the pigmentation is usually visible to the naked eye. Neuromelanin may also be found in the dorsal motor nucleus of the vagus, dorsal root ganglia, sympathetic ganglia, the tegmentum of the brain stem, and in scattered neurons in the roof of the fourth ventricle. In children the pigmentation in the substantia nigra and the locus ceruleus is pale, but histochemical methods can demonstrate the presence of neuromelanin. With development, pigmentation increases but becomes less obvious in aged brains due to neuronal loss.

One must be careful to distinguish between neuromelanin and true melanin as seen in skin and in the iris of the eye. Melanin granules are distinctly different at the fine structural level and are confined to melanophores. Within the central nervous

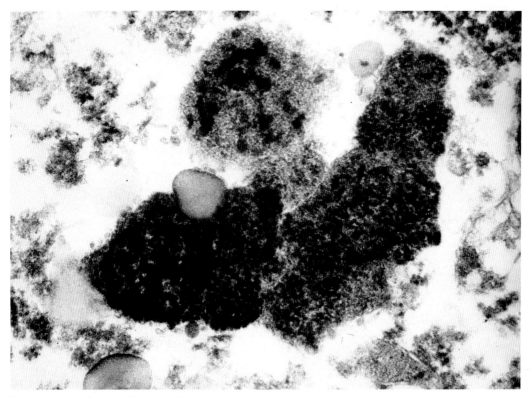

Figure 1.14.   Neuromelanin in the substantia nigra. (Original magnification ×59,000.) (From A. Hirano (67).)

system these melanophores are found only in the leptomeninges, especially in areas covering the high cervical cord. These areas are more pigmented in the darker skinned races and are pale in albinos who, however, retain the neuromelanin of the substantia nigra and locus ceruleus. These melanophores are believed to be the source of primary melanomas of the central nervous system (83).

GRANULOVACUOLAR BODIES

Granulovacuolar bodies were first described by Simchowicz in 1911. They are vacuoles, approximately 3–5 μm in diameter, with dense cores of about 1–2 μm in diameter. The core is argentophilic and stains blue with H&E. Histochemical analysis of the granulovacuolar body has not been rewarding. At the ultrastructural level, the granulovacuolar bodies consist of an outer limiting membrane enclosing a vacuole which contains a granular central core (92) (Fig. 1.15).

These bodies are common in elderly people and in young patients with Down's syndrome. The number of granulovacuolar bodies normally increases with age and much more so in Alzheimer's disease (4).

There may be a few or many granulovac-

uolar bodies within a single neuron. The involved neurons are almost always the pyramidal cells of Sommer's sector and adjacent areas. The topographic specificity as well as the exact origin of these structures are still mysterious.

ABNORMAL LIPID INCLUSIONS

Inborn genetic defects involving the loss or diminution of specific enzymes important in lipid metabolism may result in various lipidoses (1, 125, 224, 233, 245). The resulting inclusions usually appear similar in optical microscope preparations (Fig. 1.16), but, frequently, fine structural differences can be detected.

The details of changes associated with specific lipidoses will be described in Chapter 8. In addition to inborn conditions other insults such as certain intoxications have been shown to result in intracytoplasmic inclusions similar to those seen in lipidosis (103) (Figs. 1.17–1.19).

Neurofibrils

NORMAL

"Neurofibril" is the somewhat anachronistic term which has been used to refer to

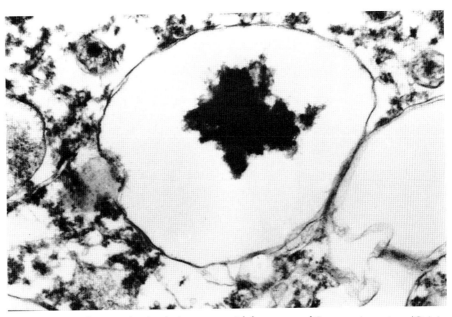

Figure 1.15. A granulovacuolar body in a pyramidal neuron of Sommer's sector. (Original magnification ×36,000.) (From A. Hirano et al. (92).)

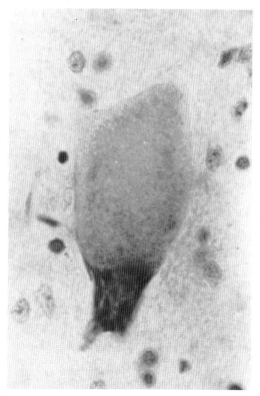

Figure 1.16. A distended motor neuron in the hypoglossal nucleus in gargoylism. Nissl stain. (Original magnification ×720.)

at least three different structures with fibrillar configurations found in the normal neuron. These are the microtubules, the neurofilaments, and the microfilaments (Figs. 1.20 and 1.21) (11, 158, 175). Among these three only the neurofilaments appear to be unique to the neuron.

Microtubules, sometimes referred to as neurotubules, are long, unbranched structures which are apparently indistinguishable from the microtubules seen in other organs. They are about 25 nm in diameter and contain a lucent core which often contains a 5-nm dense granule. The walls consist of helically arranged dense granules, about 5 nm in diameter, with 13 particles per turn of the helix.

The major protein associated with microtubules is tubulin which is a dimer consisting of an α form of 57,000 daltons, and a β form of 54,000 daltons (11). The microtubules are apparently in dynamic equilibrium with free tubulin in the living cell.

The function of the microtubules is not clear. They are usually thought to play

some role in intraneuronal transport and maintenance of cell shape.

Neurofilaments are narrower than microtubules. They are only 10 nm in diameter but have also been shown to contain a narrow, lucent core. Their length is indeterminate, and they show fine side arms. Their size places them among the so-called "intermediate filaments."

The protein associated with neurofilaments is distinct from that of other intermediate filaments, such as those seen in muscle, epithelium, fibroblasts, or even glial cells (158). In vertebrates it consists of three major polypeptides with molecular weights of 200,000, 150,000, and 68,000 daltons (127, 158). In addition to differences in molecular weights, immunohistochemical studies have shown that neurofilament protein is distinct from glial fibrillary acidic protein (158). This difference between the intermediate filaments of neurons and glia comes as no surprise to the morphologist who has long recognized the greater thickness of neurofilaments as compared to glial filaments.

The function of the neurofilament is not clear. They are believed to be part of the cytoskeleton of the cell and may be involved in intracellular transport.

Intraneuronal microfilaments are approximately 5 nm in diameter (175) and are apparently identical to the microfilaments seen in virtually all animal cells. In neurons they are most obvious in the growth cone where they form a network of anastomosing filaments.

The protein associated with microfilaments is actin with a molecular weight of 42,000 daltons (11).

The interrelationship between the various fibrillary elements among themselves, as well as to the plasma membrane and other organelles, is currently under intense investigation. The concept of a cytoskeleton responsible for the shape of the cell, the movement of organelles, and materials within the cell as well as the position of the subcellular components is slowly evolving.

PATHOLOGY

Accumulation of 10-nm Neurofilaments

The abnormal accumulation of 10-nm neurofilaments may be observed after a

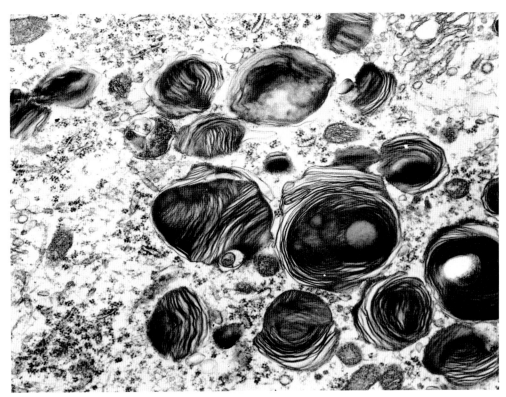

Figure 1.17. Part of the perikaryon of an anterior horn cell in the spinal cord of an aleutian mink with Chediak-Higashi disease. Dense laminated structures, essentially identical to membranous cytoplasmic bodies (233), are seen in human Tay-Sachs disease. (Original magnification ×30,000.) (From A. Hirano (67).)

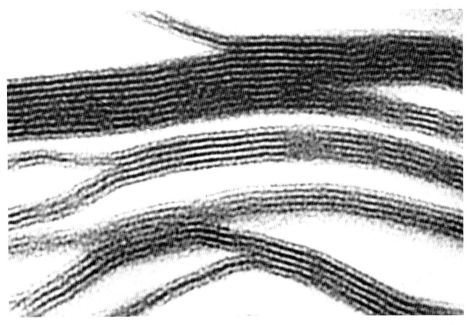

Figure 1.18. Higher magnification of a membranous cytoplasmic body. Two-nanometer lamellae are fused resulting in 3-nm dense lines separated by 2-nm intervals. (Original magnification ×360,000.) (From A. Hirano et al. (125).)

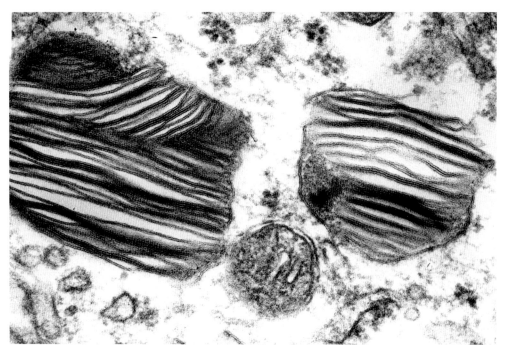

Figure 1.19. Zebra bodies in an anterior horn cell of an aleutian mink with Chediak-Higashi disease. (Original magnification ×150,000.) (From A. Hirano (67).)

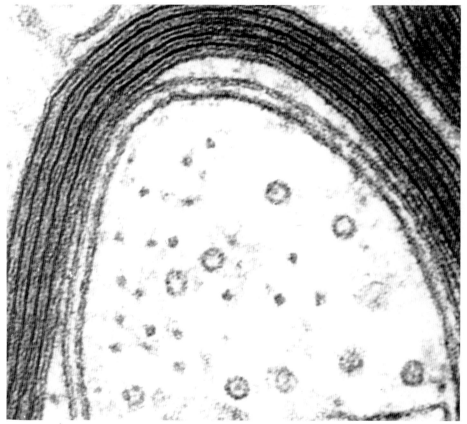

Figure 1.20. A portion of a myelinated axon in the edematous white matter of a rat. Cross-sections of microtubules and neurofilaments are visible. (Original magnification ×260,000.) (From A. Hirano (66).)

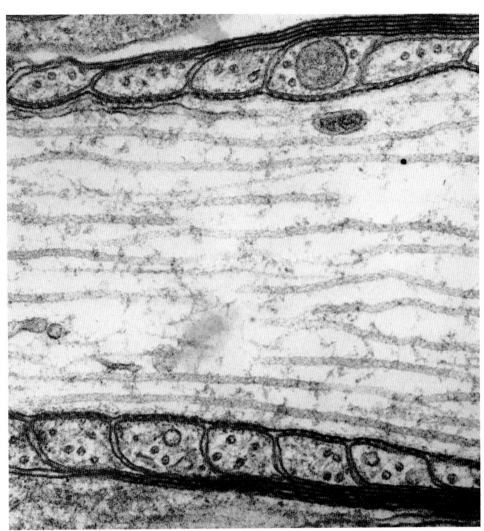

Figure 1.21. A longitudinal section through the paranodal area of a myelinated axon in cerebral white matter of a rat. Longitudinal sections of microtubules and neurofilaments are seen. (Original magnification ×97,000.) (From A. Hirano and H. M. Dembitzer: *Journal of Cell Biology* 34:555, 1967.)

number of pathological alterations (254) (Fig. 1.22). After experimental aluminum (232) or maytansine intoxication (47) large accumulations of filaments may be found in the soma and in the proximal portion of the neurites, especially dendrites. Administration of β-β'-iminodipropionitrile (IDPN) results in the accumulation of neurofilaments in the proximal portion of the axon (28). The latter are reminiscent of the so-called spheroids which may be seen in both the proximal portion of the axon (19, 100) and the cell bodies of anterior horn cells in certain cases of motor neuron disease (98).

Vinca alkaloids are mitotic spindle inhibitors that, when administered to experimental animals, result in the loss of nonciliary microtubules and the formation of a honeycomb-like, hexagonal crystalloid (66, 119) (Fig. 1.23). In addition, accumulations of 10-nm neurofilaments accompany these changes. Colchicine has similar effects except that crystalloids are not formed.

Alzheimer's Neurofibrillary Changes

Alzheimer first described neurofibrillary changes in a single case of presenile dementia. They were later observed in senile dementia of Alzheimer type and, to a lesser

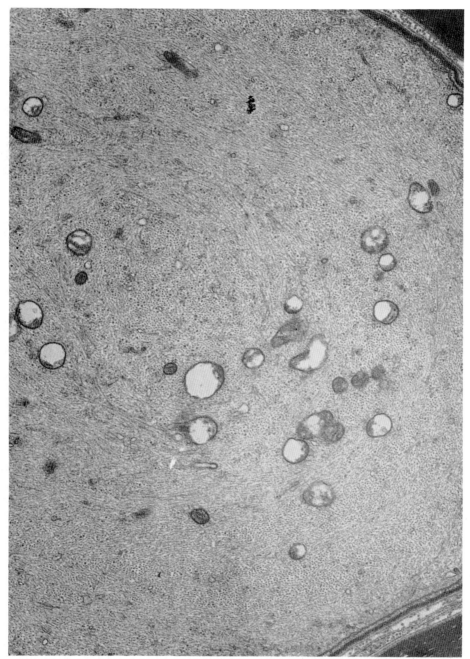

Figure 1.22.   A portion of a distended peripheral myelinated axon in a Syrian hamster with hindleg paralysis. (Original magnification ×15,000.) (From A. Hirano (79).)

degree, in normal aged patients. More recently, they have been observed in a number of conditions (17, 31, 115, 129, 255), including postencephalitic parkinsonism (57, 67), and are particularly abundant among the Chamorro population on Guam where parkinsonism-dementia complex (Fig. 1.24) and amyotrophic lateral sclerosis are particularly common (69, 108, 109, 164).

Although there is a certain degree of topographic predisposition depending on the underlying condition, the usual sites of pre-

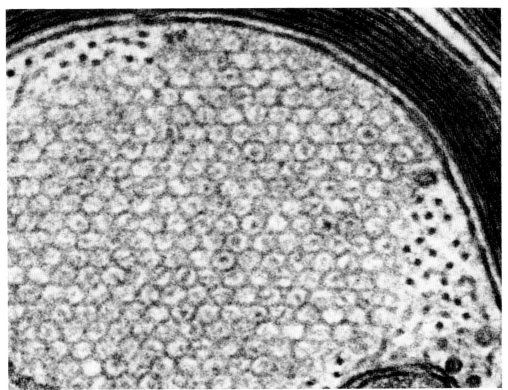

Figure 1.23. A cross-section of a myelinated axon in the white matter of a rat 4 days after implantation of vinblastine sulphate. The axoplasm contains a hexagonal crystalloid structure. (Original magnification ×170,000.) (From A. Hirano (66).)

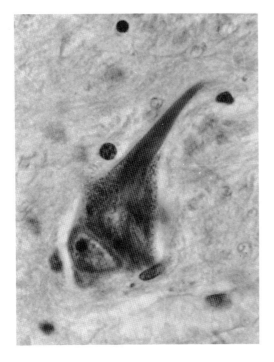

dilection are the hippocampus, especially the pyramidal cells in Sommer's sector and the glomerular formation of the parahippocampal gyrus; the frontotemporal cerebral cortex; various hypothalamic nuclei; the substantia innominata; the amygaloid nucleus; the periaqueductal gray matter, including the oculomotor nuclei; the median raphe; the substantia nigra, the locus ceruleus; the reticular formation of the brain stem; the dorsal motor nucleus of the vagus; the inferior olivary nucleus of the medulla; the dentate nucleus of the cerebellum; and the intermediate gray matter of the spinal cord. They are rarely found in the anterior horn cells of the spinal cord. Purkinje cells of the cerebellum and neu-

Figure 1.24. A pigmented neuron in the substantia nigra with Alzheimer neurofibrillary tangles. Parkinsonism-dementia complex on Guam. H&E. (Original magnification ×720.)

rons of the lateral geniculate bodies, spinal root ganglia, and sympathetic ganglia fail to reveal neurofibrillary changes (116).

The tangles are most easily visualized after silver impregnation (Fig. 1.25) but may also be seen in H&E preparations where they tend to be blue, but may be weakly eosinophilic in later stages. They are also effectively visualizable with thioflavine S.

The apparent shape of the tangle depends on its location. They are pyramidal or flame-shaped in the pyramidal neurons of the cerebral cortex but are globose in the basal ganglia or brain stem.

Electron microscopic study of Alzheimer neurofibrillary tangles reveals a characteristic morphology. When the tangles are viewed in longitudinal section fibrillar structures are seen with distinct, regular constrictions (Fig. 1.26). The constrictions usually occur at 80-nm intervals (229), but these may vary and intervals as short as 50 nm have been seen. At the constrictions the fibrils appear 10-nm wide, and they are 25-nm wide midway between the constrictions. The fundamental architecture is unclear. The fibril was originally considered to be a twisted tubule (229). Occasional circular profiles, 15 nm in cross-section, tended to support this view (92). Other

sections of the tangles revealed characteristic arciform profiles (229) (Fig. 1.27). Another view of the fundamental structures is that the "fibrillar" elements of the tangles are composed of paired 10-nm filaments twisted around one another in a helical fashion (146, 252). Any view of the fundamental structure of Alzheimer's neurofibrillary tangles must also take into account the fact that in addition to "constricted" elements one often observed straight tubules (Fig. 1.28) 15 nm in diameter (92, 132, 215, 236, 258). The straight tubules may sometimes constitute the entire tangle, or they may coexist with the constricted form.

The significance of Alzheimer's tangles is not clear. A relationship between 10-nm neurofilaments and the tangles has been suggested (181, 205). If true, however, the relationship is not a simple matter of transformation, since Alzheimer tangles have, so far, been observed only in humans, only in certain neurons, and only in certain parts of the neurons, while the 10-nm neurofilaments are widely distributed (82). Similar, but not identical, tangles have been seen in certain experimental animals (104, 251). The subject of Alzheimer neurofibrillary tangles is currently under intensive study and will be discussed in Chapter 16.

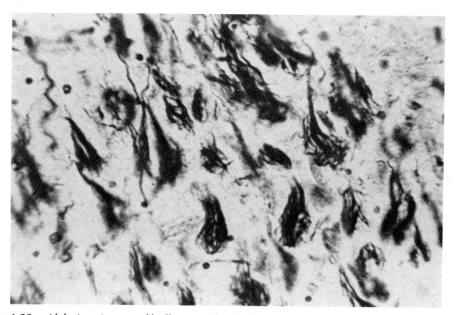

Figure 1.25. Alzheimer's neurofibrillary tangles in Sommer's sector of a Chamorro patient on Guam. Silver impregnation. (Original magnification ×500.) (From A. Hirano (64).)

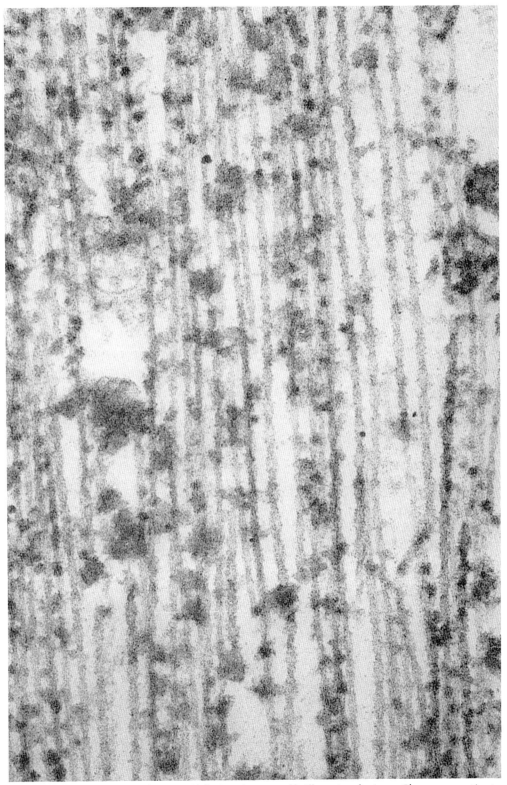

Figure 1.26. Filaments within an Alzheimer's neurofibrillary tangle in a Chamorro patient on Guam. Regular constrictions are evident. (Original magnification ×112,000.)

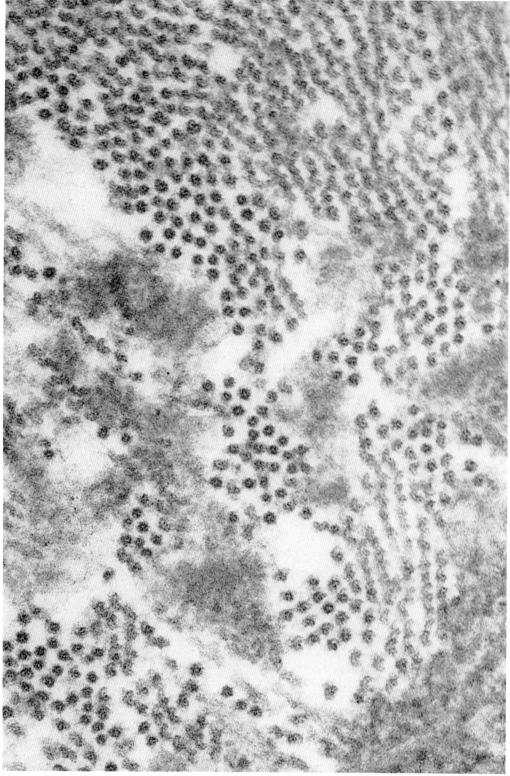

Figure 1.27. A cross-section of filaments within an Alzheimer's neurofibrillary tangle. Circular and arciform profiles are visible. (Original magnification ×160,000.)

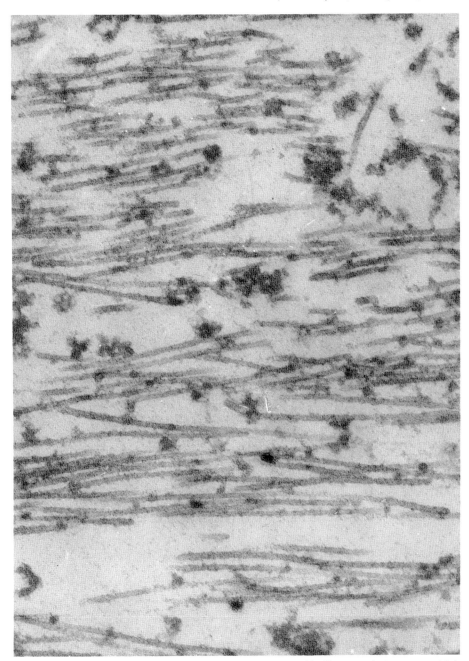

Figure 1.28. Straight 15-nm tubules in an Alzheimer's neurofibrillary tangle in a pyramidal neuron of a 91-year-old patient. (Original magnification ×88,000.)

Other Neurofibrillary Changes

Accumulations of 12-nm tubules arranged in wavy and parallel, or straight and random, groups have been observed in a case of quadriplegia of unknown etiology (154). These argentophilic fibrillary inclusions were found in almost the entire motor neuron system and in certain other neurons as well.

Other, abnormal, fibril-containing structures will be described below in the section dealing with intracytoplasmic inclusion bodies.

Mitochondria

Neuronal mitochondria are fundamentally similar to those of other cells. They are surrounded by an outer, smooth, membrane, and the interior cristae arise from the folds of an interior membrane.

The overall size and shape of the mitochondria differ, depending on their position within the cell and on the neuronal type in which they reside (186). They are known to branch. Most often, perikaryal mitochondria are sausage-shaped, about 0.1 μm wide and 1.0 μm long. The mitochondria assume a highly elongate shape in axons and dendrites but are globoid in synaptic terminals. They are absent, however, from dendritic spines. Most often, the long mitochondria contain longitudinally oriented, shelf-like cristae (Fig. 1.29). As in other tissues, in addition to cristae, the mitochondria contain dense "matrix granules" which have been associated with calcium phosphate accumulation (186).

Mitochondria, as well as other small organelles, are motile structures, and when living preparations are viewed they are found to be in continuous motion within the perikaryal cytoplasm between Nissl bodies and in the neurites.

Under pathological conditions mitochondria may show a variety of changes. They show a dramatic increase in size and number in the perikarya of Purkinje cells in kinky hair disease (44, 259) (Fig. 1.30) and in focal regions of the axon in Wallerian degeneration (118, 246) among other conditions (Figs. 1.31 and 1.32). Swollen or vacuolized mitochondria may result from ischemia which may reflect an underlying pathology or which may be the result of preparation artifacts. Under certain conditions presumably calcareous matrix granules may accumulate in abnormally large numbers. In the Gunn rat, which is an experimental model for bilirubin encephalopathy, glycogen granules are found within membrane-bounded vacuoles in the matrix of the neuronal mitochondria (141, 212). In some degenerative diseases the mitochondria appear shrunken and may have an unusually dense matrix (Figs. 1.31 and 32). Various mitochondrial alterations have been described in the neurons of the spinal ganglia of aged rats (243).

Intracytoplasmic Inclusions

PICK BODIES

Pick's disease is characterized by progressive dementia in middle age and circumscribed, profound lobar cerebral atrophy. Alzheimer, using the Bielschowsky stain, first identified argentophilic intraneuronal inclusions in a single case of Pick's disease. He referred to these structures as neurofibrillary tangles despite differences between Pick bodies and the tangles seen in Alzheimer's disease.

It is important to note that in a significant proportion of cases of lobar atrophy no Pick bodies may be found. When present

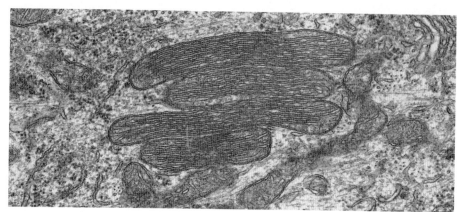

Figure 1.29. Mitochondria in a dorsal root ganglion cell of a Syrian hamster with hindleg paralysis. The direction of the cristae is parallel to the long axis of some of the elongated mitochondria. (Original magnification ×34,000.) (From A. Hirano (79).)

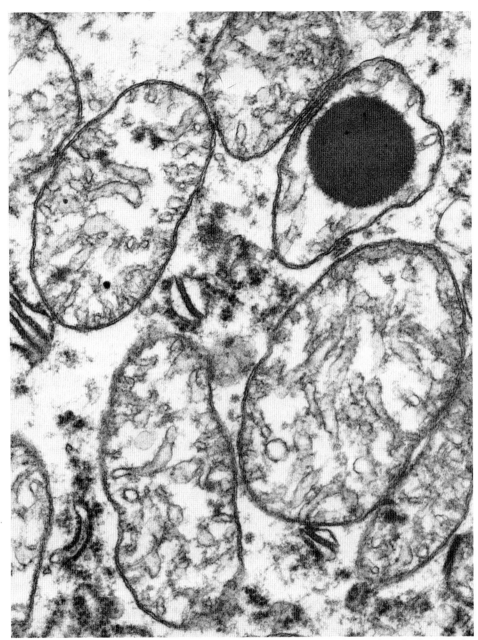

Figure 1.30. Large mitochondria in a Purkinje cell of a patient with Menkes' kinky hair disease. One of the mitochondria contains a round electron-dense deposit. (Original magnification ×45,000.) (From A. Hirano (79).)

they are most common in the pyramidal neurons of Sommer's sector and in the small neurons of the fascia dentata where they appear singly. They are single argentophilic structures (Fig. 1.33) and, because of their mild hematoxylinophilia, can be easily identified in ordinary H&E prepara-tions (Fig. 1.34). Pick bodies are approxi-mately the size of neuronal nucleus and are usually found in the apical area of the cell at a constant, narrow, but distinct distance from the nucleus. Frequently, granulovac-uolar bodies are found within or, more of-ten, surrounding the Pick body. The nearby

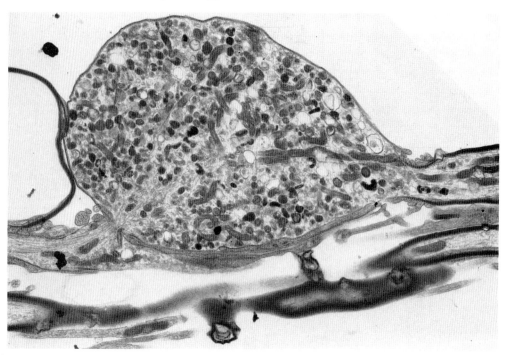

Figure 1.31. A swollen myelinated internode of an axon in the callosal radiation of a rat subjected to cyanide intoxication 4 months previously. The swollen segment of the axon is filled with numerous organelles including mitochondria. (Original magnification ×13,000.) (From A. Hirano et al. (118).)

neuropil of Sommer's sector usually contains eosinophilic rod-like structures.

Fine structural studies (15, 250) have revealed that Pick bodies consist of cytoplasmic areas containing large accumulations of fibrillary components including neurofilaments and microtubules as well as other organelles. More recently, the fibrillary material within the Pick body has been shown to have a tubular structure distinct from neurofilaments but similar to the straight tubules seen in Alzheimer-type neurofibrillary tangles (182). Two types of straight tubules were described. A slender 13- to 14-nm diameter, less electron-dense tubule as well as a thicker, denser tubule with a diameter which varied between 15 and 23 nm (182).

LEWY BODIES

These cytoplasmic inclusions were first described by Lewy in the substantia innominata and the dorsal motor nucleus of the vagus in a patient with idiopathic Parkinsonism. Lewy bodies have since been observed in the substantia nigra, locus ceru-

leus, and in certain pigmented and nonpigmented neurons in the brain stem and in the spinal cord as well as in the sympathetic ganglia and are considered to be a characteristic feature of idiopathic parkinsonism (178). Lewy bodies, in small numbers, have been associated with aging as well as with some cases of postencephalitic parkinsonism. In the latter they are usually accompanied by neurofibrillary tangles. Lewy bodies have also been observed in a small fraction of patients with parkinsonism-dementia complex on Guam. In these cases, too, the Lewy bodies are associated with neurofibrillary tangles, the main feature of the disease. In rare instances, Lewy bodies and neurofibrillary tangles have been seen within the same cell (79).

Most often Lewy bodies appear as single, round inclusions in the neuronal perikaryon or process (Fig. 1.35). In some cases they may be multiple, and they may be sausage-like or elongated and curve around the nucleus and extend into the cell process. Their size is variable, and they may be larger than the nucleus. Typically, they ap-

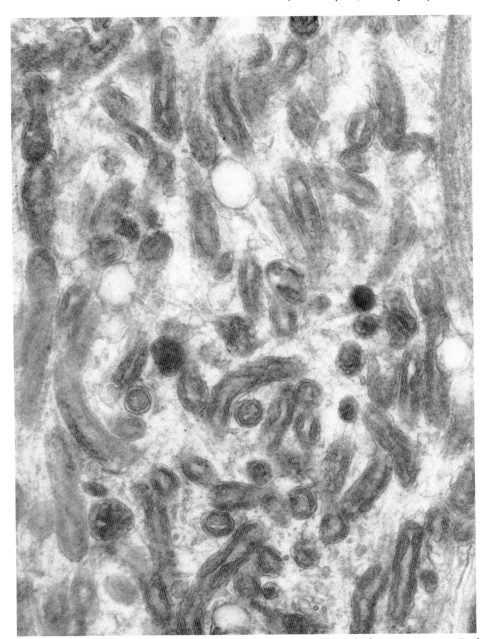

Figure 1.32. Higher magnification of an area similar to that illustrated in Figure 1.31. Dark and shrunken mitochondria are seen. (Original magnification ×45,000.) (From A. Hirano (79).)

pear as a core surrounded by a less dense amorphous halo. Sometimes they show a concentric lamellar structure.

Their staining patterns are distinct from other inclusions. Nissl stains do not stain the Lewy bodies which appear pale and empty in these preparations. Under these same conditions Lafora bodies appear blue. On the other hand, the cores of Lewy bodies are eosinophilic and are bright red after Masson's staining and are blue in Holzer preparations.

Despite the clear cut demarcation between the core and halo and between the halo and cytoplasm seen in the light microscope, fine structural study has failed to reveal any associated limiting membranes. The core consists of a tangle of 7- to 8-nm

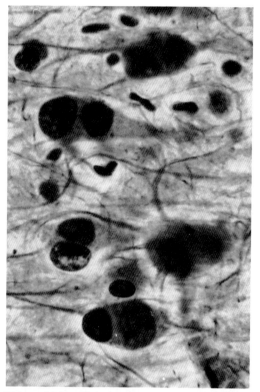

Figure 1.33. Pick bodies in Ammon's horn. Silver impregnation. (Original magnification ×720.)

filaments sometimes associated with occasional interspersed small vesicles (38, 202, 206). At the boundary between the core and the halo the filaments are arranged in a radial pattern and become less densely packed.

LAFORA BODIES

Lafora's disease is a rare neurological disorder of children. By 1973, only 64 cases had been reported in the world literature (133). It is a familial, progressive disease clinically manifested by myoclonic jerks, and it has sometimes been referred to as myoclonic epilepsy.

The characteristic pathological feature of the disease is the presence of intraneuronal, spherical Lafora bodies over widespread areas of the nervous system (Fig. 1.36). They are especially conspicuous in the substantia nigra and in the dentate nucleus of the cerebellum, where they are often larger than the nucleus, but are reportedly absent in the mammilary bodies and subthalamic nuclei (133).

Lafora bodies in neurons may appear either singly or multiply. Most often they are in the soma, but they may sometimes be seen in neuronal processes including synaptic endings.

In contrast to neurofibrillary tangles or Lewy bodies, Lafora bodies are easily recognized in Nissl preparations by their conspicuous blue color. They are also PAS-positive. PAS-positive inclusions are seen in cardiac muscle and in hepatic cells in patients with Lafora's disease (171).

Fine structural studies of nervous tissue from patients with Lafora's disease reveal that Lafora bodies consist of accumulations of short, fine filaments interspersed with finely granular material. No limiting membrane is present.

The fine structure of intraneuronal Lafora bodies is virtually identical to that of the corpora amylacea seen in astrocytes in adult and aged nervous systems. Similar structures have also been seen in axons rather than cell bodies in another neurological disease; adult polyglucosan body axonopathy (200). In addition, they have been

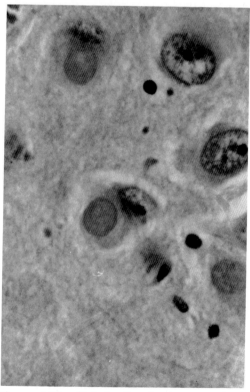

Figure 1.34. Pick bodies in Ammon's horn. H&E. (Original magnification ×720.)

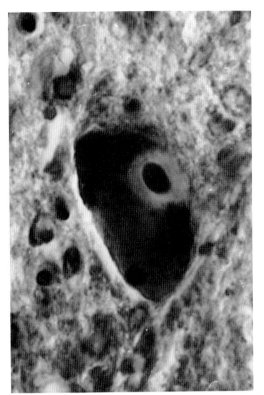

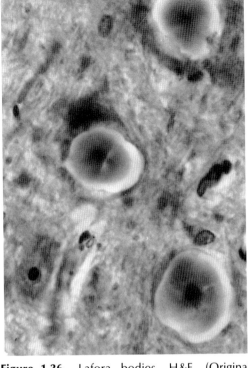

Figure 1.35. A Lewy body in a pigmented neuron of the locus ceruleus. Masson's stain. (Original magnification ×1080.)

Figure 1.36. Lafora bodies. H&E. (Original magnification ×720.)

identified in large numbers in a strain of dogs which has been used as a model for Lafora's disease (128).

INTRACYTOPLASMIC HYALINE (COLLOID) INCLUSIONS

Distinctly eosinophilic intracytoplasmic hyaline inclusions with sharply defined borders are occasionally found in the hypoglossal nuclei (Fig. 1.37) (256) and/or large anterior horn cells of elderly patients who may be apparently free of neurological disease (226). Their size is variable but may sometimes be great enough to fill and distend the soma. Other features of the cell appear normal. They are rare in children. Fine structural studies reveal that the inclusions are surrounded by ribosome-bearing membranes and that they actually consist of greatly distended portions of the rough endoplasmic reticulum (174).

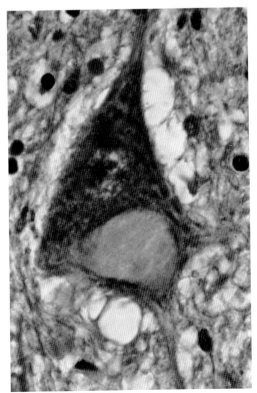

Figure 1.37. Intracytoplasmic hyaline (colloid) inclusions. H&E. (Original magnification ×720.)

BUNINA BODIES

Bunina bodies are small eosinophilic granules, a few microns wide, which were reported by Bunina in the anterior horn cells of patients with familial amyotrophic lateral sclerosis (16). Their presence was later confirmed in a number of cases of amyotrophic lateral sclerosis, including both sporadic and familial forms, as well as in patients from Guam (64, 100, 237). The granules may appear singly, or there may be several in a single cell and they are sometimes arranged in a chain.

Most workers (2, 60, 98, 180, 238) report that the fine structure of Bunina bodies consists of irregularly shaped, dense, granular material whose poorly defined border is associated with nearby organelles including the rough endoplasmic reticulum, vesicles, mitochondria, etc (Fig. 1.38). Small islands of scattered filaments are sometimes found in the interior. In addition to these structures some workers have reported the simultaneous presence of annulate lamellae (180, 238).

While originally suspected to be viral in nature the fine structural studies have not confirmed this view. It is worth pointing out that a number of other small eosinophilic inclusions have been reported in anterior horn cells in nonvirus-related conditions. These include Chediak-Higashi disease in Aleutian mink (125), vinca alkaloid intoxication (119), and neurolathyrism (106). Fine structural study has not revealed viral particles in any of these inclusions, and all are distinct from the Bunina bodies (100).

NEGRI BODIES

Patients with rabies display one to several spherical, eosinophilic Negri bodies in the cytoplasm of pyramidal cells in Ammon's horn or in the Purkinje cells. They are usually approximately as large as nucleoli, but their size is variable.

Fine structural study has revealed that they consist of tubular-shaped viral particles identical to those observed in animals infected with rabies (169).

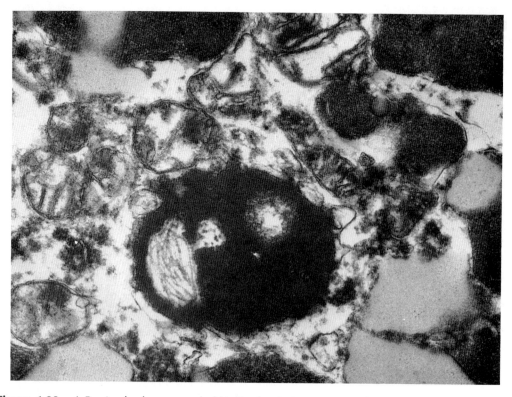

Figure 1.38. A Bunina body surrounded by lipofuscin in an anterior horn cell of an amyotrophic lateral sclerosis patient. (Original magnification ×35,000.) (From A. Hirano and K. Inoue (98).)

EOSINOPHILIC ROD-LIKE STRUCTURES

In 1965 (64) and 1966 (108) eosinophilic rod-like structures were first described in Ammon's horn of Guamanian patients with

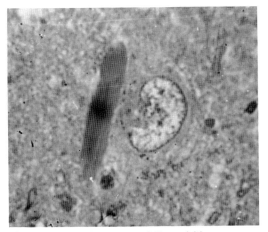

Figure 1.39. An eosinophilic rod-like structure in Ammon's horn. Epon-embedded, toluidine blue stain. (Original magnification ×1080.)

amyotrophic lateral sclerosis and parkinsonism-dementia complex (Fig. 1.39). Shortly thereafter they were described in Ammon's horn in a patient with Pick's disease and referred to as "Hirano bodies" (209).

Eosinophilic rod-like structures are best seen in H&E preparations where they appear highly refractile. They are rod-like in longitudinal section and circular or ovoid in cross-section. At high magnification they often show longitudinally oriented streaks.

Hirano bodies are particularly prominent in the electron microscope due to their characteristic fine structure which resists postmortem changes (92). They consist of highly organized, osmiophilic crystalloid arrays of interlacing filaments which display either a lattice-like or "herringbone" configuration (Fig. 1.40). Homogeneous, electron-dense material may sometimes appear as patches permeating the fibrillar structure (94). An analysis of the three-dimensional structure has been offered by Schochet and McCormick (210) and by To-

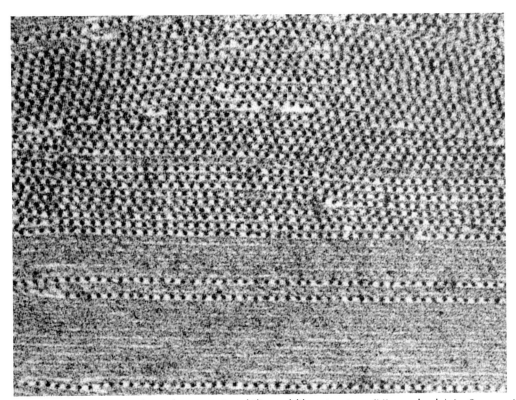

Figure 1.40. A section through an eosinophilic rod-like structure (Hirano body) in Sommer's sector of a Chamorro patient on Guam. (Original magnification ×165,000.) (From A. Hirano et al. (92).)

monago (235). They conclude that the fundamental structure consists of interesting arrays of parallel filaments. On the other hand, O'Brien et al. (176) have proposed that Hirano bodies are "stacked sheets of membrane-bound ribosomal particles derived from partially degraded rough endoplasmic reticulum or Nissl substance." Histochemical studies suggest that they are mostly proteinaceous and contain little lipid or carbohydrate (235).

Despite some contrary views (49), fine structural studies have suggested that Hirano bodies are usually intraneuronal in distribution. They have been found within processes which show synaptic contact with other neuronal elements, and Alzheimer-type neurofibrillary tangles have been identified within processes containing Hirano bodies.

Eosinophilic rod-like inclusions have been seen in a variety of human conditions and sites. It should be emphasized that they are almost exclusively confined to Sommer's sector of Ammon's horn and adjacent areas. This topographic distribution corresponds roughly to that of granulovacuolar bodies. This site also seems to be an area of high predilection for Alzheimer-type neurofibrillary tangles and even more so for Pick bodies.

Hirano bodies have been described in Pick's disease (209), Alzheimer's disease, and in Creutzfeldt-Jakob disease (161). They have also been seen rarely in the anterior horn cells (29, 207), and in axons (26) in certain motor neuron diseases. Perhaps more significantly, eosinophilic rod-like inclusions are found to be increased in Ammon's horn in the normal aged individual (50, 92, 177).

Identical structures have been observed in the cerebral cortex of aged primates (251). Other animals have shown similar inclusions, but these have usually been observed only in electron microscopic preparations and were not described in H&E-stained material (7, 179, 259). They have been seen in kuru-infected chimpanzees and in scrapie-infected animals, as well as in a number of other experimental disease conditions (69, 88). They have also been observed in the inner loops of myelin-forming oligodendroglia in rats (22). They are present in the inner loops of myelin sheaths

in the anterior roots of hamster mutants with hindleg paralysis (88), where they seem to be related to demyelination (73). In the hamster they are large and frequent enough to be identified both in H&E preparations as well as in the electron microscope.

Another abnormal eosinophilic inclusion, distinct from the Hirano body described above, has been observed in the apical dendrite of otherwise unremarkable pyramidal cells in the hippocampus in a woman who died of apparently nonneurological disease (142). The fine structure of these concentric, globular, and argentophilic inclusions consisted of an annulus-like arrangement of fine fibrils.

SMALL EOSINOPHILIC GRANULES OF THE PIGMENTED NEURONS OF THE SUBSTANTIA NIGRA AND LOCUS CERULEUS

The melanin-containing neurons of the substantia nigra and locus ceruleus sometimes contain clusters of small eosinophilic granules of unknown significance. They have been observed in apparently normal nervous tissue and in individuals of various ages.

Their fine structure has been reported to consist of groups of parallel 8.5-nm filaments connected by fine filaments (211). Similar structures are also observed within swollen cisternae of the rough endoplasmic reticulum. Others, however, regard the eosinophilic granules as altered mitochondria (214).

EOSINOPHILIC INCLUSIONS IN THALAMIC NEURONS

Small intraneuronal eosinophilic inclusions in the thalamus were originally described in a case of myotonic dystrophy (33, 249). They have since been observed in normal brain and are regarded as a phenomenon of normal aging (190).

Earlier fine structural studies suggested that these inclusions consisted of distended elements of the rough endoplasmic reticulum (33). Since then structures similar to those described in the pigmented neurons of the substantia nigra and locus ceruleus (211) have been seen in both aged human (190, 249) and murine thalami (40).

EOSINOPHILIC ROD-LIKE INCLUSIONS IN THE CAUDATE NUCLEUS

Nonspecific, rod-like inclusions with tapering ends have been described in the caudate nuclei of both normal individuals as well as some with various neurological and nonneurological conditions (144, 147). Three to ten of the 5- to 13-μm long inclusions were found within the cytoplasm of a single large neuron. They are brightly red in H&E preparations but are negative with the PAS or Bodian techniques.

Their fine structure (144) is similar to the eosinophilic inclusions seen in the pigmented neurons of the substantia nigra and locus ceruleus (211) and in the thalamus of aged humans and mice (190). It has been suggested that the eosinophilic inclusions of the caudate nucleus are age-related changes (144).

Dendrites

NORMAL

Ordinary light microscopic preparations are usually not adequate for the proper appreciation of the nature and extent of the dendrites. Most often only the major dendritic trunks are visualized. The best methods for staining the dendrite involve metallic impregnation techniques. Even these, however, are limited. The Bielschowsky silver impregnation method does, indeed, stain some dendritic branches, but apparently, only to the extent that appreciable numbers of fibrillar elements are present (Fig. 1.41). The fine distal branches are, therefore, not seen. The Golgi methods are greatly superior and are essential for the proper study of the dendrites, especially the smaller branches, but they are also limited (138). The Golgi-Cox method, which is reasonably consistent, does not usually allow visualization of the smallest branches or the spines. In addition, only about 1–5% of the neurons are impregnated, apparently at random. The rapid Golgi method does, indeed, seem to stain even the smallest branches, including the spines, but is not consistent and can result in a number of useable sections. Despite these difficulties the meticulous and patient work of neuroanatomists have allowed us a reasonably deep insight into the structure of the den-

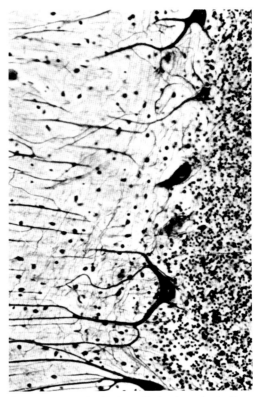

Figure 1.41. Purkinje cells in the cerebellum. Celloidin section. Silver impregnation. (Original magnification ×75.)

dritic tree. Additional information is being acquired by the application of newer techniques in which tracer substances such as fluorescent dyes or horseradish peroxidase is injected directly into the neurons by means of micropipettes (138).

The dendrites arise from the cell body and repeatedly branch, often resulting in a spectacular array. In pyramidal cells the dendritic trunks may arise from either the apical or basal portions of the cell. The apical dendrite, however, is always the most conspicuous and actually is a continuation of the cell body. The trunks branch into progressively narrower processes and, in certain neurons, finally produce the tiny dendritic spines. Purkinje cells and the pyramidal cells of the cerebral cortex are especially well endowed with dendritic spines, whereas the cerebellar basket cells and the motor neurons of the spinal cord show relatively few (186).

The extensive arborization of the dendritic tree results in an enormous expansion of the neuronal cell surface, which is, in large measure, devoted to synaptic contact. Synapses may be formed on the smooth dendritic processes themselves, as well as on the dendritic protrusions, especially the spines (Figs. 1.42 and 1.43). Thus, the shape and extent of the dendritic tree to a great extent defines the particular neuron's role in the organization of the nervous system as a whole, since it determines the field from which it will receive its input.

Those portions of the dendritic surface not involved in synaptic contact are, in certain neurons such as Purkinje cells, covered by "satellite cells," usually astrocytic sheet-like processes. These processes sometimes apparently serve to segregate individual or small groups of synapses.

Within the larger dendritic trunks the neuronal cytoplasm is essentially the same as the neuronal cell body. As the dendrites branch, however, the contents change. The Golgi apparatus does not usually extend much beyond the first branching. Eventually the contents become limited to microtubules, neurofilaments, mitochondria, and occasional elements of the smooth endoplasmic reticulum. The dendritic spines are even devoid of mitochondria, neurofilaments, and microtubules.

The dendrites form relatively late in the development of the neurons. They are always preceded by the outgrowth of the axon, and it seems quite certain that the axon has already formed its connections before the dendrites begin their differentiation (138). Eventually, however, the dendrites come to constitute over 90% of the postsynaptic surface of the neurons (138).

PATHOLOGY

The difficulty in visualizing the dendrites described above has resulted in relatively little attention being paid to the pathology of this important part of the neuron. Nevertheless, some important pathological alterations are known (148). In various lipidoses (39), as well as in a number of other conditions such as granule cell type cerebellar degeneration, kinky hair disease (137, 166), and organic mercury poisoning (130), so-called "stellate bodies" or "cacti" are found on the dendrites of Purkinje cells. These are focal expansions of the dendritic processes which may sometimes attain the size of the cell body itself. The stellate bodies themselves often display numerous radiating processes.

Reduction of dendritic arborization in cortical neurons is a well-known change seen in normal aging as well as in senile dementia of Alzheimer type (167, 204). The orientation of the dendritic tree of cerebral neurons is severely distorted and shrunken in dementia paralytica due to syphilis. In kinky hair disease and in certain other genetic disorders the dendrites of the Purkinje cells become seriously diminished and distorted (75). Several murine mutants show similar alterations of the dendritic tree of the Purkinje cells. An interesting experimental model for the loss of spines on pyramidal cells has been demonstrated by raising mice in the dark (242). A partial recovery of the spines follows return to the light.

Axons

NORMAL

While some exceptions are known, most neurons have a single axon (186). It usually arises from a specialized region of the soma, the axon hillock. That portion of the axon between the axon hillock and the first myelin segment is the "initial segment." In the anterior horn cell the initial segment narrows distally until it widens to its definitive caliber at the first myelin segment (30) or its first branch point (186). The axon then maintains its width throughout its length until it branches into finer processes at its target (186). Branches are not common but are known to occur as so-called "collaterals." They generally arise at almost right angles from the main axon (186). Athough it stains faintly blue in H&E preparations the axon is best demonstrated at the optical level by certain silver impregnation methods, after which they appear dense and black.

A great deal of our current understanding of the structure of the axon is the result of fine structural studies (68, 80, 89, 192). The axon hillock is basically an extension of the soma but has special characteristics of its own (187). The Nissl substance diminishes distally to become replaced by conspicuous fibrillary elements and clusters of free ribosomes. Mitochondria and elements of the

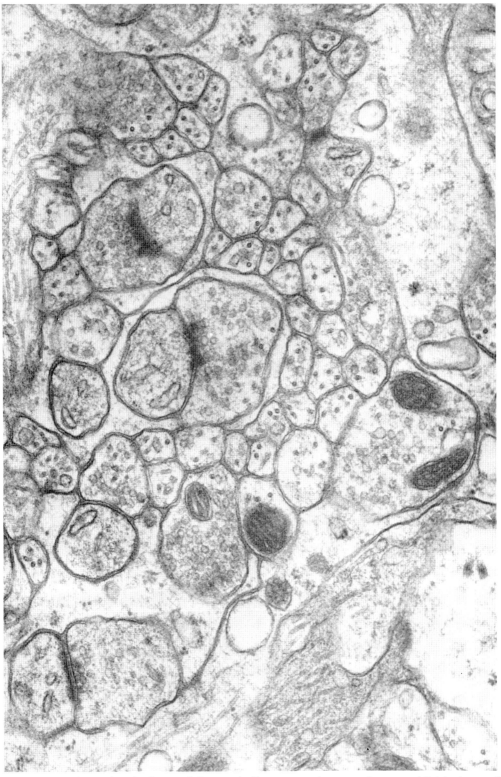

Figure 1.42. The molecular layer of the cerebellar cortex of a normal mouse. (Original magnification ×40,000.)

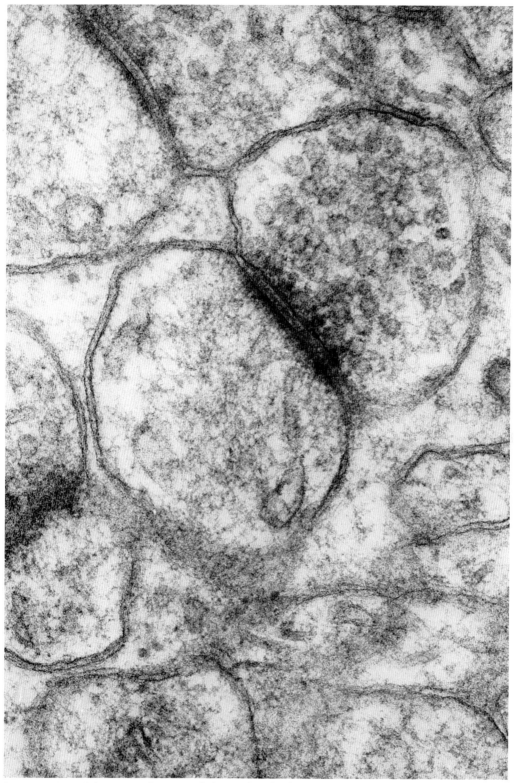

Figure 1.43. Higher magnification of the molecular layer of the mouse cerebellum. Synapses between the parallel fibers and the dendritic spines of Purkinje cells are seen. Synaptic vesicles in a presynaptic element and a postsynaptic element with a prominent postmembranous thickening are visible. The synapse is surrounded by astrocytic processes. (Original magnification ×111,000.) (From N. Malamud and A. Hirano (163).)

smooth endoplasmic reticulum are all present. Neurofilaments are a consistent feature and are oriented towards the axon. Microtubules are arranged in similarly oriented fascicles of 3 or 4 to 20 or more (186). Within the fascicles the parallel microtubules are connected by fine filaments.

The initial segment, in either myelinated or unmyelinated axons (187), is similar and contains no Nissl substance or Golgi apparatus. Clusters of free ribosomes are present. Other elements such as mitochondria and smooth endoplasmic reticulum are also seen. The fibrillary elements such as microtubules and neurofilaments constitute the most conspicuous organelles, and they are arranged as they are in the axon hillock (187, 193).

The axon itself has a relatively simple fine structure. Its characteristic organelles are the neurofilaments and microtubules as well as elements of the smooth endoplasmic reticulum. The ratio of neurofilaments to microtubules depends on the caliber of the axons. While neurofilaments are more numerous in large axons, the microtubules become more common in the small axons. Elongated mitochondria are present, but ribosomes are usually not seen beyond the first myelinated segment (186). A very fine filamentous material apparently connecting all of the axonal organelles including the plasma membrane has been described.

As in the rest of the neuron, the axon, the initial segment, and the axon hillock are surrounded by a typical plasma membrane (187). These three areas, however, are characterized by the presence of a finely filamentous material closely subjacent to the inner leaflet of the plasma membrane. This "undercoating material" is continuous beneath the plasma membrane of the axon hillock and the initial segment, but in the axon it is limited to those areas beneath the node of Ranvier. Interestingly, those areas in which undercoating material is present have been implicated in the generation and propagation of action potentials.

The conspicuousness of cytoskeletal elements in the axon has for some time suggested that they are involved in axonal flow. It has been shown that materials originating in the soma proceed toward the periphery at either a fast (100–1,000 mm/d) or a slow (1–10 mm/d) rate (138). Ex-

ogenous tracer material applied to target organs such as muscle can be traced to the proximal portion of the axon and the cell body. Tracers which have been used to study retrograde flow include horseradish peroxidase, tetanus toxin, nerve growth factor, and certain viruses (138, 149, 150). Apparently, the smooth endoplasmic reticulum provides a pathway for the rapid flow of materials in both anterograde and retrograde directions (35, 36).

In general, the slow moving proteins which have been localized by means of electron microscopic autoradiography have been found in bundles of neurofilaments, microtubules, mitochondria, and plasma membranes (138). Of all the slow moving proteins less than 5% apparently reach the nerve endings (35). In contrast, most of the fast moving components reach the axon terminals. They have been localized en route to the terminals in the plasma membrane, smooth endoplasmic reticulum, and certain storage granules (138).

The subject of axonal flow is large and complex. The reader is referred to appropriate texts for further information.

PATHOLOGY

Most axons have only a limited repertoire of reactions that may occur regardless of the underlying pathology. Among these changes is focal axonal swelling with concomitant loss of organelles (68). This change may be induced artifactitiously, or it may represent an anoxic insult to the living tissue. It has been produced experimentally by cyanide intoxication in rats (107).

In contrast to the loss of organelles, under some circumstances, there may appear an abnormal increase in certain elements. Increases in 10-nm neurofilaments have already been described in the section dealing with neurofilaments (Fig. 1.22). It is particularly commonplace in axons where neurofilaments are so prominent. Besides an increase in number, the neurofilaments may also lose their usual parallel, longitudinal orientation, and bundles of filaments assume a distorted, tangled configuration.

In cerebellar degeneration, or normal aging, "torpedoes," argentophilic focal enlargements of the proximal portions of Purkinje cell axons, are seen which are consti-

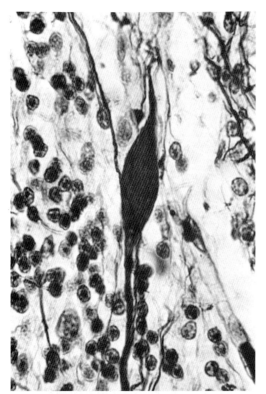

Figure 1.44. A torpedo in the granule cell layer of the cerebellum. Paraffin section. Silver impregnation. (Original magnification ×720.)

tuted of large accumulations of 10-nm neurofilaments (Fig. 1.44). Accumulations of neurofilaments, referred to as spheroids, have also been observed in the axons and cell bodies of anterior horn cells in a number of cases of ALS (19, 98). Similar structures have been induced experimentally in anterior horns and other areas by intoxication with β,β'-iminodipropionitrile (28). Filamentous accumulations in the distal portion of the axon are seen in giant axonal neuropathy of peripheral nerves (2) and after a number of experimental procedures (220).

In addition to filament accumulation, increases in mitochondria (246), vesicles, and dense bodies are also common axonal reactions (68, 155) (Figs. 1.31, 1.32, and 1.45). These, too, tend to be segmental in nature and, often, may be associated with filamentous accumulations. In these cases, the accumulation of membrane-bound organelles and disoriented or circumferentially arranged filaments are sometimes at the pe-

riphery of the axon surrounding a central core of longitudinally oriented, parallel filaments.

The smooth endoplasmic reticulum, too, is subject to pathological change. This may be reflected in an abnormal proliferation of the smooth endoplasmic reticulum in focal regions of the axon (Fig. 1.46). The membrane may assume a bizarre, whorl-like or lamellar structure in neuraxonal dystrophy or in experimental triorthocresyl phosphate or vitamin E intoxication (68, 155). Another possible configuration of the smooth endoplasmic reticulum is the formation of the so-called "honeycomb-like tubular structures" (112, 113) (Fig. 1.47). Under normal circumstances they are, for the most part, seen in the granule cell layer of the cerebellum in myelinated axons which are thought to be recurrent axons of the Purkinje cells. They have also been reported in axons in vestibular nuclei of normal rats (219). They have been described in both myelinated and unmyelinated axons of the cerebellum (113), and even in the cerebrum of experimental animals (102).

Another structure whose relationship to normal axonal components is not completely apparent is the "tubulovesicular structures" (68). These structures consist of an accumulation of branching and interconnected tubules and vesicles and may be derived from the smooth endoplasmic reticulum. They are characteristically seen in synaptic terminals (see synapses), but have also been observed within the internodal portions of the axon.

Small numbers of structures which are indistinguishable from Lafora bodies have been reported within the myelinated axons of the spinal cord and peripheral nerves of patients with various neurological diseases as well as in apparently normal aged individuals (2). These "polyglucosan bodies" have been shown to occur in larger numbers in a progressive neurological disorder of adults, termed adult polyglucosan body disease, where they are found in astrocytes and in axons in both the central and peripheral nervous system (200).

Various inclusions, obviously derived from outside the cell, have been seen within axons. Infectious organisms have been described in axons, and hematogenous edema

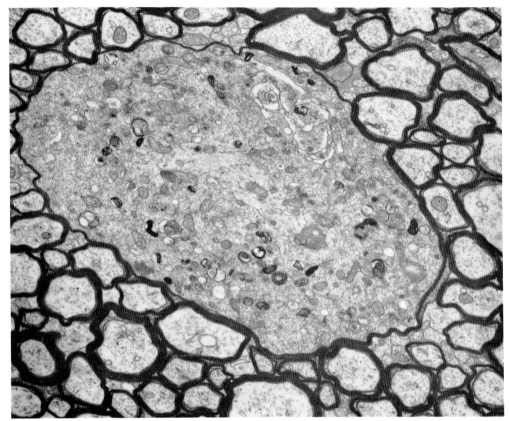

Figure 1.45. A distended myelinated axon in the corpus callosum of a rat with experimental brain injury. The axoplasm is filled with organelles. (Original magnification ×17,000.) (From A. Hirano (67).)

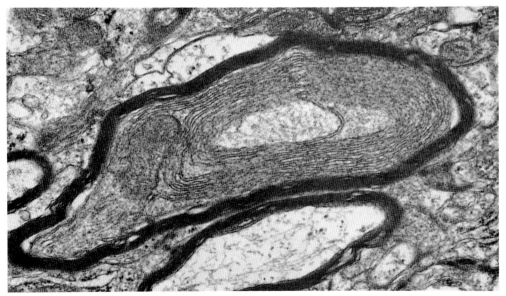

Figure 1.46. A myelinated axon in the cerebellum of a normal littermate of a jimpy mouse. A compactly arranged whorl of endoplasmic reticulum is visible within the axon. (Original magnification ×27,000.) (From A. Hirano et al. (113).)

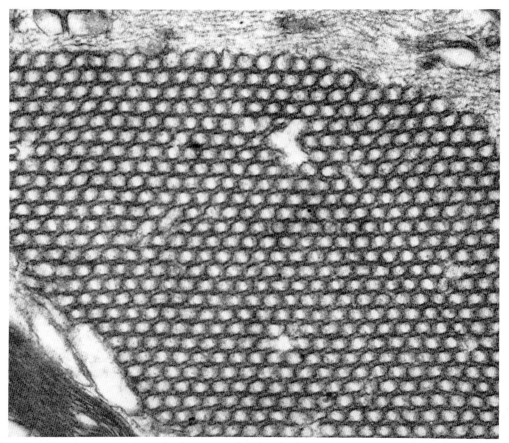

Figure 1.47. A cross-section of a honeycomb-like tubular structure in a myelinated axon in the granule cell layer in the cerebellum of a chimpanzee infected with kuru. (Original magnification ×58,000.) (From A. Hirano et al. (112).)

fluid has been identified in cases of stab wound injury associated with cerebral edema (68).

Under certain circumstances the normal relationship between the axolemma and the apposing glial or Schwann cell membrane may become severely distorted. While the distance between the two membranes is usually remarkably well maintained, the membranes are sometimes deeply invaginated into the axoplasm (68). These phenomena are sometimes seen in apparently normal tissue but become more pronounced and frequent under various pathological conditions. The paranodal area is apparently a site of predilection for these changes. Despite these sometimes drastic distortions it is noteworthy that the periaxonal space, i.e., the extracellular space between the outer leaflets of the axolemma and the plasma membrane of the myelin-

forming cell, maintains its original dimensions over most of the internodal axonal surface. Some separations do occur, but these are most often small and focal and, even when large, the axon tends to retain its original contact with the myelin-forming cell, at least over some portion of its periphery (80).

Many of the above described morphological alterations are seen in Wallerian degeneration. Wallerian degeneration occurs as the result of the transection of the axon (2, 8, 138). The anterograde effect consists of the degeneration of the distal portion of the axon. The myelin sheath of the axon distal to the injury disintegrates, and changes in the target organs, such as muscle, become evident. Eventually macrophages invade the area. Regeneration usually occurs especially in the peripheral nervous system where Schwann cell proliferation is pronounced. Changes also occur in that part of the axon proximal to the injury, although these are usually limited to the immediate vicinity of the section. During regeneration in the peripheral nervous system the proximal stump undergoes axonal sprouting and subsequent remyelination. Reactive changes in the soma and surrounding glial elements have already been described (see above, p. 5).

In addition to actual section, the axon is also subject to degenerative changes as the result of neurological disease. Motor neuron disease, spinocerebellar degeneration, intoxication, and certain metabolic disorders are all good examples of these conditions. In some of these conditions, especially certain intoxications (21, 23, 139, 220) and perhaps in certain degenerative disorders (21), the first visible lesions have been reported to be in the more distal portion of the axon, but initially, at least, not involving the synaptic terminal (distal axonopathy). Apparently the changes progress in a retrograde fashion. Despite this apparent "dying back" process (21) or distal axonopathy (220) the cell body may appear to remain intact.

Neuroaxonal dystrophy seen primarily in the nucleus gracilis of some elderly individuals as well as in infantile neuroaxonal dystrophy (41, 140, 230), in children with prolonged mucoviscidosis (221) or congenital biliary atresia (222), and in experimental vitamin E deficiency (155) may be considered as a special form of axonal degeneration. In this case, however, the changes are confined to the most distal portion of the axon, i.e., the presynaptic terminal and its immediate vicinity. Neuroaxonal dystrophy is recognizable by the appearance of scattered 15- to 120-μm spheroids or ovoids. When examined by electron microscopy these structures show a number of pathological changes characteristic of axonal change. These include enormous accumulations of organelles, tubulovesicular structures, large numbers of disarranged 10-nm neurofilaments, altered mitochondria, dense bodies, as well as concentric or lamellar accumulations of membranes presumably derived from the smooth endoplasmic reticulum (Fig. 1.48).

Another example of a process in which the axon may show a number of the morphological alterations described above is segmental demyelination as seen in multiple sclerosis or experimental allergic encephalomyelitis among many other conditions. In this case the underlying pathomechanisms affect the myelin sheath or myelin-forming cell, and the axonal changes are presumably a reaction to the alterations of the sheath.

Synapses

NORMAL

The synapse is that region of apposition between two neurons at which action potentials are transmitted. Most often it occurs between an axon and a dendrite or an axon and a cell body. The typical vertebrate synapse is "chemical" in nature in that the impulses are transmitted by means of a chemical transmitter which transverses the distance between the cells.

These are the kinds of synapses we shall discuss here. However, the reader should be aware of various other kinds of synapses which have been described, but usually in only limited examples. Chemical synapses have been described between axons and other axons, between two dendrites, between dendrites and a cell body, and even between two cell bodies. "Electrical" synapses, which are morphologically distinct from the chemical synapse, are usually features of invertebrates and certain of the lower vertebrates as well as in a few regions of the mammalian nervous system (189). There are, in addition, contacts between neurons and the nonneural target cells, usually a muscle or gland. The latter, of course, are characteristic features of the vertebrate nervous system but are almost completely confined to the peripheral nervous system and are outside the scope of this volume.

Synapses may be classified among the cell junctions. They differ, however, from most other junctions by virtue of their functional polarity, which is reflected in a morphological asymmetry. According to the physiologists, action potentials are propagated in all directions along a membrane, but they are transmitted across a synapse in one direction only. Morphologically the synapse can be divided into three distinct elements. The presynaptic terminal con-

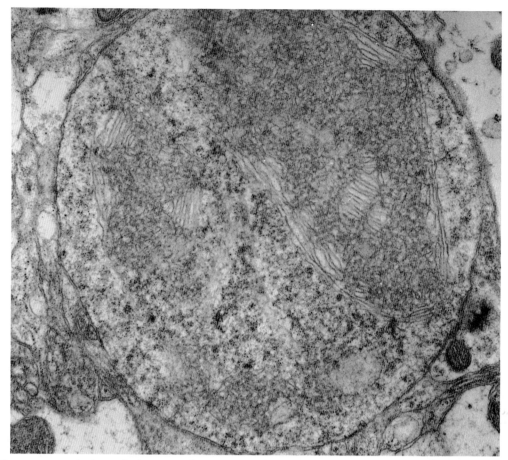

Figure 1.48. A distended neuronal process in the cerebral cortex of a patient with infantile neuroaxonal dystrophy. Tubulovesicular material virtually fills the interior. (Original magnification ×30,000.) (From A. Hirano and H. M. Zimmerman (120).)

taining synaptic vesicles, mitochondria, and a dense submembranous material, the synaptic cleft between the two cells which is characteristically filled with an electron-dense material, and the postsynaptic terminal which features a well-developed complex submembranous dense structure.

On the basis of the orientation of the pre- and postsynaptic elements it is usually easy to determine the afferent and efferent components in a neural network. In a limited number of specific cells as well as in some experimental settings, however, so-called "reciprocal" synapses have been reported in which two synapses with opposite polarities exist side by side joining the same two neurons (186).

Despite the common use of the term "terminal" or "ending" many synaptic elements

are not at the end of the neurite. Some are, indeed, located at the surface of terminal swellings of the axon or "boutons terminalis." Others, however, the so-called "en passant" synapses, are found on the shaft of the neurite arranged in a chain-like fashion.

Most synapses have been classified into two categories on the basis of morphological criteria. According to Gray the type 1 synapse may be found on dendritic spines as well as on smooth neuronal surfaces. The synaptic vesicles are spheroid and 20–60 nm in diameter. They are surrounded by a unit membrane. A dense, submembranous material may be visualized by the use of ethanolic phosphotungstic acid or bismuth iodide staining. Those synaptic vesicles at the surface of the terminal are embedded in triangular or hexagonal lacunae in this meshwork.

Presumably, when an impulse is to be transmitted the membrane of the synaptic vesicle fuses with that of the presynaptic terminal, and the neurotransmitter is released into the synaptic cleft across which it diffuses to reach the postsynaptic surface. The nature and mode of action of the neurotransmitter is outside the scope of this volume, and the reader is referred to appropriate texts of neurophysiology and neurochemistry. In type 1 synapses (55) the cleft is approximately 20 nm wide, somewhat wider than nearby extracellular spaces, and is filled with a poorly defined dense material whose nature and function is unknown.

The postsynaptic terminal in type 1 synapses is characterized by a dense, osmiophilic submembranous material which also stains with bismuth iodide or ethanolic phosphotungstic acid. The postsynaptic element may occur on a smooth portion of the dendrite or cell body or may be at the short protrusion. Most characteristically, these protrusions consist of dendritic spines which are devoid of any organelles except for fine filaments and occasional elements of the smooth endoplasmic reticulum. In some of the pyramidal neurons of the cerebral cortex ordered stacks of cisterns of smooth endoplasmic reticulum separated by a characteristic dense substance are present and form the so-called "spine apparatus." These cisterns are connected to the smooth endoplasmic reticulum of the shaft of the dendrite by means of connecting tubules (186). In other dendritic spines, however, notably in the Purkinje cells of the cerebellum, only occasional elements of the smooth endoplasmic reticulum are present, and no spine apparatus is seen.

As mentioned earlier the presynaptic ending of an axon sometimes abuts a nonneuronal target cell. In many of these cases a basal lamina intervenes between the axon and its target. Best known among these is the neuromuscular junction, but even within the central nervous system these configurations may be seen in the area postrema and median eminence. In these areas presynaptic terminals are found at the basal lamina surrounding the perivascular space of fenestrated capillaries.

In general, one may use the presence of a synapse as a reliable guide to the identification of a neuron, especially in the normal adult. However, one should be aware of the fact that during development astrocytes will sometimes show submembranous densities which appear similar to postsynaptic elements (61).

The fundamental architecture of the type 2 synapse (55) is essentially the same as that of the type 1. Several important distinctions, however, can be drawn. Type 2 synapses are found at the surface of the dendritic shafts or cell bodies rather than on spines. In some kinds of glutaraldehyde-fixed preparations their synaptic vesicles sometimes appear elliptical rather than spheroid (241). The significance of this shape is uncertain (186). The synaptic cleft in type 2 synapses is narrower than in type 1 synapses and retains the same dimensions as nearby extracellular spaces or may even be somewhat narrower. The dense submembranous structure of the postsynaptic terminals is less dense than those seen in type 1 synapses and is more similar to the presynaptic density.

An interesting correlation between structure and function has been drawn with regard to the type 1 and type 2 synapses. In the cerebellum, at least, type 1 synapses appear to be excitatory in nature, while type 2 synapses are apparently inhibitory.

On the other hand, this correlation has not yet been demonstrated in other regions of the central nervous system. Furthermore, not all synapses are easily classifiable as either type 1 or type 2. Some have widened clefts but symmetrical densities, whereas in others there are narrow clefts and asymmetric densities (186).

Another problem with regard to the clear-cut classification of synapses arises from the fact that in some cases the synaptic vesicles contain dense cores. These are substantially larger vesicles, approximately 100 nm in diameter, and are more characteristic of the peripheral nervous system and certain hypothalamic nuclei. For more information with regard to the nature of the neurotransmitter substances associated with dense core vesicles and their differences from the electron-lucent vesicles the reader is referred to appropriate texts on neurophysiology and neurochemistry.

PATHOLOGY

Among the most common examples of presynaptic pathology is the empty swelling of these structures which, if prominent enough, is visible in the light microscope and recognized as a "spongy" state. One must be cautious in the interpretation of these changes, however, since they may be induced artifactitiously. On the other hand, they represent true pathological alterations in cases of anoxia and have been induced experimentally by certain toxic agents (79).

Synaptic swelling is one of the elements contributing to "spongiform encephalopathy" seen in Creutzfeld-Jakob and kuru disease (54, 95, 156). Similar changes are seen in scrapie and other so-called "slow" virus infections in animals (45).

In some conditions the presynaptic terminal may lose most or all of its synaptic vesicles, especially those at the synaptic surface. Otherwise the terminal appears normal (82). It is not obviously swollen, and the presynaptic mesh as well as the postsynaptic ending are well developed and unremarkable.

Axonal or neuronal damage eventually may lead to atrophy and degeneration of the synaptic terminal. In some of these cases the degeneration of the presynaptic terminal is associated with an accumulation of filaments to the extent that argentophilia may be observed (56). Eventually the remains of the degenerated presynaptic terminal is removed by phagocytic cells.

The reaction of a postsynaptic terminal to the loss of its presynaptic mate is variable. Most often the postsynaptic ending is resorbed by its process and, indeed, sometimes the entire transsynaptic neuron may degenerate. On the other hand, the postsynaptic terminal may be maintained in an apparently normal process for substantial periods of time. This phenomenon may be significant for the process of reinnervation.

Tubulovesicular structures (Fig. 1.48) have been observed in presynaptic terminals as well as in axons as described above. Indeed, they were first reported in distended presynaptic terminals of cortical neurons in an infant with convulsions, mental retardation, and cortical blindness (53). Since then presynaptic terminals containing tubulovesicular structures have been observed in infantile neuronal dystrophy (Seitelberger's disease) (203), as well as in other conditions (120). In Alzheimer's

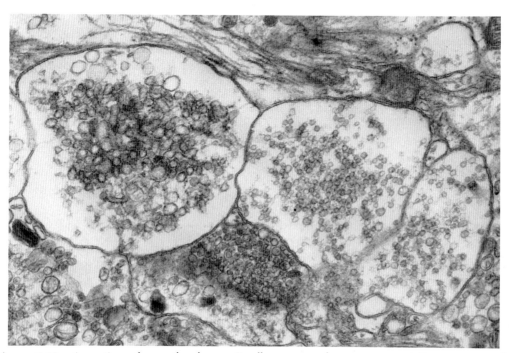

Figure 1.49. A portion of a senile plaque. Swollen neuronal processes contain many synaptic vesicles. (Original magnification ×33,000.) (From A. Hirano (79).)

disease and other conditions occasional presynaptic terminals as well as axons may contain tubulovesicular structures along with other changes.

Altered synaptic terminals are one of the important features of senile plaques. Within the plaques the synaptic terminals as well as other neuronal processes contain a variety of abnormally accumulated structures. These include mitochondria, dense bodies, synaptic vesicles (Fig. 1.49), tubulovesicular structures, neurofilaments, microtubules, and Alzheimer's neurofibrillary tangles (51, 231, 253).

Aberrant synaptic development is associated with certain known neurological diseases as well as with some experimental conditions and animal mutations. In the granule cell type of cerebellar degeneration the dendritic arborization of the Purkinje cell is severely distorted and depressed as the result of the failure of the granule cells to develop properly. In addition to some apparently normal synapses, many dendritic spines are found on the large dendritic trunks of the Purkinje cells rather than on the tertiary branchlets (90). These spines are not attached to presynaptic endings since their usual afferents, the parallel fibers of the granule cells, are missing. Instead they are covered by voluminous astrocytic processes. In other respects, however, the unattached spines appear identical to their normal counterparts, at least with regard to their histochemical and fine structural features. Similar unattached

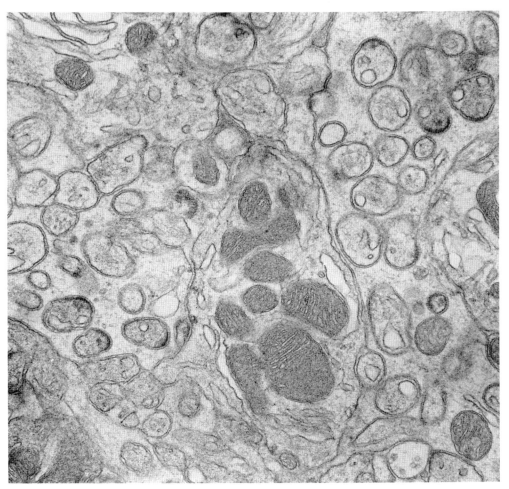

Figure 1.50. The cerebellar cortex of a weaver mouse. Many unattached Purkinje cell dendritic spines are visible within a matrix of widened astrocytic processes. Note the paucity of small caliber axons of granule cells. (Original magnification ×30,000.) (From A. Hirano and H. M. Dembitzer (84).)

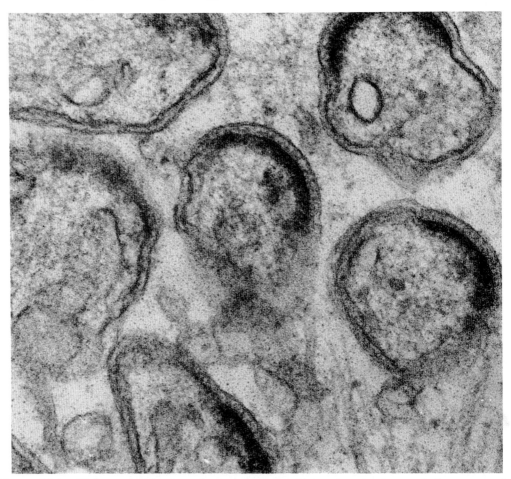

Figure 1.51. Higher magnification of unattached dendritic spines in the cerebellar cortex of a weaver mouse. Postmembranous densities and cleft material are present. The extracellular space abutting the region of the postmembranous density is wider than the other, nearby, extracellular spaces. (Original magnification ×112,000.) (From A. Hirano and H. M. Dembitzer (84).)

dendritic spines have been observed on the Purkinje cells of patients with Menkes' kinky hair disease (105).

The occurrence of apparently identical unattached spines (Figs. 1.50 and 1.51) in several experimental model systems has allowed the elucidation of the development of these structures (71). Even in normal animals rare, unattached spines may be seen (93), but when large numbers of granule cells either fail to descend or degenerate shortly after as the result of a number of conditions such as genetic defect (85, 86), intoxication (91), infection or x-irradiation, many unattached spines appear. The unattached spines are found on the distorted dendritic tree of the Purkinje cell, even though there is no immediate contact of a

potential presynaptic mate. Often, under these conditions, the usual precise alignment of the Purkinje cells is distorted.

The similar ability of presynaptic terminals for independent development has also been suggested. Fine structural studies of certain cases of neuroblastoma have revealed tumor cell processes complete with synaptic vesicles and submembranous densities in areas devoid of postsynaptic elements (77, 114) (Fig. 1.52). Similar results have been reported in certain mutant animals (218).

Other Neuronal Changes

NEURONAL LOSS

Neuronal loss is a prominent feature of

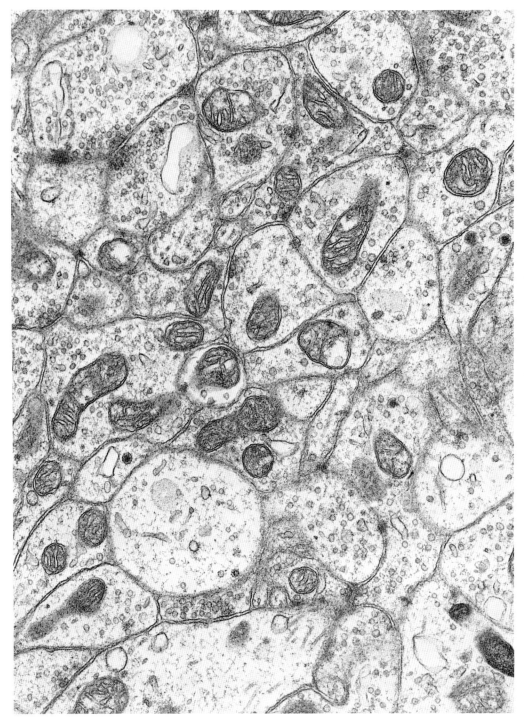

Figure 1.52. A cross-section of cell processes in a cerebellar neuroblastoma. Many synaptic vesicles are seen in almost all of the processes. Some processes demonstrate peripheral aggregates of vesicles, but no corresponding postsynaptic density is apparent. (Original magnification ×33,000.) (From A. Hirano (77).)

a number of neurological diseases. Since the neuron is incapable of division, once lost, it is not replaced.

Under some conditions the evidence of neuronal loss is clear. In Wednig-Hoffmann disease, for example, the position of the lost large anterior horn cell may be recognizable as an "empty cell bed." In olivopontocerebellar degeneration and other cerebellar degenerative diseases the former position of the Purkinje cell can be detected in silver impregnation preparations by the presence of "empty baskets." These are formed by the neurites of the basket cells which remain in place surrounding the now empty region of the Purkinje cell layer.

In many other conditions, however, neuronal loss is not marked by such obvious changes. Instead one must rely on certain other clues. Gross atrophy or shrinkage of the region as well as changes of the neuropil texture and glial scar formation are all common signs of neuronal loss. Ideally, of course, the true extent of neuronal loss in, for example, the substantia nigra in parkinsonism or the anterior horns in amyotrophic lateral sclerosis, should be evaluated by comparison with control sections.

The pattern of neuronal loss can often suggest the underlying pathomechanism. In some conditions, entire neuronal systems are involved so that in motor neuron disease, for example, the motor neurons are the primary target while other nearby neurons are spared (136). In other conditions, however, such as inflammation or infarct, all the neurons in the region are affected regardless of their function. A similar focal, plaque-like area of neuronal loss is seen in healed anterior poliomyelitis (70, 134).

Neuronophagia may precede neuronal loss. In acute poliomyelitis or Werdnig-Hoffmann disease neuronal loss may be accompanied by the accumulation of phagocytic cells around the site of the neuron. Neuronophagia, however, is quite exceptional in more long-standing cases of motor neuron disease, such as amyotrophic lateral sclerosis or in healed poliomyelitis.

FERRUGINATION

The formation of mineral deposits, including iron, at the site of a dead neuron, or "ferrugination," is uncommon but has been observed in various conditions such as Japanese B encephalitis and in old infarcts, among others. These deposits assume the shape of the neuron including the dendritic trunks and appear homogenous and dark blue in H&E or Nissl preparations.

DARK AND SHRUNKEN NEURONS

Dark, hyperchromatic and shrunken neurons are frequently seen in H&E or Nissl preparations of such chronic diseases as Alzheimer's disease, amyotrophic lateral sclerosis, and other conditions associated with neuronal loss. This phenomenon has been referred to as "simple neuronal atrophy" or "chronic nerve cell degeneration." Similar, artifactitiously induced, dark and shrunken neurons are sometimes seen in apparently normal cerebral cortex adjacent to such lesions as deep seated brain tumors and in poorly preserved material from experimental animals (18).

ISCHEMIC NEURONS

Systemic anoxia or localized circulatory disturbances result in characteristic pathological changes within a few days after the insult. These are especially prominent in the pyramidal neurons of Sommer's sector or the Purkinje cells of the cerebellum after systemic anoxia.

In H&E preparations, the nuclei of the neurons appear uniformly blue, and the cytoplasm is red. Both the perineuronal and perivascular areas appear vacuolated due, in great measure, to the swelling of the astrocytic process which invests these areas.

TRANSNEURONAL DEGENERATION
(32, 48, 198, 239)

Neuronal degeneration may follow the loss of either afferent (anterograde degeneration) or efferent (retrograde degeneration) connections. Its extent and incidence are highly variable, depending on the species, the age, and the neuronal system involved. Very little is known concerning this phenomenon in the human except for the visual system, the central tegmental tract-inferior olive connection, and some parts of the limbic system, as well as a few others. In experimental animals transneuronal degeneration is more likely to occur in younger animals and after a long period of time following substantial denervation.

SHAPE CHANGES

As already described, the shape and distribution of the dendritic tree may be altered significantly in certain conditions. The soma, too, may change as the result of pathological processes. In certain conditions, such as Menkes' kinky hair disease, the soma of the Purkinje cells shows numerous "somatic sprouts" (44, 166, 196). These consist of short, radiating cell processes visible in the light microscope (Fig. 1.53). Electron microscopic study has revealed the presence of spines at the cell surface, some of which form a synaptic connection with afferent fibers, while others appear unattached (105). Somatic sprouts similar to those described in Menkes' disease have been reported as a transient phenomenon in normal embryonic development of experimental animals as well as in certain murine mutants (71, 77).

In certain lipidoses as well as some other conditions large expansions of the basal pole of the neuron, probably including the axon hillock and initial segment of the axon, appear as so-called "meganeurites" (195). These, too have been shown to bear sprouts similar to the somatic sprouts or cactus-like dendritic expansions.

NEOPLASMS

Neuronal neoplasms within the central nervous system are extremely rare. They may be identified by the presence of a synaptic terminal at the surface of the tumor cell or synaptic vesicles within the cytoplasm. Most often the synaptic vesicles are of the dense core variety similar to those seen in neuroblastomas of the peripheral nervous system. In some cases of cerebellar neuroblastoma the tumor cells show frequent synaptic vesicles, a preponderance of which are clear rather than dense-cored (216). Many of the tumor cell processes in these cases show examples of immature presynaptic elements apparently unattached to any postsynaptic element.

Paragangliomas have been reported in the cauda equina of the central nervous system. They are morphologically identical to the paragangliomas outside the central nervous system. Like these, the paragangliomas of the central nervous system con-

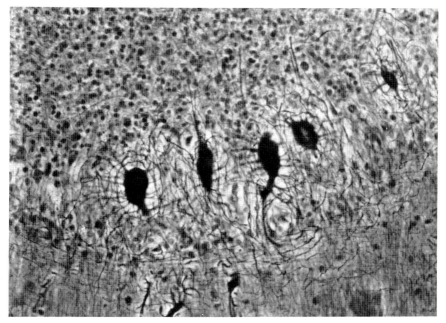

Figure 1.53. The cerebellar cortex of a patient with Menkes' kinky hair disease. Five Purkinje cells showing somatic sprouts are seen. Bielschowsky stain. (Original magnification ×180.)

tain dense core vesicles in the tumor cells, and the associated blood vessels of the tumor are fenestrated (72, 162).

ASTROCYTES

NORMAL ASTROCYTES

The astrocyte and the oligodendrocyte (see Chapter 2) are the two major glial cells of the central nervous system. They originate from the lining of the primitive neuroectoderm, the same embryonic source as the neuron. Astrocytes are found in all parts of the central nervous system (Fig. 1.54). Two varieties are distinguished. For the most part, the protoplasmic astrocytes reside in the gray matter, and they are often satellites of the soma of the large neurons (186). Because of their position among the interconnected neurons, these have a more delicate and sinuous morphology compared to the fibrillary astrocytes of the white matter. The fibrillary astrocytes display long, relatively straight processes and contain much more abundant glial fibrils than do the protoplasmic astrocytes.

The demonstration of the processes of either type of astrocyte requires special histological methods such as metallic impregnation. In conventional H&E or Nissl preparations only the nucleus of the normal astrocyte is easily seen. It appears as a pale bean-shaped structure surrounded by a faintly basophilic cytoplasm. The staining characteristics of the astrocyte sometimes make it difficult to distinguish between them and small neurons. One way of detecting a neuron is the presence of a prom-

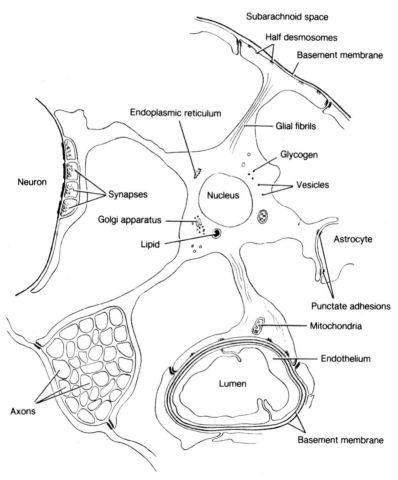

Figure 1.54. A diagram of the possible configurations of the astrocytic processes. (From A. Hirano (79).)

inent nucleolus within a clear nucleus. In contrast, the star-shaped cytoplasm of reactive astrocytes becomes very obvious due to its enlargement and increase in stainability.

As the name implies, the basic configuration of the astrocyte is star-like, with processes radiating away from the cell body (Fig. 1.55). Their morphology, however, is actually subject to considerable variation, depending on the location of the cell. For example, some astrocytes in the cerebellum are arranged with their cell bodies in the Purkinje cell layer, but most of their processes, the Bergmann fibers, are directed toward the pial surface so that the cell has a distinctly asymmetric pattern. The opposite orientation is found in subpial astrocytes where the cell body is adjacent to the pial membrane, and the processes, while radial when viewed from the pial surface, are clearly oriented toward the interior of the brain.

In general, the cytoplasmic process of the protoplasmic astrocyte consists of two parts. The proximal portion is a cylindrical, branching, tapering process. The distal part of the process, however, is more often sheet-like or laminar in shape (76, 185). Thus, in thin section the distal part of the protoplasmic astrocytic process usually does not appear circular. Instead it displays a laminar profile. The sheet-like nature of the process is especially pronounced in protoplasmic astrocytes in the neuropil.

The shape of the distal portion of the astrocytic process reflects its function as a lining or covering element. Astrocytic processes separate the neural tissue from the mesodermal elements of the central nervous system. Almost the entire surface of the central nervous system is covered by a layer of astrocytic processes interposed between the parenchyma and the pial membrane. Similarly, the surface of blood vessels is virtually covered by astrocytic foot processes (Fig. 1.56). In both of these locations the astrocytic processes are joined by punctate adhesions and occasional gap junctions, and a continuous basal lamina separates the astrocytic processes from the subarachnoid space and from the perivascular space. The presence of the perivascular or subpial astrocytes is sometimes best visualized under pathological conditions (Figs. 1.57–1.59) (65, 123). When one considers the extreme convolution of the central nervous system and the richness of its vascular bed one must be impressed by the extent of the peripheral astrocytic expansion.

In addition to the mesodermal elements

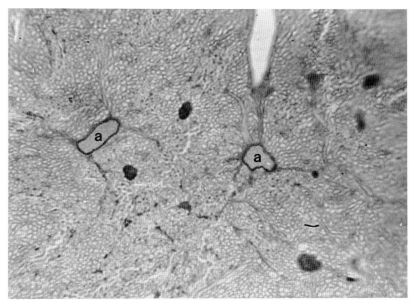

Figure 1.55. A cross-section of the optic nerve of a rat. Two astrocytes (a) are visible. Their processes are long, extending to a blood vessel in one case. Osmium-fixed Epon-embedded and silver impregnation. (Original magnification ×1,000.)

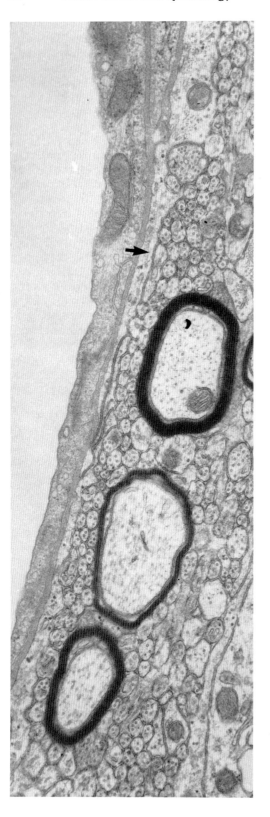

of the central nervous system astrocytic processes are also found at certain neuronal surfaces. Purkinje cells, for example, are almost completely covered by astrocytic processes. The soma as well as the dendritic arborizations, except for synaptic sites, are covered by astrocytic processes (58, 185). The synapse at each dendritic spine is closely invested by an astrocytic process (Figs. 1.34 and 1.35). Other neurons may be only partially surrounded by astrocytes. Sometimes small groups of synapses may be surrounded by an astrocytic process, almost as though it were serving as a kind of insulating element.

The function of the astrocytes may only be guessed at on the basis of their morphology and their pathological reactions. Their presence at blood vessel surfaces was at one time thought to suggest that they may serve to mediate the passage of materials from the blood vessel lumen into the neuron. However, studies with the protein tracer, horseradish peroxidase, have not borne out this suggestion (65). In addition, when the blood-brain barrier is broken, astrocytic processes, due to the lack of tight junctions between vascular foot processes are not able to prevent the penetration of the tracer which spreads into the extracellular space of the parenchyma (Fig. 1.60). Other roles such as supportive or skeletal functions have also been proposed. They are known to have a limited phagocytic ability in response to the presence of certain abnormal materials. Their presence at neuronal surfaces and synaptic sites leads to the suspicion that astrocytic processes may serve as insulators separating various types of synapses. However, no synapses are completely insulated by astrocytes, and some seem to be essentially devoid of astrocytic processes in the immediate vicinity. Conceivably, one of the principal roles of the astrocyte is to regulate the electrolyte balance, particularly potassium ion concentration, in the extracellular space, and it may also affect the concentration of certain

Figure 1.56. Thin astrocytic processes (*arrow*) intervene between the endothelial cell and underlying parenchyma. (Original magnification ×20,000.)

neurotransmitter substances in the microenvironment of certain synapses or other parts of the neuronal surface (151, 157).

The morphology of the astrocyte is characterized by the presence of many radiating processes. The latter are not easily visible in ordinary light microscopic preparation but can be detected, to some extent, after metallic impregnation. The nucleus is in the cell body and contains a small nucleolus which is difficult to discern in the light microscope but is quite distinct in the electron microscope. The perikaryon contains the usual organelles. There are a few, rather large mitochondria. Rough endoplasmic reticulum is present but sparse. Golgi apparatus is present in the perinuclear region. Small numbers of minute vesicles, lipid droplets, lysosomes, and scattered glycogen

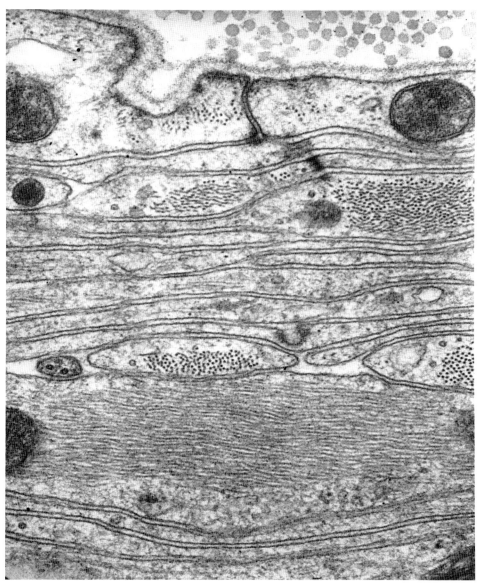

Figure 1.57. Multiple layers of astrocytic processes containing glial fibrils are present beneath the collagen-containing subarachnoid space and are separated from it by a basal lamina. (Original magnification ×64,000.)

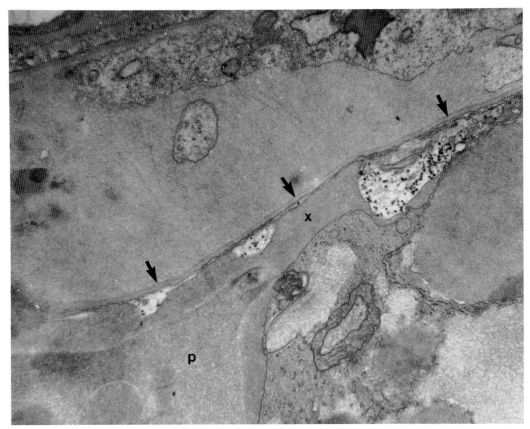

Figure 1.58. An edematous perivascular area in the brain of a rat during the acute stage after intracerebral polysaccharide implantation. The astrocytic foot processes which normally cover the perivascular space are retained but have become extremely attenuated due to the greatly distended perivascular space. The perivascular as well as the parenchymal extracellular spaces (x) are filled with edema fluid. Accumulations of polysaccharide (*p*) and a portion of a macrophage are seen in the latter space. The surface of the attenuated astrocytic layer facing the perivascular space is covered by a basal lamina (*arrows*). (Original magnification ×27,000). (From A. Hirano (65).)

granules, as well as free ribosomes, arranged in polysomes, are also observed. Freeze fracture studies of astrocytic plasma membranes have disclosed the presence of rectilinear arrays. These consist of regular arrangements of small intramembranous particles spaced at 7-nm intervals (59). They have been seen in other cell types but are most characteristic of astrocytes among the cells of the central nervous system.

The most characteristic constituent of the astrocytic cytoplasm is a class of intermediate filaments known as glial fibrils. These average 7.5-nm filaments are abundant, especially in fibrillary astrocytes (257). They are long, straight filaments with no detectable sidearms and are arranged in bundles. In cross-section the glial fibrils appear circular and have a minute clear center. Microtubules are seen in developing or reactive astrocytes but are rare in the mature cells.

Pathology of Astrocytes

NUCLEAR CHANGES

A variety of insults may lead to size and shape changes of astrocytic nuclei. These changes may result in what appear to be multiple nuclei when the relative astrocyte is reviewed in thin section in the electron microscope (Fig. 1.61). In most cases these may be assumed to be sections through a highly lobulated nucleus.

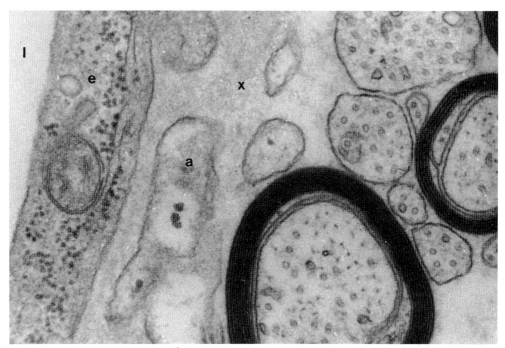

Figure 1.59. A perivascular area in the cerebral white matter during the acute stage of inflammatory edema in a rat. A wide separation between astrocytic feet (*a*) is evident in this case. A vascular lumen (*l*) and endothelium (*e*) are seen. The extracellular space (*x*) is widened. (Original magnification ×73,500.) (From A. Hirano et al. (123).)

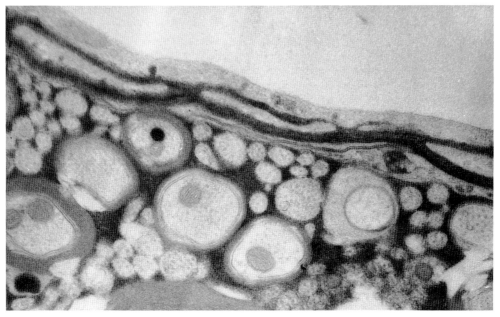

Figure 1.60. An unstained section of a rat brain which had been implanted with peroxidase. The dark peroxidase reaction product is visible between the cell processes and fills the narrow perivascular spaces. (Original magnification ×37,000.) (From A. Hirano (65).)

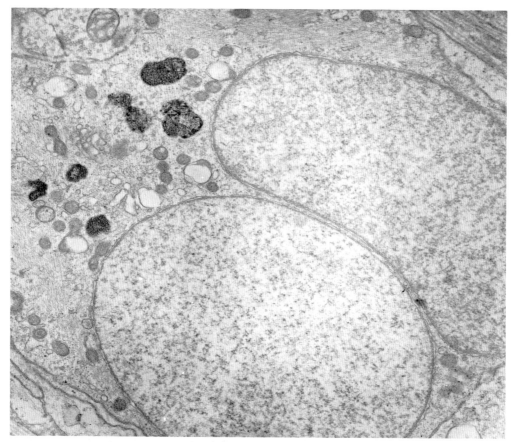

Figure 1.61. A reactive astrocyte in an injured rat brain. A bilobed nucleus as well as inclusion bodies containing electron-dense material are seen. (Original magnification ×20,000.)

"Nuclear bodies" are a common reactive change seen after a number of pathological conditions (163). These include subacute sclerosing parencephalitis and astrocytoma among others. The nuclear bodies appear as small, eosinophilic, intranuclear inclusions in the light microscope. The electron microscope reveals that they consist of spheroid accumulations of fine filaments usually accompanied by granular material (Fig. 1.62). Nuclear bodies are not confined to astrocytes but may be found in ependyma, endothelial cells, and in fibroblasts under similar pathological conditions. They have also been observed in some intracranial tumors. Filamentous inclusions arranged in rod-shaped or crystalloid patterns have also been seen within astrocytic nuclei following infection, in certain tumors as well as in some other conditions (Fig. 1.63).

Eosinophilic intranuclear inclusions have been seen in a number of viral infections. These include progressive multifocal leucoencephalopathy, subacute sclerosing panencephalitis, as well as herpes encephalitis.

Intranuclear eosinophilic inclusions, similar to those seen in kidney and liver in lead intoxication, may be found in astrocytes after experimental lead intoxication (Fig. 1.64). These astrocytic inclusions have been shown to contain lead (99, 217).

Mitotic figures in astrocytes are not seen in human postmortem material (8). They have been induced, however, in rats subjected to needle wounds but can be detected only if the tissue is fixed immediately after sacrifice (20). Anoxic encephalopathy has been reported to result in abnormal mitosis in astrocytes (34).

Nuclear shape is the basis for distin-

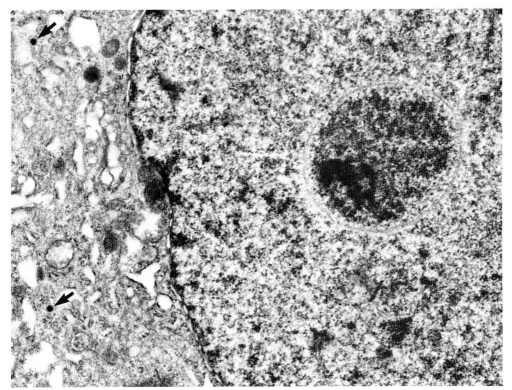

Figure 1.62. A nuclear body within the nucleus of a reactive astrocyte from a case of subacute sclerosing panencephalitis. Dense core vesicles (*arrows*) are present in the cytoplasm. (Original magnification ×20,000.) (From N. Malamud and A. Hirano (163).)

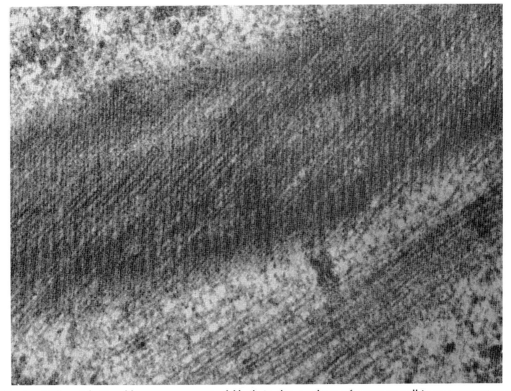

Figure 1.63. A lattice-like arrangement of fibrils in the nucleus of a tumor cell in an astrocytoma. (Original magnification ×65,000.) (From A. Hirano (79).)

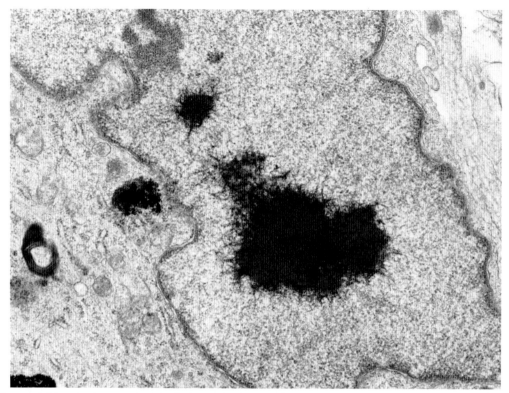

Figure 1.64. An intranuclear inclusion in a reactive astrocyte in a rat brain at the margin of an implanted pellet of lead salt. (Original magnification ×22,000.)

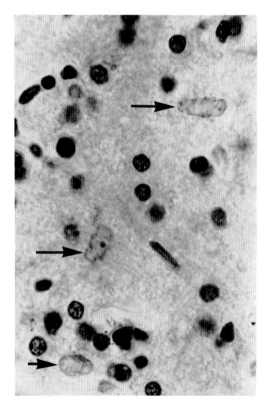

guishing Alzheimer type I and type II glia (101). Alzheimer type II glia are seen in Wilson's disease and in hepatic encephalopathy as well as in certain other conditions (Fig. 1.65). They are most common in the globus pallidus but are also found in the dentate nucleus of the cerebellum, in the cerebral cortex, as well as in other areas. The cells may be identified by large, often kidney-shaped nuclei. The nuclei appear pale in either Nissl or H&E preparations. There are only few marginal chromatin granules or nucleoli-like particles scattered at the nuclear periphery. Because the cytoplasm is usually not visualized well except for a few pigment granules this phenomenon is sometimes referred to as "naked nuclei gliosis."

The nuclei of Alzheimer type I glia, described in Wilson's disease, are also large and often lobulated. These cells are distinguished from Alzheimer type II glia by the

Figure 1.65. Alzheimer type II glia (*arrows*) in the basal ganglia of Wilson's disease. Nissl stain. (Original magnification ×720.)

presence of well-staining voluminous cytoplasm due to the presence of granular and other material.

Alzheimer type II glia have been induced in rats by experimental portocaval anastomosis (24, 173).

ASTROCYTIC SWELLING

Swelling represents one of the initial reactions of astrocytes to a variety of insults, especially hypoxia. As such it may also occur as the result of improper fixation and

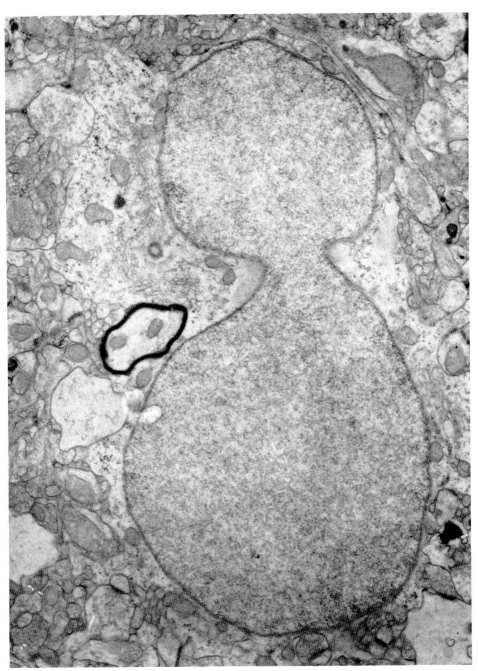

Figure 1.66. A reactive astrocyte in the cerebral cortex of a rat 12 h after stab injury. The nucleus is hourglass in shape, and the cytoplasm appears relatively clear and voluminous. Fine fibrillary material and scattered glycogen granules are distributed in the watery cytoplasm. (Original magnification ×16,000.) (From A. Hirano (122).)

must therefore be interpreted with great caution.

The swollen cytoplasm appears clear and empty in the light microscope and is described as having a "spongy" appearance. These changes are especially pronounced in perivascular and in perineuronal regions. The electron microscope reveals a pale and watery-appearing cytoplasm containing finely filamentous material (Fig. 1.66) and, often, an accumulation of glycogen granules (Fig. 1.67) (122). As might be expected the nearby extracellular spaces are narrower than normal.

Not infrequently discontinuities of the plasma membrane of swollen astrocytes may be observed in the electron micro-scope. These may sometimes be interpreted as representing ruptures of the membrane as the result of the distention of the cytoplasm. However, one must be cautious, since these changes may arise as postmortem artifacts. In well preserved tissue the plasma membrane of swollen astrocytes may also appear ruptured, but rather than simple discontinuities the edges appear to be rolled up, suggesting their elastic nature (Fig. 168A and B) (121).

In addition to the well known effects of brain edema on intracranial pressure, the concurrent changes in astrocytic morphology may be expected to have serious consequences on tissue architecture as well. The disturbance of the astrocytic processes

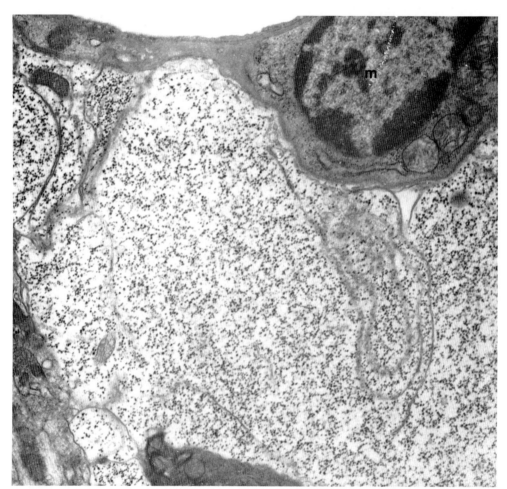

Figure 1.67. Enormously swollen perivascular astrocytic processes in a rat cerebrum are filled with numerous glycogen granules 1 d after injury. The lumen of the vessel is clear and empty. The endothelium is markedly attenuated. A mononuclear cell (*m*) is visible in the electron-dense edema fluid which fills the perivascular region. (Original magnification ×13,500.) (From A. Hirano (122).)

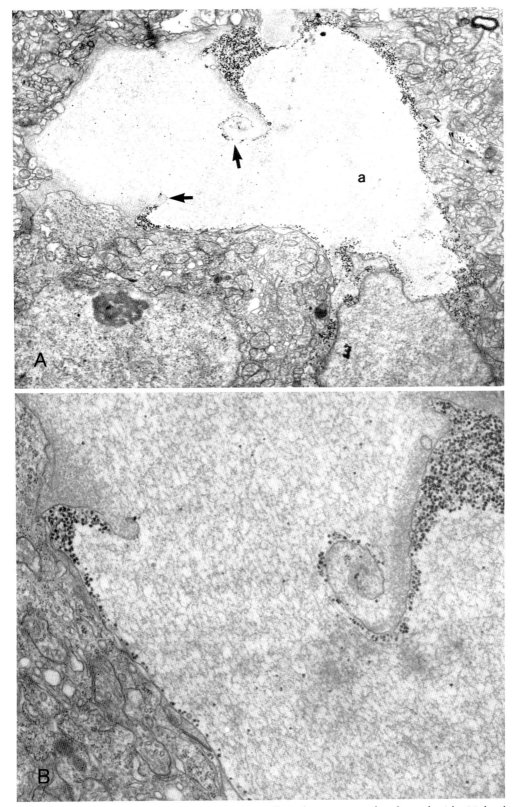

Figure 1.68. The neuropil at the margin of a pellet of cryptococcal polysaccharide 36 h after intracerebral implantation in a rat. Wide communication is evident through a ruptured plasma membrane (*arrows*) between the fluid-filled extracellular and intracellular compartment of an astrocyte (*a*). Glycogen granules are distributed at the periphery of the intracellular compartment, while finer and more compact material is seen at the periphery of the extracellular fluid. (*A*, Original magnification ×12,500; *B*, Original magnification ×30,000.) (From A. Hirano (121).)

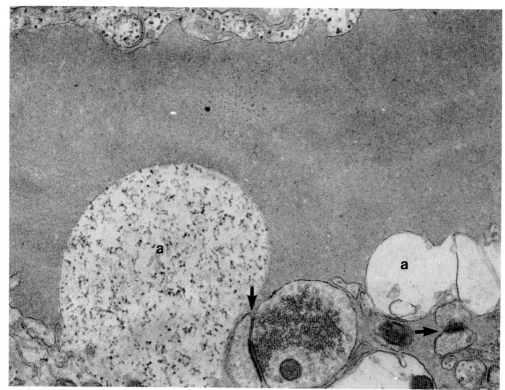

Figure 1.69.   Edematous gray matter in the forebrain of an injured rat. Edema fluid bathes the synapses (arrows). A nearby astrocyte (a) is swollen. (Original magnification ×31,000.) (From A. Hirano: *Advances in Neurology.* New York, Raven Press, 1980, vol 28, p 83.

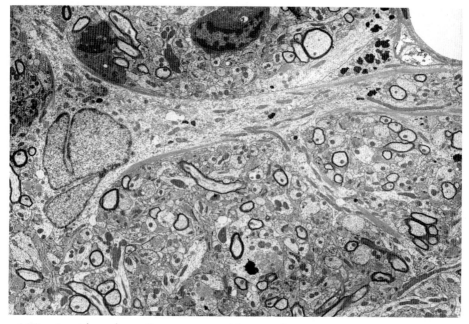

Figure 1.70.   An enlarged reactive astrocyte with several processes, including one extending to the perivascular space in the brain of an injured rat. Infolding of nucleus and prominent fascicles of glial fibrils are evident. (Original magnification ×5,000.) (From N. Malamud and A. Hirano (163).)

in relation to neuronal surfaces, especially synapses, may result in serious dysfunction of the nervous tissue (Fig. 1.69) (78).

HYPERTROPHIC ASTROCYTES

The most commonplace subacute reaction of astrocytes to various insults such as trauma, infarct, infection, or adjacent tumor is hypertrophy. It is observed within a few days after injury, becomes very pronounced in approximately a week, and depending on the condition, may taper off over several weeks or months.

Hypertrophic astrocytes appear to have eosinophilic cytoplasm and show an unusually prominent positive reaction for glial fibrillary acidic proteins. Hypertrophic astrocytes are easily distinguishable and display a clear starfish-like pattern. Fine structural studies of these cells show a cytoplasm crowded with the usual organelles, including mitochondria, vesicles, endoplasmic reticulum, Golgi apparatus, lysosomes, and especially glial fibrils which may form prominent fascicles (Fig. 1.70) or fill the background (Fig. 1.71) (119). Glycogen granules and a number of lipid-like inclusions or phagocytosed material may also be present (Fig. 1.72).

Unusually large and bizarre astrocytes, often multinucleated, may be seen in progressive multifocal leucoencephalopathy or,

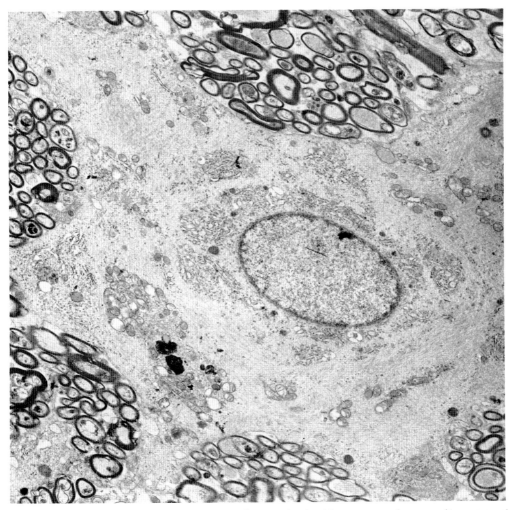

Figure 1.71.   A filament-filled astrocyte in the cerebral white matter of a rat adjacent to the implant 4 d after vinblastine implantation. (Original magnification ×5,300.) (From A. Hirano and H. M. Zimmerman (119).)

more rarely, in certain other acute demyelinating diseases. In addition, the cells of certain malignant astrocytic neoplasms, "magnocellular glioblastoma," are enormously enlarged.

FIBRILLARY GLIOSIS

Fibrillary gliosis is a reflection of a chronic condition. In these astrocytes virtually the entire cytoplasm, including the processes, becomes filled with glial filaments. They appear eosinophilic in H&E preparations, but are best stained with the Holzer stain (Fig. 1.73) or with Mallory's phosphotungstic acid-hematoxylin stain in which the glial fibrils appear blue (Fig. 1.74). Penfield's modification of the astroglial stain results in black glial fibrils and is a particularly elegant stain. The use of antibody to glial fibrillary acidic protein combined with peroxidase staining is a method of increasingly wide use for the identification of astrocytes (Fig. 1.75). The latter is more selective for astrocytes and, unlike the other methods, does not stain other tissue components. At the fine structural level the glial fibrils of reactive astrocytes, except for their numbers, are indistinguishable from those seen in normal astrocytes.

In addition to these structures, however, the so-called "Rosenthal fibers" (Figs. 1.76 and 1.77) frequently appear in long-standing lesions (63). These, too, are eosinophilic (Fig. 1.78) and appear blue after PTAH staining. They form a prominent homogenous mass and may assume an elongated or circular configuration. They are negative for glial fibrillary acidic protein. Their fine structure consists of electron-dense granular material often permeated by condensed glial filaments. Rosenthal fibers may be found in various glial scars and in astrocytomas but are especially prominent in Alexander's disease where they are widespread in the dysmyelinated areas (63, 208).

In long-standing lesions the fibrillary astrocytes may form glial "scars." However, when the lesion is especially large, such as after massive infarcts, the astrocytes may not fill the region but may leave areas of extracellular cysts. If the glial "scar" assumes the pattern of the previously existing tissue, such as in demyelinating plaques, it is referred to as "isomorphic gliosis." In other conditions, such as the focal destructive process in abscesses, the scar forms no recognizable pattern corresponding to the preexisting neural tissue and is known as "anisomorphic gliosis."

It should be pointed out that gliosis is part of normal aging. This is best seen in subpial and subependymal areas especially overlying the caudate nucleus and the fornix and floor of the fourth ventricle. The inferior olivary nucleus is another well known area prone to pronounced astrocytic proliferation even in the normal aged individual. In fact, the common occurrence of fibrillary gliosis in the inferior olive requires that caution be exercised in the interpretation of these changes. In order to be confident of a real lesion in the inferior olive one must evaluate the state of the neuronal population and may not rely solely on the presence of a high glial density.

Finally, some chronic lesions do not show particularly prominent glial reaction. For example, in Huntington's chorea, despite substantial neuronal loss, fibrillary astrocytes, while present, may be much less prominent in the region of the lesion, the caudate nucleus, than in surrounding subpial tissues.

Glial bundle formation first reported in the spinal roots of patients with Werdnig-Hoffmann disease may be classified as a special form of fibrillary gliosis. They are, for the most part, confined to the proximal portion of anterior roots and are only occasionally seen in posterior roots. They have also been described in cranial nerves. These structures were originally identified by Werdnig and Hoffmann, but their astrocytic nature was pointed out by Chou and Fakadej who named them "glial bundles." They consist of large accumulations of filament-containing astrocytic processes.

The fine structure of glial bundles (Figs. 1.79–1.81) was shown by Chou and Fakadej (27) to be identical to reactive fibrillary astrocytic processes seen in other parts of the nervous system and to be positive for glial fibrillary acidic protein. These findings were later confirmed by other investigators (81) when they were seen in both acute and chronic cases of Werdnig-Hoffmann disease. Since their original description glial bundles have been seen in a va-

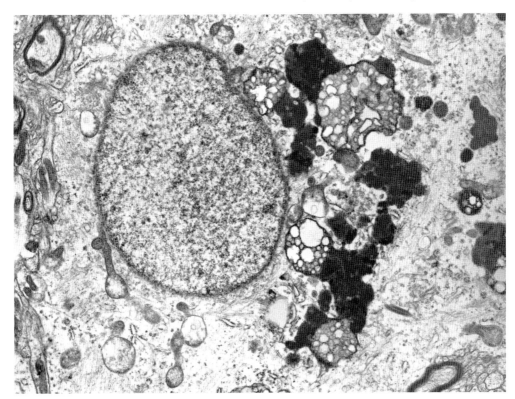

Figure 1.72. A reactive astrocyte in the white matter 1 week after polysaccharide implantation in a rat forebrain (122). Several osmiophilic lipid droplets and other membrane-bounded dense bodies are evident. (Original magnification ×11,500.)

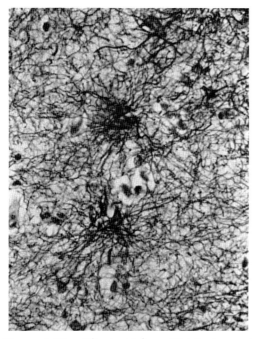

Figure 1.73. Gliosis. Holzer. (Original magnification ×360.)

riety of human diseases and in experimental conditions affecting the spinal root (81, 135).

ASTROCYTIC INCLUSIONS

Various conditions frequently result in pigmented inclusions within astrocytes. Lipofuscin is the most common and can be found after any chronic insult and in normal aged brains. In addition, astrocytes display a certain level of phagocytic activity, so that the remains of degenerated tissue may sometimes be found within them. Myelin debris may be seen within swollen astrocytes when nearby tissue is undergoing demyelination. Hemosiderin deposits often occur in association with intracranial hemorrhage. A special case of this process is "marginal hemosiderosis" or "superficial hemosiderosis" which represents accumulations of hemosiderin pigments in subpial astrocytes which may persist for long periods of time after subarachnoid hemorrhage. Various lipidoses result in the for-

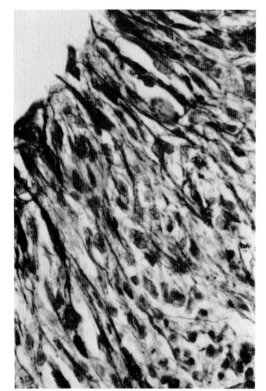

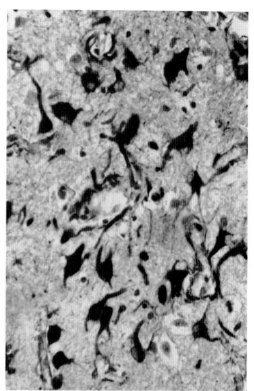

Figure 1.74. Gliosis around a blood vessel. Phosphotungstic acid hematoxylin stain. (Original magnification ×720.)

Figure 1.75. Reactive astrocytes in the cerebral cortex. Glial fibrillary acidic protein-hematoxylin. (Original magnification ×360.)

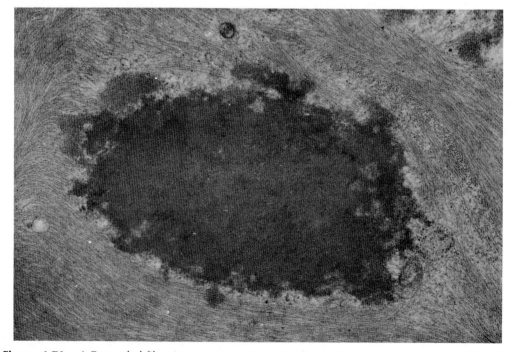

Figure 1.76. A Rosenthal fiber in a reactive astrocyte adjacent to a craniopharyngioma. (Original magnification ×25,000.) (From N. Malamud and A. Hirano (163).)

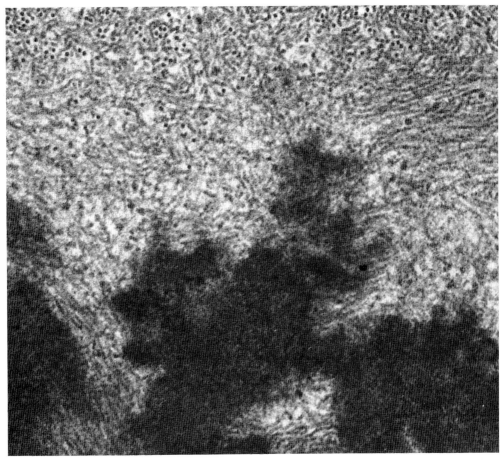

Figure 1.77.   Higher magnification of a Rosenthal fiber. (Original magnification ×96,000.) (From A. Hirano (79).)

mation of inclusions in astrocytes, although not to the extent seen in neurons.

Dense core vesicles are rather commonly found in astrocytes in various conditions including neoplasms and in subacute sclerosing panencephalitis. They were originally suspected to be viral particles or secretory granules but were later shown to be calcium-containing deposits (46). Virus-like particles have been detected in astrocytes in various other conditions.

CORPORA AMYLACEA

Corpora amylacea are invariably present in the aged brain. They are found in all individuals over the age of 40 (227). They have also been identified in aged monkeys and other animals (172). Their numbers vary widely among individuals, but they are most common in the subpial and subependymal regions, as well as in the median

portion of the lentiform nucleus, in part of Ammon's horn, and in the white matter of the spinal cord, especially the posterior column. In the latter regions they tend to be found in the perivascular areas.

The bodies are round, from 50 to 20 μm in diameter, and are basophilic, argentophilic, and PAS- positive (Fig. 1.82). They are well demarcated, amorphous structures, frequently with a denser staining, round core.

After many years of controversy as to their precise localization, fine structural studies by Ramsey (199) demonstrated corpora amylacea within astrocytic processes where they are surrounded by characteristic astrocytic components, such as glial fibrils and glycogen granules. The bodies are devoid of a limiting membrane and are composed of 6.5-nm curves and apparently branched filaments arranged in a random

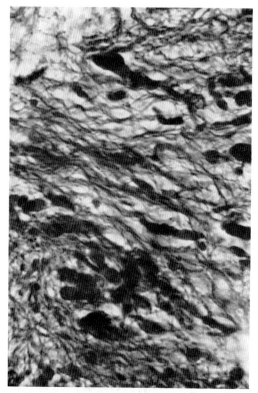

Figure 1.78. Rosenthal fibers in gliosis. H&E. (Original magnification ×720.)

fashion with some tendency to whorl formation (Figs. 1.83 and 1.84). In the central portion of the larger bodies the filaments may be more compactly arranged, and electron-dense, floccular material may be found among them.

Chemical analysis of isolated corpora amylacea indicate that they are composed largely of a glycogen-like carbohydrate mixed with small amounts of protein (3). As mentioned previously, essentially identical structures, have been described as polyglucosan bodies in axons (200) and as Lafora bodies in neurons (171).

The significance and origin of corpora amylacea is not clear. They are usually not seen in children under the age of ten (227). This is true even in children with chronic, severe gliosis, such as that accompanying leucodystrophy. Astrocytic neoplasms, either in adults or children, are also usually free of these structures. On the other hand, corpora amylacea are sometimes more frequent in very long-standing gliotic lesions in a variety of conditions in adult patients.

Recently, numerous corpora amylacea were observed in a 12-year-old child with Werdnig-Hoffmann disease. They were not only found in involved anterior horns but also within the prominent glial bundles of the anterior roots (81).

SHAPE CHANGES OF ASTROCYTIC PROCESS

Under normal conditions the sheet-like astrocytic process has a certain anatomical and functional domain. Under pathological conditions both the domain and the shape may change (71, 76). In some cases, such as in certain astrocytic neoplasms, in which the cells appear primitive, the processes are shortened sometimes to microvillous or filopodial proportions, and no domain is apparent (143). These processes tend to be cylindrical. Under other pathological conditions such as is seen in the murine mutant "weaver" or in granule cell type cerebellar degeneration, the astrocytic processes in the cerebellar cortex assume voluminous, balloon-like configurations (Fig. 1.50) and fill the parenchymal spaces (84). The tendency toward sheet-like expansion becomes more exaggerated in such conditions as the murine mutant "staggerer" and in some areas of reactive gliosis in both human and experimental conditions (Figs. 1.85–1.87). This process results in the formation of whorls of concentric lamellae of extremely flattened astrocytic processes (87). Superficially, these resemble examples of early myelination, but the absence of a central axon and their concentric rather than spiral arrangement are distinguishing features. Major dense lines are not formed, and some of the cell processes may be seen to be joined to fibril-containing larger trunks. Finally, astrocytic processes, although they remain large, may assume a purely cylindrical shape (Figs. 1.79–1.81). Frequently these processes form bundles such as in glial bundles or in glial scars in demyelinated white matter lesions or sometimes in the cortex in certain other lesions.

Neoplastic transformation of astrocytes leads to astrocytomas or malignant gliomas. In the more benign tumors many characteristic astrocytic features are retained, although they may be severely distorted. Usually the elaborate sheet-like peripheral expansions of the processes are

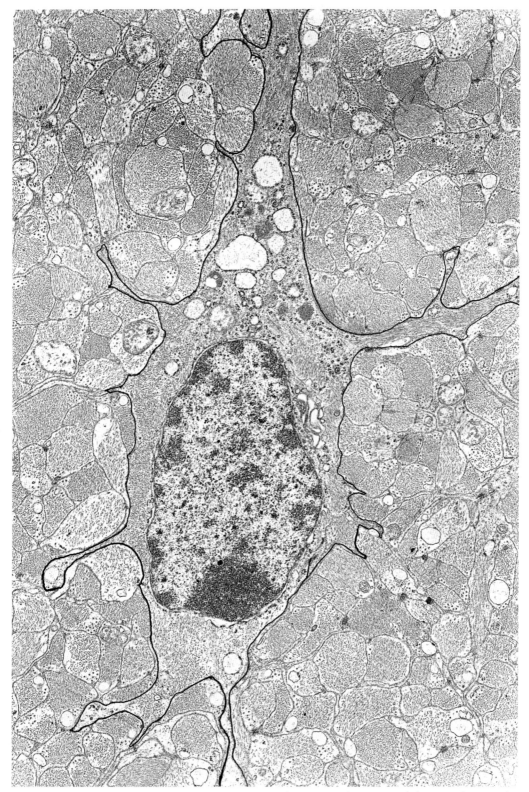

Figure 1.79. A section through a glial bundle in the proximal portion of the anterior root in a case of Werdnig-Hoffmann disease. An astrocytic cell body is seen in the center of the micrograph. It is surrounded by bundles of astrocytic processes (outlined). Glial filaments fill the processes as well as the cell body. (Original magnification ×12,000.)

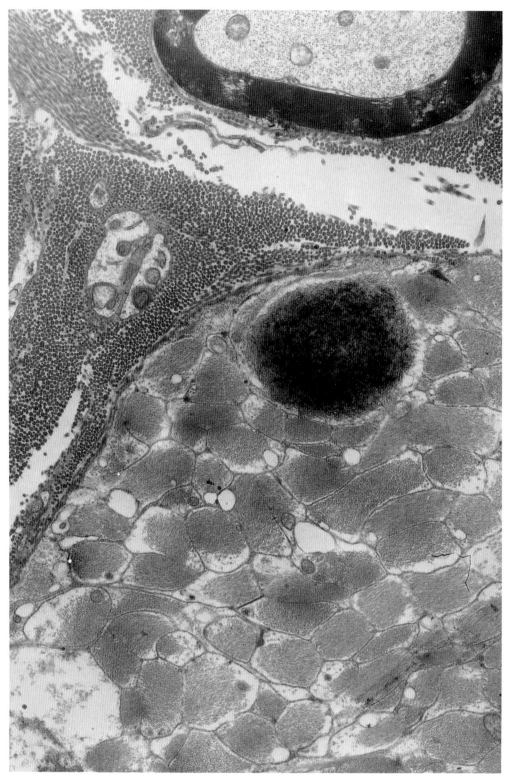

Figure 1.80.   The periphery of a glial bundle in a region similar to that illustrated in Fig. 1.79). The extracellular space contains abundant collagen fibers and a myelinated fiber. Within the glial bundle a corpus amylaceus is present within a single astrocytic process. (Original magnification ×11,000.) (From A. Hirano (81).)

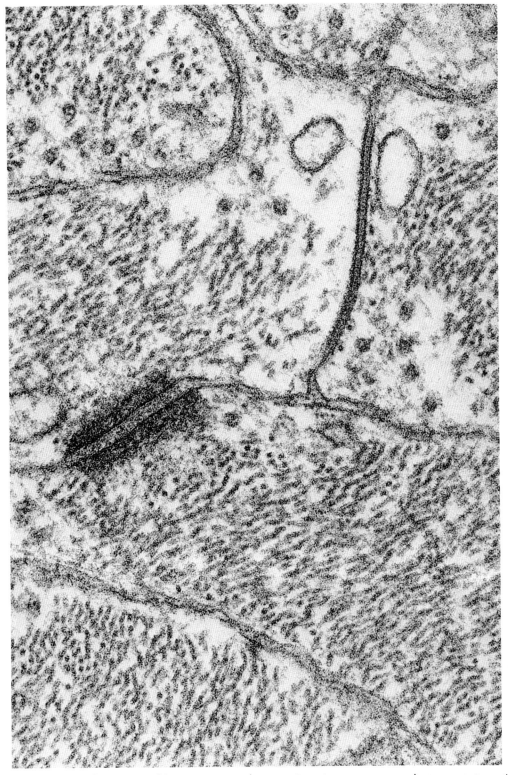

Figure 1.81. A desmosome-like junction and a gap junction are present between astrocytic processes within a glial bundle. Glial filaments and scattered microtubules are seen. (Original magnification ×120,000.) (From A. Hirano (81).)

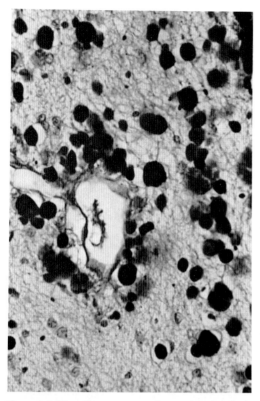

Figure 1.82. Corpora amylacea in the sub-ependymal region of the lateral ventricle. Periodic acid Schiff-hematoxylin stain. (Original magnification ×360.)

lost or diminished (143), and they lose their special relationship to the neurons.

EPENDYMA

Normal Ependyma (12, 110, 228, 248)

As seen in all other elements of the central nervous system ependymal cells arise from the embryonal neuroepithelial cells which line the primitive ventricle and central canal of the developing nervous system. Those young, proliferating cells which do not differentiate into either neuroblasts or glioblasts and which remain at the luminal surface go on to form a single ependymal layer which is virtually continuous and which lines the inner surface of the ventricle and the central canal. This process of development and differentiation goes on well after birth, so that a group of proliferating cells may be found in the subependymal region at the lateral angle of the

lateral ventricle in neonates as well as in young, mature individuals (192).

Eventually most of the mature ependyma comes to consist of a single layer of closely aligned cuboidal cells over the gray matter and somewhat more flattened over white matter (Fig. 1.88) (183). The luminal surface of the ependymal cells bears short, stubby microvillous-like processes (Fig. 1.89) which are devoid of the coating material which is so prominent on the microvilli of the luminal surface of intestinal and respiratory epithelium (96). In addition, the luminal surface of the ependyma may bear cilia which are responsible for the movement of the cerebrospinal fluid. The distribution of the cilia, which show a typical 9 + 2 arrangement of ciliary tubules (Figs. 1.90 and 1.91), varies with location and age as well as with the species (183). They have been identified in the lateral ventricle of adult humans (201).

Most often the lateral surfaces of the ependymal cell abut those of another, similar cell and form various cell junctions (Fig. 1.92), including zonulae and maculae adherentes as well as occasional gap junctions, and in areas overlying white matter (183), some interdigitation of the lateral surfaces. Zonulae occludentes are generally absent (14), except for some areas such as the area postrema and median eminence (13, 170). Interestingly, these two areas are supplied by fenestrated capillaries and are therefore devoid of the typical blood-brain barrier. Occasional coated vesicles may be seen at the lateral surface of ependymal cells.

The basal surface of ependymal cells is generally free of a basal lamina and abuts directly on the underlying parenchyma composed, for the most part, of astrocytes. In some areas, however, such as the filum terminalis, no parenchymal cells are present between the ependyma and the subarachnoid space, and a basal lamina is present at the basal surface of the ependymal cells. Hemidesmosomes are present in these areas. A similar morphology is apparent where capillaries directly abut the ependymal layer (117). In these cases, also, the basal surface of the ependymal cell may bear a basal lamina which is usually quite close to the basal lamina of the endothelial cell.

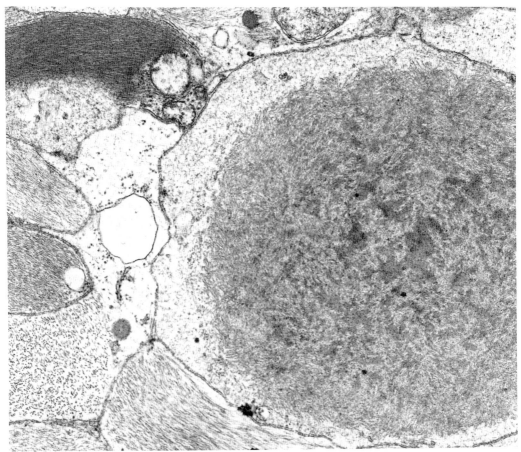

Figure 1.83. A corpus amylaceus within an astrocytic process of a glial bundle in a 12-yr-old child with Werdnig-Hoffman disease. (Original magnification ×20,000.)

In general, the interior of the ependymal cell shows a highly oriented morphology. The microvillous-like projections are filled with fine microfilaments. The apical region also contains a certain number of microtubules (Figs. 1.89 and 1.92) (117), as well as the basal bodies or blepharoplasts and associated rootlets of the cilia. The region between the nucleus and the apical surface contains a Golgi apparatus as well as lysosomal dense bodies, including lipofuscin-containing residual bodies. Mitochondria which may be present throughout the cell are more prominent in the same region. The cytoplasm is also characterized by the presence of intermediate filaments similar to those found in astrocytes. They may be scattered throughout the cytoplasm or may be found arranged in bundles.

Rough endoplasmic reticulum is sparse, but free ribosomes are found scattered in the cytoplasm, and elements of the smooth endoplasmic reticulum and occasional vesicles are seen. Small amounts of glycogen granules may occasionally be found.

The oval to round nucleus appears homogenous. It is relatively large and occupies the center of the cell. The nucleolus is not exceptionally prominent. Fibrous inclusions may sometimes be observed within the nucleus (Fig. 1.93) (117, 192). They consist of a tightly packed bundle of filaments.

In addition to typical ependymal cells, the lining of the third ventricle, especially in the region of the hypothalamus, may be punctuated by two variants. The first is the tanycyte which appears typically ependymal at the luminal surface but which extends a process to the blood vessels deep in the parenchyma or even to the pial surface in regions of thinned parenchyma (192).

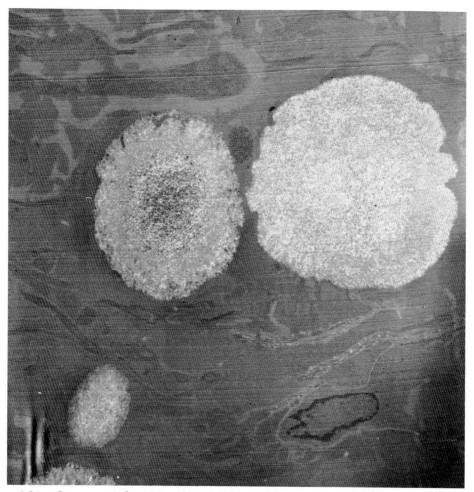

Figure 1.84. Corpora amylacea in white matter. The matrix of the bodies and nearby myelin sheaths are negative for the ethanolic phosphotungstic acid stain applied to formalin-fixed tissue. (Original magnification ×6,000.) (From A. Hirano et al. (94).)

These cells display ependyma-like features at the luminal portion, including microvillous protrusions into the lumen as well as cell junctions on those portions of the cell which abut adjacent ependymal cells. Simultaneously, the deeply penetrating processes display characteristic astrocyte-like features.

The second variant which may be found in the spinal cord as well as in the third ventricle consists of a cell process arising from a neuron (244). These processes are of two types. One penetrates between ependymal cells and forms cell junctions with their lateral surfaces. These processes bear cilia with a 9 + 0 arrangements of tubules. The other type of process also penetrates between ependymal cells and contains clear or dense-core vesicles at its luminal surface. The possibility that the cilia-bearing processes are sensory receptors responding to changes in the cerebrospinal fluid and that the synaptic vesicle-containing processes may be secretors of neuroamine has been entertained by some authors. The significance of these processes, which are especially prominent in the lower vertebrates, is obscure. Cilia are less common than at the apices of typical ependymal cells (192). Nonciliated tanycytes have been described as prominently distributed at the level of the median eminence in rats (168).

The only other cell type which may be found at the ventricular surface is the epi-

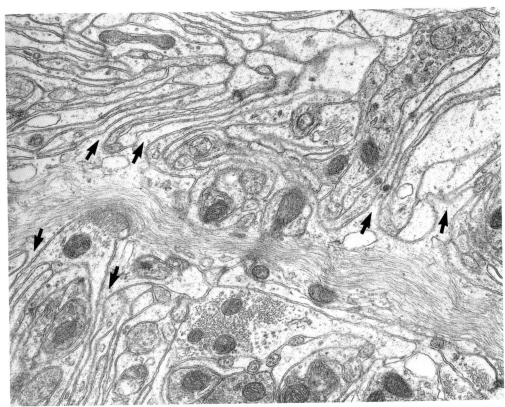

Figure 1.85. Several sheet-like processes (*arrows*) arising from a filament-filled astrocytic trunk in the cerebellum of an adult "staggerer" mouse. (Original magnification ×25,000.) (From A. Hirano and H. M. Dembitzer (87).)

thelium of the choroid plexus. These cells will be discussed elsewhere (see Chapter 5) but it should be pointed out that they vary significantly from ependymal cells with which they gradually merge at the periphery of the choroid plexus. The major difference between the two types of cells consists of the much greater size of the choroid plexus epithelium. Their luminal surfaces show no cilia, but the microvilli are considerably larger and club-shaped. The cells are joined by tight junctions, and a basal lamina separates them from an underlying connective tissue which contains fenestrated capillaries.

Pathology of the Ependyma

Ependymal cells may be affected by a variety of pathological processes which result in morphological changes. Perhaps the best known is hydrocephalus, in which the ependymal cells become stretched as the

ventricle enlarges. In severely affected areas, especially overlying white matter, the interdigitating lateral surfaces may pull apart from one another, leaving vacuole-like spaces between the plasma membranes which are still held together by cell junctions. Eventually, the junctions may break, exposing the parenchyma to the ventricular fluid (184, 247).

In chronic hydrocephalus substantial portions of the ventricle lose their ependymal lining, and underlying astrocytes form a glial scar. The glial proliferation leads to focal accumulation of reactive astrocytes which protrudes into the ventricular lumen (Fig. 1.94). Despite the absence of ependymal cells over most of these surfaces the protrusions are often referred to as "ependymal nodules." They are sometimes prominent in such chronic conditions as syphilis and tuberous slcerosis among others.

In edema, inflammation, and other in-

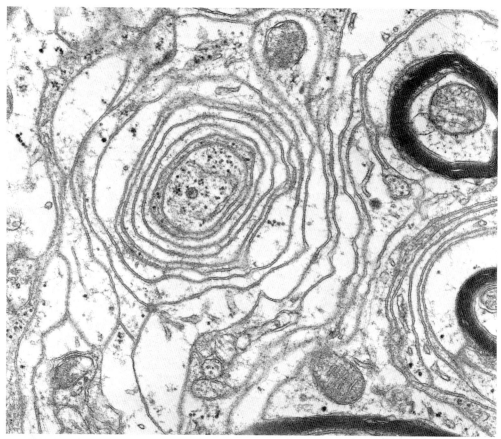

Figure 1.86. Two myelinated fibers and a cell process are surrounded by sheet-like processes of reactive astrocytes in the cerebellum of an adult "staggerer" mouse. (Original magnification ×33,000.) (From A. Hirano and H. M. Dembitzer (87).)

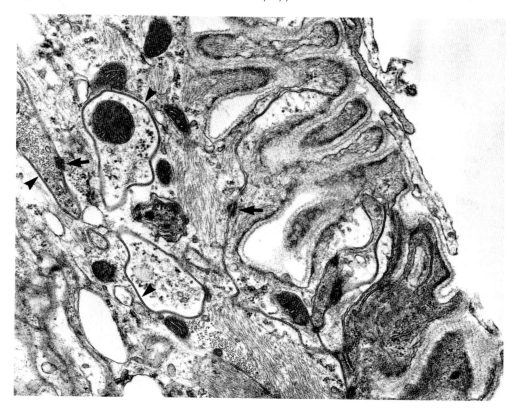

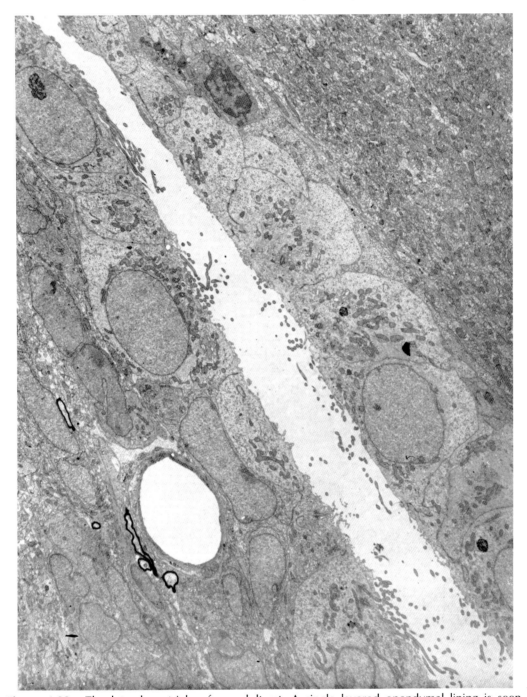

Figure 1.88. The lateral ventricle of an adult rat. A single layered ependymal lining is seen. (Original magnification ×6,000.) (From A. Hirano et al. (124).)

Figure 1.87. The infolded pial surface of an atrophic cerebellum in an adult "staggerer" mouse. Astrocytic processes are connected by both gap junctions (*arrowheads*) and desmosomes (*arrows*). (Original magnification ×25,000.) (From A. Hirano and H. M. Dembitzer (87).)

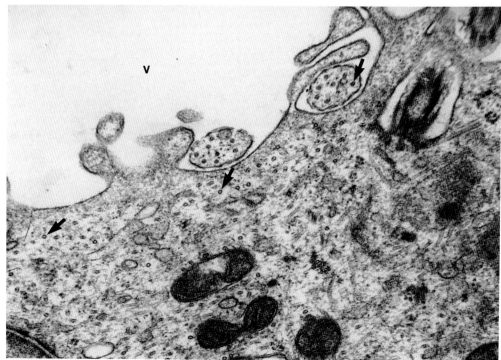

Figure 1.89. High magnification of the apical region of an ependymal cell in the adult rat. The ventricular lumen (v) is visible. Many cross-sections of microtubules may be seen (*arrows*). A cilium is seen arising from the cell surface. Microtubule-containing cell processes lie near the ependymal surface. (Original magnification ×50,000.) (From A. Hirano and H. M. Zimmerman (117).)

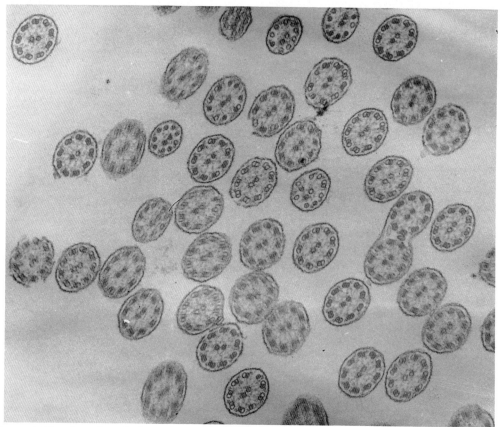

Figure 1.90. Ependymal cilia within the ventricular lumen of an adult rat. (Original magnification ×54,000.) (From A. Hirano and H. M. Zimmerman (117).)

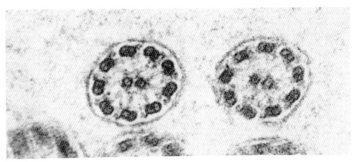

Figure 1.91. A higher magnification of ependymal cilia. (Original magnification ×110,000.) (From A. Hirano and H. M. Zimmerman (117).)

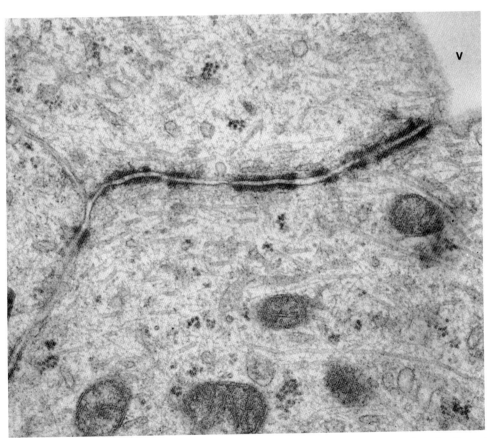

Figure 1.92. High magnification of an intercellular junction between two ependymal cells at their apical region in the adult rat. The ventricular lumen (v) is visible. Numerous longitudinal sections of microtubules are apparent. (Original magnification ×72,000.) (From A. Hirano and H. M. Zimmerman (117).)

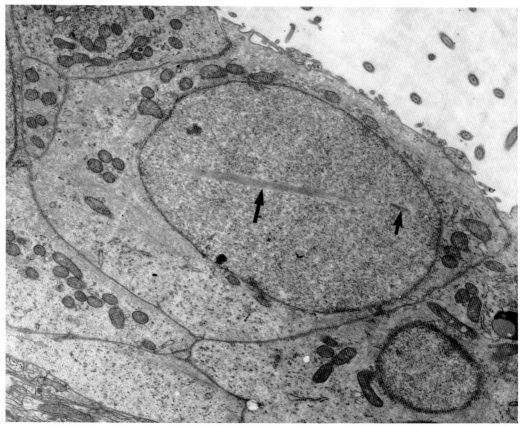

Figure 1.93. An ependymal cell lining the ventricular surface in an adult rat. One large (*large arrow*) and one small (*small arrow*) intranuclear fibrillar bundle are apparent. (Original magnification ×11,000.) (From A. Hirano and H. M. Zimmerman (117).)

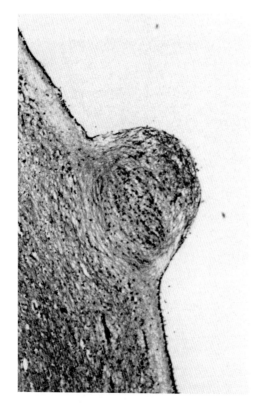

Figure 1.94. An ependymal nodule in the lateral ventricle. H&E. (Original magnification ×75.)

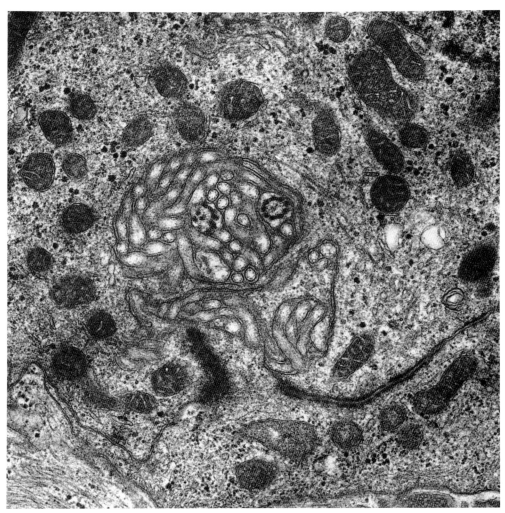

Figure 1.95. A section through an ependymoma. Compactly arranged microvilli and cilia crowd an abortive lumen. Cell junctions between tumor cells are visible. (Original magnification ×49,000.) (From T. P. Poon et al: *Electron Microscopic Atlas of Brain Tumors.* New York, Grune & Stratton, 1971.)

sults to either the underlying parenchyma or to the ependyma itself, the ependymal cells show reactive changes very reminiscent of those seen in astrocytes (124). They show a watery swelling, and there is an accumulation of glycogen granules as well as increased filament formation in the later stages. Lipid and pigment inclusions may also increase in number. The same conditions may lead to ependymal proliferation in the spinal cord (165) which can result in a multilayered accumulation of cells obliterating the central canal. Within these masses the ependymal cells often retain characteristic features such as cilia and microvillous processes which protrude into a

narrow lumen lined by cell junction-bearing cells.

Certain viral infections are known to result in pathological changes in the ependyma. In cytomegalic inclusion disease, for example, eosinophilic intranuclear and intracytoplasmic bodies are observed in ependymal as well as other types of cells.

Neoplastic transformation of ependymal cells are known as ependymomas. In the more differentiated examples the tumor cells bear the structural features characteristic of ependymal cells, albeit in a somewhat bizarre or distorted manner (97, 111). Cell junctions may be present as well as cilia and microvillous protrusions (Fig.

1.95). Sometimes they show a tendency to form a primitive lumen or canal. In benign lesions as well, it has been suggested that ependymal cells can line an expanding cystic cavity within the central nervous system (43).

ACKNOWLEDGMENT

The author is grateful to Dr. Herbert M. Dembitzer for his valuable criticism during the preparation of this manuscript.

References

1. Aleu FP, Terry RD, Zellweger H: Electron microscopy of two cerebral biopsies in gargoylism. *J Neuropathol Exp Neurol* 24:304, 1965.
2. Asbury AK, Johnson PC: *Pathology of Peripheral Nerve.* Philadelphia, WB Saunders, 1978.
3. Austin JH, Sakai M: Corpora amylacea. In: Minkler J (ed): *Pathology of the Nervous System.* New York, McGraw-Hill Book Co, 1972, vol 3, p 2961.
4. Ball MJ, Lo P: Granulovacuolar degeneration in the aging brain and in dementia. *J Neuropathol Exp Neurol* 36:474, 1977.
5. Barron KD, Dentinger MP: Cytologic observations on axotomized feline Betz cells. I. Qualitative electron microscopic findings. *J Neuropathol Exp Neurol* 38:128, 1979.
6. Batty HK, Millhouse OE: Ultrastructure of the Gunn rat substantia nigra. *Acta Neuropathol (Berl)* 34:7, 1976.
7. Beal JA: Morphogenesis of the Hirano body in neurons of the squirrel monkey dorsal horn. *J Neurocytol* 7:395, 1978.
8. Blackwood W, Corsellis JAN (eds): *Greenfield's Neuropathology,* ed 3. London, Edward Arnold, 1976.
9. Blinzinger KH, Krentzberg GW: Displacement of synaptic terminals from regenerating motoneurons by microglial cells. *Z Zellforsch Mikrosk Anat* 85:145, 1968.
10. Borit A, McIntosh GC: Myelin basic protein and glial fibrillary acidic protein in human fetal brain. *Neuropathol Appl Neurobiol* 7:279, 1981.
11. Bray D, Gilbert D: Cytoskeletal elements in neurons. *Ann Rev Neurosci* 4:505, 1981.
12. Brightman MW, Palay SL: The fine structure of ependyma in the brain of the rat. *J Cell Biol* 19:419, 1963.
13. Brightman MW, Prescott L, Reese TS: Intercellular junctions of special ependyma. In Knigger KM, Scott DE, Kobayashi H, Ishii S (eds): *Brain-Endocrine Interaction. II. The Ventricular System in Neuro-endocrine Mechanisms.* Basel, Switzerland, S Karger, 1975, p 146.
14. Brightman MW, Reese TS: Junctions between intimately apposed cell membranes in the vertebrate brain. *J Cell Biol* 40:648, 1969.
15. Brion S, Mikol J, Psimaras A: Recent findings in Pick's disease. In Zimmerman HM (ed): *Progress in Neuropathology.* New York, Grune & Stratton, 1973, vol 2, p 421.
16. Bunina TL: On intracellular inclusions in familial amyotrophic lateral sclerosis. *Korsakov J Neuropathol Psychiatry* 62:1293, 1962.
17. Burger P, Vogel FS: The development of the pathologic changes of Alzheimer's disease and senile dementia in patient with Down's syndrome. *Am J Pathol* 73:457, 1973.
18. Cammermeyer J: Nonspecific changes of the central nervous system in normal and experimental material. In Bourne GH (ed): *The Structure and Function of Nervous Tissue.* New York, Academic Press, 1972, vol 4, p 131.
19. Carpenter S: Proximal axonal enlargement in motor neuron disease. *Neurology (Minneap)* 18:84, 1968.

20. Cavanagh JB: The proliferation of astrocytes around a needle wound in the rat brain. *J Anat* 106:471, 1970.
21. Cavanagh JB: The "dying back" process. A common dominator in many naturally occurring and toxic neuropathies. *Arch Pathol Lab Med* 103:659, 1979.
22. Cavanagh JB, Blakemore WF, Kyu MH: Fibrillary accumulations in oligodendroglial processes of rats subjected to portocaval anastomosis. *J Neurol Sci* 14:143, 1971.
23. Cavanagh JB, Bennetts RJ: On the pattern of changes in the rat nervous system produced by 2, 5 hexanediol. A topographical study by light microscopy. *Brain* 104:297, 1981.
24. Cavanagh JB, Kyu MH: Type II Alzheimer change experimentally produced in astrocytes in the rat. *J Neurol Sci* 12:63, 1971.
25. Chandler RL, Willis R: An intranuclear fibrillar lattice in neurons. *J Cell Sci* 1:283, 1966.
26. Chou SM: Pathognomy of intraneuronal inclusions in ALS. In: Tsubaki T, Toyokura Y (eds): *Amyotrophic Lateral Sclerosis.* Baltimore, University Park Press, 1979, p 135.
27. Chou SM, Fakadej AV: Ultrastructure of chromatolytic motoneurons and anterior spinal roots in a case of Werdnig-Hoffmann disease. *J Neuropathol Exp Neurol* 30:368, 1971.
28. Chou SM, Hartman HA: Axonal lesions and waltzing syndrome after IDPN administration in rats. With a concept "axostatis." *Acta Neuropathol (Berl)* 3:428, 1964.
29. Chou SM, Martin JD, Cutrecht JA, Thompson HG: Axonal balloons in subacute motor neuron disease. *J Neuropathol Exp Neurol* 29:141a, 1970.
30. Conradi S: Observations on the ultrastructure of the axon hillock and initial axon segment of lumbosacral motoneurons in the cat. *Acta Physiol Scand Suppl* 332:65, 1969.
31. Corsellis JAN, Burton CJ, Freeman-Browne D: The aftermath of boxing. *Psychol Med* 3:270, 1973.
32. Cowan WM: Anterograde and retrograde transneuronal degeneration in the central and peripheral nervous system. In Nauta WJH, Ebbesson SOE (eds): *Contemporary Research Methods in Neuroanatomy.* New York, Springer, 1970, p 217.
33. Culebras A, Feldman GR, Merk F: Cytoplasmic inclusion bodies within neurons of the thalamus in myotonic dystrophy. *J Neurol Sci* 19:319, 1973.
34. Diemer NH, Klinken L: Astrocyte mitosis and Alzheimer type I and II astrocytes in anoxic encephalopathy. *Neuropathol Appl Neurobiol* 2:313, 1976.
35. Droz B, Koenig HL, DiGiamberardino L: Axonal migration of protein and glycoprotein to nerve endings. I. Radioautographic analysis of the renewal of protein in nerve endings of chicken ciliary ganglion after intracerebral injection of [³H] lysin. *Brain Res* 60:93, 1973.
36. Droz B, Rambourg A, Koenig HL: The smooth endoplasmic reticulum: structure and role in renewal of axonal membrane and synaptic vesicles by fast axonal transport. *Brain Res* 93:1, 1975.
37. Duffy PE, Kornfeld MD, Suzuki K: Neurovisceral storage disease with curvilinear bodies. *J Neuropathol Exp Neurol* 27:351, 1968.
38. Duffy PO, Tennyson VM: Phase and electron microscopic observations of Lewy bodies and melanin granules in the substantia nigra and locus ceruleus in Parkinson's disease. *J Neuropathol Exp Neurol* 24:398, 1965.
39. Fine DIM, Barron KD, Hirano A: A Central nervous system lipidosis in an adult with atrophy of the cerebellar granular layer: a case report. *J Neuropathol Exp Neurol* 19:355, 1960.
40. Fraser H, Smith W, Gray EW: Ultrastructural morphology of cytoplasmic inclusions within neurons of aging mice. *J Neurol Sci* 11:123, 1970.
41. Fujisawa K, Shiraki H: Study of axonal dystrophy. I. Pathology of the neuropil of the gracile and the cuneate nuclei in ageing a. 1 old rats. A stereological study. *Neuropathol Appl Neurobiol* 4:1, 1978.

42. Fujita S: The matrix cell and cytogenesis in the developing central nervous system. *J Comp Neurol* 120:37, 1963.

43. Ghatak NR, Hirano A, Kasoff SS, Zimmerman HM: Fine structure of an intracerebral epithelial cyst. *J Neurosurg* 41:75, 1974.

44. Ghatak NR, Hirano A, Poon TP, French JH: Trichopoliodystrophy. II. Pathological changes in skeletal muscle and nervous system. *Arch Neurol* 26:60, 1972.

45. Gajdusek DC, Gibbs CJ Jr, Alpers M (eds): *Slow, Latent, and Temperate Virus Infections.* NINDB Monograph No. 2. Washington, DC, US Department of Health, Education, and Welfare, 1965.

46. Gambetti P, Erulkar SE, Somlyo AP, Gonatas NK: Calcium-containing structures in vertebrate glial cells. *J Cell Biol* 64:322, 1975.

47. Ghetti B: Induction of neurofibrillary degeneration following treatment with maytansine in vivo. *Brain Res* 163:9, 1979.

48. Ghetti B, Horoupian DS, Wisneiwski HM: Acute and long-term transneuronal response of dendrites of lateral geniculate neurons following transection of the primary visual afferent pathway. *Adv Neurol* 12:401, 1975.

49. Gibson PH: Light and electron microscopic observations on the relationship between Hirano bodies, neuron and glial perikarya in the human hippocampus. *Acta Neuropathol (Berl)* 42:165, 1978.

50. Gibson PH, Tomlinson BE: Number of Hirano bodies in the hippocampus of normal and demented people with Alzheimer's disease. *J Neurol Sci* 33:199, 1977.

51. Gonatas NK, Anderson W, Evangelista I: The contribution of altered synapses in the senile plaque: an electron microscopic study in Alzheimer dementia. *J Neuropathol Exp Neurol* 26:25, 1967.

52. Gonatas NK, Gambetti P, Baird H: A second type of late infantile amaurotic idiocy with multilamellar cytosomes. *J Neuropathol Exp Neurol* 27:371, 1968.

53. Gonatas NK, Goldensohn ES: Unusual neocortical presynaptic terminals in a patient with convulsions, mental retardation and cortical blindness. An electron microscopic study. *J Neuropathol Exp Neurol* 24:539, 1965.

54. Gonatas NK, Terry RD, Weiss M: Electron microscopical study in two cases of Jakob-Creutzfeldt disease. *J Neuropathol Exp Neurol* 24:575, 1965.

55. Gray EG: Axo-somatic and axo-dendritic synapses of the cerebral cortex: an electron microscope study. *J Anat* 93:420, 1959.

56. Gray EG: Electron microscopy of experimental degeneration in the brain. In Caveness WH, Walker AE (eds): *Head Injury Conference Proceedings.* Philadelphia, JB Lippincott, 1966, p 455.

57. Greenfield JG, Bosanquet FD: The brain stem lesions in Parkinsonism. *J Neurol Neurosurg Psychiatry* 16:213, 1953.

58. Hama K, Kosaka T: Purkinje cell and related neurons and glial cells under high-voltage electron microscopy. In Zimmerman HM (ed): *Progress in Neuropathology.* New York, Raven Press, 1979, vol 4, p 61.

59. Hanna RB, Hirano A, Pappas GD: Membrane specializations of dendritic spines and glia in the weaver mouse cerebellum: a freeze-fracture study. *J Cell Biol* 68:403, 1976.

60. Hart MN, Cancilla PA, Frommes S, Hirano A: Anterior horn cell degeneration and Bunina-type inclusions associated with dementia. *Acta Neuropathol (Berl)* 38:225, 1977.

61. Henrikson CK, Vaughn JE: Fine structural relationships between neurites and radial glial processes in developing mouse spinal cord. *J Neurocytol* 3:659, 1974.

62. Herndon RM: Lamellar bodies, an unusual arrangement of the granular endoplasmic reticulum. *J Cell Biol* 20:338, 1964.

63. Herndon RM, Rubinstein LJ, Freeman JM, Mathieson G: Light and electron microscopic observations on Rosenthal fibers in Alexander's disease and in multiple sclerosis. *J Neuropathol Exp Neurol* 29:524, 1970.

64. Hirano A: Pathology of amyotrophic lateral sclerosis. In Gajdusek DC, Gibbs CJ Jr, Alpers M (eds): *Slow, Latent, and Temperate Virus Infections.* NINDB Monograph, No. 2. Washington, DC, US Department of Health, Education, and Welfare, 1965, p 23.

65. Hirano A: The fine structure of brain in edema. In Bourne GH (ed): *Structure and Function of the Nervous Tissue.* New York, Academic Press, 1969, p 69.

66. Hirano A: Neurofibrillary changes in conditions related to Alzheimer's disease. In Wolstenholme GEW, O'Connor M, (eds): *Ciba Foundation Symposium. Alzheimer's Disease and Related Conditions.* London, Churchill, 1970, p 185.

67. Hirano A: Electron microscopy in neuropathology. In Zimmerman HM (ed): *Progress in Neuropathology.* New York, Grune & Stratton, 1971, vol 1, p 1.

68. Hirano A: The pathology of the central myelinated axon. In Bourne GH (ed): *Structure and Function of the Nervous Tissue.* New York, Academic Press, 1972, vol 5, p 73.

69. Hirano A: Progress in the pathology of motor neuron disease. In Zimmerman HM (ed): *Progress in Neuropathology.* New York, Grune & Stratton, 1973, vol 2, p 181.

70. Hirano A: Pathology of anterior horns cells. In Bradley WG, Gardner-Medwin D, Walton JN (eds): *Recent Advances in Myology.* Amsterdam, Excerpta Medica, 1975, p 537.

71. Hirano A: Neuronal and glial processes. Form and function. In Tsukada Y (ed): *Neurobiology of Neurons and Glia.* Japan Medical Research Foundation, Modern Biology Series 32, Tokyo, Kyoritsu Shuppangaisha, 1977, p 65.

72. Hirano A: Some contributions of electron microscopy to the diagnosis of brain tumors. *Acta Neuropathol (Berl)* 43:119, 1978.

73. Hirano A: A possible mechanism of demyelination in the Syrian hamster with hind leg paralysis. *Lab Invest* 38:115, 1978.

74. Hirano A: Changes of the neuronal endoplasmic reticulum in the peripheral nervous system in mutant hamsters with hind leg paralysis and normal controls. *J Neuropathol Exp Neurol* 37:75, 1978.

75. Hirano A: Aberrant synapses in the cerebellum. *Adv Neurol Sci (Tokyo)* 22:1279, 1978.

76. Hirano A: Neuronal and glial processes in neuropathology. Presidential address to the American Association of Neuropathologists. *J Neuropathol Exp Neurol* 37:365, 1978.

77. Hirano A: On the independent development of the pre- and postsynaptic terminals. In Zimmerman HM (ed): *Progress in Neuropathology.* New York, Raven Press, 1979, vol 4, p 79.

78. Hirano A: Fine structure of edematous encephalopathy. In Cervós-Navarro J, Ferszt R (eds): *Advances in Neurology. Brain Edema.* New York, Raven Press, 1980, vol 28, p 461.

79. Hirano A: *A Guide to Neuropathology.* New York, Igaku-Shoin, 1981.

80. Hirano A: Structure of normal central myelinated fibers. In Waxman SG, Ritchie JM (eds): *Demyelinating Disease: Basic and Clinical Electrophysiology.* New York, Raven Press, 1981, p 51.

81. Hirano A: Some aspects of ultrastructure of amyotrophic lateral sclerosis. In Rowland LP (ed): *Pathogenesis of Human Motor Neuron Diseases.* New York, Raven Press, 1982, p 75.

82. Hirano A: Some aspects of the neuropathological hallmarks of neuropsychiatric disorders in the elderly. In Hirano A, Miyoshi K (eds): *Neuropsychiatric Disorders in the Elderly.* New York, Igaku-Shoin, 1983, p 1.

83. Hirano A, Carton CA: Primary malignant melanoma of the spinal cord. *J Neurosurg* 17:935, 1960.

84. Hirano A, Dembitzer HM: Cerebellar alterations in the weaver mouse. *J Cell Biol* 56:478, 1973.

85. Hirano A, Dembitzer HM: Observations on the development of the weaver mouse cerebellum. *J Neuropathol*

Exp Neurol 33:354, 1974.

86. Hirano A, Dembitzer HM: The fine structure of staggerer cerebellum. *J Neuropathol Exp Neurol* 34:1, 1975.

87. Hirano A, Dembitzer HM: The fine structure of astrocytes in the adult staggerer. *J Neuropathol Exp Neurol* 35:63, 1976.

88. Hirano A, Dembitzer HM: Eosinophilic rod-like structures in myelinated fibers of hamster spinal roots. *Neuropathol Appl Neurobiol* 2:225, 1976.

89. Hirano A, Dembitzer HM: Morphology of normal central myelinated axons. In Waxman SG (ed): *Physiology and Pathology of Axons.* New York, Raven Press, 1978, p 65.

90. Hirano A, Dembitzer HM, Ghatak NR, Fan K-J, Zimmerman HM: On the relationship between human and experimental granule cell type cerebellar degeneration. *J Neuropathol Exp Neurol* 32:493, 1973.

91. Hirano A, Dembitzer HM, Jones M: An electron microscopic study of cycasin-induced cerebellar alterations. *J Neuropathol Exp Neurol* 31:113, 1972.

92. Hirano A, Dembitzer HM, Kurland LT, Zimmerman HM: The fine structure of some intraganglionic alterations. Neurofibrillary tangles, granulovacuolar bodies, and "rod-like" structures as seen in Guam amyotrophic lateral sclerosis and parkinsonism-dementia complex. *J Neuropathol Exp Neurol* 27:167, 1968.

93. Hirano A, Dembitzer HM, Yoon CH: Development of Purkinje cell somatic spines in the weaver mouse. *Acta Neuropathol (Berl)* 40:85, 1977.

94. Hirano A, Dembitzer HM, Zimmerman HM: The fine structure of phosphotungstic acid strained neuropathologic tissue. *Acta Neuropathol (Berl)* 26:265, 1973.

95. Hirano A, Ghatak NR, Johnson AB, Partnow MJ, Gomori AJ: Argentophilic plaques in Creutzfeldt-Jakob disease. *Arch Neurol* 26:530, 1972.

96. Hirano A, Ghatak NR, Wisoff HS, Zimmerman HM: An epithelial cyst of the spinal cord. An electron microscopic study. *Acta Neuropathol (Berl)* 18:214, 1971.

97. Hirano A, Ghatak NR, Zimmerman HM: The fine structure of ependymoblastoma. *J Neuropathol Exp Neurol* 32:144, 1973.

98 Hirano A, Inoue K: Early pathological changes of amyotrophic lateral sclerosis. Electron microscopic study of chromatolysis, spheroids and Bunina bodies. *Neurol Med (Tokyo)* 13:148, 1980.

99. Hirano A, Iwata M: Neuropathology of lead intoxication. In Vinken PJ, Bruyn GW (eds): *Intoxications of the Nervous System. Handbook of Clinical Neurology,* Amsterdam, North-Holland Pub. Co., 1978, vol 36, p 35.

100. Hirano A, Iwata M: Pathology of motor neurons with special reference to amyotrophic lateral sclerosis and related diseases. In Tsubaki T, Toyokura Y (eds): *Amyotrophic Lateral Sclerosis.* Baltimore, University of Park Press, 1979, p 107.

101. Hirano A, Iwata M, Llena JF, Matsui T: *Color Atlas-Neuropathology.* New York, Igaku-Shoin, 1980.

102. Hirano A, Kochen JA: Experimental lead encephalopathy. Morphologic Studies, In Zimmerman HM (ed): *Progress in Neuropathology.* New York, Grune & Stratton, 1976, vol 3, p 319.

103. Hirano A, Llena JF: The central nervous system as a target site in toxic-metabolic states. In Spencer PS, Schaumberg HM (eds): *Experimental and Clinical Neurotoxicology.* Baltimore, Williams & Wilkins, 1980, p 24.

104. Hirano A, Llena JF: Pathology of degenerative diseases of the central nervous system. In Rosenberg RN (ed): *The Clinical Neurosciences.* New York, Churchill Livingstone, 1983, vol 3, p 285.

105. Hirano A, Llena JF, French JH, Ghatak NR: Fine structure of the cerebellar cortex in Menkes' kinky hair disease. X-chromosome-linked copper malabsorption. *Arch Neurol* 34:52, 1977.

106. Hirano A, Llena JF, Steifler M, Cohn DF: Anterior horn cell changes in a case of neurolathyrism. *Acta Neuropathol (Berl)* 35:277, 1976.

107. Hirano A, Levine S, Zimmerman HM: Experimental cyanide encephalopathy. Electron microscopic observation of early lesions in white matter. *J Neuropathol Exp Neurol* 26:200, 1967.

108. Hirano A, Malamud N, Elizan TS, Kurland LT: Amyotrophic lateral sclerosis and parkinsonism-dementia complex on Guam. *Arch Neurol* 15:35, 1966.

109. Hirano A, Malamud N, Kurland LT: Parkinsonism-dementia complex, an endemic disease on the island of Guam. II. Pathological features. *Brain* 84:662, 1961.

110. Hirano A, Matsui T, Zimmerman HM: Electron microscopic observations of ependyma. *Neurol Surg (Tokyo)* 3:237, 1975.

111. Hirano A, Matsui T, Zimmerman HM: The fine structure of ependymoma. *Neurol Surg (Tokyo)* 3:557, 1975.

112. Hirano A, Rubin R, Sutton CH, Zimmerman HM: Honeycomb-like tubular structure in axoplasm. *Acta Neuropathol (Berl)* 10:17, 1968.

113. Hirano A, Sax DS, Zimmerman HM: The fine structure of cerebella of jimpy mice and their "normal" litter mates. *J Neuropathol Exp Neurol* 28:388, 1969.

114. Hirano A, Shin YY: Unattached presynaptic terminals in a cerebellar neuroblastoma in the human. *Neuropathol Appl Neurobiol* 5:63, 1979.

115. Hirano A, Tuazon R, Zimmerman HM: Neurofibrillary changes, granulovacuolar bodies and argentophilic globules observed in tuberous sclerosis. *Acta Neuropathol (Berl)* 11:257, 1968.

116. Hirano A, Zimmerman HM: Alzheimer's neurofibrillary changes: a topographic study. *Arch Neurol* 7:227, 1962.

117. Hirano A, Zimmerman HM: Some new cytological observations of the normal rat ependyma cell. *Anat Rec* 158:293, 1967.

118. Hirano A, Zimmerman HM: Some new pathological findings in the central myelinated axon. *J Neuropathol Exp Neurol* 30:325, 1971.

119. Hirano A, Zimmerman HM: Some effect of vinblastin implantation in the cerebral white matter. *Lab Invest* 23:358, 1970.

120. Hirano A, Zimmerman HM: Aberrant synaptic development. *Arch Neurol* 28:359, 1973.

121. Hirano A, Zimmerman H, Levine S: Fine structure of cerebral fluid accumulation. V. Transfers of fluid from extracellular to intracellular compartments in a acute phase of cryptococcal polysaccharide lesions. *Arch Neurol* 11:632, 1964.

122. Hirano A, Zimmerman HM, Levine S: The fine structure of cerebral fluid accumulation. VII. Reactions of astrocytes to cryptococcal polysaccharid implantation. *J Neuropathol Exp Neurol* 24:386, 1965.

123. Hirano A, Zimmerman HM, Levine S: The fine structure of cerebral fluid accumulation. IX. Edema following silver nitrate implantation. *Am J Pathol* 47:537, 1965.

124. Hirano A, Zimmerman HM, Levine S: The fine structure of cerebral fluid accumulation. Reaction of ependyma to implantation of cryptococcal polysaccharide. *J Pathol Bacteriol* 91:149, 1966.

125. Hirano A, Zimmerman HM, Levine S, Padgett GA: Cytoplasmic inclusions in Chediak-Higashi and wobbler mink. An electron microscopic study of the nervous system. *J Neuropathol Exp Neurol* 30:470, 1971.

126. Hirosawa K: Electron microscopic studies on pigment granules in the substantia nigra and locus coeruleus of the Japanese monkey (Macca fuscata yakui). *Z Zellforsch* 88:187, 1968.

127. Hoffman PN, Lasek RJ: The slow component of axonal transport. *J Cell Biol* 66:351, 1975.

128. Holland JM, William CD, Prieur DJ, Collins GH: Lafora's disease in the dog. A comparative study. *Am J Pathol* 58:509, 1970.

129. Horoupian DS, Yang SS: Paired helical filaments in neurovisceral lipidosis (juvenile dystonic lipidosis). *Ann Neurol* 4:404, 1978.

130. Hunter D, Russel DE: Focal cerebral and cerebellar atrophy in a human subject due to organic mercury compounds. *J Neurol Neurosurg Psychiatry* 17:235, 1954.

131. Ikeda K: A study of the Marinesco body in monkey (Macaca fuscata). A comparative study to the Marinesco body in man. *Folia Psychiatr Neurol Japan* 76:778, 1974.

132. Ishii T, Nakamura Y: Distribution and ultrastructure of Alzheimer's neurofibrillary tangles in postencephalitic parkinsonism of Economo type. *Acta Neuropathol (Berl)* 55:59, 1981.

133. Iwata M: Contribution a l'etude de la maladie de Lafora. Mémoire pour le titre dássistant étranger, Université de Paris VI, U.E.R. De Médecine Pitié-Salpetrière, Paris, 1973.

134. Iwata M, Hirano A: Neuropathological study of chronic healed anterior poliomyelitis. *Neurol Med (Tokyo)* 8:157, 1978.

135. Iwata M, Hirano A: "Glial bundles" in spinal cord late after paralytic anterior poliomyelitis. *Ann Neurol* 4:562, 1978.

136. Iwata M, Hirano A: Current problems in the pathology of amyotrophic lateral sclerosis. In Zimmerman HM (ed): *Progress in Neuropathology.* New York, Raven Press, 1979, vol 4, p 277.

137. Iwata M, Hirano A, French JH: Degeneration of the cerebellar system in X-chromosome-linked copper malabsorption. *Ann Neurol* 5:542, 1979.

138. Jacobson M: *Developmental Neurobiology.* New York, Plenum Press, 1978.

139. Japanese Journal of Medical Science and Biology, Vol 28, supplement. Tokyo, National Institute of Health, 1975, p 1.

140. Jellinger K: Neuroaxonal dystrophy: Its natural history and related disorders. In Zimmerman HM (ed): *Progress in Neuropathology.* New York, Grune & Stratton, 1973, vol 2, p 129.

141. Jew JY, Williams TH: Ultrastructural aspects of bilirubin encephalopathy in cochlear nuclei of the Gunn rat. *J Anat* 124:599, 1977.

142. Katsuragi S, Eto K, Takeuchi T: A study on an eosinophilic globular inclusion body in a pyramidal cell of hippocampus. *Brain Nerve (Tokyo)* 33:725, 1981.

143. Kawamoto K, Hirano A, Matsui T: The fine structure of cell processes in astrocytoma. *Neurol Surg (Tokyo)* 6:1173, 1978.

144. Kawano N, Horoupian DS: Intracytoplasmic rod-like inclusions in caudate nucleus. *Neuropathol Appl Neurobiol* 7:307, 1981.

145. Kerns JM, Hinsman EJ: Neuroglial response to sciatic neurectomy. II. Electron microscopy. *J Comp Neurol* 151:255, 1973.

146. Kidd M: Alzheimer's disease. An electron microscopic study. *Brain* 87:307, 1964.

147. Kojima K, Ogawa H: Alcoholic hyalin-like bodies of nerve cells. *Brain Nerve (Tokyo)* 26:1000, 1974.

148. Kreutzberg GW (ed): *Advances in Neurology, Vol 12: Physiology and Pathology of Dendrites.* New York, Raven Press, 1975, vol 12.

149. Kristensson K: Retrograde axonal transport of protein tracers. In Cowan WM, Cuénoda M (eds): *The Use of Axonal Transport for Studies of Neuronal Connectivity.* Amsterdam, Elsevier, 1975, p 69.

150. Kristensson K, Olsson Y: Uptake and retrograde axonal transport of protein tracers in hypoglossal neurons. *Acta Neuropathol (Berl)* 23:43, 1973.

151. Kuffler SW, Nicholls JG: *From Neuron to Brain.* Sunderland, MA, Sinauer Associates, 1976.

152. Kumanishi T, Hirano A: Immunoperoxidase study on herpes simplex virus encephalitis. *J Neuropathol Exp Neurol* 37:790, 1978.

153. Kumanishi T, In S: SSPE: immunohistochemical demonstration of measles virus antigen(s) in paraffin sections. *Acta Neuropathol (Berl)* 48:161, 1979.

154. Kuroda S, Otsuki S, Tateishi J, Hirano A: Neurofibrillary degeneration in a case of quadriplegia and myoclonic movement. *Acta Neuropathol (Berl)* 45:105, 1979.

155. Lampert P: A comparative electron microscopic study of reactive, degenerative, regenerative and dystrophic ax-

ons. *J Neuropathol Exp Neurol* 26:345, 1967.

156. Lampert PW, Gajdusek DC, Gibbs CJ Jr: Subacute spongiform virus encephalopathies. Scrapie, Kuru and Creutzfeldt-Jakob disease: a review. *Am J Pathol* 66:626, 1972.

157. Lasek RJ (Chairman): What do glia do? In: *Society for Neuroscience, 7th Annual Meeting. Summaries of Symposia.* (BIS Conference Report 48) UXLA, Los Angeles, Brain Information Service/BRI Publication Office, 1978, p 149.

158. Lazarides E: Intermediate filaments as mechanical integrators of cellular space. *Nature* 283:249, 1980.

159. Leestma JE, Andrews JM: The fine structure of the Marinesco body. *Arch Pathol* 88:431, 1969.

160. Lieberman AR: The axon reaction: a review of the principal features of perikaryal responses to axon injury. *Int Rev Neurobiol* 14:49, 1971.

161. Llena JF, Hirano A: Abundant eosinophilic rod-like structures in subacute spongiform encephalopathy. *J Neuropathol Exp Neurol* 38:329a, 1979.

162. Llena JF, Hirano A, Rubin RC: Paraganglioma in the cauda equina region. *Acta Neuropathol (Berl)* 46:235, 1979.

163. Malamud N, Hirano A: *Atlas of Neuropathology,* ed 2. Berkeley, CA, University of California Press, 1975.

164. Malamud N, Hirano A, Kurland LT: Pathoanatomic changes in amyotrophic lateral sclerosis on Guam. Special reference to the occurrence of neurofibrillary changes. *Arch Neurol* 5:401, 1961.

165. Matthews MA, Onge MF St, Faciane CL: An electron microscopic analysis of abnormal ependymal cell proliferation and envelopment of sprouting axons following spinal cord transection in the rat. *Acta Neuropathol (Berl)* 45:27, 1979.

166. Menkes JH, Alter M, Steigleder GK, Weakley DR, Sung JH: A sex-linked recessive disorder with retardation of growth, peculiar hair, and focal cerebral and cerebellar degeneration. *Pediatrics* 29:764, 1962.

167. Mervis R: Structural alterations in neurons of aged canine neocortex: a Golgi Study. *Exp Neurol* 62:417, 1978.

168. Millhouse OE: Lining of the third ventricle in the rat. In Knigger KM, Scott DE, Kobayashi H, Ishii S (eds): *Brain-Endocrine Interaction. II. The Ventricular System in Neuro-endocrine Mechanisms.* Basel, Switzerland, S. Karger, 1975, p 3.

169. Morecki R, Zimmerman HM: Human rabies encephalitis. Fine structure study of cytoplasmic inclusions. *Arch Neurol* 20:599, 1969

170. Nakai Y, Ochiai H, Uchida M: Fine structure of ependymal cells in the median eminence of the frog and mouse revealed by freeze-etching. *Cell Tissue Res* 181:311, 1977.

171. Namba M: Lafora disease. *Brain Nerve (Tokyo)* 20:6, 1968.

172. Namba M, Yoshimura T, Kato H, Mikami Y, Mitsui H: Aging changes in the brain of Japanese monkeys (Macaca fuscata). *Seishin Yakuryo Kikin Kenkyo Nenpo* 3:27, 1971.

173. Norenberg MD, Lapham LW: The astrocyte response in experimental portal-systemic encephalopathy: an electron microscopic study. *J Neuropathol Exp Neurol* 33:422, 1974.

174. Norman MG: Hyalin ("colloid") cytoplasmic inclusions in motoneurones in association with familial microencephaly, retardation and seizures. *J Neurol Sci* 23:63, 1974.

175. Norton WT, Goldman JE: Neurofilaments. In Ralph A, Schneider DM (eds): *Proteins of the Nervous System.* New York, Raven Press, 1980, p 301.

176. O'Brien L, Shelley K, Towfighi J, McPherson A: Crystalline ribosomes are present in brain from senile humans. *Proc Natl Acad Sci USA* 77:2260, 1980.

177. Ogata J, Budzilovich GN, Gravioto H: A study of rodlike structures (Hirano bodies) in 240 normal and pathological brains. *Acta Neuropathol (Berl)* 21:61, 1972.

178. Ohama E, Ikuta F: Parkinson's disease: distribution of Lewy bodies and monoamine neuron system. *Acta Neuropathol (Berl)* 34:311, 1976.

179. Ohama E, Shibata T, Yamamura S, Ikuta F: Hirano body-like crystalline structure in the Ammon's horn induced by chronic administration of 6-hydroxydopamine. *Adv Neurol Sci (Tokyo)* 20:400, 1976.

180. Okamoto K, Hirai S, Morimatsu M, Ishida Y: The Bunina bodies in amyotrophic lateral sclerosis. *Neurol Med (Tokyo)* 13:133, 1980.

181. Oyanagi S: An electron microscopic observation on senile dementia, with special references to transformation of neurofilaments to twisted tubules and a structural connection of Pick bodies to Alzheimer's neurofibrillary changes. *Adv Neurol Sci (Tokyo)* 18:77, 1974.

182. Oyanagi S: Ultrastructural characteristics of the Pick body, as compared with those of the neurofibrillary changes in Alzheimer's disease and progressive supranuclear palsy. In Hirano A, Miyoshi K (eds): *Neuropsychiatric Disorders in the Elderly.* New York, Igaku-Shoin, 1983, p 118.

183. Page RB, Rosenstein JM, Leure-DuPree AE: The morphology of extrachoroidal ependyma overlying gray and white matter in the rabbit lateral ventricle. *Anat Rec* 194:67, 1979.

184. Page RB, Rosenstein JM, Dovey BJ, Leure-DuPree AE: Ependymal changes in experimental hydrocephalus. *Anat Rec* 194:83, 1979.

185. Palay SK, Chan-Palay V: *Cerebellar Cortex Cytology and Organization.* New York, Springer-Verlag, 1974.

186. Palay SL, Chan-Palay V: General morphology of neurons and neuroglia. In Kandel ER (ed): Section 1: *The Nervous System. Handbook of Physiology.* Bethesda, MD, American Physiological Society, 1977, vol 1, part 1, p 5.

187. Palay SL, Sotelo C, Peters A, Orband PM: The axon hillock and the initial segment. *J Cell Biol* 38:193, 1968.

188. Pannese E: Unusual membrane-particle complexes within nerve cells of the spinal ganglia. *J Ultrastruct Res* 29:334, 1969.

189. Pappas GD, Purpura DP: *Structure and Function of Synapses.* New York, Raven Press, 1972.

190. Peña CE: Intracytoplasmic neuronal inclusions in the human thalamus. *Acta Neuropathol (Berl)* 52:157, 1980.

191. Périer O, Vanderhaeghen JJ: Subacute sclerosing leucoencephalitis. Electron microscopic finding in two cases with inclusion bodies. *Acta Neuropathol (Berl)* 8:362, 1967.

192. Peters A, Palay SL, Webster H DeF: *The Fine Structure of the Nervous System. The Cells and Supporting Cells.* New York, Harper & Row, 1976.

193. Peters A, Proskauer CC, Kaiserman-Abramof IR: The small pyramidal neuron of the rat cerebral cortex. *J Cell Biol* 39:604, 1968.

194. Price D, Griffin JW: Neurons and ensheathing cells as targets of disease processes. In Spencer PS, Schaumburg HH (eds): *Experimental and Clinical Neurotoxicology.* Baltimore, Williams & Wilkins, 1980, p 2.

195. Purpura DP: Aberrant dendritic and synaptic development in immature human brain. *J Neuropathol Exp Neurol* 37:578a, 1978.

196. Purpura DP, Hirano A, French JF: Polydendritic Purkinje cells in X-chromosome-linked copper malabsorption: a Golgi study. *Brain Res* 117:125, 1976.

197. Rakic P: Mode of cell migration to the superficial layers of fetal monkey neocortex. *J Comp Neurol* 145:61, 1972.

198. Ralston HJ, Chow KL: Synaptic reorganization in the degenerating lateral geniculate nucleus of the rabbit. *J Comp Neurol* 147:321, 1973.

199. Ramsey HJ: Ultrastructure of corpora amylacea. *J Neuropathol Exp Neurol* 24:25, 1965.

200. Robitaille Y, Carpenter S, Karpati G, Dimauro S: A distinct form of adult polyglucosan body disease with massive involvement of central and peripheral neuronal processes and astrocytes. A report of four cases and a review of the occurrence of polyglucosan bodies in other conditions such as Lafora's disease and normal ageing.

Brain 103:315, 1980.

201. Roy S, Hirano A, Zimmerman HM: Ultrastructural demonstration of cilia in the adult human ependyma. *Anat Rec* 180:547, 1974.

202. Roy S, Wolman L: Ultrastructural observations in parkinsonism. *J Pathol* 99:39, 1969.

203. Sandbank U: Infantile neuroaxonal dystrophy. *Arch Neurol* 12:155, 1965.

204. Scheibel A: Structural aspects of the aging brain: spine systems and the dendritic arbor. In Katzman R, Terry RD, Bick KL (eds): *Alzheimer's Disease: Senile Dementia and Related Disorders. Aging.* New York, Raven Press, 1978, vol 7, p 353.

205. Schlaepfer WW: Deformation of isolated neurofilaments and the pathogenesis of neurofibrillary pathology. *J Neuropathol Exp Neurol* 37:244, 1978.

206. Schochet SS Jr: Neuronal inclusions. In Bourne GH (ed): *The Structure and Function of Nervous Tissue.* New York, Academic Press, 1972, vol 4, p 129.

207. Schochet SS Jr, Hardman JM, Ladewig PP, Earle KM: Intraneuronal conglomerates in sporadic motor neuron disease. *Arch Neurol* 20:548, 1969.

208. Schochet SS Jr, Lampert PW, Earle KM: Alexander's disease. A case report with electron microscopic observations. *Neurology (Minneap)* 18:543, 1968.

209. Schochet SS Jr, Lampert PW, Lindenberg R: Fine structure of the Pick and Hirano bodies in a case of Pick's disease. *Acta Neuropathol (Berl)* 11:330, 1968.

210. Schochet SS Jr, McCormick WF: Ultrastructure of Hirano bodies. *Acta Neuropathol (Berl)* 21:50, 1972.

211. Schochet SS Jr, Wyatt RB, McCormick WF: Intracytoplasmic acidophilic granules in the substantia nigra. *Arch Neurol* 22:550, 1970.

212. Schutta HS, Johnson L, Neville HE: Mitochondria abnormalities in bilirubin encephalopathy. *J Neuropathol Exp Neurol* 29:296, 1970.

213. Seite R, Mei N, Couinean S: Modification quantitative des bâtonnet intranucléaires des neurones sympathiques sous l'influence de la simulation electrique. *Brain Res* 34:277, 1971.

214. Sekiya S, Oyanagi S, Tanaka M, Hayashi S, Nakamura Y: Mitochondria as Acidophilic Granules within the Substantia Nigra and Locus Ceruleus (author's translation). Abstract, the 22nd annual meeting, Japanese Neuropathological Association, 1981, p 67a.

215. Shibayama H, Kitoh J: Electron microscopic structure of the Alzheimer's neurofibrillary changes in case of atypical senile dementia. *Acta Neuropathol (Berl)* 41:229, 1978.

216. Shin W-Y, Laufer H, Lee Y-C, Aftalion B, Hirano A, Zimmerman HM: Fine structure of the cerebellar neuroblastoma. *Acta Neuropathol (Berl)* 42:11, 1978.

217. Shirabe T, Hirano A: X-ray microanalytical studies of lead-implanted rat brains. *Acta Neuropathol (Berl)* 40:184, 1977.

218. Sotelo C: Permanence and fate of paramembranous synaptic specialization in "mutant" and experimental animals. *Brain Res* 62:345, 1973.

219. Sotelo C, Palay SL: Altered axons and axon terminals in the lateral vestibular nucleus of the rat: possible example of axonal remodeling. *Lab Invest* 25:653, 1971.

220. Spencer PS, Schaumburg HH: *Experimental and Clinical Neurotoxicology. A Textbook of Environmental Neurobiology.* Baltimore, Williams & Wilkins, 1980.

221. Sung JH: Neuroaxonal dystrophy in mucoviscidosis. *J Neuropathol Exp Neurol* 23:567, 1964.

222. Sung JH, Stadlan EM: Neuroaxonal dystrophy in congenital biliary atresia. *J Neuropathol Exp Neurol* 25:341, 1966.

223. Suzuki K, Johnson AB, Marquet E, Suzuki K: A case of juvenile lipidosis: electron microscopic, histochemical and biochemical studies. *Acta Neuropathol (Berl)* 11:122, 1968.

224. Suzuki K: Metabolic diseases. In Johannessen JV (ed): *Electron Microscopy in Human Medicine.* New York, McGraw-Hill, 1979, vol 6, p 3.

225. Suzuki Y, Atoji Y, Suu S: Microtubules observed within the cisterns of RER in neurons of the aged dog. *Acta Neuropathol (Berl)* 44:155, 1978.

226. Takei Y, Mirra SS: Intracytoplasmic hyaline inclusion bodies in the nerve cells of the hypoglossal nucleus in human autopsy material. *Acta Neuropathol (Berl)* 17:14, 1971.

227. Takeya S: *Introduction to General Neuropathology*. Tokyo, Igaku-Shoin, 1970.

228. Tennyson VM, Pappas GD: Ependyma. In Minckler J (ed): *Pathology of the Nervous System*. New York, McGraw-Hill, 1968, vol 1, p 518.

229. Terry RD: The fine structure of neurofibrillary tangles in Alzheimer's disease. *J Neuropathol Exp Neurol* 22:629, 1963.

230. Terry RD: Ultrastructural alterations in senile dementia. In Katzman R, Terry RD, Bick KL (eds): *Alzheimer's Disease: Senile Dementia and Related Disorders. Aging.* New York, Raven Press, 1978, vol 7, p 375.

231. Terry RD, Gonatas NK, Weiss M: Ultrastructural studies in Alzheimer's presenile dementia. *Am J Pathol* 44:269, 1964.

232. Terry RD, Pena C: Experimental production of neurofibrillary degeneration. *J Neuropathol Exp Neurol* 24:200, 1965.

233. Terry RD, Weiss M: Studies in Tay-Sachs disease. II. Ultrastructure of the cerebrum. *J Neuropathol Exp Neurol* 22:18, 1963.

234. Tomlinson BE: The ageing brain. In Smith WT, Cavanagh JB (eds): *Recent Advances in Neuropathology*. Edinburgh, Churchill Livingston, 1979, p 129.

235. Tomonaga M: Ultrastructure of Hirano bodies. *Acta Neuropathol (Berl)* 28:365, 1974.

236. Tomonaga M: Ultrastructure of neurofibrillary tangles in progressive supranuclear palsy. *Acta Neuropathol (Berl)* 37:177, 1977.

237. Tomonaga M: Selective appearance of Bunina bodies in amyotrophic lateral sclerosis. *J Neurol* 223:259, 1980.

238. Tomonaga M, Saito M, Yoshimura M, Shimada H, Tohgi H: Ultrastructure of the Bunina bodies in anterior horn cells of amyotrophic lateral sclerosis. *Acta Neuropathol (Berl)* 42:81, 1978.

239. Torch WC, Hirano A, Solomon S: Anterograde transneuronal degeneration in the limbic system: clinical-anatomical correlation. *Neurology (Minneap)* 27:1157, 1977.

240. Towfighi J, Baird HW, Gambetti P, Gonatas NK: The significance of cytoplasmic inclusions in late infantile and juvenile amaurotic idiocy. An ultrastructural study. *Acta Neuropathol (Berl)* 23:32, 1973.

241. Uchizono K: *Excitation and Inhibition Synaptic Morphology*. Tokyo, Igaku Shoin, 1975.

242. Valverde F: Rate and extent of recovery from dark rearing in the visual cortex of the mouse. *Brain Res* 33:1, 1971.

243. Vanneste J, van den Bosch de Aguilar Ph: Mitochondrial alterations in the spinal ganglion neurons in the aging rats. *Acta Neuropathol (Berl)* 54:83, 1981.

244. Vigh B, Vigh-Teichman I: Comparative ultrastructure of the cerebrospinal fluid-contacting neurons. *Int Rev Cytol* 35:189, 1973.

245. Volk BV, Aronson SM: *Sphingolipids, Sphingolipidosis and Allied Disorders*. New York, Plenum Publishing Corp, 1972.

246. Webster H DeF: Transient, focal accumulation of axonal mitochondria during the early stages of Wallerian degeneration. *J Cell Biol* 12:361, 1962.

247. Weller RO, Wisniewski H, Shulman K, Terry RD: Experimental hydrocephalus in young dogs. Histological and ultrastructural study of the brain tissue damage. *J Neuropathol Exp Neurol* 30:613, 1971.

248. Westergaard E: *The Lateral Cerebral Ventricles and the Ventricular Walls*. Doctoral dissertation, University of Aarhus. I. Pommission hos Andelsbog trykkeriet i Odense, 1970.

249. Wiśniewski HM, Berry K, Spiro AJ: Ultrastructure of thalamic neuronal inclusions in myotonic dystrophy. *J Neurol Sci* 24:321, 1975.

250. Wiśniewski HM, Coblentz JM, Terry RD: Pick's disease. A clinical and ultrastructural study. *Arch Neurol* 26:97, 1972.

251. Wiśniewski HM, Ghetti B, Terry RD: Neuritic (senile) plaques and filamentous changes in aged Rhesus monkeys. *J Neuropathol Exp Neurol* 32:566, 1973.

252. Wiśniewski HM, Narang HK, Terry RD: Neurofibrillary tangles of paired helical filaments. *J Neurol Sci* 27:173, 1976.

253. Wiśniewski HM, Terry RD: Re-examination of the pathogenesis of the senile plaque. In Zimmerman HM (ed): *Progress in Neuropathology*. New York, Grune & Stratton, 1973, vol 2, p 1.

254. Wiśniewski H, Terry RD, Hirano A: A neurofibrillary pathology. *J Neuropathol Exp Neurol* 29:163, 1970.

255. Wiśniewski K, Javis G, Moretz RC: Alzheimer's neurofibrillary tangles in diseases other than senile and presenile dementia. *Ann Neurol* 5:288, 1979.

256. Wisotskey HM, Moossy J: Hyaline ("colloid") cytoplasmic inclusions in neurons of human hypoglossal nuclei. *Arch Pathol* 93:61, 1972.

257. Wuerker RB: Neurofilaments and glial filaments. *Tissue Cell* 2:1, 1970.

258. Yagishita S, Ito Y, Nan Wang, Amano N: Reappraisal of the fine structure of Alzheimer's neurofibrillary tangles. *Acta Neuropathol (Berl)* 54:239, 1981.

259. Yajima K, Suzuki K: Neuronal degeneration in the brain of the brindled mouse. An ultrastructural study of the cerebral cortical neurons. *Acta Neuropathol (Berl)* 45:17, 1979.

260. Zeman W: Studies in the neuronal ceroid-lipofuscinoses. *J Neuropathol Exp Neurol* 33:1, 1974.

CHAPTER 2

Oligodendrocytes and Central Nervous System Myelin

CEDRIC S. RAINE, Ph.D., D.Sc.

HISTORY

Although well-characterized today as astrocytes and oligodendrocytes, glial cells were for many years a *pot pourri* of unclassified elements considered of secondary importance to the nerve cells which they subserved. For the oligodendrocyte, the major subject of this section, its recognition began at a time when glia were still regarded as a syncytium. Ford Robertson in 1897 and 1899 (52, 53) (reviewed by Penfield (40) and Bunge (9)) separated from the neuroglia—the "nerve glue" of Virchow (67)—a cell type which he named "mesoglia." Robertson's criteria were based upon impregnation with platinum, and his choice of nomenclature stemmed from the marked dissimilarity between these cells and the commonly accepted neuroglial cell. In 1904 and 1905, Hardesty (18, 19) further developed Robertson's observations in studies of fetal pig spinal cord (teased preparations and sections) and reported the presence of "signet-ring" cells which were associated with myelinated (medullated) fibers. Similarity was noted between these cells and Schwann cells of the peripheral nervous system (PNS) and suggested that they may be functionally related to the formation of the framework of the myelin sheath, rather than myelin itself. Their presence could not be documented before the appearance of myelin, and their numbers and cytoplasmic staining were greatest during the period of active myelination and decreased when myelination was complete. In the adult,

these cells were flattened along nerve fibers, and Hardesty believed them to have no role in the investment of the axon.

In the following decade, Cajal (13) conclusively separated the astrocyte from other neuroglia using his still applied gold sublimate method. Thus, after neurons, astrocytes became the second element of the central nervous system (CNS), leaving behind a "third element" composed of a large body of small, incompletely stained cells. The term "mesoglia" of Robertson, having received brief attention at the turn of the century, thus appeared to have slipped into obscurity. However, with the development of a silver carbonate technique, Del Rio-Hortega (14, 15) was able to separate "oligodendroglia" from the third element of the CNS, a cell type believed to correspond to Robertson's mesoglia. Since the recognition of the oligodendrocyte as a discrete glial cell type, attempts have been made to subdivide them further on the basis of numerous (usually, morphologic) criteria. Mori and Leblond (34) recognized three classes, light, medium, and dark oligodendroglia with varying proliferative activities, a terminology still in common usage (44).

DEVELOPMENT

The development of the neuroglia does not commence until neuronal division and migration have ceased when they arise from neuroepithelial (ectodermal) cells lining the neural tube. As development proceeds, they gradually withdraw their pial and ventricular attachments to become radially arranged columnar cells, known as spongioblasts (25), which then differentiate into ependymoblasts (ultimately, ependyma) and glioblasts (subependymal cells). From the latter, oligodendrocytes and astrocytes are derived (28, 53, 54). Unlike neurons, glia are capable of repeated mitotic division and migration throughout life, a feature which has important regenerative implications. While the nomenclature of the stages of glial cell differentiation might vary from author to author, spongioblasts are more commonly referred to today as glioblasts. Although glia are derived from matrix cells at the same time as neurons, they apparently remain dormant until neuronal division has ceased and migration is well-advanced (28).

In general, glial cells are programmed to provide supportive roles for neurons and consequently, follow neurons and their extensions as they migrate. Thus, cortical neurons might lack satellite oligodendrocytes early on, and fiber tracts in the spinal cord consist initially of a pure population of neurites before being subsequently separated into groups by astrocytes and, for those axons destined to be myelinated, invested by oligodendrocytes.

While it is recognized that intermediate, apparently uncommitted, oligodendrocytes, can be found in grey matter, to the neuropathologist, the oligodendrocyte really exists in two forms—satellitic oligodendroglia, applied to neuronal somata, and interfascicular oligodendroglia, located in myelinated white matter and involved in the production and maintenance of myelin. It is to these two types of oligodendrocytes that the remainder of this chapter is devoted.

MORPHOLOGY

In a routine hematoxylin and eosin (H&E) preparation, interfascicular oligodendrocytes are small cells with prominent dark rounded nuclei. Often, the cytoplasm appears swollen and clear, leaving the nucleus suspended in a vacuole-like profile—a situation brought about by poor fixation of deep white matter (Fig. 2.1). In an appropriately fixed H&E preparation (a small slice immersed fresh in fixative), a narrow rim of cytoplasm circles the small nucleus

which has a diameter of about 5 μm. In longitudinal section, the nuclei of interfascicular oligodendroglia are often aligned in rows. H&E examination of grey matter will invariably reveal one or more satellite oligodendrocytes around large neurons (Fig. 2.2). Elsewhere in H&E preparations, astrocytic nuclei can be identified by their larger size, paler staining, and irregular to elliptical shape.

Examination of oligodendroglial morphology in 1-μm thick epoxy sections stained with toluidine blue affords a more informative light microscope image in that, in glutaraldehyde/osmium-fixed preparations, satellite oligodendroglia are clearly satellitic to a wide variety of neurons (Figs. 2.3 and 2.4) and actually indent the neuronal somata. The nucleus is rounded and possesses clumped heterochromatin. The cytoplasm is sometimes barely perceptible (Fig. 2.4) but usually is more voluminous at one pole, giving the cell an ovoid profile (Fig. 2.3).

Ultrastructurally, satellite oligodendroglia are seen to reside in a small depression along the surface of the neuron (Fig. 2.5). The diameter of the entire cell ranges from about 12–16 μm. Sometimes, the cell is separated from the neuron by an interposing layer of astroglial cytoplasm (Fig. 2.6). Membrane specializations (junctions) between the oligodendrocyte and the neuron are not prominent, although they commonly occur between the oligodendrocyte and adjacent astrocytic profiles. These take the form of maculae punctata and gap junctions (Fig. 2.7). The nucleochromatin is dense and is distinctive in its possessing islands of denser chromatin (heterochromatin). The cytoplasm is moderately dense, contains a small amount of rough endoplasmic reticulum, an abundance of free ribosomes, a prominent Golgi apparatus, a few mitochondria, and an occasional dense body in the cell soma or its infrequent processes. The latter inclusion is overlooked in most textbooks but is really a feature peculiar to oligodendrocytes (Fig. 2.8). Depending upon the plane of section (seen most advantageously in the perpendicular plane), these inclusions are dome-shaped and bounded by a single membrane. The matrix consists of a cap of electron-dense material and a base of closely stacked

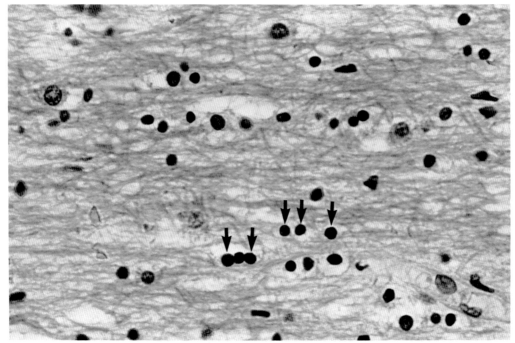

Figure 2.1.   Routine H&E preparation of longitudinally-oriented human white matter to show the small dark rounded nuclei of interfascicular oligodendrocytes surrounded by a halo of clear, swollen cytoplasm. The larger, paler stained elliptical or irregular shaped nuclei belong to astrocytes, Note how some interfascicular oligodendrocytes are aligned in rows (*arrows*). (Original magnification ×1,000.)

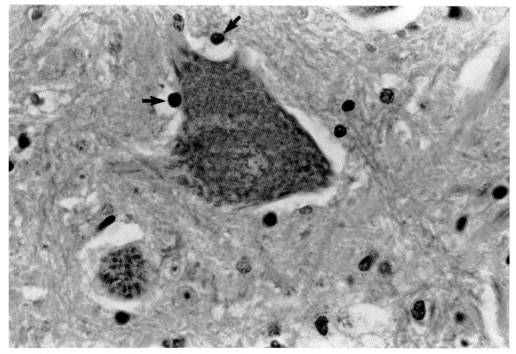

Figure 2.2.   An anterior horn cell from human lumbar spinal cord in an H&E preparation is flanked by two satellitic oligodendrocytes, the cytoplasm of which is swollen (*arrows*). Elsewhere, the elliptical nuclei of astrocytes are seen. (Original magnification ×1,000.)

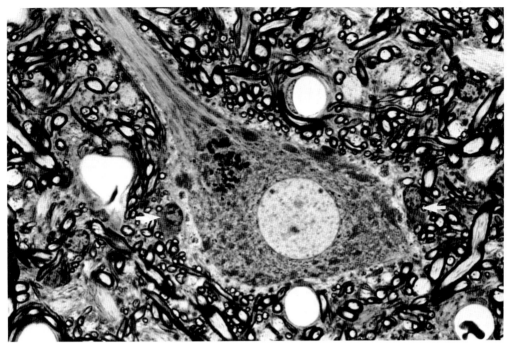

Figure 2.3. An anterior horn cell from a guinea pig spinal cord is shown in a 1-μm epoxy section stained with toluidine blue. Two satellitic oligodendrocytes with well preserved, densely staining cytoplasm are seen (*arrows*). Within the neuronal cytoplasm, clumps of Nissl substance are located peripherally, and at the base of the large dendrite (*upper left*) a collection of lipofuscin granules is seen. Elsewhere, myelinated axons are present. (Original magnification ×1,000.)

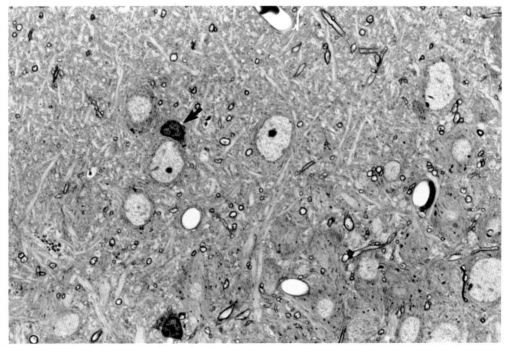

Figure 2.4. Cortical neurons from the brain of a rat are shown in a 1-μm epoxy section stained with toluidine blue. A satellitic oligodendrocyte is seen at the *arrow*. Myelinated axons are also present. (Original magnification ×1,000.)

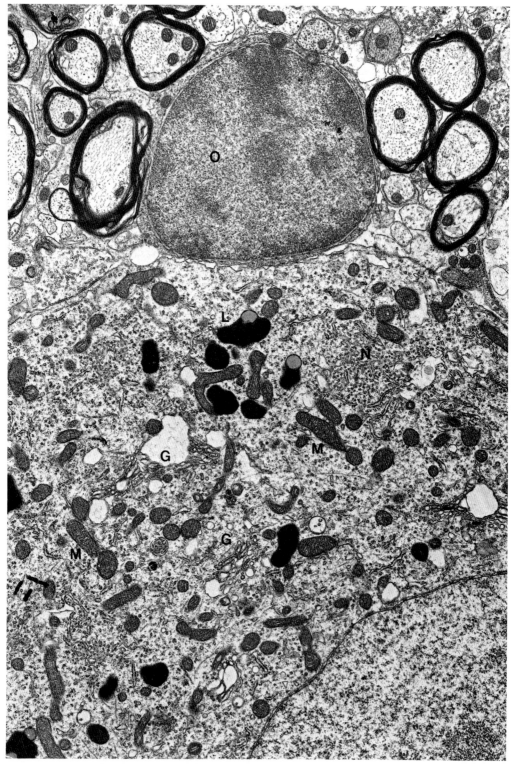

Figure 2.5. An electron micrograph from the spinal cord of a guinea pig shows a satellitic oligodendrocyte (*O*) resting upon the surface of an anterior horn cell (nucleus lower right). Note the narrow rim of oligodendroglial cytoplasm, and within the neuronal cytoplasm, Nissl substance (*N*), lipofuscin (*L*), Golgi apparatus (*G*), and mitochondria (*M*) can be discerned. (Original magnification ×12,000.)

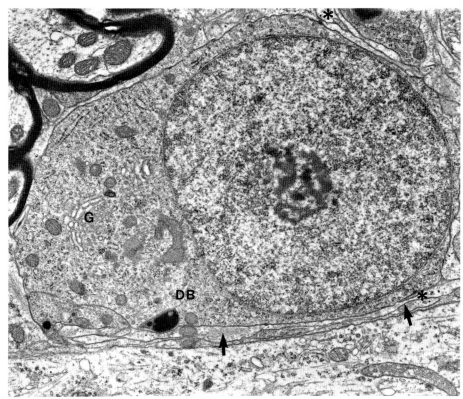

Figure 2.6. Dog lumbar spinal cord, to show a satellitic oligodendrocyte on the surface of a neuron (*below*). Between the two, several fibrous astroglial cell processes containing filaments (*arrows*) are located. Within the oligodendrocyte cytoplasm, note the prominent Golgi apparatus (*G*), the scattered fragments of rough endoplasmic reticulum, maculae punctata (*asterisks*), and the characteristic dense body (*DB*)—see text. (Original magnification ×14,300.)

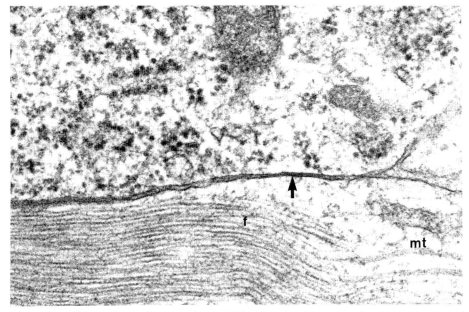

Figure 2.7. Detail from the perimeter of a satellitic oligodendrocyte to show a gap junction (*arrow*) between its plasmalemma and that of the process of a fibrous astrocyte (*below*) which contains glial filaments (*f*) and microtubules (*mt*). (Original magnification ×70,000.)

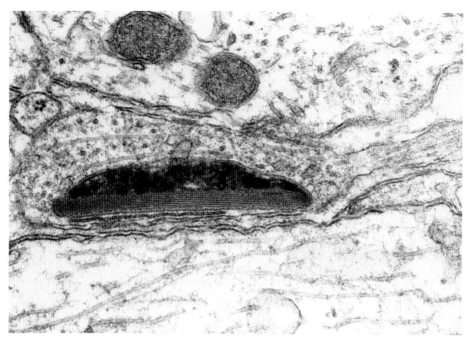

Figure 2.8. The process of an oligodendrocyte within an anterior horn of a guinea pig spinal cord contains a membrane-bound inclusion commonly seen in oligodendrocytes. Note the amorphous dense dome of the inclusion and the lamellar stacks below. Many microtubules but no intermediate filaments are also in the cell process. Above and below, neurites are located. (Original magnification ×50,000.)

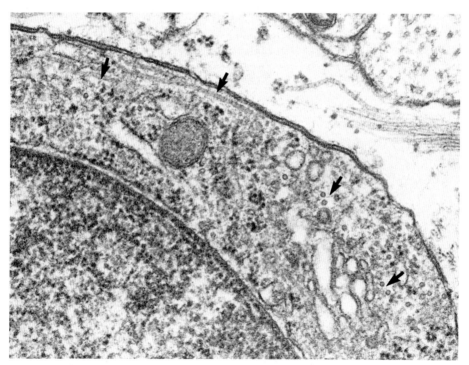

Figure 2.9. An oligodendrocyte within the white matter of a guinea pig spinal cord shows the presence of microtubules in transverse and longitudinal section (*arrows*) but no intermediate filaments. The cell is invested by an astroglial cell process containing rough endoplasmic reticulum, glial filaments, and an occasional microtubule. (Original magnification ×50,000.)

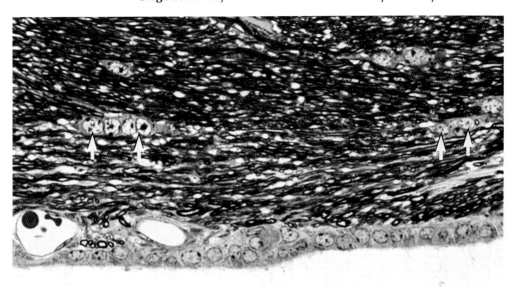

Figure 2.10.   Within the corpus callosum, rows of interfascicular oligodendrocytes are located (*arrows*) among the myelinated fibers. Ciliated ependyma are seen below. Rat brain, 1-µm epoxy section stained with toluidine blue. (Original magnification ×1,000.)

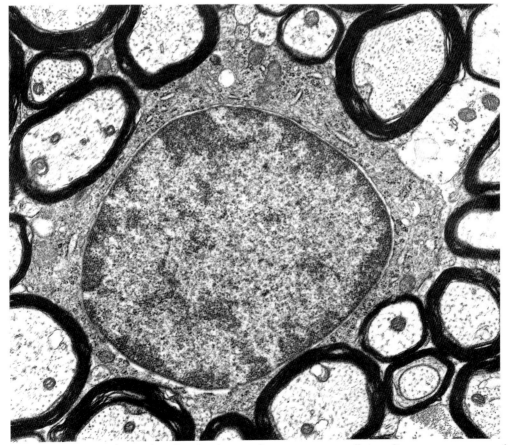

Figure 2.11.   An interfascicular oligodendrocyte from rat corpus callosum lies among transversely sectioned, myelinated nerve fibers. (Original magnification ×18,250.)

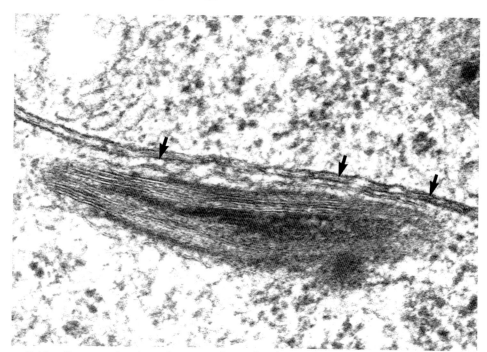

Figure 2.12. Between the plasmalemmae of two closely-apposed interfascicular oligodendrocytes, a gap junction can be discerned (*arrows*). Note also the lamellar inclusions mentioned in the text. (Original magnification ×140,000.)

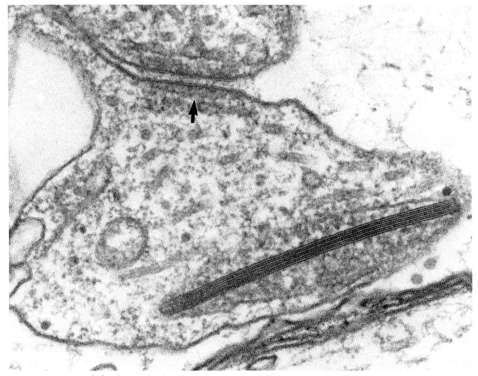

Figure 2.13. Two club-shaped oligodendrocyte processes, one of which contains a lamellar inclusion, share a small desmosome-like junction (*arrow*). Note also the many microtubules but no intermediate filaments. (Original magnification ×110,000.)

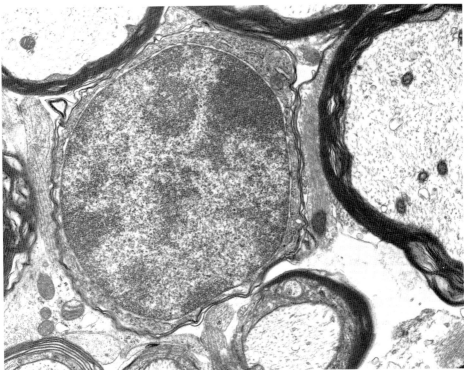

Figure 2.14.   An interfascicular oligodendrocyte is invested by several layers of myelin. (Original magnification ×13,200.)

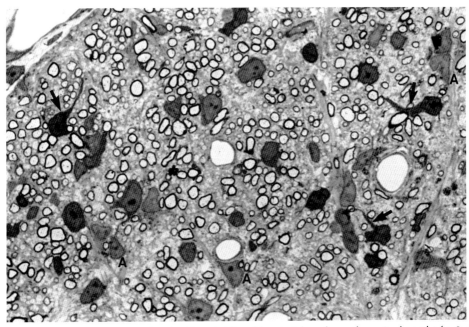

Figure 2.15.   A 1-µm section stained with toluidine blue is taken from the spinal cord of a 2-d-old kitten. Several densely staining oligodendrocytes (*arrows*) are shown with long cytoplasmic extensions to myelin sheaths. Elsewhere astrocytes (*A*) and myelinated fibers at different stages of myelination are evident. (Original magnification ×1,000.)

lamellae with a periodicity of about 4–5 nm (Fig. 2.8). These inclusions are probably tertiary lysosomes. Another important cytoplasmic property of the normal oligodendrocyte is the absence of filaments and the presence of abundant 22-nm microtubules (Fig. 2.9)—a feature first noted by Mugnaini and Walberg (35). Centrioles are rarely observed in the mature cell, except in situations where recent mitosis (e.g., during regeneration) has occurred.

Interfascicular oligodendrocytes, as the name suggests, are located between fascicles of myelinated nerve fibers where they have a tendency to form rows along the longitudinal axis (Fig. 2.10). Ultrastructural examination reveals a morphology identical to that of satellite oligodendrocytes except that the cytoplasm tends to be more dense (Fig. 2.11). Where the plasmalemmae of adjacent oligodendrocytes contact, gap junctions are frequently present (Fig. 2.12)—structures which probably have physiologic significance. In addition to gap junctions, desmosomes are sometimes seen between adjacent oligodendroglia cells and their processes (Fig. 2.13) which are easily distinguished from those of astrocytes in their possessing microtubules only. Although interfascicular oligodendrocytes are usually surrounded by or in close proximity to myelinated fibers, in the normal adult CNS, connections between the cell and its product, myelin, are rarely seen (Fig. 2.11). On rare occasions in the normal CNS, and more frequently in experimental situations, interfascicular oligodendrocytes can be seen to be surrounded by myelin (Fig. 2.14).

THE OLIGODENDROCYTE DURING MYELINOGENESIS

Although suspected for many years, a role for the oligodendrocyte in CNS myelinogenesis was not proven until the insightive analysis of Bunge and colleagues (9–12). A key observation in this work was the frequent unequivocal attachment of slender cell processes from the somata of oligodendrocytes to myelin sheaths around axons within the kitten CNS. Subsequent work from the same group documented that one cell would myelinate several axons (12). Today, many examples of connections between oligodendrocytes and CNS myelin sheaths are known (e.g., 21, 36, 47) and it is estimated that a single oligodendrocyte is capable of producing and maintaining simultaneously between 30 and 50 internodes of myelin (41).

Examination of CNS white matter during early development reveals, with relatively little effort, evidence of densely staining oligodendrocytes attached to CNS myelin sheaths by long slender, cytoplasmic processes (Figs. 2.15 and 2.16). It is now known that CNS myelination is effected when a process from an oligodendrocyte becomes flattened along a segment of an axon like a gutter. In the transverse plane, one of the lips of this process tucks under the other and moves around the axon in a spiral fashion. As the oligodendrocyte process spirals, its cytoplasmic contents become extruded until the opposite membranes meet. The two opposing inner (cytoplasmic) leaflets then become compacted and fuse to form the major dense line of the myelin sheath (Fig. 2.17). The outer leaflets of adjacent turns of myelin do not fuse but rather (except for specialized tight junctions related to the inner and outer loops of the myelin sheath) remain closely apposed and form the intraperiod line (Figs. 2.18 and 2.19). Because of the extensive expansion of the flattened oligodendrocyte process around the axon, both along and around the axon, and the maturation of the tissue, the connecting cell process becomes longer, more attenuated, and increasingly difficult to document in contact with the myelin sheath. From this point onwards, evidence of oligodendrocytic involvement is restricted to an outer loop of cytoplasm and an inner loop—the leading edge of the original flattened cell process (Fig. 2.19). Three-dimensional analysis (Fig. 2.20) shows the inner and outer loops of cytoplasm to be part of a peripherally located ridge of oligodendroglial cell cytoplasm in continuity with a lateral ridge which, when wrapped spirally, form the lateral loops flanking the node of Ranvier (Fig. 2.21 and 2.22).

At the node of Ranvier, the lateral loops are arranged in a regimented fashion, with the outermost lamella of myelin providing the most distal loop and the innermost lamella, the lateral loop most removed from

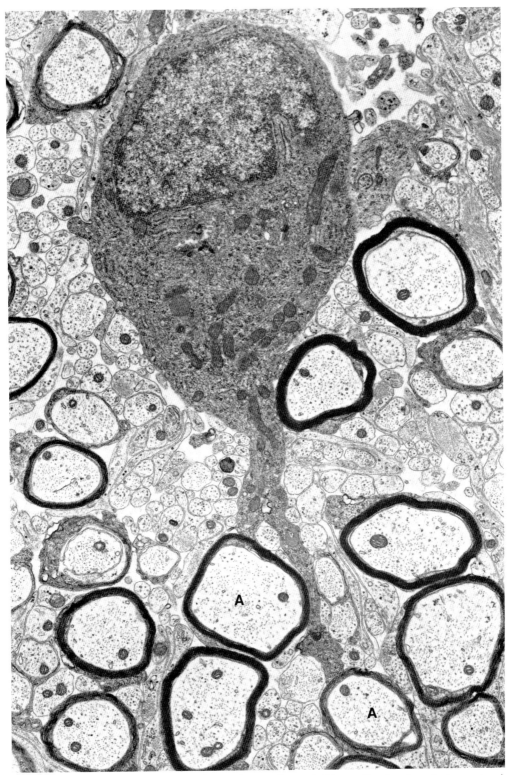

Figure 2.16.   From a preparation similar to that in Figure 2.15, an oligodendrocyte has extended a process which branches to contact the myelin sheaths of two axons (*A*). Elsewhere, note the nonmyelinated axons and fibers at different stages of myelination. (Original magnification ×16,000.)

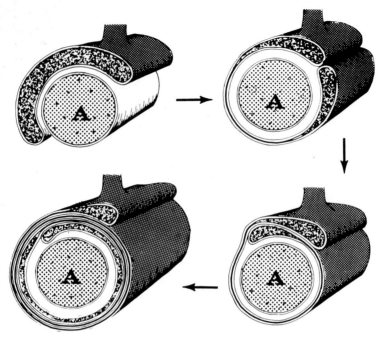

Figure 2.17. Diagrammatic representation of CNS myelination. Note how the cytoplasm of the flattened layer of oligodendroglial cytoplasm (connected to the main cell by the slender process, above) is gradually extended as myelin compaction occurs, how the major dense line is formed by the fusion of the inner leaflets of the unit membrane, and how the inner tongue apparently pulls the compacted myelin behind it as it tucks under the outer tongue and spirals around the axon (*A*). (From C. S. Raine (47).)

the node (see Fig. 2.21). Between each lateral loop and the axolemma, transverse bands (specialized spiral junctions) are located (22)—Figure 2.22. Thus, if the myelin sheath is unwrapped diagrammatically, it is seen that each myelin internode is a shovel-shaped membranous sheet with a ridge of cytoplasm connected by a narrow cell process to an oligodendrocyte (Fig. 2.21).

Since the intraperiod line of the myelin sheath is formed by the close apposition of the outer leaflets of the unit membrane of the oligodendroglial cell process, it represents a continuation of the extracellular space. This fact has several important ramifications in neuropathology, since it represents a potential point of separation (e.g., during edema) and is the surface to be first seen by the immune system. The outermost opening of the intraperiod line (beneath the outer loop) is known as the "outer mesaxon" and the innermost (over the axon), the "inner mesaxon," and at these points,

the intraperiod line forms a tight junction (Fig. 2.19).

In the PNS, an analogous situation, much simpler to analyze morphologically, presides where a Schwann cell becomes associated with a segment of axon, flattens, and spirals around it to produce PNS myelin. Unlike the situation in the CNS, the Schwann cell body forms the outer covering of the nerve fiber and is intimately connected to the sheath throughout life (Fig. 2.23). Furthermore, each Schwann cell is capable of forming only a single internode of myelin, and when more than one axon is invested, they remain unmyelinated. The Schwann cell, therefore, is much less committed than the oligodendrocyte, and while destruction of one Schwann cell will result in the loss of myelin from one segment of an axon, the death of one oligodendrocyte has the potential of producing a small demyelinated lesion. For a fuller analysis of CNS myelination see references 9, 22, 33, and 47.

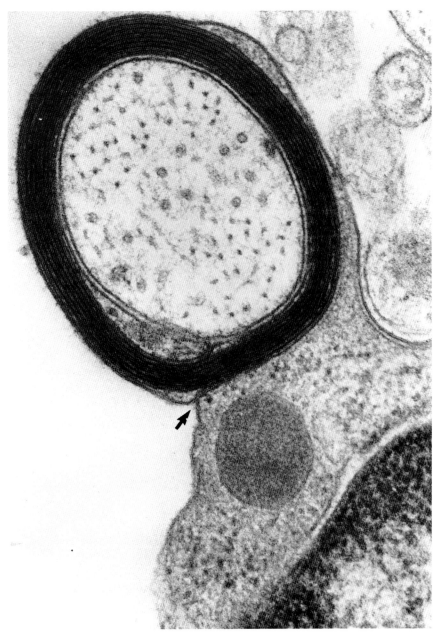

Figure 2.18. An oligodendrocyte (nucleus, *lower right*) has elaborated a process which becomes compacted to form myelin and spirals around an axon. The outer mesaxon is indicated (*arrow*). (From A. Hirano (21).) (Original magnification ×96,000.)

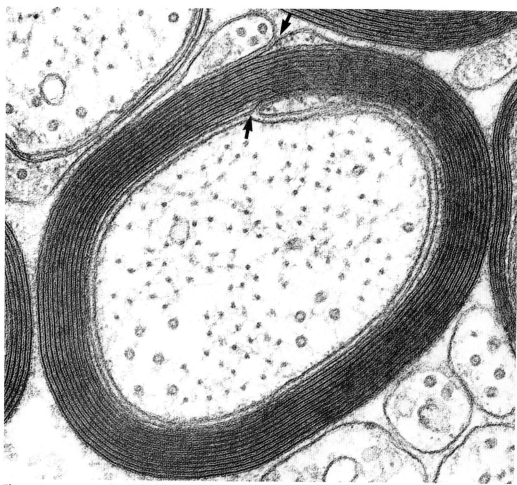

Figure 2.19. A myelinated CNS axon from the spinal cord of a dog is shown in transverse section. The outer loop lies above, and the outer and inner mesaxons are indicated (*arrows*). Note the characteristic myelin periodicity (10.6–11.0 nm between major dense lines) and beneath the outer loop, traces of a radial component in the myelin sheath (rows of tight junctions). The axon contains microtubules and cross-bridged neurofilaments. (Original magnification ×115,000.)

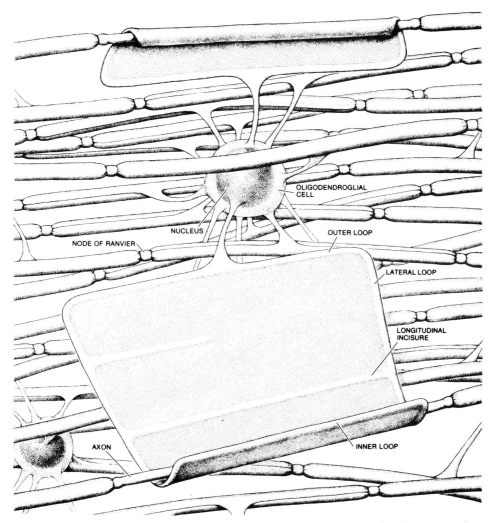

Figure 2.20. Diagrammatic representation of an interfascicular oligodendrocyte to show the relationships between its myelin internodes, partially unfurled in two cases to show the process of spiralization and origin of the inner, outer, and lateral loops, and the many axons it myelinates. (From P. Morell and W. T. Norton (33).)

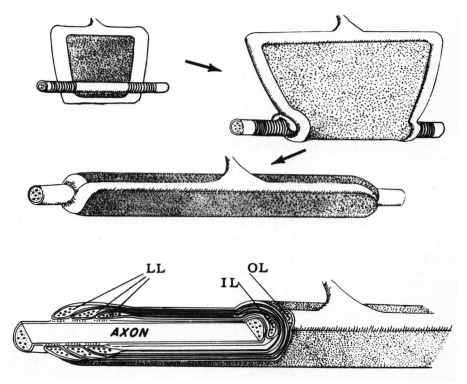

Figure 2.21. The spiralization of a shovel-shaped oligodendroglial cell process around a segment of axon to produce an internode of myelin is demonstrated diagrammatically. *LL*, lateral loop; *IL*, inner loop; *OL*, outer loop. (Modified from C. S. Raine (47).)

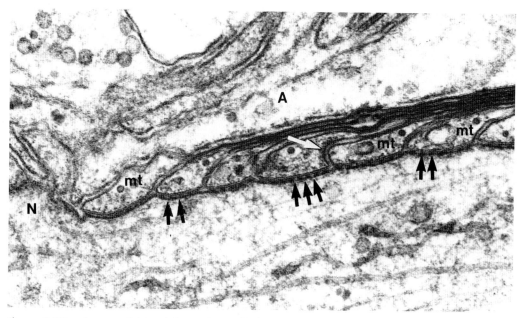

Figure 2.22. A row of lateral loops is applied to an axon in the paranodal position. Periodic transverse bands (*arrows*) can be detected between each lateral loop and the axolemma. A single microtubule (*mt*) is present in each loop, and a desmosome is present (*white arrow*). An astroglial process (*A*) meets others over the nodal axon at (*N*). (Original magnification ×80,000.)

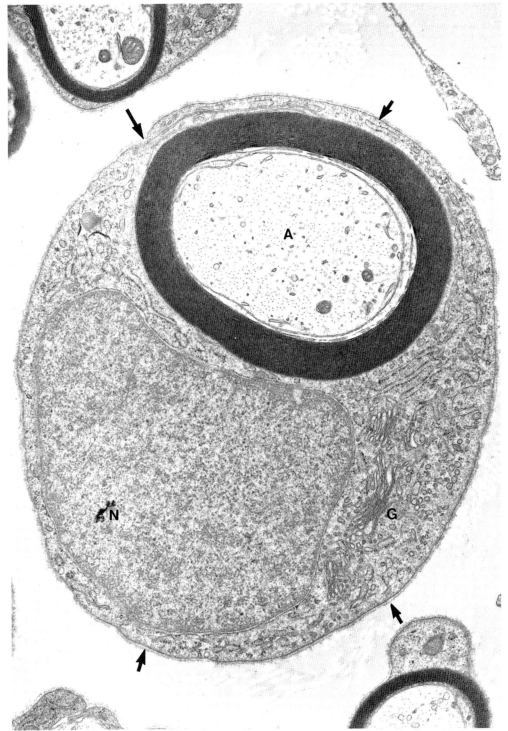

Figure 2.23. A PNS-myelinated fiber is sectioned transversely and shows the axon (*A*) surrounded by a thick myelin sheath which is elaborated by the investing Schwann cell nucleus at (*N*). The entire fiber is surrounded by a characteristic basal lamina (*small arrows*). The Golgi apparatus is seen at (*G*), the outer mesaxon at the *large arrow*. (Original magnification ×20,800.) (From C. S. Raine (47).)

RESPONSE TO DISEASE

In general, the oligodendrocyte responds poorly to pathologic insult, and as a consequence, remyelination in the CNS is often insignificant or absent. That remyelination occurs in the CNS has been known since the works of Bunge et al. (11) and Bornstein and Appel (6), and its significance in the demyelinating diseases is discussed in Chapter 11 (Raine). Stemming from the oligodendrocyte being a cell unique to the CNS, CNS myelin being a membrane with a unique biochemistry (see ref. 37), and the CNS being sequestered from the general circulation by virtue of the blood-brain barrier, both the cell and its product bear a battery of potential antigens foreign to the immune system. Furthermore, the oligodendrocyte-myelin system is highly vulnerable, since the cell is so heavily committed. Thus, if a breach occurs in the CNS vasculature, oligodendrocyte and myelin damage might ensue as a nonspecific consequence due to edema, immunologic products (immunoglobulins, lymphokines), and macrophage activity (hydrolytic enzymes). On the other hand, the biochemistry of the oligodendrocyte-myelin system depends upon a galaxy of complex enzymatic sequences. Genetic or induced perturbations in these sequences can have drastic effects upon myelination and the development of the CNS. Defects in these enzyme systems are implicated in some of the leukodystrophies and the mouse mutant models of dysmyelination (3, 62).

The oligodendrocyte is not noted for an active mitotic response subsequent to injury, and fibrillary astrogliosis has an adverse effect upon their regeneration (see Chapter 11, Raine). Nevertheless, mitotic activity has been reported after virus-induced (20), immune-mediated (51), and toxin-induced (30) demyelination. In the latter report, remyelination by satellitic oligodendroglia was a feature.

SPECIFIC MARKERS FOR OLIGODENDROGLIA AND CNS MYELIN

The following short section is not intended as a comprehensive review but merely to alert readers to the growing applicability of immunocytochemical approaches to problems related to the oligodendrocyte and its myelin. The gamut of unique biochemical properties of this cell and its membrane product (see ref. 33) has led to the development of antisera and monoclonal antibodies specific to these structures. This in turn has provided the neuropathologist with boundless new territory for exploration, using direct or indirect peroxidase labelling (2) or the Sternberger peroxidase-antiperoxidase technique (58). These markers have been applied to a variety of basic developmental and pathological problems.

At the basic level, a number of groups have produced and characterized antisera or monoclonal antibodies against whole oligodendroglia (e.g., refs. 1, 57, 65) which give specific staining of oligodendrocytes (sometimes without staining of myelin). Since both oligodendrocytes and myelin are unusually rich in the glycolipid, galactocerebroside, antisera raised against this component have been applied extensively in a number of basic (45) and disease-related (23, 64) problems where double-labeling techniques were mandated in order to distinguish cell populations with possible cross-antigenic properties. Furthermore the use of antimyelin basic protein (MBP) and antimyelin-associated glycoprotein (MAG) serum in the analysis of possible demyelination events in multiple sclerosis revealed a much more widespread loss of MAG around lesions, thus implying a primary role for this antigen in plaque development (26, 27). The application of anti-MAG and anti-MBP serum to studies on myelinogenesis has revealed changes in the localization of the antigens during myelination (59–61). For example, MAG localization appears to be more associated with oligodendroglial somata and cytoplasmic pockets around CNS fibers (Figs. 2.24A and B). On the other hand, anti-MBP serum stains oligodendrocytes prior to myelin formation, the cellular staining is most intense during myelination, and myelin sheaths are intensely stained (Figs. 2.25A and B). Immunocytochemistry of thick sections studied by light microscopy at different focal planes (Figs. 2.26A–D) after treatment with anti-MBP serum has reconfirmed the association of a single oligodendrocyte with multiple axons, some from different ana-

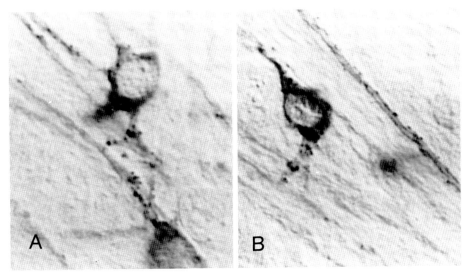

Figure 2.24.   Two examples (*A* and *B*) of oligodendrocytes attached to myelin sheaths are shown after staining with anti-MAG serum. Note the intense staining of the cell body and the globular staining along the myelin sheaths. (Original magnification ×1,000.) (From N. H. Sternberger et al. (61).)

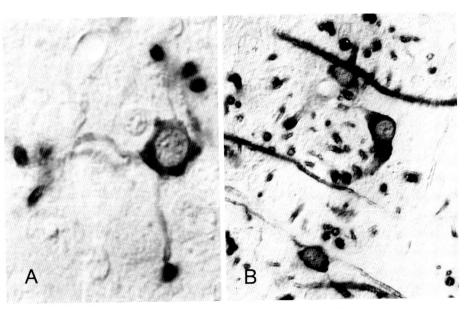

Figure 2.25.   Oligodendrocytes and CNS myelin are stained with anti-MBP serum. In *A*, an oligodendrocyte extends seven processes to surrounding myelinated axons, sectioned transversely. Newborn rat medulla. In *B*, oligodendrocytes in the pontine tectospinal tract of a 12-day-old rat show intense staining of somata and myelin sheaths, the latter seen in both the transverse and longitudinal planes. (*A*, Original magnification ×1,000; *B*, Original magnification ×600.) (*A*, From N. H. Sternberger et al. (60). *B*, From N. H. Sternberger et al. (59).)

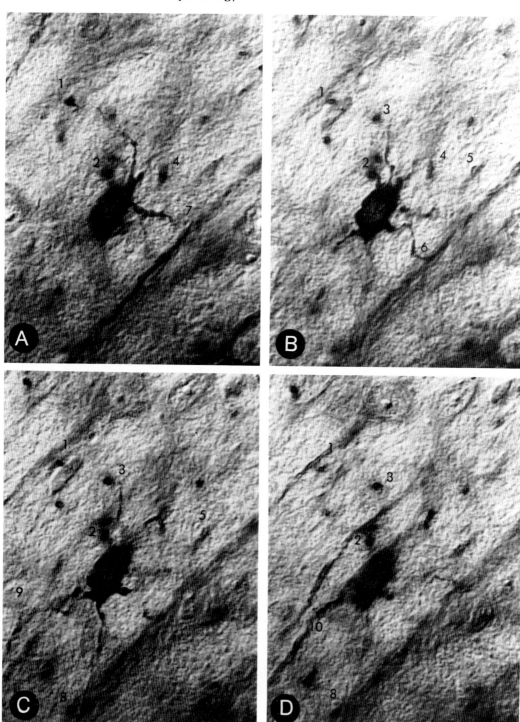

Figure 2.26. An oligodendrocyte from 5-day-old rat pons is illustrated at four levels of focus to show the extension of processes to transversely and longitudinally-oriented myelin sheaths. Anti-MBP serum staining in combination with Nomarski optics. (Original magnification ×1,000.) (From N. H. Sternberger et al. (60).)

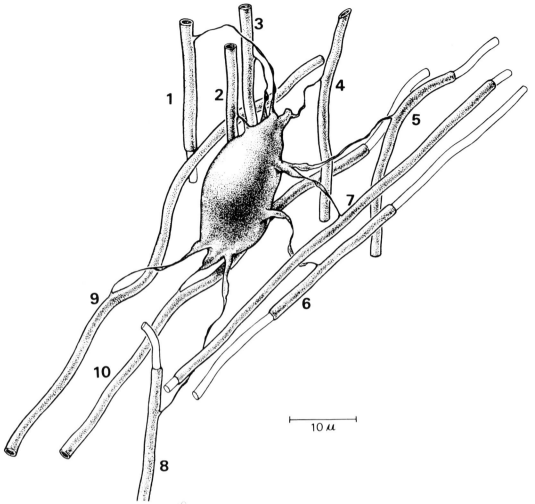

Figure 2.27. The oligodendroglial contacts with the ten myelinated fibers shown in Figure 2.26 are reconstructed diagrammatically. The six which are transversely sectioned belong to the tectospinal tract, the other four longitudinally sectioned fibers belong to the pontocerebellar tract. (From N. H. Sternberger et al. (60).)

tomical tracts (Figs. 2.26 and 2.27)—see reference 60.

In addition to proteins and lipids characteristic for myelin (either qualitatively or quantitatively) several enzymes have been shown to be specifc for the myelin membrane (e.g., carbonic anhydrase) and the oligodendrocyte body (glycerol phosphate dehydrogenase—GPDH)—see reference 66. Thus, it is not surprising that an antiserum to GPDH specifically recognizes oligodendroglia (17), thereby enlarging our armamentarium of oligodendroglial markers. Although still a controversial issue, the localization of antigens within the

CNS myelin sheath has been examined by immunocytochemistry. With a modified PAP technique and plastic-embedded material, Omlin et al. (39) have demonstrated that MBP is localized at the major dense line in the CNS. These results conflict with those of Mendell and Whitaker (32) on PNS myelin (using a different method of fixation) where MBP was claimed to be at the intraperiod line. This controversy notwithstanding, the degree of precision with which these immunologic markers can be applied to problems at the ultrastructural level is exquisitely demonstrated by such studies.

OLIGODENDROCYTES AND MYELIN IN CULTURE

Of considerable importance to neuropathology is the availability of living, in vitro preparations of oligodendrocytes and myelin. In a readily perceivable chamber, the investigator can observe and monitor chronologically by many parameters (morphology, biochemistry, immunology), changes occurring in the tissue due to a variety of causes (e.g., toxic, viral, traumatic etc.).

Most applied since their development in the 1950s have been organotypic cultures of CNS tissue (5). For this, explanted fragments of any region of the CNS neuraxis can be maintained up to months in vitro, during which time cells differentiate and CNS myelin is proliferated. For some of the applications of this system to neuropathology, the reader is referred to the reviews of Raine (46, 46). The system has been of particular value for studies on the dissection of interactions between glial cells and neurons during myelination (68), where cultures depleted of myelinating cells can be supplemented with oligodendrocytes from another source lacking neuronal influence. Also pertinent to myelination are investigations on the selective destruction of oligodendroglia during experimental demyelination in vitro (49), remyelination and sclerosis in vitro (50), inhibition of myelination (7), and the enhancement of myelin proliferation (8).

Other in vitro studies, particularly on the expression of cell-specific antigens in the CNS, have employed the use of dissociated cell cultures containing glial cells and neurons or cultures of mixed glial cells (4, 31, 45). While representing an incomplete reproduction of the in situ situation since the system lacks myelination, these investigations have had pioneer roles in establishing antigenic differences among glial cell types at different stages of development in vitro.

Yet another tissue culture system of pertinence to oligodendroglial research has emanated from neurochemical techniques which yielded bulk isolated, purified preparations of oligodendrocytes (16, 42, 43). By adopting more sterile procedures, several groups have since succeeded in maintaining these pure preparations of bulk-isolated oligodendroglia in culture for long periods (24, 29, 38, 56, 63).

CONCLUSIONS

It is apparent from multidisciplinary investigations that the oligodendrocyte interacts with the neuron to produce many segments of the insulating membrane, myelin around numerous axons. This membrane has an essential physiologic role in that its presence is necessary for rapid conduction. The nature of the neuronal signal which triggers the oligodendrocyte to associate with axons and form myelin is the subject of intensive current research. Thus, the availability of in vitro models, which permit direct visualization of oligodendrocytes in the presence and absence of neuronal components, render possible the application of highly specific markers and technologies. Furthermore, the development of a wide variety of animal models with myelin perturbations of relevance to many human conditions puts within easy reach of the neuropathologist approaches fundamental to the understanding of myelin biology and disease.

ACKNOWLEDGEMENTS

The author acknowledges with thanks the following investigators who have provided illustrative material for this chapter: Drs. William T. Norton (Albert Einstein College of Medicine) and Pierre Morell (University of N. Carolina, Chapel Hill), Figure 2.19; Asao Hirano (Albert Einstein College of Medicine), Figure 2.20; Nancy Sternberger (University of Rochester), Figures 2.26 and 2.27; and Henry deF. Webster (NINCDS), Figures 2.28 and 2.29.

Also, for their significant input into my work I would like to thank my colleagues Drs. R. D. Terry, U. Traugott, D. S. Horoupian, K. Suzuki, M. B. Bornstein, W. T. Norton, and A. Hirano; my technicians, Everett Swanson, Howard Finch, and Miriam Pakingan; and my secretary, Mary Palumbo.

Supported in part by USPHS grants NS 08952, NS 11920, and NS 07098 and by NMSS grant RG 1001-D-4.

References

1. Abramsky O, et al: Immunologic studies with isolated oligodendrocytes. *Neurology (Minneap)* 27:342, 1977.

2. Avrameas S, Ternyck T: Peroxidase labeled antibody and Fab conjugates with enhanced intracellular penetration. *Immunochemistry* 8:1175, 1971.

3. Baumann N: *Neurological Mutations Affecting Myelination.* INSERM Symp. No. 14. Amsterdam, Elsevier/North-Holland, 1980.

4. Bologa-Sandru L, et al: Expression of antigenic markers during the development of oligodendrocytes in mouse brain cultures. *Brain Res* 210:217, 1981.

5. Bornstein MB: Organotypic mammalian central and peripheral nerve tissue. In Kruse PF Jr, Patterson MK Jr (eds): *Tissue Culture Methods and Applications,* New York, Academic Press, 1973.

6. Bornstein MB, Appel SH: The application of tissue culture to the study of experimental "allergic" encephalomyelitis. I. Patterns of demyelination. *J Neuropathol Exp Neurol* 20:141, 1961.

7. Bornstein MB, Raine CS: Experimental allergic encephalomyelitis: antiserum inhibition of myelination in vitro. *Lab Invest* 23:536, 1970.

8. Bornstein MB, Raine CS: The initial structural lesion in serum-induced demyelination in vitro. *Lab Invest* 35:391, 1976.

9. Bunge RP: Glial cells and the central myelin sheath. *Physiol Rev* 48:197, 1968.

10. Bunge MB, et al: Electron microscope demonstration of connections between glia and myelin sheaths in the developing mammalian C.N.S. *J Biophys Biochem Cytol* 12:448, 1962.

11. Bunge MB, et al: Ultrastructural study of remyelination in an experimental lesion in adult cat spinal cord. *J Biophys Biochem Cytol* 10:67, 1961.

12. Bunge RP, Glass PM: Some observations on myelin-glial relationships and on the etiology of cerebrospinal fluid exchange lesion. *Ann NY Acad Sci* 122:15, 1965.

13. Cajal SR: Contribucion al concimiento de la neuroglia en el cerebro humano. *Trab Lab Inv Biol* 11:255, 1913.

14. Del Rio-Hortega P: Noticia de un nuevo y facil metodo para la coloracion de la neuroglia y del tijido conjuctivo. *Trab Lab Inv Biol* 15:367, 1918.

15. Del Rio-Hortega P: La glia de escasas radiaciones (oligodendroglia). *Bull Real Sociedad Espanola Historic Natural Tomo* 21:63, 1921.

16. Fewster ME, et al: The preparation and characterization of isolated oligodendroglia from bovine white matter. *Brain Res* 63:263, 1973.

17. Ghandour MS, et al: Double labeling immunohistochemical technique provides evidence of the specificity of glial cell markers. *J Histochem Cytochem* 27:1634, 1979.

18. Hardesty I: On the development and nature of the neuroglia. *Am J Anat* 3:229, 1904.

19. Hardesty I: On the occurrence of sheath cells and the nature of the axone sheaths in the central nervous system. *Am J Anat* 4:329, 1905.

20. Herndon RM, et al: Regeneration of oligodendroglia during recovery from demyelinating disease. *Science* 195:693, 1977.

21. Hirano A: A confirmation of the oligodendroglial origin of myelin in the adult rat. *J Cell Biol* 38:637, 1968.

22. Hirano A, Dembitzer HM: Morphology of normal central myelinated axons. In Waxman SG (ed): *Physiology and Pathobiology of Axons.* New York, Raven Press, 1978.

23. Hirayama M, et al: Absence of expression of OKT8 antigen on cultured human, calf and rat oligodendrocytes. *Nature* 301:152, 1983.

24. Hirayama M, et al: Long-term culture of oligodendrocytes isolated from rat corpus callosum by Percoll density gradient. *J Neuropathol Exp Neurol* 42:16, 1983.

25. His W: Die Neuroblasten und deren Entstehung im embryonalen Mark. *Abhandl Kgl Sachs Ges Wiss Math Phys Kl* 15:313, 1889.

26. Itoyama Y, et al: Immunocytochemical method to identify myelin basic protein in oligodendroglia and myelin sheaths of the human nervous system. *Ann Neurol* 7:157, 1980.

27. Itoyama Y, et al: Immunocytochemical observations on the distribution of myelin-associated glycoprotein and myelin basic protein in multiple sclerosis lesions. *Ann Neurol* 7:167, 1980.

28. Jacobson M: *Developmental Neurobiology,* ed 2. New York, Plenum Press, 1978.

29. Lisak RP, et al: Long-term culture of bovine oligodendroglia isolated with a Percoll gradient. *Brain Res* 223:107, 1981.

30. Ludwin SK: The perineuronal satellite oligodendrocyte. A role in remyelination. *Acta Neuropathol (Berl)* 47:49, 1979.

31. McCarthy KD, De Vellis J: Preparation of separate astroglial and oligodendroglial cell cultures from rat cerebral tissue. *J Cell Biol* 85:890, 1980.

32. Mendell JR, Whitaker JM: Immunocytochemical localization studies of myelin basic protein. *J Cell Biol* 76:502, 1978.

33. Morell P, Norton WT: Myelin. *Sci Am* 242:88, 1980.

34. Mori S, Leblond CP: Electron microscopic identification of three classes of oligodendrocytes and a preliminary study of their proliferative activity in the corpus callosum of young rats. *J Comp Neurol* 139:1, 1970.

35. Mugnaini E, Walberg F: Ultrastructure of neuroglia. *Ergeb Anat Entwicklungsgesch* 37:193, 1964.

36. Nagashima K: Ultrastructural study of myelinating cells and subpial astrocytes in developing rat spinal cord. *J Neurol Sci* 44:1, 1979.

37. Norton WT: Biochemistry of myelin. In Waxman SG, Ritchie JM (eds): *Demyelinating Diseases: Basic and Clinical Electrophysiology.* New York, Raven Press, 1981.

38. Norton WT, et al: The long term culture of bulk-isolated bovine oligodendroglia from adult brain. *Brain Res* 270:295, 1983.

39. Omlin FX, et al: Immunocytochemical localization of basic protein in major dense line regions of central and peripheral myelin. *J Cell Biol* 95:242, 1982.

40. Penfield W: Neuroglia: normal and pathological. In *Cytology and Cellular Pathology of the Nervous Tissue.* New York, Hoeber, 1932, vol 2.

41. Peters A, Proskauer CC: The ratio between myelin segments and oligodendrocytes in the optic nerve of the adult rat. *Anat Rec* 163:243, 1969.

42. Pleasure D, et al: Oligodendroglial glycerophospholipid synthesis: incorporation of radioactive precursors into ethanolamine glycerophospholipids by calf oligodendroglia prepared by a Percoll procedure and maintained in suspension culture. *J Neurochem* 37:452, 1981.

43. Poduslo SE, Norton WT: Isolation and some chemical properties of oligodendroglia from calf brain. *J Neurochem* 19:727, 1972.

44. Privat A: Morphological approaches to the problems of neuroglia. Some comments. In Schoffeniels E, et al (eds): *Dynamic Properties of Glia Cells.* Oxford, England, Pergamon Press, 1978.

45. Raff MC, et al: Galactocerebroside is a specific cell-surface antigenic marker for oligodendrocytes in culture. *Nature* 274:813, 1978.

46. Raine CS: Ultrastructural applications of cultured nervous system tissue to neuropathology. In Zimmerman HM (ed): *Progress in Neuropathology.* New York, Grune & Stratton, 1973, vol 2.

47. Raine CS: Morphological aspects of myelin and myelination. In Morell P (ed): *Myelin.* New York, Plenum Press, 1977.

48. Raine CS: Pathology of demyelination. In Waxman SG (ed): *Physiology and Pathobiology of Axons.* New York, Raven Press, 1978.

49. Raine CS, Bornstein MB: Experimental allergic encephalomyelitis: an ultrastructural study of experimental demyelination in vitro. *J Neuropathol Exp Neurol* 29:177, 1970.

50. Raine CS, Bornstein MB: Experimental allergic encephalomyelitis: a light and electron microscope study of remyelination and "sclerosis" in vitro. *J Neuropathol Exp*

Neurol 29:552, 1970.

51. Raine CS, Traugott U: Chronic relapsing experimental autoimmune encephalomyelitis: ultrastructure of the CNS of animals treated with combinations of myelin components. *Lab Invest* 48:275, 1983.

52. Robertson WF: The normal histology and pathology of the neuroglia. *J Ment Sci* 43:73, 1897.

53. Robertson WF: On the new method of obtaining a black reaction in certain tissue elements of the central nervous system (Platinum Method). *Scott Med Surg J* 4:23, 1899.

54. Skoff RP, et al: Electron microscopic autoradiographic studies of gliogenesis in rat optic nerve. I. Cell proliferation. *J Comp Neurol* 169:291, 1976.

55. Skoff RP, et al: Electron microscopic autoradiographic studies of gliogenesis in rat optic nerve. II. Time of origin. *J Comp Neurol* 169:313, 1976.

56. Snyder DS, et al: The bulk isolation of oligodendroglia from whole rat forebrain: a new procedure using physiologic media. *J Neurochem* 34:1614, 1980.

57. Sommer I, Schachner M: Monoclonal antibodies (01-04) to oligodendrocyte cell surfaces: an immunocytological study in the central nervous system. *Dev Biol* 83:311, 1981.

58. Sternberger LA: *Immunocytochemistry*, ed 2. New York, John Wiley & Sons, 1979.

59. Sternberger NH, et al: Myelin basic protein demonstrated immunocytochemically in oligodendroglia prior to myelin sheath formation. *Proc Natl Acad Sci* 75:2521, 1978.

60. Sternberger NH, et al: Immunocytochemical method to identify basic protein in myelin-forming oligodendrocytes of newborn rat CNS. *J Neurocytol* 7:251, 1978.

61. Sternberger NH, et al: Myelin-associated glycoprotein demonstrated immunocytochemically in myelin and myelin-forming cells of developing rat. *Proc Natl Acad Sci USA* 76:1510, 1979.

62. Suzuki K: Biochemistry of myelin disorders. In Waxman SG (ed): *Physiology and Pathobiology of Axons.* New York, Raven Press, 1978.

63. Szuchet S, et al: Maintenance of isolated oligodendrocytes in long-term cultures. *Brain Res* 200:151, 1980.

64. Traugott U, et al: Monoclonal anti-T cell antibodies are applicable to the study of inflammatory infiltrates in the central nervous system. *J Neuroimmunol* 3:365, 1982.

65. Traugott U, et al: Characterization of antioligodendrocyte serum. *Ann Neurol* 4:431, 1978.

66. Varon S: Macromolecular glial cell markers. In Franck G, et al (eds): *Dynamic Properties of Glia Cells.* Oxford, England, Pergamon Press, 1978.

67. Virchow R: Uber das granulirte ansehen der wandungen der gehrin ventrikel. *Allgem Zeitscher Phychiat* 3:242, 1846.

68. Wood P, et al: The use of networks of associated dorsal root ganglion neurons to induce myelination by oligodendrocytes in culture. *Brain Res* 196:247, 1980.

CHAPTER 3

Microglia

CLARISSE L. DOLMAN, B.A., M.D., F.R.C.P.(C), F.R.C.Path.

INTRODUCTION

Microglia was defined as an entity and named by Rio-Hortega in 1919 (69). This name was chosen to conform to Virchow's neuroglia, "Nervenkitt," the glue in which lie embedded the neurons. Before Rio-Hortega, in 1900, Robertson (71) had impregnated with platinum a group of supporting cells in the brain which he called mesoglia, whose shape varied from adendritic globule to bipolar with processes, and which could become phagocytic. Hatai (28) suggested in 1902 that one type of neuroglia was mesoblastic and originated from meninges and endothelial cells. In 1913, Ramon y Cajal (68) stated that the brain contained other cells, "el tercer elemento," in addition to neurons and astrocytes (68). Rio-Hortega succeeded in staining the cytoplasm of this third element with a weak silver carbonate solution, decided that it comprised two types of cells, and divided them according to their morphology into the oligodendroglia and microglia.

Between 1919 and 1932 Rio-Hortega fully characterized the microglia and gave a detailed description of morphology, life cycle, and function (70), the essence of which is as follows: Microgliocytes originate from primitive meningeal polyblasts, to a lesser extent from vessels, and invade the brain just before and after birth as ameboid cells. These come to rest in the neuropil, anchored there by cytoplasmic branches which sprout from the perikaryon. The "resting" microglia is thus a normal component of the brain after birth. Microglial cells are responsible for eliminating catabolic products. Damage to the nervous system initiates a transformation of the resting to "progressive" microglia.

The cytoplasmic processes retract; the cells revert to the amebic form and move towards the injury. They may elongate into rod cells or become phagocytic and, by ingesting debris and fat, turn into scavenger or fat granule cells.

Rio-Hortega's painstaking work was widely accepted, but it was based by necessity on the light microscopic observation of static morphology. New methodologies have uncovered facts which conflict with the classic concept. There is, moreover, little concensus and much speculation on many aspects of this cell type, and the microglia has become the most controversial element of the central nervous system. Indeed its very existence is in doubt. The material, therefore, is not presented in a didactic fashion, but rather as an analysis of the literature tempered by personal views. Since Rio-Hortega's thesis forms the basis for the whole question of the microglia, it will be used as framework for the discussion. The word "microglia" has always caused some difficulty. In Rio-Hortega's terminology it denotes a system of cells, which individually are called microglial cells or microgliocytes, corresponding to the astroglia and astrocytes and the oligodendroglia and oligodendrocytes. Modern authors frequently employ the term "microglia" as synonymous with microglial cells.

RESTING MICROGLIA

Characteristics

MORPHOLOGY IN SILVER IMPREGNATION

By light microscopy, the resting microglia can be identified reliably only by impregnation with Rio-Hortega's silver carbonate method or one of its modifications. These metallic impregnations are difficult and capricious, however, even in skilled hands, and are not specific for the microglia; oligodendrocytes and macrophages are impregnated, occasionally also pericytes and astrocytes. Many cells outside the brain, but resembling microgliocytes, are intensely argyrophilic (15). There is a marked species difference in microglial affinity for silver (15), those of the rabbit staining best, while poor or negative results are recorded for man (18). Nearly all the work on the microglia has been carried out in rodents. The illustrations in this chapter are from human material only.

When properly impregnated, the resting microgliocytes are uni-, bi- or multipolar with a slightly elongated, sometimes triangular perikaryon and broad processes which rapidly become attenuated and divide into secondary and tertiary branches, decorated with fine, right-angled spines (15, 70) (Fig. 3.1). The cytoplasm may contain tiny vacuoles. The outline of the cells is molded by the surrounding neuropil. Cammermeyer (15) describes stellate, elongated, or bulblike shapes, depending on the configuration of the adjacent cells (15).

TOPOGRAPHY

The microglia is ubiquitous in the central nervous system (15, 70). The number and arrangement of microgliocytes varies, depending on the anatomical location (70) and the animal species (15). They are more numerous in gray than in white matter. In the rat, for example, they constitute 18% of the glia of the neocortex (88), 19% of the hippocampus (37), but only 6% of the corpus callosum (58). Blinzinger and Hager (9) found them to be extraordinarily rare in the cortex of the gold hamster (9), and Feigin (18) had difficulty locating them in normal human cortex, although activated microglial cells in the same preparation were plentiful and impregnated well (18).

RELATION TO OTHER CELLS

The cells are distributed diffusely in the neuropil and do not make contact with each other (70). Nevertheless, the extent of the arborization is remarkable and extends to neurons, other glia, and vessels (15). The microgliocytes are particularly prominent as satellites of neurons, which they embrace with their branches or rest in the crown of the apical dendrite, as basilar, cell body, or apical satellites (15, 70). Another favored position is said to be around vessels (58, 70, 77), but Cammermeyer considered them rare in this location (15). They lie free as interstitial cells (58) or underneath the pia (5, 64). They have been described as numerous in the subependymal area (15, 61, 66), while others have commented on the paucity of microgliocytes near the ventricles (87).

MORPHOLOGY WITH ANILINE DYES

Rio-Hortega (70) stated that microglial cells were also easily identified in paraffin sections stained with aniline dyes, since the microgliocytes had the smallest, darkest, and most irregular nuclei of all the brain cells. Their outline could be round, oval, elongated, or twisted into C or S shapes. However, when factors such as nuclear distortion or cuts through the ends rather than the center of nuclei are taken into consideration, microglial cells are not readily recognizable in aniline-stained sections. Mori and Leblond (58) felt that in such material identification had to remain tentative. According to Cammermeyer (15), gallocyanin chrome alum and methyl green pyronin stain oligodendrocytes more intensely than microgliocytes, while the aging microglia, unlike the oligodendroglia, accumulates PAS-positive granules. In our experience, lipofuscin can be found in all aging human glial elements.

In plastic embedded semithin sections stained with toluidine blue, microglial nuclei are described as small, round, elongated, or irregular, with dark chromatin masses contrasting with the pale nucleoplasm. The same problems are encountered here as with paraffin sections. It is easy to find dark small irregular nuclei, but difficult to be certain that these represent a separate cell type and not merely distorted or tangentially cut oligodendroglial or even astrocytic nuclei.

ULTRASTRUCTURE

When the brain was first examined with the electron microscope, the resting mi-

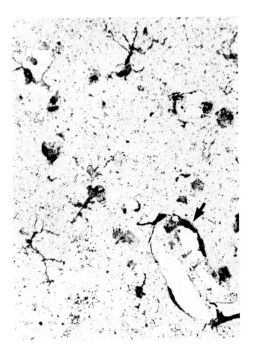

Figure 3.1. Silver-impregnated resting microgliocytes. Their cytoplasm is bipolar and divided into several processes. An *arrow* points to a ring of microglial cells around a capillary, but within the neuropil. Autopsy specimen of normal brain, stained by McCauley's modification of Rio-Hortega's silver carbonate method. (Original magnification ×320.)

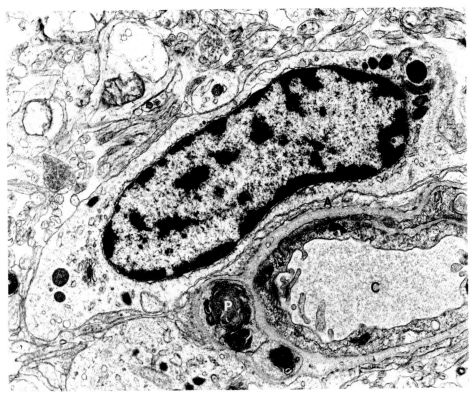

Figure 3.2. Perivascular resting microglial cell. The nucleus is elongated and the cytoplasm contains only a few organelles, amongst them black lysozomes. An astrocytic process (*A*) intervenes between the cell and the capillary (*C*). A pericyte (*P*), filled with electron-dense debris, lies enfolded within the capillary basement membrane. Electron micrograph of normal brain biopsy. (Original magnification ×14,640.)

croglia proved embarrassingly elusive. Early reports of microglial ultrastructure (29, 52) were later discounted as descriptions of oligodendroglia or "dark" neurons (58, 59). Some electron microscopists were unable to find microgliocytes and suggested that the cells seen with the light microscope were a type of oligodendroglia (35, 43, 54). Blinziger and Hager (9) blamed the difficulty in finding the microglia on the small size of the sample and the low percentage of this cell type. In 1970, Peters et al. (64) concluded that either microgliocytes did not exist as a separate entity, or if they did, could not be distinguished from the oligodendroglia. In 1976, in the second edition of their book, these authors acknowledged the existence of the microglia and provided an illustrated description of the ultrastructure.

Methods were finally devised to mark the microglial cells with silver carbonate prior to examination with the electron microscope and thus to identify them (37, 58, 89). During the last few years, many accounts of the ultrastructure of resting microgliocytes have appeared (5, 7, 9, 12, 23, 26, 34, 37, 50, 66, 77, 86, 87). The nuclei are reported as elongated, flattened, or angulated, containing heavy dark peripheral blocks of chromatin, which contrast with the lighter nucleoplasm. The resemblance to oligodendrocytes is close, but the chromatin is heavier and darker (64). Mori and Leblond (58) and Boya (12) emphasize a diagnostic crescentic nucleolus, but others mention only small nondescript nucleoli (9).

The perikaryon is slender and is described variously as dense like that of the oligodendroglia (9, 64, 66), or medium dense (7, 87), or distinctly lighter (37, 51). Spine-like processes arising at a right angle have been noticed. Small mitochondria, centrioles, a few stacked Golgi profiles, and strands of endoplasmic reticulum, often long and irregularly studded with ribosomes, rare tubules, and free ribosomes constitute the modest complement of organelles. Occasionally abundant ribosomes and a well developed Golgi area are mentioned. Of special importance are dense lysosomes, which are said to exceed in number those in the oligodendroglia, while microtubules are much less common. Glyco-

gen granules and glial filaments, characteristic of astrocytes, are absent.

The above descriptions are based on animal material. Foncin examined human biopsies and concluded that most neuronal satellites are oligodendrocytes, but he also described microglial cells with a longer, less dense nucleus, marginated chromatin, a clearer cytoplasm, many ribosomes in rosettes, dense mitochondria, and no tubules (21). Figure 3.2 illustrates a cell from a normal human biopsy, which meets the criteria established in the literature for resting microgliocytes. There are, however, no definite nuclear or cytoplasmic features which distinguish such a cell from an oligodendrocyte, and without it being so stated, an elongated shape appears to be the major criterion for identification of the microglia.

In addition to cells within the neuropil, pericytes have been described as "perivascular" or "pericytal" microglia (5, 12, 13, 58, 81). These will be discussed later. Suffice it to say here that pericytes are cells within the basement membrane of capillaries, while glial cells lie in the neuropil (Fig. 3.2).

CYTOCHEMISTRY AND IMMUNOLOGY

Resting microgliocytes contain few enzymes. They exhibit adenosine triphosphatase and uridine diphosphatase activity (31) which is shown also by other glial cells. They are negative for monocytic markers such as nonspecific esterase (61), and neither the mouse nor the human microglia from postmortem material is equipped with specific Ig Fc receptors, as tested by rosetting with sensitized sheep cells (92). Phagocytic assays with heat-killed yeast indicate that the resting microglia is incapable of nonimmunological phagocytosis. The immune peroxidase technique gives negative results with antilymphocyte, antimonocyte, and anti-B2-microglobulin sera (62), and immune fluorescence is negative with antimacrophage serum (63, 92).

The Nature of Resting Microglia

The resting microglia was initially defined on purely morphological grounds by the appearance of the cells after weak silver carbonate impregnation, which was deemed to be different from that of the equally argyrophilic oligodendroglia. Recognition by means of aniline stains is considered uncertain by most. The identification with the electron microscope has been fraught with difficulties. Descriptions vary, and even those observers who are very certain in their convictions that microgliocytes are easily identifiable ultrastructurally do not quote any specific features which unequivocally separate the microglia from the oligodendroglia. Both cell types have perikarya which impregnate with weak silver carbonate, dense chromatin in the nuclei, and scanty organelles in the cytoplasm. Perineural, interstitial, and perivascular positions are assumed by both. The subtle points of difference seem to be an elongated nucleus, with less microtubules and more lysosomes in the microglia. Cytochemically and immunologically the resting microglia behaves like the macroglia. These cells have been shown conclusively to be unrelated to the mononuclear phagocyte system. The concept of this system has superseded, but extensively overlaps Aschoff's reticuloendothelial system, to which Rio-Hortega had assigned the microglia.

PROGRESSIVE OR ACTIVATED MICROGLIA

Macrophages

HISTORY

Necrotic brain tissue liquefies and must be removed; hence, scavenger cells play a very important part in many disease processes of the central nervous system. Gluge (1841) noted "Entzündungskugeln" (inflammation globules) in encephalitis, and Virchow (1867) described fat-filled "foam cells." Stroebe (1894) pioneered in creating wounds in the spinal cord of animals, where he observed an exudation of polymorphonuclear leucocytes, soon followed by phagocytic "granule cells" (80). Pick (1904) suggested that such cells could originate from the bloodstream, endothelial cells, adventitial tissue, and the local glia. Nissl (1904) introduced the term "Gitterzelle," lattice cell, because of the lattice-like framework of the cytoplasm around ingested fat. Rio-Hortega classified these cells as progressive microglia, transformed from the resting microglia normally resident in the brain. He

described transition forms, intermediate in shape between the dendritic microgliocyte and the rounded phagocyte filled with lipid droplets or iron. The mobilized cells became ameboid, migrated toward lesions, and there proliferated. Rio-Hortega suspected that they might eventually dump their load of ingested debris into vessels and either degenerate or retreat back into the neuropil. Like the parent resting microglia, all the intermediary forms of the progressive microglia were strongly argyrophilic, and this, in Rio-Hortega's view, further confirmed the identity of the two cell types.

MORPHOLOGY BY LIGHT MICROSCOPY

The fully developed phagocytic cells are often called cerebral macrophages, since they are identical to macrophages in other parts of the body. In contrast to the "resting microglia," macrophages are recognizable at a glance in paraffin sections and with routine stains (Fig. 3.3). Their nuclei are round, oval, or indented and vary in density. Their cytoplasm is rounded and well defined, and their phagocytic prowess is made evident by diverse engulfed materials, most often lipid droplets—hence the name fat granule cell—but also fragments of myelin sheaths, red cells or hemosiderin, yeasts, pyknotic cells, and other debris.

ULTRASTRUCTURE

Ultrastructurally, the nuclei have a lighter chromatin than lymphocytes. The cytoplasm is distended by numerous membrane-bound phagosomes (Fig. 3.4A), free ribosomes, long strands of rough endoplasmic reticulum, and abundant Golgi profiles (9, 38). Hyaloplasmic rims lie under the surface which often contains filopodia (Fig. 3.4B) (33) or blunt cytoplasmic processes, the so-called ruffles (Fig. 3.4C) (23, 61).

EARLY MACROPHAGES

Before the cells have become phagocytic, they are less voluminous, with an eosinophilic, nonvacuolated cytoplasm and smaller, denser nuclei. They may assume irregular amebic shapes. At that stage, they have ultrastructurally long slender processes, free ribosomes, and only a few cister-

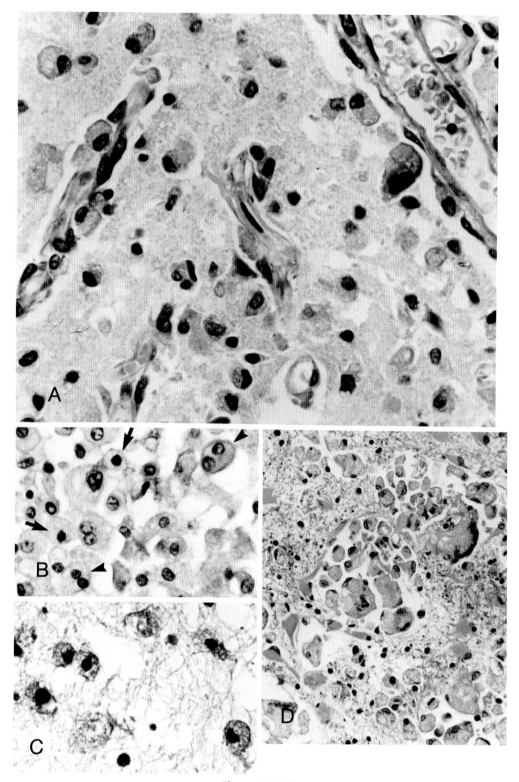

Figure 3.3*A–D*

nae of irregularly dilated rough endoplasmic reticulum (90).

NECROSIS AND INFARCTS

Macrophages are encountered in a great variety of conditions, whenever breakdown of tissue has occurred. There is hardly a disease of the central nervous system where they do not participate. In infarcts they make their appearance 2–3 days after the insult, in the subarachnoid space and within brain substance, particularly around vessels (Fig. 3.3A). Although macrophages are said to have a limited capacity for division (24), mitoses may be numerous in early infarcts (Fig. 3.3B). The flood of scavenger cells which soon fills the area of necrosis therefore consists of both new arrivals and locally proliferated cells. When the necrotic tissue has been devoured, the cells with their ingested debris gradually disappear. However, if the infarct is large, this process may take many months, and a few macrophages may persist in very old cystic softenings.

Macrophages do not visibly degenerate in lesions such as infarcts, despite some contrary claims (23). According to Furth (24), they wander away to the regional lymph nodes to die (24). Oehmichen (61) traced cerebral macrophages labeled with ferritin or colloidal iron from brain wounds to cervical lymph nodes, and Baumgarten (6) found that macrophages which had been loaded with artificial melanin and then injected into the ventricles penetrated the neuropil and entered the lumen of subependymal vessels, suggesting removal through the bloodstream.

Around hemorrhages or traumatic lesions, the cells contain hemosiderin. Infections which cause tissue death, such as necrotizing encephalitis or brain abscesses, also stimulate the influx of macrophages.

DEMYELINATING DISEASE

Demyelination alone is sufficient to provoke a macrophage response which is prominent in the acute plaque of multiple sclerosis (Fig. 3.3C). In leucodystrophies these cells often store abnormal catabolic products. The phagocytosis of such substances may influence the appearance of the cells. For example, the angular globoid cells in Krabbe's disease owe their ground glass appearance to the content of galactocerebroside (Fig. 3.3D). This compound induces the macrophages to fuse into characteristic multinucleated giant cells (61). Pathognomonic tinctorial properties, like the specific metachromasia encountered in metachromatic leucodystrophy, may be conveyed by the ingested material.

WALLERIAN DEGENERATION

In Wallerian degeneration, macrophages enter the tissue during the time of myelin breakdown in order to consume degenerate myelin sheaths and axons. Their fat content then becomes stainable in frozen sections.

CYTOCHEMISTRY AND IMMUNOLOGY

Cerebral macrophages are remarkably rich in enzymes. They contain acid phosphatase, naphthol adenosine diphosphatase and dehydrogenase, adenosine triphosphatase and uridine diphosphatase (31), triphosphopyridine nucleotide diaphorase (76), diphosphopyridine diaphorase, 5 nucleotidase, nonspecific esterase (41, 42), L-naphthyl acetate, naphthol AS acetate esterase, and L-naphthol AS-D chloroacetate esterase (61). Granules within the cytoplasm are peroxidase-positive (11).

Oehmichen implanted glass coverslips into the brains of rabbits and found that

---

Figure 3.3. (A) Large and small rounded macrophages in recent infarct of brain. Many are concentrated around vessels. Autopsy specimen stained with hematoxylin and eosin. (Original magnification ×520.) (B) Mitotic (arrows) and binucleated (arrowheads) macrophages in 2-week-old cerebral infarct indicate local proliferation. Autopsy specimen stained with hematoxylin and eosin. (Original magnification ×360.) (C) Diffusely scattered rounded macrophages in an acute plaque of multiple sclerosis contain punctate myelin debris. Brain biopsy stained with hematoxylin and eosin (Original magnification ×490.) (D) Macrophages have fused to form angular multinucleated opaque globoid cells in the brain stem of a patient with globoid leucodystrophy. Autopsy specimen stained with hematoxylin and eosin (Original magnification ×220.)

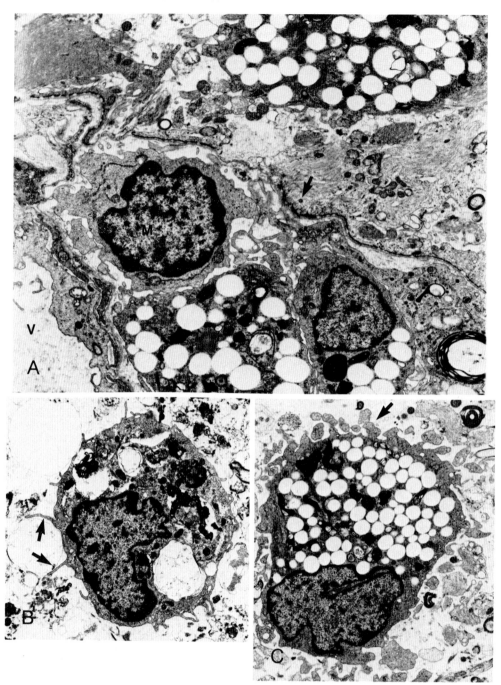

Figure 3.4. (A) Macrophages crowd the perivascular space between a venule (V) and the glia limitans (arrow) in herpes simplex encephalitis. Their cytoplasm is distended by clear vacuoles and electron-dense lipid. One cell (M) is as yet unburdened. The macrophage in the upper right hand corner has penetrated the neuropil. Electron micrograph of brain biopsy. (Original magnification ×6650.) (B) Fine cytoplasmic processes, "filopodia" (arrows), of a macrophage in a recent infarct, finger necrotic tissue, in preparation for phagocytosis. Electron micrograph of brain biopsy. (Original magnification ×9460.) (C) Blunt cytoplasmic "ruffles" wreath an engorged macrophage (arrow) in herpes simplex encephalitis. Electron micrograph of a brain biopsy. (Original magnification ×8034.)

the macrophages adhering to the coverslips were able to engulf both sensitized sheep erythrocytes and sheep erythrocyte-antibody complexes, which had been sensitized with complement 3 (3). This indicates that the cells have receptors for immunoglobulin Fc (IgFc) and complement (C3). Cerebral macrophages have been shown with the immune fluorescent technique to react with specific macrophage antibody serum (23, 63).

This reaction, the presence of surface receptors for IgFc and C3, the content of nonspecific esterase, peroxidase, and 5'-nucleotidase, and the ability to phagocytose large particles are markers for cells belonging to the mononuclear phagocyte system. Hence cerebral macrophages are members of this cell system.

Lamellar and Rod Cells

According to Rio-Hortega (70), fat granule cells are not the only form of progressive microglia. Mild stimuli do not provoke metamorphosis of resting microgliocytes to foam cells, but induce proliferation of "lamellar cells" or hypertrophy to "rod cells."

LAMELLAR CELLS (GLIAL NODULES)

Rio-Hortega applied the term "lamellar cells" to certain inflammatory cells in rabies encephalomyelitis. Small ameboid cells with kidney-shaped, twisted, or crescent-shaped nuclei, and without the abundant cytoplasm of macrophages, are the major reacting element in a variety of viral infections. In the acute phases, they appear to wriggle out from vessels (Fig. 3.5A) and swarm through the neuropil, assemble into small knots, stars, or shrubs (Strauchwerk), or congregate as glial nodules around degenerating neurons, engaging in neuronophagia (Fig. 3.5B). They are distinct from the lymphocytes and plasma cells which may surround vessels. Similar cells occur in certain other situations, for example, in incomplete infarcts.

ROD CELLS

Rod cells (Stäbchenzellen) were first observed and are most prominent in the cortex of syphilitic paretics (Fig. 3.5C). Nissl (1899) had been impressed with these "sausage or rod-shaped" cells, sometimes of "as-

tounding length," whose nuclei were occasionally as long as the height of a pyramidal cell layer (60). Rod cells tend to line up at right angles to the surface and frequently contain small cytoplasmic fat droplets or iron.

General paresis of the insane has largely disappeared, but we still see rod cells, though of more modest proportions, in other nonfulminating encephalitides, such as subacute sclerosing panencephalitis (Fig. 3.5D).

RETROGRADE NEURONAL DEGENERATION

Deafferentation of neurons results in an increase in perineuronal microglial satellites (15, 41). Blinzinger and Kreutzberg (10) observed with the electron microscope that activated microglial cells detached boutons from the damaged neurons by inserting cytoplasmic processes into the synaptic cleft. Kerns and Hinsman (34) confirmed this and also noted many mitotic cells around ventral horn cells, beginning 2 d after sciatic neurectomy. The synaptic boutons were displaced but not phagocytosed. Such descriptions are reminiscent of the accounts of experimental allergic demyelination, in which macrophagic cytoplasmic processes peel off layers of myelin (44). Matthews and Kruger (53) found aggregations of cells, thought most likely to be monocytes, but which they cautiously only called "M" cells, in the thalamus of animals after cortical ablation as a reaction to transsynaptic degeneration.

Other Areas of Activity

SENILE PLAQUES

A further area of microglial activity is the senile plaque (70). Cells, their plump bodies containing PAS positively staining lysosomal material, but with argyrophilic processes characteristic of microglia, often radiate around the center of the mature plaque (Fig. 3.5E)

MICROGLIAL SWELLING

Using electron microscopic autoradiography on silver-impregnated material from the rat hippocampus, Kitamura et al. (38) concluded that resting microglial cells undergo marked swelling in response to brain

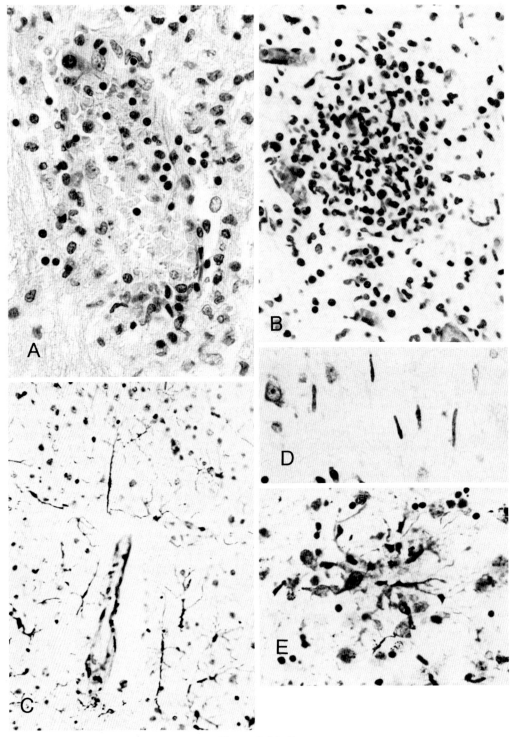

Figure 3.5*A–E*

injury. The swollen cells appeared 20 h after a stab wound and increased in number while the number of ordinary resting microglia decreased, and they were therefore considered to be derived from the microglia. Swelling of glial cells in early brain damage is a well known phenomenon, but is usually attributed to the oligodendroglia. Fujita et al. (23) saw transition forms between the swollen microglial cells and a special type of fibrous astrocyte with an indented nucleus and suggest that the microglia serves as a reserve for reactive astrocytes.

Microgliomatosis

The concept of the microglia as the representative of the reticuloendothelial system in the brain quite naturally led to the assumption that primary lymphoreticular tumors of the central nervous system arose from the microglia. Thus were born the terms microglioma and microgliomatosis, the latter because of the often diffuse nature of the neoplasm. The impression of the microglial origin of these tumors appeared to be confirmed by the frequent argyrophilia of the cells. Such neoplasms are today classified as extranodal malignant lymphomas and are known to encompass the whole spectrum of these tumors. The term microglioma has become inappropriate, and the subject will not be discussed here any further. Reactive macrophages may be prominent in some cerebral lymphomas.

Origin of Progressive Microglia

MACROPHAGES IN NECROTIC LESIONS

Rio-Hortega believed that the progressive microglia was almost exclusively derived from the resting microglia and that any contributions from the bloodstream or vessel walls were negligible. Feigin (18) supported this view, emphasizing that macrophages appeared diffusely in damaged nervous tissue and therefore had to originate from cells already existing disseminated throughout the neuropil. Others, by contrast, stated that macrophages were first seen around vessels and that this indicated migration from the bloodstream and vessel wall (4). Russell (73) noted monocytes in rat brains 12 h after a puncture wound had been made, and within 48 h these cells had become transformed into typical Gitter cells. Matthews and Kruger (53), in an ultrastructural study, actually caught monocytes in diapedesis halfway through vessel walls.

Kinetic Studies

A considerable step forward in solving the question of the origin of the progressive microglia was the application to this problem of the technique of radioactive labeling by Adrian and Walker (2) and Kosunen et al. (40). Radioactive tritiated (^{3}H) thymidine, detectable by radioautography, is a precursor of desoxyribonucleic acid (DNA) and is selectively taken up by premitotic cells synthesizing DNA. The progeny of these labeled cells will contain lesser amounts of ^{3}H-thymidine. Incorporation of the nucleotide thus indicates mitotically active, proliferating cells. The above investigators concluded that the reactive phagocytes were derived from mononuclear blood cells. This was confirmed in more extensive experiments by Konigsmark and Sidman (39) who could trace two-thirds of the macrophages which appeared in stab wounds in the brains of mice to ^{3}H-thymi-

Figure 3.5. (A) Cells with oval or twisted nuclei work their way out of a venule into the brain substance in herpes simplex encephalitis. Autopsy specimen stained with hematoxylin and eosin. (Original magnification ×220.) (B) Reactive cells with round or twisted nuclei gather to form a "glial" nodule in the spinal cord of a patient with poliomyelitis. Autopsy specimen stained with hematoxylin and eosin. (Original magnification ×220.) (C) Rod cells line up in the cerebral cortex of a syphilitic patient who died with active general paresis of the insane. Autopsy specimen stained with Cone and Penfield's modification of Rio-Hortega's silver carbonate method. (Original magnification ×170.) (D) The nuclei of rod cells in subacute sclerosing panencephalitis are also oriented at right angles to the pial surface. Autopsy specimen stained with cresyl violet. (Original magnification ×320.) (E) Microglial cells radiate around the center of a senile plaque in Alzheimer's disease. Autopsy specimen impregnated by Naoumenko and Feigin's modification of Rio-Hortega's silver carbonate method. (Original magnification ×320.)

dine-labeled hematogenous monocytes. The source of the remaining third remained undetermined but was thought most likely to be from the resting microglia.

Adrian and Schelper (1) found that after spinal cord injury only some cells contained sodium fluoride-sensitive nonspecific esterase and decided therefore that two types of macrophages were present, derived from both endogenous and exogenous sources. They postulate that glial cells might become labeled by reutilizing radioactive material from degenerated macrophages. Huntington and Terry (30) suspected from their work that the bulk of macrophages came from monocytes and doubted that the microglia participated at all. They found that there was a time-limited invasion of monocytes around a stab wound, no further labeling occurring 6 d after the wound was inflicted. Roessman and Friede (72) collected monocytes from bone marrow, labeled them radioactively in vivo or in vitro with ^{3}H-thymidine or uridine, and injected them intravenously into other animals with brain damage; labeled macrophages appeared in the lesions, proving that the injected monocytes rather than endogenous microglia had become transformed into macrophages. Since then, many similar experiments have been carried out (3, 7, 20, 32, 38, 57, 61, 79, 83, 85). Other techniques employed are labeling with colloidal carbon, which utilizes the phagocytic activity of macrophages (49), and parabiotic experiments, in which two animals are sutured together. The tagged monocytes of one animal penetrate to the brain wound of the other animal, whose bone marrow is depressed by radiation of the legs (81). All of these experiments confirmed that at least a large number of the cerebral macrophages are monocytes, attracted to the lesion from the bloodstream.

VIRAL INFECTIONS

Radioactive labeling indicated a monocytic origin also for the reactive cells in viral infections such as herpes simplex encephalitis (61, 72), Japanese B encephalitis (22), and poliomyelitis (91). Kitamura (36) was able, in experimental Japanese encephalitis, to follow labeled monocytes into glial nodules and prove their transformation to rod cells. Wolinsky et al. (91) observed in mice, experimentally infected with murine poliomyelitis, isotope-labeled cells turn into neuronophages, congregate to glial nodules, and metamorphose to rod cells. Blinzinger et al. (11) found peroxidase-positive granules, characteristic of monocytes, in the brains of mice infected with yellow fever. Kitamura (36) contended that even the cells in the so-called lymphocytic cuffs are monocytes. However, lymphocytes and plasma cells undoubtedly may be present, as shown by both light and electron microscopy.

DEMYELINATING DISEASE

Radioactive labeling and electron microscopy have demonstrated the "activated microgliocytes" in experimental allergic encephalomyelitis to be blood-borne mononuclear cells (40, 44). Radioactive labeling has also proved that multinucleated globoid cells, induced by intracerebral injection of galactose cerebroside, consist of fused phagocytic monocytes (61).

RETROGRADE DEGENERATION

Experiments designed to define the origin of cells appearing as cell clusters around neurons undergoing retrograde degeneration have had variable and contradictory results. The methods used to produce retrograde degeneration include crushing or transection of the sciatic (34, 72), facial (22, 4, 63, 77, 85), or hypoglossal nerve (3, 83), or roots of the cervical plexus (50). Transsection of nerve can lead to death of the neuron and causes a greater accumulation of microglial cells than crushing (84, 85). These satellite nodules are composed of cells which can be labeled with ^{3}H-thymidine (3, 34, 41, 49, 72), indicating a monocytic origin. Carbon particles injected intravenously, intraperitoneally, or intraventricularly, however, were not taken up by the satellites, which suggested to Stenwig (79) and Sumner (83) that their source was intrinsic and not from the bone marrow. Adrian and Schelper (1) noted many radioactively labeled cells around degenerating hypoglossal neurons, but most of these were esterase-negative and therefore were thought not to be monocytes. Persson et al. (63), on the other hand, using the immune fluorescent technique, found the satellite cells around neurons in the facial nucleus after facial nerve transsection to react with antimacrophage serum and not with antibody to the brain-specific S100 protein.

WALLERIAN DEGENERATION

Various theories have been proposed for the origin of phagocytic cells in Wallerian degeneration. The most commonly used model is the optic nerve after enucleation of the eye and to a lesser extent tract degeneration following a wound in the spinal cord. Macrophages in Wallerian degeneration are labeled by ³H-thymidine, indicating monocytic origin (48, 49), but they fail to engulf carbon particles (79). Cook and Wisniewsky (17) claimed that in degenerating optic nerve the oligodendroglia rather than the microglia became phagocytic. Skoff (75) and Vaughn and his co-workers (86–88) attributed the increase in cells to a proliferation of primitive "multipotential glia" which could then develop not only into astrocytes and oligodendrocytes but also into Gitter cells. Privat and his group (67) were unable to come to any definite conclusion but thought that after enucleation at first pericytes and then microglial cells became activated.

GRADED RESPONSE

There is concensus that at least some of the reactive or progressive microglia stems from monocytes which have recently left the bone marrow. The majority of investigators (1, 33, 50, 85) believe that there is a significant and at times a major contribution from resident brain cells. Vaughn and Skoff (87) put forth the concept of a "graded response," involving hematogenous and endogenous elements, the proportion of which depends on the type of stimulus. Severe insults provoke a bone marrow response, whereas mild damage results in a local reaction only.

Cells Postulated as Related to the Microglia

Other cells which show phagocytic activity and are thought to be related to the microglia are macrophages lying in ventricles and subarachnoid and perivascular spaces.

EPIPLEXUS CELLS

Supraependymal or epiplexus cells, first described by Kolmer in 1921, are found on the surface of normal ependyma and choroid plexus and phagocytose intraventricular debris (6, 8). Their morphology by light, transmission, and scanning electron microscopy, their phagocytic capability, and their content of nonspecific esterase and IgGFc surface receptors (16, 56, 61) mark them as true macrophages, members of the mononuclear phagocyte system. These cells have been reported to arise from the subependymal microglia (8, 56) or to migrate to the ventricles from subependymal perivascular tissue (16).

Cerebrospinal fluid contains mononuclear cells of which, in the first milliliters taken, 70% are lymphocytes and 30% monocytes. In successive samples, the percentage of monocytes rises. An origin from the pia or arachnoidal cells (55) or from pluripotential members of the reticuloendothelial system in the leptomeninges has been postulated, but it appears more likely that they are hematogenous. Pfeiffer and Schwartz examined histochemically cells of the cerebrospinal fluid and pial and arachnoidal cells obtained from neurosurgical operations and found the enzyme reactions of the monocytes and lymphocytes to correspond to those of mononuclear cells of the bloodstream and not to those of arachnoidal and adventitial cells (65). Damage to the nervous system elicits an outpouring of macrophages in the fluid compartments, as well as in the parenchyma of the brain. Macrophages are occasionally observed in apparently normal subarachnoid and perivascular spaces. In the elderly, lipopigment containing macrophages are common around vessels.

PERICYTES

These cells need a special note because several authors equate pericytes with perivascular microglial cells (5, 51, 57, 81), whereas others (13, 27) maintain that under certain circumstances they move into the neuropil and become phagocytes. Pericytes were discovered by Eberth in 1871, and the names of two later investigators, Rouget and Zimmermann, are often associated with them. They are confined to capillaries and lie on the outside of the endothelial cells, but within two layers of the basement membrane (Fig. 3.6A). Rouget ascribed to them contractile activity, and they have been reported to contain actin and myosin (45). At the metarterial level, their place is taken by the muscular precapillary sphincter and in venules and arterioles by smooth muscle cells, but these lie beyond the basement membrane of the vessel, though they are invested by their own basement membrane. Stensaas (77) describes in the brain under the name pericytes type II and III, cells in the walls of venules and arterioles, which are clearly adventitial fibroblasts (Fig. 3.6B).

Sturrock (81) argues that pericytes are the source of the microglia, since in developing fetal mouse brains, microglial cells begin to be noticeable in the neuropil shortly after pericytes have made their appearance around vessels. Baron and Gallego (5) noted astrocytes in close association with pericytes and speculated that astrocytes assist pericytes to turn into microglial cells.

Maxwell and Kruger (54) observed swelling of pericytes after low dose irradiation of the brain. A high dose of radiation caused disappearance of the capillary basement membrane and the pericytes, and since this coincided with the emergence of phagocytes in the tissues, the pericytes were assumed to have moved away from the capillaries and to have become macrophages. Many investigators concur with the opinion that pericytes change into macrophages after the basement membrane is dissolved by some disease process or destroyed by the pericytes themselves (5, 12, 13, 15, 26, 27, 58, 81). Stensaas (77) and Sumner (83) opposed these views, emphasizing that microgliocytes lie outside the vascular basement membrane and have a different ultrastructure. Oehmichen (61) considered pericytes to be a transformation stage of hematogenous monocytes. Fujita and Kitamura (22) noted that monocytes on their way through the capillary wall can temporarily occupy the position of the pericyte, a possibility previously suspected by Mori (57). The electron microscopic appearance of these monocytes differs from that of pericytes, in that they have a denser cytoplasm and the basement membrane often does not

fit as snugly around them (22). Wolinsky et al. (91), in a study of experimental murine poliomyelitis using radioactive labeling, found the pericytes to remain unlabeled, while the inflammatory "activated microglial cells" incorporated the radioactive substance, confirming the different nature of these two cell types.

Figure 3.6C shows a pericyte in a human biopsy from a recent infarct. The pericyte is degenerating, while the endothelial cell has remained intact. This suggests that pericytes perish easily and are unlikely to be the source of reactive cells. Moreover, a healthy mononuclear cell lies just outside the capillary, morphologically quite distinct from the pericyte. The disappearance of pericytes after radiation (54) therefore probably indicates their destruction, and the influx of phagocytes is independent and from the blood.

The function of pericytes is not known. Perhaps they assist endothelium in transport mechanisms between blood and parenchyma. There is no evidence that they belong to the mononuclear phagocyte system, which would be required to make them the precursors of macrophages.

The Nature of Progressive Microglia

Cerebral macrophages are acknowledged to be identical in morphology, cytochemistry, immunologic markers, and functional activity to macrophages elsewhere in the body. Epiplexus cells and free subarachnoid cells in the ventricles, the subarachnoid space, and the perivascular sleeves are also macrophages.

Numerous experiments, utilizing radioactive or carbon labeling, have proved that most of the macrophages engaged in phagocytosis of necrotic tissue after severe brain damage are derived from monocytes of bone marrow origin and that the monocytes are attracted to the scene by chemotactic stimuli, reach the central nervous system from the bloodstream by diapedesis through vessel walls, and by ingesting debris assume the shape of macrophages. The cerebrospinal fluid macrophages have a similar source.

Many authors continue to assert that indigenous cells contribute to the population of macrophages. The resting microglia, however, does not have monocyte markers

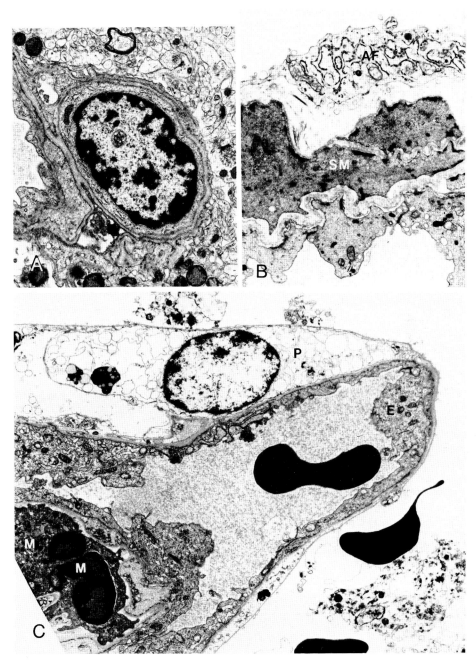

Figure 3.6. (*A*) A pericyte is enclosed by layers of the capillary basement membrane. Electron micrograph of normal brain biopsy. (Original magnification ×7280.) (*B*) An adventitial fibroblast (*AF*) around a venule contains cisternae within long profiles of rough endoplasmic reticulum. A heavy basement membrane separates the endothelium from the smooth muscle cells (*SM*), which are invested by their own thin basement membranes. Electron micrograph of normal brain biopsy. (Original magnification ×9460.) (*C*) A pericyte (*P*) in a recent infarct is dying, its cytoplasm watery and devoid of organelles except residual bodies. The capillary basement membrane is dissolving. The endothelium is intact, and a healthy monocyte (*M*) lies adjacent to the capillary. Electron micrograph of brain biopsy. (Original magnification ×4320.)

and thus cannot be parent to macrophages. The hypothetical participation of pericytes and pial or arachnoidal cells is not supported by fact. That monocytes during diapedesis may transiently occupy the pericytic space within the basement membranes of the capillary explains adequately the radioactive labeling and outward passage of an occasional seemingly pericytic cell.

Radioactive labeling experiments have established that the progressive microglial cells with oval or twisted nuclei, which congregate in viral infections to form glial nodules, are also blood-derived monocytes. They can be readily observed by light microscopy to emerge from the lumen of venules and capillaries. "Rod" cells, which seem to be gliding through the neuropil, have also been shown to be monocytes (91). Nissl applied the term "rod cell" specifically to the tremendously long cells in the cerebral cortex of patients with active general paresis of the insane. Fujita and his coworkers (23), who firmly advocate the monocytic origin of the activated microglial cells in acute viral inflammation, maintain, on the basis of electron microscopic observation of formalin-fixed tissue, that syphilitic rod cells are true glial elements of ectodermal origin. These cells have not yet been examined for glial or monocytic markers, and fresh material on active general paresis is not readily available. However, the rod cells of subacute sclerosing panencephalitis which closely resemble those of syphilis appear to be derived from monocytes rather than glial elements. They lie in relation to blood vessels in addition to lining up in the cortex like syphilitic rod cells, and also their ultrastructure suggests monocytic rather than glial origin (Fig. 3.7A–C).

The microglial response in Wallerian degeneration of neurons after axonotomy remains a disputed question, since particularly carbon labeling experiments have given results which appear to negate monocytic participation in these events. On the other hand, experiments utilizing labeling with radioactive substances have proved incontrovertibly that here again the mobilized cell is of monocytic origin. Moreover, such activities as detaching boutons by inserting cytoplasmic processes and large scale phagocytosis of myelin and other breakdown products are very typically those of macrophages.

The question of microglial cells in senile plaques has not been investigated. In PAS stains they resemble small macrophages incorporating lysosomal PAS-positive debris, and it seems reasonable to assume that they too are of monocytic origin.

AMEBOID OR NASCENT MICROGLIA

Rio-Hortega's Theory

Rio-Hortega (70) stated that microgliocytes develop from polyblasts or embryonic cells of the meninges during late fetal life and the first postnatal days, chiefly from the fold entering the choroidal fissure. Major sources are the tela choroidea over the thalami and the pia mater covering the cerebral peduncles, the pial lining and the white surfaces of the cerebellum, the bulbocerebellar fold which constitutes the inferior tela choroidea, and the pial sheaths of medium and large blood vessels. From these "fountains," large numbers of argyrophilic microgliocytes stream into the brain substance and are transformed into the branched resting microglia.

Recent Studies

Studies on histogenesis indicate that there is an outpouring of immature cells into the white matter just after birth. This appears to correspond to the so-called "myelination gliosis" (25), a rapid multiplication of the oligodendroglia in preparation for myelination. Several investigators have confirmed the presence at that time of ameboid cells which they believe to be the precursors of the microglia. Stensaas and Reichert (78) found in brains of neonatal rabbits numerous round or ameboid argyrophilic cells, rich in cytoplasmic organelles, which aggregated in areas of loose structure with large extracellular spaces. Many had in the cytoplasm vacuoles which ultrastructurally were empty or contained floccular or lamellar material. Ling (46) considers ameboid microglial cells to be normal constituents of the neonatal brain and equates them with Virchow's "Körnchenzellen." As the ameboid cells diminish in number the microgliocytes become visi-

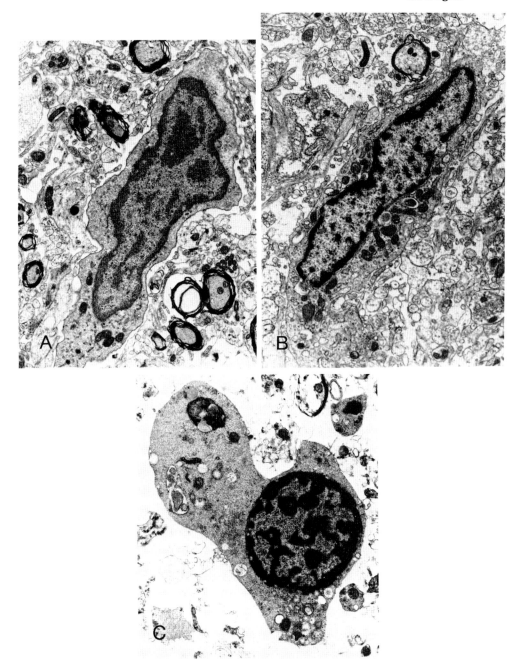

Figure 3.7. (A) This rod cell has a crisply defined cell membrane, distinctly separate from the adjacent brain tissue. The biopsy is from the same patient with subacute sclerosing panencephalitis as the autopsy specimen in Figure 3.5D. (Original magnification ×7280.) (B) An elongated interstitial microgliocyte from a normal brain biopsy resembles in shape the cell in A, but the nucleus and cytoplasm are lighter and the cell makes contact with surrounding cell processes and seems part of the neuropil. Electron micrograph of normal brain biopsy. (Original magnification ×7280.) (C) A young amebic macrophage from a recent infarct differs in shape from the rod cell in A but has a similar sharp cell outline, cytoplasmic density, and coarse nuclear chromatin. Electron micrograph of brain biopsy. (Original magnification ×7280.)

ble, suggesting a metamorphosis from one to the other. In rat corpus callosum, these cells have ultrastructurally round to oval nuclei, fairly abundant vacuolated cytoplasm, and active organelles, including an extensive Golgi system, a few filaments and microtubules, and elliptical secretory granules. The cells contain acid phosphatase, aryl sulfatase, adenosine triphosphatase, NADPH dehydrogenase, and nonspecific esterase inhibited by sodium fluoride, indicating monocytic origin (19, 46, 47). Intravenously injected carbon particles appeared successively in intravascular monocytes, perivascular macrophages, ameboid cells, and microglia (47). Imamoto and Leblond (32, 33) describe similar cells, which constitute 7% of the cell population in the corpus callosum in 5-day-old rats, including transition forms to typical microglia. The ameboid cells had disappeared by 19 d. According to these authors, blood monocytes permeate the brain in the early postnatal period, become at first monocytic ameboid cells, then somewhat macrophagic ameboid cells, of which about two-thirds degenerate and the remainder evolves into the resting microglia. While Imamoto and Leblond (33) believe that only monocytes give rise to the microglia, Ling (50) considers a dual origin possible, from monocytes and the meninges. Sturrock (81, 82) did not describe any ameboid cells in neonatal mouse anterior commissure. He did observe macrophages in the ventricles of 11-d postconception mice, at the site of the developing choroid plexus, near degenerating cells. Their numbers increased and then declined, coincident with the appearance of the microglia. Sturrock concluded that these macrophages migrated from plexus capillaries to the ventricles, where they appeared as epiplexus cells, and that they finally invaded the brain to develop into the microglia.

These views and observations are not universally shared. Caley and Maxwell (14) had noted with the electron microscope "polycystic cells" in postnatal rat cortex and white matter which they interpreted as spongioblasts. Vaughn and Peters (86) found in adult and developing optic nerve of rats no ameboid cells but a cell intermediate between astrocytes and oligodendrocytes, and this, the "third neuroglial type," later named the "multipotential glia," was thought to give rise to the macro- and microglia (87). Rio-Hortega postulated a mesenchymal and therefore meningeal origin for the microglia as opposed to the neuroectodermal microglia which developed in the subependymal primitive germ cell layer. Privat and his coworkers (66, 67) were unable to determine whether microgliocytes were totally or in part derived from subependymal cells. Fujita et al. (23) believe that the resting microglia is of ectodermal origin.

The observations summarized above are contradictory. One group demonstrates in small mammals an invasion of the perinatal brain by monocyte-derived phagocytic cells, yet these were not observed by others. Human fetal and neonatal brain parenchyma ordinarily does not contain monocytes or macrophages, although it can muster such cells quite early under pathologic conditions. Gilles (25) describes macrophages in the normal cavum septi pellucidi during the third gestational month. It remains to be determined whether macrophages ever play a part in the modelling of brain structures during normal development.

SUMMARY AND CONCLUSIONS

The preceding account of the literature reveals a bewildering divergence of opinions about the nature of the microglial cells. They are stated to be of pial, pericytic, monocytic, or glial ectodermal origin, or a combination of any of these. It is claimed that they enter the brain only perinatally, yet hematogenous monocytes and macrophages, having invaded the brain after injury even in adult life, are said to revert to resting microgliocytes. Conflicting views are expressed on whether or not the resting microglia is the main or at least the partial source of the macrophages which clean up necrotic brain tissue. Nor is there any agreement on whether or not the microglia plays a role in viral infections and syphilis or in retrograde and Wallerian degeneration. Some hypotheses propose that microgliocytes are really reserve cells for reacting astrocytes, or multipotential glia, the progenitors of both macroglia and Gitter cells.

Modern methods have not been able to demonstrate a resident cell population in the brain related to the mononuclear phagocyte system. Only occasional monocytes meander through normal brain. Theories of a mesenchymal origin of the microglia, and of its function as a reticuloendothelial defense unit stationed in the central nervous system, are therefore untenable.

The conclusion must be reached that the "progressive microglia" consists of monocytes of bone marrow origin which migrate to the central nervous system through the bloodstream when needed. There they may form "glial," now better called "monocytic" nodules, and cluster around degenerating neurons and senile plaques. Specific circumstances induce their metamorphosis to plump macrophages, elongated rod cells, or multinucleated globoid cells. There is no concrete evidence that any cells intrinsic to the brain participate in these activities.

Immunologic, cytochemical, and light and electron microsopic studies have failed to delineate at separate cell type corresponding to the "resting microglia." The perineuronal and interstitial microgliocytes are not clearly distinguishable from elongated oligodendrocytes. Both perivascular neuroglial cells and pericytes have been included under the term "perivascular microglia."

Despite some contradictory reports, the "ameboid" or "nascent" microglial cells described in the developing brain are almost certainly immature neuroectodermal elements. Since the most pronounced multiplication occurs at the time of "myelination gliosis" and in loose areas awaiting myelination, many are probably differentiating oligodendrocytes.

There is thus no relationship between resting, progressive, and nascent microgliocytes, and the term "microglia," which implies a single distinct cell system, is misleading and no longer applicable.

References

1. Adrian EK, Schelper RL: Microglia, monocytes, and macrophages. *Progr Clin Biol Res* 59A:113, 1981.
2. Adrian EK Jr, Walker BE: Incorporation of thymidine-H^3 by cells in normal and injured mouse spinal cord. *J Neuropathol Exp Neurol* 2:597, 1962.
3. Adrian EK Jr, et al: Fine structure of reactive cells in injured nervous tissue labeled with ^{3}H-thymidine injected before injury. *J Comp Neurol* 180:815, 1978.
4. Baggenstoss AH, et al: The healing process in wounds of the brain. *Am J Clin Pathol* 13:333, 1943.
5. Baron M, Gallego A: The relation of the microglia with the pericytes in the cat cerebral cortex. *Z Zellforsch* 128:42, 1972.
6. Baumgarten HG, et al: Accumulation of 14 C-5, 6-dihydroxytryptamine-melanin in intrathecal and subependymal phagocytes in the rat CNS and possible routes of their elimination from brain. *Prog Clin Biol Res* 59A:187, 1981.
7. Blakemore WF: The ultrastructure of normal and reactive microglia. *Acta Neuropathol [Suppl]* 6:273, 1975.
8. Bleier R, et al: Macrophages of hypothalamic third ventricle. I. Functional characterization of supra-ependymal cells in situ. *J Neuropathol Exp Neurol* 41:315, 1982.
9. Blinzinger K, Hager H: Elektronmikroskopische Untersuchungen über die Feinstruktur ruhender und progressiver Mikrogliazellen im Säugetiergehirn. *Beitr Pathol Anat* 127:173, 1962.
10. Blinzinger K, Kreutzberg G: Displacement of synaptic terminals from regenerating motor neurons by microglial cells. *Z Zellforsch Mikrosk Anat* 85:145, 1968.
11. Blinzinger K, et al: Ultrastructural cytochemical demonstration of peroxidase-positive monocyte granules. An additional method for studying the origin of mononuclear cells in encephalitic lesions. *Acta Neuropathol* 43:55, 1978
12. Boya J: Contribution to the ultrastructural study of microglia in the cerebral cortex. *Acta Anat* 92:364, 1975.
13. Boya J: An ultrastructural study of the relationship between pericytes and cerebral macrophages. *Acta Anat* 95:598, 1976.
14. Caley DW, Maxwell DS: An electron microscopic study of the neuroglia during postnatal development in the rat cerebrum. *J Comp Neurol* 133:45, 1968.
15. Cammermeyer J: The life history of the microglial cells: a light microscopic study. *Neurosci Res* 3:44, 1970.
16. Cohn P, et al: Macrophages of hypothalamic third ventricle. II. Immunological characterization of supra-ependymal cells in culture. *J Neuropathol Exp Neurol* 41:330, 1982.
17. Cook RD, Wisniewski HM: The role of oligodendrocytes in Wallerian degeneration. *J Neuropathol Exp Neurol* 32:160, 1973.
18. Feigin I: Mesenchymal tissues of the nervous system. The indigenous origin of brain macrophages in hypoxic states and in multiple sclerosis. *J Neuropathol Exp Neurol* 28:6, 1969.
19. Ferrer I, Sarmiento J: Nascent microglia in the developing brain. *Acta Neuropathol* 50:61, 1980.
20. Ferrer I, Sarmiento J: Reactive microglia in the developing brain. *Acta Neuropathol* 50:69, 1980.
21. Foncin JF: Microglia in the human cortex: an ultrastructural study. *Prog Clin Biol Res* 59A:171, 1981.
22. Fujita S, Kitamura T: Origin of brain macrophages and the nature of the microglia. In Zimmerman HM (ed): *Progress in Neuropathology, Vol. III.* New York, Grune & Stratton, 1976.
23. Fujita S, et al: Origin, morphology, and function of the microglia. *Prog Clin Biol Res* 59A:141, 1981.
24. Furth R Van: Cells of the mononuclear phagocyte system. Nomenclature in terms of sites and conditions. In Van Furth R (ed): *Mononuclear Phagocytes, Functional Aspects, Part I.* The Hague, Netherlands, Martinus Nijhoff, 1980.
25. Gilles FH: Myelination in the neonatal brain. *Hum Pathol* 7:244, 1976.
26. Hager H: Pathologie der Makro- und Mikroglia im elektronmikroskopischen Bild. *Acta Neuropathol [Suppl]* 4:86, 1968.
27. Hager H: E. M. Findings on the source of reactive microglia on the mammalian brain. *Acta Neuropathol [Suppl]* 6:279, 1975.
28. Hatai S: On the origin of neuroglia tissue from the mesoblast. *J Comp Neurol* 12:291, 1902.
29. Herndon RM: The fine structure of the rat cerebellum. II. The stellate neurons, granule cells and glia. *J Cell Biol*

23:277, 1964.

30. Huntington HW, Terry RD: The origin of the reactive cells in cerebral stab wounds. *J Neuropathol Exp Neurol* 25:646, 1966.

31. Ibrahim MZM, et al: The histochemical identification of microglia. *J Neurol Sci* 22:211, 1974.

32. Imamoto K: Origin of microglia: cell transformation from blood monocytes into macrophagic amoeboid cells and microglia. *Prog Clin Biol Res* 59A:125, 1981.

33. Imamoto K, Leblond CP: Radioautographic investigation of gliogenesis in the corpus callosum of young rats. II. Origin of microglial cells. *J Comp Neurol* 180:139, 1978.

34. Kerns JM, Hinsman EJ: Microglial response to sciatic neurectomy. I. Light microscopy and autoradiography. *J Comp Neurol* 151:237, 1973.

35. King JS: A light and electron microscopic study of perineuronal glial cells and processes in the rabbit neocortex. *Anat Rec* 161:111, 1968.

36. Kitamura T: Hematogenous cells in experimental Japanese encephalitis. *Acta Neuropathol* 32:341, 1975.

37. Kitamura T, et al: Electron microscopic features of the resting microglia in the rabbit hippocampus, identified by silver carbonate staining. *Acta Neuropathol* 38:195, 1977.

38. Kitamura T, et al: Initial response of silver-impregnated "resting microglia" in stab wounding in rabbit hippocampus. *Acta Neuropathol* 44:31, 1978.

39. Konigsmark BW, Sidman RL: Origin of brain macrophages in the mouse. *J Neuropathol Exp Neurol* 22:643, 1963.

40. Kosunen TV, et al: Cellular mechanisms in delayed hypersensitivity. *J Neuropathol Exp Neurol* 22:367, 1963.

41. Kreutzberg GW: Über perineuronale Mikrogliazellen. Autoradiographische Untersuchungen. *Acta Neuropathol [Suppl]* 4:141, 1968.

42. Kreutzberg GW, Barron KD: 5-Nucleotidase of microglial cells in the facial nucleus during axonal reaction. *J Neuropathol* 7:601, 1978.

43. Kruger L, Maxwell DS: Electron microscopy of oligodendrocytes in normal rat cerebrum. *Am J Anat* 118:411, 1966.

44. Lampert P, Carpenter S: Electron microscopic studies on the vascular permeability and the mechanism of demyelination in allergic encephalomyelitis. *J Neuropathol Exp Neurol* 24:11, 1965.

45. Lebeux YJ, Willemot J: Actin- and myosin-like filaments in rat brain pericytes. *Anat Rec* 190:811, 1978.

46. Ling EA: Some aspects of amoeboid microglia in the corpus callosum and neighbouring regions of neonatal rats. *J Anat* 121:29, 1976.

47. Ling EA: Light and electron microscopic demonstration of some lysosomal enzymes in the amoeboid microglia in rat neonatal brain. *J Anat* 123:637, 1977.

48. Ling EA: Brain macrophages in rats following intravenous labelling of mononuclear leucocytes with colloidal carbon. *J Anat* 125:101, 1978.

49. Ling EA: Evidence for a hematogenous origin of some of the macrophages appearing in the spinal cord of the rat after dorsal rhizotomy. *J Anat* 128:143, 1979.

50. Ling EA: The origin and nature of microglia. In Fedoroff S, Hertz L (eds): *Advances in Cellular Neurobiology*. New York, Academic Press, 1981, vol 2.

51. Ling EA, et al: Investigation of glial cells in semithin sections. I. Identification of glial cells in the brain of young rats. *J Comp Neurol* 149:43, 1973.

52. Luse SA: Electron microscopic observations on the central nervous system. *J Biophys Biochem Cyt* 2:531, 1956.

53. Matthews MA, Kruger L: Electron microscopy of nonneuronal cellular changes accompanying neural degeneration in thalamic nuclei of the rabbit. I. Reactive hematogenous and perivascular elements within the basal lamina. II. Reactive elements within the neuropil. *J Comp Neurol* 148:285, 313, 1973.

54. Maxwell DS, Kruger L: Small blood vessels and the origin of phagocytes in the rat cerebral cortex following heavy particle irradiation. *Exp Neurol* 12:33, 1965.

55. Merchant RE, Low FN: Scanning electron microscopy of the subarachnoid space in the dog: evidence for a nonhematogenous origin of subarachnoid macrophages. *Am J Anat* 156:183, 1979.

56. Mestres P, Breipohl W: Morphology and distribution of supraependymal cells in the third ventricle of the albino rat. *Cell Tissue Res* 168:303, 1976.

57. Mori S: Uptake of (^{3}H) thymidine by corpus callosum cells in rats following a stab wound of the brain. *Brain Res* 46:177, 1972.

58. Mori S, Leblond CP: Identification of microglia in light and electron microscopy. *J Comp Neurol* 135:57, 1969.

59. Mugnaini E, Walberg F: "Dark cells" in electron micrographs from the central nervous system of vertebrates. *J Ultrastruct Res* 12:235, 1965.

60. Nissl F: Ueber einige Beziehungen zwischen Nervenzellenerkrankungen und gliösen Erscheinungen bei verschiedenen Psychosen. *Arch Psychiat* 32:656, 1899.

61. Oehmichen M: Mononuclear phagocytes in the central nervous system. *Schriftenr Neurol—Neurology Series 21*, 1978.

62. Oehmichen M, et al: Immunological analysis of human microglia: lack of monocytic and lymphoid membrane differentiation antigens. *J Neuropathol Exp Neurol* 38:99, 1979.

63. Persson LT, Rönnback L, Rosengren LE: Identification of reactive cells in the injured brain. *Acta Neurol Scand [Suppl]* 67:245, 1978.

64. Peters A, et al: *The Fine Structure of the Nervous System.* Philadelphia, WB Saunders, 1st edition, 1970, 2nd edition 1976.

65. Pfeiffer J, Schwartz EW: Beitrag zur Enzymhistochemie der Liquor—und Leptomeningealzellen. *Nervenarzt* 42:267, 1971.

66. Privat A: Postnatal gliogenesis in mammalian brain. *Int Rev Cytol* 40:281, 1975.

67. Privat A, et al: Proliferation of neuroglial cell lines in the degenerating optic nerve of young rats. *J Neuropathol* 40:46, 1981.

68. Ramon Y Cajal S: Contribucion al conocimiento de la neuroglia del cerebro humano. *Trab Lab Invest Biol Univ Madrid* 11:255, 1913.

69. Rio-Hortega P del: El tercer elemento de los centros nerviosos. i. La microglia en estado normal. ii. Intervencion de la microglia en los procesos patologicos. iii. Naturaleza probable de la microglia. *Bol Soc Espan Biol* 9:69, 1919.

70. Rio-Hortega P del: Microglia. In Penfield W: *Cytology and Cellular Pathology of the Nervous System*. New York, Paul Hoefer, 1932, vol 2.

71. Robertson, FW: A microscopic demonstration of the normal and pathological histology of mesoglia cells. *J Ment Sci* 46:724, 1900.

72. Roessman U, Friede AL: Entry of labeled monocytic cells into the central nervous system. *Acta Neuropathol* 10:359, 1968.

73. Russell GV: The compound granular corpuscle or gitter cell: A review, together with notes on the origin of this phagocyte. *Tex Rep Biol Med* 20:338, 1962.

74. Schultz RL, et al: Electron microscopy of neurons and neuroglia of cerebral cortex and corpus callosum. *Am J Anat* 100:369, 1957.

75. Skoff RP: The fine structure of pulse labeled ^{3}H-thymidine cells in degenerating rat optic nerve. *J Comp Neurol* 161:595, 1975.

76. Smith B, Rubinstein LJ: Histochemical observations on oxidative enzyme activity in reactive microglia and some macrophages. *J Pathol Bacteriol* 83:572, 1962.

77. Stensaas LJ: Pericytes and perivascular microglial cells in the basal forebrain of the neonatal rabbit. *Cell Tissue Res* 158:517, 1975.

78. Stensaas LJ, Reichert WH: Round and amoeboid microglial cells in the neonatal rabbit brain. *Z Zellforsch* 119:147, 1971.

79. Stenwig AE: The origin of brain macrophages in traumatic

lesions, Wallerian degeneration and retrograde degeneration. *J Neuropathol Exp Neurol* 31:696, 1972.

80. Stroebe H: Experimentelle Untersuchungen über die degenerativen und reparatorischen Vorgänge bei der Heilung von Verletzungen des Rückenmarks, nebst Bemerkungen zur Histogenese der sekundären Degeneration im Rückenmark. *Beitr Pathol Anat* 15:383, 1894.

81. Sturrock RR: Histogenesis of the anterior limb of the anterior commissure of the mouse brain. III. An electron microscopic study. *J Anat* 117:37, 1974.

82. Sturrock RR: A developmental study of epiplexus cells and supraependymal cells and their possible relationship to microglia. *Neuropathol Appl Neurobiol* 4:307, 1978.

83. Sumner BEH: The nature of the dividing cells around axotomized hypoglossal neurons. *J Neuropathol Exp Neurol* 33:507, 1974.

84. Torvik A: Phagocytosis of nerve cells during retrograde degeneration. An electron microscopic study. *J Neuropathol Exp Neurol* 31:132, 1972.

85. Torvik A: The relationship between microglia and brain macrophages. Experimental investigations. *Acta Neuropathol [Suppl]* 6:297, 1975.

86. Vaughn JE, Peters A: A third neuroglial cell type. An electron microscopic study. *J Comp Neurol* 133:269, 1968.

87. Vaughn JE, Skoff RP: Neuroglia in experimentally altered central nervous system. In Bourne GH (ed): *The Structure and Function of Nervous Tissue.* New York, Academic Press, 1972, vol 5.

88. Vaughn DW, Peters A: Neuroglial cells in the cerebral cortex of rats from young adulthood to old age: an electron microscopic study. *J Neurocytol* 3:405, 1974.

89. Vogel FS, Kemper L: Modification of Hortega's silver impregnation methods to assist in the identification of neuroglia with electron microscopy. *Proceedings of the 4th International Congress of Neuropathology* 1962, p 66.

90. Wagner HJ, et al: Penetration and removal of horseradish peroxidase injected into the cerebrospinal fluid. Role of cerebral perivascular spaces, endothelium and microglia. *Acta Neuropathol* 27:299, 1974.

91. Wolinsky JS, et al: Hematogenous origin of the inflammatory response in acute poliomyelitis. *Ann Neurol* 11:59, 1982.

92. Wood GW, et al: The failure of microglia in normal brain to exhibit mononuclear phagocyte markers. *J Neuropathol Exp Neurol* 38:369, 1979.

93. Young MB: H³-labeled blood cells in the CNS. Response to axonotomies at various times after isotope injection. *J Neuropathol Exp Neurol* 36:465, 1977.

CHAPTER 4

The Meninges and Their Reactions to Injury

MICHAEL L. DYER, M.D.
JOSEPH C. PARKER, JR., M.D.

MORPHOLOGY (5, 7, 16, 24, 27, 41)

The meninges are mesodermal derived connective tissue coverings that invest and protect the brain and spinal cord. This mesoderm condenses into a membrane which then separates into two distinct layers by 6 weeks gestation. The inner layer becomes the pia-arachnoid membrane, or leptomeninges, and the outer layer becomes the dura mater or pachymeninx. The arachnoid membrane contains epithelium-lined villous structures that protrude into the venous dural sinuses and veins in the spinal canal and, occasionally, into the subdural spaces which serve as a pathway for resorption of cerebrospinal fluid. The brain and spinal cord are enclosed in a tight, bony compartment. Folds of dura mater envelop the brain and separate the cranial cavity into compartments. Herniation of neural tissue from one compartment into another may occur with cerebral edema but may not develop if the dural openings are anatomically limited to allow only the normal neural tissue to pass snugly through. Any intracranial mass from any cause may be associated with cerebral edema. The pia mater is a thin mesothelial membrane that is attached intimately to the neuroparenchyma. Adjacent basement membrane with adherent astrocytic foot processes creates a morphologic barrier known as the cerebrospinal-fluid-pial-brain barrier, analogous to the blood-capillary-brain barrier. Histolog-ically, the pia mater consists of fibrous tissue with a thin mesothelium. Pial blood vessels extend into the neural parenchyma, creating spaces with CSF known as Virchow-Robin spaces.

The arachnoid is positioned between the pia mater and overlying dura mater (Figs. 4.1 and 4.2). It is a thin connective tissue membrane covered by a layer of mesothelial cells and separated from the pia by the fluid-filled subarachnoid space. Fibrous trabeculae traverse the subarachnoid space along with blood vessels. The subarachnoid space surrounds all cranial and spinal nerves, providing access to these structures by any agent in the CSF. Any increase in subarachnoid or CSF pressure will compress the central vein in each optic nerve, decreasing venous return from the retina. This results in edema of the retina and optic disc, producing papilledema.

In some areas, there is a discrepancy between the curvature of the brain and the course of the arachnoid, creating a space or cistern (Fig. 4.3). The cisterna magna is found at the junction of the cerebellum and medulla oblongata; the pontine cistern, beneath the pons; the interpenduncular cistern, around the midbrain; and the small optic cistern, beneath the optic chiasm. The large lumbar spinal cistern extends from the second lumbar vertebra to the second sacral vertebra and contains the cauda equina.

The outermost fibrous membrane cover-

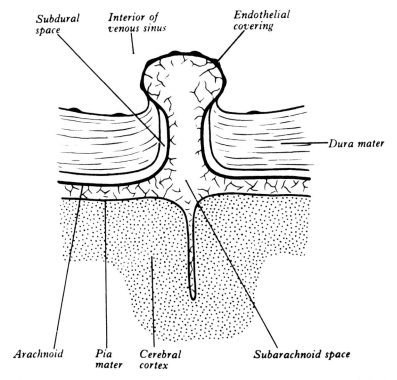

Figure 4.1. The meninges. (From P. L. Williams and R. Warwick (6).)

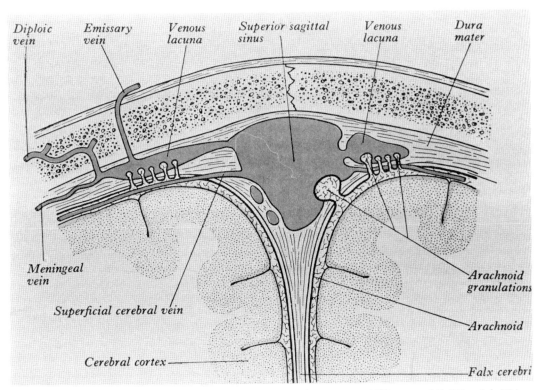

Figure 4.2. Coronal section through the meninges. (From P. L. Williams and R. Warwick (6).)

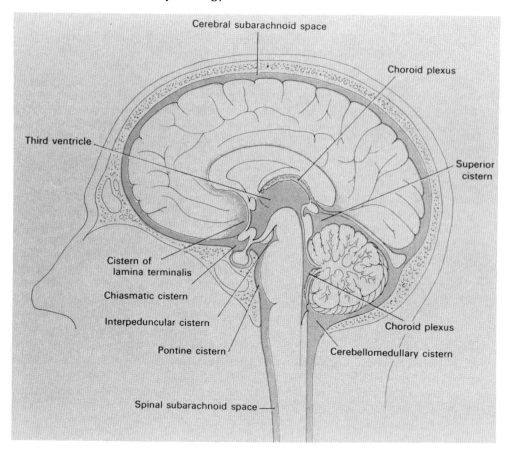

Figure 4.3. Subarachnoid cisterns. (From M. B. Carpenter (1).)

ing the brain and spinal cord is the dura, which serves as the inner periosteum of the skull and is firmly attached to the bone, particularly in infants and the elderly. The dura gives rise to folds that divide the cranial cavity into compartments. The falx cerebri is the largest septum and divides the two cerebral hemispheres (Figs. 4.4 and 4.5). The tentorium cerebelli is a dural septum that forms a roof over the posterior fossa. The free borders of the tentorium cerebelli create the tentorium incisure—the only opening between the supratentorial and infratentorial compartments. The dura forms endothelium-lined venous sinuses, which collect blood from the cerebral, meningeal, and diploic veins. Arachnoidal granulations, which project into the dural sinuses, transport CSF from the subarachnoid space into these sinuses. Arterial supply of the meninges includes three major vessels—the anterior, middle, and posterior

meningeal arteries. Meningeal veins closely follow these arteries. Sensory nerves of the dura are derived from all three divisions of the trigeminal nerves, as well as the vagal and hypoglossal nerves.

REACTIONS TO INJURY INVOLVING THE MENINGES (1, 4, 13, 20–22, 26)

The meninges have the capacity to react to various insults. For example, a subdural hematoma may result from tearing of the bridging veins. The extravasated blood stimulates a fibroblastic response by the mesothelial lining cells and perivascular fibroblasts. A mild infiltration of neutrophilic leukocytes is observed during the first 24 to 48 h. By the 5th day, a mononuclear cell infiltration of monocytes and lymphoid cells is observed with engulfment of cellular debris. The hematoma ulti-

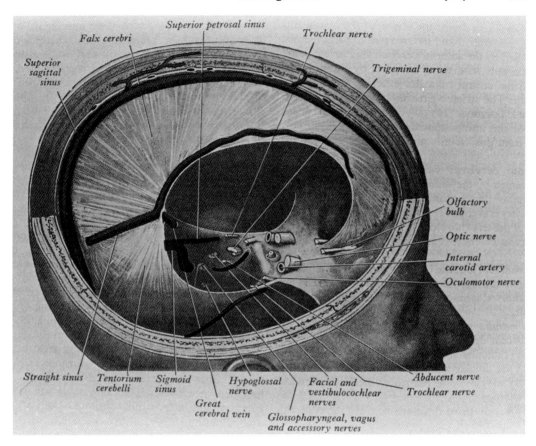

Figure 4.4. The cerebral dura and duplication. (From P. L. Williams and R. Warwick (6).)

mately becomes encapsulated in a pseudo-membrane. Breakdown of blood leads to an increased osmotic gradient, resulting in enlargement of the hematoma by accumulation of fluid. Between the 10th and 20th day, most erythrocytes are degenerated. Capillaries along with increased fibroblasts create granulation tissue. Three months after the hemorrhagic trauma, the membranous wall of the hematoma is firm, and an occasional artery may be seen. Nuclei of the newly formed connective tissue membrane become smaller, and collagenous fibers increase. Phagocytes with hemosiderin may be seen. Sometimes, the hematoma is reabsorbed, but it may continue to expand as it accumulates fluid by osmosis. The thin-walled blood vessels in the membrane act as semipermeable conductors, allowing plasma to flow from the intravascular space into the hypertonic membranous sac.

Bacteria within the subarachnoid space usually elicit a reaction, characterized by an infiltration of neutrophils in the first 24 h. Grossly, the leptomeninges become opaque and reveal vascular congestion over the base and superior surfaces of the brain. Chemical mediators from plasma and tissues, such as vasoactive amines, plasma proteins, prostaglandins, and leukocyte products contribute to the inflammatory reaction. Prostaglandins are synthesized by neutrophilic lysosomal phospholipase acting on the phospholipids of injured cell membranes. They are vasodilators and potentiate histamine-induced vascular permeability. Arachnoidal and pial cell nuclei become vesicular with a rim of chromatin adjacent to the nuclear membrane. In animal models, the arachnoidal and pial cells may actually phagocytose bacteria. Ultrastructurally, these leptomeningeal cells are similar to macrophages with scattered cytoplasmic membrane-bound inclusions. Within 3 to 5 days, inflammation consists of mononuclear cells and pial and arach-

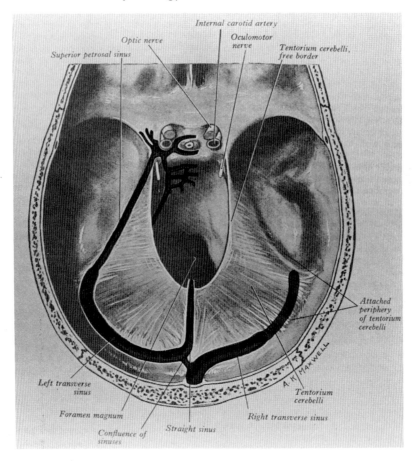

Figure 4.5. The cerebral dura and duplications. (From P. L. Williams and R. Warwick (6).)

noidal cells look like fibroblasts. Ultimately, fibrosis and thickened meninges develop with adhesions between the pia and arachnoid. Adhesions and fibrosis of the arachnoidal granulations and other areas of the leptomeninges may result in decreased resorption and/or flow of cerebrospinal fluid with eventual hydrocephalus.

A granulomatous reaction involving the meninges is usually caused by mycobacteria or fungi. Mononuclear cell infiltration is seen with scattered granulomas containing Langhans multinucleated giant cells. The granulomas appear as grey-white nodules throughout the meninges. A necrotic yellow-white, cheesy exudate may be seen along the base of the brain with encasement of cranial nerves. Foreign material implanted in the leptomeninges causes an initial, neutrophilic cellular infiltration, followed by a mononuclear cellular reaction. Dura mater shows a reaction similar to that elicited by blood, and fibroblastic prolifer-

ation tends to encapsulate the foreign material.

Trauma to the meninges may be associated with tears resulting in hemorrhage and a perivascular fibroblastic proliferation of meningeal mesothelial cells. Blood monocytes and mesothelial cells become phagocytic cells that engulf red blood cells and cellular debris. Eventually, hemoglobin is degraded into the insoluble iron protein complex, hemosiderin. Loose scar tissue forms at the site of injury and progressively thickens.

The meninges also react to tumor cells. Meningeal carcinomatosis occurs when sheet-like infiltrates of malignant cells grow along the leptomeninges around the brain and spinal cord. Grossly, the leptomeninges have a grey, fibrotic thickening similar to the aged leptomeninges. Histologically, a mild infiltration of mononuclear cells is associated with a fibroblastic reaction by the leptomeningeal mesothelial cells and perivascular fibroblasts. Tumor cells grow in nests and strands separated by dense, fibrous connective tissue and tend to collect around blood vessels and cranial nerves and in subarachnoid cisterns. The more common tumors to metastasize to the meninges include cancers from the breast, lung, skin (melanoma), prostate, and hematologic system. Tumor metastases involving the spinal column may enter Batson's venous plexus, which extends the entire length of the spinal column and communicates with basilar, occipital, and sigmoid sinuses and emissary skull veins. Metastatic tumors to the vertebral column gain entrance into Batson's venous plexus and then invade the skull and meninges. Metastases may also extend through capillary channels in the choroid plexi by traversing its endothelium. Leukemia metastasizes to the meninges directly from adjacent involved bone marrow in the skull. Another route into the meninges is direct invasion through cranial or spinal nerves.

The meninges react not only to various insults but also to aging. For instance, arachnoidal granulations become more fibrotic and develop focal calcifications. Arachnoidal cap cell hyperplasia occurs with focal meningothelial whorls. Osseous metaplasia can develop in the falx cerebri, which may be visualized radiologically. The aged dura develops fibrosis and becomes densely adherent to the inner table of the skull. Fibrocalcific plaques occurring on the arachnoid over the lower thoracic and lumbar spinal cord in older adults may hinder lumbar punctures. Changes also occur in the meningeal and neuroparenchymal blood vessels, which include reduced elasticity and ferruginous calcific deposits. Areas of brightly eosinophilic amyloid in the vascular media occur with increased frequency in elderly people. This amyloid angiopathy causes weakening of vessel walls which may lead to spontaneous and lethal intracranial hemorrhages, particularly in unusual locations as compared to hypertensive intracerebral hemorrrhages.

CEREBROSPINAL FLUID (CSF) (2, 8, 10, 14, 15, 23, 35–37, 40)

In the adult, the entire cavity with the brain and spinal cord contains 150 ml of CSF. About 840 ml of the CSF are produced each day, the majority of which are reabsorbed. Seventy percent of the CSF is produced by the choroid plexi, while the remaining 30% is formed by blood vessels in the leptomeninges and near the ependyma. Fluid formed in the lateral ventricles passes into the third ventricle through the foramina of Monro, enters the fourth ventricle through the aqueduct of Sylvius (Fig. 4.6), and then exits through the single central foramen of Magendie and two lateral foramina of Lushka into the subarachnoid space. CSF is reabsorbed by arachnoidal granulations that project into the dural venous sinuses. The major functions of the CSF are to provide protection for the brain and spinal cord and to act as a modified lymphatic system, since no lymphatics are found in the central nervous system (CNS).

Formation of CSF results from a combination of ultrafiltration and active transport of plasma products. Elevation of ion concentrations in the CSF by active ion transport within the choroid plexus produces a strong osmotic force, causing water to diffuse into it. CSF extends along the perivascular spaces of Virchow-Robin in the neuroparenchyma. Blood-CSF and CSF-brain parenchyma barriers provide a physical buffering protection mechanism and regulate the concentration of solutes in the CNS. Glucose in CSF is about 70% of the fasting blood level, and total proteins vary from 15 to 45 mg/dl. Sodium concentration is 7% greater than in extracellular fluids. CSF concentrations of calcium, hydrogen, magnesium, and potassium depend on active transport across the blood-brain barrier and are maintained within narrow concentrations.

The CSF and neural parenchyma are separated from blood by a distinct morphologic and physiologic blood-brain barrier. This barrier consists of unique capillary endothelial cells that differ from systemic capillary endothelium by possessing:

1. Tight junctions between adjacent endothelial cells
2. Decreased pinocytotic vesicles
3. Receptors for glucose and certain amino acids
4. Thickened basement membranes that are one-fourth the thickness of the endothelial cells

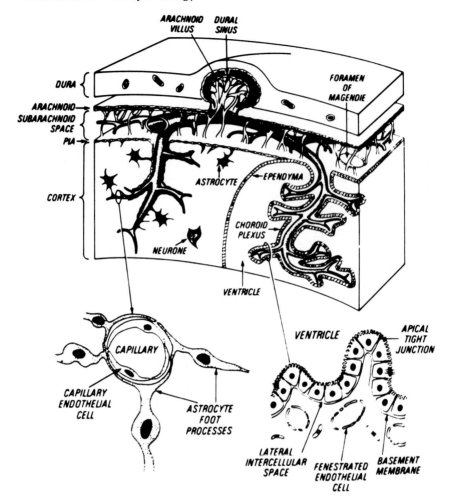

Figure 4.6. Blood-brain barrier. (From N. J. Zvaifler and H. G. Bluestein: *Arthritis and Rheumatism* 25:862, 1982.)

5. Increased (three-to-five times) mitochondria
6. Absent perivascular collagen
7. Abutting astrocytic foot processes covering about 80% of the capillary surfaces in the CNS.

The CSF-brain barrier includes pia-mesothelioid cells and ependyma interfacing with subjacent basement membranes and astrocytic foot processes. Diffusion across the subarachnoid space into the brain parenchyma depends on the lipid solubility of a substance, with lipid-soluble substances possessing greater ability to diffuse across this barrier.

REACTIONS TO INJURY INVOLVING CEREBROSPINAL FLUID (3, 6, 9, 11, 12, 17–19, 25, 28–34, 38, 39, 42)

Noncellular reactions to injury can be analyzed by examination of CSF for electrolytes, glucose, protein, enzymes, and pressure, along with other specialized substances. Pressure changes in the CNS are between 50 and 180 mm of water and may increase with increased CSF volume, decreased fluid reabsorption, and increased mass effect. Removal of CSF from a patient with increased intracranial pressure is hazardous and can result in herniations of neural tissue through the tentorial notch and foramen magnum and below the falx cerebri. Herniation or compression may result in brain stem ischemia, due to reduced venous return, resulting in cardiorespiratory arrest. Such problems can be avoided if increased intracranial pressure is recognized before a lumbar puncture is performed. (See Chapter 5.)

CSF is normally clear and has the viscosity of water. Turbidity may be caused by increased cells, microorganisms, and lipids. Increased viscosity may occur secondary to increased γ-globulin and fibrinogen which may be secondary to inflammatory processes. Clotting of blood occurs with CSF traumatic spinal taps, whereas this is not found in subarachnoid bleeds. A traumatic spinal tap usually shows gradual clearing of blood. Xanthochromia is a pale, pink-to-yellow or orange CSF supernatant indicating previous hemorrhage. This abnormal color is due to a breakdown of hemoglobin in the CSF and may persist for a month.

Glucose is transported between blood and CSF through facilitated diffusion and active transport. Acute bacterial infections may cause a marked reduction of CSF glucose which can result from metabolism of glucose by the bacteria, decreased transport, or both. Glucose levels below 50 or 80 mg/dl can be observed in primary and metastatic neoplastic diseases and in infections due to bacteria, fungi, or parasites. Viral infections are associated with normal to increased glucose levels; however, 25% of patients with mumps meningoencephalitis have decreased CSF glucose. Lactic acid levels may be associated with reduced oxygen in the CSF. Lactic acid may be increased by bacterial infections, intracranial hemorrhage, stroke, status epilepticus, or neoplasms. Normal protein in CSF measures 15–45 mg per dl. Decreased CSF protein can be caused by increased filtration through arachnoidal granulations, with increased intracranial pressure and hyperthyroidism. Increased total protein can occur with increased permeability of the CSF-blood barrier, as seen in meningitis and in endocrine, metabolic, and toxic conditions. Decreased absorption of protein by arachnoidal granulations can result in increased CSF protein. Increased immunoglobulin

fractions of protein can be detected by protein electrophoresis and may occur with lymphoproliferative diseases in the CNS. In some hereditary degenerative conditions of the CNS, increased proteins in the CSF are observed. Since albumin is not produced in the CNS, a CSF-to-serum-albumin ratio indicates the integrity of vascular permeability in the brain and reabsorption of CSF.

Cytological examination of CSF is important in the recognition of infectious diseases, neoplasms, and noninfectious processes. CSF cells are first concentrated by either ultracentrifugation or Millipore filtration and are placed on a slide and stained appropriately for screening. Neutrophils are not normally found in the CSF and, when present, indicate either infections due to almost any viable agent or noninfectious processes, such as bleeding, invasive malignancy, or chemical irritations. A most important test in the diagnosis of bacterial meningitis is the Gram stain, which is aided by countercurrent immunoelectrophoresis of CSF. Other inflammatory cells in the CSF imply certain etiopathogenetic processes. Increased lymphocytes are associated with CNS infections due to bacteria, fungi, leptospira, and viruses. Even though lymphocytes found within the CSF usually denote an inflammatory response with some element of chronicity to the irritant, they are prevalent in acute viral infections of the CNS. Eosinophils occur with bacterial, fungal, parasitic, or allergic conditions, or after intrathecal injections of foreign proteins. Basophils may be seen with chronic granulocytic leukemia. Ependymal and pia-arachnoid cells are often associated with other inflammatory cells in virtually any infection in the CNS. Macrophages may be observed with phagocytosed debris, as in hemosiderin-laden macrophages after an intracerebral bleed, macrophages containing melanin in patients with primary or metastatic malignant melanoma, and lipid-filled macrophages in remote brain damage or lipid storage diseases. Cytological evaluation of the CSF is necessary to evaluate leukemic infiltrates, neuroectodermal tumors, and metastatic carcinoma and should be utilized whenever the CSF is analyzed.

In summary, the meninges play a significant role in protecting and maintaining a proper environment for the CNS. They react to irritants like other tissues of the body and are altered obviously by maturation and aging. Tissue changes, which have been considered insignificant and "just due to aging," now appear to have clinical implications and to alter meningeal reactions to insults. How significant these aging changes are and what can be done to prevent them are challenges for the future.

ACKNOWLEDGMENTS

The authors gratefully acknowledge the assistance of Ms. Martha Childs and the staff of the Preston Medical Library, Ms. Jeanette Dean and Ms. Lisa Mary for their secretarial support, Ms. Lucille Simpson for word processing, and Mr. Rich McCoig for photographic assistance.

References

1. Apfelbaum RI, et al: Experimental production of subdural hematomas. *J Neurosurg* 40:336–346, 1974.
2. Barr ML: *The Human Nervous System: An Anatomical Viewpoint.* New York, Harper & Row, 1972, pp 358–368.
3. Brook I, et al: Measurement of lactic acid in cerebrospinal fluid of patients with infection of the central nervous system. *J Infect Dis* 137:384–390, 1978.
4. Burger PC, Vogel FS: *Surgical Pathology of the Nervous System and Its Coverings.* New York, John Wiley, 1976, pp 130–132.
5. Carpenter MB: *Human Neuroanatomy,* ed 7. Baltimore, Williams & Wilkins, 1976, pp 1–20.
6. Check W: CSF lactic acid levels, an aid to diagnosis. *JAMA* 241:781–784, 1979.
7. Copenhaver WM, et al: *Bailey's Textbook of Histology,* ed 16. Baltimore, Williams & Wilkins, 1971, pp 292–296.
8. Dyken PR: Cerebrospinal fluid cytology: practical clinical usefulness. *Neurology* 25:210–217, 1975.
9. Feinbloom RI, Alpert JJ: The value of routine glucose determination in spinal fluid without pleocytosis. *J Pediatr* 75:121–123, 1969.
10. Felgenhauer K: Protein size and cerebrospinal fluid composition. *Klin Wochenschr* 52:1158–1164, 1974.
11. Gilroy J, Meyer JS: *Medical Neurology,* ed 2. New York, Macmillan, 1975, pp 62–65.
12. Greenawald KA, et al: Glucose content in cerebrospinal fluid: a comparison with glucose levels in serum as determined by copper reduction and hexokinase methods. *Am J Clin Pathol* 59:518–520, 1973.
13. Griffiths RA, et al: Congophilic angiopathy of the brain: a clinical and pathological report on two siblings. *J Neurol Neurosurg Psychiatry* 45:396–408, 1982.
14. Guyton AC: *Textbook of Medical Physiology,* ed 4. Philadelphia, WB Saunders, 1971, pp 459–464.
15. Hammock MK, Milhorat TH: The cerebrospinal fluid: current concepts of its formation. *Ann Clin Lab Sci* 6:22–26, 1976.
16. Harvey SC, Burr HS: The development of the meninges. *Arch Neurol Psychiatry* 15:545–567, 1926.
17. Henry JB, et al (eds): *Clinical Diagnosis and Management by Laboratory Methods,* ed 16. Philadelphia, WB Saunders, 1979, vol 1, pp 635–679.
18. Kjellin KG, Söderström CE: Diagnostic significance of CSF spectrophotometry in cerebrovascular diseases. *J Neurol Sci* 23:359–369, 1974.
19. Kjellin KG, Steiner L: Spectrophotometry of cerebrospinal fluid in subacute and chronic subdural hematomas. *J Neurol Neurosurg Psychiatry* 37:1121–1127, 1974.
20. Lee SS, Stemmermann GN: Congophilic angiopathy and cerebral hemorrhage. *Arch Pathol Lab Med* 102:317–321, 1978.
21. Lindenberg R: Trauma of meninges and brain. In Minckler J (ed): *Pathology of the Nervous System.* New York, McGraw-Hill, 1971, vol 2, pp 1705–1765.
22. Loeb GE, et al: Histological reaction to various conductive and dielectric films chronically implanted in the subdural space. *J. Biomed Mater Res* 11:195–210, 1977.
23. Mathios AJ, et al: Cerebrospinal fluid cytomorphology: identification of benign cells originating in the central nervous system. *Acta Cytol* 21:403–412, 1977.
24. Moore KL: *The Developing Human: Clinically Oriented Embryology.* Philadelphia, WB Saunders, 1973, p 310.
25. Nanlkervis GA: Bacterial meningitis. *Med Clin North Am* 58:581–592, 1974.
26. Olson ME, et al: Infiltration of the leptomeninges by systemic cancer. A clinical and pathologic study. *Arch Neurol* 30:122–137, 1974.
27. Pernhkopf E: *Head and Neck. Atlas of Topographical and Applied Human Anatomy.* Philadelphia, WB Saunders, 1963, vol 1, pp 29–66.
28. Previne H, Gardner P: The gram-stained smear and its interpretation. *Hosp Pract* 9:85–91, 1974.
29. Roost KT, et al: The formation of cerebrospinal fluid xanthochromia after subarachnoid hemorrhage: enzymatic conversion of hemoglobin to bilirubin by the arachnoid and choroid plexus. *Neurology* 22:973–977, 1972.
30. Rosenthal MS: Viral infections of the central nervous system. *Med Clin North Am* 58:593–603, 1974.
31. Rytel MW: Counterimmunoelectrophoresis in diagnosis of infectious disease. *Hosp Pract* 10:75–82, 1974.
32. Siesjo BK: The regulation of cerebrospinal fluid pH. *Kidney Int* 1:360–374, 1975.
33. Smith AL: Diagnosis of bacterial meningitis. *Pediatrics* 52:589–592, 1973.
34. Smith DH: The challenge of bacterial meningitis. *Hosp Pract* 11:71–80, 1976.
35. Smith LH Jr, Thier SO: *Patholophysiology: The Biological Principles of Disease.* Philadelphia, WB Saunders, 1981, pp 476–484.
36. Sornas R: The cytology of the normal cerebrospinal fluid. *Acta Neurol Scand* 48:313–320, 1972.
37. Tietz NW: *Fundamentals of Clinical Chemistry,* ed 2. Philadelphia, WB Saunders, 1976, pp 368–376.
38. Walton JN: *Brain's Diseases of the Nervous System,* ed 8. Oxford, Oxford University Press, 1977, pp 121–131.
39. Ward PC: Cerebrospinal fluid data. I. Interpretation in intracranial hemorrhage and meningitis. *Postgrad Med* 62:181–186, 1980.
40. Westergaard E: The blood-brain barrier to horseradish peroxidase under normal and experimental conditions. *Acta Neuropathol* 39:181–187, 1977.
41. Williams PL, Warwick R (eds): *Gray's Anatomy,* ed 36. Philadelphia, WB Saunders, 1980, pp 1045–1052.
42. Woodruff KH: Cerebrospinal fluid cytomorphology using cytocentrifugation. *Am J Clin Pathol* 60:621–627, 1973.

Choroid Plexus, Cerebrospinal Fluid, Hydrocephalus, Cerebral Edema, and Herniation Phenomena

J. GORDON, McCOMB, M.D.
RICHARD L. DAVIS, M.D.

CHOROID PLEXUS

The choroid plexus, the major source of cerebrospinal fluid (CSF), is found in the lateral ventricles; the third ventricle, including the suprapineal recess; and the fourth ventricle with an extension of this tissue out of the lateral foramina of Luschka into the cerebellopontine angles.

The choroid plexus (Fig. 5.1) consists of numerous villi, each with a single layer of cuboidal epithelium which is a modified ependyma covering a stromal core derived from a layer of pia. Microvilli and a few cilia cover the apical or ventricular surface of these epithelial cells, while on the basal side lateral infoldings interdigitate with neighboring cells. Tight junctions are present at the apical side of the cells. The cells lay on a basement membrane beneath which is a stromal space containing collagen, fibroblasts, and nerve fibers. A capillary, with endothelium of the fenestrated type and devoid of tight junctions, is at the center of each villus. A blood-CSF barrier results from the presence of tight junctions at the apical end of the choroid epithelium, rather than at the capillary endothelium of the villus (12). This is in contradistinction to the capillaries of the parenchyma, in which tight junctions between the endothelial cells constitute the blood-brain barrier (Fig. 5.2).

In the infant the epithelial cells are small with dark nuclei and scanty cytoplasm. With time the cells become larger, and the nuclei become vesicular (121). A number of changes occur in the choroid plexus with aging, the most common of which is hyalinization of the blood vessels. Almost as frequently are psammoma-like bodies that contain calcium as the dominant mineral and some iron. They have been reported to be present as early as 2 months of age and, rarely, may develop a center of ossification (122). Evidence for recent and remote hemorrhage within this tissue may also be seen and consists of hemosiderin deposits, cholesterol crystals, lipid-laden macrophages, lymphocytes, and even giant cells (122). These later changes may be of such an extent that they produce small usually asymptomatic masses that have been called "xanthogranulomas" (3, 52, 64, 73, 98, 124, 127). Another characteristic finding of the aging process is the presence of "neuroepithelial" cysts, as has been described by Shuangshoti et al. (124).

The stroma of the choroid plexus, like the meninges, is derived embryologically from mesenchyme. This explains the ubiquitous presence of meningeal rests within

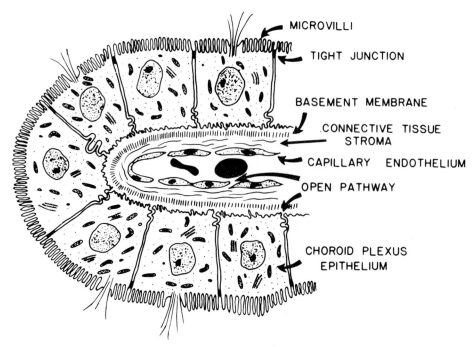

MICROVILLI

TIGHT JUNCTION

BASEMENT MEMBRANE

CONNECTIVE TISSUE STROMA

CAPILLARY ENDOTHELIUM

OPEN PATHWAY

CHOROID PLEXUS EPITHELIUM

Figure 5.1. Diagrammatic representation of the choroid plexus. The capillary endothelium is of the attenuated fenestrated type that allows an ultrafiltrate of plasma to reach the basal side of the epithelial cells. Tight junctions at the apical or ventricular side of the epithelial cells restrict molecular movement and constitute the blood-CSF barrier. (From JG McComb *Cerebrospinal Fluid Formation and Absorption*. In: *Pediatric Neurosurgery: Surgery of the Developing Nervous System.* New York, Grune & Stratton, 1982.)

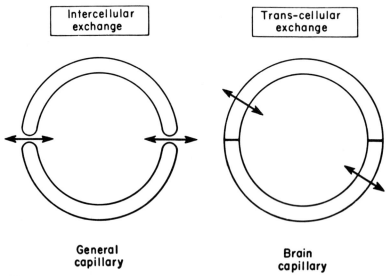

Intercellular exchange

Trans-cellular exchange

General capillary

Brain capillary

Figure 5.2. Diagrammatic representation of the differences between the general and brain capillaries. General capillaries allow all small molecules to diffuse through clefts between adjacent endothelial cells, i.e., extracellular. In contrast, the brain capillary only permits exchanges through the cells, i.e., transcellular. (From Oldendorf WH: Blood brain barrier. In: Bito LZ, Davson HM, Fenstermacher JD (eds): *The Ocular and Cerebrospinal Fluids.* New York, Academic Press, 1977.)

the choroid plexus which are, most certainly, the source of meningiomas within the ventricles and some of those located at the cerebellopontine angle. Histochemical studies of the choroid plexus have shown the presence of immunoglobulin deposits associated with various autoimmune diseases (61). Another study has shown the presence of melanin deposits to such an extent that they were grossly visible (123), and yet another shows diffuse "oncocytic" transformation (56).

CEREBROSPINAL FLUID

Function

The cerebrospinal fluid (CSF) serves several main functions: protection and support, maintenance of the normal homeostasis, elimination of metabolic wastes, and transport within the central nervous system (CNS). CSF suspends the brain and spinal cord in a watery medium and cushions the CNS from external forces applied to the skull or vertebral column. When floating in CSF the brain weighs only 50 g, reflecting the difference between the specific gravity of the brain (1.040) and that of CSF (1.007) (21). The volume of CSF fluctuates reciprocally with the intracranial blood volume and markedly dampens the moment to moment pressure changes associated with respiration, arterial pulse, arterial pressure, and posture. The blood-brain and blood-CSF barriers together allow for the development and maintenance of a specialized fluid environment, the stability and constancy of which is essential to normal CNS function. Changes in serum ion concentrations of such substances as Na, K, Ca, Mg, Cl, are buffered by the homeostatic processes which are different for each and include various transport mechanisms both into and out of the CNS by the parenchyma and/or choroid plexus (21, 27, 55, 143). CSF also functions as a lymphatic-like system, as it allows for passive removal of metabolic wastes and macromolecules by the sink action of the CSF since continual CSF drainage will keep the concentration of various substances low, producing a gradient by which they are cleared (96). CSF within the ventricular cavities and subarachnoid space (SAS) is in continuity with and similar to the fluid in the extracellular spaces, there being no restriction to free exchange of any of its constituents (Fig. 5.3). That CSF participates in neuroendocrine activity has been shown by a predictable effect on pituitary function following injection of biogenic amines into the cerebral ventricles (103). Although still speculative, it is suspected that CSF serves to distribute neuroactive transmitters within the parenchyma.

Formation

It is generally agreed that most CSF is formed in the ventricular system. Possible sites of origin include the choroid plexus, the ependyma, and the parenchyma. A method has not been developed to separate the function of the ependyma from that of the remainder of the parenchyma, so the role of the ependyma in bulk CSF formation is not known, although from morphologic considerations, its contribution is likely to be insignificant.

The choroidal epithelium has the histologic features characteristic of epithelia specialized for the transcellular transport of solutes and solvent (27, 30). The choroid plexus has been compared to the proximal renal tubule, as it can both secrete and absorb a number of substances (21, 27, 143). The discussion that follows will be limited solely to bulk secretion of CSF.

Results from isolated choroid plexus preparations would indicate that 80% or more of CSF production was from this source alone (90, 139). Perfusion of a portion of the ventricular system devoid of choroid plexus has demonstrated that 30–60% of CSF is produced from a nonchoroidal source (87, 101), whereas perfusion of the isoated spinal cord has failed to show any formation of CSF (71). Acetazolamide (Diamox), a carbonic anhydrase inhibitor, can abolish CSF formation in isolated choroid plexus preparations (139) while in vivo it causes only a 50–60% reduction (102). This fact suggests the existence of a substantial source of extrachoroidal CSF formation or, alternatively, that unblocked carbonic anhydrase is available in the non-isolated choroid plexus preparation to maintain some CSF formation. This may explain the failure of choroid plexectomy in the clinical setting to adequately control progressive hydrocephalus (89). It may be

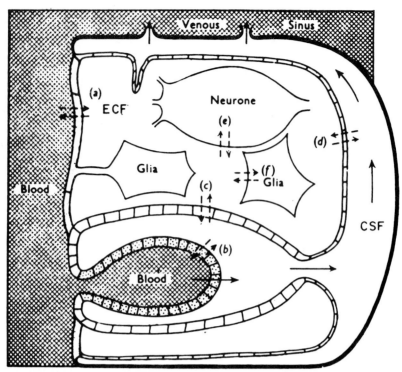

Figure 5.3. Diagrammatic representation of the blood-brain-CSF system. With a fixed intracranial volume, any increase in one component results in a decrease in the other two, i.e., the Monro-Kellie doctrine. Restrictive barriers special to the central nervous system reside at the brain capillary endothelium, at the epithelium of the choroid plexus, and within the arachnoid membrane to form the blood-brain-CSF barriers. *Solid arrows* show bulk flow of CSF from the site of major production, the choroid plexus, within the ventricles to the subarachnoid space (SAS) and then back to the vascular system. Not shown is a significant drainage pathway into the lymphatics. A free exchange occurs between the extracellular fluid and the CSF within the ventricles and SAS, with the ependyma and pia being no barrier. (From H Davson and MWB Bradbury *Symposia of the Society for Experimental Biology* 19:349, 1965.)

added that this operative procedure removes the choroid plexus only from the lateral ventricles, not from the third or fourth ventricles. The contribution of the remaining intact choroid plexus to the formation of CSF and whether or not it can compensate for that portion of the choroid plexus removed is not known.

The various lines of evidence showing the extracellular space (ECS) to be approximately 15% of the brain volume have been summarized by Welch (139). If this space were negligible, as earlier reports would indicate, the presence or absence of communication, free or restricted, between the ECS and the CSF would be irrelevant. The established presence of a substantial ECS, the lack of ependymal resistance to free exchange between the fluid in the ECS and

the CSF, and the similar composition of extracellular fluid and CSF have a direct bearing on the possibility that the parenchyma may be the main source of nonchoroidal CSF formation (12, 13, 104, 139). Support for the brain substance as the principal source of extrachoroidal CSF, amounting to possibly 10–20% of the total CSF production, has been shown in several studies: extracellular markers introduced into the parenchyma move toward the ventricles or SAS at a rate independent of their molecular weights, indicating a flow of fluid in these directions (18, 19, 110, 20). Thus, it appears that normally about 80–90% of CSF secretions derive from the choroid plexus, with the remaining portion most likely originating from the parenchyma. The obvious candidate for the parenchymal source is the capillary endothelium, as its high content of mitochondria could provide the metabolic energy required for such a function (95).

The first step in the formation of CSF is the passage of an ultrafiltrate of plasma through the nontight junctioned choroidal capillary endothelium by hydrostatic pressure into the surrounding connective tissue stroma beneath the epithelium of the villus. The ultrafiltrate is subsequently transformed into a secretion (namely, CSF) by an active metabolic process within the choroidal epithelium via a mechanism that is largely speculative (27, 139). Using the information available, a model constructed on the "standing gradient" hypothesis of Diamond and Bossert (29) has been constructed (Fig. 5.4) which assumes local osmotic forces within the cell to be responsible for the movement of water (142, 118). Sodium-potassium-adenosine triphosphatase (Na-K-ATPase) pumps sodium into the basal side of the cell, with water entering by the osmotic gradient created. Chloride may be coupled with this process or may enter the cell separately (144). Carbonic anhydrase catalyzes the formation of bicarbonate inside the cell, with the hydrogen ion being fed back to the sodium pump as a counter ion with potassium (76). In a manner analogous to that involving the

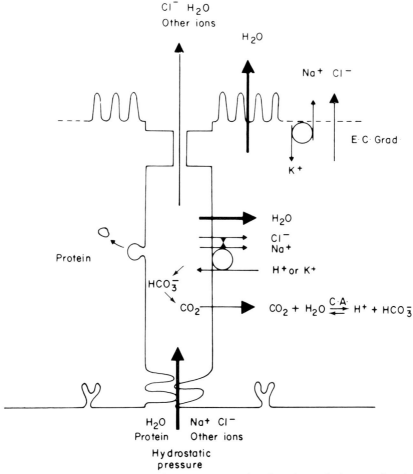

Figure 5.4. Diagrammatic summary of CSF secretion by the choroid plexus. The direction and location of the metabolic pumps are speculative, although their presence is documented. An ultrafiltrate of plasma enters the basal side of the choroid plexus epithelial cell, whereupon it is modified by metabolic processes to produce a secretion at the apical or ventricular side. (From MB Segal and M Pollay (118).)

basal side of the epithelium, Na-K-ATPase located in the microvilli on the apical surface extrudes sodium into the ventricle, followed by osmotically drawn water. Since the cells do not swell or shrink, the sum of the two processes must be in balance (117).

Under normal physiologic conditions, CSF formation can be considered independent of pressure (23, 44, 113) and averages of 20 ml/h or 500 ml/d. Approximately a three-fold turnover of CSF occurs daily as the total volume of the CSF in the ventricles and SAS averages 150 ml. Markedly elevated intraventricular pressure will reduce CSF formation by diminishing the quantity of ultrafiltrate from the choroidal capillary. The effect of temperature on CSF production in patients is not known and probably has little relevance, except in marked hypothermia. Although the data are very limited, CSF production in infants as well as in older patients is reported to be in the normal adult range (23, 67, 68). Neurogenic control of CSF formation has only recently been investigated, as previously it was not possible to separate the effects of choroidal blood flow from direct neurogenic stimulation of the choroidal epithelium. Studies purport that stimulation of adrenergic fibers can acutely diminish CSF flow by 30% (65), whreas stimulation of cholanergic pathways will increase CSF production by as much as 100% without altering blood flow in the choroid plexus (43).

Although it has long been suspected that oversecretion of CSF occurs in the presence of a choroid plexus papilloma, unequivocal evidence for this has been documented twice (33, 88). Evidence for overproduction of CSF in the absence of the choroid plexus papilloma does not exist. Through its presumed action on cyclic adenosine monophosphate, cholera toxin has been reported to double the flow of the CSF (35), a finding which has not been confirmed by another investigation (50). This latter study indicates that the apparent increase in CSF formation may result from plasma entering the ventricles following a breakdown of the blood-brain barrier rather than an increased CSF secretion rate. Drugs that reduce CSF formation do so by interfering with the entire cellular metabolic process or specific transport mechanisms. The ac-

tion of Diamox on CSF production has been extensively studied. This agent decreases CSF production by interfering with the function of carbonic anhydrase and appears to significantly diminish CSF formation in man both acutely and chronically (23, 111). Cutler et al. (23) have noted that, due to the nature of formation versus absorption curve, reduction of normal CSF production by one-third would drop the intracranial pressure by only 1.5 cm of water. This explains why Diamox, or other agents that reduce CSF formation, have not proven to be useful in the control of hydrocephalus. These conclusions have focused investigations into the pathogenesis of hydrocephalus on CSF absorption.

Absorption

The absorption of CSF and its constituents depend upon bulk flow in addition to passive or facilitative diffusion and active transport of specific solutes. The rate of CSF absorption is pressure dependent and relatively linear over a fairly wide physiologic range (23, 44, 111). The resistance to flow diminishes at higher than normal physiologic pressures (25, 74) and may relate to the opening of channels not available at lower pressures. The only proven force responsible for CSF absorption is that of a hydrostatic gradient (139).

Key and Retzius (58) and Weed (134) firmly established that arachnoid villi drain CSF. Those villi that are grossly visible, termed "arachnoid granulations" or "Pacchionian bodies," are functionally similar to those which are not. Controversy remains regarding the structure of the arachnoid villus as to the existence of open channels connecting the arachnoid side with the venous side, for the presence or absence of such channels would mean a basic physiologic difference in the manner in which CSF and its constituents drain. The open villus model would be solely pressure-responsive and would allow for passive escape of macromolecules, whereas a villus covered by a continuous tight-junctioned endothelial membrane would add the factors of osmosis, diffusion, and filtration, and macromolecules would require an active transport process to cross this barrier. The various anatomic studies are fairly evenly divided between these two possibilities. Discrepancy in morphologic findings may relate in part or in whole to the manner in which the villus is prepared for histologic study: a zero pressure gradient between the arachnoid and venous sides of the villus during fixation would allow for its collapse and, as a result, open channels would not be apparent. This explanation is supported by the findings a recent study (63). Another possible mechanism that could bridge the gap between the open versus the closed channel theory of CSF drainage has been proposed by Tripathi (129). He reported the presence of a dynamic transendothelial vacuolization process that temporarily creates an open channel through the villus endothelium, during which CSF and its constituents can flow from the SAS to the blood (128). The size of the passageways in the arachnoid villus is only pertinent if this site is virtually the exclusive location for bulk egress of CSF into the blood stream. If a significant fraction of CSF and its constituents drain elsewhere, the size and nature of the channels in the arachnoid villus is less relevant.

Until recently, the fact that CSF might drain at sites other than the arachnoid villus under normal physiologic conditions has been given scant consideration. If an alternate route is postulated, it is usually associated with the hydrocephalic brain.

In studying the CSF circulation, Schwalbe (115) in 1869 contended that the lymphatic channels were the major drainage pathways for CSF. Key and Retzius (58) took exception to this and proposed the villus as the major absorptive site, although these authors did observed that a small amount of their injected colored gelatin passed along the cranial nerves into the lymphatic system. Weed (134), in examining the work of Key and Retzius, noted that many of the arachnoid villi draining the emulsions in their cadaver preparations were ruptured by the high injected pressure (60 mm Hg), and he cautioned that such high pressures produce artifactual drainage routes. The genius of Weed's experiment was in his use of two true noncytotoxic isotonic solutions, containing ammonium citrate and potassium ferrocyanide, that subsequently precipitated granules of Prussian blue when the carotid arteries of the experimental animals were perfused with an acidified formalin mixture (134). In this way, he avoided the introductions of particulate matter into the SAS, which could possibly have led to plugging of the normal drainage pathways. He also carefully controlled the pressures at which the solutions were introduced into the SAS to keep within physiological limits (130–180 mm H_2O). This work firmly established the arachnoid villus as a major site for bulk CSF outflow. It is rarely mentioned, though, that Weed acknowledged that some of his injected solutions drained into the mucosa of the paranasal sinuses, nasal mucosa, cranial nerve root sheaths, and cervical lymph nodes; he thought that these routes were accessory. The idea that a portion of the CSF could and did drain via the lymphatic system was gradually relegated to obscurity and, for more than a generation now, standard texts and teaching have limited CSF drainage solely to the arachnoid villus. Recent laboratory investigations would indicate that a significant quantity of CSF, and under certain circumstances even the majority, can drain via the lymphatics (7–10, 69, 80, 82, 83). Ultrastructure of how CSF gains access to the lymphatics has only recently been studied. Shen et al. (120) have shown that macromolecules injected into the SAS will rapidly appear in the arachnoidal trabecular meshwork at the dural-scleral junction. The tracer then traverses the arachnoid barrier layer via microcanals to reach the intraorbital connective tissue and, subsequently, the lymphatics. This confirms previous physiologic studies (80, 83, 82). Presently no studies show to what extent lymphatic drainage of CSF exists in man, but some support for this concept comes from the clinical observation, that parents of children with CSF diverting shunts occasionally report nasal congestion and periorbital or facial swelling when their child's shunt becomes obstructed. The lymphatic drainage of CSF seems likely to play a role in the pathophysiology of hydrocephalus, either as an alternative pathway of drainage or as a cause, in cases of impaired access to the lymphatic system.

A question debated for sometime is whether or not CSF can be absorbed by the brain. The penetration of substances into

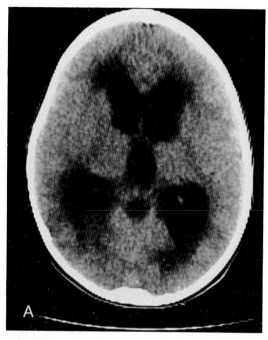
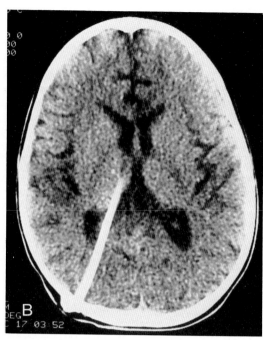

Figure 5.5. (A) Computerized tomographic (CT) scan of a child with an obstruction of the fourth ventricle producing acute noncommunicating hydrocephalus. The hypodense areas in the periventricular white matter are a result of CSF migrating from the dilated ventricles into the parenchyma in response to increased intraventricular pressure. No sulci are visible. (B) CT scan of the same child after a CSF diverting shunt has been inserted. The ventricles have markedly diminished in size, no periventricular hypodensity is evident, and the sulci are clearly visible.

the periventricular region of the hydrocephalic animal has been well documented (53, 141). With the advent of computerized tomographic (CT) scanning, periventricular hypodensity may be noted in the presence of hydrocephalus (Figs. 5.5A and B) and has been shown to be the result of CSF migrating into the area surrounding the ventricles in the face of increased intraventricular pressure (47). CSF in the parenchyma, indicative of migration, however, does not necessarily equate with absorption. Bulk flow of CSF is usually measured via the clearance of various reference macromolecules, such as albumin, which by necessity would have to enter the lumen of the blood vessel and be removed by the systemic circulation. It has been shown that cerebral capillaries have a very low permeability to albumin, and that most of any given quantity of albumin injected into the brain can be recovered from the lymph and CSF, with very little being lost to the blood (8). Zervas et al. (145) have found that horseradish peroxidase (HRP), which

has nearly the same molecular weight as albumin, could penetrate to the basal lamina of the capillary endothelium but not beyond. In addition to the impermeability of the capillaries to various reference markers, the clearance of which is the measure of CSF absorption, Welch (139) has pointed out that, as absorption occurs in response to a pressure drop, it would require a higher pressure outside the lumen of the capillary than inside, which obviously would lead to its collapse and preclude absorption. The extracellular space in the brain, which amounts to 15%, readily allows fluid flow in the parenchyma. This flow of fluid within the parenchyma is present under normal physiologic conditions (110), and its velocity and direction are responsive to changes in hydrostatic (109) and osmotic pressure gradients (110).

Macromolecules injected into the CSF of the ventricles or SAS have been observed to readily penetrate the extracellular spaces of the parenchyma, and vice versa (12, 16, 145). Evidence thus supports the contention that the brain, rather than absorbing CSF, is acting as a conduit for fluid to move from the ventricles to the SAS or into the prelymphatic channels of the blood vessels.

The choroid plexus, normally thought to be the major site of CSF production, might also possibly be involved in the absorption of CSF. Ventricular fluid can enter the subependymal extracellular space (20); once there it could flow into the stroma of the choroid plexus, where absorption could take place at the choroidal capillaries since these capillaries are fenestrated and do not have tight junctions like those in the parenchyma. The role of choroid plexus CSF absorption in hydrocephalus is not known.

As discussed above, CSF drainage appears to take place from the SAS surrounding nerve root sleeves, with subsequent entry into the lymphatic system; however, questions remain as to whether the arachnoid membrane itself can absorb CSF. Physiologic (6, 135) and electron microscopic studies (93) indicate that under normal physiological conditions the arachnoid membrane serves as an effective barrier to large molecules, that is, it functions as a blood-CSF barrier in this location. At higher than normal pressures the barrier layer apparently can be disrupted, with the resultant penetration of macromolecules into the extracellular space of the dura mater and dural lymphatic channels (15). At unphysiologically high pressures, disruption of this arachnoid barrier layer may allow for significant absorption of CSF.

Circulation

The multiple functions of CSF, coupled with its fairly rapid turnover, indeed make CSF "third circulation," as first referred to by Cushing (22). CSF circulation throughout the CNS is maintained primarily by the hydrostatic difference between the newly formed CSF within the ventricles and parenchyma and that at its sites of drainage. Less important are factors associated with pulsations of the brain and choroid plexus from the arterial tree, respiratory variations, changes in bodily position, and ciliary action.

CSF is produced in all four ventricles, although by far the majority emanates from the lateral ventricles consistent with the larger amount of choroid plexus tissue present in the lateral, as compared with the midline ventricle. The lateral ventricles are joined together at the anterior superior aspect of the third ventricle by the foramina of Monroe, each of which measures less than 1 cm at its greatest diameter. Obstruction to CSF flow can occur at one or both of these foramina by a fairly small mass. The third ventricle, normally only 3–5 mm in width, drains into the aqueduct of Sylvius, the diameter of which normally measures only 2 mm. The relatively long and narrow aqueduct makes it the most frequent site of obstruction within the ventricular system. The volume of CSF entering the fourth ventricle from the aqueduct of Sylvius is increased by that produced by the choroid plexus in the fourth ventricle, all of which exists through the midline foramen of Magendie and the perilateral foramina of Luschka into the cisterns at the base of the brain. Although the cisterns receiving the CSF are of ample volume, the three outlet foramina are quite small and can be a site of obstruction to CSF drainage. It appears that extracellular fluid is also produced by a process of secretion at the capillary-glial complex. This extracellular fluid volume then flows through the parenchyma along the intracellular clefts between brain cells or via the perivascular (Virchow-Robin) spaces to empty into either the CSF within the ventricles or the CSF within the SAS.

CSF circulation occurs in all areas of the SAS, with some regions more active than others. Although significant variation occurs, fluid egressing from the midline foramen of Magendie flows into the cisterna magna and then is distributed into the SAS surrounding the cerebellar hemisphere, the spinal SAS, and the cisterns anterior to the medulla and pons. The fluid draining from the lateral foramina of Luschka into the cerebellopontine and prepontine cisterns is added to the fluid draining from the foramen of Magendie. From the basilar cisterns, fluid flows either through the interpeduncular and prechiasmatic cisterns into the Sylvian fissure and callosal cisterns or via the ambient and precerebellar cisterns to pass into the SAS about the medial and posterior aspects of the cerebral hemispheres. Composition of CSF varies from one region to the other, as indicated by the presence of only 10 mg of protein within the ventricular fluid, 15–20 mg at the cisterna magna, and 30–45 mg at the lumbar subarachnoid space. Possible sites of CSF absorption have been previously discussed (see Absorption).

HYDROCEPHALUS

Introduction

Hydrocephalus is a net accumulation of cerebrospinal fluid (CSF) and occurs following an inbalance between CSF formation and absorption. Hydrocephalus results from an alteration of a normal physiologic process and has multiple etiologies. In almost all instances hydrocephalus develops after an increase in the resistance of CSF absorption, and at some point the CSF pressure is elevated, which may or may not be maintained, depending upon subsequent compensatory forces. With the one very rare exception of CSF overproduction from a choroid plexus papilloma, all hydrocephalus is obstructive. Therefore the terms obstructive and nonobstructive hydrocephalus have been supplanted by those of communicating and noncommunicating hydrocephalus. By definition, noncommunicating hydrocephalus indicates impairment of CSF flow within the ventricular system, while in communicating hydrocephalus the obstruction is distal to the ventricles. Improved methods of treating hydrocephalus have made the distinction between the two types less essential, but significant etiologic differences exist. Noncommunicating hydrocephalus results from such lesions as aqueductal occlusion, from obstruction of the outlets of the fourth ventricle, from masses within or adjacent to the ventricular system, and from hemorrhage and infection within the ventricular system. Communicating hydrocephalus is usually associated with subarachnoid hemorrhage, meningitis, and spread of tumor within the SAS. Occasionally, extra-axial masses encroach upon the SAS directly or indirectly increasing the resistance to CSF absorption, thereby producing a communication type of hydrocephalus. Obstruction of the venous drainage from the brain alone most likely does not produce hydrocephalus. Hydrocephalus can also be classified as con-

genital or acquired, but such a distinction has no meaning in terms of the pathophysiologic process.

Etiology

The incidence of congenital hydrocephalus occurring alone is about 1/1000 live births while hydrocephalus associated with spina bifida cystica (myelomeningocele) is present in 1–3/1000 live births. Most causes of congenital hydrocephalus are not known while a small number appear to result from maternal infection (cytomegalic virus, toxoplasmosis and, possibly, mumps, rubella, varicella, etc.), nutritional disorders (experimentally produced by hypo- and hypervitaminosis A), teratogenesis (radiation, lysergic acid dielthylamide), and genetic factors (X linked). The X-linked form of congenital hydrocephalus occurs only in males and accounts for approximately 1–2% of the total number not associated with neural tube defects. There appears to be a slightly increased risk of isolated congenital hydrocephalus being present in subsequent siblings, as compared to the general population. A much higher incidence of risk is associated if the hydrocephalus is related to spina bifida cystica. Acquired forms of hydrocephalus result from infection, tumors, trauma, and vascular lesions.

CSF Production

Production of CSF in hydrocephalus is either normal or near normal (62, 66, 68). In compensated hydrocephalus the rate of absorption must equal the rate of formation or approximately 500 ml/day, and in the uncompensated state only a small fraction of the total amount secreted is retained; thus, the overwhelming majority of CSF output is still absorbed. As CSF formation is relatively constant, the change in resistance to absorption determines the CSF pressure and whether or not the hydrocephalus is progressive. Impairment of CSF absorption in communicating hydrocephalus could occur at some or all of the following sites: the arachnoid villus; the lymphatic channels associated with the cranial and spinal nerves; lymphatic channels in the adventitia of the cerebral vessels; or the arachnoid membrane. If CSF outflow from the ventricles is blocked, (i.e., noncommunicating hydrocephalus), the passage of CSF could still proceed along blood vessel adventitia or through the ECS of the parenchyma to reach the brain surface. In addition, it is possible that absorption of CSF could occur in the stroma of the choroid plexus through the fenestrated capillaries at this location. Assuming complete ventricular block, which is not always the case (114), additional ways for CSF to exit the ventricles would be via the dilated spinal cord central canal (92, 138) or through a fistulous opening created by a rupture of the ventricular system (81, 82) into the SAS at such regions as the lamina terminalis or suprapineal recess.

Arachnoid Villi

The observation that several laboratory animals and infants have arachnoid villi but no arachnoid granulations was sited by Dandy and Blackfan (24) as an argument against these structures having an important role in CSF absorption. Subsequent investigations have shown that the arachnoid villi and granulations are anatomically and functionally the same, the only difference being that arachnoid granulations are visible to the unaided eye (17, 35). If the arachnoid villi are the major sites of CSF absorption, their numbers and individual structure should have some bearing on the development of hydrocephalus. That the number and size of arachnoid granulations increase with age need not have any implications, as there does not appear to be any relationship between those villi that are visible, namely, granulations, and their ability to absorb CSF. Few investigators have studied the villus in hydrocephalus, and those who have done so have mainly concentrated on villi associated with the superior sagittal sinus (SSS), since the greatest concentration of these structures per volume of dural sinus exists at this region (17, 40, 136), although villi are present along all of the other major sinuses, some of the major cerebral veins, and veins associated with intracranial and spinal nerves (17, 58, 79, 119, 137). Winkelman and Fay (140) examined the arachnoid granulations in 200 autopsied cases associated with preexisting convulsive disorders, and reported these structures to be absent in 14 and diminished in 28 instances. Clin-

ical correlation found hydrocephalus to be presnt in only three cases in the group with aplasia and none with hypoplasia. Gilles and Davidson (40) examined only the SSS region for arachnoid villi in an infant and a child at autopsy, each with communicating hydrocephalus. In one case no villi were present, and in the other only a few displastic villi were found. In a more thorough postmortem study Gutierrez et al. (41) examined the superior sagittal, straight and lateral sinuses of two children, searching for arachnoid villi. No villi were found in one child who had communicating hydrocephalus, and only two small patches containing a few villi were found in the second child, who did not have hydrocephalus. In spite of the near or complete lack of observed villi, CSF was being absorbed somewhere, albeit inadequately, in three of these four cases. Obviously CSF could have been absorbed at villi elsewhere within the CNS at sites not studied, or at locations without villi. Examining the entire CNS for villi would be an arduous task, and it seems to have been done rarely, if at all.

In the clinical setting, spontaneous subarachnoid hemorrhage can lead to hydrocephalus (38). Experimental studies of the arachnoid villi following the introduction of blood into the SAS have shown a variable degree of villus distention and trapping of the red blood cells (RBCs) within (1, 34). That RBC's can fill the villus following entry of blood into the SAS and can be associated with hydrocephalus does not necessarily imply that the villus is the sole or main site of CSF absorption, as the RBC's could affect all of the routes of drainage that have been previously considered. The same argument will also hold true for those instances of hydrocephalus associated with elevated levels of protein within the CSF (28, 37).

Morphologic Changes

The rate of ventricular enlargement will depend upon to what degree the resistance to absorption has increased and the distensibility of the ventricular system. That part of the ventricular system that enlarges first and reaches the largest size is surrounded by the least structural resistance (85). The temporal horn and body of the lateral ventricle dilates slower than the remainder of this cavity, as the basal ganglia offers more resistance to enlargement than does the white matter adjacent to the frontal and occipital horns. The fourth ventricle enlarges less readily than the lateral ventricles but may eventually become quite dilated. The structure least likely to dilate is the aqueduct of Sylvius. Experimental acute complete obstruction of the fourth ventricle in primates produces a rapid dilatation proximal to the site of blockage in the first 3 h, followed by a 3-h period of less rapid enlargement. After 6 h the ventricles only slowly increase in size, reaching a gross steady state in a few days (85). Ependymal cells lining the ventricles become thin and disrupted, periventricular edema develops, and tracers placed into the ventricular CSF migrate into the periventricular white matter (86). Changes secondary to hydrocephalus effect almost exclusively the white matter, especially that surrounding the ventricles, with the grey matter of both the cortex and deep nuclear masses being spared. The severity and duration of the elevated pressure within the ventricles determines the chronic changes that follow, which include progressive axonal disintegration, secondary myelin degeneration and, finally, reactive gliosis (113) which lead to irreversible tissue damage and atrophy. Clinical experience, as documented by CT scanning (Figs. 5.5*A* and *B*) and from animal studies (112) has shown that decompressing the dilated ventricular system in acute hydrocephalus will result in a very rapid reconstitution of the cortical mantle (rebulking of the parenchyma). The mechanism by which this occurs is poorly understood.

Most forms of congenital hydrocephalus are of the noncommunicating type, with obstruction at the aqueduct of Sylvius accounting for more than two thirds of this group (89). Most obstructions at the aqueduct, usually referred to as aqueductal stenosis, are characterized by either gliosis or forking of this structure. In aqueductal gliosis an overgrowth of the subependymal glia occurs and, although the cause is most often not known, it may be the result of a postinflammatory ependymitis. A forked aqueduct divides into several blind channels surrounded by normal brain, without an increase of subependymal glial tissue.

Aqueductal forking is more frequently noted in conjunction with other congenital anomalies, i.e., myelomeningocele, and is more likely developmentally related. The frequency of the site at which obstruction occurs within the ventricular system corresponds well to the anatomical locations where it is narrowed. Since the aqueduct of Sylvius is the most constricted region, it follows that it has the highest incidence of blockage. In decreasing order of frequency, obstruction also occurs at the outlets of the fourth ventricle, the intraventricular foramen of Munro, the third ventricle and, lastly, a portion of the lateral ventricles, such as a trapped temporal horn. Obstruction may occur at more than one location, as may be the case with myelomeningocele, since the *ever present* Chiari II malformation may impede CSF flow at the aqueduct, the outlets of the fourth ventricle, or in the basal cisterns of the posterior fossa. Following intraventricular hemorrhage or meningitis and ventriculitis, obstructions can develop both within and outside of the ventricles, and often a combination of both occurs. It has also been suggested that dilatation of the ventricular system in communicating hydrocephalus might compress the SAS, thereby producing a secondary block to CSF absorption as well.

CEREBRAL EDEMA

Blood-Brain and Blood-CSF Barriers

In order to better understand cerebral edema, it was first helpful to review the structure and function of the blood-brain and blood-CSF barriers. Ehrlich (31) introduced the term blood-brain barrier after observing that vital dyes given intravenously into laboratory animals produced staining of tissues throughout the body but were excluded from the brain. Although it had long been speculated that the blood-brain barrier occurred at the cerebral capillary level, it was not until the advent of electron microscopy (EM) that the tight junctions between capillary endothelial cells were noted to constitute this barrier (Fig. 5.6*A*) (11, 106). In addition to tight junctions, the capillary endothelium has but few vesicles, a high density of mitochondria, and several enzymes not found elsewhere which serve to differentiate these

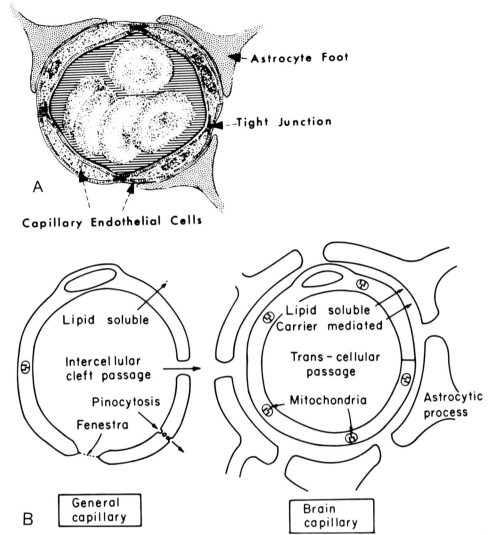

Figure 5.6. Normal cerebral capillary. Tight intercellular junctions are present. Astrocytic end-feet surround the capillaries. (From RA Fishman (36).)

capillaries from general capillaries (Fig. 5.6B). It is the inductive influence of the astrocytic end-feet which determine the special nature of the capillary endothelium (125). The main function of the capillary endothelium is to determine and closely regulate the composition of the extracellular fluid (ECF) bathing the neurons. Contrary to what was previously thought, the astrocytic end-feet do not nourish the neurons, as adequate substrates can freely diffuse in the ECF between the astrocytic end-feet (97). The endothelium may also be the site for the majority, if not all, of the extrachoroidal formation of CSF (95).

The central nervous system (CNS) would not have its protective environment if there were a barrier at the capillary endothelium alone unless CSF is also restricted from free exchanges at the choroid plexus and arachnoid membrane. Subsequent studies have shown that tight junctions at the apical end of the choroid epithelium (12) and within the arachnoid membrane (93) complete the barrier and together help to inhibit any net changes in the chemical composition of the CSF and ECF, as compared to what happens in other organs. The barrier differs depending on the nature of the substance in question and is influenced by its configuration, polarity, whether or not it is bound to plasma proteins, its lipid solubility, and the presence or absence of specific transport systems. Osmotic differences between the blood and brain, however, are only sustained for brief periods, as the barrier is readily permeable to water, and thus the brain and CSF osmolality vary directly and rapidly with changes in plasma osmolality.

Definition

The first correct hypothesis as to what constituted vasogenic edema, the most common form of cerebral edema, was made by Andral (2) in 1883, who suggested that a disturbance in the blood vessels led to a secondary accumulation of a serous exudate. That cerebral edema was associated with an increased water content was first noted by Magendie (72) following dry weight determinations of edematous brain. The modern definition of cerebral edema, which can be used interchangeably with cerebral swelling, is an increase in brain volume due to a localized or diffuse abnormal accumulation of water and sodium. Cerebral edema is different from cerebral engorgement, as engorgement results from an increase in blood volume on the basis of either vasodilatation or impairment of venous outflow. If severe enough, brain engorgement can subsequently lead to cerebral edema.

Morphologic Changes

From a gross neuropathologic standpoint, a diffusely edematous brain at autopsy is soft, large, and heavier than anticipated, with flattened gyri, narrowed sulci, and slit-like ventricles. If edema is severe enough, various forms of herniation can be observed (see below, Central Nervous System Herniations). However, from an histologic standpoint the changes that constitute cerebral edema are quite meager, a fact that kept the concept of cerebral edema from being understood for a considerable period of time. With the introduction of EM it was thought that at last it would be possible to define the ultrastructural changes that occur with cerebral edema. However, the early EM findings proved to be at variance with what could be seen

grossly and with light microscopy and indicated virtually no extracellular space, with only a 200-Å gap between the glial cell processes (70). These initial EM findings also differed from studies of extracellular markers (26) and electrical impedance (133), which indicate an extracellular space of approximately 15%. This discrepancy was subsequently resolved by showing that during routine chemical fixation for EM, fluid redistribution occurs, reducing the extracellular space (131). The use of freeze substitution methods, rather than chemical fixation techniques, eventually demonstrated conclusively by EM that an appreciable extracellular space was indeed present (5, 130, 132), thereby reconciling the differences between morphology and physiology. The EM changes associated with the vasogenic type of cerebral edema include disruption of tight junctions and the presence of an increased number of cytoplasmic vesicles within the endothelial cells (46).

Jaburek (51) was the first to observe that certain regions of the brain were more edema prone than others, especially the white matter. Morphologic studies have shown that the white matter has parallel bundles of unattached myelinated fibers with a surrounding, loose extracellular space while the gray matter has a much higher cell density with many connections between cells which reduce the number of direct linear pathways and render the extracellular space in the gray matter much less subject to swelling. Hallervorden (42) proposed a hydromechanical theory of edema spread which hypothesized that edema fluid flowed via pressure gradient along the pathways of least resistance, findings which have been substantiated by experimental work (77). Thus, the morphologic and physiologic findings help to explain why the white matter is much more edema prone.

Classification

Cerebral edema was first classified as to whether it was associated with necrosis, radiation, tumor, inflammation, granulocytic response, ischemia, toxins, osmotic disturbance or hydrocephalus. Further understanding of the pathophysiology of cerebral edema came with the division of cerebral into vasogenic and cytotoxic types by Klatzo (59) (Table 5.1). Vasogenic edema, present with brain tumors, abscesses, hemorrhage, infarction, and contusion, is the most common form seen from a clinical standpoint and results from breakdown of the blood-brain barrier. The increased permeability of the capillary endothelium leads to an extravasation of fluid and plasma proteins, of which albumin is the major constituent. The EM of vasogenic edema shows defects in the endothelial tight junctions as well as increase in the number of vesicles within the endothelial cytoplasm (Fig. 5.7).

The other type of cerebral edema described by Klatzo (59) (Table 5.1) cytotoxic edema, is characterized by swelling of all cellular elements, endothelial, glial, and neuronal, with a subsequent reduction in extracellular space (Fig. 5.8). Fishman (37) prefers the term cellular edema to cytotoxic edema because the changes are not necessarily toxic in nature and can result from conditions in which energy depletion interferes with the normal metabolic processes.

Anoxia or ischemia results in rapid failure of the adenosine triphosphate (ATP)-dependent sodium pumps within cells, allowing intracellular sodium to accumulate, with water following to maintain osmotic equilibrium. In cellular edema, capillary permeability is not effected as indicated by normal CSF protein, negative radiopharmaceutical brain scans, and no contrast enhancement seen with CT, as can be seen with vasogenic edema. Hypo-osmolality secondary to acute dilutional hyponatremia, inappropriate antidiuretic hormone secretion or acute sodium depletion can also produce cellular edema. Osmotic disequilibrium associated with hemodialysis or diabetic ketoacidosis can also lead to the same type of edema. The edema which follows acute arterial occlusion is initially cellular in nature, as it results from failure of the ATP-dependent sodium pumps. If the arterial occlusion is maintained, cerebral infarction occurs, and vasogenic edema, secondary to breakdown of the blood-brain barrier, will develop hours to days later after overlapping with the initial cellular

Table 5.1
Classification of Cerebral Edema[a]

	Vasogenic	Cellular (cytotoxic)	Interstitial (hydrocephalic)
Pathogenesis	Increased capillary permeability	Cellular swelling— glial neuronal, endothelial	Increased brain fluid due to increased resistance of CSF absorption
Location of edema	Chiefly white matter	Gray and white matter	Chiefly periventricular white
Edema fluid composition	Plasma filtrate including plasma protein	Increased intracellular water and sodium	Cerebrospinal fluid
Extracellular fluid volume	Increased	Decreased	Increased
Capillary permeability to macromolecules (plasma proteins)	Increased	Normal	Normal
Clinical disorders	Brain tumor Abscess Infarction Trauma Hemorrhage Lead encephalopathy Ischemia	Hypoxia Hypo-osmolality due to water intoxication Disequilibrium syndromes Ischemia Purulent meningitis (granulocytic edema) Reye's syndrome	Hydrocephalus Pseudotumor (?) Purulent meningitis (granulocytic edema)

[a] Adapted from Klatzo (59), Manz (75), and Fishman (36).

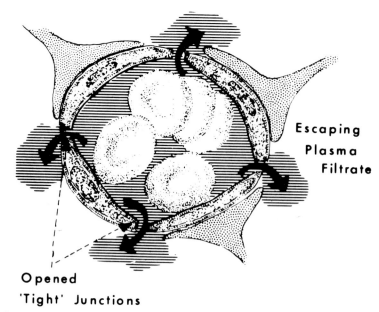

Escaping

Plasma

Filtrate

Opened

'Tight' Junctions

Figure 5.7. Alterations associated with vasogenic edema. Intercellular tight junctions allow passage of a plasma filtrate. Also present are an increased number of pinocytic vesicles which may be responsible for increased passage of macromolecules as well. (From RA Fishman (36).)

edema. That this sequence of events occurs is confirmed by the observation of the infarction not enhancing with radiopharmaceutical brain scanning techniques nor with CT scanning contrast infusion until a week or more after the event.

A third type of edema called interstitial or hydrocephalic edema has been added and is seen in hydrocephalic conditions (36, 75) (Table 5.1). This type of edema develops when CSF migrates into the periventricular white matter, increasing the ECF volume in response to an elevation in intraventricular pressure.

Mechanisms

The understanding of the mechanisms of cerebral edema has slowly evolved through physical, chemical, histologic, and physiologic studies, most of which are suited to use only in the laboratory. The advent of CT scanning has made it possible to have the opportunity to dynamically assess the process in a clinical setting. The changes associated with diffuse cerebral swelling on the CT scan include areas of hypodensity and decrease in the volume of the subarachnoid space and ventricles. If the edema is localized, mass effect may be present, as indicated by displacement of contiguous structures. White matter edema can easily be seen on CT with typical finger-like projections of hypodense areas and can indicate an increase in water content (Fig. 5.9). Another advantage of CT scanning is that serial studies can show the progression or regression of the edema.

Since the brain's expansion is limited by being confined to a rigid cranial container, the significance of cerebral edema lies in the increased brain volume that results. At first, the changes in brain volume are compensated by a decrease in CSF and blood volume which maintains normal intracranial pressure and blood flow. Progressive swelling will exceed compensatory mechanisms and intracranial pressure will begin to rise. If intracranial pressure becomes high enough, cerebral perfusion pressure will decrease interfering with cerebral blood flow, although the relationship between the two is not necessarily linear. In addition to reducing the necessary substrates for normal brain function, i.e., oxygen, glucose, and amino acids, progressive brain swelling, be it focal or diffuse, will eventually result in herniation of cerebral tissue, producing additional local ischemia and interfering with neurologic function. At times,

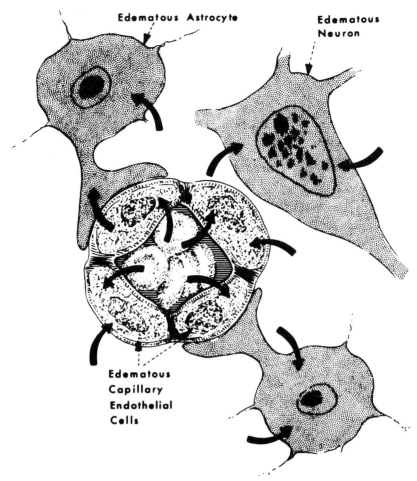

Figure 5.8. Cellular or cytotoxic edema. Neurons, glia, and endothelial swell as a result of increased volume of intracellular fluid. (From RA Fishman (36).)

the progression of edema appears to be disproportionate to the causative insult. Reasons for the progression of edema are not fully understood but it appears, particularly in vasogenic edema, that the fluid entering the parenchyma includes harmful factors released at the site of injury which are augmented by additional plasma born noxious materials. Glutamate, serotonin, fatty acids, products of the kallikrein-cli-ninogen-kinin system, free radicals, lysosomal enzymes, etc., are substances which may extend the damage over the surrounding areas distant from the site of initial damage (4, 91).

Neurologic Function

Does cerebral edema in and of itself cause neurologic dysfunction if there is no sig-

nificant increase in intracranial pressure, decrease in cerebral blood flow, or herniation of cerebral tissue? Hossmann et al. (48), using a brain tumor model with a purely vasogenic form of edema, showed no change in cerebral blood flow, in autoregulation, or in the EEG if the intracranial pressure remained normal. Marshall et al. (78) found that mice poisoned with triethyltin, producing a cytotoxic form of cerebral edema, remained neurologically normal if the intracranical pressure was not elevated. Rapoport and Thompson (105), using hyperosmotic solutions, opened the blood-brain barrier in monkeys. Even though a vasogenic form of cerebral edema was created, no neurologic abnormalities or changes in behavior of the primates were noted. Recent studies using serial CT scans in patients showed that no abnormal neu-

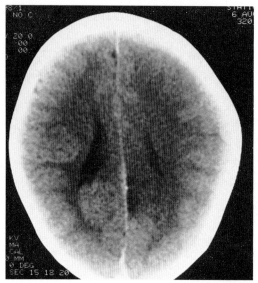

Figure 5.9. Computerized tomographic scan without enhancement of a patient with cerebral edema. The effacement of the lateral ventricle on the right side indicates mass effect. Extensive hypodensity is present in the white matter on the right side, as compared to the left side.

rologic findings or changes in EEG were related to focal white matter edema (99). Thus evidence would indicate that cerebral edema in and of itself does not measurably alter brain function, assuming no herniations of cerebral tissue, if intracranial pressure and cerebral blood flow remain within the normal range.

Resolution

The progression of vasogenic edema will be governed by the area of blood-brain barrier damage, arterial pressure, tissue hydrostatic pressure, oncotic pressure, and elastic properties and architecture of the tissue involved (14). The edema progresses until an equilibrium is reached whereby the amount of fluid escaping is equal to that being cleared and is determined by the resistance to fluid flow in the surrounding tissue. The driving force for the clearance of edema fluid is solely a pressure gradient (77), with much of the edema fluid being cleared into the CSF (109). Tissue resistance to movement of fluid is decreased in the edematous brain, as compared to the normal brain, enhancing the removal of the edema fluid (108). Klatzo et al. (60) contend that clearance of the edema is also related

to the intraglial uptake of osmotically active serum proteins, thereby releasing water to be reabsorbed. In the vasogenic form of edema, the blood-brain barrier eventually begins to reestablish itself, and the quantity of fluid and protein in the extracellular space gradually returns to normal. Homeostasis once again is established when all the abnormal fluid volume and macromolecules have been removed from the site of injury.

CENTRAL NERVOUS SYSTEM HERNIATIONS

There are a number of different herniation phenomena involving the central nervous system that are of importance to both clinician and pathologist as they treat and deal with disease of the CNS. All mass-increasing lesions of the CNS may result in one or more of these herniations. This section will discuss the various herniations and their results both clinically and pathologically. It must be emphasized at the outset that care must be exercised in the diagnosis of central nervous system herniations. They are easily and commonly overdiagnosed because of a lack of knowledge of the variations of normal, and such diagnosis may lead to unfortunate results (49).

Fungus Cerebri

One of the least common herniations as seen in civilian situations is the herniation of the brain through a defect in the skull as the result of trauma or surgery. This herniation, the so-called "fungus cerebri," is rarely seen in this day of steroid therapy, at least in civilian situations. It is more common in battlefield hospitals where massive trauma under less controlled situations occurs. Rarely, it is seen following massive cerebral injury, either traumatic or otherwise, followed by surgery with a large craniotomy defect, with subsequent herniation of swollen brain through the defect (Fig. 5.10). It must be remembered that though the term "fungus" is used, it has nothing to do with an infection, but rather the appearance of the herniating brain growing like a fungus, a mushroom, through the skull defect. As might be expected from the causes, this is most often a fatal phenomenon, or is at least most commonly associated with a fatal outcome (146).

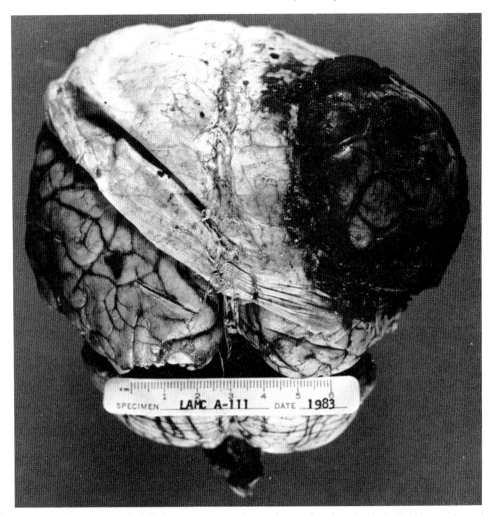

Figure 5.10. Fungus cerebri. This autopsy specimen shows the sharply delimited area of cerebrum that has herniated through a craniotomy defect. Courtesy of Dr. John S. Daniel, III, Letterman General Hospital.

Subfalcial Herniation

A more common type of herniation phenomenon is subfalcial herniation. This may occur with any lesion that is one-sided in the hemispheres with a mass increase, thus laying the way open to herniation from one side to the other. Very often, the medial surface of the herniating hemisphere is pressed against the rigid midline falx cerebri and is forced to herniate under the sharp edge of that structure, resulting in the herniation (Fig. 5.11.). The injury is most often to the cingulate gyrus or the supracingulate gyrus, but the exact area injured depends on the vagaries of individual anatomy. Again, since this phenomenon is most commonly seen with large hemispheric lesions, it is most commonly associated with a fatal outcome, and the clinical parameters are not well defined (100).

Transtentorial Herniation

The most important of the herniation phenomena from the standpoint of frequency, clinical definition, and our occasional ability to ameliorate, prevent, or rescue a patient from the almost surely fatal consequences of the herniation, is the combination of events called "transtentorial herniation." In this scenario the anatomy of the individual is as important as the causative pathologic process. This hernia-

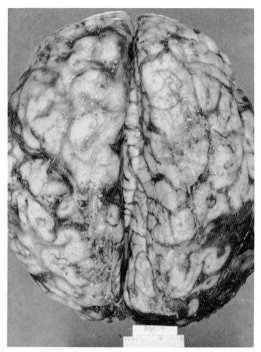

Figure 5.11. Subfalcial herniation. The sharp line of compression of the cingulate gyrus is seen, with partial herniation of this structure under the falx toward the left side.

tion may be the result of any mass-increasing lesion above the tentorium. It is usually the result of lateralized lesions but probably only because they are most frequent. Midline lesions may also result in the herniation (49, 57, 84, 100, 107, 116, 126).

Transtentorial herniation is or may be a combination of lesions, again depending on individual anatomy and the specific location of the pathologic process and its rapidity of evolution. In order to understand the several phenomena it is probably best to examine them individually.

With lateralized lesions very often quite early one sees evidence of herniation of the anteromedial part of the hippocampus over the edge of the tentorium, the so-called "uncal herniation." Caution must be exercised in making a pathologic diagnosis of this herniation, lacking a reasonable pathologic substrate, since many of us have a degreee of "physiologic" notching of our unci, even unsymmetrically. For that reason such notching must be interpreted with caution. However, this herniation is seen with greater frequency in patients with lateralized cerebral lesions and under these

circumstances must be considered a significant lesion (116).

With continued herniation of the medial temporal lobe over the edge of the tentorium, there is increasing possibility of compression of the posterior cerebral artery between the herniating temporal lobe and the crus cerebri (Fig. 5.12). This compression may compress local branches, causing local medial temporal lobe (hippocampal) infarction, complete or incomplete (Fig. 5.14), or may result in medial occipital lobe infarction, almost always hemorrhagic, resulting in a visual field defect (Fig. 5.15). The local effect of the herniation is a contusion of the medial temporal lobe where it impinges on the tentorium (Fig. 5.13). At this time, too, there is the increasing probability of compression of the third nerve by the herniating temporal lobe. This possible compression may transiently result in irritation of the parasympathetic fibers with pupillary constriction but is more commonly manifest as parasympathetic paralysis and resultant unopposed sympathetic stimulation with pupillary mydriasis. It may be unilateral, under which circumstances it is frequently localizing as to side of lesion, but it is often not recognized until it is bilateral (49, 100, 116, 126).

Compression of the posterior cerebral ar-

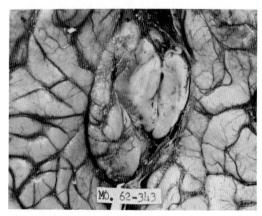

Figure 5.12. Transtentorial herniation. The hippocampus on the left of the photograph (the right hippocampus) has herniated through the tentorial notch, pushing the midbrain toward the patient's left. The notching of the inferior surface of the hippocampus is evident. AFIP negative 62-2730-5. Used with permission of the Director, Armed Forces Institute of Pathology, Washington, D.C. 20306.

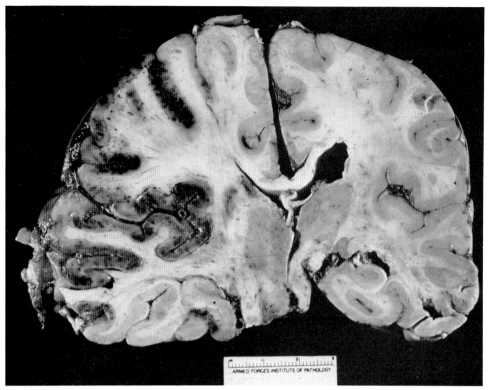

Figure 5.13. Transtentorial herniation. This coronal section demonstrates one of the complications of this herniation. The inferior surface of the temporal lobe on the left can be seen to be notched by the herniation through the tentorium. This has resulted in local hemorrhage and shift of the midbrain structures. This patient had a massive middle cerebral artery distribution infarction resulting in enough mass effect to cause this herniation. The same patient also had bilateral posterior cerebral artery distribution infarcts from the herniation. AFIP negative 62-6872-5. Used with the permission of The Director, Armed Forces Institute of Pathology, Washington, D.C. 20306.

tery may also occur contralateral to the herniating medial temporal lobe. In this circumstance the posterior cerebral artery is compressed between the midbrain, being pushed contralaterally by the herniating temporal lobe, and the contralateral temporal lobe. This again results in medial occipital lobe infarct, again almost always hemorrhagic, and thus, if the lesions are bilateral, it may result in total cortical blindness if the patient should recover (Fig. 5.15) (100, 146).

The contralateral motion of the midbrain also may result in another curiosity of this complex of movements. In this circumstance the compressed and herniating midbrain impinges on the contralateral edge of the tentorium cerebelli, compressing the crus cerebri and damaging the descending corticospinal and corticobulbar pathways and resulting in a contralateral (to the compression) paresis or paralysis, with paresis or paralysis on the same side as the lesion. This "false localizing" sign, in period before the use of CT scanning, occasionally resulted in surgery on the wrong side of the brain. The notching of the midbrain produced by this compression against the edge of the tentorium was first described by Kernohan and Woltman, and this "notch" has thus been called "Kernohan's" notch (57, 100).

With the downward movement of the midbrain and the tortional effects of the lateralized motions, there is the additional factor of compression and twisting of the aqueduct of Sylvius, with the resultant narrowing or occlusion of this iter. The resulting hydrocephalus of the third and lateral ventricles only adds to the mass effect already too apparent in the supratentorial compartment and increases the herniation

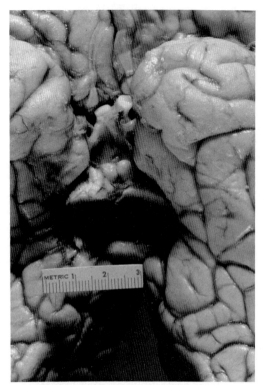

Figure 5.14. Remote transtentorial herniation. The grooving and atrophy of the hippocampus on the left side of the photograph is the evidence of the remote herniation resulting in local infarction.

effect. With primary midbrain lesions this may be the major mechanism of transtentorial herniation, and it is significantly additive to other causes (100).

Finally, as the midbrain descends through the incisura, the arterial channels, more attached to the bony and dural structures than to the brain itself, become stretched as the relatively sharply angulated upper branches of the basilar artery come under tension from the descending midbrain and brainstem. As postmortem angiographic studies have demonstrated, the arterial channels within the midbrain and upper pons begin to shear and tear, resulting in the well-known herniation hemorrhages often called "Duret hemorrhages" (Fig. 5.16). These hemorrhages most frqeuently are associated with death, although survival for some period has been recorded (49, 100, 126).

The complex of transtentorial herniation can result in a very confusing clinical pic-

ture, and even the unwary pathologist may wonder at the pathogenesis of the pathologic findings (100).

Upward Transtentorial Herniation

Probably the least common of the herniation lesions is the reverse of downward transtentorial herniation as just discussed, which is upward herniation through the tentorium cerebelli. This is almost always the result of a posterior fossa mass lesion, most frequently in the cerebellum. In this situation, the mass forces the superior cerebellum and upper pons upward through the incisura, compressing the midbrain from below and forcing the upper pons forward against the clivus and upward following the midbrain (Fig. 5.17). In this situation, perhaps even more commonly than in downward transtentorial herniation, there is distortion of the aqueduct, with compression and twisting leading to hydrocephalus of the supratentorial ventricular system. The clinical features of this herniation are much less well defined than those of the downward transtentorial herniation (32, 100).

Cerebellar Tonsillar Herniation

The best known of the herniation complexes to the general medical profession is "tonsillar herniation." The herniation of the cerebellar tonsils through the foramen magnum results in compression of the medulla oblongata by the herniating cerebellum, with dysfunction of the vital centers of respiration and cardiac rhythmic control. Again, knowledge of normal variations is essential in evaluating specific cases. There are large variations in the anatomy of the foramen magnum and of the inferior aspect of the cerebellum. Many brains have prominent cerebellar tonsils and may even show some "molding" of the inferior aspect by a relatively small foramen magnum. Others have vast foramens magnum and almost vestigial cerebellar tonsils. As has been suggested by the foregoing, care must be exercised in the interpretation of the anatomic findings at the time of autopsy (49, 100, 146).

The most common cause of cerebellar tonsillar herniation is a mass lesion in the posterior fossa, but less commonly a supra-

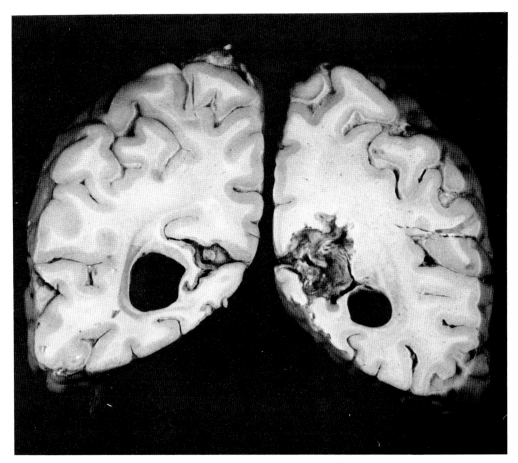

Figure 5.15.   Remote transtentorial herniation. This patient suffered bilateral infarcts in the distribution of both posterior cerebral arteries as the result of a subdural hematoma secondary to trauma. He survived for some months. The loss of cortex and some white matter in the calcarine cortical areas is evident. (Courtesy of Boyd G. Stephens, M.D., Chief Coroner-Medical Examiner, San Francisco, CA.)

tentorial mass lesion may cause tonsillar herniation, usually after or with transtentorial herniation. This is more common with midline supratentorial masses (100, 146).

With true tonsillar herniation there is almost always softening of the herniated tissue, more clearly evident after fixation than before (Fig. 5.18). Furthermore, the compressed medulla oblongata is swollen and may be either softened or firm, depending on the severity of the edema and the time that has elapsed after the impairment of tissue viability. Histologically, the herniated cerebellar tissue shows the early changes of infarction, and the medullary tissues show edema or more advanced stages of tissue death. The histologic

changes seen depend on the time of survival after herniation, and histologic changes can be minimal and not separable from postmortem changes. Under these circumstances, the gross findings may be the most reliable findings present.

Clinically, tonsillar herniation may be a most dramatic event, even if rarely encountered. It is seen most often after a lumbar puncture in an individual in whom the presence of a mass lesion intracerebrally is not expected. In these days of CT scans this is unusual, except in locales lacking such equipment. The symptoms may be varied, although sudden cardiorespiratory collapse is commonly seen. Actually, the onset of symptoms may be delayed hours or even a day or two and, although dramatic, may not

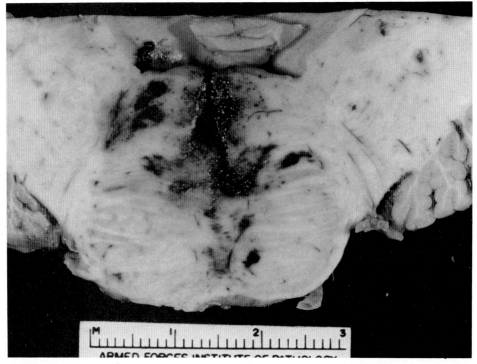

Figure 5.16. Transtentorial herniation. The recent hemorrhages present in the upper pons are the end result of the transtentorial herniation phenomenon and very often are the cause of death in these patients. Their irregular shape, often with a linear array, has led to the terms "splinter" or "flame-shaped" hemorrhages. AFIP negative 62-6872-2. Used with permission of The Director, Armed Forces Institute of Pathology, Washington, D.C. 20306.

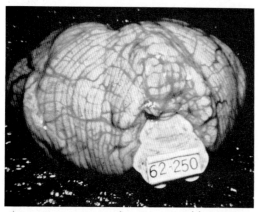

Figure 5.17. Upward transtentorial herniation. The grooving of the upper surface of the cerebellar hemispheres indicates where the tentorial edges impinged on the cerebellar tissue. This is a black and white copy of photograph number 19 in the Bailey-Riggs Teaching Set on brain tumors of the Armed Forces Institute of Pathology, and is used with the permission of The Director, Armed Forces Insitute of Pathology, Washington, D.C. 20306, Dr. Orville T. Bailey, Chicago, IL, and of Dr. Lucy B. Rorke, Philadelphia, PA, the photographer.

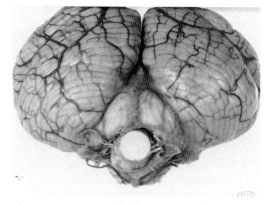

Figure 5.18. Cerebellar tonsillar herniation. This photograph shows the appearance of bilateral tonsillar herniation, with grooving of both tonsils by the edges of the foramen magnum. Such tonsils are softened, swollen, and compress the adjacent medulla oblongata, causing the cardiorespiratory complications that actually cause the death of such patients. The medullary structure is usually also soft and swollen. AFIP negative 62-2730-3. Used with the permission of The Director, Armed Forces Institute of Pathology, Washington, D.C. 20306.

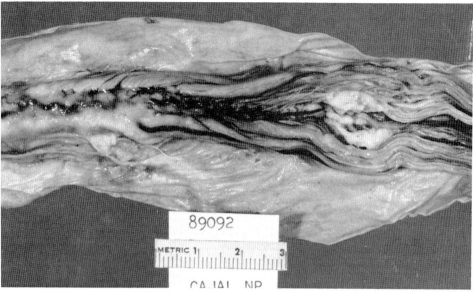

Figure 5.19. Subarachnoid cerebellar tissue emboli. This spinal cord shows masses of cerebellar tissue in the subarachnoid space over the lower cord and cauda equina. This patient had been on a respirator following a cerebral catastrophe and had had cerebellar tonsillar herniation. Some of the herniated cerebellar tissue broke through into the subarachnoid space and was "pumped," partially by the respirator's action, down into the spinal subarachnoid space.

be so sudden as to pass clinical notice. However presenting, the situation is ominous, and not many recoveries from long-standing tonsillar herniation are recorded (49, 100).

"Chronic" Tonsillar Herniation

"Chronic" cerebellar tonsillar herniation has been reported in association with the Arnold-Chiari (Chiari type II) malformation in adults and was interpreted as being the cause of death in infants and children with this malformation. With this phenomenon there is grooving of the tonsils, with atrophy of the herniated cerebellar tissue (30).

Subarachnoid Cerebellar Tissue Emboli

One of the interesting results of cerebellar tonsillar herniation, at least to the pathologist, is the subarachnoid embolization of herniated cerebellar tissue into the spinal SAS. This is probably the result of the rupture of herniated necrotic cerebellar tissue through the pia, with subsequent movement as a result of artificial respiratory ventilation, and is most often seen in

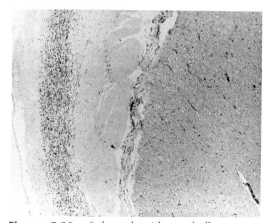

Figure 5.20. Subarachnoid cerebellar tissue emboli. This medium power photomicrograph shows the cerebellar tissue in the spinal subarachnoid space. ×10, H&E. AFIP negative 62-2418. Used with the permission of The Director, Armed Forces Institute of Pathology, Washington, D.C., 20306.

patients with "brain death." Under these circumstances cerebellar tissue is seen, either grossly or microscopically, in the spinal SAS. Cerebellar tissue has been found as far down the spinal cord as the cauda equina (Figs. 5.19 and 5.20). Most cases have been on a respirator for some days, and most have suffered a cerebral catastrophe as their initial presentation (45).

References

1. Alksne JE, Lovings ET: The role of the arachnoid villus in the removal of red blood cells from the subarachnoid space. An electron microscope study in the dog. *J. Neurosurg* 36:192–200, 1972.
2. Andral G: *Vorlesungen uber die Krankheiten der Nervenheerde*. Christian E. Leipzig, Kollmann, 1838, p 260
3. Ayers WW, Haymaker W: Xanthoma and cholesterol granuloma of the choroid plexus. *J Neuropathol Exp Neurol* 19:280–295, 1960.
4. Baethmann A, Oettinger W, Rothenfuber W, et al: Brain edema factors: current state with particular reference to plasma constituents and glutamate. In: Cervos-Navarro J, Ferszt R (eds): *Advances in Neurology*. New York, Raven Press, 1980, pp 171–195, vol 28.
5. Bondareff W, Pysh JJ: Distribution of the extracellular space during postnatal maturation of rat cerebral cortex. *Anat Rec* 160:773–780, 1968.
6. Bowsher D: Pathways of absorption of protein from the cerebrospinal fluid: an autoradiographic study in the cat. *Anat Rec* 128:23–39, 1957
7. Bradbury MWB, Cole DF: The role of the lymphatic system in drainage of cerebrospinal fluid and aqueous humour. *J Physiol (Lond)* 299:353–365, 1980.
8. Bradbury MWB, Cserr HF, Westrop RJ: Drainage of cerebral interstitial fluid into deep cervical lymph of the rabbit. *Am J Physiol* 240:F329–F336, 1981.
9. Bradbury MWB, Westrop RJ: Factors influencing exit of substances from cerebrospinal fluid into deep cervical lymph of the rabbit. *J Physiol (Lond)* 339:519–534, 1983.
10. Bradbury MWB, Westrop RJ: Lymphatics and the drainage of cerebrospinal fluid. In Shapiro K, Marmarou A, Portnoy H (eds): *Hydrocephalus*. New York, Raven Press, 1984, pp 69–82.
11. Brightman MW, Reese TS: Junctions between intimately opposed cell membranes in the vertebrate brain. *J Cell Biol* 40:648–677, 1969.
12. Brightman MW: The intracerebral movement of proteins injected into blood and cerebrospinal fluid of mice. *Prog Brain Res* 29:19–40, 1968
13. Brightmann MW, Reese TS, Feder N: Assessment with the electron microscope of the permeability to peroxidase of cerebral endothelium and epithelium in mice and sharks, In: Crone C, Lassen NA (eds): *Capillary Permeability*. Alfred Benzon Symposium II. Copenhagen, Munksgaard, 1969, pp 468–476.
14. Bruce DA, Ter Weene C, Kaiser, et al: Mechanisms and time course for clearance of vasogenic cerebral edema. In: Popp AJ, Bourke RS, Nelson LR, et al (eds): *Neural Trauma*. New York, Raven Press, 1979, pp 155–172.
15. Butler A: Correlated physiologic and structural studies of CSF absorption. In Shapiro K, Marmarou A, Portnoy H (eds): Hydrocephalus. New York, Raven Press, 1984, pp 41–58.
16. Casley-Smith R, Foldi-Borcsok E, Foldi M: The prelymphatic pathways of the brain as revealed by cervical lymphatic obstruction and the passages of particles. *Br J Exp Pathol* 57:179–188, 1976.
17. Clark WEL: On the Pacchionian bodies. *J Anat* 55:40–48, 1920.
18. Cserr HF, Cooper DN, Milhorat TH: Flow of cerebral interstitial fluid as indicated by the removal of extracellular markers from rat caudate nucleus. *Exp Eye Res* 25 (Suppl):461–473, 1977.
19. Cserr HF, Cooper DN, Suri PK, et al: Efflux of radiolabeled polyethylene glycols and albumin from rat brain. *Am J Physiol* 240:F319–F328, 1981.
20. Cserr HF: Convection of brain interstitial fluid. In: Shapiro K, Marmarou A, Portnoy H (eds): *Hydrocephalus*. New York, Raven Press, 1984, pp 59–68.
21. Cserr HF: Physiology of the choroid plexus. *Physiol Rev* 51:273–311, 1971.
22. Cushing H: *The Third Circulation*. London, Oxford University Press, 1926.
23. Cutler RWP, Page L, Galicich J, et al: Formation and absorption of cerebrospinal fluid in man. *Brain* 91:707–720, 1968.
24. Dandy WE, Blackfan KD: Internal hydrocephalus. An experimental, clinical and pathological study. *Am J Dis Child* 8:406–482, 1914.
25. Davson H, Hollingsworth G, Segal MB: The mechanism of drainage of the cerebrospinal fluid. *Brain* 93:665–678, 1970.
26. Davson H, Kleeman CR, Levin R: Blood-brain barrier and extracellular space. *J Physiol (Lond)* 159:67P–68P, 1961.
27. Davson H: *Physiology of the Cerebrospinal Fluid*. London, J & A Churchill, 1967.
28. Denny-Brown D: The changing pattern of neurologic medicine. *N Engl J Med* 246:839–846, 1952.
29. Diamond JM, Bosert WH: Stand-gradient osmotic flow. A mechanism for coupling of water and solute transport in epithelia. *J Gen Physiol* 50:2061–2083, 1967.
30. Dohrmann GJ: The choroid plexus in experimental hydrocephalus. A light and electron microscopic study in normal, hydrocephalic, and shunted hydrocephalic dogs. *J Neurosurg* 34:56–69, 1971.
31. Ehrlich P: Zur therapeutischen Bedeutung der Substituirenden Schwefelsauregruppe. *Ther Mh* 1:88–90, 1887.
32. Ecker A: Upward transtentorial herniation of the brainstem and cerebellum due to tumor of the posterior fossa. *J Neurosurg* 5:51–61, 1948.
33. Eisenberg HM, McComb JG, Lorenzo AV: Cerebrospinal fluid overproduction and hydrocephalus associated with choroid plexus papilloma. *J Neurosurg* 40:381–385, 1974.
34. Ellington E, Margolis G: Block of arachnoid villus by subarachnoid hemorrhage. *J Neurosurg* 30:651–657, 1969.
35. Epstein MH, Feldman AM, Brusilow SW: Cerebrospinal fluid production: stimulation by cholera toxin. *Science* 196:1012–1013, 1977.
36. Fishman RA: Brain edema. *N Engl J Med* 293:706–711, 1975.
37. Fishman RA: *Cerebrospinal Fluid in Diseases in the Nervous System*. Philadelphia, WB Saunders, 1980.
38. Foltz EL, Ward AA Jr: Communicating hydrocephalus from subarachnoid bleeding. *J Neurosurg* 13:546–566, 1965.
39. Friede RL, Roessmann U: Chronic tonsillar herniation. An attempt at classifying chronic herniations at the foramen magnum. *Acta Neuropathol (Berl)* 34:219–235, 1976.
40. Gilles FH, Davidson RI: Communicating hydrocephalus associated with deficient dysplastic parasagittal arachnoidal granulations. *J Neurosurg* 35:421–426, 1971.
41. Gutiérrez Y, Friede RL, Kaliney WJ: Agenesis of arachnoid granulations and its relationship to communicating hydrocephalus. *J Neurosurg* 43:553–558, 1975.
42. Hallervorden J: Uber Spatfolgen von Hirnschwellung and Hirnoedem. *Psychiatr Neurol Wochenschr* 41:1–4, 1939.
43. Haywood JR, Vogh BP: Some measurements of autonomic nervous system influence on production of cerebrospinal fluid in the cat. *J Pharmacol Exp Ther* 208:341–346, 1979.
44. Heisey SR, Held D, Pappenheimer JR: Bulk flow and diffusion in the cerebrospinal fluid system of the goat. *Am J Physiol* 203:775–781, 1962.
45. Herrick MK, Agamanolis DP: Displacement of cerebellar tissue into spinal canal. A component of the respirator brain syndrome. *Arch Pathol* 99:565–571, 1975.
46. Hirano A: Fine structure of edematous encephalopathy. In Cervos-Navarro J, Ferszt R (eds): *Advances in Neurology*. New York, Raven Press, 1980, vol 28, pp 83–97.
47. Hiratsuka H, Tabata H, Tsurouka S, et al: Evaluation of periventricular hypodensity in experimental hydro-

cephalus by metrizamide CT ventriculography. *J Neurosurg* 56:235–240, 1982.

48. Hossmann KA, Bloink M, Wilmes F, et al: J experimental peritumoral edema of the cat brain. In: Cervos-Navarro J, Ferszt R (eds): *Advances in Neurology.* New York, Raven Press, 1980, vol 28, pp 323–340.

49. Howell DA: Upper brain-stem comparison and foraminal impaction with intracranial space-occupying lesions and brain swelling. *Brain* 82:525–550, 1959.

50. Hyman S, McComb JG, Weiss MH, et al: Blood-CSF barrier breakdown following ventricular administration of cholera toxin. Presented at The American Association of Neurological Surgeons, San Francisco, CA, April 8–12, 1984.

51. Jaburek L: Uber das Gewebsluckensystem des Grobhirns und sein Bedeutung fur die Ausbreitung verschiedener pathologischer Prozesse. *Arch Psychiatr Nevenkr* 165:121–169, 1936.

52. Jaer O, Loken AC, Nesbakken R: Hydrocephalus due to xanthogranuloma. Case report. *J Neurosurg* 39:659–661, 1973.

53. James AE Jr, Strecker EP, Sperber E, et al: An alternative pathway of cerebrospinal fluid absorbtion in communicating hydrocephalus. Transependymal movement. *Radiology* 111:143–146, 1974.

54. Johnson RT, Yates PO: Clinicopathological aspects of pressure changes at the tentorium. *Acta Radiol* 46:242–249, 1956.

55. Katzman R, Pappius HM: *Brain Electrolytes and Fluid Metabolism.* Baltimore, Williams & Wilkins, 1973.

56. Kepes JJ: Oncocytic transformation of choriod plexus epithelium. *Acta Neuropathol (Berl)* 62:145–148, 1983.

57. Kernohan JW, Woltman HW: Incisura of the crus due to contralateral brain tumor. *Arch Neurol Psychiatry* 21:274–287, 1929.

58. Key EAH, Retzius MG: *Studien in der Anatomie des Nervensystems und des Bindegewebes.* Stockholm, Samson and Walin, 1875.

59. Klatzo I: Neurpathological aspects of brain edema. *J Neuropathol Exp Neurol* 26:1–14, 1967.

60. Klatzo I, Chui E, Fugiwara K et al: Resolution of vasogenic brain edema. In: Cervos-Navarro J, Ferszt R (eds): *Advances in Neurology,* New York, Raven Press, 1980, vol 28, pp 359–373.

61. Lampert PW, Oldstone MBA: Pathology of the choroid plexus in spontaneous immune complex disease and chronic viral infections. *Virchows Arch A Pathol Anat Histol* 363:21–32, 1974.

62. Levin VA, Milhorat TH, Fenstermacher JD, et al: Physiological studies on the development of obstructive hydrocephalus in the monkey. *Neurology* 21:238–246, 1971.

63. Levine JE, Povlishock JT, Becker DP: The morphological correlates of primate cerebrospinal fluid absorption. *Brain Res* 241: 31–41, 1982.

64. Liber AF, Lisa JR: Stromal tumors of the choroid plexus. *Am J Clin Pathol* 10:710–735, 1940.

65. Lindvall M, Edvinsson L, Owman C: Sympathetic nervous control of cerebrospinal fluid production from the choroid plexus. *Science* 201:176–178, 1978.

66. Lorenzo AV, Bresnan MJ, Barlow CF: Cerebrospinal fluid absorption deficit in normal pressure hydrocephalus. *Arch. Neurol.* 30:387–393, 1974.

67. Lorenzo AV, Bresnan MJ: Deficit in cereobrospinal fluid absorption in patients with symptoms of normal pressure hydrocephalus. *Dev Med Child Neurol* 15 (Suppl 29):35–41, 1973.

68. Lorenzo AV, Page LK, Watters GV: Relationship between cerebrospinal fluid formation, absorption and pressure in human hydrocephalus. *Brain* 93:679–692, 1970.

69. Love JA, Leslie RA: The effects of raised ICP on lymph flow in the cervical lymphatic trunks in cats. *J Neurosurg* 60:577–581, 1984.

70. Luse SA, Harris B: Brain ultrastructure in hydration and dehydration. *Arch Neurol* 4:139–153, 1967.

71. Lux WE Jr, Fenstermacher JD: Cerebrospinal fluid formation in ventricles and spinal subarachnoid space of the rhesus monkey. *J Neurosurg* 42:674–678, 1975.

72. Magendie E: Vorlesungen uber das nervensystem und sein Krankheiten (German translation). Leipzig, Kollmann, 1841.

73. Manlove CH, McLean AJ: Cholesteatomas of the choroid plexus of the lateral ventricle. *West J Surg* 44:422–427, 1936.

74. Mann JD, Butler AB, Johnson RN, et al: Clearance of macromolecular and particulate substances from the cerebrospinal fluid system of the rat. *J Neurosurg* 50:343–348, 1979.

75. Manz HJ: The pathology of cerebral edema. *Hum Pathol* 5:291–313, 1974.

76. Maren TH: Bicarbonate formation in cerebrospinal fluid: role in sodium transport and pH regulation. *Am J Physiol* 222:885–899, 1972.

77. Marmarou A, Takagi H, Shulman K: Biomechanics of brain edema and effects on local cerebral blood flow. In: Cervos-Navarro J, Ferszt R (eds): *Advances in Neurology.* New York, Raven Press, 1980, vol 28, pp 345–358,

78. Marshall LF, Bruce DA, Graham DI, et al: Alterations in behavior, brain electrical activity, cerebral blood flow, and intracranial pressure produced by triethyl tin sulfate induced cerebral edema. *Stroke* 7:21–25, 1976.

79. McComb JG, Davson H, Hollingsworth JR: Attempted separation of blood-brain and blood-cerebrospinal fluid barriers in the rabbit. *Exp Eye Res* (Suppl)25:333–343, 1977.

80. McComb JG, Davson H, Hyman S, et al: Cerebrospinal fluid drainage as influenced by ventricular pressure in the rabbit. *J Neurosurg* 56:709–797, 1982.

81. McComb JG, Hyman S, Weiss MH: CSF drainage following acute obstruction of the fourth ventricle in the rabbit. *Concepts Pediat. Neurosurgery* 4:90–101, 1983.

82. McComb JG, Hyman S, Weiss MH: Lymphatic drainage of cerebrospinal fluid in the cat. In Shapiro K, Marmarou A, Portnoy H (eds): *Hydrocephalus.* New York, Raven Press, 1984, pp 83–98.

83. McComb JG, Hyman S, Weiss MH: Lymphatic drainage of CSF in the primate. Presented at the American Association of Neurological Surgeons. Washington, D.C. April 24–28, 1983.

84. Meyer A: Herniation of the brain. *Arch Neurol Psychiatry* 4:387–400, 1920.

85. Milhorat TH, Clark RG, Hammock MK: Experimental hydrocephalus. Part 2. Gross pathological findings in acute and subacute obstructive hydrocephalus in the dog and monkey. *J Neurosurg* 32:390–399, 1970a.

86. Milhorat TH, Clark RG, Mammock MK, et al: Structural, ultrastructural and permeability changes in the ependyma and surrounding brain favoring equilibration in progressive hydrocephalus. *Arch Neurol* 22:397–407, 1970b.

87. Milhorat TH, Hammock MK, Chandra RS: The subarachnoid space in congenital obstructive hydrocephalus. Part 2. Microscopic findings. *J Neurosurg* 35:7–15, 1971.

88. Milhorat TH, Hammock MK, Davis DA, et al: Choroid plexus papilloma. I. Proof of cerebrospinal fluid overproduction. *Child's Brain* 2:273–289, 1976.

89. Milhorat TH: *Hydrocephalus and the Cerebrospinal Fluid.* Baltimore, Williams & Wilkins, 1972.

90. Miner LC, Reed DJ: Composition of fluid obtained from choroid plexus tissue isolated in a chamber *in situ. J Physiol (Lond)* 227:127–139, 1972.

91. Mrsulja BB, Djuricic BM, Cvejic V, et al: Biochemistry of experimental ischemic brain edema. In: Cervos-Navarro J, Ferszt R (eds): *Advances in Neurology.* New York, Raven Press, 1980, pp 217–230.

92. Murthy VS, Deshpande DH: The central canal of the filum terminale in communicating hydrocephalus. *J Neurosurg* 53:528–532, 1980.

93. Nabeshima S, Reese TS, Landis DMD, et al: Junctions in the meninges and marginal glia. *J Comp Neurol* 164:127–170, 1975.

94. Needham CW, Bertrand G and Myles ST: Multiple cranial nerve signs from supratentorial tumors. *J Neurosurg* 33:178–183, 1970.

95. Oldendorf WH, Cornford ME, Brown WJ: The large apparent work capability of the blood-brain barrier: a study of the mitochondrial content of capillary endothelial cells in brain and other tissues of the rat. *Ann Neurol* 1:409–417, 1977.

96. Oldendorf WH, Davson H: Brain extracellular space and the sink action of cerebrospinal fluid. *Arch Neurol* 17:196–205, 1967.

97. Patlak CS, Fenstermacher JD: Measurements of dog blood-brain transfer constants by ventriculocisternal perfusion. *Am J Physiol* 229:877–884, 1975.

98. Pearson GHJ: Xanthoma of the choroid plexus. *Arch Pathol* 6:595–597, 1928.

99. Penn RD, Kurtz D: Cerebral edema mass effects, and regional blood volume in man. *J Neurosurg* 46:282–289, 1977.

100. Plum F, and Posner JB: *The Diagnosis of Stupor and Coma.* Philadelphia, FA Davis, 1972, ed 2.

101. Pollay M, Curl F: Secretion of cerebrospinal fluid by the ventricular ependyma of the rabbit. *Am J Physiol* 213:1031–1038, 1967.

102. Pollay M, Davson H: The passage of certain substances out of the cerebrospinal fluid. *Brain* 86:137–150, 1963.

103. Porter JC, Ben-Jonathon N, Oliver C, et al: In: Knigge KM et al (eds): *Brain-Endocrine Interactions. II. The Ventricular System in Neuroendocrine Mechanisms.* Basel, S Karger, 1975, pp 295–305.

104. Rall DP: Transport through the ependymal linings. *Prog Brain Res* 29:159–167, 1968.

105. Rapoport SI, Thompson HK: Osmotic opening of the blood-brain barrier in the monkey without associated neurological deficits. *Science* 180:971, 1973.

106. Reese TS, Karnovsky MJ: Fine structural localization of a blood-brain barrier to exogenous peroxidase. *J Cell Biol* 34:207–217, 1967.

107. Reid WL, Cone WV: The mechanism of fixed dilatation of the pupil resulting from ipsilateral archral compression. *JAMA* 112:2030–2034, 1939.

108. Reulen HJ, Tsuyumu M, Prioleau G: Further results concerning the resolution of vasogenic brain edema. In Cervos-Navarro J, Ferszt R (eds): *Advances in Neurology.* New York, Raven Press, 1980, vol 28, pp 375–381.

109. Reulen HJ, Tsuyumu M, Tack A, et al: Clearance of edema fluid into cerebrospinal fluid. A mechanism for the resolution of vasogenic brain edema. *J Neurosurg* 48:754–764, 1978.

110. Rosenberg GA, Kyner WT, Estrada E: Bulk flow of brain interstitial fluid under normal and hyperosomolar conditions. *Am J Physiol* 238:F42–F49, 1980.

111. Rubin Rc, Henderson ES, Ommaya AK, et al: The production of cerebrospinal fluid in man and its modification by acetazolamide. *J Neurosurg* 25:430–436, 1966.

112. Rubin RC, Hockwald GM, Tiell M, Epstein F, Ghatuk N, Wisniewski H. III: Hydrocephalus. Reconstitution of the cerebral cortical mantle following ventricular shunting. *Surg Neurol* 5:179–183, 1976b.

113. Rubin RC, Hockwald GM, Tiell M et al: I. Hydrocephalus: histological and ultrastructural changes in the pre-shunted cortical mantle. *Surg Neurol* 5:109–114, 1976a.

114. Russell DS: Observations on the Pathology of Hydrocephalus. Medical Research Council Special Report Series No. 265. London, His Majesty's Stationery Office, 1949.

115. Schwalbe G: Der Arachnoidalraum ein Lymphraum und sein Zusammenhang mit den Perichoriodalraum. *Zentralbl Med Wiss* 7:465–467, 1869.

116. Schwartz GA, Rosner AA: Displacement and herniation of hippocampal gyrus through the incisura tentorium: a clinicopathologic study. *Arch Neurol Psychiatry* 46:297–311, 1944.

117. Segal MB, Burgess AMC: A combined physiological and morphological study of the secretory process in the rabbit choroid plexus. *J Cell Sci* 14:339–350, 1974.

118. Segal MB, Pollay M: The secretion of cerebrospinal fluid. *Exp Eye Res* 25 (Suppl):127–148, 1977.

119. Shantaveerappa TR, Bourne GH: Arachnoid villi in the optic nerve of man and monkey. *Exp Eye Res* 3:31–35, 1964.

120. Shen JY, Kelly DE, Hyman S, et al: Intraorbital cerebrospinal fluid outflow and the posterior uveal compartment of the hamster eye. *Cell Tissue Res*, in press, 1984.

121. Shuangshoti S, Netsky MG: Histogenesis of choroid plexus in man. *Am J Anat* 118:283–316, 1966.

122. Shuangshoti S, Netsky MG: Human choroid plexus: morpholoci and histochemical alterations with age. *Am J Anat* 128:73–96.

133. Shuangshoti S, Paisuntornsook P, Netsky MG: Melanosis of the choroid plexus. *Neurology* 26:656–658, 1976.

124. Shuangshoti S, Phonprasert C, Suwanwela N, Netsky MG: Combined neuroepithelial (colloid) cyst and xanthogranuloma (xanthoma) in the third ventricle. *Neurology* 25:547–552, 1975.

125. Stewart PA, Wiley MJ: Developing nervous tissue induces formation of blood-brain barrier characteristics in invading endothelial cells: a study using quail chick transplantation chimeras. *Dev Biol* 84:183–192, 1981.

126. Sunderland S: The tentorial notch and complications produced by herniations of the brain through that aperture. *Br J Surg* 45:422–438, 1958.

127. Szper I, Oi S, Leestma J, Kim KS, Wetzel NE: Xanthogranuloma of the third ventricle. Case report. *J Neurosurg* 51:565–568, 1979.

128. Tripathi BJ, Tripathi RC: Vacuolar transcellular channels as a drainage pathway for cerebrospinal fluid. *J Physiol (Lond)* 239:195–206, 1974.

129. Tripathi RC: Ultrastructure of the arachnoid matter in relation to outflow of cerebrospinal fluid. A new concept. *Lancet* 2:8–11, 1973.

130. Van Harreveld A, Crowell J, Malhotra SK: A study of extracellular space in central nervous tissue by freeze-substitution. *J Cell Biol* 25:117–137, 1965.

131. Van Harreveld A, Khattab FI: Perfusion fixation with glutaraldehyde and post-fixation with osmium tetroxide for electron microscopy. *J Cell Sci* 3:579–594, 1968.

132. Van Harreveld A, Steiner J: Extracellular space in frozen and ethanol substituted central nervous tissue. *Anat Rec* 166:117–129, 1970.

133. Van Harreveld A: The extracellular space in the vertebrate central nervous system. In: GH Bourne (ed): *The Structure and Function of Nervous Tissue.* New York, Academic Press, 1972, vol 4, pp 447–511.

134. Weed LH: Studies on cerebro-spinal fluid. III. The pathways of escape from the subarachnoid spaces with particular reference to the arachnoid villi. *J Med Res* 31:51–91, 1914

135. Weed LH: The absorption of cerebrospinal fluid into the venous system. *Am J Anat* 31:191–221, 1923.

136. Welch K, Friedman V: The cerebrospinal fluid valves. *Brain* 83:454–469, 1980.

137. Welch K, Pollay M: The spinal arachnoid villi of the monkeys *Cercopithecus aethiops sabaeus* and *Macaca irus. Anat Rec* 145:43–48, 1963.

138. Welch K: Selected topics relating to hydrocephalus. *Exp Eye Res* 25 (Suppl):345–375, 1977.

139. Welch K: The principles of physiology of the cerebrospinal fluid in relation to hydrocephalus including normal pressure hydrocephalus. In: Frielander WJ (ed): *Current Reviews. Advances in Neurology.* New York, Raven Press, 1975, vol 13, pp 247–332.

140. Winkelman NW, Fay T: The Pacchionian system. Histologic and pathologic changes with particular reference to the idiopathic and symptomatic convulsive states. *Arch Neurol Psychiatry* 23:44–64, 1930.

141. Wislocki GB, Putnam TJ: Absorption form the ventricles in experimentally produced internal hydrocephalus. *Am J Anat* 29:313–320, 1921.

142. Wright EM: Active transport of iodide and other anions across the choroid plexus. *J Physiol (Lond)* 240:535–556, 1974.

143. Wright EM: Mechanism of ion transport across the choroid plexus. *J Physiol (Lond)* 226:545–571, 1972.

144. Wright EM: Trasnport process in the formation of the cerbrospinal fluid. *Rev Physiol Biochem Pharmacol* 83:1–34, 1978.

145. Zervas NT, Liszczak TM, Mayberg MR, et al: Cerebrospinal fluid may nourish cerebral vessels through pathways in the adventitia that may be analogous to systemic vasa vasorum. *J Neurosurg* 56:475–481, 1982.

146. Zulch KJ: *Atlas of Gross Neurosurgical Pathology.* New York, Springer-Verlag, 1975.

CHAPTER 6

Congenital Malformations of the Nervous System

SAMUEL K. LUDWIN, M.B., B.Ch., F.R.C.P.(C)
MARGARET G. NORMAN, M.D., F.R.C.P.(C)

INTRODUCTION

Of all congenital malformations those of the central nervous system are among the most common and have assumed increasing importance in recent years due to sophisticated diagnostic procedures and the possibilities for genetic counselling and therapy. The term congenital malformation indicates only that an individual is born with a defect or abnormality of some portion of the body. The term itself indicates nothing of the cause of the deformity. Malformations may be primary or secondary, and this chapter will deal almost exclusively with primary malformations. These have been defined by an international working group (291) as a "morphological defect of an organ, part of an organ or larger region of the body resulting from an intrinsically abnormal developmental process." Primary malformations are here distinguished from secondary malformations or disruptions which are defects of an organ resulting from the breakdown or interference with an originally normal developmental process. Most disruptions are due to perinatal vascular accidents, infections, and chemicals.

The distinction between primary and secondary malformations is extremely important for both genetic counselling and treatment. Although secondary malformations (disruptions) are unlikely to recur, knowledge of their cause may lead to means of future prevention. On the other hand, many of the underlying causes of primary malformations are genetic or chromosomal in origin, and a detailed attempt must be made to define them for future genetic counselling. At the same time, it is not always easy to distinguish between primary and secondary malformations. The development of the fetal brain followed by its growth in late fetal and childhood life is a continuous process. It therefore becomes clear that an etiological agent acting in early development may lead to a primary malformation, whereas the same agent may act after the brain is formed to result in what we may recognize as a disruption. In early embryogenesis, it may not be possible to determine the cause or mechanism or even that a disruption has occurred because the embryo is too immature to mount the inflammatory and reparative changes recognized as a reaction to injury. The presence of necrosis, macrophages, dystrophic calcification, and gliosis, by which disruptive events can be recognized, usually only occurs by 17 to 18 weeks gestation, and without such evidence it may be difficult to determine whether the abnormality is a primary malformation or a disruption. A complete diagnosis in a case of deformed brain requires that in addition to the morphology, an attempt to determine etiology must be made which will involve family history and karyotyping, as well as studies of anomalies in the rest of the body.

A good working knowledge of the embryology of the central nervous system is essential, as it is only through an understanding of the mechanisms and timing of normal formation of structures of the brain that a meaningful analysis of the mechanisms and timing of the malformation can be made. Such a knowledge of embryology facilitates the understanding of the complex morphologic features, which are often poorly understood by neuropathologists. Throughout this chapter, therefore, reference will be made to normal development, and at all times attempts will be made to relate the various anomalies to disturbances in normal development.

The study of malformations in any part of the body (teratology) is guided by six principles (318).

1. The genetic structure of the individual is the setting within which outside factors operate, and the degree to which they interact varies.
2. The less mature the organism, the more susceptible it is to change, and therefore the timing of the teratogenic event can be more critical in nature. It follows from this that the earlier in development an event occurs, the more serious and widespread will be its sequelae.
3. Teratogenic agents act in a way which begins an abnormal train of events (mechanisms). These mechanisms include mutation, chromosomal nondisjunction and breaks, mitotic interference, altered nucleic acid integrity or function, lack of precursors or substrates for biosynthesis, altered energy sources, enzyme inhibitors, osmolar imbalance, and altered membrane characteristics. It is evident that as many of these mechanisms may be produced by many agents, the agents themselves may act in a relatively nonspecific way.
4. Abnormal development may vary from death, through malformations and growth retardation, to functional disorders not detectable at a morphological level.
5. Environmental agents gain access to developing tissues either by directly traversing the maternal body or by being transmitted indirectly through it.
6. The severity of abnormal develop-

ment is often proportional to dosage of the agent concerned.

The problem in examining malformed brains is that there is no simple, constant, one to one relationship between a "cause" and the final malformation, and the mechanism by which a cause works to effect the final deformity is frequently unknown. Different causes may act through the same mechanism, and the same cause may act through different mechanisms, leading to a final morphological malformation that may be the same or different both for any given single cause or for different etiological agents (318) (Table 6.1). In this regard again the timing of the agent is of critical importance. The developing organism has a limited ability to respond so that the final morphologies are limited. This is well demonstrated in the case of holoprosencephaly (217) in which it should be noted that the severity of the condition varies in both dominant and recessive forms.

Prenatal life is divided into three periods (134). The first ends with the implantation of the blastocyst. During organogenesis which lasts from the beginning of the 4th week to the end of the 8th week, there is rapid growth and differentiation of the organs of the body. The fetal period extends from the end of the 2nd month to birth. In the human, the migration of neuroblasts and axons to their destination occurs after the 8th week (283), with a final maturation continuing for months, even years after birth. The detailed description of various embryological events will be given in the sections relevant to each group of malformations. Briefly, however, the following is an outline of these events. The neural tube forms by neuralation from the neural plate, starting at about the 22nd day of gestation in the human, and being completed by days 26–28. Once the neural tube is formed, differential rates of growth produce transformation into various areas of slower growth, forming the flexures by about day 32. Bilateral growth of the cerebral hemispheres causes evagination and the beginning of the formation of the hemispheres at about day 33. Throughout this time migration of primitive neurons from around the neural tube lumen to the central nuclei and cortex takes place (281, 283). These migrations

Table 6.1
Diagram of the Successive Stages on the Pathogenesis of a Developmental Defect, Beginning with the Initial Types of Changes in Developing Cells or Tissues (the Mechanism) and Continuing to the Final Defect.[a,b]

Mechanisms	Pathogenesis	Common pathways	Final defect
Initial types of changes in developing cells or tissues after teratogenic insult: 1. Mutation (gene) 2. Chromosomal breaks, nondisjunction, etc. 3. Mitotic interference 4. Altered nuclei and integrity or function 5. Lack of normal precursors, substrates, etc. 6. Altered energy sources 7. Changed membrane characteristics 8. Osmolar imbalance 9. Enzyme inhibition	Ultimately manifested as one or more type of abnormal embryogenesis: 1. Excessive or reduced cell death 2. Failed cell interactions 3. Reduced biosynthesis 4. Impeded morphogenetic movement 5. Mechanical disruption of tissues	1. Too few cells or cell products to effect localized morphogenesis or functional maturation 2. Other imbalances in growth and differentiation	

[a] From J. G. Wilson (318).
[b] One or more mechanisms is initiated by the teratogenic cause from the environment. This leads to changes in the developmental system which become manifested as one or more types of abnormal embryogenesis. This in turn leads into pathways that seem often to be characterized by too few cells or cell products to effect morphogenesis functional maturation, but the suggestion that this is a single or common pathway for all developmental defects is conjecture.

continue long after the period of organogenesis; neurons are still moving into the pulvinar at about 21 to 22 weeks of gestation (256). In general, neurons must form synapses to survive. Often during migration they move past cells with which they ultimately form synapses, and those which fail to form synapses die. Experimentally it has been shown that when neurons die during the modelling process because they have not received input from the first neuron in the chain, they usually do so without any significant vascular or glial reaction (76). Axons continue to grow throughout the system for a long period of time. Axons of the anterior commissure cross the midline from the 10th to 12th week of gestation, and the corticospinal tract reaches the midthoracic level at about 17 weeks (283). Migration of these cells is guided by local conditions, such as the Bergmann glia, and by the segregation of neurons into class-specific laminae (53). Interference with any of these events may result in malformations.

Some generalizations that can be made about brains with congenital malformations is that most are small and that they represent an arrest in development. Except for megalencephaly, most malformed brains are small; this may be because their cell multiplication is not sufficient or that cells fail to grow large enough. The cells may die or atrophy, or there may be abnormalities of the dendritic tree, as has been shown in Down's syndrome, (251) (Fig. 6.1). The second generalization is that because growth and development is a continual process, malformations of the brain represent an arrest in development and present a continuous spectrum of abnormality. Cyclopia (determined sometime before day 24) and holoprosencephaly with a single ventricle and hemisphere (determined at about day 33) are the severest expression of malformations in the frontal part of the brain, of which arrhinencephaly revealed by absence of the olfactory nerves is the least severe. Lissencephaly, a smooth brain with no gyri and abnormalities of lamination of cortical neurons, is determined at about 11–15 weeks gestation, whereas micropolygyria, another migration defect but with multiple small gyri, probably develops from an arrest later in fetal development.

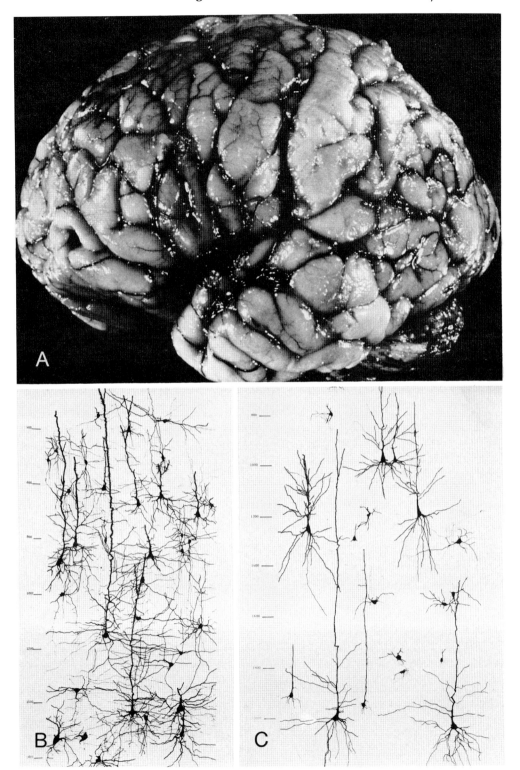

Figure 6.1. Down's syndrome. (*A*) Brain showing shortened anterioposterior diameter, gaping Sylvian fissure, and narrow superior temporal gyrus. (*B* and *C*) Camera lucida drawings of Golgi-stained occipital cortex. (*B*) Normal; (*C*) Down syndrome showing loss of dendrites and spines. (Courtesy of Dr. L. E. Becker.)

Clinical symptomatology in congenital malformations is nonspecific; terms such as mental retardation or cerebral palsy do not refer to pathological entities and may be found in patients with a variety of primary malformations or perinatal injuries. The degree of mental retardation is not always reflected in the morphology.

The Examination of Central Nervous System Malformations

When examining a case of congenital malformation, the neuropathologist should try to determine the morphological definition of that malformation and also give some idea how that malformation was caused.

In the clinical setting the task is practical—to separate what is genetically determined from that environmentally determined. In the former situation genetic counselling and antenatal diagnosis with perhaps even termination of abnormal pregnancies are possible. In particular, attempts must be made to separate malformations with a monogenic or chromosomal abnormality from those where genetic and environmental factors act, such as in neural tube defects. Where the condition is environmentally determined, an attempt must be made to distinguish recurrent from nonrecurrent causes for purposes of prevention. In the majority of cases, no cause will be found. It should also be remembered that secondary destruction can occur in the setting of a primary malformation, further complicating the picture.

In all cases a family history must be taken to trace affected members, and the pregnancy history to determine exposure to any teratogen, particularly during the critical period, should be reported. The placenta should be examined to determine pathogenesis; inflammation of the villi may indicate prenatal infection, whereas triploidy may produce cystic alteration of the villi. All other congenital anomalies, both external and internal, should be described and photographed. Some of these are consistently associated with central nervous system malformations (such as the craniofacial dysmorphoses). Extensive catalogues listing the anomalies seen in each of numerous syndromes exist and should be consulted for aid in diagnosis (145). Chromo-

some studies are important and should be done on all cases. Frequently x-rays should be performed, and to correlate with in vivo studies, an ultrasound examination should be conducted where appropriate (12). Tissues such as brain and serum should be taken where appropriate, for investigation for common perinatal infections and enough material to exclude metabolic disorders should be removed, should this be necessary.

Head circumference and body length and weight should be measured and plotted on standard growth curves to see if there are disproportions between the head and the rest of the body. The relationship between brain and calvarium should be noted. If the brain is smaller than the calvarium and it is not a collapsed hydrocephalic brain, destruction of the brain should be suspected because the calvarium grows congruent to the brain. The brain should be weighed, if necessary with the cerebellum and cerebrum separately. Cysts should be photographed and described prior to their removal, as they are fragile.

The overall proportions of the brain should be noted, and any tendency towards disproportion measured if possible. Normally the brain is smooth at 18–20 weeks, and gyri develop progressively. The gyral pattern should be carefully noted and compared with the normal pattern for gestational age (85). Gyral abnormalities will only begin to be evident at about the 28th week. The base of the brain should be examined and in particular careful note made of the olfactory nerves, which tear easily in premature infants. The presence of a residual stump and the olfactory groove in a baby in which there is no olfactory nerve suggests that it is artefactually missing. The vessels at the base of the brain should be observed; an anterior cerebral artery may be missing in cases of forebrain growth abnormalities. On section of the brain, the presence, bulk, and symmetricality should be noted in all internal structures. Where conditions such as Arnold-Chiari syndrome and agenesis of the corpus callosum are suspected, the brain may be cut sagittally instead of coronally. Careful note should be made of the size of the ventricles. Although blunting may indicate obstruction to outflow, it should be remembered that in the fetus the ventricles are proportionately large compared to the cerebral mantle. If the brain parenchyma fails to grow this state may persist, a condition known as *colpocephaly*—a nonspecific finding. The surface of the ventricles should be noted for any protrusions which may indicate either heterotopias or the tuberous sclerosis lesions of "candle-guttering." The latter are firmer and less smooth than those of heterotopias. All cranial nerves should be examined, and the presence and size of the corticospinal tracts should be noted.

Incidence

Approximately 3% of newborns have major malformations (169, 170), and of these approximately a third are malformations of the central nervous system (178). Approximately 0.062% of all neonates have chromosomal abnormalities. In trying to determine incidence of the varying malformations, there is a wide variation, depending on the population surveyed and the type of examination performed (178). Ethnic and geographic factors are important, especially for neural tube defects. Because infants with chromosomal abnormalities and severe malformation are frequently aborted, their incidence at term is much less than that seen earlier in gestation, as these malformations are incompatible with survival beyond the neonatal period, and therefore tables which survey the incidence in children and adults (200) have a lower incidence of neural tube defects which are strikingly prominent in younger patients. In addition, anencephaly is easy to diagnose and requires no specific dissection, and therefore the figure for its incidence will be higher than those for conditions requiring autopsy and histological study, such as migration defects in the cerebral convolutions. A high incidence of midline telencephalic defects was noted in some series (158), but this incidence was compiled at a center providing sophisticated neuropathological examination. These remarks also refer to many of the older classifications of congenital anomalies present in the literature (24, 168, 200).

ETIOLOGY OF CONGENITAL MALFORMATIONS

Although the largest group of congenital malformations, about 60%, are of unknown cause, about 20% are due to interactions between the hereditary tendencies and nongenetic, usually undefined factors (107). Approximately 7.5% of congenital malformations have a monogenic basis, and up to 6% of patients with congenital malformations have major chromosomal anomalies (169, 329). The remaining 12% are due to major environmental causes such as maternal infections and illness, environmental toxins, occupational hazards, pharmaceutical drugs, and nutritional problems (169, 170).

Chromosomal Abnormality

The human has 46 chromosomes, of which 22 pairs are autosomes and 2 are sex chromosomes. Fluorescent staining of chromosomes bands with quinacrine mustard (50) and Giemsa banding has aided in identification of chromosomal aberrations. Chromosomal material may be lost or gained, but loss is more deleterious, leading in almost all cases (apart from XO chromosome genotype) to fetal death in utero. Additional chromosomal material may be produced by nondisjunction resulting in either trisomy (if there is extra chromosomal material) or monosomy (if there is a missing chromosome), anaphase lag leading to mosaicism in the sex chromosomes, and fertilization of one egg by two sperms or an abnormal sperm leading to triploidy with 69 chromosomes (153).

Chromosome material may break and rearrange between one chromosome and another by means of reciprocal translations, centrifusion, and insertion. Chromosome material may be lost by deletions, and this includes ring chromosomes. Other aberrations include inversions, isochromosomes, and recombination of chromosome material (153). The mechanism of production of a malformation by chromosomal abnormalities is unknown; it has been suggested (100) that trisomies operate through a gene dosage effect which leads to an increased output of enzymes or protein. Increased proteins might be inserted into a membrane which could alter the interaction.

Since the discovery of an extra chromosome 21 in Down's syndrome (trisomy 21), numbers of articles have described morphological anomalies associated with chromosomal abnormalities. In spite of the fact that all anomalies are increased in chromosomal syndromes, no morphological abnormality is unique for any chromosomal anomaly, and it is a grouping of anomalies rather than the presence of a single malformation which allows us to distinguish syndromes of chromosomal abnormalities (28, 121, 144, 284). Thus, diagnosis by chromosome karyotyping is mandatory in every case. Trisomy 21 may be produced by three chromosomal abnormalities: 95% are due to primary trisomy of chromosome 21, 4% by translocation between chromosome 21 and one of the D or G group chromosomes, and 1% are mosaics making karyotyping essential for genetic counselling, for there is a different rate of recurrence depending on the type of trisomy 21.

Two-thirds of the brain of large series of children and fetuses with chromosomal anomaly have no pathological changes (128).

DOWN'S SYNDROME—TRISOMY 21

In Down's syndrome the brain is small and approximately three-fourths normal weight (26, 289). The skull shape is often abnormal. The shape of the brain is abnormally foreshortened (Fig. 6.1), but this is not specific and is seen in other cases with mental retardation. The frontal lobes are small, the orbital gyri slanted, and the occipital lobes flattened, reducing the anteroposterior diameter. The skull shape is often abnormal. The brain stem and cerebellum are small (66) and the gyral pattern is often abnormal, although the changes are not specific. Sometimes the pattern is simplified with coarse broad convolutions. These changes may be asymmetric. A striking feature often seen is narrowing of the superior temporal gyrus both externally and on cutting the brain. Histological examination reveals few specific anomalies. Abnormal neurons, decrease and increase of cells, delayed myelination, and a small centrum semiovale are all frequently seen. To some these features have suggested delayed ontogeny (131). In the cerebellum there may be a tuber flocculus, a bilateral accumulation of undifferentiated cells in the medial part of the peduncle of the flocculi. Other minor changes include abnormally differentiated Purkinje cell layers, asymmetry of the inferior olive, and failure of separation of the nuclei of Clarke's column. Of great

interest is the recent finding of reduced numbers in complexity of dendritic spines as demonstrated in Golgi stains (293) (Fig. 6.1B and C).

Premature aging (13) as shown by increased Alzheimer neurofibrillary tangles, plaques, and loss of pyramidal neurons is frequent in Down's syndrome individuals, dying after 30 years of age (262). The relationship between the extra chromosomal material and plaques and tangles is unknown. In addition, the distribution of these plaques in the dentate gyrus differs from the general distribution in senile dementia of the Alzheimer type. As more sophisticated linear genetic maps (175) are drawn, more enzymes and diseases will be assigned to specific loci on human chromosomes. It has been suggested that Down's syndrome is associated with one-third of the long arm of chromosome 21 (21 q), and the occurrence of triple doses of gene products on this chromosome (276) may have some influence on premature aging. Decreased myelin, possibly due to an abnormality of myelin structure, has been reported (14), but the significance of this is unclear.

TRISOMY 13–15 (TRISOMY E OR PATAU SYNDROME)

Trisomy 13 is associated particularly with anomalies of the forebrain. The morphology of the brain varies from alobar and semilobar holoprosencephaly with cyclopia to arrhinencephaly. In some of this trisomy the brain may be normal but often is decreased in size. Small cerebellar heterotopias (which are described in greater detail under cerebellar malformations) are common but not specific for trisomy 13 (298).

TRISOMY 17–18 (EDWARDS SYNDROME)

The main pathological characteristics of this syndrome include gyral abnormalities, as well as dysplasias of the hippocampus and inferior olive. Again cerebellar heterotopias, absence of the corpus callosum, and even holoprosencephaly may occur in this syndrome (298).

Environmental Agents

Congenital malformations may be caused by a variety of environmental agents acting either alone or in the setting of a susceptible genetic basis.

Viral infections generally cause destructive lesions (although rubella may cause microcephaly alone); leptomeningeal inflammation, necrosis, and mineralization usually are indications of a disruptive rather than malformative process. Cytomegalovirus and toxoplasmosis may show extensive necrotizing lesions. Maternal diabetes has been associated with holoprosencephaly and recently the caudal regression syndrome (16, 74). Maternal hyperthermia (169) has been blamed for neural tube defects. Although microcephalic and mentally retarded infants have been born to mothers with phenylketonuria (273), further pathologic findings have not yet been described in these cases. Organic mercury has been shown to be teratogenic for the human fetus (56, 209). The pathological findings in these cases of fetal methyl mercury poisoning were microcephaly and abnormal gyrations, with foci of heterotopia in the leptomeninges, disturbances of cortical lamination with bizarre, irregularly grouped neurons, and heterotopic neurons in the cerebellum. Because of the presence of gemistocytic astrocytes it was suggested by Choi et al. (56) that a disturbance of the neuroglia-neuronal relationship during migration was present. The presence of methyl mercury poisoning in the mothers of these children in Mimamata (Japan) and Iraq strengthens the case that a well known poison may be teratogenic when administered to a fetus.

Whether *fetal alcohol syndrome* exists as a true entity must remain an open question (170). Numerous anomalies have been described in this syndrome. These include microencephaly, hydrocephaly, leptomeningeal heterotopias, cerebral and cerebellar dysraphia, and brain stem disorganization (59), dysraphia, arrhinencephaly, agenesis of the corpus callosum, meningocele, syringomyelia, and olivary nuclei dysplasias. One of us (M.G.N.) has seen a Dandy-Walker malformation and in another case agenesis of the corpus callosum, heterotopias, and hyperplasia of the cerebellum. Whether the alcohol directly causes the malformation, or whether additives or contaminants, poor nutrition, or hypoglycemia are the causative agents is not clear. It is also clear that not all fetuses of alcoholic mothers have this syndrome, which occurs only in the heavier drinkers.

Finally, malformations may occur with the administration of pharmaceutical drugs. Abnormal midfacial disorders and microcephaly occur with hydantoin ingestion in the mother (138), and late gestational malformation and hemorrhages may occur with anticoagulant use during pregnancy (132).

DISRUPTIVE (DESTRUCTIVE) CONDITIONS OFTEN RESEMBLING PRIMARY MALFORMATIONS

Because CNS development continues long after the formal period of organogenesis, agents acting after the 10th to 12th week of gestation may result in brain lesions which are clearly destructive. The brain at birth is structurally abnormal, and these destructive lesions are therefore congenital malformations (that is a "structural abnormality of prenatal origin present at birth that seriously interferes with viability or physical well being") (169). The destructive nature of these lesions may be recognized, many of which are due to failures of perfusion either arising from a placental or a maternal problem or from some other environmental destructive cause. Many of these lesions are not observed by pathologists until months after they occur, and when only an old scar is evident, and it may be impossible to determine the original cause.

Porencephaly and Schizencephaly

Porencephaly as originally described in 1859 by Heschl designated cysts extending from the surface of the cerebrum to the ventricle, but the term has now come to be very loosely used and now indicates almost any cyst occurring in an infant's brain (Fig. 6.2). Yakovlev and Wadsworth (327, 328) originally divided porencephaly into *encephaloclastic* (following destructive or vascular insults) and developmental (or schizencephalic types, which were thought to be primary in nature). They differentiated the two types on the basis of the bilaterality of the developmental lesions and the presence of micropolygyria at the margins of the defect. Although there may conceivably be some instances of developmental porencephaly, we believe that almost all of these

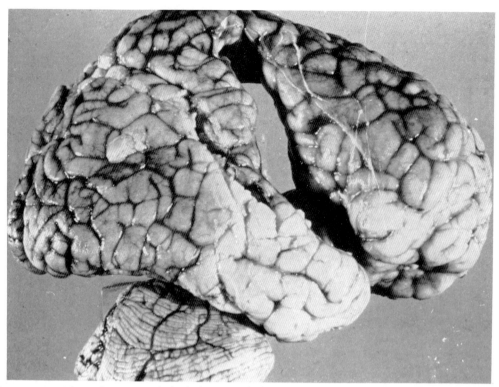

Figure 6.2. Bilateral porencephaly (schizencephaly) showing defects in territory of the middle cerebral arteries.

cysts result from necrosis of brain tissue, whether of hypoxic-ischemic, viral, or other unknown causes. It is becoming increasingly recognized (75, 190, 210, 314) that vascular insults occurring at the 24th week or later may produce a pattern of polymicrogyria. Therefore, if the lesion occurs while neurons are still migrating, a migration defect may occur at the cortical borders of the cyst, whereas after this migration, laminar cortical necrosis may occur. It is probably preferable to refer to these lesions as cavitated infarcts, and based on the morphology of the cysts to try to estimate the age at which they occurred, as well as to attempt to speculate about the agent causing the necrosis.

Schizencephaly was originally used by Yakovlev and Wadsworth to designate bilateral clefts in the brain. The term is probably no longer useful, as probably all such clefts are due to some type of destructive lesion occurring in utero (231). These defects may be diagnosed clinically and radiologically (237).

Hydranencephaly

Etiologically and morphologically, hydranencephaly represents a more severe form of porencephaly (67, 285). There is virtual absence of the cerebral hemispheres (Fig. 6.3) except for the basal parts, the temporal and occipital lobes (68), whereas in some instances cortical remnants contain cerebral cortex (133). There is a large membranous sac occupying the cranial cavity and containing cerebrospinal fluid, which is usually in continuity with the lateral ventricles but may be separate. The membrane consists of pia-arachnoid overlying a glial layer. The skull vault is normal or enlarged, with indentations on the inner aspect indicating the prior presence of brain tissue. The basal ganglia are usually normal but may be hypertrophied and distorted (327, 328). We believe that all of these cases result from destructive processes occurring in utero, and the changes depend on the time at which the insults occurred and on whether there is an asso-

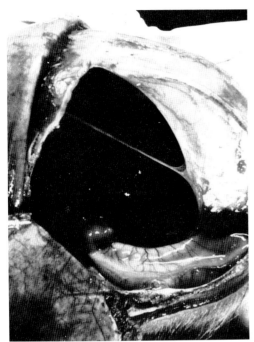

Figure 6.3. Hydranencephaly. View of the empty cranial cavity with part of the skull removed. The falx is fenestrated but present. An arc of tissue consisting of basal ganglia and remnants of occipitotemporal cortex is seen inferiorly.

ciated obstructive hydrocephalus following aqueductal stenosis. In many cases the destruction is centered around the middle cerebral artery, although it can extend well beyond that. The finding of polymicrogyria in other areas of the cortex and adjacent to the cyst area has been used as an argument that these are developmental in nature, but the same arguments that applied above to porencephaly are applicable to hydrancephaly. Experimentally, hydranencephaly can be induced in a variety of conditions (230), including monkeys after carotid artery ligation (224, 225), and we have observed this in mice exposed to the toxin cuprizone.

Other Conditions

Multicystic encephalomalacia, ulegyria, and status marmoratus (aberrant glial myelin scars occurring in basal ganglia and cortex), although superficially resembling some malformations, are clearly destructive in nature. The former represents probably an extreme degree of periventricular infarc-

tion, and the latter is well recognized as being due to perinatal hypoxia-ischemia.

NEURAL TUBE DEFECTS

Neural tube defects (NTD) is a term used to designate defects in which some part of the neural tube or its coverings are not closed. It encompasses a wide variety of defects, ranging from the most severe form of anencephaly, which is lethal, to the least severe which is spina bifida occulta consistent with a completely normal life. Other forms of neural tube defect include encephalocele, myelo- and meningomyeloceles, spinal dysraphism, some aspects of the Arnold-Chiari malformation, and tectocerebellar dysraphism (11). In order to fully appreciate the pathogenetic mechanisms involved in NTD, review of the embryology of the development of the neural tube must be considered.

The neural plate begins as a thickening in the ectoderm overlying the notochord late in the presomite stage in the human. Neurulation transforms the neural plate into the neural tube, although the mechanism inducing this is unknown (268). Elevation of the neural folds on either side of the central groove results in fusion of these folds starting at the 22nd day of gestation at the 2nd to 7th somite level, and extending rostrally and caudally from there. The anterior neuropore closes at about day 24, the posterior neuropore later, between day 26 and day 28 (240). Neurulation depends on the ability of the cells of the neural plate to change their shape due to the contractile action of microfilaments and microtubules (173, 174, 272). In addition, the surrounding ectoderm and lateral mesodermal cells contribute forces which help shape and elevate the neural folds. The intimate relationship between ectoderm, mesoderm, and the neural plate is thus established at a very early stage. Neural tube formation also depends on the presence of strong intercellular adhesions and intermediate junctions and desmosomes between the cells (137). The neural crest is formed from cells that lie just under the superficial epithelium and lateral to the neural tube, and these proliferate and migrate laterally (223). The final act is the separation of the superficial ectoderm from the neural tube with ingrowth of mesodermal derivatives between them. The fusion of the posterior neuropore concludes the process of neurulation (149), and the subsequent growth of the rostral brain has already been outlined earlier. It is thought that in the human, caudal elongation of the cord occurs through incorporation into the neural tube of new cells from a caudal blastema (tail bud), consisting of small cells surrounding separate small cavities beyond the central canal. This irregular canalization of the caudal zone of the neural tube is irregular and uneven (185) and may persist in the postfetal human equinal cord (188). The intervertebral disc at L1 to L2 is the embryological 25th or 1st lumbar somite and marks the level at which the formation of the spinal cord changes from formation by neurulation to differentiation from the tail bud or caudal blastema. Experimental extirpation of the tail bud of the chick regularly results in neural tube defects (270), and this area is obviously critical in the pathogenesis of spinal dysraphism at the thoracolumbar area. Extensive radiological and anatomical dissection of dysraphic infants (18) has emphasized the importance embryologically of this area in the production of spinal dysraphism.

Until the posterior neuropore closes, the contents of the neural tube are bathed by amniotic fluid. With closure a protein-rich fluid appears in the tube before the formation of the choroid plexus. Fluid then escapes from the canal through the semipermeable rhombic roof to cause formation of the subarachnoid space.

Etiopathogenesis of Neural Tube Defects

Although there are some special situations that occur in neural tube defects affecting the cranium and the spinal cord, in general much of the discussion on etiopathogenesis refers to both these situations.

Epidemiologically, neural tube defects have been studied extensively and have shown marked variations in prevalence rate, geographically, in different ethnic groups, over long periods of time (secular trends), and seasonally (93, 202). For example, there is approximately three-fold greater incidence in Belfast than in Lon-

don, and a gradient of decreasing prevalence from east-west in Canada and the United States. Marked differences in ethnic groups have been noted in Quebec, and prevalence differences in blacks and whites have also been noted. Although it has been claimed recently that vitamin treatments prior to conception reduce the incidence of abnormalities (286), there is now a spontaneous decline in the incidence of neural tube defects which must be considered in studying the effect of any therapy (233, 324).

Anencephaly is more prevalent in low socioeconomic groups, leading to the suggestion that maternal nutrition may be a factor. Maternal age, infection, multiple births, and other factors have all been studied without definite conclusions.

The etiological heterogeneity of neural tube defects (122, 144, 198, 308) (Table 6.2) makes elucidation of the cause difficult. Multifactorial causation of neural tube defects is well established. In addition, it was suggested (177) that neural tube defects with no other recognized causes could be divided into "singles," where there was no other malformation, and "multiples," where the neural tube defect occurred with other defects. The "singles" have the well-known epidemiological characteristics of neural tube defects: marked predominance of females and whites, geographic variation with an east-west gradient, and a decrease over time, factors not present in the "multiples." The multiples had a 0% precurrence rate and the singles a 2%. However, in another series of cases, siblings of children with tracheal dysraphism, extrophy of the bladder, and other congenital malformations had a somewhat increased risk of neural tube defects (108).

Numerous studies have indicated that these conditions may be diagnosed prenatally by the presence of raised α-fetoproteins (139, 275) (although this is not specific for NTD) and by ultrasonography (Fig. 6.4E).

Controversy has long existed over the pathogenetic mechanism of neural tube defects. Most evidence seems to favor the hypothesis that it represents a failure of closure of the neural tube due to primary failure either in neuroepithelium or in the surrounding mesoderm. The other theory

Table 6.2
Recognized Causes of Neural Tube Defects[a]

Multifactorial inheritance—anencephaly, meningomyelocele, meningocele, and encephalocele

Single mutant genes:
   Meckel syndrome—autosomal recessive
      (phenotype includes occipital encephalocele and rarely anencephaly)
   Median-cleft face syndrome—possible autosomal dominant
      (phenotype includes anterior encephalocele)
   Robert's syndrome—autosomal recessive
      (phenotype includes anterior encephalocele)
   Syndrome of anterior sacral meningomyelocele and anal stenosis—dominant, either autosomal
      or X-linked

Chromosome abnormalities:
   13 trisomy
   18 trisomy
   Triploidy
   Other abnormalities, such as unbalanced translocation and ring chromosome

Probably hereditary, but mode of transmission not established:
   Syndrome of occipital encephalocele, myopia, and retinal dysplasia
   Anterior encephalocele among Bantus and Thais

Teratogens:
   Aminopterin/amethopterin (phenotype includes anencephaly and encephalocele)
   Thalidomide (phenotype includes, rarely, anencephaly and meningomyelocele)

Specific phenotypes, but without known cause:
   Syndrome of craniofacial and limb defects secondary to aberrant tissue bands (phenotype
      includes multiple encephaloceles)
   Cloacal exstrophy (phenotype includes myelocystocele)
   Sacrococcygeal teratoma (phenotypes include meningomyelocele)

Other (unclassified)

[a] From L. B. Holmes et al. (144).

is that of reopening of the neural tube due either to a primary neuroepithelial breakdown or to increased intraluminal pressure. A large amount of experimental work has been performed to solve this problem, and this tends to favor failure of closure as a mechanism. Irradiation, administration of trypan blue, hypervitaminosis, salicylates, and antimetabolites, and maternal hyperthermia are among the agents that have produced various types of neural tube defects. Agents like colchicine (137), papaverine (183), and caffeine (184), all of which are important in microtubular and microfilamentous function, have been shown to cause neural tube abnormalities. These presumably act by interfering with cell shape change during neuralation. Many mutant mouse strains such as curly tail (274), splotch (316), and looped tail mouse (317)

all present with primary failure of closure of neural tube. The mechanisms in these also involve primary failures of the neuroepithelium through the interference with proper cell contact or failure to provide proper gap junctions. Vascular abnormalities, although once invoked (306), are not now thought to be of significance.

Marin-Padilla (205, 206) has proposed that neural tube defects result from primary mesodermal failure. From experiments using hypervitaminosis A, he suggested that primary axioskeletal defects lead to various degrees of neuroectodermal dysraphism. Alternatively, from studies of human anencephaly other authors have concluded that skull morphology in human anencephaly is the result of abnormal development of the brain and is thus a secondary phenomenon which does not indi-

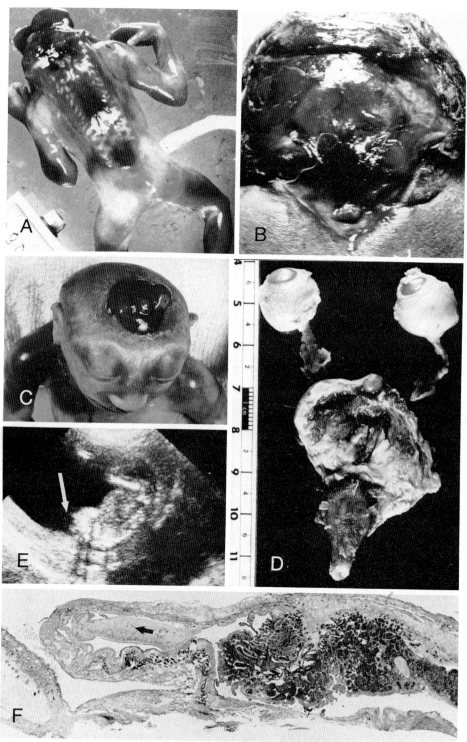

Figure 6.4. Anencephaly. (*A*) Complete rachischisis. (*B*) Holoanencephaly with intact spinal cord. (*C*) Meroanencephaly with localized defect. (*D*) Intact eyes and optic nerves terminating in the amorphous area cerebrovasculosa. The lower brain stem and spinal cord are intact. (*E*) Depiction of an anencephalic fetus in utero by ultrasound. The body and femur are well seen, but cranial vault is not visualized at expected site (*arrow*). (F) Area cerebrovasculosa. The mass of tissue consists of congested choroid plexus (*right*), connective tissue, a neuroglial plate (*arrow*), and ependymal-lined cavities covered by epidermis. Hematoxylin and eosin.

cate what the primary failure is (102, 120, 219). These two points of view are not incompatible, because a primary failure of neuroepithelium could coexist with a primary failure of chordomesoderm.

Some authors have favored secondary opening of the neural tube, although there is little clinical or experimental evidence for this. Padget (234, 235, 236) showed some clefts in the neural tube (neuroschisis) with overlying blebs of edema fluid in the mesoderm and ectoderm of some human and animal embryos. In addition, Gardner (115–119) has postulated that hydrostatic pressure from a persistence of the embryonic state of physiological hydrocephalus is responsible for forcing open the previously closed tube.

Anencephaly

Anencephaly is the most extreme example of defects in closure of the neural tube. This is a condition that has been known since ancient times and has been found in an Egyptian mummy. The term cranioschisis refers to all specimens of cranial opening with scalp defects, whereas the term rachischisis refers to an open defect in the dorsal spine leading to exposure or destruction of the underlying cord. Cranioschisis and rachischisis may occur together (Fig. 6.4A) or separately. Anencephaly with acrania (loss of skull vault) has usually been classified (186) into merocrania (meroanencephaly), in which there are large but incomplete defects of the cranial vault with alteration and protrusion of the brain through the defect, and holoacrania (*holoanencephaly*), in which there is total absence of the cranial vault with more or less complete destruction of the contents.

Anencephaly is a striking malformation. In holoacrania (Figs. 6.4A and B) no cranial vault exists at all, although in meroacrania (Fig. 6.4C), the cranial vault may be more formed. The frontal bone and the squamous portions of the parietal and occipital bone are rudimentary, the base of the skull is small, and the anterior and middle cranial fossae are decreased in size or absent. The sella turcica is shallow or absent, and the craniopharyngeal canal may be open. The cranial nerve foramina are patent, and although the orbital apertures may be set far apart and the palate cleft, the face is usually formed and eyes relatively normal. The spine is abnormally curved anteriorly and the vertebrae may be irregular. Rachischisis, ranging from total (Fig. 6.4A) to spina bifida cystica or even occulta, may be associated. A spinal defect may be associated with absence of the spinal cord (amyelia), in which case the spinal meninges are found within the defect. The eyes, which are of normal size, are prominent and seem to protrude from the junction of the brow and the base of the skull. The brain in holoanencephaly is replaced by a small disc-shaped mass of hemorrhagic tissue, the *area cerebrovasculosa* (Fig. 6.4D, F), which sits on the base of the skull and is usually covered by a thin smooth lobulated membrane. The amount of neural tissue varies greatly; the more complete the absence of the vault, the less neural tissue is present. Microscopic sections of the area cerebrovasculosa (Fig. 6.4F) show a mixture of abnormal vessels, fibrous tissue, neuroglial tissue in which neurons can only rarely be identified, and choroid plexus which may be infiltrated with extravasated blood. The superficial covering may show some squamous epithelium; at the edge where the mass becomes continuous with the skin, the skin is abnormal, lacking appendages. In cases of meroanencephaly, the brain may not be completely absent, and those structures that are preserved are usually those of the hindbrain. In cases where the brain stem is present (Fig. 6.4D), various cranial nerve nuclei may sometimes be identified (221); the cranial nerves may be rudimentary and end blindly in the mass. Even though the brain stem may be apparently preserved, the cerebellum is usually not preserved, only occasional remnants being seen. Even when the vertebral canal is closed, the cord usually is thin (*micromyelia*), with gliosis of the white matter and loss of neurons in the grey matter. The spinal cord may show numerous abnormalities (186), of which absence of corticospinal tracts is constant. This is not a primary defect but is consequent on the loss of cerebral hemispheres. Nodules of immature neural tissue occur in the spinal subarachnoid space (23), and subarachnoid striated muscle heterotopia have been described (8). The presence of the eyes indicates that the optic vesicles have formed and grown out of the brain, a process starting at about the 4th week of gestation. The eyes usually lose their connection to the remnant of the brain, but the optic nerves may end blindly in the area cerebrovasculosa (Fig. 6.4D). Derivatives of the neural crest are present in complete rachischisis, as evidenced by the finding of peripheral nerve and dorsal root ganglia. Peripheral muscle is normal.

There are other associated defects in anencephaly. The anterior pituitary is usually present but is small and normally shaped and may be displaced. The hypothalamus is missing (6), as is the pituitary stalk (186). In spite of the absence of the hypothalamus, TSH and ACTH can be produced using releasing hormones, suggesting their production in the pharyngeal hypophysis (212). The adrenals show absence or atrophy of the fetal zone and atrophy of the adult cortex (227), although they have been shown to be normal up to 17 to 20 weeks in anencephalics. Presumably until the normal portohypophyseal circulation is finally completed at the 20th week of gestation (160) the pituitary is under the influence of the placenta or other factors. The thyroid looks normal but may be functionally inactive (6), and the lungs, perhaps due to secondary atrophy of the diaphragm with arrest of growth and maturation, become hypoplastic (312). Nodules of neural tissue may be found in the lungs of anencephalics as an incidental finding (54). The thymus gland may be enlarged secondary to hypoadrenalism (186).

Encephaloceles (Meningoencephaloceles) and Cranial Meningocele

An encephalocele is a herniation of brain tissue outside of the cranial cavity. Although analogous to spina bifida and myelomeningocele, it is far less frequent (208), but both morphologically and in a familial sense it is related to anencephaly and spina bifida (308). Although some authors (Emery and Kalhan, 1970) have thought that these lesions represent blow-outs from overlying mesodermal defects (95) or from hydrocephalic forces acting on infarcted brain (52), they are generally felt to be true neural tube defects.

Eighty to ninety percent of encephaloceles occur in the occipital region (216) (Fig. 6.5), where they protrude through either the dorsal foramen magnum or the squamous occipital bone. The fossae at the base of the skull are small, and the frontal

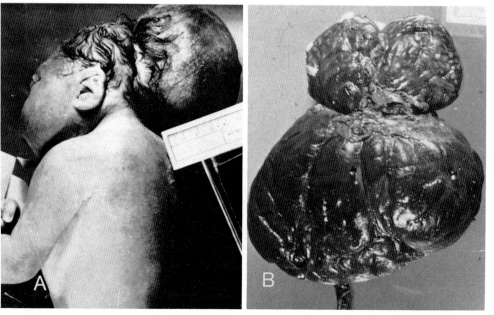

Figure 6.5. Occipital encephalocele. (A) The encephalocele is covered by intact scalp. (B) The encephalocele (bottom) contains more tissue than the normally situated brain (top).

bones may slope backward, depending on how much brain is herniated into the sac. Parietal or vertex encephaloceles may be present at the posterior fontanel (95) or rostral to it (214). Frontal encephaloceles may be associated with facial deformities, and a high incidence of these has been reported in Thailand (295). Nasal encephaloceles pass through the defect of the cribriform plate into the nasopharynx, whereas transphenoidal encephaloceles may pass through a cleft palate and protrude into the pharynx (182, 208, 249). Encephaloceles may appear in the orbit through the orbital fissures (308).

The falx and tentorium in these cases are usually small. The scalp over encephaloceles is usually intact (Fig. 6.5), and underlying it there is dura and leptomeningeal tissue. Varying amounts of brain can be found in encephaloceles. This varies in each case, and they may contain varying degrees of cerebellum (see under Arnold-Chiari malformations), brain stem, and portions of cerebral hemispheres. The amount of cerebral hemispheres in the sac on both sides is asymmetric. The herniated brain tissue enters the encephaloceles through an opening narrower than the diameter of the encephalocele; this results in varying degrees of hemorrhage, frank infarction, and sclerosis of the encased brain tissue due to pressure on vessels as they cross the encephalocele. There may be distortion and abnormalities of the brain remaining in the cranial cavity secondary to this herniation. The ventricles may be abnormal, being compressed together or dilated due to obstruction. Agenesis of the anterior commissure, septum pellicidum, and the fornical system has been described in four of five cases by Karch and Urich (172), and encephaloceles may be associated with holoprosencephaly (152). The brain stem may be extremely distorted, and normal structures may be difficult to identify. The cerebellum may be unidentifiable, rudimentary, or sclerotic. Vermal aplasia may be present with encephalocele together with other tectal abnormalities (110). Abnormal fetal vasculature may surround the brain stem and cord (172), and masses of bundles of neuroglia tissue may be found at the ventricular cavities. Ependyma and choroid plexus may also be present in the enceph-

alocele. Secondary hydrocephalus may be caused by obstruction to CSF flow. Microcephaly and mental retardation are common (129), and the presence of brain in the sac is of serious prognostic consequence.

Cranial meningoceles are usually situated over a small bony defect and contain subarachnoid fluid. Histologically they may contain leptomeninges, dura, and connective tissue.

Spinal Neural Tube Defects (Spina Bifida, Meningocele, and Myelomeningocele)

Like other neural tube defects, spinal dysraphias involve covering ectoderm, mesoderm, and neural structures and are of varying degrees of severity.

The least severe is *spina bifida occulta* which is found in anything from 1 to 24% of normal people (110), depending on age examined (156), to complete rachischisis which has been described above. The spinal neural tube defects are among the most common congenital malformations in man. Similarly, the clinical symptomatology may range from asymptomatic lesions, possibly associated with deformities and gait abnormalities, to myelomeningoceles which have profound neurological deficits, both motor and sensory; total rachischisis is incompatible with life. The familial incidence is strong in this group of disorders; 4.1 to 2% of siblings of individuals treated neurosurgically for spinal dysraphism had a sibling with neural tube malformation (49).

The majority of lesions occur in the thoracolumbar area, which may be related to the susceptibility of the caudal blastema in this area as has been discussed above. Bone changes are striking and indeed may be the only manifestation. The vertebral arches may be absent or unfused (Fig. 6.6C) with lateral displacement of the pedicles and widened spinal canal. There may be associated bony or cartilaginous spur formation, suggestive of associated diastomatomyelia (Fig. 6.41), and a variety of other associated bony changes may be found (18).

In spina bifida occulta, there is failure of the bone to fuse, but the underlying spinal cord does not usually show dysraphia. However, numerous cases show some form of fibrous traction bands between the bone

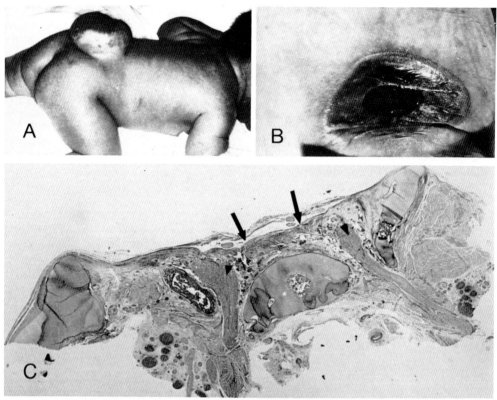

Figure 6.6. Myelomeningocele. (*A*) Lumbar spina bifida cystica. (*B*) This thoracolumbar myelomeningocele has undergone necrosis and appears as a flat open defect. (*C*) Microscopic section of a myelomeningocele. The dorsal arches are absent. The dorsal root ganglia and spinal nerves (*arrowheads*) emerge ventrally through the foramen between the pedicles and the vertebral body. Dorsal to the vertebral body, the area medullovasculosa (*arrows*) consists of vascular connective tissue and neuroglia.

and the spinal cord which require surgical intervention, and there is a high degree of diastomamyelia (42% in some series) (150, 155, 156). A variety of minor abnormalities have been described under the skin in association with spina bifida occulta, the commonest of which is surgically excised lipoma (96). A dermal sinus may be present, and frequently these lesions are marked by the presence of a cutaneous vascular malformation or hypertrichosis.

SPINA BIFIDA CYSTICA

These conditions which are associated either with meningocele or myelomeningocele consist of a cystic defect protruding on the skin (Fig. 6.6A).

If the meninges alone protrude into this defect the lesion is called a *meningocele*, and this occurs in approximately 10–20% of cases. The cyst is connected to the ver-tebral canal by a narrow channel and is composed of skin dura and arachnoid. The cord itself is often abnormal.

The other 80–90% of spina bifida cystica consists of *myelomeningoceles* (Fig. 6.6A) which are usually dome-shaped with a central red wet oozing area (*area medulla-vasculosa*) (Fig. 6.6C) which usually becomes epithelialized after birth. Eighty to 90% of these cases occur in the lower thoracolumbar region, but the bone defect usually extends all the way down to the sacrum (18). The cyst may be filled with fluid and sealed by arachnoid and is often fused to the cord remnants. Peripheral nerves traverse the cyst and end either in the cord remnants or blindly within the mass of the area medulla-vasculosa (Fig. 6.6C). Microscopic examination reveals vascularized connective tissue, with leptomeninges and irregularly disposed glial neuronal tissue containing motor neurons and ependyma. Studies of the cord both in and around the cystic lesion (97) have revealed hydromyelia and syringomyelia proximal to the myelocele in 29 and 14% of cases, respectively. Within the meningomyelocele, there was an open neural plate in 35%, and total or partial diastomatomyelia in 36%, together with compression of the cord by arachnoid cyst. Distal to the main lesion, diastomatomyelia was found in 25% and double or multiple spinal cord canals in 29%. Peripheral nerve and dorsal root ganglia and other neural crest derivatives are easily found in the mesoderm adjacent to the cyst. The cyst may also contain keratin, dermoid cysts, and hair.

Both meningoceles and myeloceles may ulcerate and become the source of infective meningitis. Secondary necrosis in utero may destroy the entire neural plate in severe cases of spina bifida cystica or rachischisis, leaving only the underlying osseous bed (Fig. 6.6B). After birth meningitis may produce the same effect.

Spina bifida cystica may occur in association with numerous other congenital malformations of the nervous system. Its most common association is with hydrocephalus and the Arnold-Chiari syndrome which will be discussed below. Why this association should be present is not known, but Warkany and O'Toole (309) have suggested that as in animal experiments, the spina bifida complex may be a multifocal abnormality developing independently owing to a common noxious influence that affects many sites simultaneously.

VENTRAL SPINAL DEFECTS

Various ventral defects may occur and are sometimes referred to as anterior meningomyelocele. These consist of neurenteric (enterogenic) cysts, anterior sacral meningoceles, and teratomas. *Neurenteric cysts* probably arise early in embryogenesis when the endoderm and ectoderm are close together. Mesoderm grows between and separates endoderm and notochord about the end of the 3rd week, and failure of separation may lead to the formation of these cysts. The cysts are intraspinal, ventral to the cord, and occur in the cervicothoracic region; they may be intramedullary, attached to the meninges or to the vertebra. There are sometimes various vertebral defects which allow the cysts to communicate with intrathoracic cysts and be lined with various types of epithelium (esophagus, stomach, or small intestine).

Anterior sacral meningocele is a protrusion of a sac of dura and leptomeninges through a defect in the sacrum. It is said to have been inherited as an X-linked dominant; however, in one family 11 individuals in three generations with male to male transmission had partial sacral agenesis and anterior sacral meningoceles or teratomas, or both, suggesting an autosomal dominant transmission of this family (330). Cystic *teratomas* of the spinal cord have also been described (258).

DISORDERS OF FORMATION OF STRUCTURES DERIVING FROM THE ANTERIOR TELENCEPHALIC WALL

Many previous reports have ascribed malformation in this group to failure of cleavage of the forebrain, but we prefer to regard them as a failure of the normal outgrowth of the telencephalic vesicles, rather than an absence of the dynamic act of cleaving. Because of the common derivation from the anterior telencephalic wall, the frequent association of these malformations with others in the same group, and the frequent incidence in defined syndromes and chromosomal abnormalities, they should be regarded as representing a spectrum of disorders, caused by growth disturbances of different severity or occurring at different periods of time, affecting the geographical area of the anterior telencephalic wall either wholly or in part.

The normal embryological development of the anterior telencephalic wall is depicted diagrammatically to facilitate an understanding of the mechanisms of pathogenesis (Fig. 6.7). During the 5th week of development the telencephalic vesicles which are the future cerebral hemispheres arise as paired lateral evaginations of the single prosencephalic cavity (134) (Fig. 6.7A). At first the cavities of the telencephalic vesicles are continuous widely with the primary vesicle. By the 7th to 8th week, however, the choroid plexus invaginates the dorsal medial aspect of each lateral cavity.

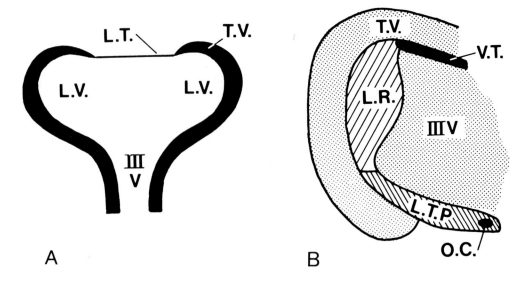

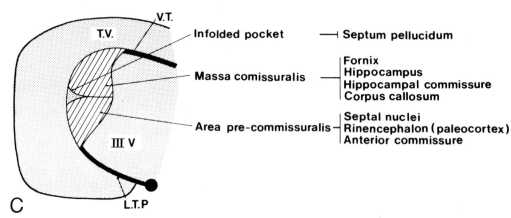

Figure 6.7. Diagrammatic representation of embryogenesis of the anterior telencephalic wall. (*A* and *B*) Dorsal and medial sagittal views at 5 weeks. (*C*) Medial sagittal view after differentiation of the lamina-reuniens. *L.V.*, lateral ventricle; *IIIV*, third ventricle; *T.V.*, telencephalic vesicle; *L.T.*, lamina terminalis; *L.T.P.*, lamina terminalis proper; *L.R.*, lamina reuniens; *O.C.*, optic chiasm; *V.T.*, velum transversum.

At the same time the backward growth of the lateral vesicles results in the formation of the two cerebral hemispheres. During this time the connections between the cavities of the telencephalic vesicles with the primary prosencephalic cavity become narrowed, forming the foramina of Monro. The remaining midline prosencephalic cavity and the diencephalic cavity with which it is continuous form the 3rd ventricle. In the meantime the anterior telencephalic wall, which originally began as the wall of the prosencephalic cavity, undergoes develop-

ment (159, 197, 257). From this area, which is known as the lamina terminalis, originate the forebrain commissures and related structures. The lamina terminalis extends from the optic chiasm up to the velum transversum. According to Rakic and Yakovlev (257) there are two distinct parts to the anterior wall of the lamina terminalis (Fig. 6.7*B*).

1. The lamina terminalis proper, the ventral portion which eventually becomes the adult lamina terminalis at the ante-

rior aspect of the 3rd ventricle and which is a relatively acellular and inert structure.

2. The dorsal part, known as the lamina reuniens of His which is highly cellular and thickened.

After evagination and growth of this telencephalic vesicle, this dorsal part of the lamina reuniens infolds in between the growing vesicles and forms a median groove (called the sulcus medianus telencephali medii). The banks of this groove then fuse forming the massa commissuralis. The lamina reuniens is therefore made up of two separate parts: the ventral part lying above the lamina terminalis proper (the area precommissuralis) and the dorsal part consisting of the fused massa commissuralis (Fig. 6.7C). From this dorsal massa commissuralis develop the primordia of the hippocampus and archicortex, the corpus callosum, the hippocampal commissure, and the fibers of the fornix. The ventral area precommissuralis gives rise to the septal nucleus, the rhinencephalon (paleocortex), and the anterior commissure. In addition, when the lamina reuniens infolds, a small sac appears under the anterior border of the massa commissuralis. This breaks down further and becomes the cavum septi pelluci between the banks of the sulcus medianus telencephali medii. Dorsally it becomes sealed by the growth of the rostrum of the corpus callosum.

At about 9–10 weeks of embryonic life, the fibers of the anterior commissure grow into the area precommissuralis, and the hippocampal commissure develops about a week or two later. The first fibers of the corpus callosum appear in the massa commissuralis at about the 11th to 12th week. The corpus callosum grows in a caudal direction with the growth of the hemisphere and assumes an adult configuration by the 20th week.

The olfactory bulb appears at 6 weeks as a cortical formation; it is thought that its development is induced by nerve fibers from the olfactory epithelium of the nasal fossa. The narrow stemmed olfactory peduncle connects with the septal and amygdaloid nuclei and the peripheral cortex. The hippocampal formation becomes differentiated anteriorly with evagination of the

hemispheres and during development proceeds back to the posterior end of the cerebral hemisphere, extending caudally, with the more rostral part disappearing as caudal parts develop. Rotation of the various structures ensues, leading to the characteristic adult relationship of the dentate gyrus to the rest of the hippocampus. The hippocampus assumes its adult configuration and position by approximately the 14th to 16th week.

Considering these details aids considerably in the understanding and pathogenesis of the various malformations. It becomes clear that a major early injury to the anterior telencephalic wall will lead to holoprosencephaly, arrhinencephaly, and failure of formation of the commissures. More localized insults can cause lack of development of specific structures. A defect in the entire lamina reuniens may result in total agenesis of the corpus callosum, the anterior commissure, and the hippocampal commissure. Should the defect be more dorsally localized, the anterior commissure could be spared but the corpus callosum totally absent. Focal posterior midline arrest late in morphogenesis, resulting perhaps from a cyst or mass, may cause partial agenesis of the corpus callosum alone (197, 290). More ventrally situated defects would affect preferentially the development of the rhinencephalon and the olfactory bulbs and tracts.

In addition it becomes important to consider the relationship between the neural tube and the surrounding mesenchymal tissue of the anterior embryo. The principle of mesenchymal induction of neural differentiation in development is well established and can take place in cell-free suspension (301). The forebrain appears to be induced by the prechordal mesenchyme around the dorsal lip of the foregut. This prechordal mesoderm evolves into the facial bone (the hindbrain and spinal cord may be induced by the mesenchyme of the notochord). A disturbance of this prechordal mesoderm will not only cause malformations of its derivative structures but may also influence its inductive capabilities on forebrain structures (79, 197, 239, 326).

The pathogenesis and etiology of this group of conditions have attracted a large amount of interest in recent years because of the frequency of association with chromosomal abnormality, existence in familial forms (80, 218), and the association with environmental agents. Anomalies have been reported in their most striking manifestations not only as part of trisomy 13–15 (Patau syndrome) (67, 239, 287, 300) but also in trisomy 17–18 (Edwards syndrome) (211, 294). A wide variety of other chromosomal abnormalities have been associated with this group of malformation (such as 13q syndrome, ring 13 and 18 p syndrome, monosomy-G mosaicism, and ring 18 syndrome monosomy and triploidy). Holoprosencephaly has been described in both monozygotic and dizygotic twins (44) and in nontwin siblings (21), as well as in a father and son (201).

Occurrence in children of diabetic mothers (74) and other environmental factors such as maternal rubella, toxoplasmosis, fetal alcohol syndrome, and drug treatment have been implicated (159). Experimentally cyclopia and prosencephaly have been reported in lambs which ingested the plant "veratrum californicum" on grazing pastures in Idaho (33).

Holoprosencephaly

This term has been used to designate the most severe form of anterior telencephalic wall failure and implies the tendency of prosencephalon to remain "holistic." Although the terms holotelencephaly, arrhinencephaly, and olfactory hypoplasia have all been used interchangably, they should be kept apart because, although they often exist together, they may be found separately. As can be understood from the discussion on embryology and general comments on pathogenesis, the degree of involvement depends on timing, location, and severity of the insult. The patient with severe forms are usually stillborn, but may survive and show mental retardation, motor abnormalities, spasticity, and disturbances in temperature regulation (229). It is important to try to estimate the severity, and this can be assessed, not only clinically, where some guide is given by the severity of facial anomalies (see below) but also by specialized investigation with ultrasonography and CT scanning (44, 81, 265). This diagnosis can also be made antenatally using ultrasound (35). The importance of ac-

curate assessment of the degree of central nervous system involvement for the purpose of clinical-pathological correlation must be stressed.

DeMyer and coworkers (78, 79) have classified the holoprosencephalies into alobar, semilobar, and lobar forms. In all these forms there may be shortening and narrowing of the skull, with absence of lamina cribrosa and the crista Galli. Depending on the degree of involvement of the face, there may be hypoplasia or absence of bones around the nasal cavity. The pituitary fossa may be shallow, and most holoprosencephalic brains are small. Although cases of so-called *aprosencephaly* (complete absence of the forebrain) have been reported in the radiological literature (3), in the absence of pathological examination this entity remains suspect.

In *alobar prosencephaly* (Figs. 6.8A–C), the telencephalon is not separated into hemispheres or recognizable lobes, and there is a single mass with a single large ventricle (Fig. 6.8A). The dorsal part of the mass consists of a transverse convolution representing the remnant of the cingulate gyrus, which is horseshoe-shaped when seen from behind (Figs. 6.8A–C, 6.9) and overlies an arch of white matter which lies adjacent to the common ventricle. The common ventricle may balloon dorsally in the form of a cyst, and its thin covering is the roof plate of the telencephalon median together with remnants of telachoroidea (326). This cyst occupies the space between the hemispheres and the caudally displaced tentorium and cerebellum. Choroid plexus may still be found in the cyst. This cyst may be disrupted on removal of the brain (Fig. 6.8A). Detailed architectonic studies (326) have shown that although parietal and occipital lobes appear to be lacking, these are present laterally, and that the deficiencies in the cortex lie within the frontal lobe. The cortex bordering the opening of the common ventricle has the architectonic structure of the hippocampus and rhinencephalon. The rhinencephalon and its associated structures, such as corpus callosum, anterior commissure, central nuclei, and hippocampus may be absent. Aplasia of the olfactory bulb and tracts may be seen (Fig. 6.12). The blood supply to the mass comes from bilateral middle cerebral

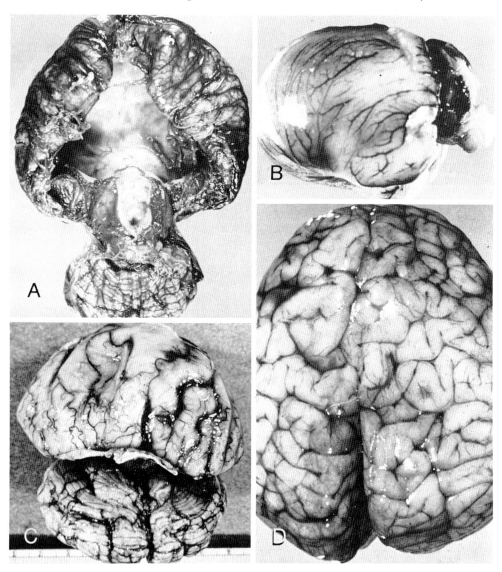

Figure 6.8. Holoprosencephaly. (*A*) Alobar holoprosencephaly viewed from above. The single large ventricle is exposed dorsally. (*B*) Alobar holoprosencephaly in a fetal brain (approximately 17 weeks). (*C*) Alobar holoprosencephaly. The brain is extremely small; in this case the dorsal surface is intact. (*D*) Lobar holoprosencephaly. Separation into two hemispheres has only occurred posteriorly.

arteries, although the anterior cerebral artery may be single. The degree of involvement of the optic tract depends upon the degree of eye deformities, which may range from a single optic nerve in the case of cyclopia (Fig. 6.11) to aplasia of the nerve. The basal ganglia shows varying degrees of abnormality, with fusion of the thalami (Fig. 6.9) and corpus striatum (Fig. 6.10) being commonest and complete absence of the corpus striatum occurring rarely.

In *semilobar prosencephaly*, separation of the hemispheres is indicated by a narrow longitudinal sulcus that extends along the dorsal surface towards the frontal pole but never onto the orbital surface. Lobar structure is rudimentary. The corpus callosum is often absent or may be suggested by some commissural fibers (Fig. 6.10). The rhinencephalon may be absent, and the thalami and basal ganglia may be fused.

In *lobar holoprosencephaly* (Fig. 6.8*D*) the

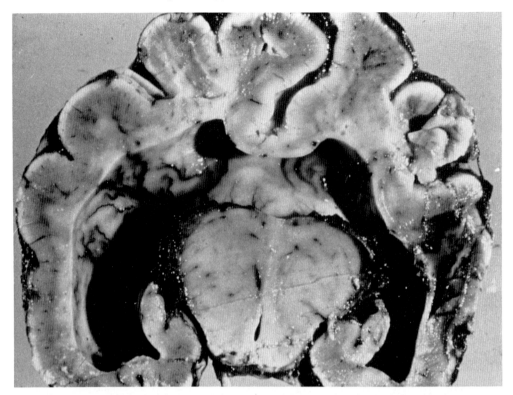

Figure 6.9. Semilobar holoprosencephaly. The cingulate gyrus is transversely curved and is continuous across the apparent longitudinal fissure. No corpus callosum is seen. The ventricle is single and large. The thalami are fused.

separation of the hemispheres is usually complete except anteriorly. The two hemispheres may remain connected at the base of the longitudinal cerebral fissure by a plate of grey and white matter remnant of the telencephalon medium. This may resemble the corpus callosum which, however, cannot form in these circumstances. Although there may be communication between the bodies of the lateral ventricles, the occipital and temporal horns are separated. The corpus callosum may be absent, or when the hemispheres are not joined by the telencephalon medium, it may be incomplete or present. The rhinencephalon may be absent, rudimentary, or complete. The thalami and basal ganglia (Fig. 6.10) may be fused broadly, but when the hemispheres are fully separated a thick interthalamic adhesion may be the mildest expression of this pattern of malformation (176). The brains in these cases may show hypoplasia of frontal lobes with the anterior portions being pointed. The pituitary may be absent, and endocrine abnormalities especially hypopituitarism may be present (21, 142, 326).

Of great importance in this group of conditions is the coexistence of facial abnormalities (78, 79). As has been discussed above, these usually derive from disturbances to the prechordal mesenchyme and are presumably caused by the same agents that interfere with the growth of the anterior telencephalic wall. The most severe of these conditions is *cyclopia* (Fig. 6.11) (2, 90), in which the orbits are fused and in which the eyeballs are either set very close together or are completely fused. In these instances a small nasal protuberance is present above the orbits. The optic tract may be single or absent. In less severely deformed cases, the orbits are abnormally close together (*hypotelorism*), and there is microphthalmia. The nose may be flattened. This is similar to *cebocephaly* where there are two eyes and orbits but a flattening of the nasal area. Medial cleft lips and palates without a philtrum represent still less severe forms of involvement, and some-

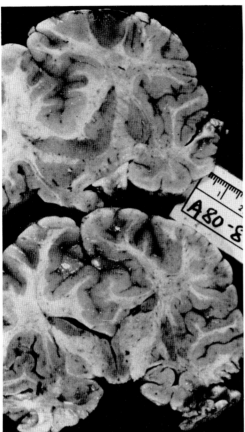

Figure 6.10. Lobar holoprosencephaly. Fusion of the caudate is seen, and the ventricles are almost obliterated anteriorly (*top*). Posteriorly (*bottom*) the ventricles are formed, and the caudate nuclei are unfused.

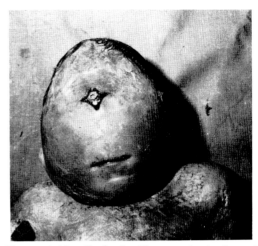

Figure 6.11. Cyclopia. The eye is single and the nose missing.

times there is a pointing of the forehead similar to that seen in the brain itself, called *trigonocephaly*. Frontonasal dysplasia (in which there is ocular hypertelorism, a wide nasal bridge, and hypoplasia and clefting of the upper lip) is usually not associated with holoprosencephaly and has been considered opposite in nature to holoprosencephaly (110). This median cleft face syndrome may occasionally be present as an expression of holoprosencephaly (265).

The frequency of associated malformations in holoprosencephaly is of great importance, not only in understanding etiopathogenesis but also for clinicopathological correlation and prognosis. These have been reviewed (159). Craniofacial dyplasias were present in 92% of cases (most frequently microcephaly, hypertelorism, hy-

potelorism, and cleft formations). Associated CNS malformations were present in 93% of cases (migration disorders, displaced hippocampus, fusion of basal ganglia, hydrocephalus, cysts, and dysraphic lesions). Holoprosencephaly has been associated also with occipital encephalocele and aqueduct stenosis (152). Malformations outside the nervous system have been found frequently including musculoskeletal, genitourinary, cardiovascular, and gastrointestinal defects. In general it may be stated that the severity of the craniofacial defect and the presence of associated organ malformations mirror the severity of the malformation of the brain (79, 130, 159), although the correlation is not always accurate in the individual case. In general, too, it may be stated that the more severe the CNS malformation (and therefore the craniofacial defect) the more likely the possibility that the underlying etiology is that of a chromosomal disorder (159). Patients with holoprosencephaly and normal karyotypes (34, 80) often do not have the extracranial anomalies.

Olfactory Aplasia (Arrhinencephaly)

This may occur as an incidental finding (Fig. 6.12), representing a very mild form of anterior telencephalic wall malformation, or else it may occur as part of holoprosencephaly, or in association with agenesis of the corpus callosum or other anterior telencephalic wall derivatives. There may

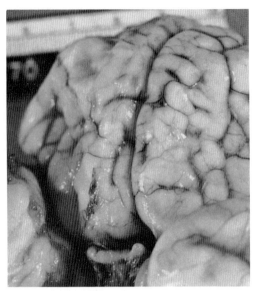

Figure 6.12. Olfactory aplasia (arrhinencephaly). The olfactory nerves are absent, and the olfactory sulci unformed.

be absence of the olfactory bulbs, tracts, the trigone, and the anterior perforated area. If the anomaly is isolated, the rest of the limbic system and hippocampus is normal.

Agenesis of the Corpus Callosum

The general pathogenetic aspects of this lesion have been discussed above. This condition may occur as an isolated malformation. The corpus callosum is always absent in holoprosencephaly. These defects may be present in patients with mental retardation or else be found incidentally at autopsy (38). They have been associated with relapsing hypothermia (229). The diagnosis may be made radiologically (73, 201).

Besides the associated defects which are commonly found with loss of the corpus callosum, a few more well defined syndromes have been described. In the *Aicardi syndrome* there is agenesis of the corpus callosum with associated mental retardation, seizures, vertebral anomalies, and the characteristic ocular finding of chorioretinitis (30). An *acrocallosal syndrome* (228) in which agenesis of the corpus callosum, mental retardation, and polydactyly are present has also recently been described.

In agenesis of the corpus callosum there is either partial (218) or complete (Fig.

6.13) replacement of the corpus by a thin fibrous membrane. Usually the posterior part is more severely affected when the agenesis is partial. The 3rd ventricle may open directly onto the surface of the brain. Rarely a lipoma, meningioma, or cyst (290) in the base of the median fissure may not only indicate the site of the absent corpus, but may also be implicated in its causation. The 3rd ventricle is often dilated dorsally (Fig. 6.13*A* and *B*). A thick longitudinal bundle of myelinated fibers (*Probst's bundle*) is often found (Fig. 6.13*C*), originating in the white matter of the frontal lobe and terminating in the occipital lobe. Its nature is uncertain, but it is thought to contain misdirected fibers intended for the corpus callosum (although fibers of the strial lancii and the fornical systems may also be present). The volume of fibers in this bundle is usually less than that of a normal corpus callosum. These bundles usually exist on the superior surface of the lateral ventricles, lateral to the midline membranous roof. They may sometimes also appear as short stumps of white matter. In coronal sections the cerebral hemisphere shows ventricles with pointed upper corners (Fig. 6.13*C*) (so-called bat-wing ventricular shape) which may be recognizable on pneumoencephalogram.

The gyral pattern on the medial aspect of the hemispheres may be abnormal. The supracallosal gyri are arranged radially (Fig. 6.13*A*) in the areas where the corpus callosum is absent, and the parietooccipital and calcarine sulci fail to intersect. The cingulate gyrus is absent. There may be associated cortical abnormalities such as polymicrogyria. Anterior to the foramen of Monro which is widely elongated, a band of grey and white matter consisting of the central nuclei extends from the paraolfactory cortex up to the bundle of Probst. Further back this band becomes thinned into the septum pellucidum, which joins the fornices to the longitudinal Probst bundle. The leaves of the septum pellucidum are widely separated and incline sharply laterally instead of vertically (Fig. 6.13*C*), sometimes resembling a membranous ventricular roof. In some instances the septum pellucidum is absent. The absence of the splenium leads to abnormal dilatation of the trigone of the lateral ventricle. The

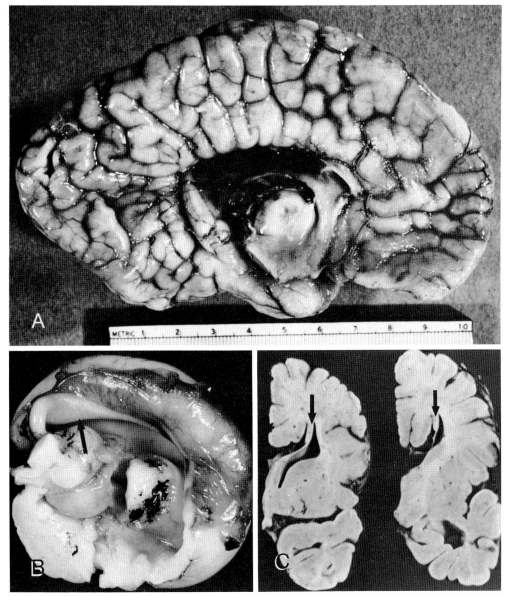

Figure 6.13. Agenesis of corpus callosum. (A) The absence of the corpus callosum is accompanied by an absence of the cingulate gyrus. There is a radial arrangement of gyri around the ventricle on the medial surface of this hemisphere. (B) Agenesis of the corpus callosum in a 24-week-old fetus. The hippocampus (*arrow*) has failed to migrate posteroinferiorly, and the temporal lobes are poorly formed. (C) The ventricles are pointed (bat-wing shape), and the leaves of the septum pellucidum incline laterally from the fornix and septal nuclei up to Probst's bundle (*arrows*).

hippocampal commissure may be absent. The fornices themselves while inherently normal may be displaced laterally.

Agenesis of the corpus callosum may be associated with numerous other malformations. Nine of 11 cases reported by Parrish et al. (238) had associated malformations of the central nervous system, and 8 were associated with malformations of the rest of the body. In Jellinger's series (158) 88% of cases of agenesis of the corpus callosum had associated CNS malformations, of which hydrocephalus, migration disturbances, rhinencephalic defects, and other abnormalities were common.

Malformations of the Septum Pellucidum

The formation of the septum pellucidum from the anterior telencephalic wall has already been described above. Various malformations arising from disturbances of this structure at various stages may be found. Absence of the septum pellucidum may be seen associated with other telencephalic wall defects, such as holoprosencephaly (Fig. 6.8), and some cases of agenesis of the corpus callosum. This absence can be clearly seen on radiological investigation and at autopsy. It must be distinguished from cases of secondary destruction of the septum pellucidum following hydrocephalus (Fig. 6.16C). In these cases small stumps or remnants of the septum may be seen. In some instances the septum may be partially fused with the caudate nucleus (232, 303). Another syndrome has been described linking absence of the septum pellucidum with porencephalies and other developmental defects (4).

SEPTOOPTIC DYSPLASIA

This midline malformation of the brain consists of agenesis of the septum pellucidum (Fig. 6.14) and hypoplasia of the optic pathways (77). There is hypoplasia of the optic nerve and discs, which have double-contoured papillae.

CAVUM SEPTI PELLICUDI AND CAVUM VERGAE

The cavum septi pellucidi and its posterior extension, cavum vergae, are normal embryological cavities which generally become obliterated after the 39th week (189, 278). In the infant they are lined by glia (321). Persistence of the cavum septi pellucidi is common (12% of adolescents), when they may be lined by ependyma (196). Very rarely, cavum vergae may be present without a cavum septi pellucidi. They are usually asymptomatic, but some can exist as large cysts (70), which may become symptomatic by blocking the foramen of Monro and causing internal hydrocephalus or other symptoms (247, 151, 189, 278).

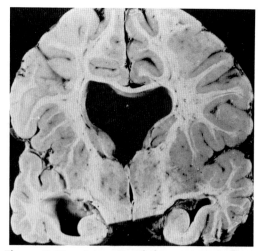

Figure 6.14. Agenesis of the septum pellucidum from a case of septooptic dysplasia. The lateral ventricles are not separated. The ventral surface of the corpus callosum is smooth (compare with Fig. 6.16C).

ARNOLD-CHIARI MALFORMATION

Although Cleland in 1883 first described an infant with a myelomeningocele, herniation of the vermis, and deformities of the medulla and tectal plate, the entity now known as the Arnold-Chiari syndrome was first delineated by Chiari in 1891 (55), and then again in 1896. In 1894 Arnold described a case of an infant with myelomeningocele and other truncal and limb deformities, together with herniation of the cerebellum, and it was his colleagues Schwalbe and Gredig in 1907 who linked his name with Chiari's to define the malformation. Although these authors attempted to subdivide the malformation into the cerebellar herniation (Arnold) and the brain stem deformity (Chiari), most authorities do not distinguish these two entities.

Chiari originally described three types of lesion, which have been widely accepted since his reports.

Type I consists of herniated cerebellar tonsils with minimal displacement of the brain stem.

Type II is a defect conforming to the description of the classical Arnold-Chiari malformation discussed in detail below.

Type III consists of cervical spina bifida with herniation of the cerebellum through the bony defect forming an encephalocele.

In addition in 1896 Chiari included as a fourth type a case of cerebellar hypoplasia, which, however, is clearly a different entity.

Type III is better considered as a form of rostral neural tube defect. It is very rare (245) and may be present together with abnormalities of the neck, such as the Klippel-Feil syndrome (48) and iniencephaly.

Although type I has classically been considered part of the Arnold-Chiari malformation (51, 232), especially the adult types (241), there are good reasons for supporting the view that most cases are really examples of chronic tonsillar herniation (see below). Most of the cases occur in adults and older children, are usually asymptomatic, and are not associated with myelomeningocele or hydrocephalus. The cerebellar herniations arise from the tonsils (indicating a later embryological origin than would occur with the vermis), and in spite of Norman's assertion (232) that the nerve roots angled upwards and the brain stem was displaced, this is not found in most cases. Indeed examination of Chiari's original drawing shows no upward displacement of the nerve roots and no displacement of the medulla (48). Fibrovascular adhesions may occur in any longstanding displacement. Cases of *convincing* adult Arnold-Chiari malformation should therefore at least have some features of the type II as described by Chiari (see below) to be so considered, which includes herniation of the cerebellar vermis with or without the tonsils, deformities of the lower brain stem, and associated spina bifida.

PATHOLOGY

The pathological findings have been well described (46, 47, 72, 110, 124, 232, 244, 245, 303). The hallmark of the disease is displacement of the cerebellum and distal brain stem through the foramen magnum where they become tightly packed in the upper cervical canal (Figs. 6.15 and 6.16). The herniated cerebellar tissue usually arises from the inferior vermis, but the tonsils may also be involved. Daniel and Strich (72) found involvement of the uvulus, nodules, and pyramis in that order. The herniated cerebellar tissue usually overlies

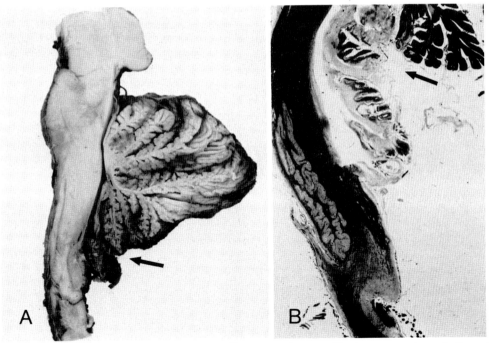

Figure 6.15.   Arnold-Chiari malformation. Midline sagittal view of brain stem and cerebellum. (*A*) Autopsy specimen, (*B*) Microscopic section stained with Loyez. Displaced, distorted sclerotic cerebellar tissue is seen below the site of the edge of the foramen magnum (*arrows*). The fourth ventricle and brain stem nuclei are also displaced, and there is a dorsal kink of medulla over the cervical cord in *B*.

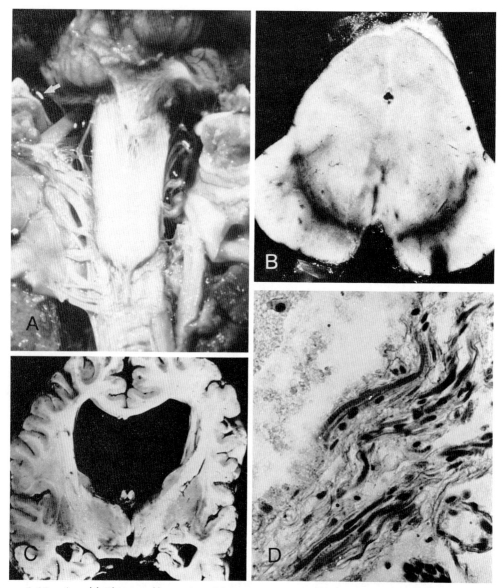

Figure 6.16. Arnold-Chiari malformation. (*A*) Posterior view of herniated brain stem and cerebellar tissue beneath the edge of the foramen magnum (*arrow*). The upper cervical nerve roots are angled upwards. (*B*) Beaking of the tectum due to fusion of the colliculi. (*C*) Hydrocephalus with destruction of septum pellucidum. Note residual septal stumps on ventral surface of corpus callosum. (Compare with Fig. 6.14). (*D*) Striated muscle within a leptomeningeal glial heterotopia.

the dorsal medulla in the form of a peg or strand (Fig. 6.15) and is often tightly bound to it by fibrovascular adhesions of the leptomeninges. The herniated tissue may be firm and gliotic, and there is a dorsal groove rostral to it, caused by the edge of the foramen magnum (Fig. 6.15*A*). Histological examination of the herniated cerebellar tissue shows gliotic folia (Fig. 6.15*B*), in which there is loss of Purkinje and granular cells

with Bergmann glial proliferation. Some of the folia may contain dysplastic changes suggestive of polymicrogyria. Heterotopias may be present in the cerebellar white matter. The medulla oblongata is usually displaced caudally into the upper cervical cord, in conjunction with an elongated fourth ventricle and its choroid plexus (Fig. 6.15). On 50% of cases there is an s-shaped curve, "or kinking," caused by a lump on the lower medulla, which overlies the dorsal cervical cord (Fig. 6.15b). The bend occurs caudal to the gracile and cuneate nuclei which lie within the medulla. Although the brain stem and cerebellar vermis are usually displaced together, there may be preferential or sole displacement of either. In addition, although the inferior vermis usually covers the dorsal roof of the elongated fourth ventricle, it may come to lie intraventricularly; in some cases it may be covering only the upper part of the elongated ventricle, while in other cases there is only a thick glial roof to the fourth ventricle. The fourth ventricle may show cystic dilatation, and there may be ventricular clefts extending deep into the cerebellar white matter, lined by gliotic tissue (thus distinguishing them from true ependymal-lined diverticulae).

The leptomeninges are fibrotic, and there is vascular engorgement caused by chronic venous congestion; in some instances there is vascular proliferation so severe that it resembles a vascular malformation. Heterotopic glial and mesenchymal tissue, including striated muscle, may be found in the meninges (Fig. 6.16D) (8).

The posterior fossa is smaller than normal, not only due to bony abnormalities (see below) but also because of a low peripheral attachment of the tentorium cerebelli. The tentorial notch is widened as a result of poor development of the leaves, and these may cause a grooving of the upper surface of the cerebellum.

The displacement of the caudal brain stem results in upward angulation of the rostral cervical spinal roots (Fig. 6.16A), instead of their normal lateral or downward course. This appearance, however, disappears within about the first five segments, and the thoracic and lumbar roots have a normal course.

The Arnold-Chiari malformation as defined above is almost always associated with a myelomeningocele as described earlier, and indeed, it is questionable whether it occurs without it. Peach (243) described one such case with a normal spine, and there probably exist other cases, in which the spinal pathology is of a lesser degree. Most described cases have occurred in chronic tonsillar herniation (see below) and have previously been labeled "Arnold-Chiari-Type I" (241). High cervical myelo-

meningoceles are more frequently associated with occipital encephaloceles (so-called Chiari type III). On the other hand, not all cases of myelomeningocele have the Arnold-Chiari malformation. The incidence of the Arnold-Chiari malformation in infants born with myelomeningocele varies from 40–90% in different series, being found most commonly in the thoracolumbar and lumbar types (110). In addition the severity of the lumbar lesion frequently mirrors the severity of the posterior fossa lesion.

Hydrocephalus is frequently associated with the malformation (Fig. 6.16C), although may not always be present. It is frequently seen in fetuses with Arnold-Chiari, as early as 18–24 weeks (22). The degree is highly variable, and besides being responsible for clinical symptoms, the hydrocephalus may cause superadded pathological features, such as flattening and deformity of the cerebellum, herniation of the occipital lobes into the posterior fossa, or upward herniation of the cerebellum. The cause of the hydrocephalus is not clear but may be related to obliteration of the cisterna magna, to blockage of the foramen of Magendie by glial tissue, or to coexistent obstruction to the aqueduct of Sylvius.

Numerous other malformations have been found associated with the Arnold-Chiari malformation. A common finding is beaking of the tectum (Fig. 6.16B), formed by fusion and elongation of the inferior colliculi, which is directed backwards and downwards. Although up to 50% of cases have aqueductal stenosis, with shortening or lateral compression, almost all are anatomically patent (94). This feature may be secondary to the hydrocephalus (207, 215). The aqueduct stenosis may be stenosed or forked or may even show gliosis, suggesting that in some cases postnatal infection may play a role. An enlarged massa intermedia and hypoplasia and fenestration of the falx may often be seen (46, 47, 245, 246). Cerebral heterotopias may be found and often project into the lateral ventricles. Although cerebral microgyria has frequently been described, true four-layered polymicrogyria is less common, although it is seen in half the cases (245) in one series. More commonly, a complexity of gyral architecture caused by folding and resulting in small gyri may be seen, which has a normal cortical architectural lamination. These are often found in cases where hydrocephalus is present (Fig. 6.17).

Anomalies of the spinal cord are common in the form of hydromyelia, syringomyelia with the cavity forming caudal to the cervicomedullary junction, and diastematomyelia.

Of some importance are the associated skeletal defects, many of which are useful in radiological diagnosis and which have not always received full attention in the literature (205, 206). The commonest of these defects are craniolacunae, basillar impression, shortness of the posterior fossa, and occipitoatlantoaxial abnormalities, as well as concavity of the clivus. Craniolacunae are found in up to 55% of series of patients with myelomeningocele. They consist of variations in thickness of the squamous bones of the skull, with areas of erosion of the inner table at times so severe that there is a defect covered by fibrous tissue alone. These defects are more easily seen following transillumination of the bone. Craniolacunae are not related to any intracranial structures, and although are

often associated with hydrocephalus, may occur in its absence.

Another associated skull anomaly is basilar impression. This may be noted radiologically by depression of the base of the skull with protusion of the cervical spine into the anterior rim of the foramen magnum. Narrowing and distortion of the foramen may be present, whereas in other cases it has been shown to be large. Besides the spina bifida already described, hemivertebrae and other abnormalities of the vertebral bodies may be found.

PATHOGENESIS

Because of the complexity and associated defects of the Arnold-Chiari malformation, the detailed pathogenesis is the subject of great controversy. In view of the absence of any single causative developmental defect, the precise stage at which the lesion forms in embryonic life is also difficult to determine. Because the defect has been observed in early embryos and is usually associated with myelomeningocele, its production has been thought to take place in the 4th or 5th week of embryonic life (114); however, this does not preclude the possibility that the

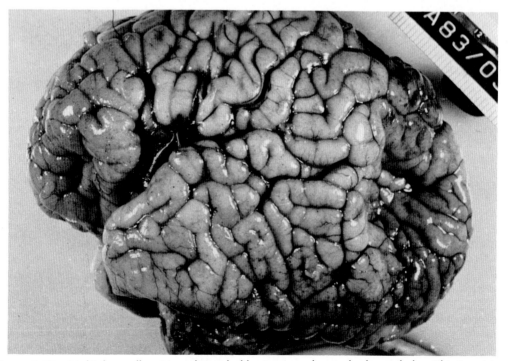

Figure 6.17. Multiple small gyri in a distended brain secondary to hydrocephalus. This is not true micropolygyria (See Fig. 6.21A).

induction of the lesion could take place over a larger time period and may not be due to a single episode. A consideration of numerous theories of causation and their relation to the observed pathological features are of importance. It should be emphasized that no *single* theory has explained not only the Arnold-Chiari malformation itself but also all the associated anomalies (spinal, brain stem, migrational), and therefore all current theories are unsatisfactory.

1. One of the earliest theories postulated that a tethering of the lower spinal cord by myelomeningocele produced traction of the hindbrain and displaced it caudally (191, 193, 248). The chief objection to this theory is that the malformation may take place in the absence of a cord lesion (243, 299). Also the malformation may develop in fetuses before the time of the relative ascent of the cord, which would be expected to cause the traction (17, 89). In addition, the traction theory would imply that all nerve roots should be directed downward, which is not the case as has been described above. This theory also does not explain the upward herniation of the cerebellum, beaking of the tectum, and kinking of the medulla. In addition, the malformation is not seen in other cases where the spinal cord is tethered, such as in lipomas or spina bifida occulta.

2. Increased hydrostatic pressure with downward flow of the CSF into the cord is another traditional theory that has been invoked as a basis for the Arnold-Chiari malformation. The increased pressure was held accountable for forcing the hindbrain contents into a craniocaudal direction. More recently, Masters (207) compared the degree of hydrocephalus with the cross-sections of various compartments, and came to the conclusion that the hindbrain prolapse was secondary to the hydrocephalus. Gardner (115–119) who has been one of the leading exponents of this theory stated that the cause of this increase in pressure is loss of permeability to CSF in the rhombic roof which leads to persistence of the normal embryonal state of encephalohydromyelia and establishes a high caudal pressure. Besides causing the cranial abnormalities, the increased pressure might rupture the neural tube. With rupture, neuroschitic blebs and associated dysraphic

state such as myelomeningocele may form (234–236). No experimental evidence relates all these changes to pressure disorders, however (114), and hydrocephalus does not always lead to Arnold-Chiari malformation and spina bifida (101). Moreover, the Arnold-Chiari malformation may be present without hydrocephalus (245, 246), and a patient has been described who had a closed central canal and spina bifida in which the medulla was placed distally (40, 41). The presence of vernicomyelia (154) suggested to some authors that the flow of CSF could be inwards, not necessarily outwards. Some experimental evidence (204) has shown that hydrocephalus induced by the *Reovirus* can result in the induction of the Arnold-Chiari malformation.

3. Most of the postulated theories on the Arnold-Chiari malformation now revolve round some disturbance in the normal growth of the contents of the posterior fossa relative to the development of the fossa itself. It has been suggested (72) that elongation of the medulla is caused by overgrowth of the hindbrain with subsequent displacement. Experimentally (315) interference with the notochord may cause such overgrowth and hydrocephalus. Clinically (10, 98) there has been no confirmatory evidence. Daniel and Strich (72) as well as Peach (246) also suggested that brain stem dysgenesis caused by failure of the pontine flexure to develop may also give rise to this abnormality. This postulated failure in normal straightening of the pontine flexure, however, has not been accompanied by disorganized nuclear groups in the brain stems of patients with Arnold-Chiari malformation. Although Barry et al. (17) suggested that the cerebellum had undergone an "overgrowth" generally, the cerebellum itself is relatively small. Recent observations by Jennings et al. (162) in an early case of fetal Arnold-Chiari malformation suggested a dyssynchrony between the neuroectoderm and mesodermal components resulting in a caudal displacement of the brain stem. They postulated that early aberration of neural folding resulted in displacement of the normal brain stem/spinal cord transitional zone and stressed the importance of the presence of the mesoderm in inducing this normal formation of the

neural tube. Similarly, Marin-Padilla and Marin-Padilla (206) in their experiments using vitamin A pointed out the formation of axial defects including underdevelopment of the occiput, which then caused secondary neurological changes. The importance of these early inducing events needs to be further examined.

Chronic Tonsillar Herniation

This is a term used by Friede (110) to designate a group of cases in which there is protrusion of the cerebellum below the foramen magnum, but without the other stigmata of the Arnold-Chiari syndrome described above. This has caused much controversy, because previously most cases have been considered examples of what was called "Arnold-Chiari Type I" (241). Classically these cases occur in older children or adults and are not associated with myelomeningocele. The other reasons for not considering them to be part of the Arnold-Chiari malformation have been described above. In addition, herniations indistinguishable from the "Chiari I" deformity have occurred after establishment of spinal subarachnoid shunt, suggesting that many examples of the so-called "Chiari I malformation" may also be acquired disorders rather than malformations. It would therefore be reasonable to designate all those cases in which cerebellar herniation usually of the tonsillar type is the *only* malformation, as chronic tonsillar herniation, perhaps following some acquired disorder (279).

In chronic tonsillar herniation, microscopic examination usually reveals the presence of sclerotic folia. Although many of these cases are asymptomatic, the condition is not without clinical importance, as we have observed a few cases where patients with this condition have died after relatively minor trauma to the skull. It is thought that the impaction of the structures in the foramen magnum renders these patients more susceptible to damage.

Anomalies in the Formation of Convolutions

After fusion of the neural tube between the 3rd and 4th week of embryonic development and formation of the major divisions of the tube, neuronal migration begins. The fate of the neuroepithelial cells, all of which take part in early cell generation (280), has been traced with autoradiography and Golgi methods (282, 283). From about the 7th week, cell migration takes place, with postmitotic ventricular cells migrating outwards and accumulating at the junction of the intermediate and marginal zones (the cortical mantle), where they form the neocortical plate. This increases in thickness and compacts during the 10th to 11th week, the major wave of migration, and beneath this plate the intermediate zone consisting of spongioblasts and glial fibers contains fewer cells (Fig. 6.18).

Controversy exists as to when the cortex has a full complement of neurons. Although it is felt by some that this is complete in the middle of gestation (83), it is not clear whether the cells remaining in the ventricular and intermediate zones in late pregnancy contribute to the cortex. The importance of radial glial fibers in guiding migrating neurons has been established (253–255). Successive migrating neurons along a given fiber leapfrog over more established cells and become oriented in a vertical radial column. Horizontal stratification and the formation of normal cortical laminations start occurring in the archicortex and insular and sensory motor areas. Typical six-layered isocortex is only seen at about 26–28 weeks (181), although some cells in the fourth layer appear larger by 24 weeks in the frontal cortex. The external surface of the hemispheres is usually smooth up to the 24th week, except for the presence of the earlier sulci, the Sylvian, the hippocampal, olfactory sulcus, and parietooccipital fissure. By the 24th week, Rolandic and callosomarginal fissures and the calcarine sulcus become evident, which deepen by the 28th week. These represent the primary sulci; the secondary sulci start to develop after the 24th week, continuing till birth. They first appear as pits that gradually transform into sulci. The more detailed analysis of cortical sulcal and gyral formations has been reported elsewhere (85). The cellular migration in the cerebellum will be considered under the cerebellar malformations.

Anomalies in the formation of cerebral

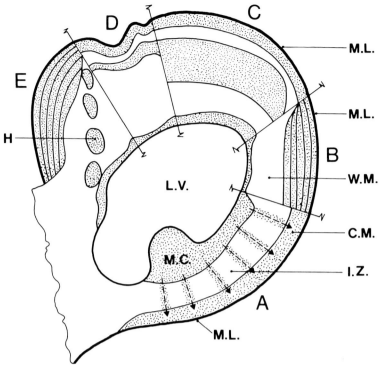

Figure 6.18. Diagrammatic depiction of the pathogenesis of convolutional migration disorders. (A) Normal fetal migration (12 weeks). (B) Normal six-layered mature cortex. (C) Four-layered pachygyric cortex. (D) Four-layered micropolygyric cortex. (E) Heterotopic cortex. Stippled lines depict neuronal layers. Analogous layers in different groups are depicted in continuity. *M.L.*, molecular layer; *W.M.*, white matter; *C.M.*, cortical mantle; *I.Z.*, intermediate zone; *M.C.*, matrix cells; *H*, heterotopias; *L.V.*, lateral ventricle.

gyri, fissures, and sulci are the result of a combination of failure of neuroepithelial cell migration from the periventricular germinal layer to the cortical mantle, a failure of maturation once they have reached this area, and in many cases there is probably either a failure of adequate cell proliferation or increased cell death, as many of these brains are small. Traditionally these malformations have been considered to occur early during the migration process. That malformations may be produced by interference with neuronal maturation has been demonstrated in various experimental animals. Convolutional anomalies specific for the gestational age of the experimental subject have been caused at various fetal ages by irradiation of mice (41). There are certain cerebellar mutant strains of mice (reeler, stagger, and weaver), which manifest cerebellar cortical abnormality caused by disordered migration patterns (282). Human instances of microgyria have been related to intrauterine infection with cytomegalovirus (64, 67, 226); microgyria in humans has also been reported following exposure to radiation and coal gas (135).

It is now recognized that some of the disorders of cortical lamination which were once regarded as migration disorders are attributable to neuronal necrosis following vascular or anoxic insults occurring at a much later stage than has previously been ascribed to be of importance in neuronal migration deficiencies (190, 210, 231, 314). In all of these cases vascular insufficiency and anoxia occurred in the third trimester, suggesting that the malformations occurred at least to some degree as a result of necrosis rather than a failure of normal growth.

Agyria-Pachygyria (Lissencephaly)

These terms have been used interchangeably for the most severe form of the neuronal migration defects, characterized by a simplified convolutional pattern in which there are a few broad gyri separated by only the primary fissures and sulci. Lissencephaly refers to the extreme form and applies to those brains that are small, and where the smooth agyric cortex is present diffusely throughout the brain (Fig. 6.19). A short oblique Sylvian fissure with an exposed insula and operculum may be the only fissure seen. The brains of these patients resemble those of immature fetuses. Lesser degrees of this condition may exist, referred to as a pachygyria or agyria (Fig. 6.20A and B), and the anomaly may be focal, bilateral, diffuse, or generalized. The brain may be normal in weight, but more often is microcephalic, and the lateral ventricles are dilated. Although true hydrocephalus may sometimes be present, in many cases the lateral ventricle dilatation recalls the situation seen in normal fetal development, a condition known as *colpocephaly*. The abnormal gyration most commonly affects the central areas of the cortex symmetrically, and these patients may present with cerebral diplegia which may

be spastic (232) or atonic (87). Asymmetric involvement may cause hemiplegia. The involvement often coincides with the distribution of one or both middle cerebral arteries or even with the distribution of one of the smaller branches of these vessels.

On cut sections, the grey matter is abnormally thick and may extend almost to the ventricular wall (Fig. 6.20). There is a marked reduction of white matter, usually reflected in diminution of pyramidal tracts. If the condition is focal the affected gyri may resemble the tubers of tuberous sclerosis (67). Classically the pachygyric cortex contains four layers microscopically (63, 67). The first outer layer resembles the normal molecular layer of the cortex. The second contains nerve cells more densely packed than normal. In the deeper parts of the second layer large somewhat bizarre-appearing neurons may be found. This layer has been thought to be analogous to the normal cortex. It represents cells that have arrived and matured earliest, before the rest of the migrating neurons were prevented from reaching their normal position

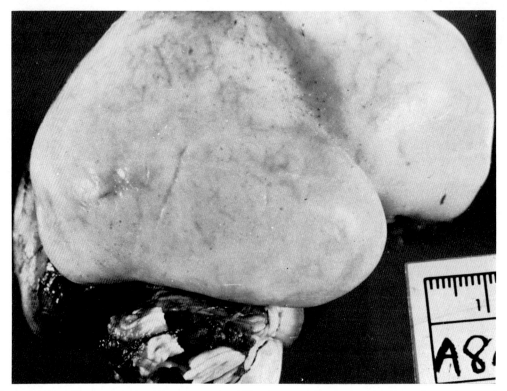

Figure 6.19. Lissencephaly. The cortex is diffusely smooth, and only the Sylvian fissure has formed.

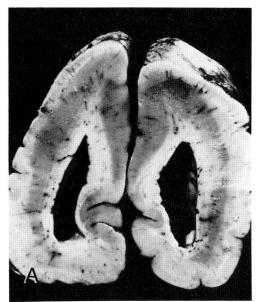

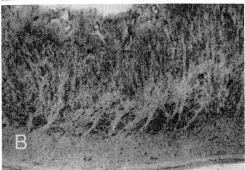

Figure 6.20. Agyria/pachygyria. (A) Cut surface showing a smooth agyric cortex superiorly, with scattered poorly formed gyri. A thick band of grey matter extends from the cortex almost completely through the white matter. (B) Nissl stain of a pachygyric cortex. The band of neurons extends from the surface (*top*) to thin layer of white matter adjacent to the ventricle (*bottom*). On the right there is a suggestion of four-layered cortex.

(135). The third layer is relatively acellular and consists of axons, in which special stains may demonstrate myelinated fibers resembling the arcuate fibers. It has been suggested that a migration arrest has permitted development of the axons in the third layer to create a barrier against later migration of neurons destined for the superior layers (63, 67). Williams et al. (314) demonstrated in Golgi-stained material that this third layer contains dense glial scars, a reaction to laminar necrosis during

cell migration, and suggested that it would also act as a barrier against further migration. The fourth layer is often the thickest and contains nerve cells and fibers. It is thought to represent neurons arrested in migration. Beneath the grey matter, the white matter is thinned, gliotic, and often contains heterotopic nodules of neurons impinging on the ventricular surface. At the junction between normal and pachygyric cortex, the first and second layers of the pachygyric cortex can be seen to be merging with the normal cell layers of the adjacent cortex.

At a practical level it should be pointed out that in most cases this four-layered cortex is not found. Commonly a large thick relatively homogeneous layer of cells is present in which it is difficult to distinguish laminae (Fig. 6.20*B*).

The presence of associated lesions often demonstrates disordered migration diffusely in the brain. Nodules of heterotopic neurons may be seen in the cerebellum, and there may be cerebellar polymicrogyria. Another finding is that of dysplasia of the inferior olive (Fig. 6.30), with heterotopic nodules lying in the dorsolateral medullary tegmentum, which represent olivary neurons which have been arrested in their migration from the rhombencephalic lip to the ventral medulla. They resemble olivary neurons and often contain myelinated fibers similar to that found around the main olivary nuclei (see below). Overall, it is felt that pachygyria-lissencephaly represents a migration defect occurring far earlier than that of polymicrogyria (see below).

Polymicrogyria

Polymicrogyria is far more common than pachygyria (62, 67). Many features of its pathogenesis in development resemble those of pachygyria, although some differences are present. The two conditions have been described to be found together, although this has been questioned (67). Polymicrogyria may also occur focally, in which it is often found as an incidental finding, as well as in a more diffuse fashion, when it may be associated with mental retardation, seizures, and either hemiplegia or diplegia. True polymicrogyria depends not only on the typical gross observations, but also on the demonstration of convincing histological changes (see below). It must be distinguished from a far more frequent phenomenon, which is the demonstration of apparently multiple small gyri seen usually in hydrocephalic brains often associated with the Arnold-Chiari malformation (Fig. 6.17). In this latter instance the gyral complexity may be secondary to growth of the cerebral mantle over a spherical area greater than normal due to hydrocephalus; histologically, normal laminated cortex is found.

Whether focal or generalized, true polymicrogyria is composed of an abundance of small closely packed miniature gyri which create an appearance on the surface which has been traditionally described as "cobblestone" or "moroccan leather" (Fig. 6.21A). The molecular layers of different gyri may fuse, forming shallow or absent sulci which can be appreciated only on cut surface. Like pachygyria, the polymicrogyria may be either unilateral or bilateral, diffuse, or occur in irregular patches. Like pachygyria, it may be confined to a single vascular distribution, which is most often the middle cerebral. Cut sections reveal a convoluted pattern of grey matter forming finger-like festooned ribbons of cells. Certain areas of the cortex are traditionally said to be spared, such as the cingulate, calcarine, and hippocampal gyri. It is possible that this reflects the earlier development of these areas (285) and may suggest a time of causation of polymicrogyria later than has been previously thought.

If severe, microcephaly may be present. The micropolygyria may be associated with nodular heterotopias, as well as colpocephaly. It is commonly associated with the Arnold-Chiari malformation, and cerebellar polymicrogyria and heterotopias may be also seen.

The cortical pattern varies histologically from area to area (Fig. 6.21B). A four-layered cortex, the basic constituents of which are similar to that seen in pachygyria, is commonly seen, and it is difficult to make the diagnosis of true polymicrogyria without seeing some areas of this disordered lamination. In other areas, milder forms of cortical dysplasias, such as radial columns of cells (Fig. 6.23) often with gland-like structures (62), may be the only

signs. In other areas the cortex appears normal, but the neurons appear immature. In contrast to agyria, inferior olivary heterotopias are less common, lending further weight to the suggestion that polymicrogyria occurs later than agyria-pachygyria. In some areas a two-layered cortex, in which a single band of nerve cells underlies a normal molecular layer, may be found. This has been suggested (210) to represent a more severe form of damage. The leptomeninges may show abnormal vessels or lipomatosis.

Although polymicrogyria has traditionally been thought to occur as a malformation resulting from a failure of migration, there are certain features of this condition which may suggest a linkage with the encephoclastic disorders. First of all the lesion usually occurs in the 4th to 5th month, and indeed has been reported following vascular, toxic, or anoxic ischemic lesions from the 6th month onwards (190, 210, 231, 261). The lesions are often in a vascular distribution (232), and the vasculature may be abnormal (29). It has always been argued that the finding of polymicrogyria in the wall of a porencephalic cyst is evidence that the latter is a malformative rather than an encephaloclastic condition. It may very well be that the cyst represents the more central manifestations of a destructive phenomenon, with the surrounding polymicrogyria representing a less severe manifestation of the same incident. This was certainly suggested by McBride and Kemper (210) who noted polymicrogyria in the center of a pair of bilateral lesions in the distribution of the middle cerebral artery. In this case the two-layered form of micropolygyria was present in the central part of the lesions, with the four-layered type of cortex being in a peripheral location. This suggested to the authors that polymicrogyria could exist in different morphological forms, depending on the severity. In this latter case it was felt that the insult had occurred approximately 16–20 weeks of age.

Whether polymicrogyria is malformative or postdestructive, it occurs in the second or early third trimester and should be distinguished from the pre- or perinatal conditions of "sclerotic microgyria" or "ulegyria," which almost certainly always occurs from anoxia, ischemia, or hypoperfusion.

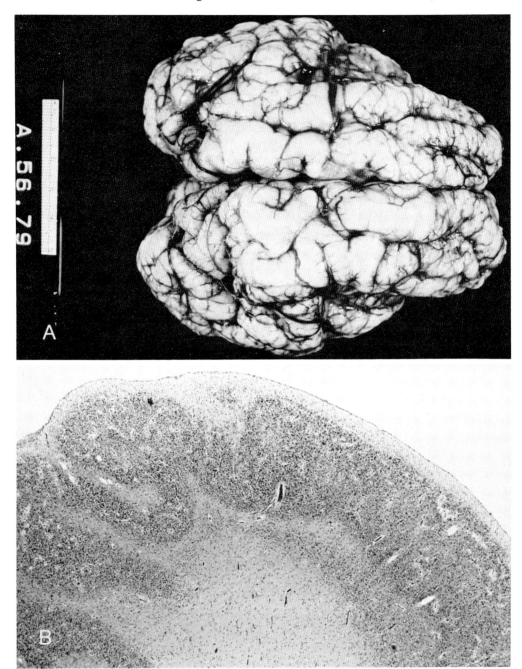

Figure 6.21. Micropolygyria. (*A*) Small wrinkled gyri are present diffusely laterally except for the dorsomedial frontoparietal cortex. The brain is small. (*B*) Complex undulating micropolygyric cortex blends gradually with normal cortex (*right*). In places four layers are discernible (middle), whereas in the rest only two layers can be seen. Hematoxylin and eosin.

Heterotopias

Heterotopias consist of displaced masses of nerve cells found in the white matter anywhere on the path from the original site of periventricular neuronal production to the final migration destination in the cortex. In the most common form, they consist of nests of ectopic neurons which may be close to the walls of the lateral ventricles

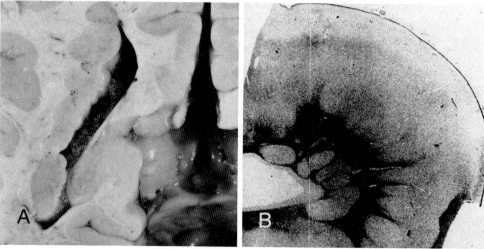

Figure 6.22. Cerebral heterotopias. (A) Cut section of brain showing a lamina of grey matter heterotopias protruding into the ventricle. (B) Microscopic section of cerebral hemisphere showing periventricular heterotopias lying in the white matter. The cortex is also pachygyric. Loyez stain for myelin.

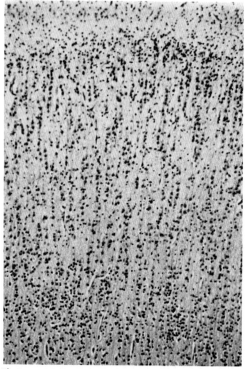

Figure 6.23. Microscopic section of cortex from a term neonate demonstrating a columnar arrangement of the neurons. Hematoxylin and eosin.

(Fig. 6.22). In these instances there are no gross convolutional abnormalities. The nests may be diffuse or focal; if focal they are common adjacent to the anterior and posterior horns of the ventricle. They may be situated adjacent to the basal ganglia but may also be subcortical in situation. When they project as small nodules into the lateral ventricle (Fig. 6.22A), there is no associated calcification or gliosis, distinguishing them from the subependymal nodule of tuberous sclerosis. This may be difficult to distinguish on gross examination in the neonate, and the diagnosis may have to be determined microscopically. They may also be found in cerebellar white matter (see under disorders of cerebellum), and may be found in conjunction with polymicrogyria, pachygyria, or microcephaly. They may be symmetrical. They are found in both cerebrum and the cerebellum in trisomy D and E (67, 294). They may also be found in the cerebrohepatorenal syndrome of Zellweger (307).

In other forms of heterotopias, frequently bilateral, the ectopic neurons exist in diffuse laminae in the deep white matter. In this form they often resemble the fourth layer of a pachygyric cortex, lending weight to the suggestion of a block in migration.

Other Less Common Forms of Cerebral Dysplasias

A rare anomaly is the so-called *nodular cortical dysplasia* (110) which has also been termed "status verrucosus simplex" or "brain wart" (65, 125). These are rare dysplasias and consist of superficial round cortical nodules comprised of nerve and glial cells which are irregularly oriented and gliotic. The hallmark of the nodule is the presence of a central core containing myelinated fibers and a blood vessel. The brain wart may be associated with polymicrogyria, microencephaly, and periventricular heterotopias. They may be single but are commonly multiple, occurring mainly in the frontal lobe.

A frequent finding in many premature brains and in many brains with other malformations is the finding of nerve cells arranged in *radial columns* (Fig. 6.23). This appearance recapitulates the fetal arrangement whereby nerve cells migrate along the radially arranged columns of glial fibers. The significance of this lesion is poorly understood, as it may occur entirely incidentally in the absence of any other malformations. It has been described frequently in Down's syndrome.

Numerous other minor findings may be found in brains with malformations or incidentally at autopsy. These include the finding of three-layered entorrhinal cortex in areas where a neocortical arrangement is expected. *Leptomeningeal heterotopias* consisting of glia, neurons, fibrous tissue, and in rare instances skeletal muscle are common (Fig. 6.16*D*) (8), particularly in diseases such as Arnold-Chiari malformation and those associated with trisomies.

Cortical dysplasias and all forms of migration defects have been described in the *cerebrohepatorenal syndrome of Zellweger* (42, 307). This condition, though rare, is of theoretical importance, because metabolic defects both in mitochondria and in long chain fatty acids have been described. It therefore points out the possibility that many of these diseases may be caused by a persisting metabolic abnormality, presenting first in fetal development.

Malformations of the Cerebellum

After the neural tube has formed, the pontine flexure develops at about 4 weeks gestation. This results in the neural tube becoming widest at the level of the rhombencephalon, leading to attenuation of the roof of the rhombencephalon, as well as flaring of the alar plates. The formation of the pontine flexure leads to a transverse crease in the roof of the rhombencephalon, wherein develops the choroid plexus. The major part of the cerebellum develops from that portion of the rhombencephalon anterior to this crease. The lateral edges of the alar plates become greatly thickened by the end of the 4th week due to intense neuroblast proliferation and become the paired rhombic lips (Fig. 6.24, *left*). From the cells of the rhombic lips develop most of the anlage of the cerebellum, as well as some of the brain stem nuclei, such as the inferior olivary nuclei. The rhombic lips

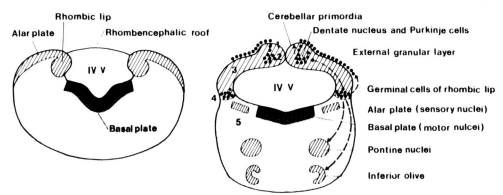

Figure 6.24. Diagrammatic representation of the development of the rhombencephalic roof at early (*left*) and later (*right*) stages. Normal migration patterns are shown by *arrows*. An arrest at *1* might prevent the rhombic lips from fusing leading to vermal agenesis. An arrest at *2* may lead to cerebellar heterotopias and cortical dysplasias. An arrest at *3* or *4* may lead to vermal or neocerebellar agenesis; if at *4*, pontine nuclear or inferior olivary hypoplasia may also result. A block at *5* leads to inferior olivary heterotopias.

grow dorsomedial and eventually reach the apex of the roof of the fourth ventricle between 5 and 6 weeks of gestation. Fusion of the two lips starts at about 7½ weeks and continues past the 12th week when the vermis forms (Fig. 6.24, *right*). This growth occurs anterior to the transverse crease marked by the choroid plexus. The roof of the rhomboencephalon posterior to the crease remains thin and relatively acellular. Anterior to the insertion of the choroid plexus there is a small anterior membranous portion which is briefly permeable to the passage of CSF during development (61, 311). This rapidly becomes incorporated into the vermis. The cerebellar primordia thus form as paired structures. Although initially the cerebellar anlagen lie within the ventricle, by the 3rd month they begin to grow extraventricularly. The flocculonodular fissure separates the flocculi of the hemispheres and the nodule of the vermis (the archicerebellum) from the rest of the cerebellum. This is the first subdivision to occur. By approximately 12 weeks the primary fissure dividing the anterior lobe of the cerebellum from the posterior lobe becomes established, and by 15–16 weeks the main fissures of the anterior and posterior lobes of the vermis are demarcated. Although the posterior lobe eventually grows larger than the anterior lobe, the growth of the vermis occurs earlier, and its fissures and lobules are completed approximately 4–8 weeks earlier than those of the hemispheres (neocerebellum).

There is virtually no mitotic activity occurring in the midline; the cells in the cerebellum derive from migration from the rhombic lips. The external granular layer migrates outwards along the external surface from the rhombic lips, whereas the deep cerebellar nuclei and the Purkinje cells derive from cells that migrate internally closer to the ventricular surface.

The caudal inert roof membrane perforates eventually, giving rise to the foramen of Magendie (319). The foramen of Magendie may be opened by 8 weeks, whereas the lateral foramen of Luschka opens only after 8 weeks (40, 236, 311). The cerebellar hemispheres normally start fusing before the opening of the lateral apertures (114). A later date of opening of the apertures has been postulated by other authors.

It is thus obvious (Fig. 6.24) that interruption to growth can occur at various times and stages along the path of development of rhombic lip neurons, giving rise to varying combinations of cerebellar and brain stem abnormalities.

The Dandy-Walker Syndrome

The term Dandy-Walker syndrome refers to a group of hindbrain malformations in patients of all ages characterized by aplasia or hypoplasia of the vermis, cystic dilatation of the fourth ventricle, and a large posterior fossa with upward displacement of the torcula and sinuses (7, 296). Hydrocephalus is frequently associated (25, 110). Extensive pathological accounts have been published (25, 69, 140). Although the diagnosis is frequently made during infancy and childhood, cases of Dandy-Walker syndrome in adults (195) have been found. Familial cases are described, and the occurrence of Dandy-Walker syndrome in identical twins has been reported (161). Modern methods of ultrasound and CT scanning have led to early diagnosis (Figs. 6.25 and 6.26), and the diagnosis has been made in a fetus of 33 weeks gestation by ultrasound (103).

The first criterion of the Dandy-Walker syndrome is a malformation of the cerebellar vermis (Figs. 6.27 and 6.28). In a significant number of cases, up to 25%, the vermis is entirely absent. Usually, however, greater or lesser degrees of hypoplasia, including distortion or rotation, are present. Often only the nodule of the vermis is present. Partial aplasia of the vermis usually involves the posterior part of the vermis more than the anterior. In continuity with this hypoplastic vermis is the most obvious feature of the syndrome, the posterior fossa cyst (Figs. 6.27 and 6.28). The cyst membrane is formed in continuity with both the remnants of the vermis in the midline and the cerebellar hemispheres laterally. It is attached to the normal roof of the fourth ventricle (Figs. 6.27 and 6.28) and is lined on its internal aspect by ependyma and externally by a layer of pia-arachnoid. Glial tissue is incorporated in the membrane. Within the cyst wall, especially laterally, there are remnants of cerebellar tissue; calcification may occur. The size of the cyst

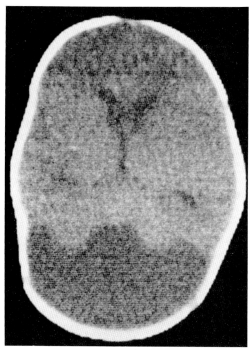

Figure 6.25. CT scan of a large posterior fossa cyst in the Dandy-Walker malformation.

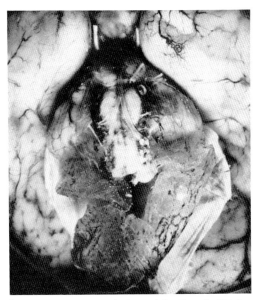

Figure 6.27. Ventral view of the Dandy-Walker malformation in a neonate. The brain has been photographed under water, distending the posterior fossa cyst which balloons dorsally in the midline between the cerebellar hemispheres.

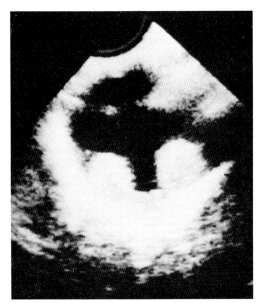

Figure 6.26. Ultrasound representation of the posterior fossa cyst in the Dandy-Walker malformation.

Figure 6.28. Coronal sections of the brain stem and cerebellum in the Dandy-Walker malformation. Posteriorly (*top*) the vermis is absent, and a large cavity in continuity with the fourth ventricle separates the cerebellar hemispheres. Anteriorly (*bottom*) a small fragment of vermis is present. The cyst wall is in continuity with the cerebellar hemispheres.

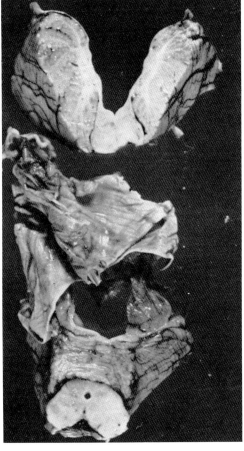

varies considerably and does not always correlate with the degree of vermal hypoplasia. Hypoplasia of the cerebellar hemispheres, as well as heterotopias or other cortical dysplasias, are often seen.

Although hydrocephalus is often the presenting feature of the Dandy-Walker syndrome, the degree of ventricular dilatation varies considerably. In some instances hydrocephalus is barely detectable, but in others it can lead to thinning of the cortical mantle. Although the extent does not correlate with either the size of the posterior fossa cyst or the degree of vermal hypoplasia, the severity of hydrocephalus is of great importance, as it determines the prognosis more than any other factor (104, 114).

The posterior fossa is considerably enlarged, with thinning of the bones which may be detectable on radiological examination. The torcular herophili, the lateral and straight sinuses, and the tentorium, are elevated. Of some importance is the frequent association of other cerebral anomalies, which are present in approximately two-thirds of cases (140, 297). A very common associated feature is agenesis of the corpus callosum (25, 57, 114, 252, 269). In addition, there are other midline cranial abnormalities, which include infundibular hamartomas and brain stem lipomas (140). Malformations and ectopias of the inferior olives are frequently seen (Fig. 6.30) (136, 140, 157), and occipital encephaloceles have been reported (271). In addition, the syndrome has often been associated with other systemic anomalies, many of them of midline origin (140), and polydactylsm and syndactylysm are occasionally noted.

Historically the status of the outlet foramina of the fourth ventricle has been the source of controversy. It was originally felt that these were obstructed leading to hydrocephalus. Complete obstruction of the foramina was only found in one case of D'Agostino et al. (69) and in 5 of 21 cases described by Hart et al. (140) (see also refs. 71, 296). In addition, besides the finding of patent foramina in most cases, the theory is also untenable, because normally the foramina open only after the anterior membrane area has involuted and the cerebellar anlage have fused in the midline.

A far more likely pathogenesis involves a disturbance in the development of the rhombic lips and the roof of the fourth ventricle (Fig. 6.24, *right*). Acceptance of this theory explains the cerebellar vermal aplasia sometimes involving the hemispheres, the dorsal cerebellar cyst, as well as some of the associated features in the brain stem, such as the dysplastic olivary nuclei, which are also derivatives of the rhombic lip. Additional evidence has been provided experimentally. In a strain of hydrocephalic mouse with defective development of the vermis, the bulging of the rostral membranaceous area of the roof of the fourth ventricles was present before the opening of the ventricular apertures (37). Persistence of this rostral membranaceous area with development of hydrocephalus and agenesis of the corpus callosum has also been induced in mice by the administration of galactoflavin (167). A similar early disturbance in the anterior membranaceous area which fails to become permeable and incorporated into the vermis could also explain the hydrocephalus in the Dandy-Walker syndrome. The associated brain stem abnormalities involving displacement and dysplasia of several nuclear groups of the medulla (157) also imply a disturbance of neuroblast proliferation and migration from the rhomboencephalic lip with a persistent anterior membrane. Although some authors have tried to link the Dandy-Walker syndrome and the Arnold-Chiari malformation through a common mechanism of cleavage of the neural tube (82, 236), comparison of the associated findings in the two conditions (114) does not support this unitary view. Hart et al. (114) surmised the timing of the defect to be at about the 6th to 7th week of embryonic life, judging from the coexistence of polydactyly. The finding of the defect in identical twins is of great interest (161), but does not lend conclusive additional information as to whether the defect can be environmentally or genetically acquired.

The cysts of the posterior fossa have to be distinguished from retrocerebellar arachnoid or ependymal cysts which may displace the brain stem but usually are not associated with malformation. The Dandy-Walker malformation must also be distinguished from those cases of true atresia of the outlet foramina which lack the other malformative stigmata of the syndrome.

Atresia of the Cerebellar Foramina

Friede (110) has correctly separated this very rare entity from consideration with the Dandy-Walker syndrome, in view of the finding that atretic foramina are by no means an integral part of the Dandy-Walker syndrome. The development of the foramina of the fourth ventricle has already been discussed, but it should be pointed out that a relatively large amount of cerebrospinal fluid can be drained through a relatively small channel such as the aqueduct; to become symptomatic, foramenal atresia must be relatively severe, involving at least two, and maybe even all three of the outlet foramina of the fourth ventricle. Occasional finding of atresia of any of the foramina is common at autopsy. When examined histologically the foramina are covered by a glial membrane lined with ependyma. This should distinguish them from postinfectious, posthemorrhagic, or traumatic fibrosis of the leptomeninges. This distinction may in individual cases be difficult to make. Although atresia may be found in some cases of Dandy-Walker syndrome (140), cases where the other features of the syndrome are absent have been described (25). In those rare cases where all three foramina are atretic, obstructive hydrocephalus may be present.

Disorders of Cerebellar Hemispheres

The embryological development of the cerebellum has already been discussed. It is obvious that either the *paleocerebellum* (the vermis and the flocculi) or the *neocerebellum* (the hemispheres) can be aplastic. These disorders are not mutually exclusive, and both forms of aplasia can be combined. In addition, at times the aplasia may effect the anterior lobes more than the posterior lobes or vice versa. It is possible that these differences are related to both the timing of the lesions (as the vermis develops before the hemispheres) or perhaps the spatial organization of the cerebellum. (See Fig. 6.24). Rare cases of complete agenesis of the cerebellum have been reported (250, 331).

APLASIA OF THE VERMIS

Aplasia of the vermis is presumably related to a failure of correct fusion of the cerebellar anlage in the midline. It has been well described (110, 111, 112, 166). Although some cases are sporadic, Joubert et al. (166) described familial cases and also described a peculiar breathing pattern of tachypnea followed by apnea (*Joubert's syndrome*). Aplasia of the vermis usually results in a small cerebellum in which the flocculi may or may not be identifiable. The two cerebellar hemispheres may be bridged by a membrane, or else they may be fused together (220). The absence of a midline cyst and of a high position of the torcular and tentorium distinguishes this from the Dandy-Walker syndrome. If any part of the vermis is still present it is usually the anterior part. The roof nuclei are usually absent, and the dentate nuclei may be fused in the midline. Of great interest has been the association of midline vermal hypoplasia with abnormalities of other midline structures. Friede (111) has described the occurrence of dysraphia of the tectum with a triangular shape to the midbrain, and an unsegmented midbrain tectum has been described by Calogero (45) in a case of vermian agenesis. In addition, Michaud et al. (220) have described vermal aplasia with septooptic dysplasia and other associated abnormalities in the case of an infant whose mother had taken phencyclidine in the first 6 weeks of pregnancy. The dating of the tectal lesion (which begins to segment in the normal human at about 6 weeks) and the final fusion of the cerebellar plate at about the 8th to 9th week could produce affectations of widespread midline structures. Further evidence uniting the midline cerebellar structures with those of the anterior telencephalic wall is seen in a case by Friede and Briner (113) in which they report a case of hyperplasia of the vermis with a dorsal hyperplastic fornix over the corpus callosum.

NEOCEREBELLAR APLASIA (PONTONEOCEREBELLAR APLASIA)

This condition is characterized by hypoplasia or absence of one of the cerebellar hemispheres (Fig. 6.29). In these cases the vermis may be normal or small, and the flocculi are commonly persistent. In some

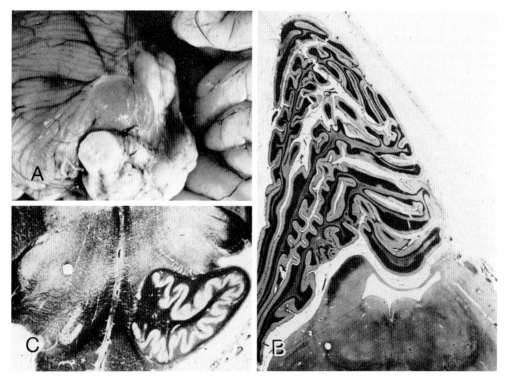

Figure 6.29. Unilateral cerebellar agenesis. The right cerebellar hemisphere is absent (*A* and *B*), as is the right superior cerebellar peduncle (*B*), while the left inferior olive is hypoplastic (*C*). (*B* and *C*) Loyez stain for myelin.

cases the vermis may be partially aplastic as well (Fig. 6.29*B*). In areas where the cerebellum is hypoplastic, there may be normal cortex adjacent to areas where the white matter extends to the surface. In other areas there is disorganization of the normal cortex with heterotopias. The dentate nuclei may be absent or disorganized into islands of heterotopias. The contralateral inferior olive (Fig. 6.29*C*), as well as the homolateral superior cerebellar peduncle (Fig. 6.29*B*), may be decreased in size or absent.

Abnormalities of the olivary nuclei are frequently associated with cerebellar aplasias. This is not surprising in view of the common origin of cerebellar anlage and inferior olivary nucleus from the rhombencephalic lip. The most common abnormalities in the inferior olive are those of disorganization of all or part of the nucleus (136) and the presence of olivary heterotopias, seen lying in the path of migration from the rhombencephalic lip to the final position of the nucleus (Fig. 6.30). In cases of complete cerebellar agenesis of one side,

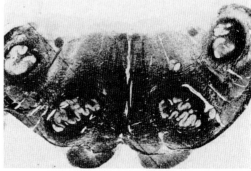

Figure 6.30. Inferior olivary heterotopias. Bilateral heterotopias resembling the inferior olive and surrounded by white matter bundles lie in the dorsolateral medullary tegmentum in the path of migration from the rhombencephalic lip (see Fig. 6.24). Loyez stain for myelin.

the inferior olive may be totally lacking or decreased on the contralateral side (Fig. 6.29*C*). The pontine nuclei may be absent as well. Other associated abnormalities include those associated with anterior telencephalic wall malformations, such as arrhinencephaly and agenesis of the corpus callosum.

There may be *aplasia of the fourth ventricle* (Figs. 6.31 and 6.32), in which this structure is either totally obliterated or in which there are few residual nests of ependymal cells to mark the previous existence of the central canal. Occipital encephalo-

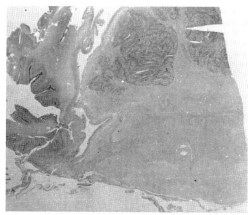

Figure 6.31. Aplasia of the fourth ventricle. A mass of central heterotopic cerebellar tissue lies dorsal to the pons. No fourth ventricle is present. The lateral cerebellar hemisphere folia are hypoplastic. Hematoxylin and eosin.

cele may also be coexistent (111). The fact that this entity has been described in familial instances (116, 304, 331), as well as in cases of presumed toxicity, points to a complex pathogenesis and also helps to emphasize the multifactorial and perhaps temporal nature of the induction of these lesions.

MIGRATION DISORDERS OF THE CEREBELLAR HEMISPHERES

The cells of the cerebellum derive from the ventricular zone of the rhombencephalic lip and adjacent alar plate. At about 9 weeks, cells migrate out towards the rhombencephalic roof and the cerebellar anlage, destined to form the deep cerebellar nuclei and the Purkinje cells. Small neuroblasts from the rhombic lip also migrate out to the external surface and over the cerebellum forming the external granular layer, which starts at about 8 to 9 weeks, and covers the entire cortex by 14 weeks (187) (Fig. 6.24, *right*). These cells are highly mitotic, and on reaching the cerebellum migrate inward along the path of the radial glia of the cerebellum to occupy a final destination in the internal granular layer. With migration of these

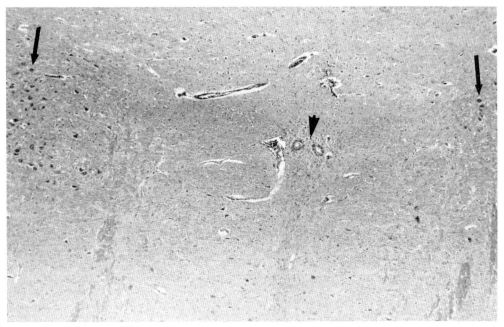

Figure 6.32. Aplasia of the fourth ventricle. Microscopic section of pons from Figure 6.31. The abducens nuclei (*arrows*) with existing nerve fibers are seen bilaterally, while centrally only a few ependymal canals represent the 4th ventricle (*arrowhead*). Hematoxylin and eosin.

cells inward, the external granular layer diminishes in thickness and usually disappears postnatally after variable times. The intimate relationship of the migrating neurons to the radial glia, which guides these cells, has been well reviewed (254, 280). Numerous congenital mouse mutants species have been described showing various aberrations of cerebellar architecture (283). Some of these have been related to defects in the neuroblasts, whereas others have been related to defects in the glial composition with consequent architectural abnormalities.

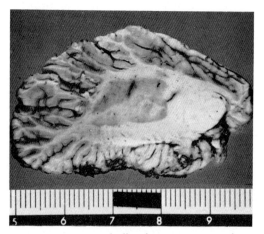

Figure 6.33. Cerebellar heterotopia. A large grey matter mass is present adjacent to the dentate nucleus in the white matter.

Because development in the cerebellum occurs in different places at different times and continues over an extremely long period of time, agents that interrupt normal growth may have different effects. Some lesions are caused by focal disruption of neuroblast migration early in development, and these lead to localized cortical dysplasias and heterotopias. On the other hand, if an agent acts after the Purkinje cells have matured but while the granular cell is both dividing and migrating, more diffuse lesions affecting the entire granular layer will ensue.

Heterotopias

Rorke et al. (263) have described numerous minor abnormalities in up to 85% of normal infants. These include clusters of granular cells in the dentate nucleus (110), sometimes admixed with large cells resembling Purkinje cells, localized heterotopias containing layered Purkinje cells and granular cells. It should be emphasized that these need to be distinguished from aberrantly directed normal folia which have been cut in tangential or cross-section. Many of these abnormalities appear to involute with age (109).

Large heterotopias are less common (Fig. 6.33) and may be found both as isolated incidental findings or in conjunction with other malformations such as Arnold-

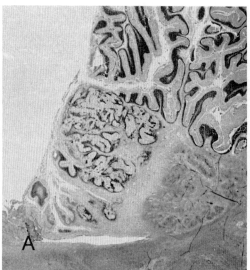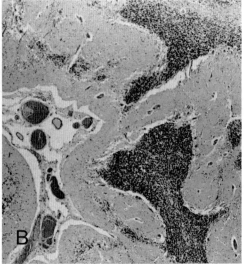

Figure 6.34. Cerebellar polymicrogyria. (A) A localized mass of multiple small cortical cerebellar gyri are present. (B) An undulating complex cortical pattern of molecular and granular layers replaces the normal folial architecture.

Chiari, Dandy-Walker malformation, and other cerebellar hypoplasias. They are relatively common in trisomy 13–15 (see above). In general, cerebellar heterotopias exist in the white matter of the hemispheres and consist of nests of large cells at times resembling Purkinje cells, which may or may not have an admixture of granular neurons. Other heterotopias appear to be more highly organized with lamination of Purkinje cells and granular cells lying in a correct relationship to the molecular layer (300).

Cerebellar Polymicrogyria (Focal Cortical Dysplasia, Heterotaxis, Agyria, and Pachygyria)

These lesions are grouped as they probably represent disturbances in cerebellar migration occurring focally. While the gyri are not always small and multiple (110), in some instances an excessive folding and small gyri are seen. Micropolygyrias are usually well defined (Fig. 6.34A) and affect any portion of the cerebellar cortex singly, multiply, unilaterally, or bilaterally. The cortex is thicker than normal, and there are interwoven layers containing both granular cells and what appears to be normal molecular layers (Fig. 6.34B). Purkinje cells are often displaced. Depending on the smoothness of the surface, the term agyria or pachygyria may be applied, although there seems little merit in so doing. These lesions are frequently associated with other malformations.

Other Cerebellar Lesions

The time span available for susceptibility to teratogenic agents is extremely long in the cerebellum. There is a group of congenital cerebellar atrophies, affecting mainly the granular cell layer but sometimes including Purkinje cells as well, which are diffuse and which have been considered by some to be destructive lesions and by others to be malformations. These are probably caused by agents acting at a later period than most of these other malformations, and we would prefer not to include them with the malformations, as the basic structure of the cerebellum remains intact. Full descriptions of these degenerations of the granular layer (granular aplasia, congenital atrophy of granular layer with or without

loss of Purkinje cells, cerebrocerebellar atrophy) can be found in the literature (110, 303).

Similarly, the entity of diffuse hypertrophy of the cerebellar cortex (Lhermitte-Duclos' disease), although of uncertain origin, behaves as a neoplasm and will not be considered further. The reader is referred elsewhere (267) for a full description.

DISORDERS OF THE CEREBRAL AQUEDUCT

The normal cerebral aqueduct develops beneath the tectal plate from the lumen of the neural tube. From the second fetal month to the time of birth, the size of the aqueduct relative to that of the midbrain decreases. According to Woollam and Millen (322), this decrease is accomplished by thickening of the developing neural tissue which compresses the canal. These authors also have shown considerable variation in the degree of folding of the ependyma, wedging of the lumen, and luminal narrowing which can still be considered within the range of normality. These same authors found the narrowest portion of the normal adult aqueduct to measure approximately 8 mm^2, with a range of 4–15. In children the mean figure was 5 mm^5. Because of the wide variation in size and configuration of the lumen, the point at which the aqueduct becomes obstrutive to the flow is difficult to define (20, 99); the complexity is unsuitable for precise mathematical analysis. According to Russell (266) the normal aqueductal lumen narrows towards the center of the superior colliculi, widens, narrows again at the level of the inferior colliculi, and finally widens into the fourth ventricle. Because of its short length and the narrowness of the aqueduct, this area is extremely susceptible to obstruction.

Obstruction of the Aqueduct (Stenosis)

Classically obstructive anomalies of the aqueduct have been classified into: stenosis, forking or atresia, and membrane formation (226). The fourth group, gliosis, was considered by Russell to be postinflammatory and therefore not a developmental lesion. Although this classification has largely been accepted (232, 303), the separation of the etiological and pathological features of various groups into completely distinctive entities is uncertain (20, 86). The ability of the fetal brain to heal after an acquired insult leaving little trace of the destructive process is well known. This has been experimentally confirmed following infections with mumps virus in hamsters (165). In these animals aqueductal stenosis and hydrocephalus developed without any residual histological evidence of inflammation. These experiments have therefore cast doubt on the simple division of anomalies of the aqueduct into developmental and destructive conditions. Stenosis of the aqueduct is often found associated with other congenital malformations, such as hydrocephaly, the Arnold-Chiari malformation, and in cases of holoprosencephaly (152, 199). In recent years, some evidence has accumulated suggesting that in many cases the aqueduct stenosis may develop secondarily to hydrocephalus rather than causing it (180, 215, 313). These authors have suggested that the aqueduct is blocked by the lateral compression of the midbrain between the occipital and temporal lobes by enlarged lateral ventricles. Further elucidation of this point must await more detailed pathological studies of the relationship between aqueduct stenosis and hydrocephalus at early stages.

STENOSIS OF THE AQUEDUCT

This is a rare condition, the only abnormality present being a decrease in the diameter (as compared with a normal aqueduct at the same level). The aqueduct itself may not even be visible on gross inspection (Fig. 6.35). Microscopically, no gliosis is seen in the subependymal layers. Clusters of ependymal cells may be seen forming short channels around the stenosed and narrowed aqueduct. In addition, complete absence (atresia) may be present for varying lengths. Stenosis of the aqueduct may occur as a familial sex-linked trait affecting males only (31, 92, 310). Flexed adducted thumbs are noted in some of these cases. Although this condition has been noted in approximately 32 families (1, 148, 180), actual pathological examinations have been rare. Indeed in one of Landrieu's cases, not subject to pathological examination, the aq-

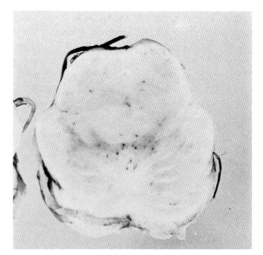

Figure 6.35.   Aqueduct stenosis. The aqueduct cannot be visualized on gross examination.

ueduct appeared patent on radiological examination.

FORKING OF THE AQUEDUCT

In this condition more than one main channel of reduced dimension can be found separated by glial tissue. The ventral channel is usually a slit, whereas the dorsal canal is forked and irregular with surrounding ependymal ductules. These channels may communicate with each other or may enter the ventricle. The colliculi may be fused as an associated malformation.

SEPTUM FORMATION

This occurs at the caudal end of the aqueduct and causes obstruction by a thin glial membrane (Fig. 6.36). Some of the septa have been associated with infection.

GLIOSIS OF THE AQUEDUCT

In this condition a narrow lumen is surrounded by a gliotic reaction, with the outline of the original aqueduct marked by a disrupted layer of ependymal cells. This condition is thought to result from widespread ependymal infection and is therefore strictly speaking not a true malformation. In many individual cases, however, it is not clear morphologically whether cases fall into this or the malformative category.

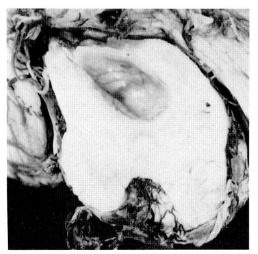

Figure 6.36. Aqueduct septum (membrane). The aqueduct is grossly dilated following obstruction by this glial septum.

GENERALIZED DISTURBANCES IN THE GROWTH OF THE NERVOUS TISSUE

This group of diseases is characterized by conditions in which growth disturbances are diffuse. Etiologically this is an extremely wide group of diseases, being associated with familial, chromosomal, and environmental factors. In addition sporadic cases occur. Many of these conditions occur in association with chromosomal or genetic syndromes and are also commonly found in association with other more specific extraneural congenital malformations. This area is controversial, because frequently the normal range of variations is difficult to define precisely, and the degree of abnormality may not be estimated accurately.

Microcephaly

Microcephaly, which in a strict sense refers to a decrease in the size of the head, should be differentiated from the term *microencephaly,* which denotes a small size of the brain. In common practice and in the literature, the terms are often used interchangeably, but this practice should not preclude accurate description of both brain and skull. The small size of the head is usually secondary to cerebral abnormality. A decrease in the size of the head and of the brain is the most common abnormality

in the mentally retarded patient. The normal weight of the brain ranges widely; a mature brain that weighs less than 900 g is generally regarded as abnormal (232, 303). Microcephaly and microencephaly in the developing child has been defined as either a head size or a brain size smaller than the mean for age and sex by more than 3 standard deviations.

It should be pointed out at the outset that microcephaly and microencephaly are not pathological entities. They may be of diverse etiological origin and may be associated with degenerative, destructive, or malformative conditions. They may follow congenital infections (e.g., rubella, toxoplasmosis cytomegalic contusion disease, and meningitis), toxins, irradiations, phenylketonuria, or Tay-Sachs disease (232). They are common in chromosomal abnormalities (308). In this section only microcephaly that is presumably malformative in origin will be discussed. No mention will be made of those cases of microcephaly that occur secondary to destructive or metabolic lesions. Microcephaly is frequently associated with other congenital malformations, such as disorders of cell migration (lissencephaly, microgyria, heterotopias) or with holoprosencephaly and absence of the corpus callosum. In addition, as will be seen below, microcephaly may be associated with lesser degrees of congenital malformations; where these become a major part of the overall picture, the overall diagnosis should reflect the preponderance of either the microcephaly or the associated malformations.

Microcephaly is generally found in the context of mental retardation, although some cases of true microcephaly are seen in apparently normal individuals. The degree of associated features such as seizures, motor disorders, and basal ganglia disorders depend on the individual case. Microcephaly has been induced in experimental animals by irradiation (141), with chemical agents using cell mitotic inhibitors, ethylnitrosourea, and hypophysectomy. Malnutrition is thought to be a cause of microcephaly, but this is controversial.

The bones of the cranium are small and combine with the normal size of the facial bones to give peculiar appearances to many of these infants and children. In most instances all parts are small (Fig. 6.37), although the frontal and temporal lobes may be affected more than the others. The insula may be exposed and the parietooccipital sulcus enlarged. Colpocephaly is common. A small cord (*micromyelia*) may be present. The gyral pattern varies tremendously. In some instances it may be simplified with coarse gyri (Fig. 6.37), whereas in other cases there is a pattern of increased gyral complexity. The centrum semiovale is small. The basal ganglia are generally unaffected and may appear disproportionately large. Nonspecific minor abnormalities of architecture are frequent. The cortical nerve cells are often arranged in radial columns. They have been described by some authors as being separated by myelinated fibers, but this is rare, and the specificity of such an arrangement has been questioned (67). Heterotopias and occasional true polymicrogyrias and pachygyrias may be seen in many of these cases.

In some cases a decrease in neurons is evident histologically. In others the neuronal content appears normal; perhaps future Golgi studies will reveal a decrease in dendrites accounting for the microcephaly.

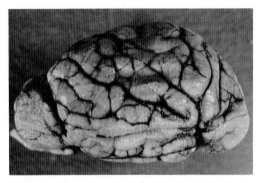

Figure 6.37. Microcephaly. The brain is abnormally small, with a pointed shape and a coarse simplified gyral pattern.

FAMILIAL MICROCEPHALY

This is not a single entity but refers to many different genetic syndromes. A form

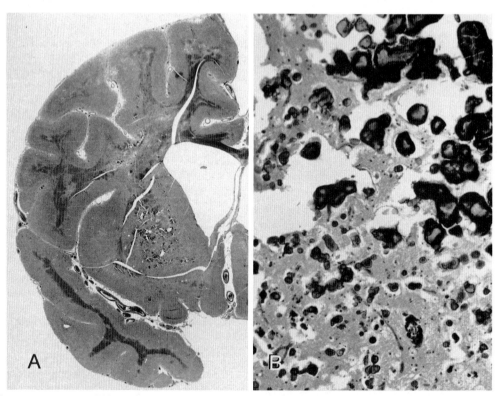

Figure 6.38. Familial microcephaly with calcification. Brain from a patient with Cockayne's syndrome. (*A*) Cut section showing coarse simplified gyri, large ventricles, decreased white matter, and dark staining (mineralization) of basal ganglia. Hematoxylin and eosin. (*B*) Microscopic section of basal ganglia showing calcospherites and mineralization of neurons and blood vessels. Hematoxylin and eosin.

described by Norman (232) as a mendelian recessive displays a small cranium with a receding forehead and furrowed scalp. In these cases the brain may be extremely small (500–600 g). The convolutional pattern was described as simplified, with coarse gyri resembling an anthropoid brain. Other cases of familial microcephaly have been described with ocular (213) or facial (146) abnormalities.

In some cases massive calcification is a feature of familial microcephaly (163). Although the degree of gyral atrophy is not extreme, the ventricles are large (Fig. 6.38A). The putamen, globus pallidus, and dentate nucleus contain large amounts of mineral deposits, which have been shown to be a mixture of calcium and iron (Fig. 6.38B). Many of these deposits are seen in the walls of blood vessels. The relationship of this entity to Fahr's disease is unclear. A further example of familial microcephaly with calcifications occurs in *Cockayne's syndrome* (60, 222, 288). These authors have all described microcephaly and cerebral calcification especially in the basal ganglia, as well as dwarfism, mental retardation, sunken eyes and a prominent nose, pigmentary retinal degeneration, and deafness. Numerous other abnormalities have

also been described. In one instance (288) neurofibrillary tangles and bizarre astrocytes were also found in these cases, suggesting that the degeneration in these instances was primary and not secondary to blood vessel involvement. An interesting feature in these cases has been atrophy of white matter, with patchy demyelination which in the past has been confused with Pelizaeus-Merzbacher disease.

Other isolated familial instances of microcephaly and various facial and white matter anomalies have also been described. It is obvious that many of these cases represent different entities, and a true definition of their etiopathogenesis may be revealed by future genetic or metabolic studies.

Megalencephaly

The term megalencephaly covers a wide variety of conditions, all of which are characterized by an excessive brain weight (Fig. 6.39). The definition of an megalencephalic brain is also unclear. Brain weights over 1600 g (232, 303) and 1700 g (285) have been quoted, though weights of this magnitude are often found in apparently normal looking brains. Megalencephaly has

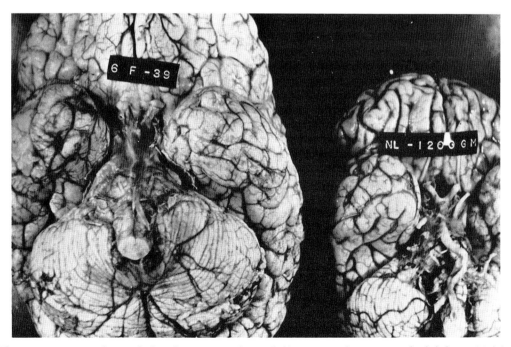

Figure 6.39.   Megalencephaly. The increased size (*left*) compared to a normal adult brain (*right*) is well seen.

been found on occasions in some individuals of superior intelligence (Tolstoy was reputed to have had a markedly enlarged brain), but more frequently they are found in mentally retarded patients. Megalencephaly frequently results from nonmalformative processes (for example, Tay-Sachs disease in its early stages, Hunter-Hurler disease, Alexander's disease, spongy sclerosis of Canavan). A further category of megalencephalic brains occurs in those associated with proliferative conditions such as tuberous sclerosis.

The malformative conditions associated with megalencephaly usually include disorders of migration, such as polymicrogyria and heterotopias and syringomelia (43, 91). Although the cortical thickness and white matter are usually increased, the corpus callosum is variable and may even be thinned. Longitudinal callosal bundles with absence of olfactory tracts have also been described by Urich (303). In these cases megalencephaly may be associated with a chromosomal anomaly, such as Klinefelter's syndrome (43).

Megalencephaly may be unilateral (32, 203, 302). In these instances, the neuronal and glial cells may appear cytologically abnormal and bizarre. Manz et al. (203) found that there was an increase in neuronal and glial DNA, as well as proteins, in an megalencephalic hemisphere which suggested heteroploidy of chromosomal DNA. Others such as Friede (110) have suggested that the cells are indeed diploid and that megalencephaly is due to an initial overproduction of cells. He postulated that the normal bionecrosis that exists during development does not occur, and a surplus of neurons results.

The patients with unilateral megalencephaly may have associated overgrowth of face, limbs, or an entire body half, which is usually homolateral rather than contralateral to the megalencephaly.

It should be pointed out that in many of these instances where the neurons or the glia are bizarre, the possibility of a forme fruste of tuberous sclerosis or von Recklinghausen's disease should be ruled out.

Arachnoid Cysts

These cysts are malformations of the meninges (9, 292). Although they are most common in the sylvian fissure, they also occur in the parasaggital area, over the convexity, and in the posterior fossa (Fig. 6.40), and next to the spinal cord (58). They lie between the layers of the arachnoid or between the dura and the arachnoid. Their origin has been attributed to maldevelopment of the leptomeninges. Although they are thought to communicate with the subarachnoid space at an early stage, it is postulated by Starkman et al. (292) that closure of the connecting channels traps fluid in the cyst. The mature cysts usually show no connection with the ventricles or the subarachnoid space either radiologically or grossly. The cysts contain clear colorless fluid. Their walls are thicker than arachnoid but thinner than dura and usually smooth. There is usually no epithelial lining. The presence of old hemorrhage, inflammation, and fibrosis may tend to exclude the diagnosis of congenital arachnoid cyst, in favor of a localized subdural or subarachnoid pathological process result-

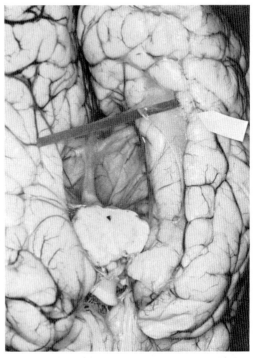

Figure 6.40. Arachnoid cyst of the posterior fossa. The cyst lies dorsal to the midbrain at the incisural notch; the midbrain has been distorted. The *arrowhead* points to the site of attachment to the basal leptomeninges.

ing in a localized loculation of fluid. In addition, these cysts have to be distinguished from so-called "glial ependymal" cysts which contain glia in their walls and presumably derive from glial heterotopias in the subarachnoid space (7). Some association between different kinds of cysts may be present. Although cysts are often asymptomatic, they may cause the signs and symptoms of space-occupying lesions, and the posterior fossa cysts have caused hydrocephalus by obstruction at the incisura of the tentorium. The spinal arachnoid diverticula have been associated with symptoms of pain, weakness, and sensory changes, suggestive of nerve root involvement.

MALFORMATIONS OF THE SPINAL CORD

Amelia is usually found only in anencephalic monsters, where it is part of the rachischisis component of craniorachischisis. It has been dealt with under anencephaly. Spina bifida has already been discussed under neural tube defects.

Diastematomyelia, Dimyelia, and Diplomyelia

Cases of duplication of the spinal cord are not common. Although they are usually grouped together under the term diastematomyelia, Hori et al. (147) have differentiated cases under these three headings:

Dimyelia shows complete duplication of the spinal cord in which there may be medial hypoplasia, but each cord has a complete set of roots.

In *diplomyelia*, an isolated accessory spinal cord lies either ventral or dorsal to the normal cord and lacks nerve roots.

Diastematomyelia describes a more common situation, in which there is lateral bifurcation of the spinal cord into two separate structures (Fig. 6.41). The degree of differentiation in this condition varies from a cord in which there are four sets of columns and roots, through those in which there is hypoplasia of the medial roots, to those in which the columns and roots are present on one-half of the cord alone. Diastematomyelia is frequently associated with other malformations of the cord (see under

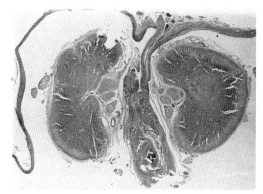

Figure 6.41. Diastematomyelia. The two cords are separated by two dural sacs, containing a small fragment of bone. The two cords have rotated medially, and the anterior sulci with their anterior spinal arteries face each other. Half of each cord is hypoplastic. Hematoxylin and eosin.

spina bifida) (47, 84, 97). Typical cases of diastematomyelia are associated with either a bony or fibrous septum at the site of the lesion, complete division of the spinal canal into two, or other local conditions favoring dysraphia such as neurenteric cyst (147). In typical cases there is rotation of both components of the diastematomyelia so that the anterior sulci face the midline. The degree of separation also determines what invests the two halves of the cord. If a separate bony canal or septum is present, each half of the cord has its own dural sheath as well as pial sheath. If no septum is present, although individual pial sheaths are present, the dural and arachnoid sheaths are shared. Although these various forms of duplication of the cord have been thought to be caused by failure of the neural tube to close, it has also been suggested (88) that duplication may occur as a consequence of faulty canalization of the medullary cord in the tail region. Although these duplications often represent severe anomalies, duplication and/or dorsal extension of the central canal and other minor duplications of localized areas of the cord may occur with lesser consequences. It has been emphasized (147) that it is important to distinguish between true diplomyelia and diastematomyelia, as the surgical treatment of the former involved excision of the accessory cord which has no connection to the normal cord, whereas the treatment of the latter involves removal of the spinal fibrous, bony, or cartilagenous spur.

Hydromyelia

Hydromyelia is dilatation of the central canal. In many instances this appears to be a continuation of the fetal situation, but it is frequently seen in association with many of other anomalies involving the brain stem and cord, such as myelomeningocele, diastematomyelia, and the Arnold-Chiari syndrome. If longstanding, the ependymal lining may be replaced by a wall of gliosis. Its association with syringomyelia will be discussed below.

Syringomyelia

This is defined as a tubular cavitation of the spinal cord extending over many segments (Fig. 6.42). In its most common form it is seen as a secondary phenomenon after trauma, ischemia, tumor, or arachnoiditis (15, 106). Many authors have considered it to be an entity separable from hydromyelia (127). The distinction, however, is not altogether clear, as a hydromyelic cord may develop diverticula which track up and down the cord forming syringomyelic cavities. In addition, the central canal may be connected with the syringomyelic cavity and develop an ependymal lining. Increased intracranial and CSF pressure may aid in the formation of syringomyelic cavities from a dilated central canal (105, 115–119). Syringomyelia is most common in the cervical cord, and grossly the cord appears fluctuant and collapses on being cut. The syrinx is seen as a transverse slit (Fig. 6.42) which may be asymmetrical, destroys the grey commissure, and extends through the dorsal column to reach the pia near the dorsal roots. Although classically regarded as having a malformative origin in some situations, this is not altogether clear, and it is inserted in this chapter for the sake of completion.

In *syringobulbia*, slits are seen in the medulla passing ventrolaterally from the floor of the fourth ventricle or along the median raphe and between the pyramid and inferior olive.

Other Abnormalities of the Spinal Cord

Several other less important anomalies of the spinal cord may be found incidentally or in association with other malformations.

MICROMYELIA (HYPOPLASIA)

Hypoplasia of the cord is relatively common in conjunction with other malformations. Isolated hypoplasia appears to be an extremely rare occurrence.

DISTURBANCES IN DECCUSSATION OF THE PYRAMIDAL TRACTS

These may be seen (305) with the corticospinal tracts descending in the anterior columns (Fig. 6.43), and the lateral columns may be very small and lack corticospinal fibers. Ultimately the fibers do cross but at local levels in the spinal cord. This situation is normally found in the small mammal *Procavia capensis*. Failure of deccusation of the corticospinal tract may sometimes fol-

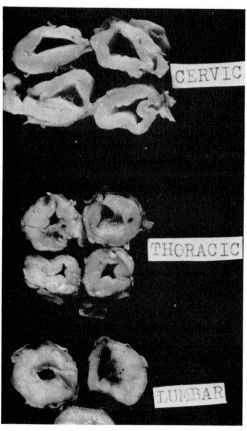

Figure 6.42.   Syringomyelia. In this instance the cavity extends from the cervical to the lumbar cord.

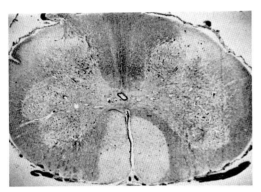

Figure 6.43. Nondecussation of the pyramidal tract. The corticospinal tracts have not crossed and descend in the anterior columns. They are readily apparent as they are unmyelinated in the neonate. No lateral corticospinal tracts of significance can be seen. Loyez stain for myelin.

low unilateral destruction of this tract early in development or follow any other event which may interfere with crossing which usually occurs in the medulla at about the 16th week.

LATERAL SPINAL CORD SULCI

In any situation where the corticospinal tracts fail to develop properly, an infolding may occur giving a characteristic sulcus (Fig. 6.44). Although these changes are undoubtedly of secondary nature, their presence often gives some clue that there has been a malformation in development of these tracts. Generally they do not form when previously normal tracts undergo degeneration.

Various aplasias affecting the dorsal columns, in sacral agenesis, and in various other isolated reports have been reviewed by Friede (110).

PROLIFERATIVE CONDITIONS ASSOCIATED WITH MALFORMATIONS

A few disorders which show features of proliferation, neoplasia, and malformation are included in this chapter for the sake of completeness, on the assumption that they represent fundamental disturbances at an embryonic and often genetic level.

Because they involve skin and nervous system simultaneously, they have been called *neuroectodermal dysplasias* (325), and this close relationship has been ex-

plained by the wide distribution of neural crest derivatives throughout the body (36). The old alternative term *phakomatosis* refers to the small flat retinal tumor seen in tuberous sclerosis.

Neurofibromatosis (Von Recklinghausen's Disease)

Neurofibromatosis is included in this section as an example of a disease in which there is a combination of malformative, hyperplastic, and neoplastic processes. Extensive reviews covering the biology, genetics, and clinical manifestations of the disease have recently been published (259, 260), and detailed descriptions of the neoplasms can be found elsewhere (267). It is a relatively common disease (1:3000) but has a wide range of expressivity. It is inherited as an autosomal dominant with a high degree of penetrance. The mutation rate is very high, accounting for new cases. Genetically and clinically, there may be many forms of the disease, of which the classical and the acoustic or central forms are the most common.

Because of the dysgenetic growth of numerous elements having a common origin in the neural crest, neurofibromatosis has been labeled as *neurocristopathy* (36). The general clinical manifestations include café au lait spots and skin neurofibromas. Tumors of the peripheral and autonomic nerves and the spinal (Fig. 6.45A) and cranial nerve roots take the form of neurilemmomas (schwannomas) and neurofibromas and are often multiple. In the central form the vestibulocochlear and trigeminal

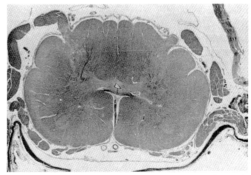

Figure 6.44. Bilateral lateral column sulci indicate the site of decreased or nonformation of the corticospinal tracts. Hematoxylin and eosin.

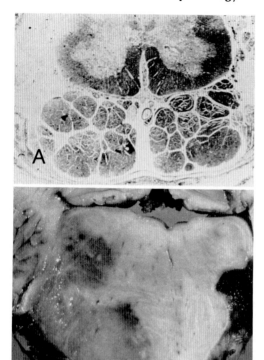

Figure 6.45. Neurofibromatosis. (*A*) Diffuse neurofibromatous change in ventral spinal roots. Loyez stain for myelin. (*B*) Cerebellopontine angle neurofibrosarcoma invading the brain stem.

seen (260). Histologically, heterotopias of neurons, astrocytes, and ependymal cells may be found, and the cortical architecture may be disturbed.

Numerous dysgenetic, hamartomatous, and/or proliferative lesions have been seen in neurofibromatosis (126, 259, 260). These include schwannosis (in the form of invasion of Schwann cells into the dorsal root entry zones of the cord or of proliferation of nerve sprouts around the vessels in the brain or the cord), meningiomatosis, angiomatosis, and glial nodules in the cortex or white matter. In some cases there is a diffuse proliferation of both nerves and vessels around the vessels in the brain parenchyma and the leptomeninges (Fig. 6.46).

In general the mechanism underlying the pathological changes is unknown, although a generalized involvement of the neural crest derivatives has been invoked. Increased levels of nerve growth factor have

nerves (often bilaterally) are more commonly involved. The pathology of these tumors is described elsewhere (267). Malignant transformation in peripheral nerve tumors is well described; 50% of all malignant schwannomas occur in neurofibromatosis, as do almost all neurofibrosarcomas (Fig. 6.45*B*). Other central nervous system tumors often found include meningiomas (often multiple), optic nerve gliomas, pilocytic astrocytomas of the third ventricle, and diffuse cerebral gliomas. Extraneural malignancies found more commonly in neurofibromatosis include Wilms' tumor and leukemia.

Large numbers of patients with neurofibromatosis have varying degrees of mental deficit; many of these patients have macrocephaly or megalencephaly (259), although this seems to be often of postnatal onset. Pachygyria, polymicrogyria, and heterotopias may be found (264). Meningoceles, often thoracic, and syringomyelia may be

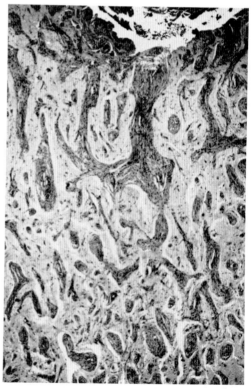

Figure 6.46. Cerebral cortex in neurofibromatosis. Diffuse infiltration of meninges and perivascular spaces by proliferating nerve elements (Schwann cells and axons), vessels, and smooth muscle.

been reported in some forms of the disease (259, 260), but the role of this substance remains speculative.

Tuberous Sclerosis (Bourneville's Disease, Epiloia)

Tuberous sclerosis is a striking disease which is usually familial, being transmitted as a mendelian dominant. Numerous sporadic cases exist, and *formes frustes* are thought to be relatively common. Prevalence rates are between 1:100,000 and 1:170,100. The subject of tuberous sclerosis has been covered in a recent review (123).

The most common presenting symptom is seizures, which occurrs in 88% of all patients. On examination, however, the skin lesions are found in 91%, and mental retardation (60%) and retinal hamartomas (50%) are frequently seen.

The skin lesions are extremely common and consist of facial angiofibromas (adenoma sebaceum), hypomelanotic macules, and shagreen patches, which are connective tissue hamartomas. Other cutaneous lesions such as fibromas and café au lait spots are also common (194). Involvement of the viscera is frequent. One of the most characteristic lesions in tuberous sclerosis is the retinal hamartoma (phakoma) which is a flat grey oval shaped astrocytic hamartoma, often obscuring a blood vessel or lying on the optic nerve head. Sometimes the lesions may be nodular. Rhabdomyomas of the heart are found in 30% of all cases, and angiomyolipomas and cysts are found in the kidneys. Other manifestations include pulmonary lymphangiomyomatosis, hemangiomas of the spleen and the liver, gingival fibromas, and fibrous dysplasia in the bones. An interesting aspect of this disease is the reported association of cases with neurofibromatosis and Sturge-Weber facial angiomatosis.

The brain is the organ most frequently involved, and this may be microcephalic, megalencephalic, or normal in weight. The characteristic feature of the disease is the presence of multiple tubers over the cortical surface (Fig. 6.47A). When the brain is fresh and unfixed, they stand out as firm nodules and are easily palpable. After fixation, especially after removal of the leptomeninges, they are readily visible and can

vary from microscopic size up to 2–3 cm in diameter. The cortical tubers typically involve the crest of the gyri and may be more pale in color than the surrounding cortex. They may involve only one gyrus or cross over to adjacent gyri obscuring the sulcal markings. They may be multiple, the number varying in a given case up to more than 40. A central dimple may often be found. Pelizzi described two forms: (1) a hard blanched and widened gyrus with a smooth crown and (2) a rounded flattened well circumscribed nodule with a dimpled center. On cut section, the lesion may be easily seen (Fig. 6.47B). Characteristically the tuber obscures the normal grey white margin and often greatly expands the normal gyrus. Additional cortical lesions may be seen in the depths of sulci. Other nodules containing heterotopic collections of cells may be found in the white matter.

Histologically the tubers consist of numerous cells distorting the normal architecture of the cortex. There may be bizarre multinucleated hypertrophied astrocytes and groups of giant cells, many of which are abnormal bizarre neurons which have irregularly oriented processes and abnormal shapes. It is sometimes difficult to determine whether a cell is an astrocyte or a neuron. Dense fibrillar gliosis may be present. Neurofibrillary tangles, argentophilic globules, and granulovacuolar degeneration have been seen in these cells (143). Collections of cells may be seen in the white matter as well. Within the ventricular system, the most striking lesions are nodular protruberances seen subependymally (Fig. 6.48). These are often seen in the vicinity of the thalamostriate vein and sulcus terminalis. These give rise to the characteristic "candle guttering" appearance. They are sometimes found in the 3rd and 4th ventricle and even in the aqueduct. They are firm, often extremely hard, and may become calcified, in which case they may be visualized on radiological examination. Although slow growing they may obstruct the foramen of Monro and cause hydrocephalus. Microscopically, the nodules consist of hyperplastic fibrillary astrocytes and aggregations of large atypical astrocytes with many nuclei and long processes. They are in many respects analogous to the glial retinal hamartoma or nodule (phakoma) described

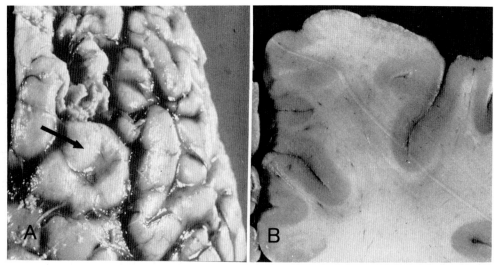

Figure 6.47. Tuberous sclerosis. (*A*) Surface view of rounded cortical tuber (*arrow*). (*B*) Cut surface showing a tuber which has expanded the gyrus and obliterated the grey-white junction.

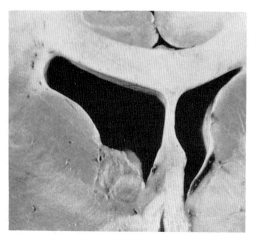

Figure 6.48. Subependymal glial nodule in tuberous sclerosis protrudes into the lateral ventricle.

above. The subependymal nodule may become a glioma (267), in which case it displays characteristic strap-like neoplastic astrocytes. Other cases show neoplasia of other elements, with a picture that has been called a spongioneuroblastoma (164). Occasional cerebellar tubers are found, containing abnormal Purkinje cells. As in neurofibromatosis, heterotopias, polymicrogyria, and other disorders of cortical architecture are frequently found. Tuberous sclerosis may occur in the fetus (277), the neonate (19), and in early life (242). These findings indicate that the disease is truly a

genetic developmental anomaly, although many of the lesions require time to develop to their fullest extent. Formes frustes of tuberous sclerosis may cause difficulty in diagnosis (27, 179) and should always be suspected and ruled out in cases of megalencephaly or mental retardation with seizures.

Encephalofacial Angiomatosis (Sturge-Weber Disease)

This is a rare nonfamilial disease, which is often associated with mental deficiency. In its full form, the syndrome includes both facial and cranial hemangiomatoses. Although formes frustes have been described with only cerebral (192) or dermal (194) involvement, the existence and significance of these have been questioned (5). The diagnosis may also be made if there is an angioma of the choroid of the eye.

The facial lesion is called a "port-wine stain" (nevus flammeus), and this is generally confined to one side of the face. The localization within the territory of one or more branches of the trigeminal nerve is of some significance, as some authors have stated that the ophthalmic branch is always involved (5, 232, 303). Indeed it has been claimed that cerebral changes are never found if the ophthalmic branch is not involved. The lesion may sometimes extend across the midline or involve the buccal mucosa.

The striking feature in the brain is the presence of leptomeningeal angiomatosis, usually involving the parietooccipital cortex, although the entire hemisphere may be involved. The veins of the pial hemangioma are dilated and tortuous and lie in folds in the subarachnoid space. Most of these vessels appear to be veins, and even when they have a thick muscular coat, the elastic lamina is missing. Occasionally this angiomatosis extends into the brain, where calcified hamartomatous veins in the cortex and subcortical white matter may be found. This, however, is relatively rare.

Beneath this leptomeningeal angiomatosis, cerebral calcification and atrophy are striking features. At times the cortex can be entirely replaced by calcification and none of the normal landmarks made out. In the less severe cases, calcification of either the outer cortical layers or less commonly the deeper layers may be seen. The calcifications in the cortex, made up of calcium phosphate and carbonate salts as well as iron, range from small amorphous globules around capillaries or large vessel sheaths to large mulberry-shaped masses. Involvement of the vessels in the underlying white matter may also be present. Secondary anoxic or ischemic changes may occur in the form of laminar necrosis of the cortex. In these areas of necrosis there is often evidence of calcium salt deposition. The profound venous stasis in the leptomeninges is thought to cause secondary stasis of the cerebral capillary bed, and the altered cerebral metabolism in the blood-brain barrier leads to deposition of iron and calcium. No doubt the vast cerebral anoxia caused by the vascular changes induces the neuronal loss, atrophy, and gliosis that are present. It is tempting to attribute the resulting mental deficiency to these changes, but this is not at all clear. In some cases, angiomatosis does not cause calcification but merely arrests development of the hemisphere, producing a hemiatrophy or lobar atrophy. The calcification of the cortex produces a characteristic radiological pattern, called "railroad tracking." Angiomatous lesions may be found in the other viscera, although there are few additional changes in the nervous system. Enlargement of the gasserian ganglion, with proliferation of capsule cells and ectopic ganglion cells, have been reported (320), and Sturge-Weber disease has been reported in association with tuberous sclerosis.

The connection between the facial and brain angiomatosis has been attributed to the embryological continuity of the vascular supply of the telencephalic vesicles, the eye, and the overlying skin. Only later with the posterior growth of the occipital poles do the vascular plexuses separate. Thus an embryonal vascular malformation of the plexus easily explains the separated lesions of the face and the occipitotemporal cortex. However, the occasional occurrence of contralateral cerebral lesions and the lack of dural and diploic involvement have never been satisfactorily explained (232).

Neurocutaneous Melanosis

Normally there are melanin-containing cells derived from the neural crest in the pia mater, especially over the ventral aspect of the brain stem. At times these pigmented cells may proliferate and become a predominant feature. Frequently the proliferation of melanin-containing cells in the meninges occur together with similar proliferation in the skin. In the Touraine syndrome, inherited as a mendelian dominant disease, patches of pigmentation are grossly visible in the pia mater associated with cutaneous pigmented nevi. In other syndromes, the pigmented lesions may sometimes occur without the skin manifestations and may be sporadic and not familial occurrences. In these cases the pigmentation may be diffuse (Fig. 6.49) and the cellular infiltrate deposited widely in the leptomeninges and

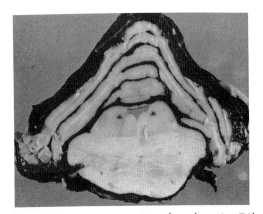

Figure 6.49. Leptomeningeal melanosis. Diffuse thickening and infiltration of the meninges over the brain stem and between the cerebellar folia by black melanoma tissue.

perivascular spaces. At times these cells may undergo neoplastic transformation and become melanomas. These may rarely metastasize other organs (171, 267).

Von Hippel-Lindau Disease

This disease is included in the present discussion because of the involvement of the central nervous system, as well as retinal, pancreas, kidney, and skin (39). These areas may show capillary hemangioblastomas, which in the brain are characteristically in the cerebellum but may also be found in the medulla, area postrema, spinal cord, and retina (267). The skin is a rare site for tumors. Cysts may be found in the pancreas and kidney, and hypernephromas may be seen. The disease is dominantly inherited.

ACKNOWLEDGMENTS

The authors thank Drs. L. E. Becker, L. J. Rubinstein, and E. Sauerbrei and the Stanford University Pathology Department for their generosity in providing illustrative material, and Mrs. P. Scilley for typing the manuscript.

Mr. B. Gubbins and Ms. M. Chiong provided excellent technical assistance.

References

1. Adams C, Johnston WP, Nevin NC: Family study of congenital hydrocephalus. *Dev Med Child Neurol* 24:493–498, 1982.
2. Adelmann HB: The problem of cyclopia. *Q Rev Biol* 11:161–284, 1936.
3. Adkins WN, Kaveggid EG: Sporadic case of apparent aprosencephaly. *Am J Genet* 3:311–314, 1979.
4. Aicardi J, Goutieres F: The syndrome of absence of the septum pellucidum with porencephalies and other developmental defects. *Neuropediatrics* 12:319–329, 1981.
5. Alexander GL, Norman RM: The Sturge-Weber syndrome. Bristol, England, John Wright & Sons, 1960.
6. Allen JP, Greer MA, McGilvra R, Castro A, Fisher DA: Endocrine function in an anencephalic infant. *J Clin Endocrinol Metab* 38:94–98, 1974.
7. Alvord EC Jr, Marcuse PM: Intracranial cerebellar meningoencephalocele (posterior fossa cyst) causing hydrocephalus by compression at the incisura tentorii. *J Neuropathol Exp Neurol* 21:50–69, 1962.
8. Ambler MW: Striated muscle cells in the leptomeninges in cerebral dysplasia. *Acta Neuropathol* 40:269–271, 1977.
9. Anderson FM, Landing BH: Cerebral arachnoid cysts in infants. *J Pediatr* 69:88–96, 1966.
10. Ariens-Kappers J: Developmental disturbance of the brain induced by German measles in an embryo of the 7th week. *Acta Anat* 31:1–20, 1957.
11. Auer RN, Gilbert JJ: Cavum vergae: without cavum septi pellucidi. *Arch Pathol Lab Med* 106:462–463, 1982.
12. Baldwin VJ, Kalousek DK, Dimmick JE, Applegarth

DA, Hardwick DF: Diagnostic pathologic investigation of the malformed conceptus. In Rosenberg HS, Bernstein J (eds): *Perspectives in Pediatric Pathology.* 1982. New York, Masson, 1982, vol 7, pp 1–63.
13. Ball MJ, Nuttall K: Neurofibrillary tangle, granulovacuolar degeneration and neuron loss in Down's syndrome: quantitative comparison with Alzheimer dementia. *Ann Neurol* 7:462–465, 1980.
14. Banik NL, Davison AN, Palo J, Savolainen H: Biochemical studies on myelin isolated from the brains of patients with Down's syndrome. *Brain* 98:213–218, 1975.
15. Barnett HJM, Foster JB, Hudgson P: Syringomyelia. Philadelphia, WB Saunders, 1973.
16. Barr M Jr, Hanson JW, Currey K, Sharp S, Toriello H, Schmickel RD, Wilson GN: Holoprosencephaly and caudal regression are increased in infants of diabetic mothers. *J Pediatr* 102:565–568, 1983.
17. Barry A, Patten RM, Stewart BH: Possible factors in the development of the Arnold-Chiari malformation. *J Neurosurg* 14:285–301, 1957.
18. Barson AJ: Spina bifida: the significance of the level and the extent of the defect to the morphogenesis. *Dev Med Child Neurol* 12:129–144, 1970.
19. Batstone CF, Cole AP, Sandry SA: A case of tuberose sclerosis in the newborn. *Acta Pediatr Scand* 60:349–352, 1971.
20. Beckett RS, Netsky MG, Zimmerman HM: Developmental stenosis of the aqueduct of Sylvius. *Am J Pathol* 26:755–771, 1950.
21. Begleiter ML, Harris DJ: Holoprosencephaly and endocrine dysgenesis in brothers. *Am J Med Genet* 7:315–318, 1980.
22. Bell JE, Gordon A, Maloney AFJ: The association of hydrocephalus and Arnold-Chiari malformation with spina bifida in the fetus. *Neuropathol Appl Neurobiol* 6:29–39, 1980.
23. Bell JA, Gordon A, Moloney AFJ: Abnormalities of the spinal meninges in anencephalic fetuses. *J Pathol* 133:131–144, 1981.
24. Benda CE: *Developmental Disorders of Mentation and Cerebral Palsies.* New York, Grune & Stratton, 1952.
25. Benda CE: The Dandy-Walker syndrome or the so-called atresia of the foramen Magendie. *J Neuropathol Exp Neurol* 13:14–29, 1954.
26. Benda CE: Mongolism. In Minckler J (ed): *Pathology of the Nervous System.* New York, McGraw-Hill, 1971, vol 2.
27. Berg JM, Crome L: A possible case of atypical tuberous sclerosis. *J Ment Defic Res* 4:24–31, 1960.
28. Bergsma D: *Birth Defects: Atlas and Compendium.* National Foundation, March of Dimes. Baltimore, Williams & Wilkins, 1973.
29. Bertrand J, Gruner J: The status verrucosus of the cerebral cortex. *J Neuropathol Exp Neurol* 14:331–347, 1955.
30. Bertoni JM, Von Loh S, Allen JR: The Aicardi syndrome: report of 4 cases and review of the literature. *Ann Neurol* 5:475–482, 1979.
31. Bickers DS, Adams RD: Hereditary stenosis of the aqueduct of Sylvius as a case of congenital hydrocephalus. *Brain* 72:246–262, 1949.
32. Bignami A, Palladini G, Zapella M: Unilateral megalencephaly with nerve cell hypertrophy; an anatomical and quantitative histochemical study. *Brain Res* 9:103–114, 1968.
33. Binns W, James LF, Shupe JL, Thacker EJ: Cyclopian-type malformation in lambs. *Arch Environ Health* 5:106–108, 1962.
34. Bishop K, Connolly JM, Carter CH, Carpenter DG: Holoprosencephaly. A case report with no extracranial abnormalities and normal chromosome count and karyotype. *J Pediatr* 65:406–414, 1964.
35. Blackwell DE, Spinato JA, Hirsch G, Giles HR, Sackler J: Antenatal ultrasound diagnosis of holoprosencephaly: a case report. *Am J Obstet Gynecol* 14:848–849, 1982.

36. Bolande RP: The neurocristopathies. A unifying concept of disease arising in neural crest maldevelopment. *Hum Pathol* 5:409–429, 1974.

37. Bonnevie K, Brodal A: Hereditary hydrocephalus in the house mouse. IV. The development of the cerebellar abnormalities during foetal life with notes on the normal development of the mouse cerebellum. *Skr Norske Vidensk Akad* 4:1–60, 1946.

38. Bossy JG: Morphological study of a case of complete, isolated and asymptomatic agenesis of the corpus callosum. *Arch Anat Histol Embryol* 53:289–340, 1970.

39. Bourdillon PJ, Hickman RC: Von Hippel-Lindau's disease presenting at an early age. *J Neurol Neurosurg Psychiatry* 30:559–562, 1967.

40. Brocklehurst G: The development of the human cerebrospinal fluid pathway with particular reference to the roof of the fourth ventricle. *J Anat* 105:467–475, 1969a.

41. Brocklehurst G: A quantitative study of a spina bifida foetus. *J Pathol* 99:205–211, 1969b.

42. Brown FR, McAdams AJ, Cummins JW, Konkol R, Singh I, Moser AB, Moser HW: Cerebro-hepto-renal (Zellweger) syndrome and neonatal adrenoleukodystrophy: similarities in phenotype and accumulation of very long chain fatty acids. *Johns Hopkins Hosp Med J* 151:344–351

43. Budka H: Megalencephaly and chromosomal anomaly. *Acta Neuropathol (Berl)* 43:263–266, 1978.

44. Burk U, Hayek HW, Zeider U: Holoprosencephaly in monozygotic twins—clinical and computer tomographic findings. *Am J Med Genet* 9:13–17, 1981.

45. Calogero JA: Vermian agenesis and unsegmental midbrain tectum. Case report. *J Neurosurg* 47:605–608, 1977.

46. Cameron AH: The Arnold-Chiari and other neuroanatomical malformations associated with spina bifida. *J Pathol Bacteriol* 73:195–211, 1957a.

47. Cameron AH: Malformations of the neuro-spinal axis, urogenital tract and foregut in spina bifida attributable to disturbances of the blastopore. *J Pathol* 73:213–221, 1957b.

48. Carmel PW: The Arnold-Chiari malformation. In *Pediatric Neurosurgery: Surgery of the Developing Nervous System*. New York, Grune & Stratton, 1982, pp 61–77.

49. Carter CO, Evans KA, Till A: Spinal dysraphism: genetic relation to neural tube malformation. *J Med Genet* 13:343–350, 1976.

50. Caspersson T, Farber S, Goley GE, Kudynowski J, Modest EJ, Simonsson E, Wahg U, Zech L: Chemical differentiation along metaphase chromosomes. *Exp Cell Res* 49:219, 1968.

51. Caviness VS Jr: The Chiari malformations of the posterior fossa and their relation to hydrocephalus. *Dev Med Child Neurol* 18:103–116, 1976.

52. Caviness VS Jr, Evrard P: Occipital encephalocele. A pathologic and anatomic analysis. *Acta Neuropathol* 32:245–255, 1975.

53. Caviness VS Jr, Rakic P: Mechanisms of cortical developments: a review from mutations in mice. *Ann Rev Neurosci* 1:297–326, 1978.

54. Chen WJ, Kelly MM, Shaw C-M, Mottet NK: Pathogenic mechanisms of heterotopic neural tissue associated with anencephaly. *Hum Pathol* 13:179–182, 1982.

55. Chiari H: Ueber Veranderungen des Kleinhirns infolge von Hydrocephalie des Grosshirns. *Dtsch Med Wochenschr* 17:1172–1175, 1891.

56. Choi BH, Lapham LW, Amin-Zaki L, Saleem T: Abnormal migration, deranged cerebral cortical organization, and diffuse white matter astrocytosis of human fetal brain: a major effect of methyl mercury poisoning in utero. *J Neuropath Exp Neurol* 78:719–733, 1978.

57. Chun RWM, Wesenberg RL, Annis BL, Chou SM: Dandy-Walker and absence of the corpus callosum; associated syndromes (abstr). *Neurology* 16:324, 1966.

58. Cilluffo JM, Gomez MR, Reese DF, Onofrio BM, Miller RH: Idiopathic ("congenital") spinal arachnoid diverticula. Clinical diagnosis and surgical results. *Mayo Clin Proc* 56:93–101, 1981.

59. Clarren SK, Alvord EC Jr, Sumi SM, Streissguth AP, Smith DK: Brain malformations related to prenatal exposure to alcohol. *J Pediatr* 92:64–67, 1978.

60. Cockayne EA: Dwarfism with retinal atrophy and deafness. *Arch Dis Child* 21:52–54, 1946.

61. Cohen H, Davies S: The morphology and permeability of the roof of the fourth ventricle in some mammalian embryos. *J Anat* 72:430–455, 1938.

62. Crome L: Microgyria. *J Pathol Bacteriol* 64:479–495, 1952.

63. Crome L: Pachygyria. *J Pathol Bacteriol* 71:335–352, 1956.

64. Crome L: Cytomegalic inclusion-body disease. *World Neurol* 2:447–458, 1961.

65. Crome L: Brain warts. *J Ment Defic Res* 13:60–65, 1969.

66. Crome L, Cowie V, Slater E: A statistical note on cerebellar and brain-stem weight in mongolism. *J Ment Defic Res* 10:69–72, 1966.

67. Crome L, Stern J: *Pathology of Mental Retardation*, ed 2. Edinburgh, Churchill-Livingstone, 1972.

68. Crome L, Sylvester PE: Hydranencephaly (hydrencephaly). *Arch Dis Child* 33:235–245, 1958.

69. D'Agostino AN, Kernohan JW, Brown JR: The Dandy-Walker syndrome. *J Neuropathol Exp Neurol* 22:450–470, 1963.

70. Dandy WE: Congenital cerebral cysts of the cavum septi pellucidi (fifth ventricle) and cavum vergae (sixth ventricle); diagnosis and treatment. *Arch Neurol Psychiatry* 25:44–46, 1931.

71. Dandy WE, Blackfan KD: Internal hydrocephalus: an experimental, clinical and pathological study. *Am J Dis Child* 8:406–482, 1914.

72. Daniel PM, Strich SJ: Some observations on the congenital deformity of the central nervous system known as the Arnold-Chiari malformation. *J Neuropathol Exp Neurol* 17:255–266, 1958.

73. Davidoff LM, Dyke CG: Agenesis of the corpus callosum; its diagnosis by encephalography. *Am J Roentgenol Radium Ther* 32:1–10, 1934.

74. Dekaban A: Arhinencephaly in an infant born to a diabetic mother. *J Neuropathol Exp Neurol* 18:620–626, 1959.

75. Dekaban A: Large defects in cerebral hemispheres associated with cortical dysgenesis. *J Neuropathol Exp Neurol* 24:512–530, 1965.

76. DeLong GR, Sidman RL: Effects of eye removal at birth on histogenesis of the mouse superior colliculus: an autoradiographic analysis with tritiated thymidine. *J Comp Neurol* 118:205–224, 1962.

77. DeMorsier G: Etudes sur les dysraphies cranio-encephaliques; agenesie du septum lucidum avec malformation du tractus optique. La dysphasic septo-optique. *Schweiz Arch Neurol Psychiatr* 77:267–292, 1956.

78. DeMyer W, Zeman W: Alobar holoprosencephaly (arhinencephaly) with median cleft lip and palate; clinical, electroencephalographic, and nosologic considerations. *Confin Neurol* 23:1–36, 1963.

79. DeMyer W, Zeman W, Palmer CG: The face predicts the brain: diagnostic significance of median facial anomalies for holoprosencephaly (arhinencephaly). *Pediatrics* 35:256–263, 1964.

80. DeMyer W, Palmer CG: Familial alobar holoprosencephaly (arhinencephaly) with median cleft lip and palate. Report of patient with 46 chromosomes. *Neurology* 13:913–918, 1963.

81. Derakshan I, Sabouri-Deylami N, Lotfi J: Holoprosencephaly computerised tomographic and pneumographic findings with anatomic correlation. *Arch Neurol* 37:55–57, 1980.

82. De Reuck J, vander Eecken H: Transitional forms of Arnold-Chiari and Dandy-Walker malformations. *J Neurol* 210:135–141, 1975.

83. Dobbing J, Sands J: Timing of neuroblast multiplication in developing human brain. *Nature* 226:639–640, 1970.

84. Doran PA, Guthkelch AN: Studies in spina bifida cystica. I. General survey and reassessment of the problem. *J Neurol Neurosurg Psychiatry* 24:331–345, 1961.

85. Dorovini-zis K, Dolman CL: Gestational development of brain. *Arch Pathol Lab Med* 101:192, 1977.

86. Drachman DA, Richardson EP Jr: Aqueductal narrowing, congenital and acquired; a critical review of histologic criteria. *Arch Neurol* 5:552–559, 1961.

87. Druckman R, Chao D, Alvord EC Jr: A case of atonic cerebral diplegia with lissencephaly. *Neurology* 9:806–814, 1959.

88. Dryden RJ: Duplication of the spinal cord: a discussion of the possible embryogenesis of diplomyelia. *Dev Med Child Neurol* 22:234–243, 1980.

89. Duckett S: Foetal Arnold-Chiari malformation. *Acta Neuropathol* 7:175–179, 1966.

90. Duke-Elder WS: Congenital deformities. In *Normal and Abnormal Development*, part 2. *System of Ophthalmology*. St. Louis, CV Mosby, 1964, vol 3.

91. Dyggve H, Tygstrup I: Megalencephaly. *Dev Med Child Neurol* 6:581–584, 1964.

92. Edwards JH, Norman RM, Roberts JM: Sexlinked hydrocephalus. Report of a family with 15 affected members. *Arch Dis Child* 36:481–485, 1961.

93. Elwood JM, Elwood JH: *Epidemiology of Anencephalus and Spina Bifida*. Oxford, England, Oxford University Press, 1980.

94. Emery JL: Deformity of the aqueduct of Sylvius in children with hydrocephalus and myelomeningocele. *Dev Med Child Neurol* 16(Suppl 32):40–48, 1974.

95. Emery JL, Kalhan SC: The pathology of exencephalus. *Dev Med Child Neurol* 12(Suppl 22):51–64, 1970.

96. Emery JL, Lendon RG: Lipomas of the cauda equina and other fatty tumours related to neurospinal dysraphism. *Dev Med Child Neurol* 11(Suppl 20):62–70, 1969.

97. Emery JL, Lendon RG: The local cord lesion in neurospinal dysraphism (meningomyelocele). *J Pathol* 110:83–96, 1973.

98. Emery JL, Naik D: Spinal cord segment lengths in children with meningiomyelocele and the "Cleland-Arnold Chiari" deformity. *Br J Radiol* 41:287–290, 1968.

99. Emery JL, Staschak MC: The size and form of the cerebral aqueduct in children. *Brain* 95:591–598, 1972.

100. Epstein CJ, Epstein LB, Weil J, Cox DR: Trisomy 21: mechanisms and models. *Ann NY Acad Sci* 396:107–118, 1982.

101. Erdohazi M: A clinical and pathological study of 43 cases of hydrocephalus not associated with spina bifida. *Dev Med Child Neurol* 11(Suppl 20):31–37, 1969.

102. Fields HW Jr, Metzner L, Garol JD, Kokich VG: The craniofacial skeleton in anencephalic human fetuses. I. Cranial floor. *Teratology* 17:57–66, 1978.

103. Fileni A, Colosimo C, Mirk P, deGaetano AM, Rocco CD: Dandy-Walker syndrome: diagnosis in utero by means of ultrasound and CT correlations. *Neuroradiology* 24:233–235, 1983.

104. Fischer EG: Dandy-Walker syndrome: an evaluation of surgical treatment. *J Neurosurg* 39:615–621, 1973.

105. Foster JB, Hudgson P: The pathology of communicating syringomyelia. In Barnett HJM, Foster JB, Hudgson P (eds): *Syringomyelia*. Philadelphia, WB Saunders, 1973a.

106. Foster JB, Hudgson P: The radiology of communicating syringomyelia. In Barnett HJM, Foster JB, Hudgson P (eds): *Syringomyelia*. Philadelphia, WB Saunders, 1973b.

107. Fraser FC: Relation of animal studies to the problem in man. In Wilson JG, Fraser FC (eds): *Handbook of Teratology*. New York, Plenum Press, 1977, vol 1, pp 75–96.

108. Fraser FC, Czeizel A, Hanson C: Increased frequency of neural tube defects in sibs of children with other malformations. *Lancet* 2:144–145, 1982.

109. Friede RL: Dating the human cerebellum. *Acta Neuropathol* 23:48–58, 1973.

110. Friede RL: *Developmental Neuropathology*. Berlin, Springer-Verlag, 1975.

111. Friede RL: Uncommon syndromes of cerebellar vermis aplasia. II. Tectocerebellar dysraphia with occipital encephalocele. *Dev Med Child Neurol* 20:764–772, 1978.

112. Friede RL, Boltshauser E: Uncommon syndromes of cerebellar vermis aplasia. I. Joubert syndrome. *Dev Med Child Neurol* 20:758–763, 1978.

113. Friede RL, Briner J: Midline hyperplasia with malformation of the formical system. *Neurology* 28:1302–1305, 1978.

114. Gardner E, O'Rahilly R, Prolo D: The Dandy-Walker and Arnold-Chiari malformations. Clinical, developmental and teratological considerations. *Arch Neurol* 32:393–407, 1975.

115. Gardner WJ, Breuer AC: Anomalies of heart, spleen, kidneys, gut and limbs may result from an overdistended neural tube: a hypothesis. *Pediatrics* 65:508–514, 1980.

116. Gardner WJ: Myelomeningocele: the result of rupture of the embryonic neural tube. *Cleve Clin Q* 27:88–100, 1960.

117. Gardner WJ: Hydrodynamic mechanism of syringomyelia: its relationship to myelocele. *J Neurol Neurosurg Psychiatry* 28:247–259, 1963.

118. Gardner WJ: Myelocele: rupture of the neural tube? *Clin Neurol Proc Congr Neurol Surg* 15:57–79, 1967.

119. Gardner WJ: The dysraphic states, from syringomyelia to anencephaly. Amsterdam, Excerpta Medica Foundation, 1973.

120. Garol JD, Fields HW Jr, Metzner L, Kokich VG: The cranio-skeleton in anencephalic human fetuses. II. Calvarium. *Teratology* 17:67–74, 1978.

121. Gilbert EF, Optiz JM: Developmental and other pathologic change in syndromes caused by chromosome abnormalities. In: *Perspectives in Pediatric Pathology*. New York, Masson, 1982, vol 7, ch 1, pp 1–63.

122. Giroud A: Causes and morphogenesis of anencephaly. In Wolstenholme GEW, O'Connor CM (eds): *Ciba Foundation Symposium on Congenital Malformations*. Boston, Little, Brown & Co, 1960.

123. Gomez MR (ed): *Tuberous Sclerosis*. New York, Raven Press, 1979.

124. Gooding CA, Carter A, Hoare RD: New ventriculographic aspects of the Arnold-Chiari malformation. *Radiology* 89:626–632, 1967.

125. Grcevic N, Robert F: Verrucose dysplasia of the cerebral cortex. *J Neuropathol Exp Neurol* 20:399–411, 1961.

126. Greene JF Jr, Fitzwater JE, Burgess J: Arterial lesions associated with neurofibromatosis. *Am J Clin Pathol* 62:481–487, 1974.

127. Greenfield JG: Syringomyelia and syringobulbia. In Blackwood W, McMenemy WH, Meyer A, Norman RM, Russell DS (eds): *Greenfield's Neuropathology*, ed 2. London, Edward Arnold, 1971.

128. Gulotta F, Rehder H, Gropp A: Descriptive neuropathology of chromosomal disorders in man. *Hum Genet* 57:337–344, 1981.

129. Guthkelch AN: Occipital cranium bifidum. *Arch Dis Child* 45:104–109, 1970.

130. Habedank M, Thomas E: Clinical and neuropathological investigations of four cases of holoprosencephaly with arhinencephaly. *Neuropaediatrie* 2:144–163, 1970.

131. Hall B: Delayed ontogenesis in human trisomy syndromes. *Hereditas* 52:334–344, 1965.

132. Hall JG, Pauli RM, Wilson KM: Maternal and fetal sequelae of anticoagulation during pregnancy. *Am J Med* 68:122–140, 1980.

133. Halsey JH, Allen N, Chamberlin HR: The morphogenesis of hydranencephaly. *J Neurol Sci* 12:187–217, 1971.

134. Hamilton WJ, Mossman HW: Nervous system. In Hamilton WJ, Mossman HW (eds): *Human Embryology*, ed 4. Baltimore, Williams & Wilkins, 1972.

135. Hanaway J, Lee SI, Netsky MG: Pachygyria: relation of findings to modern embryologic concepts. *Neurology* 18:791–799, 1968.

136. Hanaway J, Netsky MG: Heterotopias of the inferior olive: relation to Dandy-Walker malformation and correlation with experimental data. *J Neuropathol Exp*

Neurol 30:380–389, 1971.

137. Handel MA, Roth LE: Cell shape and morphology of the neural tube: implications for microtubular function. *Dev Biol* 25:78–95, 1971.

138. Hanson JW, Myrianthopoulos NC, Harvey MAS, Smith DW: Risks to the offspring of women treated with hydantoin anticonvulsants, with emphasis on fetal hydantoin syndrome. *J Pediatr* 89:662–668, 1976.

139. Harris R, Jennison RF, Barson AJ, Laurence KM, Ruoslahti E, Seppala M: Comparison of amniotic-fluid and maternal serum alpha-fetoprotein levels in the early antenatal diagnosis of spina bifida and anencephaly. *Lancet* 1:429–433, 1974.

140. Hart MN, Malamud N, Ellis WG: The Dandy-Walker syndrome: a clinicopathological study based on 28 cases. *Neurology* 22:771–780, 1972.

141. Hicks S, D'Amato CJ: How to design and build abnormal brains using radiation during development. In Fields WS, Desmond NM (eds): *Disorders of the Developing Nervous System*. Springfield IL, Charles C Thomas, 1961.

142. Hintz RL, Menking M, Sotos JF: Familial holoprosencephaly with endocrine dysgenesis. *J Pediatr* 72:81–87, 1968.

143. Hirano A, Tuazon R, Zimmerman HM: Neurofibrillary changes, granulovacuolar bodies and argentophilic globules observed in tuberous sclerosis. *Acta Neuropathol* 11:257–261, 1968.

144. Holmes LB, Driscoll SG, Atkins L: Etiologic heterogeneity of neural tube defects. *N Engl J Med* 294:365–369, 1976.

145. Holmes LB, Moser HW, Halldorsson S, Mack C, Pant SS, Matzilevich B: Mental retardation: an atlas of diseases with associated physical abnormalities. New York, MacMillan, 1972.

146. Hooft C, de Hauwere R, van Acker KJ: Familial noncongenital microcephaly, peculiar appearance, mental and motor retardation, progressive evolution to spasticity and choreo-athetosis. *Helv Pediatr Acta* 23:1–12, 1968.

147. Hori A, Fischer G, Dietrich-Schott B, Ikeda K: Dimyelia, diplomyelia, and diastematomyelia. *Clin Neuropathol* 1:23–30, 1982.

148. Howard FM, Till K, Carter CO: A family study of hydrocephalus resulting from aqueduct stenosis. *J Med Genet* 18:252–255, 1981.

149. Hughes AF, Freeman RB: Comparative remarks on the development of the tail cord among higher vertebrates. *J Embryol Exp Morphol* 32:355–363, 1974.

150. Hughes JT: Developmental disorders. In *Pathology of the Spinal Cord*. London Lloyd-Luke (Medical Books), 1966.

151. Hughes RA, Kernohan JW, Craig WM: Caves and cysts of the septum pellucidum. *Arch Neurol Psychiatry* 74:259–266, 1955.

152. Hutchinson JW, Stooring J, Turner DT: Occipital encephalocele with holoprosencephaly and aqueduct stenosis. *Surg Neurol* 12:331–335, 1979.

153. Hsu LYF, Hirschorn K: Numerical and structural chromosome abnormalities. In Wilson JG, Fraser FC (eds): *Handbook of Teratology*. New York, Plenum Press, 1977, vol 2, ch 3, pp 41–79.

154. Jacobs EB, Landing BG, Thomas W Jr: Vernicomyelia: its bearing on theories of genesis of the Arnold-Chiari complex. *Am J Pathol* 39:345–353, 1961.

155. James CCM, Lassman LP: Diastematomyelia. A critical survey of 24 cases submitted to laminectomy. *Arch Dis Child* 39:125–130, 1964.

156. James CCM, Lassman LP: Spinal dysraphism: spina bifida occulta. London, Butterworth, 1972.

157. Janzer RC, Friede RL: Dandy-Walker syndrome with atresia of the fourth ventricle and multiple rhombencephalic malformations. *Acta Neuropathol (Berl)* 58:81–86, 1982.

158. Jellinger K, Gross H: Congenital telencephalic midline defects. *Neuropaediatrie* 4:446–452, 1973.

159. Jellinger K, Gross H, Kaltenback E, Grisold W: Holo-

prosencephaly and agenesis of the corpus callosum: frequency of associated malformations. *Acta Neuropathol (Berl)* 55:1–10, 1981.

160. Jenkins G, McMillen IC, Thorburn GD: The development of fetal hypothalamic-pituitary gonadal and adrenal function. *Contr Gynecol Obstet* 5:580–590, 1979.

161. Jenkyn LR, Roberts DW, Merlis AL, Royycki A, Nordgren RE: Dandy-Walker malformation in identical twins. *Neurology* 31:337–341, 1981.

162. Jennings MT, Clamen SK, Kokich VG, Alvord EC: Neuroanatomic examination of spina bifida aperta and the Arnold-Chiari malformation in a 130 day human fetus. *J Neurol Sci* 54:325–338, 1982.

163. Jervis GA: Microcephaly with extensive calcium deposits and demyelination. *J Neuropathol Exp Neurol* 13:318–329, 1954a.

164. Jervis GA: Spongioneuroblastoma and tuberous sclerosis. *J Neuropathol Exp Neurol* 13:105–116, 1954b.

165. Johnson RT, Johnson KP: Hydrocephalus following viral infection. The pathology of aqueductal stenosis developing after experimental mumps viral infections. *J Neuropathol Exp Neurol* 27:591–606, 1968.

166. Joubert M, Esenring J-J, Robb JP: Familial agenesis at the cerebellar vermis. A syndrome of episodic hyperpnoea, abnormal eye-movements, ataxia and retardation. *Neurology* 19:813–825, 1969.

167. Kalter H: Experimental mammalian teratogenesis; a study of galactoflavin-induced hydrocephalus in mice. *J Morphol* 112:303–317, 1963.

168. Kalter H: *Congenital Malformations*. Chicago, University of Chicago Press, 1968.

169. Kalter H, Warkany J: Congenital malformations: etiological factors and their role in prevention. Part I. *N Engl J Med* 308:424–431, 1983a.

170. Kalter H, Warkany J: Congenital malformations. Part II. *N Engl J Med* 308:491–497, 1983b.

171. Kaplan AM, Itabashi HH, Hanelin LG, Lu AT: Neurocutaneous melanosis with malignant leptomeningeal melanoma. A case with metastases outside the nervous system. *Arch Neurol* 32:669–671, 1975.

172. Karch SB, Urich H: Occipital encephalocele: a morphological study. *J Neurol Sci* 15:89–112, 1972.

173. Karfunkel P: The role of microtubules and microfilaments in neurulation Xenopus. *Dev Biol* 25:30–56, 1971.

174. Karfunkel P: The mechanisms of neural tube formation. *Int Rev Cytol* 38:245–271, 1974.

175. Keates B: Genetic mapping: chromosomes 6–22. *Am J Hum Genet* 34:730–742, 1982.

176. Kepes JJ, Clough C, Villanueva A: Congenital fusion of the thalami (atresia of the third ventricle) and associated anomalies in a 6 months old infant. *Acta Neuropathol* 13:97–104, 1969.

177. Khoury MH, Erickson JD, James LM: Etiologic heterogeneity of neural tube defects. II. Clues from family studies. *Am J Hum Genet* 34:980–987, 1982.

178. Kurtzke JF, Goldberg ID, Kurland LT: The distribution of deaths from congenital malformations of the nervous system. *Neurology* 23:483–496, 1973.

179. Lagos JC, Gomez MR: Tuberous sclerosis: reappraisal of a clinical entity. *Mayo Clin Proc* 42:26–49, 1967.

180. Landrieu P, Ninane J, Ferriere G, Lyon G: Aqueductal stenosis in x-linked hydrocephalus: a secondary phenomenon? *Dev Med Child Neurol* 21:637–642, 1979.

181. Larroche JC: The development of the central nervous system during intrauterine life. In Falkner F (ed): *Human Development*. Philadelphia, WB Saunders, 1966.

182. Lau BP, Newton TH: Sphenopharyngeal encephalomeningocele. *Radiol Clin North Am* 34:386–398, 1965.

183. Lee H, Nagele RG: Neural tube closure defects caused by papaverine in explanted early chick embryos. *Teratology* 20:321–332, 1979.

184. Lee H, Nagele RG, Pietrolungo JF: Toxic and teratologic effects of caffeine on explanted early chick embryos. *Teratology* 25:19–25, 1982.

185. Lemire RJ: Variations in development of the caudal

neural tube in human embryos (Horizons XIV–XXI). *Teratology* 2:361–370, 1973.

186. Lemire RJ, Beckwith JB, Warkany J: *Anencephaly*. New York, Raven Press, 1978.

187. Lemire RJ, Loeser JD, Leech RW, Alvord EC: *Normal and abnormal development of the human nervous system*. Hagerstown, MD, Harper & Row, 1975.

188. Lendon RG, Emery RL: Forking in the central canal in the equinal cord of children. *J Anat* 106:499–505, 1970.

189. Levin P, Gross SW: Cavum septi pellucidi: an illustrative case. *J Mt Sinai Hosp* 30:59–63, 1965.

190. Levine DN, Fisher MA, Caviness VS Jr: Porencephaly with microgyria: a pathologic study. *Acta Neuropathol* 29:99–113, 1974.

191. Lichtenstein BW: Distant neuroanatomic complications of spina bifida (spinal dysraphism). *Arch Neurol Psychiatry* 47:195–214, 1942.

192. Lichtenstein BW: Sturge-Weber-Dimitri syndrome cephalic form of neurocutaneous hemanigomatosis. *Arch Neurol Psychiatry* 71:291–301, 1954.

193. Lichtenstein BW: Atresia and stenosis of the aqueduct of Sylvius. *J Neuropathol Exp Neurol* 18:3–21, 1959.

194. Lichtenstein BW: Hamartomas and phakomatoses. In Minckler J (ed): *Pathology of the Nervous System*. New York, McGraw-Hill, 1971, vol 2.

195. Lipton HL, Preziosi TJ, Moses H: Adult onset of the Dandy-Walker syndrome. *Arch Neurol* 35:672–674, 1978.

196. Liss L, Mervis L: The ependymal lining of the cavum septi pellucidi. A histological and histochemical study. *J Neuropathol Exp Neurol* 23:355–367, 1964.

197. Loeser JD, Alvord EC Jr: Agenesis of the corpus callosum. *Brain* 91:553–570, 1968.

198. Lorber J: The family history of spina bifida cystica. *Pediatrics* 35:589–595, 1965.

199. Lorber J, Bassi U: The aetiology of neonatal hydrocephalus (excluding cases with spina bifida). *Dev Med Child Neurol* 7:289–294, 1965.

200. Ludwin SK, Malamud N: Pathology of congenital anomalies of the brain. In Newton TH, Potts DG (eds): *Anatomy and Pathology. Radiology of the Skull and Brain*. St. Louis, CV Mosby, 1977, vol 3, pp 2979–3015.

201. Lynn RB, Buchanan DC, Fenichel GM, Freeman FR: Agenesis of the corpus callosum. *Arch Neurol* 37:444–445, 1980.

202. MacMahon B, Yen S: Unrecognised epidemic of anencephaly and spina bifida. *Lancet* 1:31–33, 1971.

203. Manz HJ, Phillips TM, Rowden G, McCullough DC: Unilateral megalencephaly, cerebral cortical dysplasia, neuronal hypertrophy, and heterotopia: cytomorphometric, fluorometric cytochemical, and biochemical analyses. *Acta Neuropathol (Berl)* 45:97–103, 1979.

204. Margolis G, Kilham L: Experimental virus induced hydrocephalus—relation to pathogenesis of the Arnold-Chiari malformation. *J Neurosurg* 31:1–9, 1969.

205. Marin-Padilla M: Notochordal basichondrium relationships: abnormalities in experimental axial skeletal (dysraphic) disorders. *J Embryol Exp Morphol* 53:15–38, 1979.

206. Marin-Padilla M, Marin-Padilla TM: Morphogenesis of experimentally induced Arnold-Chiari malformations. *J Neurol Sci* 50:29–55, 1981.

207. Masters CL: Pathogenesis of the Arnold-Chiari malformation. The significance of hydrocephalus and aqueduct stenosis. *J Neuropathol Exp Neurol* 37:56–74, 1978.

208. Matson DD: Neurosurgery of infancy and childhood, ed. 2. Springfield, IL, Charles C Thomas, 1969.

209. Matsumoto H, Koya G, Takeuchi T: Fetal Minamata disease. *J Neuropathol Exp Neurol* 24:563–574, 1965.

210. McBride MC, Kemper TL: Pathogenesis of four-layered microgyric cortex in man. *Acta Neuropathol (Berl)* 57:93–98, 1982.

211. McDermott A, Insley J, Barton ME, Rowe P, Edwards JH, Cameron AH: Arrhinencephaly associated with a deficiency involving chromosome 18. *J Med Genet* 5:60–67, 1968.

212. McGrath P: Aspects of the human pharyngeal hypophysis in normal and anencephalic fetuses and neonates and their possible significance in the mechanisms of control. *J Anat* 127:65–81, 1978.

213. McKusick VA, Stauffer M, Know DL, Clark DB: Chorioretinopathy with hereditary microcephaly. *Arch Ophthalmol* 75:597–600, 1963.

214. McLaurin RL: Parietal cephaloceles. *Neurology* 14:764–772, 1964.

215. McMillan JJ, Williams B: Aqueduct stenosis. Case review and discussion. *J Neurol Neurosurg Psychiatry* 40:521–532, 1977.

216. Mealey J Jr, Dzenitis AJ, Hockey AA: The prognosis of encephalocoeles. *J Neurosurg* 32:209–218, 1967.

217. Melnick M: Current concepts of the etiology of central nervous system malformations. Recent advances in the developmental biology of central nervous system malformation. *Birth Defects* 25:19–41, 1979.

218. Menkes JH, Philippart M, Clark DB: Hereditary partial agenesis of corpus callosum, biochemical and pathological studies. *Arch Neurol* 11:198–208, 1964.

219. Metzner L, Garol JD, Fields HW Jr, Kokich VG: The craniofacial skeleton in anencephalic human fetuses. III. Facial skeleton. *Teratology* 17:75–82, 1978.

220. Michaud J, Miyrahi EM, Urich H: Agenesis of the vermis with fusion of the cerebellar hemispheres, septo-optic dysplasia and associated anomalies. Report of a case. *Acta Neuropathol (Berl)* 56:161–166, 1982.

221. Mizuno N, Yoshida M, Okamoto M: Helwig's triangular fasiculus in anencephalic fetuses. *J Comp Neurol* 132:167–188, 1968.

222. Moosy J: The neuropathology of Cockayne's syndrome. *J Neuropathol Exp Neurol* 26:654–660, 1967.

223. Morriss GM, Thorogood PV: An approach to cranial neural crest cell migration and differentiation in mammalian embryos. In Johnson MH (ed): *Development in Mammals*. Amsterdam, North Holland, 1978, pp 363–412.

224. Myers RE: Atrophic cortical sclerosis associated with status marmoratus in a perinatally damaged monkey. *Neurology* 19:1177–1188, 1969a.

225. Myers RE: Cystic brain alteration after incomplete placental abruption in monkey. *Arch Neurol* 21:133–141, 1969b.

226. Navin JJ, Angevine JM: Congenital cytomegalic inclusion disease with porencephaly. *Neurology* 18:470–472, 1968.

227. Naeye RL, Blanc WA: Organ and body growth in anencephaly. *Arch Pathol* 91:140–147, 1971.

228. Nelson MM, Thomson AJ: The acrocallosal syndrome. *Am J Med Genet* 12:195–199, 1982.

229. Noel P, Humbert JP, Ectors M, Franken L, Flament-Durand J: Agenesis of the corpus callosum associated with relapsing hypothermia. A clinico-pathological report. *Brain* 96:359–368, 1973.

230. Norman MG: Perinatal brain damage. In Rosenberg HS, Bolande R (eds): *Perspectives in Pediatric Pathology*. Chicago, Yearbook Medical Publishers, 1978, vol 4, pp 73–78.

231. Norman MG: Bilateral encephaloclastic lesions in a 26 week gestation fetus: effect on neuroblast migration. *J Can Sci Neurol* 7:191–194, 1980.

232. Norman RM: *Greenfield's Neuropathology*, ed 2. London, Edward Arnold, 1963.

233. Owens JR, McAllister E, Harris F, West L: 19-year incidence of neural tube defects in area under constant surveillance. *Lancet* 2:1032–1035, 1981.

234. Padget DH: Spina bifida and embryonic neuroschisis—a causal relationship. Definition of the postnatal conformations involving a bifid spine. *Johns Hopkins Med J* 123:233–252, 1968.

235. Padget DH: Neuroschisis and human embryonic maldevelopment. New evidence of anencephaly, spina bifida and diverse mammalian defects. *J Neuropathol Exp Neurol* 29:192–216, 1970.

236. Padget DH: Development of so-called dysraphism, with embryologic evidence of clinical Arnold-Chiari and Dandy-Walker malformations. *Johns Hopkins Med J* 130:127–165, 1972.

237. Page LK, Brown SB, Gargano FP, Shortz RW: Schizencephaly: a clinical study and review. *Child Brain* 1:348–358, 1975.

238. Parrish ML, Roessmann U, Levinsohn MW: Agenesis of the corpus callosum: a study of the frequency of associated malformations. *Ann Neurol* 6:349–354, 1979.

239. Patel H, Dolman CL, Byrne MA: Holoprosencephaly with median cleft lip; clinical pathological, and echoencephalography study. *Am J Dis Child* 124:217–221, 1972.

240. Pattern BM: Embryological stages in the establishing of myeloschisis with spina bifida. *Am J Anat* 93:365–395, 1953.

241. Paul KS, Lye RH, Strang FA, Duthor J: Arnold-Chiari malformation. Review of 71 cases. *J Neurosurg* 58:183–187, 1983.

242. Paulson GW, Lyle CB: Tuberous sclerosis. *Dev Med Child Neurol* 8:571–586, 1966.

243. Peach B: Arnold-Chiari malformation with normal spine. *Arch Neurol* 10:497–501, 1964a.

244. Peach B: Cystic prolongation of fourth ventricle; an anomaly associated with Arnold-Chiari malformation. *Arch Neurol* 11:609–612, 1964b.

245. Peach B: Arnold-Chiari malformation. Anatomic features of 20 cases. *Arch Neurol* 12:613–621, 1965a.

246. Peach B: Arnold-Chiari malformation. Morphogenesis. *Arch Neurol* 12:527–535, 1965b.

247. Pendergrass EP, Hodes PJ: Dilatations of the cavum septi pellucidi and cavum vergae. *Ann Surg* 101:269–295, 1935.

248. Penfield W, Cone W: Spina bifida and carnium bifidum; results of plastic repair of meningocele and myelomeningocele by a new method. *JAMA* 98:454–461, 1932.

249. Pollock JA, Newton TH, Hoyt WF: Transsphenoidal and transethmoidal encephaloceles; a review of clinical and roentgen features in 8 cases. *Radiology* 90:442–453, 1968.

250. Priestley DP: A case of complete absence of the cerebellum. *Lancet* 2:1302, 1920.

251. Purpura DP: Pathobiology of cortical neurons in metabolic and unclassified amentias: In Katzman R (ed): *Congenital and Acquired Cognitive Disorders.* New York, Raven Press, 1979, pp 43–68.

252. Raimondi AJ, Samuelson F, Yarzagaray L, Norton T: Atresia of the foramina of Luschka and Magendi: the Dandy-Walker cyst. *J Neurosurg* 31:202–216, 1969.

253. Rakic P: Guidance of neurons migrating to the fetal monkey neocortex. *Brain Res* 33:471–476, 1971a.

254. Rakic P: Neuron-glia relationship during granule cell migration in developing cerebellar cortex. A Golgi and electron-microscopic study in Macacus rhesus. *J Comp Neurol* 141:283–312, 1971b.

255. Rakic P: Mode of cell migration to the superficial layers of fetal monkey neocortex. *J Comp Neurol* 145:61–84, 1972.

256. Rakic P, Sidman RL: Telencephalic origin of pulvinar neurons in the fetal human brain. 2. *Anat Entwickl Gesch* 129:53–82, 1969.

257. Rakic P, Yakovlev PI: Development of the corpus callosum and cavum septi in man. *J Comp Neurol* 132:45–72, 1968.

258. Rewcastle NB, Francouer J: Teratomous cysts in the spinal canal. *Arch Neurol* 11:91–100, 1962.

259. Riccardi VM: Von Recklinghausen neurofibromatosis. *N Engl J Med* 305:1617–1626, 1981.

260. Riccardi VM, Mulvihill JJ (eds): Neurofibromatosis (von Recklinghausen's disease). *Advances In Neurology.* New York, Raven Press, 1981, vol 29.

261. Richman DP, Stewart R, Caviness VS Jr: Cerebral microgyria in 27 week fetus: an architectonic and topographic analysis. *J Neuropathol Exp Neurol* 33:374–384, 1974.

262. Ropper AH, Williams RS: Relationship between plaques, tangles and dementia in Down syndrome. *Neurology* 30:639–644, 1980.

263. Rorke CB, Fogelson MH, Riggs HE: Cerebellar heterotopia in infancy. *Dev Med Child Neurol* 10:644–650, 1968.

264. Roseman NP, Pearce J: The brain in multiple neurofibromatosis (von Recklinghausen's disease): a suggested neuropathological basis for the associated mental defect. *Brain* 90:829–838, 1967.

265. Roubicek M, Spranger J, Wende S: Frontonasal dysplasia as an expression of holoprosencephaly. *Eur J Pediatr* 137:229–231, 1981.

266. Russell DS: *Observations on the Pathology of Hydrocephalus.* London, Her Majesty's Stationery Office, 1949.

267. Russell DS, Rubinstein LJ: *Pathology of Tumours of the Nervous System,* ed 4. London, Edward Arnold, 1977.

268. Saxen L: Neural induction: past, present, and future. *Curr Top Dev Biol* 15:409–418, 1980.

269. Scarcella G: Radiologic aspects of Dandy-Walker syndrome. *Neurology* 10:260–266, 1960.

270. Schoenwolf GC: Effects of complete tailbud extirpation on early development of the posterior region of the chick embryo. *Anat Rec* 192:289–296, 1978.

271. Schreiber MS, Reye RDK: Posterior fossa cysts due to congenital atresia of the foramina of Luschka and Magendie. *Med J Aust* 2:743–748, 1954.

272. Schroeder TE: Neurulation in Xenopus laevis. Analysis and model based upon light and electron microscopy. *J Embryol Exp Morphol* 23:427–462, 1970.

273. Scott TM, Fyfe WM, Hart DM, Farquhar JW: Maternal phenylketonuria: abnormal baby despite low phenylalanine diet during pregnancy. *Arch Dis Child* 55:634–636, 1980.

274. Seller MJ, Adinolfi M: The curly-tail mouse: an experimental model for human neural-tube defects. *Life Sci* 29:1607–1615, 1981.

275. Seller MJ, Singer JD, Coltart TM, Campbell S: Maternal serum-alpha-fetoprotein levels and prenatal diagnosis of neural-tube defects. *Lancet* 1:429–433, 1974.

276. Shapiro BL: Down's syndrome—a disruption of homeostasis. *Am J Med Genet* 14:241–269, 1983.

277. Sharp D, Robertson DM: Tuberous sclerosis in an infant of 28 weeks gestational age. *Can J Neurol* 10:59–62, 1983.

278. Shaw CM, Alvord EC Jr: Cava septi pellucidi et vergae: their normal and pathological states. *Brain* 92:213–224, 1969.

279. Shillo J, Strand R, Fischer EG, Winston KR: Chiari 1 "malformations"—an acquired disorder? *Neurosurgery* 55:604–609, 1981.

280. Sidman RL, Miale IL: Histogenesis of the mouse cerebellum studied by autoradiography with tritiated thymidine. *Anat Rec* 133:429–430, 1959.

281. Sidman RL, Miale IL, Feder N: Cell proliferation and migration in the primitive ependymal zone; an autoradiographic study of histogenesis in the nervous system. *Exp Neurol* 1:322–333, 1959.

282. Sidman RL, Rakic P: Neuronal migration, with special reference to developing human brain: a review. *Brain Res* 62:1–35, 1973.

283. Sidman RL, Rakic P: Development of the human central nervous system. In Haymaker W, Adams RD (eds): *Histology and Histopathology of the Central Nervous System.* Springfield, IL, Charles C Thomas, 1982, vol 1, pp 3–245.

284. Smith DW: Recognizable patterns of human malformation in major problems. *Problems in Clinical Pediatrics.* Philadelphia, WB Saunders, 1982, vol 7, pp 10–75.

285. Smith JF: *Pediatric Neuropathology.* New York, McGraw-Hill, 1974.

286. Smithells RW, Sheppard S, Schorah CJ, Seller MJ, Nevin NC, Harris R, Read AP, Fielding DW: Apparent prevention of neural tube defects by preconceptional vitamin supplementation. *Arch Dis Child* 56:911–918, 1981.

287. Snodgrass GJAI, Butler LJ, France NE, Crome L, Russell A: The "D" (13–15) trisomy syndrome: an analysis of 7 examples. *Arch Dis Child* 41:250–261, 1966.

288. Soffer D, Grotsky HW, Rapin I, Suzuki K: Cockayne syndrome: unusual neuropathological findings and review of the literature. *Ann Neurol* 6:340–348, 1979.

289. Solitare GB, Lamarche JB: Brain weight in the adult mongol. *J Ment Defic Res* 11:79–84, 1967.

290. Solt LC, Deck JHN, Baim RS, TerBrugge K: Interhemispheric cyst of neuroepithelial origin in association with partial agenesis of the corpus callosum. Case report and review of the literature. *J Neurosurg* 52:399–403, 1980.

291. Spranger JM, Spranger J, Benirschke K, Hall JG, Lenz W, Lowry RB, Opitz JM, Pinsky L, Schwarzacher HG, Smith DW: Errors of morphogenesis: concepts and terms. Recommendations of an international working group. *J Pediatr* 100:160–165, 1982.

292. Starkman SP, Brown TC, Linell EA: Cerebral arachnoid cysts. *J Neuropathol Exp Neurol* 17:484–500, 1958.

293. Suetsugu M, Meharein P: Spine distribution along the apical dendrites of the pyramidal neurons in Down's syndrome. *Acta Neuropathol* 50:207–210, 1980.

294. Sumi SM: Brain malformations in the trisomy 18 syndrome. *Brain* 93:821–830, 1970.

295. Suwanwela C, Hongsaprabhas C: Fronto-ethmoidal encephalomeningocele. *J Neurosurg* 25:172–182, 1966.

296. Taggart JK Jr, Walker AE: Congenital atresia of the foramens of Luschka and Magendie. *Arch Neurol Psychiatry* 48:583–612, 1942.

297. Taly B, Freignang HG, Durity FA, Moyes PD: Dandy-Walker syndrome: analysis of 21 cases. *Dev Med Child Neurol* 22:189–201, 1980.

298. Taylor AI: Autosomal trisomy syndrome: a detailed study of 27 cases of Edwards syndrome and 27 cases of Patau syndrome. *J Med Genet* 5:227–252, 1968.

299. Teng P, Papatheodorou C: Arnold-Chiari malformation with normal spine and cranium. *Arch Neurol* 12:622–624, 1965.

300. Terplan KL, Sandberg AA, Aceto T Jr: Structural anomalies in cerebellum in association with trisomy. *JAMA* 197:557–568, 1966.

301. Toivonen S, Tarin D, Saxen L, Tarin PJ, Wartiovaara J: Transfilter studies on neural induction in the newt. *Differentiation* 4:1–7, 1975.

302. Townsend JJ, Nielsen SL, Malamud N: Unilateral megalencephaly: hamartoma or neoplasm? *Neurology* 25:448–453, 1975.

303. Urich H: Malformations of the nervous system. In Blackwood W, Corsellis JAN (eds): *Greenfield's Neuropathology*. London, Edward Arnold, 1976, pp 361–469.

304. Urich H: Cerebellar malformations: some pathogenetic considerations. *Clin Exp Neurol* 16:119–131, 1979.

305. Verhoaart WJC, Kramer W: The uncrossed pyramidal tract. *Acta Psychiatr Neurol Scand* 27:181–200, 1952.

306. Vogel FS, McClenahan JL: Anomalies of major cerebral arteries associated with congenital malformations of the brain. With special reference to the pathogenesis of anencephaly. *Am J Pathol* 28:701–711, 1952.

307. Volpe JJ, Adams RD: Cerebro-hepato-renal syndrome of Zellweger: an inherited disorder of neuronal migration. *Acta Neuropathol* 20:175–198, 1972.

308. Warkany J: *Congenital Malformations: Notes and Comments*. Chicago, Year Book Medical Publishers, 1971.

309. Warkany J, O'Toole BA: Experimental spina bifida and associated malformations. *Child's Brain* 8:18–30, 1981.

310. Warren MC, Lu AT, Ziering WH: Sex-linked hydrocephalus with aqueductal stenosis. *J Pediatr* 63:1104–1110, 1963.

311. Weed LH: The development of the cerebro-spinal spaces in pigs and in man. *Contrib Embryol* 5:41–52, 1917.

312. Wigglesworth JS, Desai R: Is fetal respiratory function a major determinant of perinatal survival? *Lancet* 1:264–267, 1981.

313. Williams B: Is aqueduct stenosis a result of hydrocephalus? *Brain* 96:399–412, 1973.

314. Williams RS, Ferrante RJ, Caviness VS Jr: The cellular pathology of microgyria: a Golgi analysis. *J Neuropathol Exp Neurol* 35:114, 1976

315. Wilson DB: Effects of embryonic overgrowth on the avian optic tectum. *Am J Anat* 135:549–560, 1972.

316. Wilson DB, Finta LA: Gap junctional vesicles in the neural tube of the Splotch (sp) mutant mouse. *Teratology* 19:337–340, 1979.

317. Wilson DB, Finta LA: Early development of the brain and spinal cord in dysraphic mice—a transmission electron microscopic study. *J Comp Neurol* 190:363–371, 1980.

318. Wilson JG: Current status of teratology. In Wilson JG, Fraser FC (eds): *Handbook of Teratology*. New York, Plenum Press, 1977, vol 1, ch 2, pp 49–62.

319. Wilson JT: On the nature and mode of origin of the foramen of Magendie. *J Anat* 71:423–428, 1937.

320. Wohlwill FJ, Yakovlev PI: Histopathology meningofacial angiomatosis (Sturge-Weber's disease): report of four cases. *J Neuropathol* 16:341–364, 1957.

321. Wolf A, Bamford TE: Cavum septi pellucidi and cavum vergae. *Bull Neurol Inst NY* 4:294–309, 1935.

322. Woollam DHM, Millen JW: Anatomical considerations in the pathology of stenosis of the cerebral aqueduct. *Brain* 76:104–112, 1953.

323. Wright S: The genetics of vital characters of the guinea pig. *J Cell Comp Physiol* 56(Suppl 1):123–151, 1960.

324. Wyndham GC, Edmonds LD: Current trends in the incidence of neural tube defects. *Pediatrics* 70:333–337, 1982.

325. Yakovlev PI, Guthrie RH: Congenital ectodermoses (neurocutaneous syndromes) in epileptic patients. *Arch Neurol Psychiatry* 26:1145–1194, 1931.

326. Yakovlev PI, Guthrie RH: Pathoarchitectonic studies of cerebral malformations. III. Arrhinencephalies (holotelencephalies). *J Neuropathol Exp Neurol* 18:22–25, 1959.

327. Yakovlev PI, Wadsworth RC: Schizencephalies: a study of the congenital clefts in the cerebral mantle. I. Clefts with fused lips. *J Neuropathol Exp Neurol* 5:116–130, 1964a.

328. Yakovlev PI, Wadsworth RC: Schizencephalies: a study of the congenital clefts in the cerebral mantle. II. Clefts with hydrocephalus and lips separated. *J Neuropathol Exp Neurol* 5:169–205, 1964b.

329. Yamamoto N, Watanabe G: Epidemiology of gross chromosomal anomalies at the early stage of pregnancy. *Contrib Epidemiol Biostal* 1:101–106, 1979.

330. Yates VD, Wilroy RS, Whitington GL, Simmons JCH: Anterior sacral defects: an autosomal dominantly inherited condition. *J Pediatr* 102:239–242, 1983

331. Yoshida M, Nakamura M: Complete absence of the cerebellum with arthrogryposis multiplex congenita diagnosed by CT scan. *Surg Neurol* 17:62–65, 1982.

CHAPTER 7

Perinatal Neuropathology

FLOYD H. GILLES, M.D.

INTRODUCTION AND GENERAL COMMENTS

The evaluation of the pathology of the late fetal brain of 20–40 weeks of gestation requires recognition of a number of potentially confusing and distracting features. The histology of the brain of the immature child differs in many substantial respects from that of the mature brain, and both the histology and the cellular reactions change during maturation. Lesions, superimposed on a changing developing brain, range in apparent complexity from simple loss of neural tissue (e.g., necrosis and cysts) to complex malformations resulting from various admixtures of developmental arrests, abnormalities of migration, and abortive attempts at repair. Developmental delay, a kind of "lesion," is unique to the fetal and neonatal brain and may be seen as general failure of growth (e.g., in weight), or as failure of the adequate acquisition of some developmental component such as myelin. Differentiation between developmental delay (in the above sense) and atrophy (loss of tissue previously acquired) is important, as the suspected etiologies of these two classes of disease are considerably different.

Misleading Notions

The impact on clinicians of the pathologist's interpretation about pathogenetic mechanisms can be abrogated by two widely held notions among pathologists, both related to the etiologic nonspecificity of morphologic abnormalities in the neonatal brain. The first notion is that acute morphologic changes in the brain of recently dead infants arise from the same constellations of antecedents as do neuronal depletions and glial scars found in the brains of children who have survived fetal or neonatal insult. Some of the acute changes may well have arisen from the systemic abnormalities that led to the death of the child. However, it is clear that children who survive an insult have a distinctly different set of antecedents than do children who die during an insult. The second notion is that pathologic changes in brains derived from neonates with common systemic illnesses reflect damage induced by those specific illnesses. This argument does not rest on firm ground until it is shown that the changes in the brain are distinctly different from the morphologic abnormalities found in dead neonates of the same gestational and survival age comparable in every way except for the systemic disease in question.

A further problem is raised by extrapolation directly from dead to living. Interpretations based on morphologic material from dead children that are to be used by the clinician in living children need more than a common event (e.g., hypoxia) to bridge the gap between the dead and the living. The associations between morphologic events in the dead and clinical events are, at best, fraught with danger for two reasons. First, there is the myriad of clinical events that antedate death; usually the strength of the association between clinical events in the living and morphologic events in the dead is not measured. Second, even clinical events with strong associations

243

with morphologic events in the dead may not have the same potential for inducing damage in living children. The strength of the association between clinical events and brain damage must eventually be tested in the living to have clinicial meaning. Finally, the pathologist and the clinician may be trapped by the same conceptual model widely used in medicine: the simple model that equates a single antecedent with a single pathologic effect. There appear to be very few diseases with single causes. Most "causes" are events that increase the likelihood of a disease, not in isolation, but in conjunction with other antecedents. Likewise, there is no single pathologic change in the brain of the neonate that is etiologically specific. Necrosis and hemorrhage, for example, each have a multitude of antecedents. Thus, physicians are obligated not to ascribe etiologic meaning to a lesion on what may be a speculative basis (for instance, not all lesions are caused by anoxia or its cogeners hypoxia or hypoxischemia).

Important Lesions

What are the clinically important lesions in perinatal neuropathology? Certainly not malformations (either as to number of brains of neonates involved by these lesions at the autopsy table or as to the frequency of the lesions that underlie most of the clinical deficits in the brains of autopsied individuals who occupied schools for the mentally retarded). The important lesions in neonatal brains are those of hemorrhage, necrosis, and infection, and are usually acquired either while in utero (after midgestation), at birth, or in the immediate postnatal period as emphasized in the recent reviews of Friede (28), Norman (63), and Rorke (75). The lesions in the brains of the older patients who had been hospitalized tend to be scars attributed to acquired, not malformative, lesions.

There is a widespread notion among neonatologists, neurologists, and neuropathologists that asphyxia is the source of most acquired abnormalities in the neonatal brain. In fact, in currently available texts of neuropathology some 28 distinct morphologic abnormalities of the neonatal brain are attributed to asphyxia, hypoxia, or anoxia. What this means is that the clinician cannot predict with specificity the abnormality to be found in the baby's brain, and the pathologist cannot predict with specificity which of the components of "asphyxia" were antecedent to the abnormality he finds in the baby brain. The term asphyxia is poorly defined, refers to a multifaceted and nonspecific outcome (the kind of brain damage), is not a unique antecedent (but includes many components such as lowered oxygen, increased carbon dioxide, lowered pH, depressed respiration, cyanosis, etc.), and clouds the search for other antecedents. As a term, it confuses three very important and distinct issues. It is often used in the sense of meaning impaired neural *function* (e.g., depressed respiration), or in the sense of being a *cause of brain damage* (in some centers, apparently the only cause), or in the sense of *the resulting brain damage* (even some neuropathologists speak superficially of necrosis or hemorrhage as being "anoxic," "ischemia," hypoxischemic," or "asphyxic" in spite of the fact that each of these terms is merely an interpretation, all too often not based on comparisons with controlled populations).

Infection will be covered elsewhere in this volume. However, the ability of inflammatory cells to respond to foreign invaders in the brain of the unborn child is acquired during gestation as it is in other organs. Plasma cells probably do not enter the brain prior to midgestation and other inflammatory cells even later. Further, some cerebral tissues become susceptible to predatory organisms only at certain stages in development (e.g., the germinal matrix and rubella interaction—germinolysis). Other gestational invaders are associated with anomalies or with caseous necrosis, etc.

The topics in this chapter are aimed at providing (a) comparative standards for fetal brains and (b) selected common pathologic lesions. The topics include sections about an approach to the neonatal brain, atlantooccipital relationships, changing norms and reaction capabilities, signs of repair or regeneration, and the important lesions of hemorrhage, necrosis and the perinatal leukoencephalopathies, delay in myelination, edema and herniation, and peri- and postnatal trauma.

AN APPROACH TO THE NEONATAL BRAIN

The infant's brain is usually approached by the modified Beneke procedure using incisions along the sutures to open the parietal and frontal bones (70). However, the difficult anatomic problems of hydrocephalus, posterior fossa tumors, posterior fossa malformations, and retrocerebellar subdural hematomas or retrocerebellar arachnoidal or ependymal cysts can be more easily studied when a suboccipital craniectomy and an upper cervical laminectomy are done before opening the cranium.

The first goal in the pathologic analysis of the neonate or infant with hydrocephalus is to delineate the reason for the hydrocephalus, the second is the search for secondary diverticuli that may distort the midbrain or cerebellum, and the third is the search for the complications of therapies, particularly shunts.

The suboccipital exposure of the posterior fossa allows direct visualization of the most frequent obstructive processes in the neonate, namely infratentorial processes (Fig. 7.1). For instance, two surgically treatable causes of infantile hydrocephalus that are easily missed with the supratentorial approach are retrocerebellar cysts and retrocerebellar subdural hematomas. Further, the suboccipital exposure enhances the evaluation of the neonate with Chiari or other malformation or the older child with a posterior fossa neoplasm.

For the suboccipital approach the occipital skin flap is loosened over the back of the head and neck down to C4 or C5. The entire procedure can usually be done without additional incisions in young infants. The supraoccipital bone and the dorsal arches of the upper cervical vertebrae lie subjacent to the upper cervical posterior muscle mass. The arches of C1 and C2 are removed, the dura is opened with a cruciate incision leaving the arachnoid intact, and the dorsal aspect of the cervicomedullary junction at the caudal border of the foramen magnum is inspected. The cerebellum is relatively small in the neonate, and the vallecula is wide. Further, the neonatal foramen magnum is relatively large, and, if there is no rhombencephalic or cranial malformation or tumor, the lower third of the fourth ventricle can be seen under the caudal cerebellum through the transparent arachnoid of the cisterna magna. Retrocerebellar cysts and subdural hematomas bulge immediately into view. Varying amounts of the lower edge of the supraoccipital bone may be ronguered away for optimal exposure, depending on the abnormality in the posterior fossa. The spinal cord is divided below the caudal end of the lesion (e.g., the caudal end of the cerebellar peg in a Chiari malformation). The cervical roots and lower cranial nerves are divided along with the vertebral arteries, and the specimen is then left in the head until later removal from above by the usual procedure.

The approach to the infant with hydrocephalus is dependent upon the degree of hydrocephalus. The goal of the approach is an intact, unruptured brain. Ventricular fluid is easily drained with a large trocar placed into the lateral ventricle through the coronal suture. The head is turned on its side and the uppermost parietal or frontal bone can be reflected, while the ventricular fluid drips out. The hydrocephalic brain slowly collapses within the skull, and bridging veins, dural adhesions, and finally cranial nerves and great vessels at the base can be divided. The brain can be poured out into the weighing pan and then poured directly into the formalin crock and suspended in the usual fashion with a heavy thread under the upper end of the basilar artery. Once suspended, any transtentorial diverticuli or other diaphanous cyst walls will float out into the formalin, particularly if the brain is shaken gently. Ventricular size can be reconstituted with fixative (as long as the fixative is injected into the ventricle and not into the paraventricular parenchyma) before the rapidly fixing narrowed cerebral mantle hardens.

Complications of therapeutic endeavors are mostly operative or shunt-related, although local ventricular diverticuli sometimes occur at the site of ventricular punctures through the lateral corner of the fontanelle. As shunt infections are a major problem, shunt tube contents must be cultured at the time of autopsy, patency determined, and evidence of past or recent inflammation should be sought at both the ventricular and distal ends. Plexitis, ventriculitis, ventricular synechiae, coarcta-

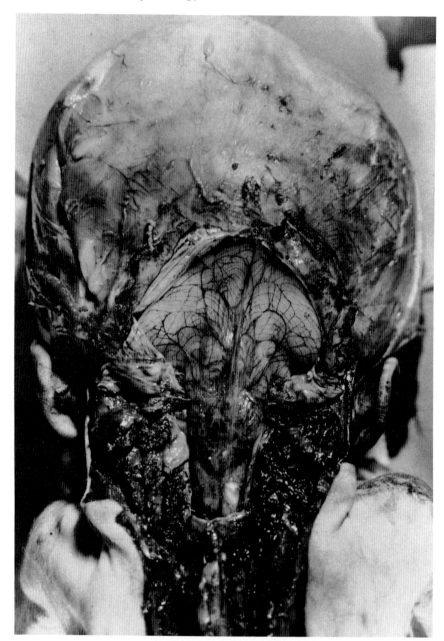

Figure 7.1. The suboccipital craniectomy and upper cervical laminectomy exposes the rhomben-cephalic and upper cervical cord malformations in an infant with a Chiari II malformation. The posterior skin flap was removed for photographic purposes; in the usual case, the same degree of exposure of neural and bony structure can be obtained within the intact posterior skin flap without additional incisions, and many processes extending through the foramen magnum can be delineated.

tion of a corner of a ventricle, or frank bands of connective tissue traversing the ventricle are often found. Loculated collections of ventricular fluid are easy to recognize and to distinguish from ventricular diverticuli. The location of the shunt tube must be identified. The point of penetration of the cerebral mantle is quickly discerned; the ventricular end can be more problematic when not in the appropriate ventricle. Location in the thalamus, septum, or hypothalamus occasionally occurs and should be brought to the attention of the surgeon. More important, though, a shunt that is buried in brain is unlikely to drain ventricular fluid adequately (particularly when it has migrated through the brain into the subarachnoid space lateral to the chiasm, into the interpeduncular fossa, or into the transverse fissure above the roof of the third ventricle). In this situation the functioning ventriculostomy is usually through the floor or roof of the third ventricle or through a diverticulum from a lateral ventricle. Clearly, portions of the study of shunt complications must await sectioning after fixation.

The relative sizes of the skull and brain give valuable information about atrophy or extracerebral processes. A brain small for the volume of the skull may be atrophic or may be separated from the skull by a subdural effusion or hematoma (the latter are often missed when loose intracranial blood is considered venous or sinus in origin). In the neonate, infant, and young child, the calvarium reflects and adjusts to the size of the growing brain (84). The volume of the cranium appears not to shrink significantly following a destructive lesion of the brain, and, consequently, the subarachnoid spaces enlarge secondarily if the brain (or a portion of it) atrophies. Conversely, lesions acquired early in developmental life are associated with a tightly fitting cranium usually of much greater thickness than normal with disproportionately small anterior and middle cranial fossae. There is a simple relationship between head circumference and brain weight (volume) in the neonate (not children or adult) throughout the second half of gestation (61) (Fig. 7.2).

Fresh brain weight $Y = 0.037X^{2.57}$

(where X = head circumference in centimeters and Y = weight of brain in grams)

Conversely, a small brain and a small head (assuming relatively normal size of the infant) implies that the brain failed to grow adequately.

The base of the skull both reflects cere-

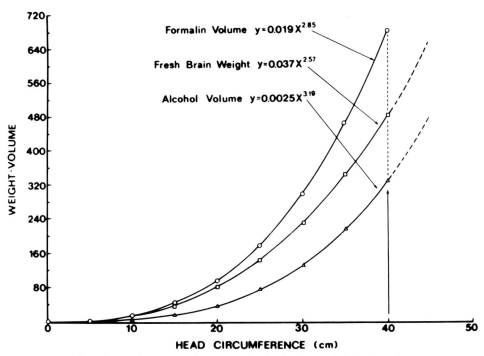

Figure 7.2. Simple relationships exist between fresh, fixed, and dehydrated brain weight and head circumference in the neonate. (Reproduced with permission from Gilles FH, Leviton A, Dooling EC: *The Developing Human Brain: Growth and Epidemiologic Neuropathology*. Littleton, MA, John Wright-PSG, Inc., 1983.)

bral anatomic abnormalities and induces cerebral distortions when malformed. Relative sizes of the three fossae, asymmetries in the skull, the distance between the lateral sinuses and the foramen magnum, and the angle between the clivus (dorsum sellae and basioccipital bones) and the line formed by the cribriform plate and upper surface of the body of the sphenoid all give clues as to the processes within the brain. Conversely, abnormalities of any of these structures will distort the brain.

ATLANTOOCCIPITAL RELATIONSHIPS IN THE NEONATE

The anatomic relationships among the components of the atlantooccipital articulation are remarkably different in the neonate than in the adult. The final modeling of this complex diarthrodial joint takes place after birth, largely during the first postnatal year. At the time of birth, the foramen magnum has attained almost its adult size, whereas the dorsal arch of the atlas (as well as other components of the atlas) must still increase more than two-

fold in size. One anatomic result of this discrepancy is that the narrowing seen from the inside of the posterior fossa in the neonate and usually called the foramen magnum is, in fact, the spinal canal within the atlas. Further, at the time of birth, the lateral mass of the atlas and the occipital condyle are very hypoplastic, and the atlantooccipital and atlantoaxial ligaments are lax (Fig. 7.3). Developmentally, the atlas "catches up" with the foramen magnum in size during the last half of the first postnatal year. The anatomic results of these developmental conditions during the first half of the first postnatal year are (a) the vertebral arteries are unprotected in their course between the bony lamina of the atlas and the bony exoccipital bone and (b) can be simultaneously compressed by mild extension of the baby's head upon its neck (Fig. 7.4), interrupting blood flow to the brainstem, cerebellum, and upper cervical spinal cord. These developmental relationships form the anatomic basis for one source of sudden unexpected death in the neonate and infant, particularly during procedures involving extension of the head upon the neck, such as inexpert intubation (31).

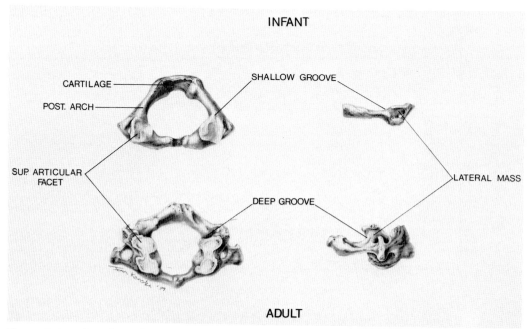

INFANT

CARTILAGE

POST. ARCH

SHALLOW GROOVE

SUP ARTICULAR FACET

LATERAL MASS

DEEP GROOVE

ADULT

Figure 7.3.   The atlas at birth contains a very small lateral mass that enlarges markedly, mainly in the first postnatal year, to reach adult size.

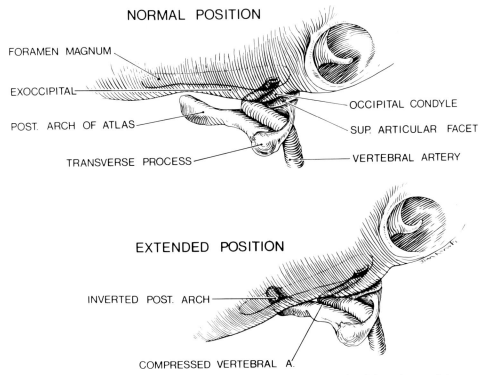

Figure 7.4. The relationships between the occipital bone, the arch of the atlas, and the vertebral artery in the infant in the normal position and when extended are indicated.

CHANGING NORMS

The developing human brain is a maelstrom of changing anatomic events, functions, and reactive capabilities. Migrating immature neurons, differentiating glial cells, sprouting capillaries with multiplying endothelial cells, and myelinating white matter (to name a few) change constantly during maturation. The cells involved in these events cannot be considered a priori to have the same vulnerabilities and reaction capabilities as their counterparts in the mature brain with the same names. Further, as the cellular patterns change during development, reaction capabilities also change. Finally, some morphologic events in the developing brain are limited to fetal development. Cellular and regional necrosis are considered abnormal in the adult brain. They are normal events at some sites or developmental stages in the developing brain. Thus, understanding of these events will give guidance to the pathology or deviations from these norms.

A caveat about "normality" is appropriate. The brains we deal with are obviously derived from infants dead for a variety of reasons. While the reference point for histologic change is an ideal, the "normal," the comments in this section apply only to the brains of dead (thus abnormal) infants, even though implying normality in some instances. What is considered "normal" is often only a judgement based on the frequency of an event.

Normative Guidelines

WEIGHT

The maximum rate of growth of the fetal brain in weight is attained at the end of gestation. The maximum acceleration in growth takes place at 24–25 weeks of gestation (61). The model

Brain weight (g)

$$= 1.065e^{-e^{(2.108-0.0498 \text{ (gest. age weeks)})}}$$

predicts fresh brain weight at each week of gestation and allows the pathologist to make a reasonable estimate of the expected size of the brain (Fig. 7.5). However, there

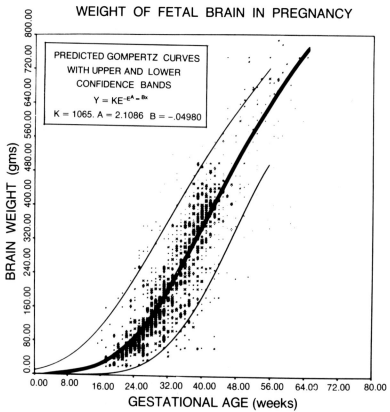

WEIGHT OF FETAL BRAIN IN PREGNANCY

PREDICTED GOMPERTZ CURVES
WITH UPPER AND LOWER
CONFIDENCE BANDS

$$Y = KE^{-E^A - Bx}$$

$K = 1065. \quad A = 2.1086 \quad B = -.04980$

BRAIN WEIGHT (gms)

GESTATIONAL AGE (weeks)

Figure 7.5. The expected weight of the brain during gestation is indicated along with the 95% confidence limits. (Reproduced with permission from Gilles FH, Leviton A, Dooling EC: *The Developing Human Brain: Growth and Epidemiologic Neuropathology.* Littleton, MA, John Wright-PSG, Inc., 1983.)

is a wide range in weight at any specific gestational age. The weight of the brain after fixation is unreliable, as fetal and term brains gain about 30% in weight during formalin fixation (Fig. 7.2).

SULCATION

Gyri appear in regular sequence on the surface of the cerebrum throughout the last half of gestation. The extent of sulcation provides a reliable estimate of the developmental age of the infant and simultaneously, provides the first clue about telencephalic abnormalities, such as small patches of sclerotic microgyria, micropolygyria, or pachygyria. For instance, the orientation of gyri adjacent to defects in the underlying cerebral mantle provides information about the gestational timing of certain destructive lesions. The gyri around defects of early gestational origin (i.e., be-

fore sulcation) tend to point into the defect in a radial fashion in contrast to those of late gestational origin that follow their normal distribution (i.e., the defect was acquired after the appropriate gyri were formed). Since the primary sulci are acquired between midgestation and the end of the second trimester, an acquired telencephalic defect merely interrupts tissue in place at the time of the damage; those gyri remaining retain a recognizable pattern, normal for the age at which the insult occurred.

In general, there are a few straightforward rules that the development of sulci seem to follow. All of the major fissures are formed by midgestation, usually, in fact, by 16–17 weeks of gestation. Thus, the Sylvian, calcarine, interhemispheric, etc., fissures should be obvious early. The primary sulci make their appearance between midgestation and the end of the second trimester. For practical purposes the primary sulci should appear by 27 or 28 weeks of gestation. Central, first temporal, first frontal, pre- and postcentral, orbital, interparietal, second frontal, and second temporal sulci should be easy to recognize at this time in gestation (Fig. 7.6). Usually, the sulci temporally develop asymmetrically in the two cerebra but are constant in location. Further, fissures and primary sulci are remarkably constant in location from brain to brain, but the differences in the order of appearance of the sulci in the left or right cerebrum are somewhat more variable.

During the third trimester, second and third order sulci appear. They subdivide primary gyri or secondary gyri in an extremely variable fashion, so variable a fashion, in fact, that the final pattern of secondary and tertiary gyri may be unique to each human brain, and, perhaps, to each cerebral half (22).

Sulci are often thought of as "indenting" previously smooth surfaced cerebra. However, during the gestational ages that primary sulcation is taking place, the fetal brain undergoes an extraordinary burst in growth, and the spurt in growth and beginning sulcation start more or less simultaneously at a time when the cerebral mantle is too close to the lateral ventricle to allow the degree of indentation of sulci implied in the above concept. In point of fact, the more likely explanation of sulcal appearance is that the cortex on either side of a prospective sulcus grows outward carrying the crests of the gyri on either side of the sulcus centrifugally, leaving the trough of the sulcus behind.

MYELINATION

Myelination of the late fetal and neonatal brain is a dramatic and important event; it provides a series of changing patterns that simultaneously allow detailed assessment of the progress of development and provide clues about delay or abortion of that progress. Almost 50 yr ago Roback and Scherer (73) noted a marked proliferation of glial nuclei at sites about to undergo myelination. They coined an unfortunate term "myelination gliosis" for this morphologic event, unfortunate because it is similar to the term "astrogliosis," a marker of abnormality. The histologic difference between the two processes is found in the cytoplasm of the cells involved. The glial cells related to myelination do not have the large plump eosinophilic cytoplasm found in "reactive" or hypertrophic astrocytes. Along with the increase in numbers of glial nuclei the cytoplasm of glial cells accumulate large quantities of premyelin lipids that are prominently sudanophilic. The accumulation of large quantities of lipid prior to the appearance of the myelin sheath has been demonstrated both biochemically and histologically. Unfortunately, these myelination changes in glial cells are easily confused with glial fatty metamorphosis, an abnormality (49), as was pointed out by Sumi (87). A local increase in the activity of several oxidative enzymes accompanies these histologic events (26), and there is a parallel increase in blood flow to the white matter (45) and in glucose utilization (46). In fact, Kennedy maintains that the metabolic requirement of myelinating white matter exceeds that of immature grey matter. As the myelin sheath is deposited around the axon, the histochemical characteristics of the tissue change, and glial nuclear density appears to diminish as the myelin sheaths enlarge displacing glial nuclei. Gradually the glial cells acquire the appearance of mature oligodendroglia. The forebrain, with multiple axonal systems myelinating at different times in gestation and postnatally, and at different rates, contains mixtures of variably myelinated fibers and sudanophilic material for the duration of the process. However, not all sudanophilic material in the fetal and neonatal brain is related to normal myelination, because, in the second half of gestation, macrophages in or near necrosis also accumulate sudanophilic material.

The evaluation of the degree of myelination of the fetal brain is important, as the process of myelination seems exquisitely sensitive to multiple stresses placed upon the developing nervous system while in utero and immediately after birth. One of the major risk factors of delayed myelination is, in fact, malnutrition, and, thus,

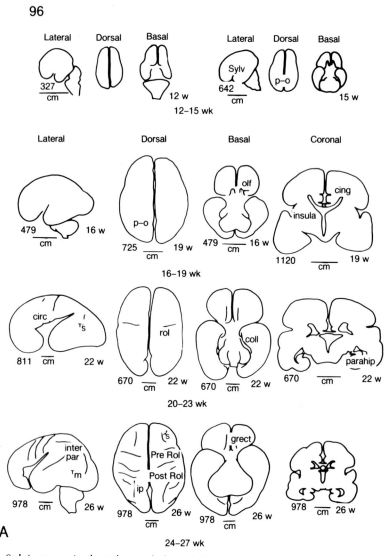

Figure 7.6. Sulci appear in the telencephalon of the human infant in a regular sequence outlined in these diagrams at selected gestational ages. (A) Through the end of the second trimester. (B) Third trimester. (Reproduced with permission from Gilles FH, Leviton A, Dooling EC: *The Developing Human Brain: Growth and Epidemiologic Neuropathology.* Littleton, MA, John Wright-PSG, Inc., 1983.)

this relatively simple evaluation may give a clue as to the circumstances within which the family lived or it may reflect an adverse systemic process within the fetus such as maternal malnutrition or some unrecognized environmental toxins.

Selected Myelin Patterns at Various Gestational Ages

The timing of myelination in the second half of gestation has been worked out in considerable detail by multiple workers (summarized in Gilles et al. (35)). The details of postnatal myelination are still largely anecdotal. For the pathologist needing a rough approximation of the timing of myelination, Table 7.1 lists the gestational ages at which 50% of neonates at a given gestational age contain small amounts of myelin (microscopic only, not discernible

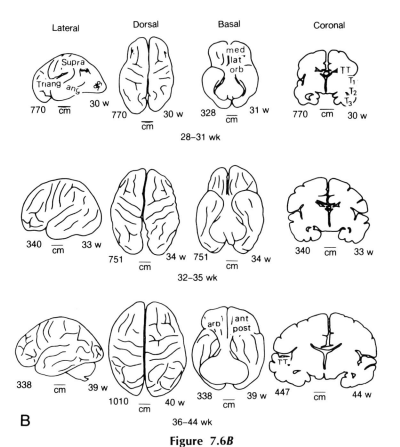

Figure 7.6B

Table 7.1
Microscopic Myelination[a]

Present at	Myelination
20 weeks	Medial longitudinal fasciculus, medulla, pons; fasciculus gracilis, lumbar, thoracic; fasciculus proprius, lumbar, thoracic, cervical; lateral spinothalamic tract, lumbar, thoracic, cervical; dorsal spinocerebellar tract, thoracic; fasciculus cuneatus
22 weeks	Medial longitudinal fasciculus, mesencephalon; dorsal spinocerebellar tract, cervical; fasciculus gracilis, cervical
23 weeks	Medial lemniscus medulla; trapezoid body
24 weeks	Inferior cerebellar peduncle; spinal trigeminal tract, medulla; lateral lemniscus, pons, midbrain
25 weeks	Medial lemniscus, mesencephalon
26 weeks	Superior cerebellar peduncle, pons, mesencephalon
27 weeks	Cerebellum, parasagitial
28 weeks	Ansa lenticularis; habenulointerpeduncular tract; amiculum, inferior olive
29 weeks	Capsule, red nucleus; optic tract
32 weeks	Internal capsule, posterior limb; optic chiasm
34 weeks	Central corona radiata; corticospinal tract, mesencephalon
35 weeks	Transpontine; middle cerebellar peduncle; corticospinal tract, pons; pyramid; corticospinal tract, cervical, thoracic
38 weeks	Cingulum; internal capsule, anterior limb; optic radiation, rostral; mesencephalic peduncle, lateral; cerebellum, hemisphere; corticospinal tract, lumbar
39 weeks	Fornix; optic radiation, occipital
46 weeks	Corpus callosum; anterior commissure; mesencephalic peduncle, medial
48 weeks	Mammillothalamic tract

[a] The degree of myelination expected in 50% of infants at selected weeks of gestation.

to the naked eye) in each of several myelinating sites.

Evaluation of Myelination in a New Fetal Brain

A practical, easy to use, method of evaluation of myelination in a fetal brain relative to a standard, called the Ridit evaluation (35), is available for the pathologist concerned with evaluating the *overall* degree of myelination in a new neonatal brain. This method uses the material in the National Collaborative Perinatal Project as a reference material and requires the pathologist to do a myelin stain on 12 easy-to-find sites within the brain. A score is calculated that is compared with the National Standard to give an estimate of the degree of myelination of the new brain for any week during the last half of gestation.

LEPTOMENINGES

The leptomeninges change as they mature throughout the last half of gestation and may appear fairly densely cellular and contain moderate numbers of macrophages. The primitive leptomeninx differentiates from mesenchymal tissue into dura, arachnoid, and pia. The creation of the arachnoidal space between the arachnoid and pia requires removal of mesenchymal tissue, leaving the arachnoidal struts. This development of the leptomeninges continues throughout most of the last half of gestation and is accompanied by leptomeningeal histiocytes and macrophages. There are two exceptions to this sequence. The leptomeninges over the superior cerebellum subjacent to the tentorium usually do not develop arachnoidal spaces completely enough to allow massive hemorrhage into the cisterna magna from an intraventricular bleed to migrate freely over the superior surface of the cerebellum. Conversely, subpial hemorrhages in the superior surface of the cerebellum may rupture into the overlying arachnoid, but often remain local arachnoidal hematomas without flow into the nearby cisterna magna.

The second variation on the general theme of leptomeningeal maturation occurs in the region of the roof of the fourth ventricle, which includes the midline and lateral foramina connecting the fourth ventricle with the subarachnoid space. The developing nervous system goes through a complex set of maneuvers to establish this connection between the cavity of the neural tube and its surrounding mesenchymal leptomeninges. The sequence of events seems similar for both the lateral and midline foramina, although they have been only studied in detail in regards to the midline foramen. The communication is established in multiple species, including birds, by a curious thinning and outpouching of the roof of the fourth ventricle that carries the dorsal wall of the fourth ventricle far out into the retro- and infracerebellar region. The ependyma thins as does the subependymal glial layer and becomes admixed with the connective tissue of the arachnoid. Thus the pouch wall (Blake's pouch (6)) contains regions of ependyma lying on a thin glial layer, as well as regions of thin connective tissue indistinguishable from the surrounding pial connective tissue. The pouch carries in its rostral surface a prominent component of the roof of the fourth ventricle, the choroid plexus. In some individuals the choroid plexus is carried far dorsally along the under and caudal surfaces of the vermis at the depths of the vallecula. In many species, including man, this dorsal pouch continues to atrophy and establishes communication with the subarachnoid space; in a few species, the final communication is never established, and Blake's pouch persists into adulthood. The lateral recesses are thought to develop in a similar fashion, but formal studies are not yet available. The subarachnoid extent of the ependyma-lined glial tube or the dorsal or lateral foramen containing choroid plexus in its dorsal wall is sometimes surprising, as it may extend either laterally to the lateralmost region of the undersurface of the cerebellum, or it may curve caudally along the lateral surface of the medulla to the cervicomedullary junction in the foramen magnum. Any one of these three choroid plexus-containing structures may occasionally become isolated from the ventricle and enlarge because of their secretory capabilities to form major space-taking cysts in the posterior fossa. They are readily treated surgically, are not associated with other malformations of the central nervous system as is the Dandy and Blackfan (16) (Dandy-Walker) malformation, and are frequently missed clinically or pathologically. They are distinct from the local arachnoidal fibroses associated with arachnoidal cysts and have a different pathogenesis.

VENTRICLES

The shape of the fetal lateral ventricles changes throughout pregnancy. Shortly after telencephalic outpouching in the second month of gestation, the lateral ventricle is almost globular except for the base which is truncated over the striatum and the ganglionic eminence. Early in gestation there is a massive burst in growth of the striatum followed later by the massive spurt in growth of the remaining portions of the telencephalic wall. During the growth of the striatum, the lateral ventricular shape in the plane of the interventricular foramen is that of an inverted teardrop. The growth of the remaining portions of the telencephalic wall lags behind, as it were, and with the growth of the base, the thalamus, the telencephalic wall, and finally the corpus callosum, the lateral ventricle gradually narrows and eventually becomes slit-like.

EPENDYMA

During the growth of the nervous system, new cells are generated in the ventricular wall in a layer variously called the germinal zone, matrix, ventricular, or the subventricular zone. Sometimes this layer is incorrectly called the ependymal zone, as though it were lined by ependymal cells. However, telencephalic ependymal cells differentiate relatively late in gestation; earlier the germinal cells or the early glia abut directly upon the ventricle. In portions of the ventricular system where the germinal tissue is consumed early in gestation the ependymal cells appear and then line the ventricular wall (e.g., the central canal, fourth ventricle, aqueduct, and third ventricle). In portions of the nervous system where the germinal mass is still active later in gestation, the differentiation and proliferation of ependymal cells occur later (e.g., the telencephalon). For parts of the telencephalic ventricle ependymal differentiation continues through to the end of gestation.

Absence of ependymal cells has often been taken as a marker of prior damage to the ventricular wall. It is clear that if the absence of ependymal cells is associated with a small granuloma, as in a granulomatous ventriculitis, or with small nodules of astrocytes, this is probably an appropriate conclusion. However, the absence of ependymal cells is probably not an adequate marker if there are no other signs of damage to the ventricular wall or subventricular tissue. There are some regions of the telencephalic ventricular wall that usually are not covered by ependyma in the neonate. There are discontinuities in the ependyma in all neonatal brains along the occipital horn and in most neonates on the undersurface of the corpus callosum in the frontal horn and over section CA_2 of the hippocampus (23). Thus, absence of ependyma at these sites is probably not a significant pathologic finding.

CHOROID PLEXUS

The choroid plexus of each of the ventricles is an anatomically complex organ throughout gestation. In most of the ventricles, it fills the ventricle, and its epithelium contains an extraordinary amount of glycogen. Small amounts of lipid are found in its stroma. As regional maturation progresses, the amount of glycogen in the choroid plexus diminishes. The loss of glycogen takes place first in the fourth ventricle, then the third, and finally, near the end of gestation the lateral ventricular plexus epithelium loses its glycogen. Only a small amount of glycogen remains after the end of the first postnatal month.

GREY MATTER

Throughout gestation and the first postnatal year the major neuronal populations of the brain are in various stages of differentiation. Immature neuroblasts appear as naked hyperchromic nuclei without distinguishing characteristics. In the usual preparations they cannot be differentiated from many kinds of glial cells as they have no Nissl substance or nucleoli. Other than karyorrhexis or failure of staining, they do not undergo the usual changes of more mature neurons following insult. Thus, during the second half of gestation, the nervous system contains a remarkable mixture of mature and immature neurons in different regions as well as considerable numbers of neurons in telencephalic white matter. As the brain matures, the white matter neurons appear to diminish in number, presumably because of increasing separation as myelinated tracts intervene. More important to the pathologist, though, is the necessity of recognizing regions containing immature neurons. For instance, sector CA$_2$ of the hippocampal gyrus (approximately Sommer's sector) normally lags behind the other portions of the hippocampal allocortex in maturation, leading to the occasional misinterpretation that these small, hyperchromic neurons are necrotic. The fact of the matter is that necrosis limited to this portion of the neonatal brain is extraordinarily rare, if it exists at all.

WHITE MATTER

Histologically complex, the white matter of the neonatal brain contains cells that are in part similar to those of the adult, and while the same names are occasionally used, these cells are different developmentally, functionally, and potentially have different vulnerabilities and reactive capabilities. Near the ventricle persistent germinal cells are present in often eccentric perivascular masses. Further peripherally, at least four classes of cells can be distinguished, based on nuclear characteristics in human material; their analogies to ultrastructurally defined cells in the developing white matter of experimental animals have not been established. In the subependymal white matter immediately adjacent to the ventricle, there is a layer of astrocytes and glial fibrils that can gradually be distinguished as the germinal layer disappears. The ventricular wall is the only location in the telencephalon during the third trimester at which hypertrophic astrocytes and glial fibrils are normally encountered. In contrast, the white matter of the brain stem and spinal cord normally contain small hypertrophic astrocytes and glial fibrils by the third trimester.

Transient Components and "Normal" Necrosis in the Human Fetal Brain

Some components of the fetal brain are normally lost during the course of development. For instance, cells of the neuronal

mass in the tuberculum olfactorium (43), the trochlear nucleus (11), the dorsal root ganglia, and the anterior horn cell columns (51, 74) are lost in part after being laid down in excess. The mass of germinal tissue linking the ventricular system is lost in its entirety along with its blood vessels. Surely, many of the cells migrate from the ventricular wall to assume positions elsewhere in the brain, but karyorrhexis of cells in the germinal mass gives mute evidence of actual cellular necrosis.

Changing Reaction Capabilities

Major cerebral insults during the first 2 or possibly 3 months of gestation are thought to result in either death or malformation. Repair and reconstitution attempts within embryonic human neural tissue are largely unrecognized. During the first few months of postconceptional life, we do not see macrophages, hypertrophic astrocytes, or glial fibrils in the embryonic or young fetal brain in response to an insult. Whether the tissue is merely resorbed (4) or whether some other heretofore unrecognized reaction takes place is unknown. A histiocytic response has been described in the early cavum septi pellucidi at about 12 weeks of gestation (72) and in the leptomeninges at about 20 weeks (15). After the 6th fetal month, the cellular response of the brain is increasingly comparable to that of the mature brain. In general, the more that regional maturation has produced neuronal and glial cells comparable to those of the adult, the more comparable will be the responses.

Different Kinds of Reactions in Perinatal Brain

In addition to cellular reactions that become increasingly similar to adult reactions with advancing gestational age, neonatal brains often contain a different class of lesions. This class of lesions is characterized by the failure of acquisition or delay in the development of some component (e.g., failure of growth in bulk, delay of myelination, or delay in sulcation). These defects may be found in isolation or in combination with evidence of other lesions in the brain.

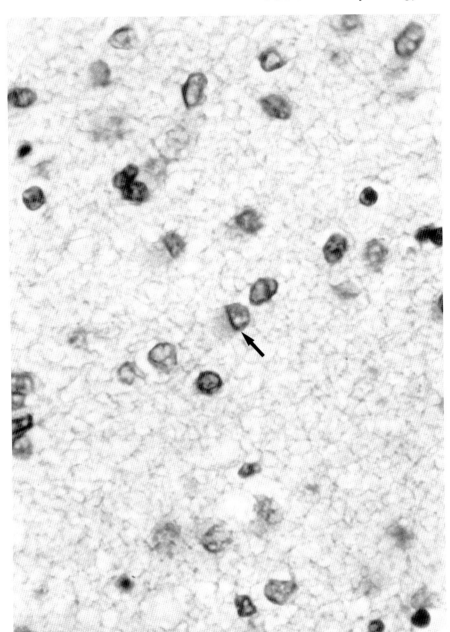

Figure 7.7. The hypertrophic astrocyte in the fetal brain is similar in most respects to its adult counterpart, except for the larger amount of eosinophilic cytoplasm in the latter. The contrast between the hypertrophic astrocyte in the neonatal brain and other glial cells is well seen in midphoto (*arrow*). Hematoxylin and eosin (H&E). (Original magnification × 950.)

Changes in Reacting Cells at the End of the Second Trimester

In the forebrain, the ability of glial cells to develop abundant cytoplasms and to construct PTAH-stainable glial fibrils is weakly, but firmly, established by the end of the second trimester (Fig. 7.7). Macrophages appear in cerebral lesions at about the same gestational age. The timing of these reactive capabilities of these cells in other regions of the brain is unknown but would presumably antedate the end of the second trimester in those regions of the diencephalon, mesencephalon, rhomben-cephalon, and spinal cord that exhibit early gestational cellular maturation. Cells responding to cerebral injury may themselves be influenced by the damaging agent as evidenced by the longer incubation periods for the first appearance of hypertrophic astrocytes and macrophages in cerebra of neonatal kittens damaged by different insults (30). We have provided guidelines for the development schedule of reacting cells in the human telencephalon in the proportions of cases at each gestational week that contain specific responses (32). Thus, hypertrophic astrocytes, macrophages, and focal necroses are unlikely before the end of the second trimester. Microglia-like cells, on the other hand, are almost always found in the forebrain by the end of the second trimester (32).

SIGNS OF REPAIR AND REGENERATION

A considerable body of experimental work has established some of the repair and response capabilities in the brains of several fetal animals (see Demeyer (19), Schneider (79), Goldman (38) for examples). Little documentation of comparable repair efforts in the human fetal brain has been provided, and the available information seems to be circumstantial. Information concerning even the most fundamental questions about human brain regrowth and regeneration capability is lacking, even though some anecdotal information is available. For instance, an extraordinary example of rebulking of the neonatal brain has been provided by infants with hydro-cephalus. The dramatic change in amount of cerebral tissue after shunting an infant with hydrocephalus has been recognized from the early years of pneumoencephalog-raphy. However, the potential amount of this increase of cerebral tissue has never been quantitated, the relationship to age of onset of the hydrocephalus, duration of hy-drocephalus, or the age at which shunts were inserted are questions that have not been studied, and the actual changes that take place to increase the apparent cerebral tissue bulk is unknown. It seems unlikely that the increase in bulk is simply increase in tissue water content because the white matter changes in density from water-rich

paraventricular white matter in acute hy-drocephalus to more normal white matter following the decrease in the ventricular size. However, no experimental work is available that touches upon these points.

HEMORRHAGE

Hemorrhage is the most common lesion the pathologist encounters in the brain of the fetus and neonate (24). The study of the etiology of intracranial hemorrhage in the newborn is sufficiently complex that distressingly few significant risk factors have been elaborated over the century and a half since neonatal intracranial hemor-rhage was depicted by Cruveilhier (14). Hemorrhages occurring at different sites and hemorrhages of different size may have different etiologies. Hemorrhages of the same size and at the same site also may result from different etiologies. Therefore, hemorrhage per se is etiologically nonspe-cific and has potentially a myriad of risk factors. To complicate matters further, experimental models of neonatal intracranial hemorrhage have been used to explore putative antecedents; unfortunately, most of these models fail to simulate in size, site, and stage of fetal development of the comparable lesions in the human neonate.

Surprisingly, the distribution of hemor-rhages in stillborn infants is similar in many respects to that in liveborn infants. For instance, large hemorrhages were found at autopsy in the leptomeninges in 56% of liveborn infants and in 43% of stillborn neonates, in the ventricular system in 20% of liveborn and 9% of stillborn neonates, in telencephalic white matter in 5% of live-born and 3% of stillborn, and in the ger-minal matrix in 19% of all liveborn and 5% of all stillborn neonates in the National Collaborative Perinatal Project (24). Sep-arate hemorrhages of microscopic size were found in the leptomeninges in 42% of live-born and 37% of stillborn infants, in the ventricular system in 41% of liveborn and 26% of stillborn, in the ganglionic eminence in 36% of liveborn and 17% of stillborn, and in the cerebral white matter in 41% of liveborn and 34% of stillborn infants. Con-sideration of these similarities between liveborn and stillborn infants lends support to the suspicion that some of the significant antecedents of intracranial hemorrhage in the neonate may antedate birth. This possibility was further supported by the identification of some risk factors of ganglionic hemorrhage antedating pregnancy.

Hemorrhage into the subarachnoid space (Fig. 7.8) or the ventricular system (Fig. 7.9) are two readily recognized lesions in the brains of neonates. Large parenchymal hemorrhages are less frequent, may rupture into either of the above sites and form the source of intraventricular or subarachnoid hemorrhage, but, rarely, if ever, seem to result from rupture from ventricular or arachnoidal accumulations of blood in a reverse direction into parenchyma. Unfortunately, little information is available about the risk factors of parenchymal hemorrhages, and they will not be dealt with extensively in this chapter. Other common sites of hemorrhage are the subpial molecular layer, falx and tentorium, and cerebellum. Hemorrhages located beneath the pia and extending various distances into the molecular layer were studied extensively by Friede (27). They are most frequently found in the isocortex of the temporal and parietal lobes or in the molecular layer of the cerebellum. Hemorrhage into the tentorium or the falx is found in most autopsied neonates. The hemorrhage lies between the two connective tissue leaves of these structures and causes little mischief unless large enough to rupture into the subdural space above or below the tentorium. The resulting subdural hematomas may be clinically significant (36). In contrast, cerebellar parenchymal hemorrhages occurred in about one-seventh of liveborn neonates in the collaborative perinatal project.

Subarachnoid Hemorrhage

Hemorrhage into subarachnoidal spaces results from rupture of vessels within the arachnoid, the parenchyma, or as a direct extension from the fourth ventricle after an intraventricular hemorrhage. Arachnoidal hemorrhages may be petechial, small, or large. Each size is potentially of different etiology, and specific etiologies should be sought in local sources such as parenchymal hematomas, subpial hemorrhages, or tear of the falx or the tentorium, or in the systemic conditions leading to bleeding diatheses. Once these etiologies have been excluded, there remains a large number of infants with petechia, small, or large subarachnoid hemorrhages.

In order to delineate the risk factors of uncomplicated subarachnoidal hemorrhage, we used for a case control study only those cases with hemorrhage in the subarachnoid space without accompanying intraventricular, parenchymal, or falcine, tentorial, or dural hemorrhage.

There were three general groups of significant risk factors that can be grouped under the umbrella terms trauma, intrapartum hypertension, and unfavorable uterine environment. There was only a small amount of support for the hypothesis that trauma contributed significantly, and it consisted of the observation that primigravidas were at greater risk of delivering a child with subarachnoid hemorrhage than were multigravidas who did not experience any late fetal wastage. The second of risk factors was intrapartum hypertension. Intrapartum hypertension was a risk factor in its own right, but it was closely associated with several other risk factors including previous fetal death. The mechanism underlying this association is unclear at present but could be subjected to a laboratory investigation. The third group of risk factors, unfavorable uterine environment, included such factors as maternal gonococcal infection, late age at menarche, intrapartum hypertension, and prior fetal wastage (53).

Intraventricular Hemorrhage

Intraventricular hemorrhage is a frequent and dramatic finding in the brains of neonates. Two major sources of hemorrhage are the germinal matrix overlying the head, body, and tail of the caudate, and the choroid plexus. Parenchymal hemorrhages often rupture into the ventricular system, but occur far less frequently. Hemorrhages extending into the ventricular system from hematomas in the transverse fissure or the velum interpositum are rare, as is their putative source, rupture of the great vein of Galen. The extensive literature is summarized in Friede (28).

Germinal Matrix

A common source of intraventricular hemorrhage is the vascular bed of the mass of germinal tissue overlying the caudate,

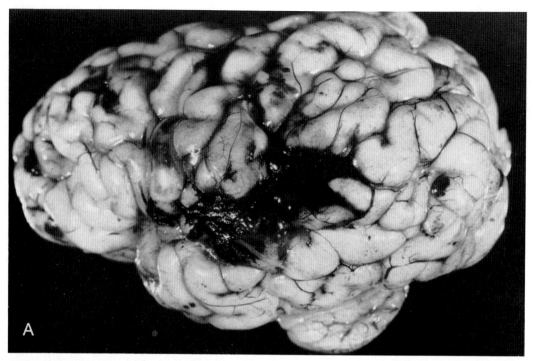

Figure 7.8. (*A* and *B*) Isolated multiple hemorrhages are present in the subarachnoid space. (*C*) They may arise from rupture of vessels within the arachnoid, from large parenchymal hemorrhages, or from multiple, minute subpial petechiae.

most commonly, within the large mass overlying the head of the caudate (ganglionic eminence) rostral to the interventricular foramen and rostral, therefore, to the thalamus and its associated thalamostriate vein (terminal vein). The blood vessels of the ganglionic eminence are capillaries or small or large endothelium-lined sinusoidal channels similar to the vascular channels in telencephalic white matter. There are no arteries or veins per se within the mass of germinal tissue. Large channels, similar in size to those lying immediately subjacent to the ventricle elsewhere, and presumably draining veins, lie at or near the interface between the germinal tissue or the ganglionic eminence and the caudate. Until the present time, the arterial supply to the large mass of germinal tissue has been unclear. The only major statement about the arterial supply is that of Hambleton and Wigglesworth (41) and Pape and Wigglesworth (65) whose claim that this anatomic structure is supplied by the recurrent branch of the anterior cerebral artery is not supported in the vascular bed they figured for this

artery. Further, they included the anterior choroidal artery as a source of supply to the caudate and germinal mass. However, this claim flies in the face of the distribution of the latter artery figured in the classic text of Stephens and Stilwell (85). The other possible arterial supply to the germinal tissue is that of the lateral striate arteries. These vessels muscularize from the base upward toward the caudate, and a small amount of muscularis can be found in the terminal branches of these vessels within the caudate lying within several hundred micra of the germinal matrix by the end of the second trimester of gestation.

The germinal tissue of the ganglionic eminence is the embryologic source of the striatum and other telencephalic anlage early in gestation. It attains its maximum absolute volume at the end of the second trimester and rapidly diminishes in size thereafter (44). The likelihood of finding germinal matrix hemorrhage is maximal during the involution phase of this germinal tissue.

Capillaries in any germinal tissue site

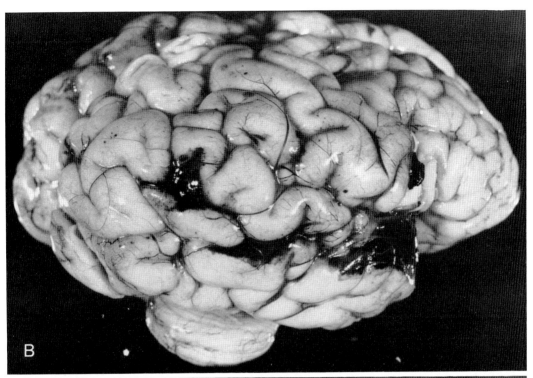

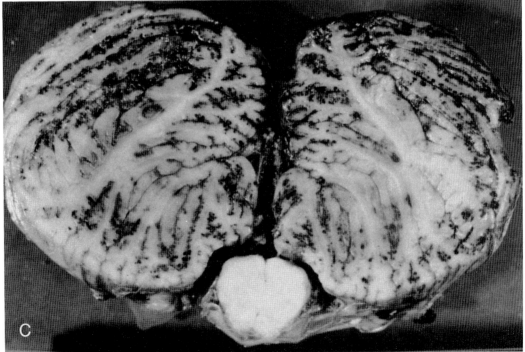

Figure 7.8 *B* and *C*

may leak, and small petechiae can be found adjacent to the lateral ventricle at most any point containing a collection of germinal tissue. Thus, the germinal tissue adjacent to any horn of the lateral ventricle, the third ventricle, or the rhombic lip of the fourth ventricle may contain petechia or larger hemorrhages at appropriate gesta-

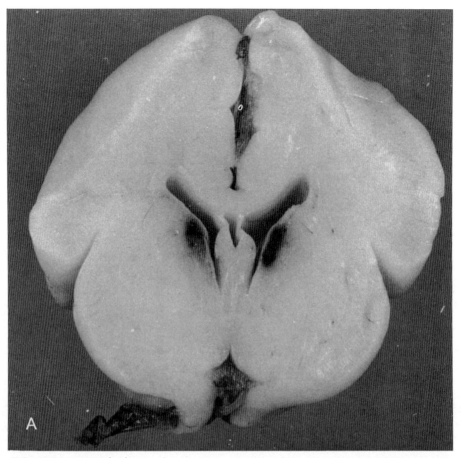

Figure 7.9. Intraventricular hemorrhage may or may not dilate the lateral ventricles and may arise from local hemorrhages in the germinal matrix (usually over the head of the caudate (*A*), choroid plexus, or within the parenchyma of the cerebrum (*B* and *C*) or the cerebellum. In the parenchymal hematomata figured in *B* and *C* it is clear that these hemorrhages are primarily parenchymal with secondary extension into the ventricular system.

tional ages. Multiplicity and bilaterality of hemorrhages in germinal tissues are the rule. Probably the reason the main bulk of the subependymal germinal matrix hemorrhage is usually located over the head of the caudate is that it reflects the mass of germinal tissue in which it occurs and the number of capillaries at risk at this point. The pathogenesis of hemorrhage in this tissue is unclear; none of the hypotheses presented to date for this very common lesion in the prematurely born infant are satisfactory. No good explanation for the processes that instigate capillary hemorrhage is available. However, once capillary diapedesis begins, there is a very good reason that a large amount of blood may extravasate. The germinal tissue of the ganglionic eminence contains a large amount

of plasminogen activator, presumably one of the proteases liberated by embryonic tissue undergoing involution or remodeling. Thus, any fibrin deposited is immediately lysed and, histologically, a fibrin-containing clot is rarely encountered in these hematomas (34).

The risk factors of ganglionic eminence hemorrhage in the dead infants in the National Collaborative Perinatal Project were largely correlates of low gestational age.

Choroid Plexus

The choroid plexus is sometimes the source of intraventricular hemorrhage (28, 39) (Fig. 7.10). It is often undervalued in the consideration of possible sources of intraventricular hemorrhage. When careful attention is paid to the choroid plexus of

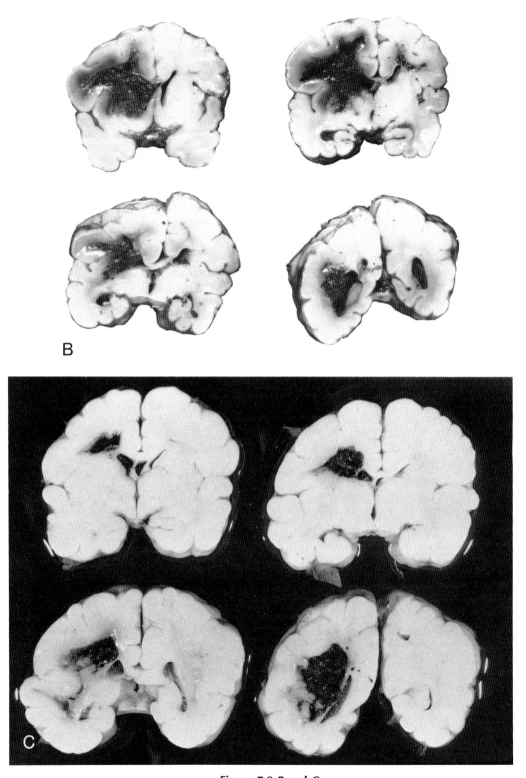

Figure 7.9 *B* and *C*

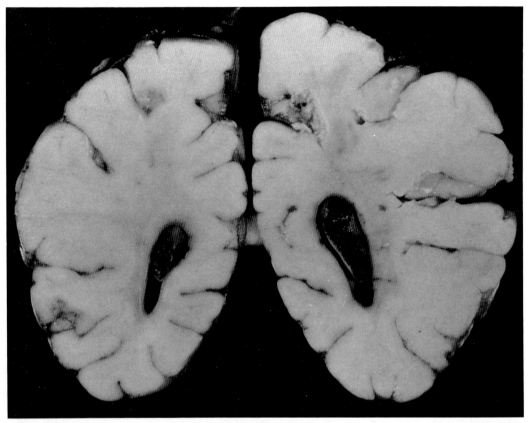

Figure 7.10. The glomus of each choroid plexus in the atrium of the lateral ventricle is filled with local hemorrhage that has not yet ruptured into the ventricular system.

the blood-filled lateral ventricle (no matter other apparent sources of ventricular hemorrhage), it will be found that intraplexus bleeding (i.e., hemorrhage into the stroma between the endothelial capillaries and the epithelium of the plexus) is present in the majority of cases at all gestational ages. Intraplexus bleeding can readily be separated from ventricular blood lying externally to the plexus epithelium. Thus, most cases with both intraventricular hemorrhage and germinal matrix hemorrhage are accompanied by intraplexus hemorrhage, and, often, the plexus seems to be the sole source of the intraventricular hemorrhage, particularly toward the end of gestation when there is no longer any appreciable germinal tissue lining the ventricle.

Intraventricular Hemorrhage: Consequences

The most frequent sequel of intraventricular hemorrhage is hydrocephalus requiring shunts. Ventricular dilatation may accompany intraventricular hemorrhage or may follow later. Some cases of recent intraventricular hemorrhage are associated with marked ventricular dilatation; others are not. The degree of ventricular dilatation presumably reflects the amount of blood released into the ventricular system, the pressure under which the blood is released, and whether the hemorrhage encounters a block in its escape into the subarachnoid space. In older individuals marked ventricular dilatation may occur after an arterial rupture into the ventricular system. In this age group there are no muscularized arteries that have been convincingly demonstrated to extend into the germinal mass at the time of greatest risk of encountering germinal matrix hemorrhage (26–31 weeks), the most frequently acknowledged source of the intraventricular hemorrhage, although the medial and lateral groups of the striate arteries are muscularized to within 100–200 μm of the germinal mass by the end of the second trimester. When the ventricles are found dilated, either a large amount of blood has been released into the ventricular system from multiple low pressure sites, or there is a block to the escape of blood from the ventricular system. The usual statement that intraventricular blood clots is based largely on the cast of the blood found in the formalin-fixed brain. Blood in a hematoma hardens, in formalin, of course, and while superficially appearing to be a clot, rarely contains fibrin on microscopic section. There is a good reason for the lack of fibrin in the intraventricular mass of blood, that is, that the choroid plexus contains a large amount of a fibrinolytic agent. Further, intraventricular blood is usually liquid at the time of autopsy and often when the lateral ventricle is drained by puncture during life. Whether the outlets of the fourth ventricle and the immature arachnoid containing potentially incompletely developed arachnoidal spaces are capable of handling the large bulk flow of blood required in this process is unknown. Certainly the blood engorges the perimedullary and prepontine cisterns after it fills the cisterna magna. It engorges the cisterna ambiens and the perichiasmatic cisterns less frequently. Blood is large amounts in the cisterna magna and the intraarachnoidal spaces is similarly liquid (the arachnoid is the source of a similar fibrinolytic agent).

These engorged basilar spinal fluid flow pathways may form a functional block to the flow of blood-filled spinal fluid if they are incompletely developed, or more peripheral subarachnoid pathways may be incompletely developed. Whether or not the intraventricular hemorrhage is associated with ventricular dilatation at the time of the hemorrhage, posthemorrhage ventricular dilatation has become the most common source of cases of hydrocephalus for some pediatric neurosurgical groups. Perinatal postintraventricular hemorrhage hydrocephalus is a major complication.

Parenchymal Hemorrhage

Clinical studies of prematurely born neonates with intracranial hemorrhage would profit considerably if they more often took into consideration the anatomic locations of the hematomas. Hemorrhages large

enough to be detected by either computer-assisted tomography or ultrasonography usually occur in the ganglionic eminence or in the deep white matter of the telencephalon; the five to ten-fold difference in the rates of hemorrhage at these two sites (National Collaborative Perinatal Project) and the gestational ages at which they most likely occur (27–31 weeks for the hemorrhages into the ganglionic eminence and throughout the last half of gestation for deep telencephalic hemorrhages) are dramatically different. Therefore, to lump hemorrhages at these two sites together, even though contiguous, denies our current knowledge of pathology and can be expected to produce confusing information about therapeutic effects, inappropriate predictions about outcome, and may well continue the confusion about the etiology of these two entities.

Parenchymal hematomas are far less commonly encountered in the brains of neonates than are subarachnoid hemorrhage, intraventricular hemorrhage, germinal matrix hemorrhage, or choroid plexus hemorrhage. They may be found alone, or in the company of any of the above hemorrhages. They may be large or small, single or multiple, unilateral or bilateral, and may or may not be associated with necrosis of cerebral tissue or focal infarcts. Large parenchymal hemorrhage disrupts cerebral tissue and may extend to the ventricular or subarachnoid space. At the present time the various etiologies are obscure.

Necrosis and the Perinatal Leucoencephalopathies

Signs of cellular and tissue necrosis are found frequently in the fetal brain. Early signs of necrosis of mature neurons include karyorrhexis, eosinophilia, loss of nuclear membrane, and failure of the nucleus or cytoplasm to stain. The hyperchromic, pyknotic neuron may be an artifact and in isolation is not a reliable criterion of neuronal necrosis (9). Nuclear, cytoplasmic, or pericellular vacuolization may reflect the mode of death as in mature brains (55) (although this phenomenon has not been studied in neonatal brains) or the difficulties of histologic preparations at these ages.

Necrotic lesions in neonatal telencephalic white matter (Fig. 7.11) have at-

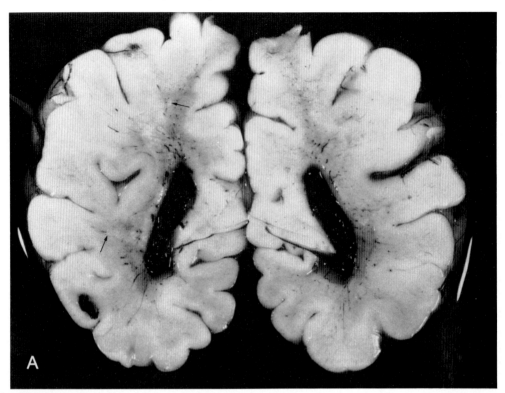

Figure 7.11.   Focal white matter necroses in the neonatal cerebrum consist of small, chalky-white opacities. They are preferentially distributed in the parieto-occipital (*A* and *B*) and frontal (*C*) white matter. Often located in deep cerebral white matter, they may extend well out of the gyral white matter cores (*A*).

tracted the attention of pathologists for over a century (66–68). The evolution of our notions of the pathogenesis of this group of lesions was nicely unraveled by Schmorl (78) and Friede (28). Friede felt that the name commonly used for these lesions "periventricular leucomalacia" was inappropriate for these small focal lesions, as the term suggests a widespread abnormality of white matter. He suggested that these small focal necroses were, in fact, small infarcts.

These lesions may be found at multiple sites in several patterns within the deep and superficial white matter located peripherally to the gyral cores (10, 50, 78) and tend to occur in frontal and parietooccipital white matter (10, 83). In contrast, they are quite infrequent in the white matter below the central sulcus containing the corticospinal system and thus seem not to form the pathologic basis for the diplegia of many neonatally brain-damaged people, particularly those with normal cerebral

function. The common location of these small lesions bilaterally in the deep parietooccipital white matter in the optic radiation and in the association pathways just lateral to the optic radiation (Fig. 7.11) might give these lesions a role in the pathologic anatomy of some children with "learning disabilities," as these association pathways are those connecting auditory and visual regions of the brain and, presumably, are those used in the manipulation of visual, auditory, and language symbols.

The risk factors of the perinatal leucoencephalopathy characterized by focal necroses are multiple but do not include markers of hypoxia, anoxia, or systemic hypotension. The risk factors include congenital anomalies, endotoxemia, as well as maternal factors which have been grouped under the rubric unfavorable intrauterine environment and a socioeconomic effect (52). Comparable lesions have been induced in neonatal kitten telencephalic white matter by transient endotoxemia (30, 33). Ad-

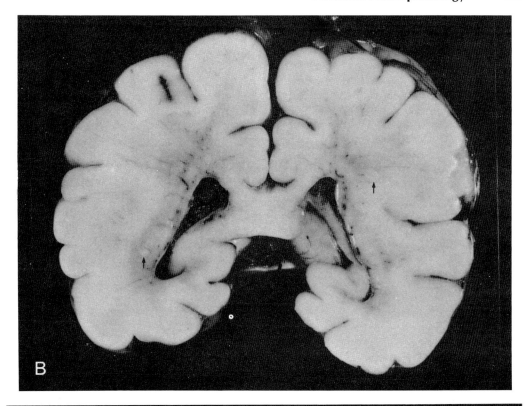

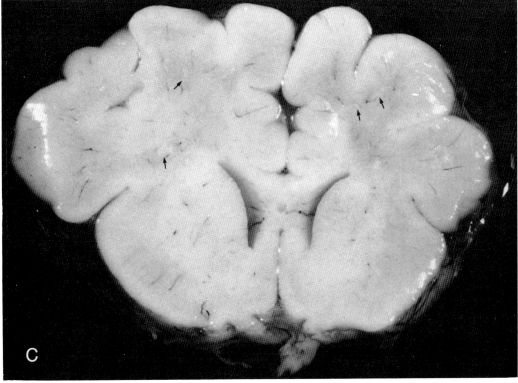

Figure 7.11 *B* and *C*

ditional points of the history of this lesion were pointed out by Landing. The focal necroses and their preponderant distribution in the deep white matter with occipital preponderance were beautifully described by Schmorl in 1903 (78). Schmorl said that these necroses, ranging in size from a point to more than linseed, are closely related to blood vessels and quoted Moebius as having made the same observation previously. Schmorl found fibrin thrombi in nearby vessels frequently, an observation we have not been able to replicate. He also quotes Hirschfeld who related these lesions to infection of the navel, an association denied by Schmorl. Further, he states that no bacteria could be demonstrated in these necroses either on culture or on stain. Perrin and Landing (69) made the suggestion that these lesions were related to transient endotoxemia, and a similar suggestion was made by Gluszcz (31) who claimed that he could stain bacteria in these lesions. I have not been able to confirm the observations about stainable bacteria in these lesions, as both fibrin and small fragments of necrotic cerebral tissue are stained in the usual bacterial stains. Even if bacteria were found in some it would not account for the large number of lesions without bacteria.

Do these focal white matter necroses occur in border zones? Large, symmetric, wedge-shaped necroses do occasionally occur in the brains of neonates. They involve the same border zones as do the comparable lesions in the adult, namely, the border zones between the anterior and middle cerebral arteries, the border zones between the superior and inferior cerebeller arteries, and, rarely, the border zones between the middle and posterior cerebral arteries. In general, they are large wedge-shaped cortical and subcortical necroses, with or without hemorrhage, with the apex pointed toward the nearest ventricle. They are not very often seen, but, when present, they are quite comparable to those in the adult. The small focal necroses under discussion have sometimes been attributed to hypothetical arterial border zones between long medullary penetrating arteries and recurrent collaterals or transventricular arteries (DeReuck (20), DeReuck and VanderEecken (21), as well as more recent authors). I have called these border zones hypothetic for

three reasons. The first is that muscularized vascular channels are nonexistent in most of the telencephalon (with the exception of the striatal arteries) until the very end of gestation when a few can be found. The second reason is that "recurrent collaterals" and transventricular arteries are either extremely rare or nonexistent in the forebrain of the human during the last half of gestation (47). The vascular bed of most of the forebrain (exclusive of the striatum) consists of a complex meshwork of endothelium-lined vascular channels throughout most of the last half of gestation. Thus, the anatomic substrate for border zone lesions in the deep white matter seems to be lacking. There is another reason to question this concept. I would agree, as mentioned above, with Shuman and Selednick (83) that these small focal necroses are found most frequently in the deep frontal and deep parietal and occipital white matter. It is hard to imagine a border zone lesion that tended to spare the central regions of the brain but simultaneously involved both poles.

Are these small focal lesions due to generalized hypoxia? Many authors have thought that hypoxia was a major etiology of these small focal necroses. They came to this conclusion because of a high frequency of hypoxic experiences in their children with focal white matter necroses. Unfortunately, they failed to compare the frequency of hypoxia in their infants with white matter necroses with the frequency of hypoxic experiences in babies without small focal white matter necroses, thus limiting the value of their observations. Further, the case-control study of Shuman and Selednick (83) indicated that low Apgar scores were not associated with focal white matter necrosis, a finding supported in the material of the National Collaborative Perinatal Project (52).

Necrosis has many potential antecedents. While hypoxia may have a role, the evidence, other than anecdotal, is not convincing. Many factors, endogenous and exogenous, have the potential of increasing the risk of necrosis. One of these risk factors, transient endotoxemia, has gained considerable epidemiologic and experimental support over recent years. Other risk factors are mentioned above. However, the pathogenesis of the microvascular or parenchymal damage implied in these associations remains unknown.

The history of the putative antecedents of these small focal necroses reveals the methodologic problems that I have alluded to. Virchow and Parrot found a general metabolic disorder in most of the neonates with this lesion. Moebius found thrombosed vessels in the majority. Vivius found that all 300 of his cases had icterus. Herschfeld found omphalitis in most of his cases. Hlava found emboli in his cases (all quoted in Schmorl (78)). Schmorl found icterus in his 280 cases, but no omphalitis. In 1924 and 1927 Schwartz (summarized in his 1961 monograph) found anoxia and birth injury in the majority of his cases and induced a long series of papers attributing these lesions to anoxia culminating in the excellent pathologic paper by Banker and Larroche (1962), who also have found anoxia in their 51 cases. The multiplicity of putative antecedents reflects either a multiplicity of actual antecedents or a methodologic problem. Each of these studies sought common clinical events among dead infants whose brains contained these lesions; each study neglected to estimate the frequency of the same clinical events in dead children without these lesions. Thus, I suspect that we will eventually find a multiplicity of antecedents that may, or may not, include some specific aspect of anoxia.

Other perinatal telencephalic leucoencephalopathies are characterized by hypertrophic astrocytes (Fig. 7.7), amphophilic globules (Fig. 7.12), and acutely damaged glial cells, alone or in combination with each other or with necrotic foci. A large body of evidence has accumulated supporting the notion that these changes in neonatal human brain are abnormal and have significant constellations of risk factors. Their relationships and risk factors are detailed in Gilles et al. (32). In dead neonates, the perinatal telencephalic leucoencephalopathies are age-related, and several groups of overlapping risk factors were identified for each. The risk factors can be grouped under the headings of endotoxin effect, unfavorable uterine environment, congenital anomaly effect, or socioeconomic effect. Of particular interest, multiple markers of maternal and neonatal endotoxemia were associated with most of the leucoencephalopathies. That these associations in dead infants may be clinically important in living children is supported by the increased risk of neurologic dysfunction in offspring of mother who have had urinary tract infections during pregnancy (8).

Less Frequent Abnormalities Following Pre- or Perinatal Insult

A wide variety of other infarcts and necroses are found in the brains of individuals surviving pre- or perinatal injury. Unilateral cystic necroses may occur relatively early or late in gestation, often are limited to the distribution of a major cerebral artery, and are assumed to have resulted from impairment of flow in that vessel. Symmetric or asymmetric patches of micropolygyria have occasionally been ascribed to lowered flow in specific arterial beds, although the anatomic distribution of these lesions has not convincingly been limited to the entirety of a single arterial bed without extension into adjacent arterial beds. Patches of micropolygyria are also seen in the cerebellum. Large bilateral losses of cerebral tissue, often with preservation of those temporal and occipital regions supplied by the posterior cerebral arteries, have been called hydranencephaly. When damage has been limited to the cortex, it is often most pronounced around the depths of sulci, leaving the remaining gyral crest with the appearance of a mushroom. The entire gyrus is often the site of extensive scarring of cortex and white matter; hence the name of sclerotic microgyria (ulegyria) for this condition. The condition of sclerotic microgyria can readily be distinguished from micropolygyria, an abnormality of cortical formation and from polygyria or multiple small gyri, a condition sometimes seen in otherwise normal brains or in association with some other abnormality of the cerebrum.

The thalamus and striatum deserve special comment. These structures are sometimes the site of bilateral acute neuronal necrosis, neuronal mineralization, or glial fibrillary scarring (77), or the curious condition of status marmoratus or marbled state. These conditions may be found in

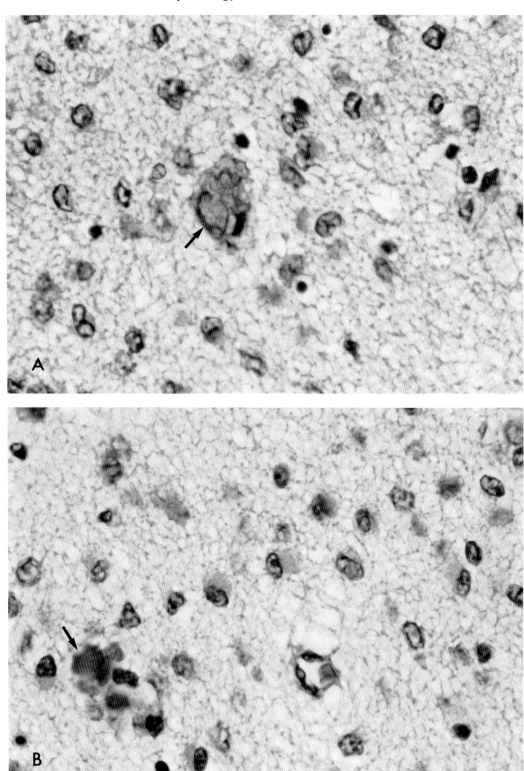

Figure 7.12. Small, mulberry-like, often multilaminated globules are frequently found in deep white matter of cerebra of neonates. In *A* a mulberry-like globule lies in midphoto, and in *B* another globule lies at the lower left. In *B* several hypertrophic astrocytes are also seen. H&E. (Original magnificiation ×950.)

isolation or with widely spread damage elsewhere in the nervous system. Status marmoratus refers to patterns of myelinated fibers bizarre for the striatum or thalamus occurring in association with neuronal loss and fibrillary gliosis (a similar condition sometimes can be seen in the damaged isocortex, but has not been described in the hippocampus). The "marbeling" of the thalamus and striatum has been found to be myelination of glial fibrils in part (5, 7), is often related to a complicated birth or to early postnatal disease in the human (59, 64), and was found in a neonatally damaged monkey (62) and in neonatally damaged kittens (29, 30).

Neuronal necrosis limited to the subiculum and the basis pontis is a curious condition in neonatal brains. Frequent in some institutions (3, 27, 58), it is rare in others. This marked difference in prevalence among institutions can either by regarded as an impediment to its study or a stimulus to the search for differing risk factors at these specific institutions. Pontosubicular necrosis has been associated with both the anoxia of respiratory distress and with hyperoxia, but the role of confounding variables in these studies is not clear.

Perinatal cardiorespiratory, umbilical cord, or placental catastrophies are sometimes followed by symmetric tegmental and tectal lesions in major neuronal aggregates in the brain stem (Fig. 7.13D), total cystic necrosis of the tegmentum, or an extraordinary astrocytosis of these structures extending upward into the thalamus with disproportionately little neuronal loss. These neonates may also have symmetric necrosis of neurons in the anterior horns of their spinal cord, particularly the lumbosacral spinal cord, or the latter may occur in isolation following such a catastrophe. Bilateral lesions in the border zones between the anterior and middle cerebral arteries are infrequent in the neonate, but may occur (Fig. 7.13C). Even more rarely encountered under these circumstances are bilateral lesions in the cerebellum in the border zones between the superior and inferior arteries.

CYSTS

Cystic lesions (Fig. 7.14) within the prosencephalon are found frequently in the brains of infants and children with neuro-

logic and intellectual deficits. Although rarely found in the context of a catastrophic event during gestation or parturition, the critical constellations of antecedents leading to the different kinds of cysts are not known.

Prosencephalic cystic lesions fall into two general categories on the basis of neuronal aggregates or glia in the neural tissue lining the wall.

Cystic Lesions with Heterotopic Neuronal Tissue

Nodules or layers of tissue containing aggregates or layers of neurons extend from ventricular to pial surface in the walls of these cysts. Usually, these lesions are associated with abnormalities of gyral pattern or lamination of adjacent cortex (17). Surrounding gyri may point into the deficit. If bilateral and symmetric in site (but not necessarily in size), the cystic lesions constitute the schizencephalic deficit of Yakovlev and Wadsworth (89) (Fig. 7.15). Occasionally, in this condition, the walls of the deficit are approximated, and nodules or layers of heterotopic neuronal tissue are spread from ventricle to surface along an "ependymal-pial" seam. Presumably, these defects are related to a time in development when the mantle was forming, and the heterotopic nodules along the wall may reflect a local disorder of migration or a disorganized result of abortive repair.

Cystic Lesions without Heterotopic Neuronal Tissues

These cystic lesions are small or large deficits in the cerebral mantle involving grey or white matter which may be single or multiple in number and symmetric or asymmetric in location (Fig. 7.14). Most are thought to have developed late in gestation and lack the heterotopic tissue along the cyst wall. Sometimes, they lie in a distribution strongly suggestive of a specific vascular bed.

Multicystic Encephalomalacia. This condition is distinctive because of the predominance of lesions in cerebral white matter. Wolf and Cowan (88) felt from their review of their cases and the literature that this was a disctinctive entity, the end stage of a destructive process that occurred relatively late in gestation. Multiple names

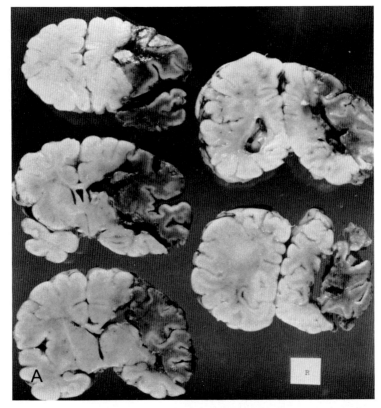

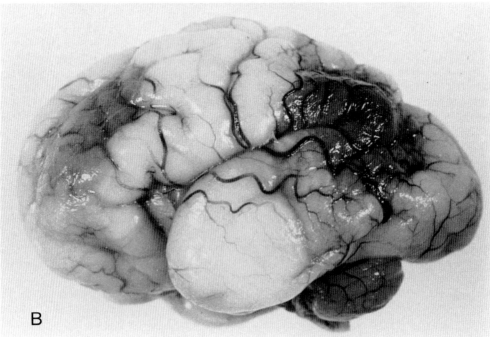

Figure 7.13. Necrosis in the late fetal and neonatal brain. Large focal necroses may occupy the beds of large vessels (middle cerebral artery (A)), their branches (B), or the border zones between arterial beds (C). Focal symmetric necrosis of tegmental and tectal neuronal aggregates reveals itself as focal brain stem discolorations D.

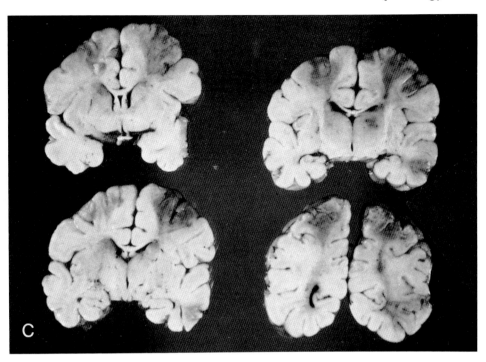

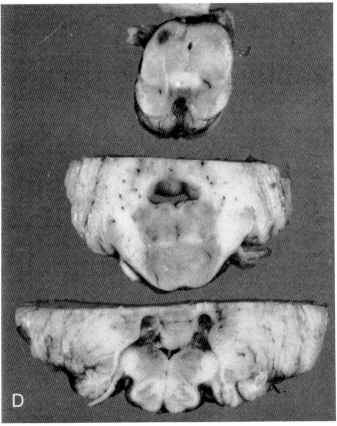

Figure 7.13 *C* and *D*

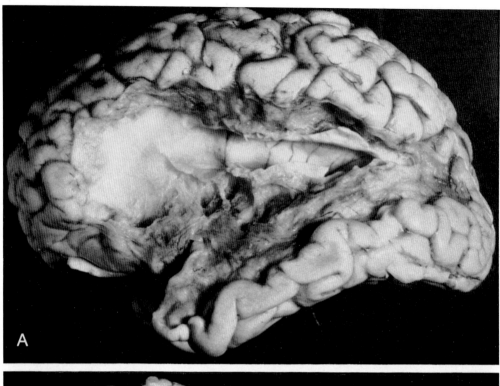

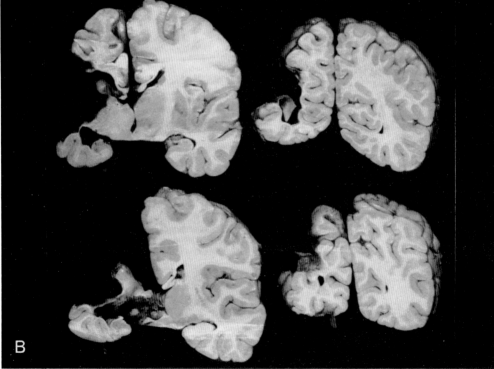

Figure 7.14. (*A*) This large cystic lesion of the left cerebrum is located entirely within the distribution of the left middle cerebral artery and is thought to have occurred late in gestation. Gyri have been interrupted by the infarcts; remaining gyri are not oriented toward the lesion. (*B*) In coronal section, the cystic infarct occupies almost all of the bed of the middle cerebral artery.

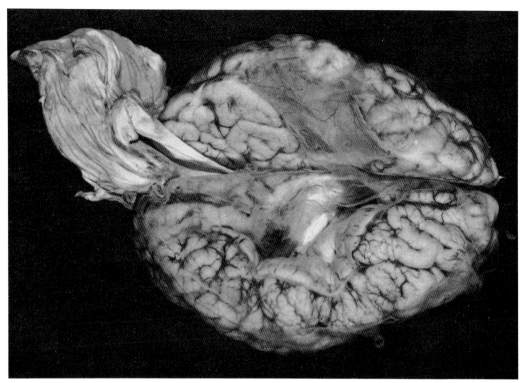

Figure 7.15.   Schizencephaly. On the *right*, the meninges have been removed, exposing a cavity extending into the ventricle lined by multiple anomalous small gyri. Surrounding gyri tend to radiate from the cyst wall. The symmetric lesion on the *left* is still covered by arachnoid.

have been applied to this condition. Some names have implied a causative relationship (e.g., parturitional porencephaly), although a cystic lesion ipso facto rarely implicates directly a specific antecedent. These lesions have been described in infants after severe birth trauma, venous obstruction, and cerebral ischemia. Crome (12) found changes in leptomeningeal vessels; whether the causative process was a vasculopathy or the vascular abnormalities resulted from diminished requirement for blood flow is not clear. Others have alluded to reduced blood flow, but were unable to account for the predominance of these lesions in cerebral white matter (1, 57, 60). Fowler and Mellor (25) described multiple cystic encephalomalacia in a stillborn infant with congenital heart disease and a hypoplastic right ventricle. They felt that it resulted from venous stagnation or stagnant anoxia. Others have found multicystic encephalomalacia after maternal carbon monoxide poisoning. The risk of developing this abnormality seems to extend through-

out the last part of gestation and parturition.

Cystic defects in the neonatal brain have a wide range in size. Maximal cystic lesions of the cerebrum are encompassed in the term hydranencephaly, a condition in which most of the dorsal aspects of both cerebral hemispheres are gone except for a thin leptomeningeal-glial membrane enclosing the cyst (13, 14, 40). Variable amounts of the basal regions of the occipital and temporal lobes and the basal ganglia are retained. The relative normality of these retained regions supports the contention that the damaging insult occurred in the last half of gestation as well as the contention, in some cases, that the damage is related to significantly lowered cerebral blood flow with failure of supply to the distal regions of all three major arterial beds.

Only a few cases of multicystic encephalomalacia were found in the NCPP material. Unfortunately, little new information can be added. All had had catastrophic events during gestation or at the time of birth, including umbilical cord knotted around the neck or neonatal asphyxia.

Cystic Lesions of the Ganglionic Eminence. Cystic degeneration of the portion of the germinal matrix overlying the striatum, the ganglionic matrix, has been recognized since the first descriptions of the congenital rubella syndrome were published in 1967 (18, 48, 76, 81, 82); it was first mentioned by Schwartz (80). These lesions are usually bilateral (Fig. 7.16) and apparently occur at a time when the mass of germinal cells of the ganglionic matrix is considerable (i.e., midgestation). The term germinolysis, proposed by Shaw and Alvord (82), is ideal in that it emphasized the premature loss of this fetal tissue by a process apparently different from that usually encountered in older brains. It also implies that the insult occurs at a gestational time when the germinal mass is voluminous. Therefore, these lesions likely occurred before the third trimester, even though the cysts may persist well after birth. The cysts, small or large, may contain glial trabeculae or nodules of germinal cells. The source of these cysts is unknown, but it seems likely a large proportion reflect an encounter between the fetus and a viral agent (82). The proportion remaining as posthemorrhagic cavities (80) must be very small, as hemosiderin-filled macrophages are uncommon in the walls of these cysts.

DEFECTS IN MYELINATION

Delay in myelination is associated with multiple factors that indicate that myelinating brain is vulnerable to many of the same factors that are antecedent to growth retardation in other organs. Small-for-dates babies are at increased risk of delayed myelination, and maternal and postnatal malnutrition may contribute to delay in myelination as has been suggested by a number of biochemical studies of the brain of malnourished children. The other risk factors are maternal cigarette smoking, third trimester uterine bleeding, and depressed maternal hematocrit (54).

EDEMA AND HERNIATION

Edema

The unmyelinated brain of the premature or term human infant contains consid-erably more water than does the myelinated brain of the older child or adult. Therapeutic clinical strategies require more information about the role of swelling or edema of the brain of the neonate. Even though the neonatal brain appears to be "wetter" than the adult brain and has the propensity of swelling during fixation (usually attaining a postfixation weight 30% greater than fresh weight), the pathologist must differentiate cerebral swelling uncomplicated by necrosis from the swelling of necrotic tissue. Unfortunately, the few pathologic studies of edema of the perinatal brain have given conflicting information, and the question remains open.

Anderson and Belton (2) estimated swelling in asphyxiated "freshly stillborn" or dead neonates of less than 1 week of age, autopsied 14–78 h after death, and felt that brain swelling did occur. Increased tension of dura, pallor, and flattening of gyri were found in only 4 of 16 infants, and it is unclear whether these infants had undergone cerebral necrosis. Pryse-Davies and Beard (71) defined brain swelling as enlargement of the cerebral hemispheres, gyral flattening, and sulcal narrowing in a careful prospective study of all neonatal autopsies in a maternity hospital. They concluded that swelling was not found under 33 weeks of gestation in the absence of intraventricular hemorrhage. By term, however, 89% of all brains were swollen. Water content in these brains was least in the most "swollen" brains, and the amount of necrosis is unclear. Experimental studies of asphyxiated neonatal animals has similarly provided conflicting information, and one group (Streicher et al. (86)) came to the conclusion that "neonatal brain does not have a tendency to edema."

Herniation

Transtentorial herniation in the neonate with local necrosis of the herniated cortex is virtually nonexistent, unless the result of extensive hemispheral necrosis (Fig. 7.17). Similarly, cerebellar herniation through the foramen magnum is rare in the absence of a space taking process in the posterior fossa.

Focal necrosis along the lower edge of the parahippocampal gyrus adjacent to the tentorial edge and along the lower edge of the cerebellum adjacent to the foramen mag-

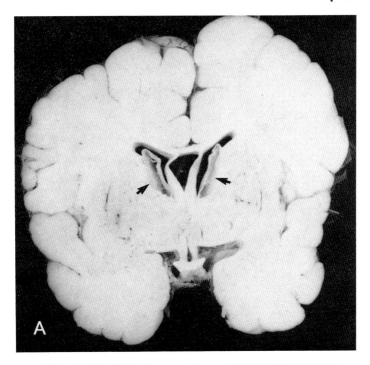

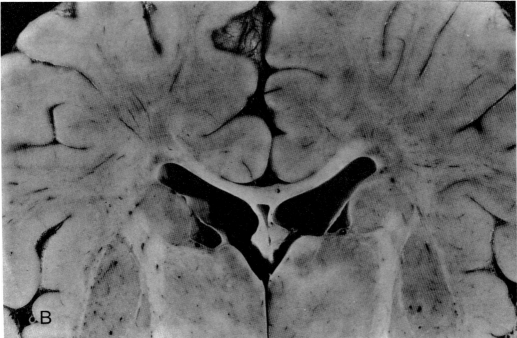

Figure 7.16. Large symmetric cysts are seen overlying and medial to the head of the caudate. (A) Late fetal brain. (B) 1 yr of age.

num was not present in the sample of the 1155 brains from the National Collaborative Perinatal Project in the absence of widespread necrosis of the cerebrum or the cerebellum.

Thus, our available information allows only the conclusions that swelling may be a manifestation of necrosis in the neonatal brain and not uncomplicated tissue fluid accumulation and that significant hernia-

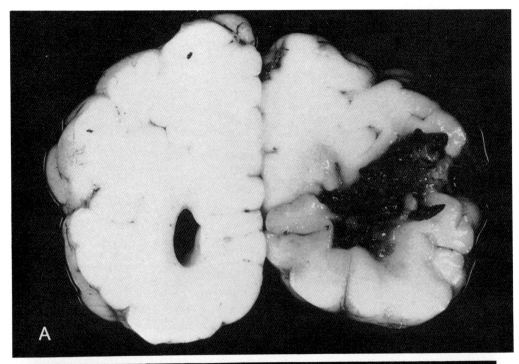

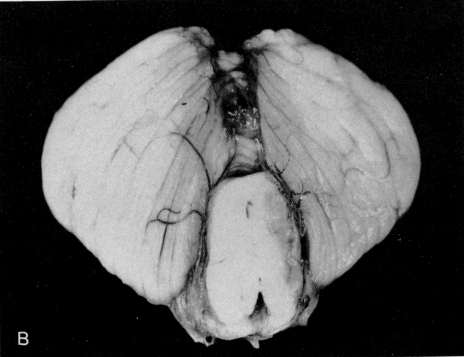

Figure 7.17.   The right cerebrum contains a large hematoma in the parietooccipital region (A). It is markedly swollen and has herniated past the tentorium, driving the opposite midbrain into the free edge of the left side of the tentorium. The left side of the midbrain is necrotic (B).

tion of the parahippocampal gyrus or cerebellum accompanied by local necrosis is very rare.

PERINATAL AND POSTNATAL TRAUMA

The problem of traumatic lesions in the neonatal and postnatal brain is sometimes vexing for the pathologist. Often, what constitutes a traumatic lesion is unclear. Obstetric trauma is extremely uncommon today compared to the kinds of lesions a pediatric pathologist encountered 50 yr ago. However, obstetric and postnatal traumatic lesions do occur, and they must be recognized, even though different from traumatic lesions of the brain in the adult. The important, though infrequent, lesions occurring during birth include tears of the cervical spinal cord, and, less frequently, tears of the brachia of the cerebellum. Tears of the free edge of the tentorium are quite uncommon, although slight separation of the upper and lower leafs of the tentorium or of the two halves of the falx must be almost universal in dead neonates. These separations may result from molding of the head during birth and, except for the associated intrafalcine or infratentorial hemorrhage (Fig. 7.18), these lesions are of little consequence unless one of the dural sheets is torn and a large quantity of blood leaks into the infratentorial or supratentorial subdural space. The latter subdural hematomas have considerable potential for creating mischief and, unfortunately, are often missed by the pathologist when their blood is regarded as being blood-derived from the lateral sinuses or cerebral veins. It is doubly important for the pathologist to recognize these subdural collections, as they are of considerable clinical importance and are easily missed even with computer-assisted tomography. Infratentorial, retrocerebellar, or supracerebellar subdural hematomas displace the cerebellum and potentially obliterate the outlets of the fourth ventricle, leading to rapidly developing hydrocephalus. When clinically recognized, they are readily removed surgically.

Linear and depressed skull fractures, usually from misplaced forceps, are associated with local subarachnoid hemorrhage, but little else, unless the dura has been torn. Tear of the dura may be followed by an enlarging fracture that results from a pulsatile outpouching of fibrotic arachnoid through the dural defect. While sometimes called a leptomeningeal cyst, this term is probably inaccurate, as no isolated or loculated cyst exists, and the surgical repair consists of only a patch across the dural rent.

In the neonate the only other significantly frequent lesions are tears of the cervical spinal cord. The tears are easy to overlook, as the ligaments and membranes around the joints of the vertebral column are quite redundant, and the vertebral column may pop back into place immediately after the dislocation with very little articular or extradural hemorrhage. However, even very small tears within the spinal cord can prove disastrous to the patient.

Traumatic lesions in the unmyelinated cerebrum of the postnatal child are quite different than those of the adult (56). In the infant, the cortex usually does not contain wedge or cone-shaped contusions following a blow or fall. In contrast to the mature brain, the white matter of the baby brain tears, usually in a linear fashion, and usually symmetrically. The white matter tears are usually located high in the parasagittal frontal white matter, although orbital, temporal, and parietal white matter may be involved singly or in combination. White matter tears of this nature are traumatic in origin.

SUMMARY

Fetal and neonatal brains of the same putative gestational age vary considerably in many developmental aspects. The variation is related to the combined effects of biologic variation, the effects of insult to the developing brain, and to error in the estimation of gestational age. His (42) recognized this variability in degree of developmental among human embryos already at a few weeks of gestational age. This variability appears to extend throughout gestation. The pathologist's attempt to eliminate the difficulties surrounding the estimate of gestational age by the elimination of cases that do not adhere to some arbitrary standard such as body weight or body length is a two-edged sword. These attempts often allow internal comparisons of considerable exactitude, but diminish the

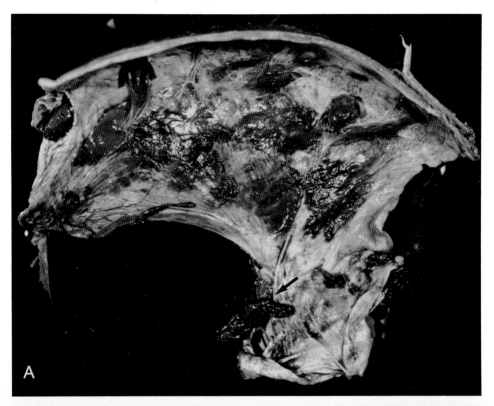

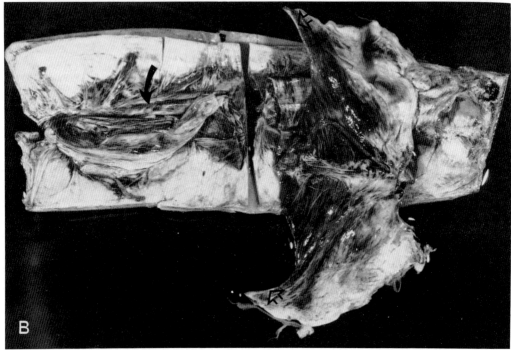

Figure 7.18.   Multiple hemorrhages and small hematomata in the falx and the tentorium. (*A*) The falx contains multiple hemorrhages and hematomata (frontal, *left*). The great vein of Galen lies below midpicture (*arrow*). Little blood is apparent within the tentorium. (*B*) The tentorium (viewed from below, frontal, *left*, *arrows* mark the free edge) contains multiple confluent hematomata. The sagittal sinus and part of the falx (*curved arrow*) lie under the sagittal suture.

likelihood of finding clinical antecedents that affect both cerebral development and the body parameter chosen for the independent variable. That is, he is less likely to find an antecedent that affects both myelination and body mass if he eliminates from his study those cases of the wrong body size.

Hemorrhage, necrosis, malformation, inflammation, and delayed acquisition of some component of the neonatal brain are each the nonspecific end stages of the interaction of a multitude of clinical risk factors. Intracranial hemorrhage does not always result from trauma; necrosis does not always result from hypoxia. To have value for the clinician or for the pathologist a putative clinical antecedent must have predictive power. A putative clinical antecedent should predict with considerable specificity the morphologic outcome, and vice-versa; the morphologic outcome should predict with considerable specificity the clinical setting. Unfortunately, some 28 specific and distinct morphologic abnormalities are attributed to neonatal asphyxia (hypoxia or anoxia) in current texts of neuropathology. The clinician who must make judgments about potential outcomes following neonatal disasters will find neither solace nor help in this kind of information.

If most morphologic abnormalities in the fetal brain are etiologically nonspecific and are the end stages of a multitude of adverse clinical conditions, then we must continue our search for the multitude of risk factors that enhance or depress the likelihood of each specific morphologic outcome.

ACKNOWLEDGMENT

This work was supported by the Burton E. Green Foundation.

References

1. Aicardi J, Goutieres F, De Verbois AH: Multicystic encephalomalacia of infants and its relation to abnormal gestation and hydraencephalcy. *J Neurol Sci* 15:357, 1972.
2. Anderson JM, Belton NR: Water and electrolyte abnormalities in the human brain after severe intrapartum asphyxia. *J Neurol Neurosurg Psychiatry* 37:541, 1974.
3. Barmada M, Moossy J, Painter M: Pontosubicular necrosis and hyperoxemia. *J Neuropathol Exp Neurol* 38:304, 1979.
4. Becker H: Uber Hirngefassausschatungen; intrakranielle Gefassverschlusse; uber experimentelle Hydranencephalie (Blasenhirn). *Dsch Ztschr Nervenh* 161:446, 1949.
5. Bignami A, Ralston HJ III: Myelination of fibrillary astroglial processes in long term Wallerian degeneration.

6. The possible relationship to "status marmoratus." *Brain Res* 11:710, 1968.
6. Blake JA: The roof and lateral recesses of the fourth ventricle, considered morphologically and embryologically. *J Comp Neurol* 10:79, 1900.
7. Borit A, Herndon RM: The fine structure of placques fibromyeliniques in ulegyria and in status marmoratus. *Acta Neuropathol* 14:304, 1970.
8. Broman SH: Perinatal antecedents of severe mental retardation in school age children. Presented at the 86th Annual Convention of the American Psychological Association, Toronto, 1978.
9. Cammermeyer J: I. An evaluation of the significance of the "dark" neuron. *Ergeb Anat Entwicklungsgesch* 36:1, 1962.
10. Clark DB, Anderson GW: Correlation of complications of labor with lesions in the brains of neonates. *J Neuropathol Exp Neurol* 20:275, 1961.
11. Cowan W, Wenger E: Cell loss in the trochlear nucleus of the chick during normal development and after radical extirpation of the optic vesicle. *J Exp Zool* 164:267, 1967.
12. Crome L: Multilocular cystic encephalopathy of infants. *J Neurol Neurosurg Psychiatry* 21:146, 1958.
13. Crome L, Sylvester PE: Hydranencephaly (hydrencephaly). *Arch Dis Child* 33:235, 1958.
14. Cruveilhier J: *Anatomie Pathologique du Corps Humain*, part 2, XVth Liv. Paris, JB Bailliere, 1829–1835.
15. Dambska M: Encephalic necrosis and inflammatory reaction in fetuses and newborn. *Pol Med J* 22:404, 1968.
16. Dandy WE, Blackfan, KD: Internal hydrocephalus: an experimental, clinical, and pathological study. *Am J Dis Child* 8:406, 1914.
17. Dekaban A: Large defects in cerebral hemispheres associated with cortical dysgenesis. *J Neuropathol Exp Neurol* 24:512, 1965.
18. DeLeon GA, Girling DG: Cystic degeneration of the telencephalic subependymal germinal layer in newborn infants. *J Neurol Neurosurg Psychiatry* 38:265, 1975.
19. Demyer WE: Development of axonal pathways after neurosurgical lesions in the septum of the fetal rat: fornix ventralis, commissure of the fornix ventralis, corpus callosum and anterior commissure. *Res Publ Assoc Res Nerv Ment Dis* 51:269, 1973.
20. DeReuck J: The human periventricular arterial blood supply and the anatomy of cerebral infarctions. *Eur Neurol* 5:321, 1971.
21. DeReuck J, VanderEecken H: Cerebral vasculature, morphology, and pathology. An embryological study of the periventricular vascularization and its clinico-pathological significance, in Meyer JS, Lechner H, Reivich M, et al (eds): *Cerebral Vascular Disease*, 6th International Conference, Salzburg, 1972. St. Louis, CV Mosby, 1974, pp 136–141.
22. Dooling EC, Chi J, Gilles, FH: Telencephalic development: changing gyral patterns. In Gilles FH, Leviton A, Dooling EC (eds): *The Developing Human Brain: Growth and Epidemiologic Neuropathology*. Boston, Wright PSG, 1983.
23. Dooling EC, Chi JG, Gilles FH: Developmental change in ventricular epithelia. In Gilles FH, Leviton A, Dooling EC (eds): *The Developing Human Brain: Growth and Epidemiologic Neuropathology*. Boston, Wright PSG, 1983.
24. Dooling EC, Gilles FH: Intracranial hemorrhage: topography. In Gilles FH, Leviton A, Dooling EC (eds): *The Developing Human Brain: Growth and Epidemiologic Neuropathology*. Boston, Wright PSG, 1983.
25. Fowler M, Mellor G: Cerebral malformation and degeneration produced in later foetal life by a primary cardiac anomaly. *J Pathol Bacteriol* 90:523, 1965.
26. Friede RL: A histochemical study of DPN-diaphorase in human white matter with some notes on myelination. *J Neurochem* 61:8, 1961.
27. Friede RL: Ponto-subicular lesions in perinatal anoxia. *Arch Pathol* 94:343, 1972.
28. Friede RL: *Developmental Neuropathology*. New York,

Springer-Verlag, 1975.

29. Gilles FH, Averill DR Jr, Kerr C: Changes in neonatally induced cerebral lesions with advancing age. *J Neuropathol Exp Neurol* 36:666, 1977.

30. Gilles FH, Averill D, Kerr CS: Neonatal endotoxin encephalopathy. *Am Neurol* 2:49, 1977.

31. Gilles FH, Bina M, Sotrel A: Infantile atlantooccipital instability. *Am J Dis Child* 133:30, 1979.

32. Gilles FH, Leviton A, Dooling EC: *The Developing Human Brain: Growth and Epidemiologic Neuropathology*. Boston, Wright PSG, 1983.

33. Gilles FH, Leviton A, Kerr CS: Endotoxin leucoencephalopathy in the telencephalon of the newborn kitten. *J Neurol Sci* 27:183, 1976.

34. Gilles FH, Price RA, Kevy SV, Berenberg W: Fibrinolytic activity in the ganglionic eminence of the premature human brain. *Biol Neonate* 18:426, 1971.

35. Gilles FH, Shankle W, Dooling EC: Myelinated tracts: growth patterns. In Gilles FH, Leviton A, Dooling EC (eds): *The Developing Human Brain: Growth and Epidemiologic Neuropathology*. Boston, Wright PSG, 1983.

36. Gilles FH, Shillito JS: Infantile hydrocephalus: retrocerebellar subdural hematoma. *J Pediatr* 76:529, 1970.

37. Gluszcz A: On the periventricular septic necroses of the brain in premature infants. In Jacob H (ed): International Congress of Neuropathology, 4th, Munich, 1961, No. III. Proceedings; in drei Banden. Stuttgart, Theime Verlag, 1962.

38. Goldman PS: Functional recovery after lesions of the nervous system. 3. Developmental processes in neuronal plasticity. Recovery of function after CNS lesions in infant monkeys. *Neurosci Res Program Bull* 12:217, 1974.

39. Grontofft O: Intracerebral and meningeal haemorrhages in perinatally deceased infants. I. Intracerebral haemorrhages. A pathologico-anatomical and obstetric study. *Acta Obstet Gynecol Scand* 32:333, 1953.

40. Halsey JH Jr, Allen N, Chamberlin HR: The morphogenesis of hydranencephaly. *J Neurol Sci* 12:187, 1971.

41. Hambleton G, Wigglesworth JS: Origin of intraventricular haemorrhage in the preterm infant. *Arch Dis Child* 51:651, 1976.

42. His W: *Anatomie Menschlichen Embryonen*. Leipzig, East Germany, 1880–1895.

43. Humphrey T. The development of the human tuberculum olfactorium during the first three months of embryonic life. *J Hirnforsch* 9:437, 1967.

44. Jammes JL, Gilles FH: Telencephalic development: Matrix volume and isocortex and allocortex surface areas. In Gilles FH, Leviton A, Dooling EC (eds): *The Developing Human Brain: Growth and Epidemiologic Neuropathology*. Boston, Wright PSG, 1983.

45. Kennedy C, Grave GD, Jehle JW, Sokoloff L: Blood flow to white matter during maturation of the brain. *Neurology* 20:613, 1970.

46. Kennedy C, Sakurada O, Shinohara M, Miyaoka M, Sokoloff L: A comparison of the rates of local cerebral glucose utilization in newborn and pubescent monkeys. *Ann Neurol* 6:176, 1979.

47. Kuban K, Gilles FH: Human telencephalic angiogenesis. *Ann Neurol* 14:356, 1983.

48. Larroche JC: Sub-ependymal pseudo-cysts in the newborn. *Biol Neonate* 21:170, 1972.

49. Leech RW, Alvord EC Jr: Glial fatty metamorphosis: an abnormal response of premyelin glia frequently accompanying periventricular leucomalacia. *Am J Pathol* 74:603, 1974a.

50. Leech RW, Alvord EC Jr: Morphologic variations in periventricular leucomalacia. *Am J Pathol* 74:591, 1974b.

51. Levi-Montalcini R: The origin and development of the visceral system in the spinal cord of the chick embryo. *J Morphol* 86:253, 1950.

52. Leviton A, Gilles FH: The epidemiology of the perinatal telencephalic leucoenphalopathy characterized by focal necroses. In Gilles FH, Leviton A, Dooling EC (eds): *The Developing Human Brain: Growth and Epidemiologic Neuropathology*. Boston, Wright PSG, 1983.

53. Leviton A, Gilles FH, Dooling EC: The epidemiology of subarachnoid hemorrhage. In Gilles FH, Leviton A, Dooling EC (eds): *The Developing Human Brain: Growth and Epidemiologic Neuropathology*. Boston, Wright PSG, 1983.

54. Leviton A, Gilles FH, Dooling EC: The epidemiology of delayed myelination. In Gilles FH, Leviton A, Dooling EC (eds): *The Developing Human Brain: Growth and Epidemiologic Neuropathology*. Boston, Wright PSG, 1983.

55. Lindenberg, R: Morphotropic and morphostatic necrobiosis; investigations on nerve cells of brain. *Am J Pathol* 32:1147, 1956.

56. Lindenberg R, Freitag E: Morphology of brain lesions from blunt trauma in early infancy. *Arch Pathol* 87:298, 1969.

57. Lindenberg R, Swanson PD: "Infantile hydranencephaly"—a report of five cases of infarction of both cerebral hemispheres in infancy. *Brain* 90:839, 1967.

58. MacAdams AJ: Pulmonary hemorrhage in the newborn. *Am J Dis Child* 113:255, 1967.

59. Malmud N: Status marmoratus: a form of cerebral palsy following either birth injury or inflammation of the central nervous system. *J Pediatr* 37:610, 1950.

60. Marburg O, Casamajor L: Plebostasis and phlebothrombosis of brain in newborn and childhood. *Arch Neurol Psychiatr* 52:170, 1944.

61. McLennan JE, Gilles FH, Neff R: A model of growth of the human fetal brain. In Gilles FH, Leviton A, Dooling EC (eds): *The Developing Human Brain: Growth and Epidemiologic Neuropathology*. Boston, Wright PSG, 1983.

62. Myers RE: Atropic cortical sclerosis associated with status marmoratus in a perinatally damaged monkey. *Neurology* 19:1177, 1969.

63. Norman MG: Perinatal brain damage. *Perspect Pediatr Pathol* 4:41, 1978.

64. Norman RM: Etat marbre of corpus striatum following birth injury. *J Neurol Neurosurg Psychiatry* 10:12, 1947.

65. Pape KE, Wigglesworth JS: *Haemorrhage, Ischemia and the Perinatal Brain*. London, Heinemann, 1979.

66. Parrot MJ: Sur las steatose viscerale par inanition chez le nouveau-ne. *C R Acad Sci [D] (Paris)* 67:412, 1868a.

67. Parrot MJ: Etude sur la steatose interstitielle diffuse de l'encephale chez le nouveau-ne. *Arch Physiol Norm Pathol (Paris)* 1:530, 662, 706, 1868b.

68. Parrot MJ: Etude sur le ramollissement de lencephale chez le nouveau-ne. *Arch Physiol Norm Pathol (Paris)* 5:59, 176, 283, 1873.

69. Perrin EV, Landing BH: "The Schmorl lesion" in jaundiced infected infants. *Am J Dis Child* 104:551, 1962.

70. Potter EL, Craig JM: *Pathology of the Fetus and the Infant*, ed 3. Chicago, Year Book, 1975.

71. Pryse-Davies J, Beard RW: A necropsy study of brain swelling in the newborn with special reference to cerebellar herniation. *J Pathol* 109:51, 1973.

72. Rakic P, Yakovlev PI: Development of the corpus callosum and cavum septi in man. *J Comp Neurol* 132:45, 1968.

73. Roback HN, Scherer HJ: Uber die feinere Morphologie des fruhkindlichen Gehirns unter besonderer Berucksichtigung der Gliaentwicklung. *Virchows Arch [Pathol Anat]* 294:365, 1935.

74. Romanes GH: Motor localization and effects of nerve injury on ventral horn cells of spinal cord. *J Anat* 80:117, 1946.

75. Rorke LB: *Pathology of Perinatal Brain Injury*. New York, Raven Press, 1982.

76. Rorke LB, Spiro AJ: Cerebral lesions in congenital rubella syndrome. *J Pediatr* 70:243, 1967.

77. Rosales RK, Riggs HE: Symmetrical thalamic degeneration in infants. *J Neuropathol Exp Neurol* 21:372, 1962.

78. Schmorl CG: Verhandl Deutsch. *Pathol. Gesellsch* 6:109, 1903.

79. Schneider GE: Is it really better to have your brain lesion early? A revision of the "Kennard principle." *Neuropsychologia* 17:557, 1979.

80. Schwartz P: *Birth injuries of the Newborn: Morphology, Pathogenesis, Clinical Pathology and Prevention.* New York, Hafner Publishing, 1961.
81. Shaw CM: Subependymal germinolysis. *J Neuropathol Exp Neurol* 32:153, 1973.
82. Shaw CM, Alvord EC Jr: Subependymal germinolysis. *Arch Neurol* 31:374, 1974.
83. Shuman RM, Selednik LJ: Periventricular leukomalacia. A one-year autopsy study. *Arch Neurol* 37:231, 1980.
84. Smith DW, Tondury G: Origin of the calvaria and its sutures. *Am J Dis Child* 132:662, 1978.
85. Stephans RB, Stilwell DL: *Arteries and Veins of the Human Brain.* Springfield, IL, Thomas, 1969.
86. Streicher E, Wisniewski H, Klatzo I: Resistance of immature brain to experimental cerebral edema. *Neurology* 15:833, 1965.
87. Sumi SM: Periventricular leukoencephalopathy in the monkey. A search for the "normal control" and the "early lesion." *Arch Neurol* 31:38, 1974.
88. Wolf A, Cowen D: The cerebral atrophies and encephalopathies of infancy and childhood. *Res Pub Assoc Nerv Ment Dis* 34:199, 1955.
89. Yakovlev PI, Wadsworth RC: Schizencephalies: a study of the congenital clefts in the cerebral mantle; clefts with fused lips. *J Neuropathol* 5:116, 1946.

CHAPTER 8

Inherited Metabolic Disease

LAURENCE E. BECKER, M.D., F.R.C.P.(C)
ALLAN YATES, M.D., Ph.D., F.R.C.P.(C)

INTRODUCTION

In general, metabolism is the sum of the chemical processes by which a living, organized substance is produced and maintained. Using this definition, most diseases have a metabolic aspect. However, in this chapter, we are using the term "metabolic diseases" in a restricted sense to include only those that are genetic, progressive and largely neurologic, and have a demonstrable or presumed inborn error of metabolism.

The pattern of inheritance in most of these diseases is autosomal recessive; in a few, the best known of which are Fabry's disease, mucopolysaccharidosis type II (Hunter syndrome), adrenoleukodystrophy, Pelizaeus-Merzbacher disease, Lesch-Nyhan syndrome, and Menkes disease, there is X-linked recessive inheritance.

The progressive aspect of our definition means that only conditions in which there is a deleterious change in status over time are included. Genetic disorders such as tuberous sclerosis and some conditions that are progressive but have no currently suspected biochemical etiology are not discussed in this chapter. However, leukodystrophies have been included, even though no enzyme deficiency has been detected in most cases, because they occur in childhood, and some of them (metachromatic leukodystrophy and Krabbe's disease) have recognized enzyme defects.

The nervous system is more often severely involved in the metabolic disorders than any other system. Therefore, most metabolic diseases could be included, but

we have restricted ourselves to conditions that are neurologic in their main expression. The emphasis is on those in which morphological alterations of nervous tissues have been well described; but, we have also included conditions that are of interest to the neurology consultant where the neuropathological findings may be nonspecific (some aminoacidurias) or even absent (Lesch-Nyhan syndrome). Just as the chemistry of the metabolic diseases is far more complex than is suggested by the simple statement of a specific enzyme defect, so the understanding of how that chemical defect is translated into cytopathological alteration and eventually clinical manifestation of disease is more complex and poorly understood in most metabolic diseases.

The result of the enzymatic defect is a disturbance of cell function that expresses itself first as an unhealthy cell, then a dying cell, and finally no cell. Depending on the disease, pathological alterations may or may not be evident and, when present, may be apparent at an early or only at a late stage. Ultimately, the classification of metabolic diseases will be based on the primary biochemical defects. However, in this chapter, we emphasize the morphological aspects to increase understanding of how the biochemical defect is translated into an abnormal organelle, abnormal cell, abnormal organ, and an abnormal patient.

In many metabolic diseases, the abnormal patient and the abnormal organ have been well described. We are now at the stage where examination of the cell and its organelles and metabolism will help provide more precise information on the pathogenesis of the cellular injury at the ultrastructural and molecular levels.

Within the cell, various metabolic processes are compartmentalized to cell membrane, mitochondrion, lysosome, or cytosol. The vast majority of inherited metabolic diseases are disorders of lysosomes, although abnormalities of mitochondria have also been suggested. While it could be worthwhile from some perspectives to discuss metabolic disease on the basis of abnormal organelle pathology, currently, such a classification is cumbersome and impractical. Therefore, we have organized this chapter into three traditional categories: storage diseases, leukodystrophies, and other metabolic diseases. Within each large category, specific diseases, as defined by the biochemical defect (when known), are discussed.

In addition to impaired nervous system function due to the direct effect of the primary enzyme defect, the brain may be damaged indirectly by the accumulation of an unmetabolized substance in extracellular fluids, the effects of metabolic malfunction of another organ (e.g., the liver), or abnormalities of vasculature due to an underlying metabolic disturbance (Menkes disease, Fabry's disease, and homocystinuria).

The clinical manifestations of a metabolic disease vary in accordance with the nature of the biochemical defect, the stage of maturation of the nervous system, dietary intake, administration of certain drugs, and the occurrence of infection. The role of maturation is particularly important in view of the tendency for certain metabolic abnormalities to become most active at different stages of maturation. For example, some diseases produce their main pathology only during critical phases of development (e.g., phenylketonuria). Once this stage is passed, the biochemical abnormality appears to be less harmful in its effects on the nervous system.

The relative importance of diagnostic methods that can be applied in a Pathology Department to patients with metabolic disease is ever changing. Because of the general interest and rapid progress in the better understanding of many of these diseases, information on diagnosis can become outdated very quickly. The success of certain screening programs combined with amniocentesis has significantly increased the rarity of many of these conditions so that in the future even fewer neuropathologists will have an opportunity to examine tissue from such patients. In circumstances where tissue from patients with rare metabolic diseases is available to the pathologist, there should be no hesitation in seeking consultation from a special laboratory so that clinical, neuropathological, and biochemical information can be correlated in the most meaningful way.

STORAGE DISORDERS

Storage disorders are characterized by genetically determined enzymatic defects, often localized to the lysosome and usually associated with an abnormal, membrane-bound inclusion on electron microscopy (EM). Lysosomal acid hydrolases are synthesized in the cytoplasm and transported into the cisternae of the endoplasmic reticulum. The Golgi apparatus packages the hydrolases into primary lysosomes that fuse with autophagic vacuoles, forming secondary lysosomes. In the secondary lysosomes the hydrolases degrade cytoplasmic constituents present in the autophagic vacuole, and constituents that cannot be degraded form so-called residual bodies. In this sequence, presumably malfunction can occur at any stage.

In lysosomal storage diseases there is defective activity of specific lysosomal enzymes with failure of catabolism, resulting in storage of the undigested material. Some disorders have a defect in more than one enzyme. For example, I-cell disease has a more generalized dysfunction of lysosomal membranes that results in reduced activity of lysosomal enzymes in tissue and cultured fibroblasts but elevated levels of enzymes in the serum or culture media.

Storage of material within a neuron may lead to cytoplasmic distension. In neuronal ceroid lipofuscinosis, stored material is easily detected, but the cytoplasm may not be obviously swollen. However, the large neuron with a ballooned rounded contour, reduced Nissl substance, and peripherally displaced nucleus is characteristic of many neuronal storage diseases.

Both paraffin-embedded and frozen sections are essential to identify stored material within the cytoplasm using histological methods. Since the lipids readily dissolve in alcohol and mucopolysaccharides in water, fresh frozen material should always be taken from autopsy and biopsy tissue. Limited special staining is suggested: for lipids, oil red O (ORO), Sudan black B (SBB), and Luxol fast blue (LFB); for glycogen and other carbohydrate-containing constituents, periodic acid-Schiff (PAS) with and without diastase; for metachromatic materials, acidic cresyl violet (Hirsch-Pfeiffer) and toluidine blue; for mucopolysaccharides, mucicarmine and Alcian blue. The same stains should also be used on paraffin-embedded tissue, because residual storage products may be present. The presence of insoluble lipofuscin and ceroid can be detected and confirmed by their autofluorescence. Before recent advances in biochemistry, rigorous histochemical examination was used to delineate the nature of the stored material. Details of the use of these staining methods are available in older publications (345).

The limitations on the specificities of these histochemical techniques suggest that direct biochemical analyses of the appropriate tissues are more valuable in terms of identifying a specific enzyme defect. Therefore, it is essential that the pathologist freeze appropriate tissues as soon as possible. In any degenerative disorder where the diagnosis is not clear, a large portion of frontal lobe must be protected from the effects of formalin. The anguish of finding an entire brain fixed in formalin because the diagnosis was assumed to be "just mental retardation" is to be avoided at all costs.

The specificity of the ultrastructural characteristics of the residual lysosomal contents is sometimes disappointing. The identification of membranous cytoplasmic bodies (MCBs), for example, may confirm the diagnosis of a storage disease but does not help identify a specific type of enzyme defect. On the other hand, the characteristic curvilinear or fingerprint bodies may help delineate specific, currently recognized categories of ceroid lipofuscinosis.

The clinical manifestations of lysosomal storage diseases are variable, although certain neurological signs may provide helpful clues to the presence of an inborn error of metabolism. Most of these diseases can interfere with normal brain development and produce developmental delay or mental retardation. Seizures, mental deficiency, and visual loss are frequently the major findings in so-called grey matter disease. In contrast, in the white matter diseases (leukodystrophies), ataxia, pyramidal tract signs, and peripheral neuropathy are more common.

The storage diseases have been divided into four large groups: lipidoses, mucopolysaccharidoses, mucolipidoses, and generalized glycogenoses. Although both metachromatic leukodystrophy (MLD) and Krabbe's disease are associated with a specific enzyme defect, for convenience in differential diagnosis they have been included under the heading of leukodystrophies.

Lipidoses

Sphingolipids are a group of hydrophobic compounds that, by definition, contain a sphingosine moiety. There are several specific types of sphingosines, but all are long, straight chain compounds containing hydroxyl groups on carbon atoms 1 and 3, and a subterminal amino group on carbon 2. In human nervous tissues most sphingosine is 18 carbons long and has a fatty acid bound to the amino group through an amide linkage forming the compound known as ceramide. The terminal hydroxyl is usually covalently linked to some other moiety (Fig. 8.1). Sphingomyelin is formed when phosphorylcholine is attached to ceramide; glycosphingolipids form a class of compounds that have at least one sugar attached to ceramide.

Several systems of nomenclature have been applied to glycosphingolipids. The simplest denotes the number of sugars extending from carbon 1 of ceramide (e.g., ceramide monohexoside (CMH), ceramide dihexoside (CDH) and ceramide trihexoside (CTH)). In addition, trivial names are commonly used in reference to some (e.g., cerebroside for CMH). Glycosphingolipids that contain a sulfate radical are referred to as sulfatides, and those with sialic acid

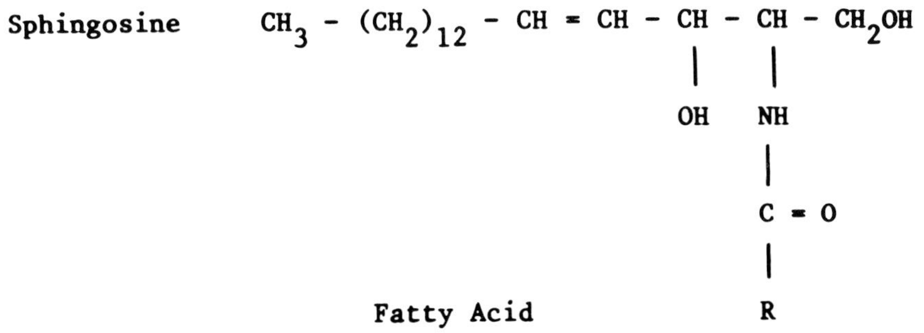

Sphingosine $CH_3 - (CH_2)_{12} - CH = CH - CH - CH - CH_2OH$

$$OH \quad NH$$

$$C = O$$

Fatty Acid   R

Figure 8.1.   Ceramide composed of sphingosine and a fatty acid (R). The latter is of variable chain length and sometimes hydroxylated.

attached to the oligosaccharide backbone are gangliosides.

The nomenclature system of Svennerholm (464) is most commonly used for gangliosides. The number of sialic acid groups per molecule is referred to by a letter or letters (M for mono; D for di; T for tri; Tet for tetra). The length of the parent oligosaccharide chain is referred to by a number. For example, the oligosaccharide glucose-galactose-N-acetylgalactosamine-galactose is designated as number 1, the oligosaccharide without the terminal galactose is 2, glucose-galactose is 3, and galactose alone is 4. The letters a and b refer to the sites of attachment to the oligosaccharide of the sialic acid groups when there is more than one (Table 8.1).

The oligosaccharide chains are synthesized by the addition of one carbohydrate group at a time (99). The first is added to ceramide to form cerebroside. Each reaction is catalyzed by a specific enzyme that transfers the carbohydrate from a nucleotide sugar to the appropriate acceptor. These enzymes are referred to as glycosyltransferases. The transferase reactions are similar to those involved in some biosynthetic reactions of glycoprotein synthesis. However, unlike glycoproteins, glycolipid oligosaccharide chains are not transferred directly to acceptors through dolichol-linked intermediates.

The catabolism of glycolipids also proceeds one sugar at a time but in the reverse direction (99). Specific glycosidase enzymes cleave the terminal sugar from the oligosaccharide chain. This progresses until ceramide is formed that in turn is split into fatty acid and sphingosine by the enzyme ceramidase. Many of the lipidoses are due

Table 8.1
Structure of Gangliosides

Ganglioside	Structure[a]
G_{M2}	Cer-glc-gal-GalNac and Glc
	NeuAc
G_{M1}	Cer-glc-gal-GalNac-gal
	NeuAc
G_{D1a}	Cer-glc-gal-GalNac and Glc-gal
	NeuAc NeuAc
G_{D1b}	Cer-glc-gal-GalNac and Glc-gal
	NeuAc
	NeuAc
G_{T1b}	Cer-glc-gal-GalNac and Glc-gal
	NeuAc NeuAc
	NeuAc

[a] Cer, ceramide (sphingosine + fatty acid); glc, glucose; gal, galactose; NeuAc, N-acetylneuraminic acid; GalNac, N-acetylgalactosamine.

to a deficiency of a specific glycosidase that results in the accumulation of its lipid substrate (Table 8.2).

GAUCHER'S DISEASE (GLUCOSYL CERAMIDE LIPIDOSIS)

In 1882, Gaucher (157) described a condition that he thought was a neoplasm of the spleen. It was later correctly identified as a storage disease with accumulation of glucosyl ceramide. Brady et al. (45) in 1965 demonstrated the deficient activity of splenic glucocerebrosidase responsible for this storage. Although the disorder has been classified into three general groups,

Table 8.2
Major Sphingolipidoses and Their Associated Enzyme Defects

Disease	Principal sphingolipid	Enzyme defect
Gaucher's	cer-| glc	β-Glucosidase
Niemann-Pick	cer-| pchol[a]	Sphingomyelinase
Krabbe's	cer-| gal	β-Galactosidase
Metachromatic leukodystrophy	cer-gal-| O-SO$_3$	Arylsulfatase A
Fabry's	cer-glc-| gal-gal	α-Galactosidase
Tay-Sachs	cer-glc-gal-| GalNac	Hexosaminidase A
Generalized gangliosidosis	cer-glc-gal-GalNac-| gal | NeuAc | NeuAc	β-Galactosidase

[a] pchol, phosphorylcholine.

there is a spectrum of clinical, morphological, and biochemical presentations, and overlap cases have occurred. All types appear to be inherited as an autosomal recessive trait and are panethnic, although ethnic preponderance does occur in some types.

Gaucher's disease, the most common sphingolipidosis, is diagnosed either by demonstrating deficient glucocerebrosidose activity in leukocytes, skin fibroblasts, or spleen, or by showing elevated levels of glucocerebroside in spleen, liver, or serum. Although levels of residual enzyme activity have been reported to correlate with the severity of the disease, this does not hold true for all cases (46, 147).

Type 1 (Chronic Nonneuronopathic or Adult Type)

The most common type of Gaucher's disease is the chronic nonneuronopathic or adult type, which occurs with a relatively high frequency in Ashkenazic Jews. These patients generally live to adulthood, often with few adverse effects of their disease, and free of neurological involvement. However, a few adult cases with neurological abnormalities have now been described (429). The abnormalities have been manifest as psychiatric behavioral disturbances, abnormalities of memory and mentation, myoclonus, asterixis, a Parkinsonian-like movement disorder, pyramidal tract signs, seizures, and abnormal extraocular movements. At least four patients have also had gliomas of the brain, but the significance of these is obscure (266).

Clinically, the disease may become apparent at any time between infancy and late adulthood, but most commonly it appears in the second decade. Splenomegaly is a frequent presentation; hypersplenism, hepatomegaly, microcytic anemia, thrombocytopenia, and thinning of the cortex of long bones may develop. Elevated serum levels of nontartrate-inhibitable acid phosphatase activity and Gaucher cells in the bone marrow help in diagnosis, but definitive diagnosis is made by demonstrating deficient glucocerebrosidase activity in leukocytes (46).

The brain is usually normal both grossly and microscopically. However, a few cases have perivascular cuffing, with mononuclear cells containing inclusions similar to Gaucher cells (429) (see below). In these rare cases, such cells are present throughout the central nervous system, but their relationship to the neurological abnormalities is unknown. Also, brain and liver have deficient glucocerebrosidase activities in such cases, but the lipid content of the brain was normal when studied (429).

The spleen is enlarged due to massive infiltration by Gaucher cells arranged in an alveolar fashion in the red pulp. These cells, which are of histiocytic origin, also infiltrate bone marrow, sinusoids of the liver, lymph nodes, and lungs.

The Gaucher cell is 20–100 μm in diameter and usually has one eccentric nucleus, although multinucleate forms can occur. With light microscopy, the cytoplasm has the appearance of "crinkled tissue paper" or "crumpled silk" (Fig. 8.2A). Rod-shaped cytoplasmic structures are visible with Nomarski interference microscopy. After dias-

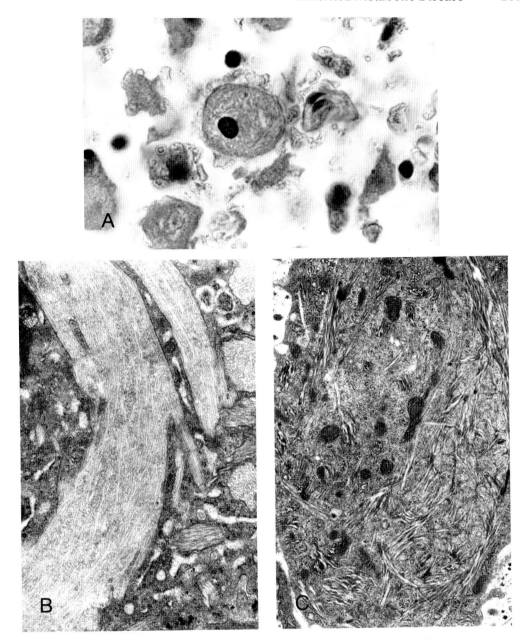

Figure 8.2. (A) A Gaucher cell from spleen showing the characteristic "crinkled tissue paper" appearance to its cytoplasm. Hemotoxylin and eosin (H&E). (Original magnification ×960.) (B and C) Galactocerebroside forming predominantly tubular structures in a liver biopsy sample, either as large aggregates (B) or as small bundles of twisted tubules (C). Electron micrograph. (B, Original magnification ×18,000; C, Original magnification × 14,000.) (Courtesy of Dr. E. Cutz.)

tase treatment, they remain positive with PAS. They sometimes stain positively for iron due to large amounts of ferritin, and for acid phosphatase. They are faintly positive with ORO and SBB and are faintly metachromatic with acidic cresyl violet (322). With scanning EM, the cell surface appears rough due to microvilli, ruffles, ridges, and blebs (112). With transmission EM, the membrane-bound cytoplasmic inclusions are rod-shaped structures with a right-hand twist. They are up to 5 μm in length and 12.75 nm in diameter (Fig. 8.2*B* and *C*). Freeze-fracture and X-ray diffraction studies have shown that the inclusions are solid and consist of series of bilayers, each about 6 nm thick (242). Chemically, they consist of 10% each of protein, cholesterol, and phospholipid, and 70% glycolipid, of which 90% is glucosylceramide (128). The major source of the stored glucosylceramide in spleen is from white and red blood cells.

Type 2 (Acute Neuronopathic or Infantile Type)

Although 10% of patients with acute neuronopathic or infantile type Gaucher's disease are abnormal at birth and a few have no problems until into the second year of life, most develop clinical abnormalities around 3 months of age. These usually consist of hepatosplenomegaly, feeding difficulties, and failure to thrive. Hypersplenism rarely occurs. At 6 months of age, neurological signs become evident, after which decline is rapid. During this phase the following occur: strabismus, dysphagia, neck rigidity, retroflexion of the head, spasticity with hyperreflexia and Babinski response, trismus, laryngeal stridor, and psychomotor regression. Serum acid phosphatase is high, and Gaucher cells are present in the bone marrow. Most patients do not live more than 2 yr, and death is usually due to pulmonary complications.

Pathological changes in the nervous system have been well described (29, 135, 322). The brain weighs less than normal, but externally there are no gross abnormalities. The cut surfaces show a thin cerebral cortex and atrophic basal ganglia with a sharp demarcation between cortex and white matter.

Neuronal cytoplasmic storage occurs predominantly in basal ganglia, thalamus, brain stem nuclei, Purkinje cells, and anterior horn cells of spinal cord, particularly in the larger neurons. The cytoplasm is only moderately distended and with PAS is positive. Staining with acidic cresyl violet shows metachromasia. Neuronophagia occurs in the same sites as neuronal storage. Neuronal loss is ubiquitous throughout the central nervous system (CNS), but is particularly noteworthy in layers 3 and 5 of the cerebral cortex and in the hippocampus,

and may be most severe in the dentate nuclei. Gaucher cells and smaller histiocytes with similar cytoplasmic staining properties occur mainly in the perivascular spaces of cerebral white and grey matter. They have also been seen lying free in layers 3 and 5 of the cerebral cortex. In addition to Gaucher cells, one case had a peculiar multifocal, astrocytic gliosis in the perivascular regions and arachnoid (245).

An electron microscopic study of cerebral cortex shows that some neurons have a prominent, dilated endoplasmic reticulum with anastomosing cisternae (2). Occasional membrane-bound inclusions similar to MCBs and zebra bodies are seen, but the typical inclusions of Gaucher's disease are extremely rare in cortical neurons. Several white matter tracts in brain stem become demyelinated (245), but the centrum ovale appears histologically normal. However, moderately low levels of cerebral galactocerebroside suggest that the myelin may be biochemically abnormal (149).

Some investigations have not found increased amounts of glucosylceramide in the brain (149), while others have found elevated levels of glucosylceramide and glucose-containing sulfatide (445) in grey and white matter. Svennerholm (463) found that in cerebrosides from the brain of a patient with infantile Gaucher's disease, two-thirds of the fatty acids were 18 carbons long. This is similar to cerebral gangliosides but different from extraneural cerebroside. Therefore, he suggested that the accumulated brain glucosylceramide was derived by cerebral ganglioside catabolism rather than from a hematogenous source. The biochemical mechanisms responsible for the cellular damage to neural cells are unknown. It does not appear that accumulating glucosylceramide is responsible. Indeed, data are still insufficient to consider it categorically as a "neuronal storage disorder." Perhaps glucosylsphingosine plays a similar role in this disorder as galactosylsphingosine does in Krabbe's disease according to the "psychosine hypothesis" of Suzuki et al. (457). The identification of glucosylsphingosine in spleen and liver from three types of Gaucher's disease supports this possibility (316).

The morphological abnormalities in spleen, liver, lymph nodes, and lung are similar to those seen in type 1. Abnormalities of bone are unusual in type 2.

Type 3 (Subacute Neuronopathic or Juvenile Type)

The most heterogeneous and least common type of Gaucher's disease is subacute neuronopathic or juvenile (type 3). Some of the younger cases in this category may be more closely related to type 2, and the older ones to type 1 patients with neurological involvement. The largest single group of type 3 patients has derived from northern Sweden, where a unique mutation is thought to have occurred several hundred years ago (120).

Age at onset varies from the first to the fourth decade, with splenomegaly being the most frequent initial sign. Patients can develop nonneurological disorders similar to type 1 patients with hepatomegaly, hypersplenism, deficiency of clotting factors, bony abnormalities, pingueculae, and pulmonary problems. Discrete white spots scattered throughout the retina have been described, but cherry red spots probably do not occur. Seizures and mental deterioration are the most common neurological abnormalities (317).

In addition, patients may have dysarthria, ataxia, myoclonus, extraocular movement disorders, trismus, laryngeal stridor, dysphagia, and pyramidal tract signs. Neurological deterioration may be accelerated by splenectomy (120, 316). The age at death has varied from late infancy to middle age.

Neurochemical and neuropathological findings have been similar to those reported for type 2. Some investigators have found elevated levels of glucosylceramide in the brain, while others have not. Morphological changes have also been variable but in general are similar to type 2 findings in the few studies available.

NIEMANN-PICK DISEASE

Niemann-Pick disease refers to a group of disorders first described in single cases clinically by Niemann (315) and morphologically by Pick (356). Klenk, in 1934 (230) demonstrated that sphingomyelin accumulates in this disorder. Detailed descriptions of 18 patients by Crocker and Farber (84) illustrated the clinical and pathological diversity within this group. The classification of patients with Niemann-Pick disease by Crocker (85) into four types, the basis of most subsequent classifications including that of Fredrickson and Sloan (147), will be used here.

Type A (Acute Neuronopathic Form)

Type A, the acute neuronopathic form, is most common and one of the best characterized forms of Niemann-Pick disease. It is an autosomal recessive disease with an increased incidence in the Jewish population. During the first 6 months of life, hepatosplenomegaly, generalized lymphadenopathy, vomiting, and failure to thrive develop in the affected child. Chest roentgenograms show a reticular-to-nodular infiltrate diffusely throughout the lung fields. Peripheral blood mononuclear cells have cytoplasmic vacuoles, and foamy histiocytes are seen in the bone marrow and cerebrospinal fluid (CSF) (72). Neurologic involvement is usually present by 1 yr of age with progressive dementia, pyramidal tract signs, and impaired hearing and vision. Cherry red spots are present in the fundi of about half the patients. Death usually occurs by 3 yr of age.

The characteristic biochemical feature of Niemann-Pick disease is accumulation of sphingomyelin, particularly in liver and spleen (20 times normal levels), cerebral grey matter (three times normal), and white matter (twice normal) (220). The first step in the catabolism of sphingomyelin is a hydrolysis reaction forming phosphocholine and ceramide. This is catalyzed by the enzyme sphingomyelinase. Brady et al. (44) first demonstrated that this enzyme is deficient in patients with type A Niemann-Pick disease. Assays for this enzyme activity in leukocytes can identify affected monozygotes as well as heterozygote carriers (153).

The brain usually is slightly atrophic, there may be severe cerebellar atrophy, and the white matter appears grossly normal (85). Microscopically, the neuronal cytoplasm is distended and stains positively with PAS, ORO, SBB, and LFB (Fig. 8.3A). Astrogliosis and histiocytosis are present throughout the grey matter, often particularly prominent in the cortical molecular layer and in the Purkinje cell layer of the

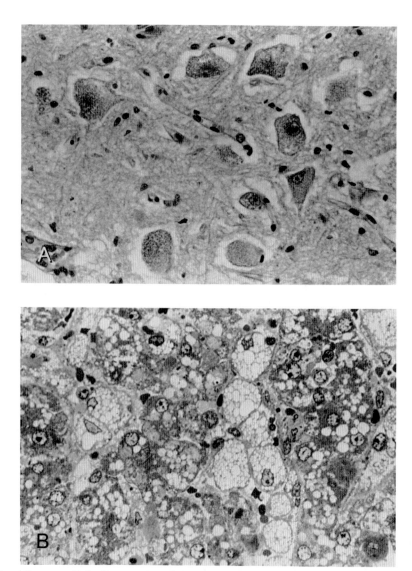

Figure 8.3. Niemann-Pick disease. (A) Thalamic neurons showing a moderate degree of cytoplasmic distension. LFB. (Original magnification ×380.) (B) Liver packed with lipid-laden phagocytic foam cells. H&E. (Original magnification ×240.)

cerebellum. Secondary to the neuronal damage, there is a varying degree of demyelination and associated astrogliosis. Both the arachnoid and choroid plexus are infiltrated with foamy histiocytes. Distended ganglion cells are found in the retina together with perivascular foamy histiocytes (327). In the peripheral nerve, demyelination and foamy histiocytes have been described (177). By electron microscopy, MCBs measuring 0.6–4 μm in diameter have been seen. The inclusions consist of multiple, concentric layers of membranous material with a periodicity of 4.5–5.5 nm (265).

Systemically, the characteristic histological feature is the foam cell, or Niemann-Pick cell (Fig. 8.3B), which has been found in most tissues of the body. Although not specific for Niemann-Pick disease, it is characteristic. It measures 20–90 μm in diameter and may be uni- or multinucleate, with 2–4 nuclei. The cytoplasm contains numerous small vacuoles or droplets that are birefringent in polarized light and fluoresce greenish-yellow in ultraviolet light. Enlargement of the spleen, liver, and lymph nodes is due to storage of sphingomyelin at those sites.

Type B (Chronic Nonneurologic Form)

Patients with type B (nonneurologic) Niemann-Pick disease develop hepatosplenomegaly within the first few years of life, followed by recurrent respiratory infections without any evidence of neurological involvement. Of particular interest is the finding of Wenger et al. (499) that the brain and liver of an affected 19-week-old fetus were completely lacking in lysosomal sphingomyelinase, unlike control samples. However, there was normal activity of a nonlysosomal sphingomyelinase in the brain. Possibly the presence of this enzyme explains the lack of neurological abnormalities in type B.

Type C (Chronic Neuronopathic Form)

Type C, the chronic neuronopathic form of Niemann-Pick disease, is a complex group probably consisting of several disease subtypes. In the five cases reported by Crocker and Farber (84), onset of clinical symptoms was in late infancy, with death occurring between 3 and 5 yr of age. There were psychomotor retardation and cherry red spots (one case) but no seizures. Patients with a similar history but a more protracted course (death occurring in the second or third decade) have also been reported (342). Characteristically, the older cases have hepatosplenomegaly and foamy histiocytes in the liver, spleen, lymph nodes, bone marrow, and lungs. Foamy histiocytes that stain sea blue with May-Grünwald-Giemsa and are autofluorescent with ultraviolet light have also been described in the bone marrow.

The basic biochemical defect is unknown. Results of total sphingomyelinase activity studies for several tissues have been variable, but generally close to normal. It is both reported and disputed that affected patients are deficient in an isoenzyme of sphingomyelinase that can be separated by isoelectric focusing (64). It has also been suggested that these patients lack a protein essential for activity of sphingomyelinase (74). Further evidence that the genetic and biochemical defects are similar in types A and B but not in type C comes from somatic cell hybridization studies (36).

On neuropathologic examination the brain is atrophic, and on coronal sections demyelination may be evident. Microscopically, a severe neuronal loss associated with astrogliosis primarily affecting the cerebral cortex is striking. The residual neurons have distended cytoplasm, and similar cells are also found in basal ganglia, brain stem, and spinal cord. The Purkinje cells usually are not distended.

The storage material is weakly positive with SBB and PAS, but does not stain with LFB. Astrogliosis has been described as more prominent in the marginal layer of the cerebral cortex than in the deeper layers (327). The molecular layer of the cerebellum is also astrogliotic and contains numerous histiocytes. Secondary demyelination is prominent and associated with dense astrogliosis. The brain stem shows relative preservation of myelin except for involvement of descending cortical spinal tracts and brachium conjunctivum cerebelli. No abnormalities of choroid plexus or leptomeninges are evident.

Ultrastructurally, Pellissier et al. (347) described multilamellar figures measuring 0.6 μm with a periodicity of 5.5 nm. They also described pleomorphic inclusions measuring 0.5–1.5 μm in diameter associated with a limiting membrane, concentric lamellae, and fine osmiophilic granules, together with small clear vacuoles that may represent lipofuscin. Sphingomyelin is only slightly increased in the liver and not elevated in either cerebral cortex or white matter (355). Gangliosides G_{M2} and G_{M3} are elevated in both grey and white matter.

Dystonic Juvenile Idiocy without Amaurosis. Another closely related group of disorders included in Crocker's type C is referred to as dystonic juvenile idiocy without amaurosis (131), adult neurovisceral lipidosis (500), juvenile dystonic lipidosis (259), and juvenile Niemann-Pick disease with vertical supranuclear ophthalmoplegia (53, 311). Age at onset has been from 5 yr through to the third decade of life. Some geographic clusters have been found, such as the Spanish-American group described by Wenger et al. (499) and the Nova Scotian group (see below). Some affected patients died in their early teens, while others survived to more than 40 yr of age.

Two neurological features are usually present in dystonic juvenile idiocy without amaurosis: voluntary vertical supranuclear ophthalmoplegia with preservation of involuntary vertical eye movements and various types of dystonic movements. Hepatosplenomegaly is also present. Two types of abnormal histiocytes have been described in the bone marrow. Type A cells have a large amount of vacuolated cytoplasm containing occasional erythrocytes and numerous inclusions that stain dark blue with May-Grünwald-Giemsa stain. They are weakly positive with PAS and SBB. They may be precursors of type B cells, which are smaller and contain small blue-grey granules that stain intensely with PAS and SBB (311).

Very little work has been done on the chemical composition of the brain in dystonic juvenile idiocy without amaurosis, but Norman et al. (327) found that levels of cholesterol and lecithin are increased in the cerebral cortex. In the spleen, elevated levels of total phospholipids, triglycerides, cerebroside, cholesterol, sphingomyelin, phosphatidylcholine, and lysobisphosphatidic acid have been described (222, 500).

The cerebrum is moderately and the cerebellum markedly atrophic (327). Cytoplasmic ballooning of the neurons is present throughout the neuraxis, but not all neurons are affected. Large axonal swellings are common. Astrogliosis is variable but not a prominent feature. Only occasional Purkinje cells and cells of the inferior olivary nucleus are affected.

The neuronal storage material varies in staining from region to region (199). Some parts are intensely positive with PAS and LFB, while others are not. White matter is frequently normal. Arachnoidal and choroid plexus cells are normal.

Ultrastructurally, the neurons contain a variety of inclusions. Membranous lamellar profiles may be either loosely arranged or more compact with the appearance of zebra bodies. The lucent lines are 1.7 nm, the dark lines 2.7 nm, and, when fused, the periodicity is about 5.5 nm (222). Dense amorphous and granular material is at the center of some of these lamellar profiles and contained within vacuoles. There is a tendency for a cell to accumulate mainly one form of inclusion (228). In one case neurons had neurofibrillary tangles composed of paired helical filaments (199).

Type D (Nova Scotia Variant)

Type D, the Nova Scotia variant of Niemann-Pick disease, is very similar to type C. In some cases the two types may be identical. However, type D is considered as a separate group because all of the patients are from families of Acadian stock, near Yarmouth, Nova Scotia, Canada. The disorder is inherited as an autosomal recessive trait, and most patients' families are derived from an Acadian who settled in that area in 1691 (373).

The affected individuals may be jaundiced and develop splenomegaly in infancy, but early development is usually normal. The onset of neurological abnormalities occurs during the first few years of life, with mental retardation and ataxia. Seizures, dysarthria, abnormal movements, tremors, paralysis of vertical gaze, and spasticity have all been reported to develop later. Death usually occurs in the second or third decade.

The bone marrow contains foamy histiocytes, and the cerebral cortex has shown a small increase of neutral glycolipid. Total ganglioside level in white matter has been described as slightly elevated, and total sphingomyelinase is elevated in liver and spleen but normal in brain, kidney, and leukocytes. A second sphingomyelinase active at pH 7.4 is said to be normal in brain (373). In the spleen, elevated levels of cholesterol, cholesterol esters, total phospholipids, sphingomyelin, and lysobisphosphatidic acid have been reported (373).

CNS neurons have ballooned cytoplasm (85), but further details of the neuropathology are lacking.

Type E (Adult Nonneuronopathic Form)

Type E Niemann-Pick disease patients may represent long-surviving patients with type B (148). They store sphingomyelin in spleen, liver, and bone marrow, but in the few cases described no neurological abnormalities have been noted.

OTHER SPHINGOLIPIDOSES

Fabry's Disease (Angiokeratoma Corporis Diffusum Universale or Hereditary Dystopic Lipidosis)

Fabry's disease is a rare, X-linked inherited disorder. Heterozygotes may be normal, but most have some attenuated clinical abnormalities. Frequently, the first clinical manifestation in hemizygotes is cutaneous angiectases in childhood, most prominently on the thighs and trunk below the umbilicus. Although a few patients have survived into the seventh decade, most die around 40 yr of age due to cardiovascular and renal disease secondary to lipid deposition (107).

The main clinical neurological abnormalities are pain and autonomic dysfunction. The origin of the pain, which is predominantly in the extremities, is uncertain. However, lipid accumulates in dorsal root ganglia, and myelinated peripheral nerve fibers are lost, two factors that may play a role in pain. Impaired autonomic function probably contributes to hypohidrosis and reduced saliva and tear formation, but glandular dysfunction due to lipid accumulation within the secretory apparatus may also be partially responsible (63, 150). Other symptoms due to autonomic dysfunction include postprandial indigestion, nausea, cramps, belching, gastric reflux, loose stools, flatus, and painful diarrhea. Because of cerebral vascular involvement, stroke syndromes also occur.

Fabry's disease is due to a generalized deficiency of α-galactosidase A activity. This enzyme normally cleaves terminal α-linked galactose from the glycolipids that accumulate in several tissues in this disorder. Ceramide trihexoside is the major accumulation product, but ceramide digalactoside and blood group B glycolipids are also elevated in some tissues.

Birefringent material in urine sediment or within blood vessels of a skin biopsy support the diagnosis of Fabry's disease, but definitive evidence is obtained only through biochemical studies. Elevated levels of ceramide trihexoside must be demonstrated in urine sediment, plasma and cultured fibroblasts. For prenatal diagnosis, deficient α-galactosidase A and B levels must be demonstrated in cultured amniotic fluid cells and the karyotype must be XY. Morphological and biochemical confirmation of the prenatal diagnosis in aborted fetuses has been obtained (322).

Abnormalities of cerebral vessels are similar to those elsewhere in the body (i.e., accumulation of lipid in endothelial, perithelial, and smooth muscle cells). In addition, hypertensive changes as a consequence of renal disease may occur. Cerebral aneurysms, thrombosis, and embolic and hemorrhagic episodes have all been reported (322).

Glycolipids also accumulate in the nervous system. The cytoplasm of affected neurons is swollen and appears foamy after paraffin embedding. Frozen sections of these cells are birefringent with polarized light and stain positively with ORO, SBB, and PAS (243, 370). Affected neurons appear to be well localized. Accumulation of these lipids has been found in the following: supraoptic and paraventricular nuclei; midline nucleus; substriatal grey, amygdaloid nucleus; presubiculum; fifth and sixth cortical layers of parahippocampus and inferior temporal gyrus; dorsal motor nucleus of the vagus; salivary nuclei; Edinger-Westphal nucleus; reticular formation of the pons and medulla; trigeminal ganglion; nonpigmented cells of substantia nigra; intermediolateral and intermedioventral (Onuf's nucleus) cell columns of spinal cord; dorsal root and sympathetic ganglia; and submucous and myenteric plexuses (370, 448, 469).

At the ultrastructural level (176), the cytoplasmic inclusions are similar to MCBs but mainly of parallel rather than concentric orientation together with lipid and poorly formed membranous material.

In the peripheral nerve some investigators have found an axonal loss, mainly in large fibers (148, 349), but others have reported the loss in small fibers (338).

Electron microscopy of peripheral nerve shows that the cytoplasm of fibroblasts and perineurial, endothelial, and perithelial cells contain lamellated inclusions up to 2 μm in diameter (338). The profiles are both parallel and concentric (45). Axonal swelling, axoplasmic rarefaction, and loss of organelles, as well as some segmental demyelination have been found, but Schwann cells are generally normal (62, 338, 349). Pleomorphic lipid inclusions have been seen in skeletal muscle fibers, endomysial capillaries, and fibroblasts, but no related clinical abnormalities have been observed (176).

Specific identification of the stored material by histochemical techniques is difficult, but Faraggiana et al. (137) found that two peroxidase-labeled lectins known to have affinity for α- and β-D-galactose were strongly reactive with the storage material on frozen sections. They also reported the occurrence of typical myelin-like inclusions in the transplanted kidney of one patient, an observation that remains unexplained.

Farber's Disease (Lipogranulomatosis)

Farber's disease is an extremely rare disorder in which ceramide accumulates in several different tissues. This accumulation is due to deficient activities of the enzyme that splits ceramide into sphingosine and free fatty acid (acylsphingosine deacylase or acid ceramidase). The deficit was first shown by Sugita et al. (446) in kidney and cerebellum. Clinical abnormalities appear in early infancy as a painful arthropathy of hands and feet. Subcutaneous nodules, nu-

tritional failure, psychomotor retardation, intermittent fever, and respiratory and swallowing problems subsequently develop (138). Most patients die before 2 yr of age, although longer survivals have occurred (122).

Diagnosis is confirmed by demonstrating deficient ceramidase activity in cultured skin fibroblasts (122). Prenatal detection of the disease in fetuses at risk is possible by determining ceramidase levels on cultured amniotic fluid cells (141). The characteristic histological abnormality in extraneural tissues is granuloma formation with variable proportions of spindle-shaped cells with foamy cytoplasm, a few lymphocytes, and collagen. With EM, the cytoplasmic inclusions appear as vacuoles filled with curvilinear bodies for which the name "Farber bodies" has been proposed (403). However, with this disorder, Farber bodies have not been found in the brain.

The main neuropathological finding is cytoplasmic accumulation of storage material in neurons of cerebellum, brain stem, anterior horn cell column, retina, dorsal root, and autonomic ganglia.

G_{M1} GANGLIOSIDOSIS

One group of disorders shares the common abnormality of an accumulation of G_{M1} ganglioside in nervous tissues. Until the nature of the accumulated material was chemically identified (170, 208, 328), cases were described under a variety of terms. It is now established that there are several different clinical patterns of this disorder (454) and that glycopeptides, neutral glycolipids, oligosaccharides, and glycosaminoglycans accumulate in both neural and extraneural tissues.

Biochemistry and Genetics

The accumulation of G_{M1} ganglioside, neutral glycolipids, glycosaminoglycans, and oligosaccharides occurs as a result of a very low activity of the enzyme G_{M1}-β-galactosidase-A, which catabolizes G_{M1} to G_{M2}. Presumably, it also catabolizes the other stored constituents, all of which have a terminal galactose. However, the oligosaccharides excreted in the urine of patients with type 1 differ from those excreted by patients with type 2 (337, 512).

Genetic complementation studies have

been performed by fusing cultured fibroblasts from patients with different phenotypic manifestations of G_{M1}-galactosidase deficiencies. On the basis of such studies, Bootsma and Galjaard (41) proposed that these patients should be subdivided into two groups. Group A (including types I and II) have defective G_{M1}-β-galactosidase as a result of a mutation in the allele coding for it. Group B patients have normal G_{M1}-β-galactosidase protein, but because of a mutation of another allele, they lack a cytoplasmic component essential for normal activity of the enzyme. Both of these abnormalities would be inherited as autosomal recessive traits.

This model is attractive, but Gravel et al. (172) emphasized that some patients with sialidosis are phenotypically very similar to those with G_{M1} gangliosidosis. Thus, it must be established with certainty that the group B patients do not have some other disorder, such as sialidosis, that is simply masquerading as G_{M1} gangliosidosis (see below). The finding of both types in one family provides further evidence that types 1 and 2 are allelic (139).

It would be reasonable to expect that the time of onset and severity of these disorders would correlate with the amount of enzyme activity measured by in vitro assays, but this has not been the case (392), probably due to the unphysiological nature of the assay conditions. However, Suzuki et al. (462) found a quantitative correlation between the radiolabeling patterns of gangliosides in cultured fibroblasts and the time of onset of the clinical disease.

Type 1 (Generalized G_{M1} Gangliosidosis)

The clinical abnormalities in type 1 G_{M1} gangliosidosis, often present from birth, are poor appetite, poor weight gain, hypotonia, and decreased activity. There is also frontal bossing, a depressed nasal bridge, low-set ears, hypertrophic gums, and hepatosplenomegaly. Cherry red spots in the macula occur in half of the patients (329). Psychomotor development is noticeably retarded by age 6 months. Bony abnormalities similar to Hurler's syndrome are apparent. Hyperreflexia, hyperacusia, and muscle weakness are also seen. Rapid deterioration oc-

curs during the 2nd year with blindness, deafness, decerebrate rigidity, and death.

The disorder is inherited as an autosomal recessive trait. In fetuses of 15–20 weeks, cells in the brain, dorsal root ganglia, and several extraneural tissues were vacuolated and contained abnormal cytoplasmic inclusions (218, 258). This demonstrates that the biochemical disorder is present and expressed before birth.

The brain is atrophic with narrowed gyri, dilated ventricles, and lighter-than-normal weight. By light microscopy, most of the surviving neurons of cerebral cortex, basal ganglia, cerebellum, thalamus, brain stem, and spinal cord have swollen cell bodies (451). Neuronal loss and astrogliosis are prominent. However, not all neurons are equally affected. Purkinje cells and neurons in the locus ceruleus may be only slightly abnormal. Even those that are markedly swollen may display variable staining with PAS, although with frozen sections, staining is more consistently positive. Axonal degeneration with myelin loss and astrogliosis is prominent in both centrum ovale and long tracts.

Electron microscopy of affected neurons shows that they contain a variety of inclusion bodies in the cytoplasm. MCBs similar to those found in other ganglioside storage diseases, varying in size between 0.5 and 3.0 μm, are the predominant findings. Glial cells contain myelin figures and lamellar material.

Liver, spleen, lymph nodes, bone marrow, lung, kidney, and colon all contain cells with foamy cytoplasm strongly positive with PAS after paraffin embedding. Clumps of these cells are present in germinal centers of the spleen and lymph nodes, in liver sinusoids, in colonic mucosa, and in alveolar spaces and septae of the lungs. The ganglion cells of the colon, rectum, and stomach are distended and contain PAS-positive granules in their cytoplasm.

Type 2 (Juvenile G_{M1} Gangliosidosis)

The onset of clinical abnormalities in type 2 (juvenile) G_{M1} gangliosidosis occurs around 1 yr of age with weakness, ataxia, and frequent falling (331). The fundi remain normal throughout the course of the illness. Facial features are generally normal, and there is no or only mild clinical hepatosplenomegaly. Subtle radiological changes indicative of dysostosis multiplex are present by 12 months of age. Clonic-tonic seizures may develop during the 2nd year, and mental and motor retardation become severe during the 3rd year of life. Recurrent infections are a problem and frequently lead to death between 3 and 7 yr of age, although some patients have lived considerably longer.

The brain is severely atrophic and may be only half the normal weight (161). The cerebral cortex and basal ganglia are small and the lateral ventricles markedly dilated. The cerebellum is only slightly atrophic. Microscopically there is extensive neuronal loss and gliosis throughout most of the cerebral cortex, deep nuclei, cerebellum, and spinal cord. The cytoplasm of remaining neurons is swollen and finely granular, with the histochemical staining characteristics of a glycolipid. The locus ceruleus, substantia nigra, cuneate nucleus, and nuclei of the inferior colliculi may be relatively spared. The neuronal inclusions are overwhelmingly MCBs similar to those of Tay-Sachs disease. There are also other lipid bodies with variously arranged lamellae.

There is slight to moderate hepatosplenomegaly, and lymph nodes are enlarged. The aortic and mitral valves are thickened and contain foamy histiocytes. Scattered throughout the kidney, liver, spleen, lymph nodes, and bone marrow are foamy histiocytes with histochemical characteristics of glycolipid.

Other Types

Several other much less common phenotypes of G_{M1} gangliosidosis have been described. Three cases are of particular interest. Ogino et al. (336) described a patient who clinically and pathologically was similar to type 2. Although G_{M1} ganglioside was stored in the parietal and occipital lobes, the frontal lobes had a normal ganglioside composition. Goldman et al. (168) reported a case of a male who died at 27 yr of age after a 23-year history of progressive dystonia. G_{M1} ganglioside was stored predominantly in the neurons of the basal ganglia, dysfunction of which was probably responsible for the movement disorder. Lowden et al. (262) described a patient with

type 2 G_{M1} gangliosidosis who died at 17 yr of age. At autopsy, there was striking neuronal accumulation of ceroid lipofuscin. They emphasized that there may be a host of rare variants in this group of disorders. These cases also demonstrate that different sets of neurons may be differently affected by a specific abnormality of a lysosomal enzyme like G_{M1}-β-galactosidase.

G_{M2} GANGLIOSIDOSES

Tay-Sachs disease was first described more than a century ago as a condition involving progressive mental and motor deterioration with onset in infancy and fatal outcome in early childhood. The ballooned neurons suggested lipid storage, which was confirmed in 1962 when Svennerholm (466) identified the storage material as a G_{M2} ganglioside. Since then other variants of G_{M2} gangliosidosis have been described, prompting considerable research interest centering on the gangliosides (139).

In general terms, G_{M2} ganglioside has a ceramide backbone to which are linked glucose, galactose, N-acetylgalactosamine, and N-acetylneuraminic acid according to the sequence shown in Figure 8.1. G_{M2} ganglioside is catabolized to G_{M3} by the enzymatic removal of N-acetylgalactosamine from the nonreducing end of the oligosaccharide. An enzyme that catalyzes a reaction of this type is called N-acetyl-β-D-hexosaminidase, of which several have been described. In man there are three lysosomal hexosaminidases (A, B, and S). Each is a dimer (i.e., is composed of two subunits), and each subunit monomer is composed of two covalently linked polypeptide chains. There are two types of polypeptides, designated α and β. Hexosaminidase A has two different subunits; one is composed of two α polypeptides ($\alpha2$), and the other of two β polypeptides ($\beta2$). Hence, it is a heteropolymer designated $\alpha2\beta2$. Hexosaminidase B is a homopolymer composed entirely of β polypeptides ($\beta2\beta2$), and hexosaminidase S, a minor component, is an α homopolymer ($\alpha2\alpha2$). Normal brain contains both major isoenzymes (A and B), but there are several disease conditions in which G_{M2} is stored due to a deficiency of one or both major enzymes.

These disorders are named according to the isoenzyme that remains. Thus, Tay-

Sachs disease, which is deficient in hexosaminidase A, is called "variant B." Sandhoff disease is called "variant O" because both isoenzymes are deficient. "Variant AB" has no endogenous hexosaminidase activity, but both enzymes are present. It is caused by the absence of an activator substance, possibly a protein (247) required for the breakdown of G_{M2}. (See Sandhoff and Christomanou (392) for an excellent review.) There are several other rare variants, and a comprehensive system of classification based on biochemical, genetic, and clinical criteria has been suggested (333).

Hexosaminidase deficiencies have also been described in several other disorders, but the role of the defect in the pathogenesis of these diseases is still uncertain. They include Ramsay Hunt's syndrome, Friedreich's ataxia, olivopontocerebellar ataxia, Menzel ataxia, Holmes ataxia, rare cases of motor neuron disease, and other miscellaneous disorders (215).

Tay-Sachs Disease

In Tay-Sachs disease (variant B), there is a marked accumulation of G_{M2} ganglioside in brain. However, there are also elevated levels of several other glycolipids and glycoproteins with N-acetylgalactosamine at the nonreducing end of the oligosaccharide (59, 206, 207).

Tay-Sachs disease is an autosomal recessive condition occurring mainly in Jewish children. Affected infants are normal at birth, but within 2 months hyperacusis (i.e., an exaggerated motor response to sound), one of the first manifestations of the disease, occurs. This is followed by axial hypotonia, and delay or regression of psychomotor development (404). Bilateral cherry red spots of the macula can appear by 2.5 months of age. This appearance is due to the contrast between the red spot at the macula, where the vascular choroid appears through the thinned retina, and the grey appearance of the surrounding fundus due to lipid storage and degeneration of the ganglion cells. This is not specific for Tay-Sachs disease. Cherry red spots also occur in G_{M1} gangliosidosis type 1, Niemann-Pick disease, late infantile MLD, Farber's disease, mucolipidosis I, and cherry-red-spot

myoclonus syndrome (sialidosis type I). Between 6 and 12 months of age, purposeful movements and spontaneous vocalization decrease, and there is a vacuous facial expression. The previously normal-sized head may become megacephalic (105), and seizures, spasticity, corticospinal tract signs, blindness, dementia, and cachexia develop. Death usually occurs within 3 to 5 yr of onset.

The size of the brain is somewhat variable, depending on the stage of the disease. In some cases, megaloencephaly occurs late in the course of the disease and is thought to be due to extensive neuronal storage and astrogliosis (479). In other cases, the brain becomes atrophic due to loss of neurons and demyelination. On coronal sectioning, the cortical ribbon is narrowed, and the margin between grey and white matter is blurred. The centrum ovale is often severely demyelinated (Fig. 8.4A). The optic nerves and cerebellum are atrophic.

Microscopically, the main abnormality is the distended cytoplasm and displaced nucleus of all neurons, particularly the largest ones (Fig. 8.4B). The material in the cytoplasm is characteristic of glycolipid (positive ORO, SBB, PAS, and LFB). In some cases, autofluorescence has been described, attributed to lipofuscin accumulation (451). With time, the neurons degenerate, and astrocytic and histiocytic reactions develop, leading to disruption of cortical cytoarchitecture. Secondary to the axonal degeneration, the myelin breaks down, often giving the brain a dramatic demyelinated and cystic appearance. In the cerebellum, Purkinje cells develop ballooned cytoplasm with antler-like distension of their swollen dendrites and torpedo-like formation of their axons. The degeneration is accompanied by progressive loss of myelin and astrogliosis. In the spinal cord, the anterior horn cells are most affected, with prominent cytoplasmic distension. There is also descending degeneration of the corticospinal tract. Neurons of autonomic ganglia and axons of peripheral nerve contain storage material (306). There is a progressive loss of ganglion cells from the retina, especially in the margins of the fovea; the remaining ganglion cells are swollen with storage material. The nerve fiber layer is thin and the optic nerve atrophic. Amacrine cells store

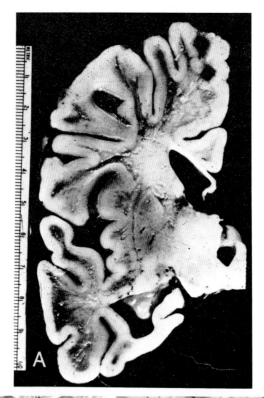

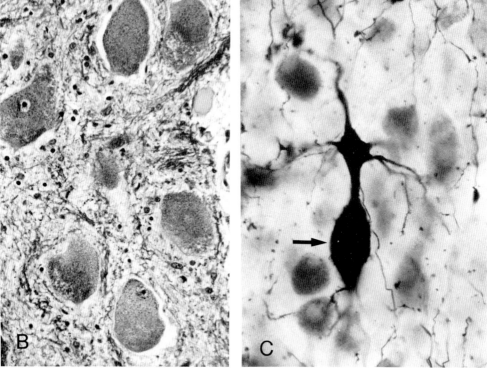

Figure 8.4. Tay-Sachs disease. (*A*) A coronal section showing prominent secondary demyelination and early cavitation from severe neuronal and axonal loss. (*B*) Anterior horn cells showing cytoplasmic distension from accumulated ganglioside with peripheral nuclear displacement. LFB. (Original magnification ×380.) (*C*) Neuron with a meganeurite (*arrow*) in the preaxonal segment. Rapid Golgi method. (Original magnification ×640.)

ganglioside, but rods, cones, and pigmentary epithelium are spared (306).

Golgi impregnations of pyramidal neurons have revealed the presence of a large neuronal process, called a meganeurite by Purpura and Suzuki (368), interposed between the cell body and axon (Figs. 8.4C and 8.5). Meganeurites, probably the torpedo-like swellings seen in conventional histological preparations, may contain spines.

The ultrastructural appearance of the storage material in Tay-Sachs disease is not diagnostic and tends to be variable in appearance. The classical MCB described in detail by Terry and Weiss (479) is a membrane-bound, oval-to-round structure measuring 0.5–2.0 μm in diameter. Most often, these structures contain electron-dense membranes arranged concentrically (Fig. 8.6A). Dense layers (2.5–3.0 nm) alternate with clear spaces (2.6 nm) for a periodicity of 5–6 nm. Some other common varieties of inclusion are a parallel arrangement of dense membranes (Fig. 8.6B), an accumulation of amorphous granular material, and large aggregates of pleomorphic lamellae. The meganeurites seen at an ultrastructural level contain large numbers of MCBs. Some of the spines on the surface of the meganeurites have postsynaptic elements in contact with presynaptic processes containing synaptic vesicles (368).

Evidence of neuronal storage in the fetus with demonstration of MCBs was seen in neurons of spinal ganglia, spinal cord, and cerebellum (92).

Visceral tissues show no major morphological abnormality, but elevated ganglioside levels (130) have been detected in several extraneural tissues and inclusion bodies described in liver (492).

Sandhoff Disease

Sandhoff et al. (391) first described the disorder in which there is an accumulation of G_{M2}, globoside (460), and several oligosaccharides in both neural and extraneural tissues (312, 442, 481). The primary defect is a total deficiency of hexosaminidase A and B. As a consequence, all of the materials stored have either N-acetylglucosamine or N-acetylgalactosamine at the nonreducing end of the oligosaccharide.

The clinical course is very similar to that of Tay-Sachs disease and includes the early development of cherry red macular spots and macrocephaly after 12 months of age. Sandhoff disease is inherited as an autosomal recessive disorder and occurs most frequently in non-Jewish families.

The cerebrum may be slightly enlarged and the cerebellum small, but frequently both brain and visceral organs appear grossly normal. Microscopically the cytoplasm of neurons in both central and peripheral nervous systems (including Auerbach's and Meissner's plexuses) is distended with storage material. Vacuolated histiocytes are present in lung, spleen, lymph nodes, thymus, and bone marrow (339). Cytoplasmic vacuolation of nonneural parenchymal cells also occurs. Dolman et al. (115) emphasized the marked vacuolation of pancreatic acinar cells. In general, the histochemical properties of the storage material are similar to those in Tay-Sachs disease.

Electron microscopy shows that most of the storage material in neurons is structurally similar to the MCBs of Tay-Sachs disease. Not surprisingly, the shape and form of the lamellae are variable; both concentric and parallel (zebra body) forms are described (115, 182, 476). Similar structures are also found in many nonneural cells. By light microscopy, only the ganglion cells of the retina appear distended with storage material. However, EM shows that MCBs, zebra bodies, and small vesicles occur in ganglion cells, inner and outer nuclear layers, endothelial cells, and pericytes (57).

Variant AB

The rare variant AB is so named because hexosaminidase A and B are both biochemically normal but G_{M2} ganglioside accumulates in the nervous system (80). Conzelmann and Sandhoff (79) found that the failure of G_{M2} catabolism is due to the deficiency of a soluble activator that promotes the interaction of hexosaminidase A with lipid substrates. Very few cases of this disorder have been reported, but there is no apparent ethnic predisposition. The clinical course is similar to that of variant B, although the time of onset and death may be a little later, and cerebellar dysfunction may be a little more prominent in variant AB.

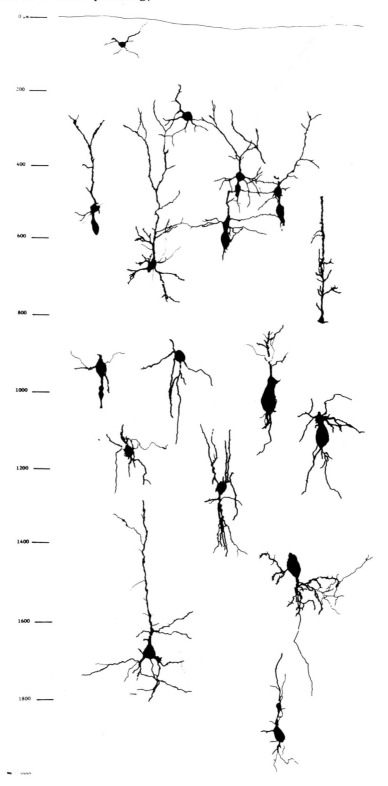

Figure 8.5. Composite camera lucida drawing from the visual cortex of a patient with Tay-Sachs disease showing numerous neurons with prominent meganeurites.

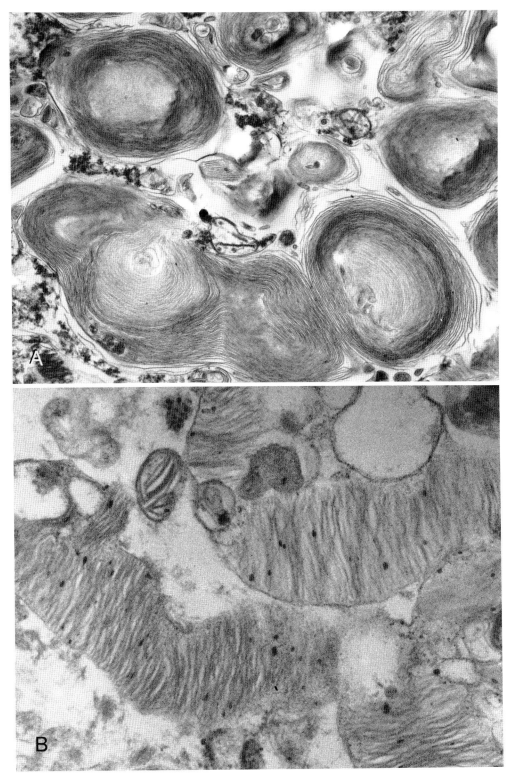

Figure 8.6. Tay-Sachs disease. (*A*) Concentric lamellar MCBs in the cytoplasm of cortical neurons. Electron micrograph. (Original magnification ×12,000.) (*B*) Parallel lamellar arrays (zebra bodies) in the cytoplasm of cortical neurons. Electron micrograph. (Original magnification ×12,000.)

Grossly the brain is either normal or slightly atrophic, but visceral organs are normal. Light microscopy demonstrates widespread neuronal storage of material, although some areas are more involved than others. The retinal macular ganglion cells are swollen, but visceral organs are not involved. With Golgi staining meganeurites with spiny processes are seen on neurons. EM shows that cytoplasm of both neurons and astrocytes contains MCBs, zebra bodies, and pleomorphic lipid bodies (168). The cerebral cortex has elevated levels of ganglioside, most of which is G_{M2}. GA2 (asialo G_{M2}), lactosylceramide, and glucosylceramide levels are also increased in brain. Serum, leukocyte, fibroblast, and cerebral cortex all have normal activities of N-acetylglucosaminidase.

Other Rare Variants

A few cases of late infantile (onset of neurological abnormalities between 2 and 4 yr of age) and juvenile (onset after 4 yr) G_{M2} gangliosidosis have been reported (54, 330). It is still not certain whether they should be considered two distinctly separate disease entities. There is no ethnic predisposition in either category. The clinical course in the late infantile cases is one of progressive dementia, ataxia, and seizures. A peculiar cherry red macular change is occasionally present. Seizures are not always seen in the juvenile patients, who may also have normal vision and fundi. Hyperacusis, hyperactive deep tendon reflexes, and cerebellar disturbances may occur. There is no organomegaly.

Morphological abnormalities are similar in both types. The brain is slightly atrophic. The neurons contain MCBs, zebra bodies, lipofuscin, and fingerprint-like profiles (296, 456). There are elevated levels of G_{M2} ganglioside in the cerebral cortex, liver, and spleen. Hexosaminidase A levels measured with artificial substrates and detergents are markedly decreased in some, but only partially decreased in others.

G_{M2} gangliosidosis has also been reported in adults. Most have been Jewish (374, 505), but one was not (340). Although neurological abnormalities appeared early in some, progression was very slow. Intellectual function may be affected, but the dominant clinical feature is progressive involvement of motor function. Spinocerebellar dysfunction is the most common manifestation, but peripheral neuropathies also occur. Hexosaminidase A levels in plasma, leukocytes, and tears are low.

The cerebrum may be slightly small, but the cerebellum is notably atrophic. Cortical neurons contain PAS- and ORO-positive granules, but few are ballooned. Subcortical neurons are most severely affected and have granules that stain positively for PAS and LFB. There are cerebellar losses of both Purkinje and granule cells. MCBs, zebra bodies, and membranovesicular bodies occur in all types of neurons, but lipofuscin is present only in the inferior olivary nucleus (374).

G_{M3} GANGLIOSIDOSIS

One case has been reported of a ganglioside metabolism disorder in which G_{M3} is the only ganglioside present in brain and liver. This has also been referred to as G_{M3} (hematoside) sphingolipodystrophy and anabolic sphingolipidosis type G_{M3}. The Jewish male patient reported in detail by Tanaka et al. (473) had seizures, delayed motor development, macroglossia, gingival hyperplasia, hypoplastic mandible, broad hands and feet, loose, coarse, hirsute skin, and bilateral inguinal hernias at 1 month of age. Fundi were normal. The child died at 14 weeks of age.

Thin-layer chromatography of the ganglioside fraction from the sample of brain obtained at autopsy showed a marked increase in G_{M3} with almost complete absence of G_{M1} and G_{M2}. G_{M3} was markedly increased in the liver. G_{M3} sialidase activity in brain and liver was normal, but G_{M3}-UDP-N-acetylgalactosaminyl transferase was completely absent. On this basis, it was suggested that the basic defect was an inability to synthesize gangliosides with oligosaccharides more complex than G_{M3} (473). This is of some interest because the suggested enzyme defect may be in an anabolic pathway, in contrast to the other storage diseases where the defect is in catabolic enzymes.

The child's brain was slightly large for age but had a normal gyral pattern. Histologically, myelinated areas were extensively vacuolated, most noticeably in the cerebral subcortical areas, globus pallidus, and brain stem; the optic nerves and spinal cord were less involved. Alzheimer type II astrocytes were also present. Ultrastructurally, the vacuoles were due to wide spaces between myelin lamellae and swollen astrocytic processes. No MCBs were seen. The neurons were normal in size and staining properties and showed no evidence of storage substances within them.

NEURONAL CEROID LIPOFUSCINOSIS

An age-related cytoplasmic pigment has been known to exist in neurons for almost 100 yr (236). It was named lipofuscin because of its dark appearance and lipid characteristics (204). The term ceroid was initially used to describe a pigment in cirrhotic rat livers (252) and also has been used in reference to the material that accumulates in several neuronal storage diseases (418).

The subcellular origins of lipofuscin and ceroid are not definitely established, but they are probably derived from several different organelles including mitochondria, lysosomes, and Golgi membranes (163). Evidence for this is the presence of lysosomal- and mitochondrial-enzyme activities demonstrated both biochemically and histochemically. Lipofuscin and ceroid are chemically complex and consist of lipids, amino acids, and an autofluorescent insoluble polymeric substance (477). The lipids include phospholipids, cholesterol, cholesteryl esters, and dolichols (508). The chemical nature of the insoluble residue is uncertain and still under active investigation. These pigments have been studied with numerous histochemical stains (201); the two most commonly used are PAS and neutral lipid stains. Ceroid and lipofuscin both give a green autofluorescence under ultraviolet light with an excitation wavelength near 350 nm.

The biological roles of ceroid and lipofuscin are not known. The association of massive accumulation of ceroid with severe neurological dysfunction suggests that it may have adverse consequences on neuronal function. Deleterious effects of neuronal lipofuscin accumulation in the elderly are still speculative (119).

The term neuronal ceroid lipofuscinosis (NCL) was used by Zeman and his colleagues (517, 518) to distinguish a group of familial cerebromacular degenerations distinctive clinically and pathologically from the gangliosidoses. In the early literature, ganglioside storage diseases were included with the NCL under the heading amaurotic familial idiocy. More recently, there has been a tendency to refer to the genetic subtypes of NCL by eponymic designation. Although Crome and Stern (90) used the term "Batten's" disease to cover the whole group of NCLs, we prefer to recognize four main syndromes. On the basis of age at onset, clinical course, and pathology, these forms are referred to as Haltia-Santavuori disease (infantile), Jansky-Bielschowsky disease (late infantile), Batten-Spielmeyer-Vogt disease (late juvenile), and Kufs' disease (adult).

Diagnosis still depends mainly on electron microscopic examination of lymphocytes (30, 114, 116, 272, 319, 408), skin (19, 20, 114, 140, 278) or conjunctival (19, 20, 511) biopsies, although rectal, sural nerve, muscle (69) and brain (169) biopsies have been used. The storage material is reasonably characteristic for each clinical type and is found within lysosomal-like bodies in neurons and retina as well as in many extraneural tissues (240), such as the anterior pituitary, pancreas, thyroid gland, sweat gland, adrenal gland, smooth muscle, distal convoluted tubules of the kidney, and histiocytes. With Romanowsky's stains, bone marrow histiocytes contain bright blue granules and qualify as sea-blue histiocytes (152).

Wolfe and his collaborators (313, 509) found that dolichols comprise a significant proportion of the lipids in the storage cytosomes isolated from brains of patients with infantile, late infantile, and juvenile neuronal ceroid lipofuscinosis. Elevated dolichol levels also occurred in cerebral cortex and urinary sediment of these same disorders (509). Therefore, measurement of dolichol levels may be a useful diagnostic test in this group of diseases. While the basic defect is unknown, they speculate that it may be in the Golgi membranes and related organelles where dolichols are involved in glycoprotein synthesis. It is interesting that dolichol levels in cerebral cortex progressively increase with age in both humans and rats (313). However, the biological significance of this is not clear.

Haltia-Santavuori Disease (Infantile)

The Haltia-Santavuori infantile form of neuronal ceroid lipofuscinosis was described in Finland by Santavuori et al. (393, 394) and Haltia et al. (188). They described 15 cases of the infantile NCL characterized by a clinical onset before 2 yr of age and a rapid course. Psychomotor deterioration, ataxia, hypotonia, microcephaly, and myoclonic jerks were prominent features. Seizures were infrequent or did not occur at all. There was blindness by 2 yr of age, with optic atrophy and brownish discoloration of the macula on funduscopic examination.

Histologically, these cases are characterized by severe neuronal loss and distension of residual neurons by granular material. However, no true cytoplasmic ballooning is seen. In some neuronal perikarya, distinct homogeneous cytoplasmic inclusions are present, with staining characteristics as described above. Often the inclusions are surrounded or indented by a vacuole. Between the cortical neurons are fields of phagocytes containing coarse granules and two or even three nuclei. There is a very prominent astrogliosis with hypertrophic astrocytes containing coarse, thick glial processes and granules similar to those of the neurons.

In the youngest patients, the myelin is fairly well preserved in the subcortical arcuate fibers, although astrogliosis is recognized. In the older patients, a striking axonal loss and demyelination are present, together with astrogliosis. The arcuate fibers are not spared. In the basal ganglia and brain stem the nerve cells are swollen, with cytoplasm containing large amounts of granular storage material. In addition, large numbers of histiocytes are present. In the cerebellum all the Purkinje as well as granular cells have disappeared and are replaced by hypertrophic Bergmann's glia and scattered histiocytes. Storage material in the nerve cells, histiocytes, and astrocytes are resistant to lipid solvents including chloroform methanol. Unstained sections show apple green autofluorescence in ultraviolet light. The granules are acid-fast and strongly PAS-positive and stain intensely black with SBB and LFB. Acid phosphatase activity is demonstrated in the granules.

On electron microscopy, the most prominent finding is the presence of electron-dense storage material in the cytoplasm of neurons as well as histiocytes, astrocytes, endothelial and perithelial cells. The deposits vary in shape and size, the average round or oval inclusion measuring 0.1–0.5 μm in diameter. On higher magnification, deposits sometimes have a concentric laminar appearance with lines about 8.5 nm thick. None of the cytosomes has curvilinear profiles or fingerprint patterns. The distinctive pathology is that of severe neuronal destruction with massive accumulation of histiocytes, some of which are multinucleated, and intense fibrillary astrogliosis associated ultrastructurally with uniform granular storage material. In the retina, there is a complete loss of ganglion and bipolar cells with demyelination of the optic nerve (393).

Jansky-Bielschowsky Disease (Late Infantile)

Jansky-Bielschowsky NCL is an autosomal recessive disorder with onset between 2 and 5 yr characterized by generalized seizures, myoclonic jerks, ataxia, spasticity, and mental deterioration. Blindness is common, and funduscopically there is macular degeneration with "rings" of pallor associated with hyperpigmentation (517).

The brain, especially the cerebellum, is atrophic. Microscopically, there is severe loss of neurons and isomorphous gliosis in the cerebellum, with preserved neurons in cerebral cortex, basal ganglia, and brain stem. The residual neurons are minimally or moderately distended by granular material that stains positively with SBB, PAS, LFB, and Ziehl-Neelsen. The granular material within the cytoplasm demonstrates green autofluorescence with ultraviolet light (Fig. 8.7). Status spongiosus of the forebrain cortex attributed to seizure-induced anoxia-ischemia has been described. Myelin loss and astrogliosis are proportional to the degree of neuronal loss. Although glial cells contain sparse amounts of ceroid lipofuscin, endothelial cells and visceral organs contain easily identified ceroid lipofuscin (113, 171, 412).

Golgi impregnation studies identify a fusiform enlargement of the proximal axon segments of most pyramidal neurons. The

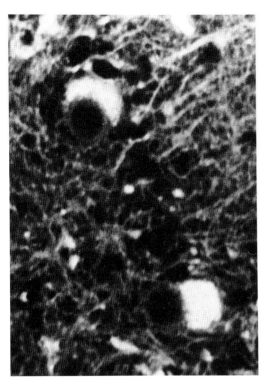

Figure 8.7. Autofluorescence of neuronal cytoplasmic lipofuscin in a patient with Jansky-Bielschowsky disease. Autofluorescence. (Original magnification ×380.)

pyramidal neurons, however, have a good complement of spines that appear to have normal morphology. Synapses on the axon hillock and dilated proximal axon segments of pyramidal neurons have been described as much reduced in number (503).

Ultrastructurally, the neuronal inclusions may be membrane-bound and irregularly contoured and may contain arciform, lamellar structures called curvilinear bodies (Fig. 8.8A), ranging from 0.2–1.0 μm in diameter. These bodies are composed of aggregates of curvilinear profiles, sometimes forming complete circles or arranged parallel to one another, producing a tubular appearance. Fingerprint-like profiles and osmiophilic granular bodies may also be identified in some cells in some cases (16, 121). The retina shows loss of rods and cones, with preservation of the outer nuclear layer. Some ganglion cells contain ceroid lipofuscin, and others are degenerated, accounting for the optic nerve atrophy.

Batten-Spielmeyer-Vogt Disease (Late Juvenile)

Batten-Spielmeyer-Vogt NCL is an autosomal recessive disease that usually begins between 5 and 10 yr of age. A decrease in visual acuity leading to blindness is usually the first sign, followed several years later by mental deterioration, dysarthria, seizures, and myoclonic jerking. After several more years, motor dysfunction occurs in the form of generalized extrapyramidal rigidity, weakness, or spasticity (142). Brain atrophy tends to be relatively mild.

The neurons are mildly to moderately distended by ceroid lipofuscin. Cerebellar granule cells are sometimes severely reduced (514). Ultrastructurally, the neuronal intracytoplasmic bodies are 1–4 μm in diameter, enclosed by a unit membrane and composed of gently curved laminar profiles called fingerprint bodies (Fig. 8.8B). The fingerprint pattern is due to a series of closely packed, paired, dense membranes each separated from the next by a clear space. The dense line measures about 2.7 nm in thickness, and the clear zone within the pairs measures 1.4–2.0 nm. The space between the pairs is 2.5 nm (453). The lysosomal origin of the inclusions is suggested by the many intermediate forms from lysosomes to fingerprint-bearing inclusions and the positive acid phosphatase they contain. Other cell constituents were not abnormal. Zeman and Donahue (515) say that curvilinear and granular bodies may also be found in this type.

In the retina, the ganglion cell layer and the optic nerve are well preserved, but the neurons contain ceroid lipofuscin. The entire neuroepithelium including the outer nuclear layer is destroyed, leading to a fusion of the pigmented epithelial layer and the membrana limitans (165).

Kufs' Disease (Adult)

The adult form of NCL is more variable. Its onset is in adulthood, usually with choreoathetosis or myoclonus. Mental deterioration may be slight or absent, and there are no seizures or retinal changes. Some cases are familial. One report of four generations being affected suggests a dominant pattern of transmission (40).

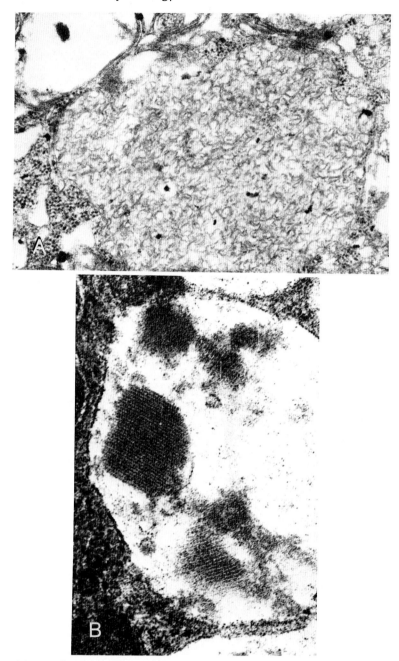

Figure 8.8. (A) Curvilinear profiles in the cytoplasm of a neuron from a brain biopsy of a patient with Jansky-Bielschowsky disease. Electron micrograph. (Original magnification ×63,700.) (B) Fingerprint-like body in the cytoplasm of lymphocyte from a patient with Batten-Spielmeyer-Vogt disease. Electron micrograph. (Original magnification ×94,000.) (Courtesy of Dr. C. L. Dolman.)

Atrophy of the brain is moderate. Nerve cell loss and accumulation of ceroid lipofuscin tends to be somewhat focal. A partial loss of cerebellar granule cells with preservation of Purkinje cells has been reported

(40, 144). Golgi studies have demonstrated enlarged axon hillocks with an absence of synaptic boutons on these swellings (143).

Ultrastructurally, the neurons contain bodies with coarse granular material associated with vacuoles. Chou and Thompson (73) used the terms lypofuscin-lipid compound body (0.5–1.2 μm) and miniature MCBs (0.2–0.3 μm) to describe the cytoplasmic inclusions they found most commonly.

No retinal lesions have been described in Kufs' disease.

Pigment Variant. A pigment variant is the term suggested by Seitelberger and Simma (411) to describe a form of cerebral ceroid lipofuscinosis with mental and neurologic deterioration, including myoclonus associated pathologically with ceroid lipofuscin and extraneuronal pigment. Although axonal spheroids are absent, a resemblance to Hallervorden-Spatz disease was suggested because of the heavy pigmentation in the zona reticularis of substantia nigra and globus pallidus. Yellow-brown pigmentation was also present in the outer layers of the cortex and leptomeninges. The nature of the extraneuronal pigment is unknown, since it has never been isolated and biochemically characterized (198).

OTHER DISORDERS INVOLVING LIPIDS

Cerebrotendinous Xanthomatosis

Cerebrotendinous xanthomatosis is a rare, autosomal recessive disease beginning in late childhood, characterized by slowly progressive dementia and cerebellar ataxia. Bilateral pyramidal tract signs, pseudobulbar palsy, cataracts, and xanthomas of tendons and lungs appear later, as the disease progresses (485). A hydroxylase defect in the synthesis of bile acid results in a decreased bile acid pool with subsequent cholesterol overproduction (389). Only part of the excess cholesterol is converted into bile acids. The rest is deposited in tissues, and some is converted to dihydrocholesterol (cholestanol). Serum cholesterol levels are normal, but cholestanol concentrations in brain, plasma, and tendon (295) are elevated.

In the case report of the autopsy findings reported by Schimschock et al. (399) gross examination of the brain revealed mild atrophy of frontal lobes and cerebellar folia. No atherosclerotic involvement of vessels at the base of the brain was found. Coronal sections did not suggest any abnormality except for the yellow, softened areas of cerebellar white matter.

Microscopically, two patterns of pathology occur: xanthomatous reaction and demyelination. The xanthomatous formation is characterized by multinucleated giant cells and foamy macrophages associated with necrosis, cystic spaces, and needle-like clefts representing the deposition of cholestanol. Crystalline deposits were sometimes seen within astrocytes. An intense foreign body reaction occurred most prominantly in the cerebellum and to a lesser degree in the upper brain stem.

The demyelination that occurs in this disease is less easily explained. Perhaps because the cholesterol in myelin is replaced by cholestanol, the myelin becomes unstable and breaks down (467). Demyelination, giant cells, astrogliosis, and perivascular lipid-laden macrophages characterize the areas of demyelination. The areas maximally involved are optic nerves, brain stem, cerebellum, and spinal cord. Within the brain stem, the pyramidal tracts, transverse pontine fibers, and superior cerebellar peduncles, and, within the spinal cord, pyramidal tracts and posterior columns are characteristically demyelinated (3). Peripheral nerves are normal. Extra-CNS xanthomas occur in tendons, lungs, and bones.

A different condition but one that may be related is the familial disease described by Jervis (214), occurring in late infancy, associated with deposition of cholesterol crystals in basal ganglia and degeneration of cortex and cerebellum.

Low-Density Lipoprotein Deficiency (Abetalipoproteinemia or Bassen-Kornzweig Syndrome)

Abetalipoproteinemia is an autosomal recessive condition associated with pigmentary retinal degeneration, a neurological disorder resembling Friedreich's ataxia, acanthocytosis (red blood cells with thorny projections), and chronic diarrhea (fat malabsorption). There is a hypocholesterolemia, with an absence of low-density lipoprotein in the serum.

Neuropathological alterations reported in two patients consisted of demyelination of spinocerebellar tracts, corticospinal tracts, and posterior columns (111, 427). In one case, a loss of neurons in the motor cortex, anterior horn cell column, and molecular layer of the cerebellum was described. In the other, lipofuscin pigment was present in anterior horn cells, but no loss of neurons was demonstrated in cord or cerebellum. Peripheral nerve demyelination with some axonal loss does occur. Ocular pathology includes absence of rod and cone processes except at the macula. Pigmented cells invade retina and are grouped around blood vessels, producing a picture of retinitis pigmentosa (493).

High-Density Lipoprotein Deficiency (Tangier Disease)

Tangier disease, named after an island on the east coast of the United States, is a rare, autosomal recessive disorder characterized by deficiency of high-density lipoprotein in plasma and storage of cholesterol esters in many tissues (tonsils, spleen, liver, bone marrow, and corneas) (28). The diagnosis is made by biopsy of the skin and rectal mucosa and the presence of low levels of plasma cholesterol with very low levels of high-density lipoproteins. Clinical expression varies from only yellow tonsillar hypertrophy to hepatosplenomegaly and severe peripheral neuropathy. Of special interest is the asymmetric loss of sensation over the scalp, face, and limbs with distal sparing. The findings by Bale et al. (28) of small terminal sensory nerves encircled by fat-containing histiocytes suggest that the unusual pattern of sensory loss may be the result of mononeuritis multiplex affecting fine nerve twigs. Ultrastructurally, cytoplasm of Schwann cells is filled with an array of clear vacuoles, myelin figures, and other cytosomes (142). Muscle biopsies confirmed a denervation pattern in several patients with Tangier disease (133). No central nervous system abnormalities have been described.

Refsum's Disease

Refsum's disease is an autosomal recessive disorder characterized by onset in adolescence or early adulthood with retinitis pigmentosa, peripheral neuropathy, cerebellar ataxia, and an elevated CSF protein. The primary defect is an absence of phytanic acid α-hydroxylase, which results in a failure of conversion of phytanic acid (a

20-carbon branched-chain acid) to α-hydroxyphytanic acid, producing phytanic acid storage disease. Since the origin of phytanic acid is exclusively dietary, clinical improvement occurs with appropriate management (377).

The CNS lesions are neither constant nor specific (65). Loss of Purkinje cells and neurons from retina, visual cortex, and dentate and from inferior olivary and red nuclei has been reported. Hypertrophic peripheral neuropathy is characteristic. The crystalline-like inclusions in Schwann cells seen on EM are thought to originate from mitochondria. Kolodny et al. (233) showed mitochondrial abnormalities in a liver biopsy, and CNS tissue cultures given phytanic acid have mitochondrial abnormalities, suggesting that mitochondrial damage occurs in this disease.

Wolman's Disease

Wolman's disease is a rare, fatal disorder that is probably inherited as a Mendelian recessive trait. It presents in the first few months of life as failure to thrive, diarrhea, steatorrhea, hepatomegaly, abdominal distension, and vomiting. The adrenals are enlarged and appear calcified roentgenologically. There is progressive anemia, and liver biopsy shows fatty change, periportal necrosis, and fibrosis (61). Mental deterioration occurs shortly after clinical onset, but this could be due to general debilitation. Death commonly occurs within several months of clinical onset.

At autopsy, the nervous system is grossly normal. However, sudanophilic droplets have been described in autonomic neurons, choroid plexus, endothelium, pericytes, ganglion cells of retina, and both neurons and glia of brain. EM examination shows that in the CNS there are lipid droplets in oligodendroglia, astrocytes, endothelial cells, and pericytes but not cortical neurons. In the peripheral nervous system, endoneurial, perineurial, and Schwann cells are involved. In all these cells, the lipid may be membrane-bound (with single or double membranes) or free in the cytoplasm. There is enlargement and yellowish discoloration of liver, intestines, adrenals, and lymph nodes. Foamy macrophages are present in lymph nodes, liver, spleen, and intestines.

Most of the stored lipid is cholesterol

ester, but several other lipids are also elevated in the involved extraneural tissues (triacylglycerols, free fatty acid, ether-linked glycerolipids) (253). It appears that one of the basic defects in this disorder is a deficiency of acid ester hydrolases. Neutral ester hydrolase is normal (195).

Mucopolysaccharidoses (MPS)

The mucopolysaccharide storage diseases are characterized by a genetic deficiency of an enzyme involved in the catabolism of mucopolysaccharides, also called glycosaminoglycans. This deficiency results in accumulation of mucopolysaccharides in several tissues. These disorders are often referred to as lysosomal storage diseases and, as seen on EM, the cellular inclusions are bound by a single membrane and stain positively for acid phosphatase (192). The term mucopolysaccharidosis was suggested by Brante (52) after the identification of increased chondroitin sulfate B (dermatan sulfate) in the livers of several patients with Hurler's syndrome. Subsequently, the demonstration of mucopolysacchariduria by Dorfman and Lorincz (117) confirmed the validity of this term.

Jeanloz (210) introduced the word glycosaminoglycan (GAG), which is more specific than mucopolysaccharide. The GAGs are large polysaccharide molecules that, in living systems, are usually covalently linked to a protein core. They are found in large amounts in skin, cartilage, bone, cornea, blood vessels, heart valves, and tendons. They are made up of repeating dimers

of an amino sugar usually linked to a hexuronic acid (e.g., β-D glucuronic or L-iduronic acid). The amino sugar is either glucosamine or galactosamine. Both of these are either acetylated or sulfated at the amino group, and both may also be sulfated at carbon 4 or carbon 6 of the hexose ring (118, 226, 350). The nomenclature and structure of the GAGs are outlined in Table 8.3 adapted from Pennock and Barnes (350) and Figure 8.9.

In general, this group of storage diseases (Table 8.4) (287) varies widely in severity, but the clinical signs are progressive. All patients with these diseases have coarse facial features, referred to as "gargoylism," some degree of skeletal involvement, called "dysostosis multiplex" and multiple organ involvement. All the disorders except the Morquio syndrome show dysostosis multiplex. Short stature is present in all except the Scheie syndrome. Arteriosclerosis develops in most of the mucopolysaccharidoses, with deposits of mucopolysaccharide in arterial smooth muscle cells. Although there is mucopolysaccharide in the brain, there is also prominent lipid accumulation. The underlying enzymatic defects are related to failure to break down dermatan sulfate, heparan sulfate, or keratan sulfate. A specific diagnosis can be established by screening urine for the presence of GAGs and then applying enzyme assays to patients who have positive urine results.

MPS I

Type I mucopolysaccharidosis consists of three clinical entities due to deficiency of

Table 8.3
Nomenclature of Glycosaminoglycans[a]

Previous name	Present name	Amino sugar	Hexuronic acid	Hexosamine sulfate
Chondroitin	Chondroitin	N-acetylgalactosamine	Glucuronic acid	None
Chondroitin sulfate A	Chondroitin-4-sulfate	N-acetylgalactosamine	Glucuronic acid	O-SO$_4$
Chondroitin sulfate C	Chondroitin-6-sulfate	N-acetylgalactosamine	Glucuronic acid	O-SO$_4$
Chondroitin sulfate B	Dermatan sulfate	N-acetylgalactosamine	Glucuronic and iduronic acid	O-SO$_4$
Heparitin sulfate	Heparan sulfate	N-acetylglucosamine	Glucuronic and iduronic acid	N-SO$_4$, O-SO$_4$
Karatosulfate	Keratan sulfate	N-acetylglucosamine	Galactose	O-SO$_4$

[a] From C. A. Pennock and I. C. Barnes (350).

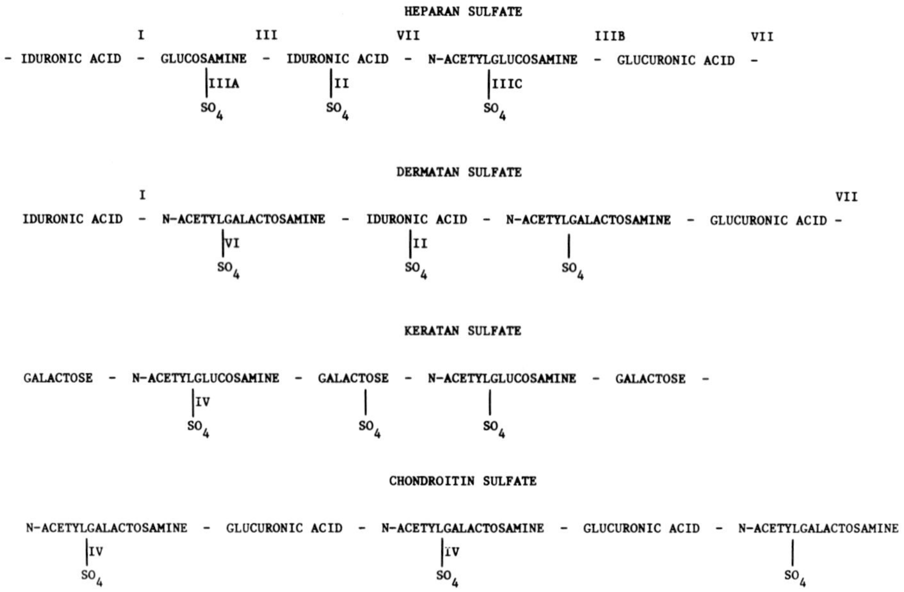

HEPARAN SULFATE

```
         I              III            VII                    IIIB              VII
 - IDURONIC ACID  -  GLUCOSAMINE  -  IDURONIC ACID  -  N-ACETYLGLUCOSAMINE  -  GLUCURONIC ACID  -
                        │IIIA            │II                   │IIIC
                        SO₄             SO₄                    SO₄
```

DERMATAN SULFATE

```
         I                                                                              VII
 IDURONIC ACID  -  N-ACETYLGALACTOSAMINE  -  IDURONIC ACID  -  N-ACETYLGALACTOSAMINE  -  GLUCURONIC ACID  -
                        │VI                       │II
                        SO₄                       SO₄                       SO₄
```

KERATAN SULFATE

```
 GALACTOSE  -  N-ACETYLGLUCOSAMINE  -  GALACTOSE  -  N-ACETYLGLUCOSAMINE  -  GALACTOSE  -
                    │IV
                    SO₄                     SO₄                  SO₄
```

CHONDROITIN SULFATE

```
 N-ACETYLGALACTOSAMINE  -  GLUCURONIC ACID  -  N-ACETYLGALACTOSAMINE  -  GLUCURONIC ACID  -  N-ACETYLGALACTOSAMINE
          │IV                                           │IV
          SO₄                                           SO₄                                          SO₄
```

Figure 8.9. Diagram showing the oligosaccharide units that accumulate in the mucopolysaccharidoses. The site of the defect is indicated by the designation of I to VII, which refers to the type of mucopolysaccharide disorder. (From A. Dorfman and R. Matalon (118).)

Table 8.4
Mucopolysaccharidoses[a]

Type	Eponym	Urinary excretion	Known enzyme deficiency
MPS I-H	Hurler	Dermatan sulfate and heparan sulfate	α-L-iduronidase
MPS I-S	Scheie	Dermatan sulfate and heparan sulfate	α-L-iduronidase
MPS I-H/S	Hurler-Scheie	Dermatan sulfate and heparan sulfate	α-L-iduronidase
MPS II	Hunter	Dermatan sulfate and heparan sulfate	Iduronate sulfatase
MPS III A	Sanfilippo	Heparan sulfate	Heparan N-sulfatase
MPS III B	Sanfilippo	Heparan sulfate	N-acetyl-α-D-glucosaminidase
MPS III C	Sanfilippo	Heparan sulfate	Acetyl CoA-α-D-glucosamini-dase-N-acetyltransferase
MPS III D	Sanfilippo	Heparan sulfate	N-acetyl α-D-glucosaminide-6-sulfatase
MPS IV A	Morquio	Keratan sulfate	Galactosamine-6-sulfate sulfatase
MPS IV B	Morquio	Keratan sulfate	β-galactosidase
MPS V		Now Type I-S	
MPS VI	Maroteaux-Lamy	Dermatan sulfate	N-acetylgalactosamine-4-sulfatase
MPS VII	Sly	Dermatan sulfate	β-glucuronidase

[a] Adapted from J. B. Stanbury et al. (438).

α-L-iduronidase, an enzyme required for degradation of both heparan sulfate and dermatan sulfate (283, 286). The most severe is MPS I-H (Hurler's syndrome) and the least severe MPS I-S (Scheie's syndrome). The intermediate form is designated MPS I-H/S (Hurler-Scheie compound).

Hurler's and Scheie's syndromes differ clinically, but in both the deficiency of α-L-iduronidase is thought to be due to homozygosity of an allele at the structural locus for iduronidase (286). All types have excessive urinary excretion of dermatan or heparan sulfate (117) and excessive accumulation of radioactive sulfated mucopolysaccharide by cultured fibroblasts (145). The reduction of this accumulation ("correction") by mixing with reference cell lines of another genotype or by addition of purified Hurler correction factor specifically identifies the type of mucopolysaccharidosis (146, 310). The allelic nature of Hurler's and Scheie's syndromes was established using this cross-correction technique (498). These tests have been superseded by assays of α-L-iduronidase activity in leukocytes or cultured fibroblasts (187).

MPS I-H (Hurler's Syndrome)

Hurler's syndrome is the classic mucopolysaccharide storage disease in which there is severe progression leading to death by 10 yr of age. It is transmitted by an autosomal recessive pattern of inheritance. Distinctive skeletal changes associated with mental retardation occur in infancy or early childhood. The constellation of skeletal abnormalities consists of a large scaphocephalic skull, shallow orbits, poorly developed sinuses, large sella turcica, spatulate ribs, thickened medial ends of the clavicles, beaked vertebrae, small pelvic ilium, shallow acetabula, and long bones with widened diaphyses. These changes are referred to as lipochondrodystrophy (175).

Patients also have marked hypertelorism, flattening of the bridge of the nose, wide nostrils, thick lips, protruding tongue, and wide-spaced teeth (gargoylism). Corneas become clouded during early life. Short neck, progressive kyphosis, protuberant abdomen, hepatosplenomegaly, and umbilical and inguinal hernias are characteristic, and prominent hirsutism is common. Progressive flexion contractures of the elbows and hands develop during the 1st year of life, and progressive hyperostosis of the skull may lead to conduction deafness. Death usually occurs from respiratory or cardiac failure, with coronary artery insufficiency a common terminal event (287).

In addition to the α-L-iduronidase deficiency, there is a partial deficiency of β-galactosidase activity (488). The latter may be due to inhibition of the enzyme by the accumulated GAG with the resultant failure of glycosphingolipid breakdown. G_{M1}, G_{M2} and G_{M3} gangliosides are elevated in the brain (102, 267, 449).

Gross examination of the brains of patients with Hurler's syndrome reveals boggy, fluid-filled, opaque, and thickened leptomeninges covering an atrophic cortex. The ventricles are enlarged, and perivascular spaces separating vessels from brain parenchyma are prominent (449).

Microscopically, the leptomeninges and perivascular spaces may show increased collagen and clusters of histiocytes (Fig. 8.10). In the cerebral cortex, thalami, and basal ganglia, the most striking feature is the ballooned appearance of the neurons with peripheral displacement of Nissl substance. The degree of neuronal enlargement

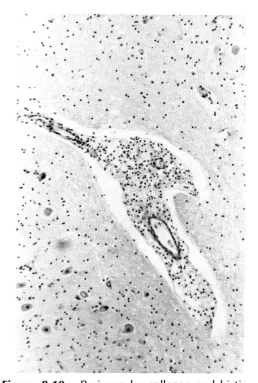

Figure 8.10. Perivascular collagen and histiocytes contributing to a prominent, clear area surrounding parenchymal vessels in a patient with Hurler's syndrome. PAS. (Original magnification ×100.)

is less in the brain stem. In the cerebellar cortex, there is Purkinje cell loss, with residual cells showing an enlarged ballooned appearance. Torpedoes are frequent. Anterior horn cells are similarly enlarged. The neuronal cytoplasm stains positively for ORO, SBB, LFB, and PAS. These stains suggest that the stored material within the cytoplasm is lipid in character.

GAGs are difficult to demonstrate histochemically unless special techniques are used, such as using frozen tissue with or without fixation in tetrahydrofuran and acetone (190). Preservation of the GAGs allows positive staining with toluidine blue, mucicarmine, Alcian blue, PAS, and colloidal iron. Such positive cells are found in the periadventitial spaces in the white matter. Faint staining can be demonstrated in some neurons, particularly Purkinje cells (104). Other changes in white matter are mild and consist of a variable degree of astrogliosis, depending on the amount of cortical damage.

Although histochemically there is little GAG in nerve cells, the amount of GAG in brains, determined by chemical methods, is signficantly increased (78). Mesenchymal elements contribute substantially to the increased content of GAG, mostly dermatan sulfate, in the brain and its coverings.

EM studies by Aleu et al. (12) showed that neurons accumulate a large number of pleomorphic bodies bounded by unit membrane measuring up to 1 μm in diameter representing ganglioside storage. These cytosomes are called zebra bodies (Fig. 8.11A) because of the arrangement of transverse lamellae forming a sequence of light and dark bands. In addition, numerous vacuoles filled with concentric lamellae are present (Fig. 8.11B and C). The lamellar arrangements merge, producing numerous intermediate forms. In occasional cerebral neurons and pericytes, and in nonneural tissue such as liver, spleen, leukocytes, and rectal mucosa histiocytes, the cytoplasm contains membrane-bound vacuoles filled with a faintly granular material (487) representing GAG (Fig. 8.11D). The ultrastructural appearance depends on the nature of the stored material: cerebral neurons, primarily ganglioside storage and hepatocytes, primarily GAG. Pathological studies of the cornea (166) show that Bowman's membrane is disrupted by clumps of vacuolated cells that stain positively with Alcian blue. The corneal lamellae are separated, and the epithelium of the basal layer is vacuolized. Ultrastructurally, these vacuoles contain fine granular densities (231).

MPS I-S (Scheie's Syndrome)

Because of its different clinical findings, Scheie's syndrome was initially classified as MPS type 5. However, it was found that a deficiency of α-L-iduronidase was present in both Hurler's and Scheie's syndromes (27). Some residual enzyme would be expected to function in vivo to explain the mild clinical picture, but this has not been convincingly demonstrated (287).

Scheie's syndrome is an autosomal recessive disorder with most of the clinical features of Hurler's syndrome, except that neurological development is normal. The corneal clouding and joint contractures are often more severe than in Hurler's syndrome. By about 10 yr of age, stiff joints, especially in the hands and feet, are noted. Life expectancy may be normal (27).

The neuropathological findings in Scheie's syndrome are very different from those of Hurler's syndrome (103). The cortical neurons are histologically normal. Ultrastructurally, the neurons contain a small number of lipofuscin-like inclusions and lipofuscin granules. The perivascular mesenchymal change is similar to that of Hurler's syndrome. Brain GAG is only slightly increased compared to its three-fold rise in Hurler's syndrome. The lesions in liver, spleen, kidneys, lymph nodes, heart, and arteries are similar to those of Hurler's syndrome.

MPS I-H/S (Hurler-Scheie Compound)

Patients with the Hurler-Scheie compound have inherited one Hurler and one Scheie gene and have a disease intermediate in severity between the Hurler and the Scheie phenotypes (441). The oldest known patient with this disorder (29 yr) had destruction of the sella turcica and cribriform plate caused by an arachnoid cyst (288). Arachnoid cysts are especially common in the MPS I-H/S syndrome.

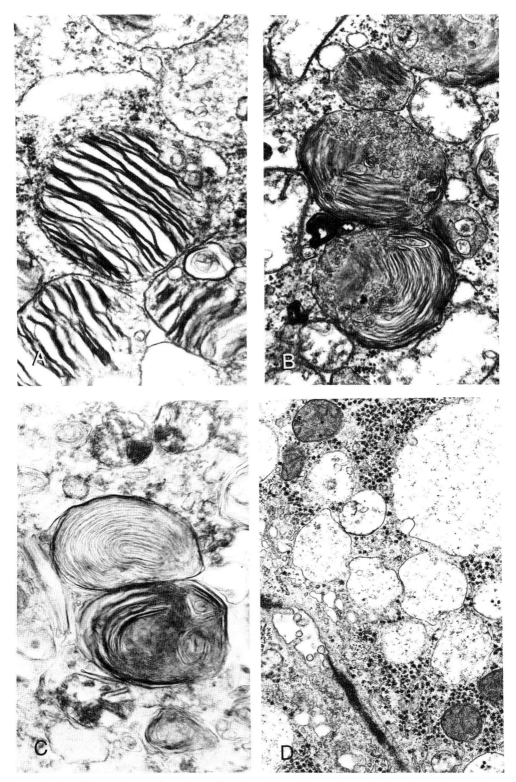

Figure 8.11. Neuronal storage of ganglioside in Hurler's syndrome in the form of cytoplasmic inclusions called zebra bodies (*A*) or MCBs (*B*), which may be somewhat pleomorphic in appearance, compared to Tay-Sachs disease. (*C*) In the liver, mucopolysaccharide (GAG) is present, and can be demonstrated in lysosomes (*D*). Electron micrographs. (*A*, Original magnification ×11,000; *B*, Original magnification ×12,000; *C*, Original magnification ×37,000; and *D*, Original magnification ×20,000.) (Courtesy of Dr. E. Cutz.)

MPS II (HUNTER'S SYNDROME)

Hunter's syndrome differs from Hurler's syndrome in several ways: slower progression of the disease, longer survival, absence of corneal clouding, and X-linked recessive inheritance. Both dermatan sulfate and heparan sulfate are excreted in excess, and the enzyme deficiency is α-iduronate sulfatase. Diagnosis is now established by direct assay of the enzyme in serum and cells (251). Severe and mild forms of the disease are described (27).

In the severe form, there is short stature, joint stiffness, coarse facial features, hepatosplenomegaly, hernias, deafness, retinitis pigmentosa, and, ultimately, cardiac failure. Neurological deterioration and loss of previous skills are gradual beginning at 4–5 yr, with death usually before 15 yr (436).

One of the mildest cases is that described by Karpati et al. (221), in which there were multiple nerve entrapments with preservation of intelligence and survival into late adulthood.

A report by Meier et al. (291) of a 23-week fetus described clear vacuoles in perineurial, endothelial, pericytic, and meningeal cells. The meninges were thickened by multivacuolated cells. EM showed membrane-bound vacuoles 0.5–1 μm in diameter containing granular material in fibroblasts, capillary pericytes, Schwann cells, meningothelial cells, and neurons. Other types of inclusions were present in better differentiated cells, such as spinal cord motor neurons and dorsal root ganglia neurons that were membrane-bound and showed a regular pattern of transverse (zebra bodies) or concentric (MCBs) lamellae. Meier et al. (291) suggested that the fine granular material represented GAG and the lamellar material ganglioside. Biochemical evidence indicated that zebra bodies and MCBs contained ganglioside (291), and most of the clear vacuoles contained acid mucopolysaccharide (282). Sural nerve biopsies have shown lamellated and granular inclusions in Schwann cells, fibroblasts, and perineural cells (468).

MPS III (SANFILIPPO SYNDROME)

Four types of Sanfilippo syndrome can be distinguished (287, 309). Enzymatic assays show that the A form is due to a deficiency of heparan N-sulfatase, the B form to an inactivity of N-acetyl-α-glucosaminidase, the C form to lack of acetyl CoA α-glucosaminidase-N-acetyltransferase, and the D form to lack of N-acetyl-α-D-glucosaminide-6-sulfatase. Sanfilippo syndrome is an autosomal recessive disorder characterized by early childhood onset of mental retardation in the absence of marked skeletal or somatic manifestations. The calvaria tends to be unusually dense, and the thoracolumbar vertebrae have a biconvex configuration. Generalized hirsutism is usually marked. Diagnosis can be established by assay of enzyme activity in fibroblasts, leukocytes, or serum (27).

Ghatak et al. (158) and others (95, 102, 134, 212, 474, 496, 507) reviewed the neuropathology of Sanfilippo syndrome. The cerebrum is atrophic without evidence of cerebellar atrophy. The leptomeninges are slightly thickened. Neuronal loss and astrogliosis are variable throughout the cerebral cortex, basal ganglia, and thalamus. In the residual neurons, the perikaryon contains material that stains with LFB and PAS, but the most prominent feature is distention of the dendrites. The ballooned dendrite is often larger than the cell body. Purkinje cell dendrites are particularly severely affected.

Ultrastructurally, material in dendrites is largely composed of MCBs, with both concentric whorls and stacks of parallel lamellae. Several authors (134, 158, 449) have described MCBs with pale, eccentric, irregular lamellae. They have also found lamellated inclusions in vacuolated ependymal, choroid plexus, pericytic, and meningeal cells. Witting et al. (507) suggested that neuronal ganglioside storage is a secondary phenomenon. That is, the mucopolysaccharides may form a complex with β-galactosidase, inactivating that enzyme and preventing breakdown of gangliosides. They found that β-galactosidase activity was reduced to 32% of normal in Sanfilippo disease. At present, there are no apparent differences in the neuropathology among the mucopolysaccharidosis subtypes (183, 279).

Storage material has been described in Kupffer cells of the liver, proximal renal tubules, splenic reticulum cells, lymph nodes, chondrocytes, heart valves, and arterial walls (507).

MPS IV (MORQUIO SYNDROME)

Morquio, in 1929 (303), described a family of Swedish extraction in which four children were affected with MPS IV. Probably the first description of this disease was that of Osler in 1897 (287), whose patients may have been related to the large number of affected French Canadians (151).

MPS IV is an autosomal recessive disorder usually diagnosed between 1 and 4 yr and associated with prominent skeletal dysplasia consisting of short trunk, pectus carinatum, and short neck. The facies is coarse, with a broad mouth and spacing between the teeth. Corneal clouding is mild, deafness common, and intelligence usually normal. Major neurologic problems are associated with the consistent feature of hypoplasia of the odontoid process. A tendency for ligament laxity leads to atloaxial subluxations and consequent cervical myelopathy that may manifest itself as acute quadriplegia (162). In the severe form, patients do not survive beyond their 30s, usually dying of cardiorespiratory insufficiency (175). This disease is due to a defect in degradation of keratan sulfate, which is normally found only in cartilage, nucleus pulposus, and cornea (175). The enzyme defect is galactosamine 6-sulfate sulfatase, which is deficient in fibroblasts, liver, and brain (237). Screening for keratan sulfate in the urine is an important test. Unlike some of the other mucopolysaccharides, gangliosides and other lipids do not accumulate in the brain.

In a single case of Morquio syndrome, Gilles and Deuel (162) showed vacuolated, somewhat enlarged but not ballooned neurons primarily in thalamus and hippocampus associated with neuronal depletion and astrogliosis. Subsequently, Koto et al. (237) showed similar PAS-positive, coarse, intracytoplasmic, globular inclusions most prominent in frontal cortex, hippocampus (resistant zones of Ammon's horn), claustrum, putamen, and thalamus (lateral nucleus). No neuronal storage was noted in the cerebellum, brain stem, or retina (237). EM shows membrane-bound cytoplasmic inclusions ranging in size from 1–5 μm,

containing stacked, straight, or tangled membranes often associated with pale, homogeneous lipid droplets ranging in size from 500–700 nm (237). The membranes are 40–60 nm wide and consist of two electron-dense lines separated by a central electron-lucent zone of 20–25 nm. Inclusions identical to MCBs or zebra bodies are rarely found. Some neurons also contain inclusions indistinguishable from lipofuscin. The chemical nature of the neuronal inclusions remains undetermined (237).

MPS VI (MAROTEAUX-LAMY SYNDROME)

Maroteaux et al. (273) described a Hurler-like condition in which there were somatic changes but normal intelligence, with mucopolysacchariduria predominantly of dermatan sulfate. Patients with the rare, autosomal recessive Maroteaux-Lamy syndrome have severe corneal clouding, skeletal abnormalities, and facial appearances similar to Hurler's syndrome patients. However, the bone changes are more severe, and intelligence is normal. Deafness may be present, and hydrocephalus is often marked. Dwarfism is noticeable by the age of 3 yr, and growth ceases by 7 yr. There is usually hepatosplenomegaly. The odontoid is hypoplastic, and atloaxial subluxation may occur as in Morquio syndrome. The most distinctive radiological features include constriction of the metaphyses and an abnormal pelvis, with small acetabula and flared ilia (175). In patients with the severe form, death usually occurs during the 20s, but milder forms have been reported (369). The enzyme defect is arylsulfatase B (N-acetylgalactosamine 4-sulfatase), resulting in accumulation and urinary excretion of dermatan sulfate. Abnormal, coarse, metachromatic granules (Reilly granules) in leukocytes are more prominent in MPS VI than in the other mucopolysaccharidoses. They are also found in cornea, conjunctiva, and skin (369). The granules, present in all leukocyte lines, are 0.5–1.5 μm in size, usually surrounded by a halo, and distributed throughout the cytoplasm. Ultrastructurally, they are membrane-bound, fibrillogranular vacuoles whose origin and nature have not been established (246).

Reports of CNS pathology are limited to

descriptions of hydrocephalus believed to be secondary to thickening of leptomeninges and cord compression occurring secondary to atloaxial subluxation (167).

MPS VII (SLY'S DISEASE)

Sly's disease is a rare, autosomal recessive mucopolysaccharidosis with dysmorphic facial and skeletal features. In the case reported by Sly et al. (425) the child had a prominent flare of the lower ribs, pigeon breast, hepatosplenomegaly, umbilical hernia, and a short trunk. Mental retardation was suspected at 30 months of age. The child had premature fusion of sagittal and lambdoid sutures, and the odontoid process was hypoplastic. Since this description, other reports have suggested a marked variation in the phenotypic expression of the disease (186). Mucopolysaccharide levels of dermatan sulfate and heparan sulfate in the urine are elevated. A deficiency of β-glucuronidase in fibroblasts, leukocytes, and serum confirms the diagnosis. This enzyme deficiency leads to failure of degradation of dermatan sulfate and heparan sulfate (186).

Neurons have been described as vacuolated and variably PAS-positive, with EM showing membrane-bound, clear, or granular vacuoles (506). Liver biopsy has shown storage material in lysosomes (186) and Reilly granules in leukocytes (354).

Mucolipidoses (Oligosaccharidosis)

Many disorders in patients with characteristics of mucopolysaccharidosis or sphingolipidosis and mucopolysacchariduria have been labeled mucolipidoses (435).

In mucolipidosis both GAGs and lipids accumulate in lysosomes as a result of a single enzyme defect. Therefore, the mechanism responsible for the lipid accumulation differs from that in the mucopolysaccharidoses, where it is secondary to GAG aggregation within the cell interfering with glycolipid catabolism. Because there is both GAG and lipid accumulation, some authors have suggested that G_{M1} gangliosidosis, Sandhoff disease, and multiple sulfatase deficiency be included as mucolipidoses (224). However, we are including only the mucolipidoses I to V, mannosidosis, and

fucosidosis. All of these disorders, except mucolipidosis IV, are associated with oligosacchariduria, which can be detected by thin-layer chromatographic methods (443).

MUCOLIPIDOSIS I (SIALIDOSIS, ACID NEURAMINIDASE DEFICIENCY)

Mucolipidosis I is a lysosomal storage disorder that results from a deficiency of an acid neuraminidase (N-acetylneuraminic acid hydrolase), with accumulation of sialic acid-rich oligosaccharides in many tissues. Some authors have used the term sialidosis to describe these disorders (126, 261).

Wide phenotypic diversity occurs within this biochemical defect. Kelly and Graetz (224) described an infant with a Hurler-like phenotype and apparently normal mental development. Others (67, 437) have described adolescents with a Hurler-like phenotype, severe neurologic disorder, and a cherry red spot in the macula. Kelly et al. (225) believe that these reports describe stages of evolution of the same disorder, that is, the cherry red spot myoclonus syndrome (34, 332, 375), which has been called type 1 sialidosis, and the dysmorphic group, type 2 sialidosis (126).

Cherry red spot myoclonus syndrome is associated with a normal physical appearance, with clinical presentation at 8 to 15 yr with myoclonus and/or decreasing visual acuity. Usually the intellect is normal. The myoclonus is severe and progressive, beginning in the limbs and induced by stimulation, movement, or emotion (332). The disorder is autosomal recessive and associated with a neuraminidase deficiency and, usually, normal levels of β-galactosidase in body fluids and urine (34, 375).

In patients with Hurler-like features type 2 sialidosis (dysmorphic type), thick lips, flattened nasal bridge, and mild hypertelorism are present. Radiographic features are similar to those in mucopolysaccharidosis, although usually milder. Cherry red spots in the macula, mental retardation, myoclonus, and ataxia are present. In juvenile-onset cases, joint stiffness and decreased visual acuity develop between 8 and 15 yr of age and slowly become worse (225). In these patients, there is urinary excretion of sialyloligosaccharides and reduced neur-aminidase activity in cultured fibroblasts (261). There may be a deficient β-galacto-sidase in body tissues and fluids (126). The mechanism responsible for the β-galacto-sidase deficiency is not clear.

In several cases (434, 440), lipid analyses of brain biopsies have been normal. Al-though no complete neuropathological ex-amination is available in the literature, bi-opsy of a sural nerve showed metachro-matic myelin degeneration (435). In liver tissue, vacuolated hepatocytes and Kupffer cells have been described. On EM, the in-clusions are limited by single membranes containing reticulogranular structures. Pe-ripheral lymphocytes are vacuolated, and bone marrow cells contain coarse granules in vacuoles (443). The nature of the storage substances is not known, but histochemical and ultrastructural studies suggest the presence of abnormal amounts of muco-polysaccharides and glycolipids (244, 434).

Analysis of a brain biopsy sample (461) revealed increases in cholesterol esters, cer-ebrosides (slight), and free amino acids. The ganglioside content and pattern were normal.

Histologically, cytoplasmic inclusion bodies are present in neurons, astrocytes, and Schwann cells, and EM shows that they contain large lysosomes with hetero-geneous material and multiple small vacu-oles with clear contents (461). In the report of a sural nerve biopsy, the presence of segmental demyelination and remyelina-tion without metachromatic material was noted. EM examination showed that the vacuolation in Schwann cells consisted of membrane-bound vacuoles containing var-ious amounts of lamellar arrays of membra-nous material mixed with lobular, electron-dense bodies (169). Inclusion bodies con-taining clear vacuoles have also been de-scribed in cultured fibroblasts, peripheral lymphocytes, Kupffer cells, kidney glomer-ular epithelium, and pericytes.

MUCOLIPIDOSIS II (I-CELL DISEASE)

Mucolipidosis II is a Hurler-like condi-tion with peculiar fibroblast inclusions (I-cells) and normal mucopolysacchariduria, first described by Leroy et al. (244). The disease is usually detected soon after birth.

There are coarse facial features, psycho-motor retardation, mild hepatosplenomeg-aly, kyphoscoliosis, restricted joint mobil-ity, unusually tight skin, and lipochondro-dystrophy. The children are dwarfed and mentally retarded. Corneas are clear. Usu-ally cardiac failure or pneumonia leads to death by age 5–6 yr.

The disorder is a lysosomal storage dis-ease due to the deficiency of several acid hydrolases. Although the basic defect is not known, it may represent an abnormality of enzyme localization. Hickman and Neufeld (193) suggested that most acid hydrolases share a common recognition marker target-ing them to lysosomes and that this marker is defective in I-cell disease. In I-cell dis-ease, the lysosomal enzymes are secreted rather than packaged in lysosomes. There-fore, intracellular storage results from the intracellular deficiency of many acid hydro-lases that are required for the catabolism of mucopolysaccharides, glycolipids, and glycoproteins.

The enzymes found at elevated levels in body fluids and partly deficient in fibro-blasts include α-L-iduronidase, iduronate sulphatase, β-glucuronidase, N-acetyl-β-hexosaminidase, arylsulfatase A, β-galac-tosidase, α-mannosidase, and α-L-fucosi-dase. These enzymes are required for the catabolism of mucopolysaccharides, glyco-lipids, and glycoproteins. Of the enzymes studied, only acid phosphatase and β-glu-cosidase are at normal levels. This multiple enzyme deficiency in fibroblasts accounts for the storage of mucopolysaccharide and glycolipid and the accumulation of exces-sive sulfated mucopolysaccharide.

With so many enzymes affected, the lab-oratory can choose which one to assay most simply and reliably. Usually screening for two- or three-fold elevations of N-acetyl-β-hexosaminidase or arylsulfatase A activity in serum is an effective test for this condi-tion. When fibroblasts are available, a char-acteristic pattern of deficiencies or of iso-enzymes can be established. The presence of inclusions is not a good diagnostic cri-terion, since inclusions can develop in nor-mal cells under certain culture conditions (175).

The brain is grossly normal, and there is no histological evidence of central neuronal storage or astrogliosis, although a few perivascular, lipid-laden macrophages are present (160, 277). In the cytoplasm of some neurons Martin et al. (277) found a small number of membrane-bound vacuoles containing a fine granular matrix, a lamellar array with a periodicity of 12.5 nm, lipofuscin granules, or a mixture of the above subcellular structures. They suggested these findings are "minimal and equivocal." More significant are the largely empty-appearing, membrane-bound vacuoles that may be prominent in fibroblasts of all tissues and in Schwann cells, peripheral neurons, and pericytes. Martin et al. (277) could not confirm histochemically the presence of glycolipids or mucopolysaccharides in the cytoplasmic inclusions. Therefore, mental retardation found in these patients cannot be satisfactorily explained on a morphological basis.

MUCOLIPIDOSIS III (PSEUDO-HURLER POLYDYSTROPHY)

Mucolipidosis III is a rare, autosomal recessive disease described as pseudo-Hurler polydystrophy (223, 274). As in I-cell disease, there are high levels of several lysosomal hydrolases in serum and low levels in fibroblasts. The disease is similar to mucolipidosis II and may be a milder form of the same biochemical defect. It has a later onset, a milder course, less mental retardation, and survival into adult life.

The onset of disease is between 2 and 4 yr of age, with joint stiffness, coarse facial features, corneal clouding, and mild mental retardation. The radiological features of lipochondrodystrophy are present.

No significant neuropathology has been described, but vacuolated plasma cells are found in bone marrow (223).

MUCOLIPIDOSIS IV

Berman et al. (35), in 1974, first reported a case of mucolipidosis IV. The absence of mucopolysaccharide excretion distinguishes this disease from the mucopolysaccharidoses and the mild clinical manifestations and lack of identifiable enzyme changes (in both serum and tissues) from mucolipidoses I, II, and III. Slowly progressive neurologic deterioration beginning in the first months of life, early childhood corneal clouding, absence of skeletal abnormality, and hepatosplenomegaly are char-

acteristic clinical findings. The disease is thought to be autosomal recessive, and most cases have occurred in Ashkenazic Jews (83).

Assays of serum, red cell leukocyte, and fibroblast enzymes have failed to identify a specific defect in mucolipidosis IV (83). In the lipid analysis reported from a brain biopsy (475) total ganglioside content was increased in the white matter, but the pattern was normal. Total phospholipids were increased. EM studies of biopsies taken from skin, conjunctiva, cornea, peripheral nerve, muscle, and liver have shown two types of inclusions (83, 227, 255, 478): membrane vesicles filled with granular material and/or MCBs. Similar inclusions have been described in the brain in both neurons and glia. Cytoplasmic storage inclusions have also been described in an abortus in cells of the brain, cornea, conjunctiva, and other epithelial tissues (232).

FUCOSIDOSIS

Fucosidosis is a rare autosomal recessive disorder caused by an absence of α-L-fucosidase resulting in accumulation of fucose-containing polysaccharides and glycosphingolipids in the liver and fucose-containing oligosaccharides in the brain (127, 489). Clinical presentation is between 2 and 4 yr of age, with delayed growth, mental retardation, Hurler-like facies, hepatomegaly, umbilical hernia, and vacuolated lymphocytes. Skeletal alterations are discrete, and urinary excretion of mucopolysaccharides is normal. Other clinical findings include cardiomegaly, nonfunctioning gallbladder, salivary gland hypertrophy, thickened skin, and respiratory tract infections.

Ultrastructural examination of the brain and liver (257) shows findings different from those seen in mucopolysaccharidosis. Dense, clear, and lamellar inclusions are present in these tissues. The lamellar profiles are either concentric or parallel and are found prominently in hepatocytes, although they are also present in the brain. Clear inclusions are by far the most numerous in the glial cells. A variety of inclusions is present in oligodendroglia, endothelial cells, and macrophages. The neurons are packed with round, clear structures, only rarely containing lamellar arrangements. Unlike the mucopolysaccharidoses, in fucosidosis the lipidic lamellar component is prominent in hepatocytes and less common in other cell types, particularly neurons where the storage appears to be almost exclusively mucopolysaccharide (257).

Several forms of fucosidosis have been described: type I with early onset, marked enzyme deficiency, and death around the age of 3 to 5 yr; type II with partial enzyme deficiency, survival to adulthood, and occurrence of angiokeratoma; and type III with severe deficiency or complete absence of α-L-fucosidase activity with survival to adulthood (156, 433).

MANNOSIDOSIS

Mannosidosis is a rare, autosomal recessive disorder that was first described by Öckerman in 1967 (334). Initial presentation is usually between 1 and 4 yr of age. The clinical characteristics are psychomotor retardation, Hurler-like facies, lipochondrodystrophy, deafness, respiratory infections, and hepatosplenomegaly. The basic defect is deficiency of α-mannosidase A and B (70) that causes accumulation of mannose-rich oligosaccharides in the brain and viscera and excessive excretion of these in the urine (320).

The brain may be grossly normal (447). Microscopically, neuronal cytoplasmic ballooning is present in cortex, basal ganglia, brain stem, and spinal cord, with maximum involvement of the large neurons. Purkinje cell dendrites have many fusiform focal swellings, but the perikarya are not distended. In contrast, ganglion cell bodies of paravertebral, sympathetic, trigeminal, and dorsal root ganglia are severely distended. Neuronal loss in cerebrum and cerebellum is associated with diffuse demyelination of centrum ovale (447). The peripheral nerves show no abnormalities (447).

EM examination of neurons reveals cytoplasmic storage of vacuoles of varied sizes (1–2 μm in diameter) enclosed by a single membrane and containing uniform, finely granular material and small lipid droplets but no lamellar structures. Astrocytes, endothelial cells, and pericytes have similar material. However, the anterior horn cells and sympathetic ganglia contain vacuoles with frequent stacks of fine fibrils (447). Systemically, PAS-positive vacuoles have been noted in lymphocytes, bone marrow cells, spleen, and lymph nodes. Ultrastructurally, hepatocytes, Kupffer cells, endothelial cells, and bile duct epithelium all contain membrane-bound cytoplasmic vacuoles. The ultrastructural similarity of the storage vacuoles in the nervous and visceral tissues is in accordance with the accumulation of mannose-rich oligosaccharides in brain and liver (335). The appearance of the vacuoles in mannosidosis is similar to that found in the neuron of fucosidosis (257). The fine stacks of fibrils found in the anterior horn cells and the ganglion cells of the peripheral and sympathetic ganglia may represent mannose-rich glycoproteins (447).

Storage vacuoles in the cerebral neurons have characteristics similar to those in the Angus cattle model of mannosidosis described by Jolly (216). Golgi studies of neurons in feline mannosidosis show meganeurities, abnormal sprouting of neurites, focal dendritic enlargement, and spine loss (495).

SALLA DISEASE

The eponym Salla disease was used by Aula et al. in 1979 (22) to identify the disease in a family from a geographically isolated area of northern Finland. This family had coarse facial features, progressive mental retardation, vacuolated lymphocytes, and large lysosomal cytoplasmic bodies within fibroblasts. Life span appears to be normal. Increased urinary free sialic acid excretion has been found in these patients, but the basic defect is unknown (378).

Glycogen Storage Diseases

As more enzyme studies are performed on patients who have glycogen storage diseases, it is apparent that deficiencies of enzymes involved in glycogen synthesis and degradation can produce a wide clinical spectrum (Table 8.5). Patients with glycogen storage disease can present with disorders primarily of the liver, heart, or musculoskeletal or nervous system. Howell and Williams (203) described eight specific enzyme deficiencies plus a group of "other possible inherited defects in glycogen metabolism." Because of conflicting naming

Table 8.5
Glycogen Storage Diseases

Type	Enzyme deficiency and disease	Major tissue involvement
I	Glucose 6 phosphatase (von Gierke's)	Liver
II	α-1,4-glucosidase (acid maltase) (Pompe's)	Muscle, CNS
III	Debrancher	Liver
IV	Brancher	Liver
V	Muscle phosphorylase (McArdle's)	Muscle
VI	Hepatic phosphorylase	Liver
VII	Muscle phosphofructo-kinase	Muscle
VIII	Hepatic phosphorylase kinase	Liver

and numbering systems, they preferred to refer to the diseases by the nature of the enzyme defect rather than by eponym or number. However, the literature, in general, tends to use both numbers and enzyme defect.

In this section we concentrate on the disorders that affect primarily brain (types II and, rarely, IV) and muscle (types II, III, IV, and VII). All the enzyme deficiencies are rare and, except types V and VII, are manifested clinically or biochemically in childhood. The inheritance is autosomal recessive, except for type VIII, which is X-linked. A definitive diagnosis is established by enzyme assays from liver, muscle, red blood cells, white blood cells, or cultured fibroblasts (203).

GLYCOGEN STORAGE DISEASE WITH MUSCLE AND BRAIN INVOLVEMENT (POMPE'S DISEASE)

The type II glycogen storage disease is called Pompe's disease or generalized glycogenosis. It includes three clinical forms (132). In the infantile form, the presenting symptom is profound hypotonia with macroglossia, cardiomegaly, cardiac failure, and death by age 1 yr. In the childhood form, the disease progresses more slowly. Limb girdle weakness is usually present, but organomegaly and respiratory muscle involvement are variable with death by the second decade. In the adult group, the presentation is myopathic, mimicking other chronic myopathies. The electromyogram may show myotonic discharges without clinically detectable myoclonia. Diagnosis is made by demonstrating a deficiency of α-1,4-glucosidase (acid maltase) (318) in fibroblasts, liver, muscle, kidney, heart, or CNS and by finding membrane-bound (lysosomal) glycogen in any of these tissues.

In the infantile form, the brain may be grossly normal (270). Histologically, distended neurons giving the cytoplasm a granular or foamy appearance and staining positively for PAS are most prominent in dorsal root ganglia, anterior horn cells, and motor nuclei of the brain stem, with a lesser involvement of other brain stem nuclei (154). Very slight to moderate storage is present in the cortical neurons and Purkinje cells by the 18th week of gestation (205). In areas of severe damage, neuronal loss and astrogliosis are evident. Glycogen-containing astrocytes are most pronounced in white matter, subpial, and subependymal regions. Myelination glia, but not mature oligodendroglia, contain glycogen. Choroid plexus epithelium, ependymal cells, arteriolar smooth muscle, and capillary pericytes also contain glycogen. In the peripheral nervous system, Schwann cells contain excessive glycogen (154, 270).

Ultrastructurally, glycogen accumulates in greatly distended lysosomes, particularly in astrocytes. Glycogen-containing vacuoles also fill the endothelial cells and pericytes. Martin et al. (276) found only two to three glycogen-filled lysosomes in the cytoplasm of most cortical neurons and none in nuclei, dendrites, axons, or synapses. Excessive free glycogen was not present in neurons or astrocytes.

Ultrastructural observations have been more frequently reported in striated muscle (68), where deposits of glycogen appear as large pools of free glycogen, and within membrane-bound lysosomes. The location of glycogen within lysosomal membranes is of diagnostic significance in this group of glycogen storage diseases.

The reasons for the differences in the three clinical forms are not apparent, since lysosomal α-1,4 glucosidase activity is deficient in all tissues in all three groups (109, 132). The small amount of residual activity of the enzyme in the adult in contrast to the infant may explain the differences in severity between these two forms of the disease (109).

At autopsy, there is massive accumulation of glycogen in most tissues including kidney, liver, and heart, as well as basophilic material digested by amylase and containing phosphate (276). In the type IV glycogenosis, McMaster et al. (289) described hypotonia, muscular atrophy, and decreased or absent tendon reflexes. They correlate these clinical findings with autopsy evidence of amylopectin accumulation.

A disease that resembles generalized glycogen storage disease with cardiomegaly, hypotonia, cerebral dysfunction, and early onset has been described (491). There is no glycogen abnormality, but tissue deposition of ethanolamine (PAS-positive) occurs due to a deficiency of ethanolamine kinase.

Glycogen storage in the CNS has not been demonstrated in the other storage diseases. However, neurological symptoms may occur in some of these other disorders secondary to hypoglycemia (203).

GLYCOGEN STORAGE DISEASE WITH MUSCLE INVOLVEMENT

The glycogen storage diseases that affect muscle include types II, III, V, and VII. In type II glycogenosis, there is marked storage of glycogen in the muscle lysosomes, most marked in the infantile form of the disease (Fig. 8.12A and B) and less marked in the adult form. In type III glycogenosis, muscle weakness and wasting have been described (50, 58, 348).

In type V glycogenosis patients complain of limitation in performing strenuous exercise because of painful muscle cramps, associated with a deficiency of muscle phosphorylase (285, 384). During ischemic exercise, there is no increase in venous lactate from the exercised limb (285). Myoglobinuria may occur. A fatal infantile form of muscle phosphorylase deficiency has been described by DiMauro and Hartlage (110). The histology of the muscle in type V shows subsarcolemmal, PAS-positive, oval glycogen aggregates. On EM, there is increased glycogen, especially in the intermyofibrillar space, causing disarray of myofibrillar structure (407).

Tarui et al., in 1965 (475), described a phosphofructokinase deficiency in skeletal muscle in three siblings with symptoms identical to those of McArdle's disease. This combination is sometimes referred to as type VII glycogenosis.

LEUKODYSTROPHIES

The leukodystrophies are a heterogeneous group of disorders (Table 8.6) that have in common extensive degenerative changes of CNS white matter. They are sometimes called dysmyelinating disorders. The historical development of the classification of the leukodystrophies is described in detail by Stam (438). The nosological term orthochromatic was originally used to distinguish leukodystrophies that did not have metachromatically staining material. Sudanophilic, orthochromatic material (mainly cholesterol ester) is produced whenever myelin is broken down in vivo regardless of the etiology. Thus, it is not surprising that a group whose distinguishing characteristics are so nonspecific should contain cases with numerous diverse clinical and neuropathological findings. For example, some cases have had a genetic or familial pattern of inheritance, but many have been sporadic.

As the biochemical abnormalities for specific leukodystrophies are elucidated, the diseases are reclassified more accurately as specific metabolic disorders (e.g., MLD, Krabbe's disease, and adrenoleukodystrophy). The number of subtypes within the original sudanophilic category will decline progressively as our understanding of them at the molecular level increases. Other types of leukodystrophies will also be reclassified when their etiologies and pathogeneses are determined. In the meantime, subclassifications of leukodystrophies on the basis of clinical and morphological data must suffice for several types.

Metachromatic Leukodystrophy (Sulfatide Lipidosis)

Metachromasia is the phenomenon of color change that some dyes undergo when they bind to other compounds. This is in contradistinction to orthochromatic staining in which the dye remains its original color after binding. In 1910, Alzheimer (235) noted metachromatic staining of nervous tissues in a case of diffuse cerebral

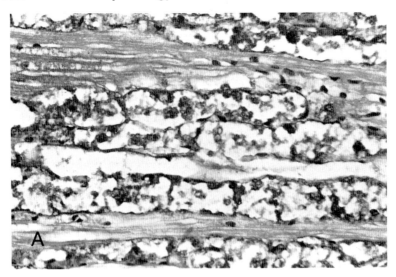

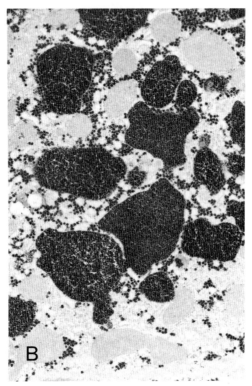

Figure 8.12. (*A*) Longitudinal section of muscle from a case of type II glycogen storage disease showing vacuolation of fibers and aggregates of PAS-positive glycogen adjacent to preserved fibers. PAS. (Original magnification ×240.) (*B*) Glycogen aggregated both within lysosomes and free in the cytoplasm. Electron micrograph (liver). (Original magnification ×8,000.) (Courtesy of Dr. E. Cutz.)

sclerosis, and, in 1957, Austin (23) found that urine sediment of patients with MLD stains metachromatically with toluidine blue. In the next 2 yr, Jatzkewitz (209) and Austin (24) independently reported that the basis for the metachromasia in cerebral tissues was the presence of large amounts of sulfatides. Subsequently, the basic defect was found to be a deficiency in the activity of the enzyme (cerebroside sulfatase) re-

Table 8.6
Leukodystrophies

Metabolic diagnosis
   Metachromatic leukodystrophy
   Krabbe's disease
   Adrenoleukodystrophy

Pathologic diagnosis
   Alexander's disease
   Canavan's disease
   Pelizaeus-Merzbacher disease
   Cockayne's disease
   Sudanophilic leukodystrophies

sponsible for cleaving the sulfate radical from sulfatide. Because this type of enzyme has been most frequently assayed using sulfate esters of phenol as the substrates, it is commonly referred to as arylsulfatase.

More than one arylsulfatase has been identified, but the one deficient in MLD is arylsulfatase A (ASA), which is normally present in brain, liver, kidney, pancreas, spleen, heart, lung, leukocytes, fibroblasts, and serum. Stumpf et al. (444), using immunological methods, found that the ASA protein is present in patients with MLD, but is enzymatically inactive. Disorders due to ASA deficiencies have been classified mainly on the basis of the age at appearance of clinical manifestations (late infantile, juvenile, and adult MLD). In addition, in multiple sulfatase deficiency, activities of other sulfatases as well as ASA are deficient. All of these diseases are autosomal recessive.

The diagnosis of the late infantile form of MLD can be highly suspected on the basis of clinical signs and symptoms. However, late presentations are easily misdiagnosed initially. Electrophysiological studies of peripheral nerve function are abnormal in all types (75), as are auditory evoked brain stem responses early in the disease (55). The definitive diagnosis is made by demonstrating deficient ASA activity. The most reliable enzyme source is leukocytes or cultured fibroblasts, but activities lower than normal have also been found in the serum and urine of patients.

Affected fetuses have been detected by assaying amniotic fluid fibroblasts. Although myelination had not yet begun, metachromatic material was present in nervous tissues of an affected fetus aborted at 23 weeks gestation (290).

Dulaney and Moser (123) discussed the problem of carrier diagnosis. Although ASA activities in patients do not overlap with those of normal controls, great caution must be exercised in the diagnosis of the carrier status, especially in fetuses. Very low ASA levels have been detected in clinically normal relatives of patients with MLD. Such persons in utero may have been diagnosed as having MLD. Therefore, both parents should be carefully studied if an amniotic cell ASA level is very low.

TYPE 1 LATE INFANTILE FORM

The late infantile form of MLD is a moderately rare, autosomal recessive disorder. Although rare congenital cases have been described, the disease usually begins between 1 and 2 yr of age with motor signs of peripheral neuropathy (flaccid weakness, hypotonia, hypoactive deep tendon reflexes), followed by intellect, speech, and coordination deterioration that is often rapid. Within 2 yr of onset, there is evidence of severe, diffuse, white matter dysfunction—decerebrate posturing, quadriplegia, and blindness.

The brain may be slightly enlarged, of normal size, or atrophic; the ventricles may or may not be dilated (49, 323). Gross appearance of the cerebral white matter in some cases is normal, but in others it is a dull, chalky white-to-grey color. In some, the cerebellum is small and firm with atrophy of the folia. Histologically, there is marked loss of cerebral and cerebellar myelin, although the cerebral arcuate fibers are generally better preserved (Fig. 8.13*A* and *B*). Axonal damage and loss are usually severe in demyelinated areas. The corticospinal tracts are severely affected, but many other brain stem tracts are only partially damaged. Some spinal cord tracts are similarly affected. Brain and Greenfield (49) thought that areas unmyelinated at birth were the most severely affected.

There is a loss of interfascicular oligodendrocytes from damaged and even from some unaffected areas. Fibrillary gliosis is heavy in demyelinated tissues, and orthochromatic lipid droplets are lightly scattered in a perivascular distribution. Throughout the damaged white matter are

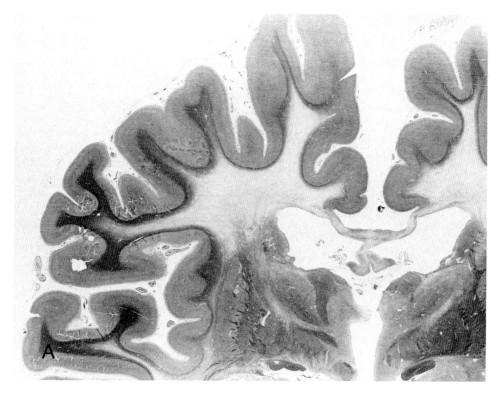

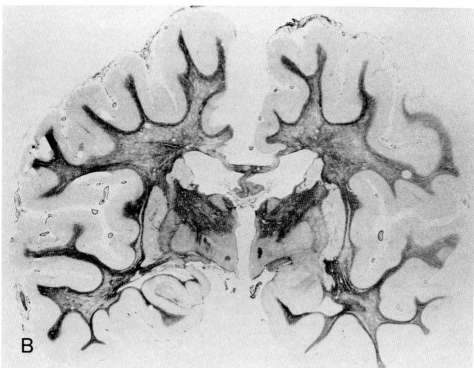

Figure 8.13.   Frontal coronal section of a patient with MLD showing (*A*) demyelination with preservation of subcortical arcuate fibers (LFB; original magnification ×1.5) and (*B*) prominent astrogliosis throughout the white matter (Holzer; original magnification ×0.7).

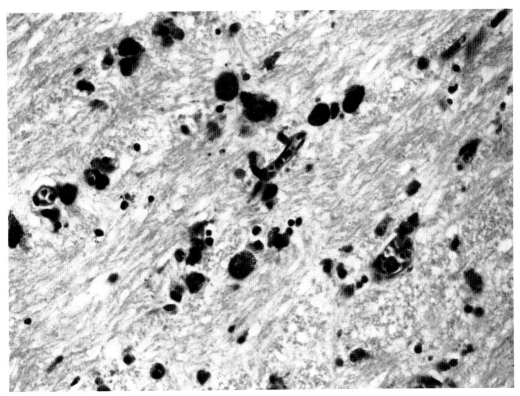

Figure 8.14. Globular deposits in the white matter of a patient with MLD. PAS. (Original magnification ×400.)

numerous granular bodies (Fig. 8.14). Some are in macrophages, but others are free in the tissues. These stain positively with SBB, PAS, Hirsch-Pfeiffer (cresyl violet acetic acid), and toluidine blue.

The cerebral cortex is histologically normal, but nerve cell loss occurs in claustrum, thalamus, globus pallidus, subthalamic nucleus, lateral geniculate, and lateral nucleus of mammillary body. Metachromatic material is present in the cytoplasm of the surviving neurons in these areas. Similar material accumulates in neurons of many brain stem nuclei and spinal cord and dorsal root ganglia (323).

With EM, the cytoplasmic inclusions are most prominent in oligodendrocytes and astrocytes, although they are also reported in neurons. They are complex, membrane-bound, and made up of variable proportions of three microstructures (Fig. 8.15): a concentrically lamellar structure with a periodicity of 56 to 58 nm; narrow, perpendicular bands with a periodicity of 100 nm

making a tuftstone or herringbone pattern that, on cross-section, produces a hexagonal arrangement; and an amorphous matrix that is probably mucopolysaccharide. The herringbone pattern of inclusions is characteristic of MLD (173, 379).

Peripheral nerve is usually severely affected. There is segmental demyelination, which accounts for slowed nerve conduction velocities. Thin myelin sheaths and loosely packed myelin suggest that attempts at remyelination occur. Schwann cells contain metachromatic granules, frequently in nodal and perinuclear regions. Ultrastructurally, these granules are dense, membrane-bound, laminated structures (351).

The eyes are also affected. At funduscopic examination, the macula is greyer than normal. Histologically, the ganglion cells of the retina are decreased in number and the remaining ones distended with metachromatic material in the cytoplasm. Ultrastructurally, this metachromatic ma-

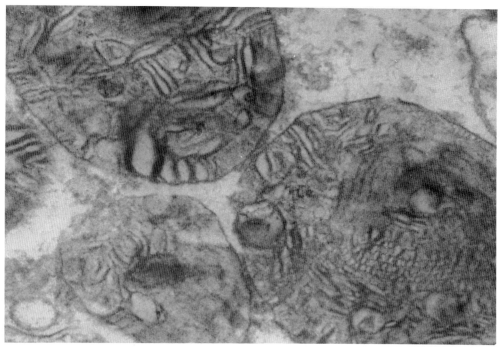

Figure 8.15. Inclusion bodies containing stacks of irregularly arranged lamellar arrays from a juvenile case of MLD. Electron micrograph. (Original magnification ×55,000.) (From S. Takashima et al. (472).)

terial is similar to that in the cerebral white matter (248).

Metachromatic material is also present in some extraneural tissues: intrahepatic bile ducts and periportal histiocytes of the liver, adrenal medulla, gallbladder epithelium, and renal tubular cells. The latter are the source of the metachromatic granules in urine sediment. With EM, the renal inclusions are similar to those in white matter, but those in liver differ somewhat (380). Multiple polypoid masses may project from the mucosa into the lumen of the gallbladder, and the mucosal cells and villi are distended with macrophages containing metachromatic material.

Results of chemical analyses of the brain are consistent with the morphological findings. In the white matter, there are decreased levels of most myelin lipids (cholesterol, cerebrosides, ethanolamine phosphoglycerides, and sphingomyelin) but a greatly elevated proportion of sulfatide. The lipid compositions of white matter, isolated myelin, and the metachromatic granules are all quite similar (452). The sulfatide that accumulates in MLD fibro-

blasts when sulfatide is added to the culture medium is ultrastructurally similar to that of the herringbone type of inclusion (388). It seems reasonable that the abnormal cerebroside to sulfatide ratio in MLD myelin contributes to the breakdown of myelin sheath (235). Poduslo et al. (360) found altered glycoproteins, suggesting a problem in myelin assembly in addition to structurally unstable myelin.

TYPE 2 JUVENILE FORM

There is a continuum in the ages at onset of clinical signs and symptoms of MLD from the neonatal period through to later adulthood. Cases beginning between 3 and 21 yr of age are considered to be the juvenile form of MLD. It becomes manifest in a variety of ways: learning difficulties, problems with concentration, emotional instability, and motor impairment. Peripheral neuropathic signs are not common initially. There is a steady progression of neurological impairment, including dementia, speech disorders, bulbar abnormalities, pyramidal tract dysfunction, ataxia, seizures, and tremors. Motor nerve conduction becomes slowed. The course of the disease lasts 3–20 yr, with death usually occurring in early adulthood (189).

Few cases of juvenile MLD have been studied at autopsy. The brain weighs less than normal and appears atrophic with dilated ventricles (181, 472). The cerebral and cerebellar white matter is reduced in amount and appears gelatinous and browny-yellow. Histological abnormalities qualitatively similar to those in the infantile form are seen in CNS white matter, peripheral nerve, liver, kidneys, and adrenals (181, 275). Neuronal accumulation of metachromatic material has been described (472). Ultrastructurally, the metachromatic granules have a multilamellated appearance, but, unlike in late infantile cases, prismatic structures are not usually found (264). Chemical analysis of cerebral white matter has shown a marked decrease of myelin constituents but a relative excess of sulfatide (181).

TYPE 3 ADULT FORM

The very uncommon patients with MLD whose clinical abnormalities begin after 21 yr of age are considered to have the adult form of MLD (25). Initially, they may be given a psychiatric diagnosis because of behavioral disturbances. Psychological testing early in the course of the disease may reveal defects in visual-spatial ability (38). Definite neurological abnormalities develop over a period of several years. The clinical course of the disease may last decades, although sometimes it is only 2 or 3 yr.

The brain is atrophic with dilated ventricles. The cerebral white matter is firm, shrunken, and yellowish. Microscopic and histochemical findings are similar to those of the late infantile form, although the amount of metachromatic material may be less in both white matter and neurons (239, 470). The ultrastructural appearance of the metachromatic granules is more diverse than in the infantile form (164, 217). Chemical composition of white matter is also qualitatively similar to the late infantile form. However, myelin lipids are more depleted, and there is less increase in sulfatide in the adult from (357).

TYPE 4 MULTIPLE SULFATASE DEFICIENCY (MUCOSULFATIDOSIS, VARIANT O, AUSTIN'S DISEASE)

Multiple sulfatase deficiency (MSD) is an extremely rare disorder that begins clinically around 1 yr of age. The symptoms resemble infantile MLD, except that Hurler-like features are present. Developmental milestones are retarded, and there is neurological regression. Seizures, nystagmoid eye movements, optic atrophy, pyramidal tract dysfunction, and evidence of motor neuropathies develop. There are bony abnormalities of chest and spine, and slight hepatosplenomegaly (235).

The chemical findings are complex. There are deficient activities of cerebroside sulfatase, steroid sulfatase, and mucopolysaccharide sulfatase. In several tissues there is decreased activity of arylsulfatase A, B, and C, phosphoadenosylphosphosulfate-sulfatase, and β-galactosidase. In brain, there are increased levels of sulfatide, cholesterol sulfate, gangliosides (G_{M3}, G_{M2}, and G_{D3}), and dermatan sulfate. Myelin has increased amounts of sulfatide (136). The liver has elevated concentrations of cholesterol sulfate and sulfated GAGs. Kidney and urine sediment has increased amounts of sulfatide and sulfated GAGs (26).

Somatic hybrid cell clones of infantile MLD and MSD restore the activity of ASA. The mutations in these two disorders responsible for the defect in ASA are nonallelic. Arylsulfatase C activity is also restored, which indicates that the MSD is not due to a common enzyme inhibitor (71).

The child with MSD originally described by Austin in 1973 (26) died at 11 yr of age. The brain was small with shrunken white matter, cortical atrophy, and dilated ventricles. Histological findings of central and peripheral nervous tissues included the abnormalities found in infantile MLD. In addition, there was marked loss of cortical neurons, and the remaining neurons were distended with metachromatic material. EM studies revealed zebra bodies, fingerprint-like profiles, and myelinoid structures (376). Histological findings in kidney are similar to those in the infantile forms, but the liver is normal.

AB Variant

One case of the AB variant of MSD has been described (185). The patient, 21 yr old at that time, had psychomotor retardation from 1 yr of age. During her teens, she was clumsy, weak, and ataxic, and between 14 and 21 yr of age she developed behavioral abnormalities and became socially withdrawn, mute, and incontinent. She had pseudobulbar affect and palsy, macular greyness, and evidence of peripheral neuropathy. A peripheral nerve biopsy had features identical to those of infantile MLD. ASA activities were normal in leukocytes and urine, as was cerebroside sulfatase in cultured fibroblasts. The authors suggest that the metabolic abnormality may be due to a deficiency of an activator protein required for cerebroside sulfatase activity.

Krabbe's Disease (Globoid Cell Leukodystrophy)

Krabbe in 1916 (238) gave the first complete description of the relatively uncommon leukodystrophy that bears his name, but Collier and Greenfield in 1924 (77) gave the name globoid to the characteristic cells present in the white matter. Suzuki and Suzuki (458) have thoroughly reviewed the literature and made major contributions to our understanding of this disorder.

Clinical onset usually occurs between 3 and 5 months of life, although a few cases with later onset have been reported (184). Affected infants are frequently normal for the first few months of life but develop intermittent fevers, sometimes accompanied by seizures, feeding problems, hyperesthesia, hyperirritability, and psychomotor regression. Dementia and motor abnormalities become dominant and rapidly progress. Optic atrophy is common. The child's head frequently remains small, and there is no visceromegaly. CSF protein is usually elevated. Evidence of peripheral neuropathy has occured as early as 7 weeks of age, but by 6 months, deep tendon reflexes are usually hypoactive (124). Death generally occurs by 2 yr of age.

The basic defect in Krabbe's disease is a deficiency of galactocerebroside β-galactosidase. To demonstrate this deficiency the enzyme activity must be assayed with the natural substrate galactocerebroside. The enzyme β-galactosidase (the enzyme deficient in G_{M1} gangliosidosis, which is assayed with synthetic substrates) is not deficient in Krabbe's disease. Conversely, in G_{M1} gangliosidosis, galactocerebroside-β-galactosidase activity is normal or slightly elevated. Galactocerebroside-β-galactosidase activity is also low in serum, leukocytes, and cultured fibroblasts of patients with Krabbe's disease (455). Affected patients are homozygous for this autosomal recessive trait. Heterozygous carriers generally have levels of galactocerebrosidase intermediate between normal controls and patients with the disease, but there is considerable overlap in these values with noncarrier controls (465).

Galactocerebrosidase activity is also very low in patients with late-onset globoid cell leukodystrophy (89). However, in one such case, cultured fibroblasts had a higher residual activity and maximum velocity and different pH optimum for galactocerebrosidase from those of a patient with the infantile form. This suggests that there may be different allelic mutations of the locus coding for this enzyme, which explains the phenotypic variability. Studies of affected fetuses have demonstrated morphological abnormalities of nervous system involvement as early as 20 weeks gestation. This indicates that irreversible neurological damage may occur even before birth (281).

Although galactocerebroside injections into brain induce globoid cells, they do not affect oligodendrocytes, the destruction of which seems to be the pivotal step in the pathogenesis of the brain lesions. Miyatake and Suzuki (299) found that the enzyme psychosine galactosidase is also deficient in brain, liver, and kidney of patients with Krabbe's disease, which is responsible for the elevated levels of psychosine. They proposed "the psychosine hypothesis" that the accumulation of psychosine, which is extremely toxic, in oligodendrocytes is responsible for their destruction, and the consequent destruction and impaired formation of myelin. It is still not certain whether galactocerebrosidase and psychosine galactosidase activities are due to the same enzyme.

In affected patients the brain is small with external evidence of cerebral atrophy. The sectioned cerebrum has the typical ap-

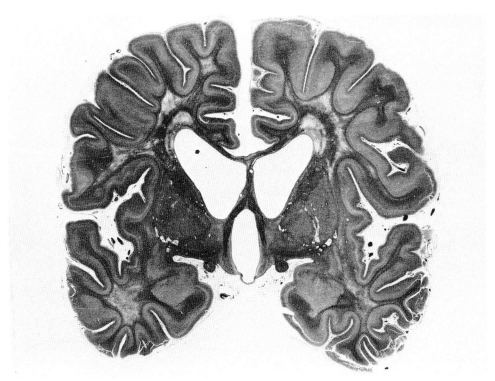

Figure 8.16. Coronal section of the brain from a case of Krabbe's disease showing ventricular dilation and both demyelination and astrogliosis. PTAH (Original magnification ×0.7.)

pearance of a leukodystrophy with greyish discoloration of the centrum ovale and corona radiata, both of which are rubbery firm. There is a tendency to spare subcortical arcuate fibers. The ventricular system is dilated (Fig. 8.16). In severely affected cases, the white matter may be a fibrous mesh, occasionally with some small cystic areas. The brain stem is small, with greyish discoloration of the pyramidal tracts. The cerebellar white matter is similarly abnormal but sometimes less severely affected (184).

Typically histological abnormalities in the brain occur in areas that are normally heavily myelinated. These demonstrate a severe lack of myelinated axons and oligodendroglia. There are numerous reactive astrocytes together with perivascular clusters of globoid and "epithelioid" cells, giving the tissue a hypercellular appearance (Fig. 8.17A). The globoid cells are 20–40 μm in diameter and have several oval nuclei. Epithelioid cells are smaller mononuclear cells with similar cytoplasm (324). The globoid and epithelial cells are thought

to be basically similar and to originate from histiocytes. The cytoplasm is moderately positive with PAS but stains only weakly with SBB. These abnormalities are most marked in phylogenetically newer areas and less pronounced in fornix, hippocampus, mammillothalamic tract, and basal ganglia. The pyramidal tracts are the most severely affected areas in spinal cord.

D'Agostino et al. (93) described the histological changes in detail. In the "early" stage, myelin and axonal loss is minimal, and PAS-positive material is present in microglia and mononuclear epithelial cells. During a more advanced stage, multinucleate globoid cells and reactive astrocytes appear, and axons are decreased in number. Myelin is absent in the late stage when globoid cells are fewer in number and tend to be perivascular. In the final stage, myelin and axons are absent (Fig. 8.17B), and there is mainly astrocytic gliosis.

The cerebral cortex is histologically normal with both conventional and Golgi stains, despite its essential isolation as a consequence of degeneration of the afferent

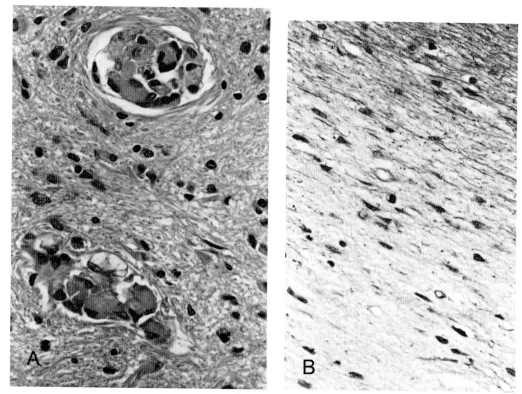

Figure 8.17. Krabbe's disease. (A) Prominent perivascular multinucleated globoid cells and epithelioid cells in a demyelinated, astrogliotic background. PAS, (Original magnification ×240.) (B) Extensive axonal loss in the late stage. Bielschowsky. (Original magnification ×380.)

axons to it from white matter (504). Except for superimposed abnormalities such as pneumonia, extraneural tissues are histologically normal. There is a marked loss of ganglion cells from retina, but the eye is otherwise normal.

EM shows that the mononuclear and multinucleated globoid cells are similar and have numerous pseudopodia and contain subplasmalemmal linear densities 0.1–1 μm in length. These findings support the suggestion that the cells are of macrophage origin (510). The cells also contain characteristic inclusions that have straight or curved tubular profiles with longitudinal striations with a periodicity of about 6 nm in width. They are of variable size but up to 5 μm in length and between 10 nm and 200 nm wide (Fig. 8.18).

In cross-sections, the cells vary from small and round to larger multilamellar contours appearing irregularly crystalloid. Some lie free in the cytoplasm; others appear to be surrounded by a limiting membrane. They appear to be either scattered among normal cytoplasmic organelles or surrounded by an electron-lucent area (17). Pure galactocerebroside crystals have a similar appearance. Less common are twisted tubules 30 nm in length, with constrictions every 200 nm (406) containing 4–5 nm longitudinal striations. Both types of inclusions have been produced by injecting galactocerebroside into rat brains (455). Astrocytes and oligodendroglial cells do not contain tubular inclusions, which are found in endothelial and perithelial cells (458).

In peripheral nerve, there is a decreased density of myelinated but not of unmyelinated fibers, mainly due to a decreased proportion of larger myelinated axons (400). Teased fiber preparations demonstrate segmental demyelination. Osmiophilic lipid droplets occur in Schwann cell cytoplasm at the paranodal region, and ORO- and SBB-positive material is present in occa-

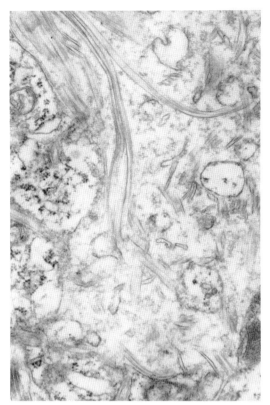

Figure 8.18. Curvilinear tubular profiles and crystalloid cross-sectional contours characterizing the cytoplasm of the globoid cells in Krabbe's disease. Electron micrograph. (Original magnification ×70,000.)

sional Schwann cells of frozen section material. EM shows that Schwann cells contain myelin debris in autophagosomes, although typical globoid cells are not found. Inclusions similar to those of globoid cells are present in Schwann cells of myelinated fibers and macrophages. Some axons are surrounded by thin, loose, myelin sheaths indicative of remyelination. Congential muscle fiber-type disproportion has been reported (100).

A few cases with later onset, between 2 and 55 yr, have been reported as late infantile or juvenile globoid leukodystrophy (89). The duration of the illness has been between 5 months and 2 yr. Early development is usually normal, but the patients show cortical blindness with optic atrophy, and pyramidal tract abnormalities. Peripheral nerve function and CSF protein levels may be normal. Morphological findings in the CNS of most cases have been similar to those of the infantile form, but globoid cells may be absent if the clinical course is prolonged (490). There are some older reports of Krabbe's disease occurring in adults, but there are no biochemically confirmed cases.

Lipids highly concentrated in myelin are markedly diminished in cerebral white matter (125). The levels of cholesterol, cerebrosides, and sulfatides are decreased to a greater extent than the total phospholipids. The proportion of the latter comprised of ethanolamine phosphoglyceride is reduced, but the choline phosphoglyceride fraction is elevated. The phospholipid fatty acid profile is similar to that found in white matter of normal, 2- to 4-month-old infants. Only minor changes in these compounds occur in cerebral cortex. The gangliosides G_{M3}, G_{M2}, and G_{D3} are elevated in both grey and white matter (125). All of these changes are probably due to the myelin deficiency and replacement with astrocytes and globoid cells. The lack of cholesterol esters correlates with the absence of sudanophilia. Although the levels of cerebroside and sulfatide are both low, the cerebroside to sulfatide ratio is significantly increased in the centrum ovale. This is due to an accumulation of cerebroside in globoid cells and not to an elevated cerebroside content of myelin. Galactosylsphingosine (psychosine) is elevated at least 100-fold in affected white matter.

Adrenoleukodystrophy

The group of patients who have CNS demyelination and abnormalities of the adrenal gland are now usually referred to by Blaw's (39) term adrenoleukodystrophy. Since the original description of Siemerling and Creutzfeld in 1923 (420), over 50 cases have been described and variously classified as orthochromatic leukodystrophy, sudanophilic leukodystrophy, diffuse sclerosis, melanodermic leukodystrophy, and Schilder's disease. Most of the cases referred to as Schilder's disease have been in young males with classic adrenoleukodystrophy (ALD). The remainder probably had some multiple sclerosis variant (321, 397). Because of this and the fact that Schilder's original three cases did not constitute a uniform group (390), the term Schilder's disease should no longer be used.

ALD is inherited as an X-linked recessive disorder and manifests itself in four clinically recognizable forms according to the classification of Moser et al. (304): classical ALD, adrenomyeloneuropathy (AMN), neonatal leukodystrophy, and symptomatic heterozygotes.

ALD and AMN may be two expressions of a common genetic and biochemical defect that should be called adrenoleukomyeloneuropathy (341). The finding of overlap cases with ALD and peripheral neuropathy supports this concept (409). The consistent biochemical abnormality found in these disorders is an increased proportion of very long chain fatty acids (especially $C_{26:0}$) in cholesterol ester, gangliosides, sphingomyelin, free fatty acids of brain and adrenal and cholesterol esters of peripheral nerve, plasma, cultured fibroblasts, and skeletal muscle (304). Obligate heterozygotes have a ratio of $C_{26:0}$ to $C_{22:0}$ in cultured fibroblasts, intermediate between normals and affected patients. Much of the hexacosanoic acid in the accumulated cholesterol ester is derived from the diet, but the basic enzymatic defect in this disorder is unknown. There is evidence of both increased synthesis (483) and impaired oxidation (423) of long chain fatty acids. Genetic studies on clones of cultured fibroblasts indicate that the disorder is X-linked, and the gene is subject to inactivation (297).

CLASSIC ADRENOLEUKODYSTROPHY

Typically, patients with ALD are in the first decade of life when clinical signs first develop. However, adult cases have been described (362), and one patient had no symptoms until 52 yr of age (254). The duration from onset to death is between 1 and 9 yr, and the course is usually steadily progressive, although relapsing and remitting courses have been reported (497). Behavioral disturbance has been the most frequent neurological presentation, often leading initially to a psychiatric diagnosis. Other features include seizures, visual loss (cortical blindness), and corticospinal tract involvement, progressing to spastic quadriparesis. CSF protein is mildly elevated in some cases. The proportion of patients who have clinical evidence of adrenal failure is uncertain, but one-third of the cases in the series of Schaumburg et al. (397) had fatigue, vomiting, and cutaneous pigmentation. Serum cortisol levels are usually normal, but adrenocorticotrophic hormone (ACTH) stimulation studies have demonstrated primary adrenocortical failure in most patients in whom they have been done.

At autopsy, there may be external evidence of cerebral atrophy and ventricular dilation, but the cerebral cortex appears normal. Abnormalities are restricted to white matter and are usually most severe in the occipital, parietal, and posterior temporal lobes. These regions are firm and appear gelatinous and brown in the fresh state (Fig. 8.19A) but grey and shrunken after formalin fixation. The less involved margins are pink and soft. As well as the centrum ovale, the fornix, hippocampal commissure, cingulum, and corpus callosum are frequently involved, but there is relative sparing of subcortical arcuate fibers and Gennari's band, especially in the less involved areas (Fig. 8.19B). The lesions may be symmetrical posteriorly but asymmetric in the frontal lobes. Secondary atrophy of the pyramidal tracts leads to a grey, shrunken appearance of the posterior limb of the internal capsule, lateral cerebral peduncles, basis pontis, pyramids, and lateral corticospinal tracts. The cerebellar white matter is variably involved, occasionally including the peduncles and the region adjacent to the dentate nucleus (321, 397).

Histologically, the cerebral cortex is normal except for mild gliosis in deeper layers. Secondary neuronal loss may occur in the mammillary bodies and some thalamic nuclei. Schaumburg et al. (397) described three histological zones in the involved white matter. The first zone was the largest region and was usually mostly posterior. This region was devoid of myelin, oligodendrocytes, and axons and consisted of dense fibrillary gliosis. There were occasional perivascular macrophages with PAS-, ORO-, and SBB-positive cytoplasm. The second zone, surrounding the first, contained numerous lipid-laden macrophages and bare axons, some myelinated axons, and a prominent perivascular infiltrate of lymphocytes and plasma cells. More extensively, in the third zone, myelin sheaths were partially disrupted, but axons were intact, and mac-

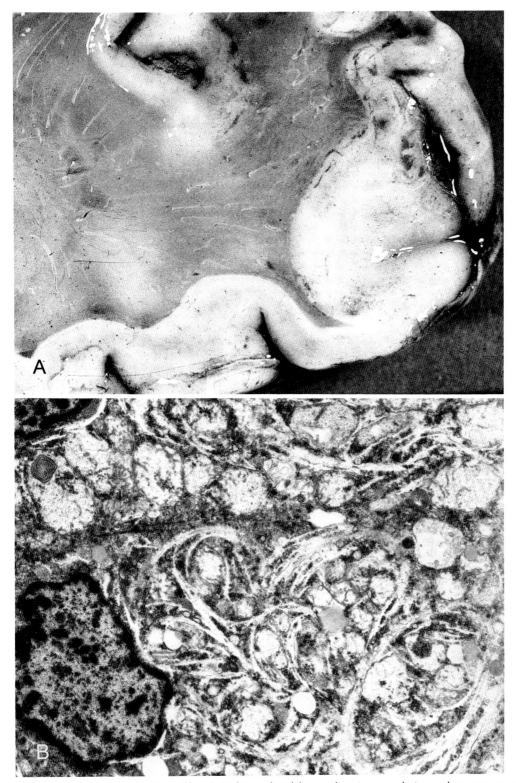

Figure 8.19.   Adrenoleukodystrophy. (*A*) The unfixed brain showing a gelatinous homogeneous loss of myelin. (*B*) Characteristic curvilinear clefts evident in the adrenal gland, although the actual membranous profiles cannot be identified. Electron micrograph. (Original magnification ×10,500.)

rophages were scattered throughout the tissue. The main involvement in brain stem and spinal cord was Wallerian degeneration of the corticospinal tract, and in cases with dentate nuclear involvement, the superior cerebellar peduncles were similarly affected.

EM shows cytoplasmic, membrane-bound inclusions in macrophages (159), consisting of linear membranous profiles with two 2.5-nm wide, electron-dense lines separated by a clear space (2–7 nm). Frequently, the actual membranous profiles cannot be identified; instead the characteristic curvilinear clefts are present (Fig. 8.19B). In severely affected areas of this white matter the amount of myelin debris in macrophages may obscure the other linear profiles. Linear inclusions are not present in astrocytes. Inclusions have also been found in Schwann cells and endoneurial macrophages of peripheral nerve.

The adrenals vary from severely atrophic to normal on gross inspection. The evolution of microscopic changes in the adrenal cortex has been studied in detail by Powers and Schaumburg (363). These abnormalities are restricted to the zonae fasiculata and reticularis. The earliest change is the appearance of birefringent cytoplasmic striations. Accumulation of this material damages the cells, causing an increase in ACTH that in turn causes cytoplasmic ballooning, striations, and vacuolar changes. The ballooned cells stain more weakly with ORO than normal cells.

Ultrastructurally, the striations consist of lamellar profiles. The lamellae vary in thickness from 0.6 to 1.2 nm and the interlamellar clear spaces from 0.1 to 0.7 nm. These are probably composed of cholesterol esters with very long chain fatty acids. Powers and Schaumburg (363) suggest that these are responsible for impairment in function and death of the adrenal cortical cells. The testes are frequently immature, but lamellar inclusions are found in the cytoplasm of presumptive Leydig's cell precursors (364). Linear inclusions have also been found in phagocytes of liver, spleen, and thymus and, occasionally, renal tubular epithelial cell (159). The diagnosis of ALD is suggested by computer-assisted tomography of the brain and confirmed by biopsies of brain, adrenals, testes, peripheral nerve, skin, or conjuctiva. Martin et al. (280) demonstrated by EM the usefulness of studying the small nerve twigs of skin or conjunctival biopsies in 11 cases of ALD and its variants.

ADRENOMYELONEUROPATHY

A few cases of peripheral neuropathy have been described in males in whom adrenal insufficiency developed in childhood with or without subsequent hypogonadism. Neurological abnormalities usually do not become evident until adulthood, when progressive spastic paraparesis, distal neuropathy and, later, cerebellar ataxia and dementia occur (174, 366). The main morphological abnormalities are severe loss of axons and myelin from the corticospinal tracts throughout the brain stem and spinal cord as well as from the fasciculus gracilis. There is mild proliferation of astrocytes in these tracts and in the white matter of the cerebrum and cerebellum. There is a loss of large, myelinated fibers from peripheral nerve, and the adrenals may be severely atrophic. With EM, lamellar profiles are seen in CNS macrophages and adrenal cortical and Leydig's cells (398).

NEONATAL ADRENOLEUKODYSTROPHY

A very rare form of ALD occurs early in infancy with failure to thrive and seizures. One patient had craniofacial abnormalities (33). Psychomotor retardation and adrenocortical failure develop, and death occurs between 2 and 7 yr. The adrenals are atrophic, and adrenocortical cells have cytoplasmic striations and lamellar-lipid inclusions. The cerebral cortex in some cases is micropolygyric, but the main neuropathological findings are in the white matter. There is loss of myelin from the centrum ovale, brain stem, and cerebellum with reactive astrocytes and fibrillary gliosis. Lamellar inclusions occur in the macrophages in brain, liver, and lymph nodes (271). Brown et al. (56) suggest that neonatal adrenoleukodystrophy may be related to Zellweger's syndrome, based on the accumulation of very long chain fatty acids in both conditions. Zellweger's syndrome is associated with facial abnormalities (high forehead, hypertelorism, epicanthal folds), hypotonia, small cortical renal cysts, and hepatomegaly. Micropolygyria and sudan-ophilic neutral lipid deposits have been noted but no adrenal abnormalities (56).

SYMPTOMATIC HETEROZYGOTE

Two families have been studied in which primary adrenal insufficiency, hypogonadism, and neurological abnormalities coexist (304, 341). The neurological disorders include spastic paraparesis, a spinal sensory level, sensorimotor neuropathy, and autonomic neuropathy. The condition has occurred in females as well as males. Therefore, it appears that some heterozygotes may be "manifest carriers."

Alexander's Disease

Alexander's disease, first described in 1949 (13), is a rare, probably autosomal recessive, progressive disorder reported in infants, juveniles, and adults (387). In the infantile group, there is psychomotor retardation and megacephaly, often with hydrocephalus, spasticity, and seizures. Those with a juvenile onset have spasticity, bulbar signs, and mental deterioration. The clinical features in adults are variable. The diagnosis can be suspected on computerized tomography by a striking frontal enhancement with contrast administration (Fig. 8.20) but can be confirmed only by brain biopsy.

At autopsy, the weight of the brain is increased, and only on coronal sectioning is the soft, grey, sometimes collapsed white matter apparent, especially in the frontal lobes. The cerebral cortex is usually white and firm. The lateral and third ventricles may be dilated. The outlines of the basal ganglia are sometimes indistinct, but no gross abnormalities of brain stem, cerebellum, or spinal cord are apparent (155).

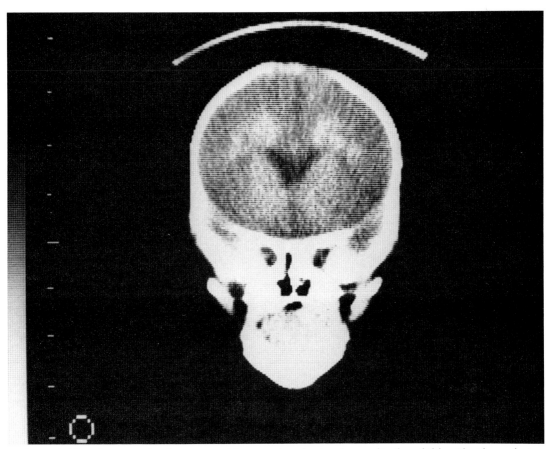

Figure 8.20. Computerized tomographic scan (contrast-enhanced) of a child with Alexander's disease. Increased densities are seen in the periventricular frontal white matter and basal ganglia.

Microscopically, the diagnostic feature is the massive accumulation of Rosenthal fibers arranged roughly perpendicular to pia (Fig. 8.21*A*), blood vessels, and ependyma in both grey and white matter (191, 415). Although they are also scattered haphazardly throughout the CNS, there is a striking sparing of cerebellar cortex. The Rosenthal fibers tend to aggregate, in particular around the cerebral aqueduct, with erosion of ependymal lining and apposition of aqueductal walls and stenosis.

Rosenthal fibers are elongated, irregularly contoured bodies of variable length (1–200 μm). The larger bodies appear to have no relationship to cells, but smaller granules are clearly seen in the cytoplasm of astrocytes. Sometimes these early granular changes are the predominant pathology, with characteristic Rosenthal fibers difficult to identify especially in a brain biopsy. The Rosenthal fibers stain red with hematoxylin and eosin, dark purple with Mallory's phosphotungstic acid hematoxylin, brownish-black with Bielschowsky, and blue with LFB. They are not birefringent, and both PAS and amyloid stains are negative. In infantile cases, the myelin loss is striking, and in these areas, astrogliosis, which is sometimes very pleomorphic, is prominent. Perivascular accumulations of lymphocytes and histiocytes are not uncommon.

Immunohistochemistry, using antiglial fibrillary acidic protein sera, shows that the Rosenthal fibers are negative (Fig. 8.21*B*), although the cytoplasm immediately surrounding the fiber is clearly positive (431). This correlates with the EM, which shows the Rosenthal fiber to be densely osmiophilic and surrounded by sheaths of astroglial fibers, some of which seem to merge with the central osmiophilic mass (Fig. 8.22 (32, 191). The antigenic and ultrastructural differences between Rosenthal fibers and glial filaments suggest that if the glial filaments are transferred into Rosenthal fibers, they must have undergone a profound change. The other possibility is that the Rosenthal fibers are unrelated to glial filaments and consist of an unidentified chemical substance. Histochemical reactions suggest that the material is a protein composed of proteolipid and containing inositol and fatty acid (415).

Sometimes there is no apparent direct relationship between myelin loss and Rosenthal fibers, but generally the number of Rosenthal fibers is related to the degree of demyelination. The severely involved areas tend to be centrum ovale, tegmental brain stem, and deep cerebellum around the dentate nuclei. Sudanophilic myelin breakdown products (cholesterol esters and other neutral lipids) are consistently present. Nerve cell loss and associated astrogliosis are present to a variable extent, often extensively involving the cerebral cortex and, to a lesser degree, basal ganglia and brain stem. Histologically, peripheral nerve and muscle are normal (431).

The cause of demyelination in a disease process that affects mainly astrocytes is not clear. Herndon and Rubinstein (191) suggested that Rosenthal fibers may result from a metabolic defect in the astrocytes in pathways responsible for formation and degradation of glial filaments. In the infantile cases, this defect may interfere with normal nutritive and supportive functions of the astrocyte, leading secondarily to demyelination. In an experimental model Horoupian et al. (200) suggested that a defect of the blood-brain barrier occurs with deposition of nickel in the perivascular space and subsequent inducement of Rosenthal fibers.

Spongy Degeneration of the Nervous System (Canavan's Disease or Canavan-van Bogaert-Bertrand Spongy Degeneration)

Canavan's disease, or spongy degeneration of the nervous system (66), was first described as a separate disease by van Bogaert and Bertrand in 1949 (486). It is an autosomal recessive condition occurring in Jewish infants. The onset is typically in the first 6 months of life and is characterized by apathy, loss of motor activity, and hypotonia. In most cases, blindness and optic atrophy are reported. Megacephaly is conspicuous. By 1 yr of age, the infant is spastic with periodic decereberation, myoclonus, and generalized seizures. Impairment of extraocular movements is not uncommon. The CSF protein may be slightly elevated. A rare, juvenile form (in patients older than 5 yr) has also been described (211). These

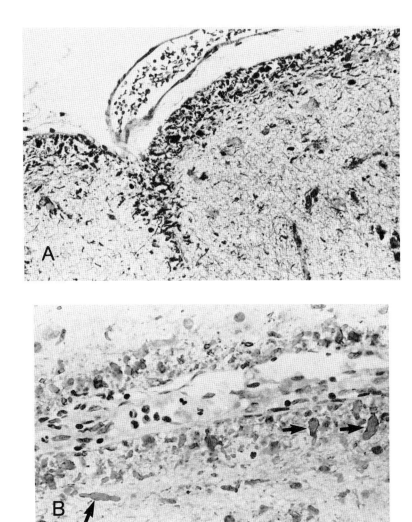

Figure 8.21.   Rosenthal fibers in Alexander's disease. (*A*) Clustered in a subpial location in the cortex. LFB. (Original magnification ×240.) (*B*) Negative for reaction against antisera to glial fibrillary acidic protein (*arrows*). Immunoperoxidase. (Original magnification ×380.)

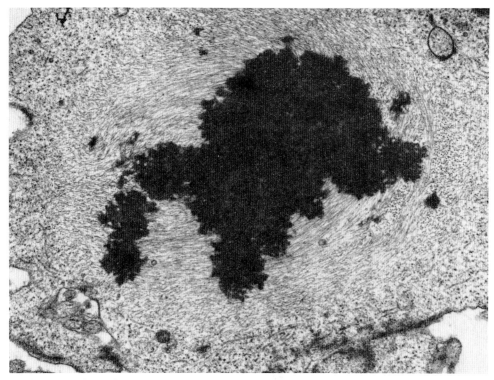

Figure 8.22. In Alexander's disease, osmiophilic masses of variable size constituting the Rosenthal fiber. A dense network of glial filaments forms the background. Electron micrograph. (Original magnification ×12,500.)

older children are not Jewish and have cerebellar signs and spasticity without mental retardation. Megacephaly has not been seen in this form.

In classic infantile spongy degeneration, the brain is heavier than normal. On coronal sections, the white matter is soft, gelatinous, and grey, with the texture of a wet sponge. The occipital lobe is more involved than the frontal and parietal areas, which are in turn more affected than the temporal lobes. The globus pallidus is severely involved, with brain stem and spinal cord less affected. The cerebellum is generally atrophic (4, 8, 196).

Microscopically, there is spongy change (Fig. 8.23A), demyelination, proliferation of Alzheimer type II astrocytes (Fig. 8.23B), and scarce fibrillary gliosis (196). Vacuolation involves the arcuate fibers and extends into the deep cortex, both cerebral and cerebellar. The vacuoles are round to oval cavities, larger than neurons. Demyelination is moderate with mild gliosis, normalappearing oligodendrocytes and little or no sudanophilic debris. In contrast to other leukodystrophies in which there is preservation of arcuate fibers, these show prominent involvement in this disorder. In the cerebellum, the vacuoles are most prominent in the junctional area between white matter and the granule cell layer of cortex. Alzheimer type II astrocytes are present, but the usual association with hepatic disease is absent. The neurons are normal in the early stages but later in the course of the disease they degenerate, and reactive astrogliosis becomes more prominent. In the retina, ganglion cell loss and vacuolation of the optic nerve have been present (196). Peripheral nerve lesions consisting of perineurial and endoneurial histiocytic infiltration together with slight demyelination and axonal swelling have been described (450).

In the white matter, ultrastructural studies indicate that the vacuoles seen by light microscopy appear to be due to both clear spaces within myelin sheaths that are splitting at the major dense lines and swelling

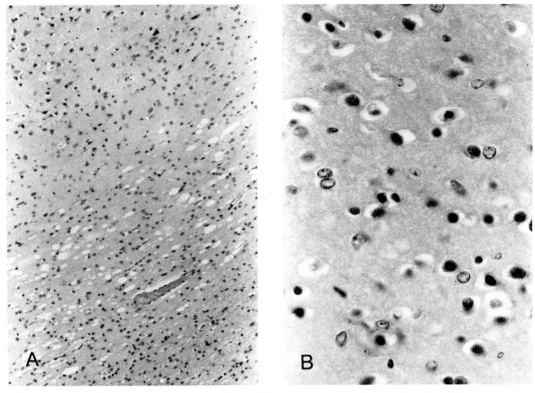

Figure 8.23. Subcortical white matter of a child with Canavan's disease showing (A) a prominent spongiform alteration and (B) Alzheimer type II astrocytes. H & E. (A, Original magnification × 100; B, Original magnification ×380.)

of astrocytic cytoplasm (4). In both grey and white matter, the astrocytic cytoplasm is distinctly watery. These astrocytes have large, pale nuclei and prominent nucleoli. The mitochondria are very elongated, measuring up to 12 μm in length with a filamentous matrix and irregular cristae (8).

Despite extensive studies, no definite biochemical basis for the vacuolation has been established. Abnormal astrocytic mitochondrial morphology and decreased or absent mitochondrial adenosine triphosphatase (ATPase) suggest that the ATPase defect may be responsible for the cellular swelling by interfering with regulation of intracellular fluid and electrolyte concentrations. Experimentally, ouabain, a powerful inhibitor of sodium-potassium-activated ATPase, produces brain vacuolation similar to that seen in this disease (81). However, Adornato et al. (8), assaying ATPase and cytochrome oxidase activities in fresh frozen biopsy tissue, found that these activities did not differ from those

seen in controls. Triethyltin, cuprizone, and certain aminoacidopathies produce spongy change, predominantly in white matter, but no abnormalities in trace-metal or amino-acid metabolism have been identified in patients with this disease.

Although the precise cause of the fluid accumulation is not known, the EM and histochemical studies suggest that the disease is due to a metabolic abnormality of astrocytic mitochondria.

Pelizaeus-Merzbacher Disease

The criteria for classifying a case in the same group as those originally described by Pelizaeus in 1885 and Merzbacher in 1910 have been debated at length (413). Zeman et al. (516) required that X-linked inheritance be demonstrated, excluding many cases considered by others (326) as belonging in this category. Based on the pattern of demyelination, Seitelberger in 1970 (413) included six subtypes but in 1981 (414), taking other aspects of the conditions into consideration, described only three subtypes of Pelizaeus-Merzbacher disease.

INFANTILE FORM (SEITELBERGER)

The infantile form of Pelizaeus-Merzbacher disease is characterized by nystagmus, extrapyramidal signs, and complete failure of psychomotor development. The duration of the disease is from several months to a few years. Chemical analyses have shown a reduction of total lipids.

Neuropathological findings consist of an atrophic brain with a striking and diffuse absence of myelin associated with astrogliosis. Brain stem and spinal cord myelin is better preserved, and peripheral nerve myelin is normal. On EM, sparse myelin lamellae can be identified. Although Seitelberger (410) considered this condition to be a neonatal variant of Pelizaeus-Merzbacher disease, others have suggested that there is a primary failure of brain myelination (405).

JUVENILE FORM (CLASSICAL TYPE)

The classical form of Pelizaeus-Merzbacher disease becomes clinically manifest in the first decade of life. It is an X-linked, recessive, very slowly progressive disorder characterized by nystagmus, intermittent shaking movements of the head, ataxia, choreoathetoid movements, and psychomotor retardation. Other than a reduction of total lipids, no specific neurochemical abnormality has been found.

The brain and often the cerebellum are atrophic, with large ventricles, normal cortex, patchy demyelination, and variable astrogliosis. The myelin around blood vessels tends to be better preserved (tigroid or leopard skin pattern of demyelination), and lipid-laden macrophages containing SBB-positive material are sparse, probably because of the slow progression of the disease. Axons tend to be fairly well preserved (414).

Chemical analyses have also been performed on brains of classical Pelizaeus-Merzbacher disease. Bourre et al. (42, 43) found that total isolatable brain myelin was only 7% of normal. In white matter the amount of cerebroside, sulfatide, and sphingomyelin was markedly decreased. In sphingolipids of white matter and isolated myelin, α-hydroxylated and very long chain fatty acids were greatly reduced. They concluded that the disorder may be due to a defect in the synthesis of these fatty acids, resulting in impaired myelinogenesis.

ADULT FORM (LÖWENBERG AND HILL)

The adult form of Pelizaeus-Merzbacher disease was first described by Löwenberg and Hill in 1933 (263). Inheritance is autosomal dominant, and clinical onset is in adulthood. Patients characteristically have predominantly psychotic features together with corticospinal tract involvement, ataxia, and speech difficulties.

The brain tends to be mildly atrophic with severe demyelination associated with astrogliosis. There is preservation of arcuate myelinated fibers and perivascular islets of myelin. Some loss of axons may be apparent. Sudanophilic material is present but not abundant, and much is perivascularly distributed (414).

Cockayne's Syndrome

The main features of Cockayne's syndrome, first described in 1936 (76), are onset in late infancy, autosomal recessive pattern of inheritance, dwarfism, deafness, cataracts, retinal pigmentation, optic atrophy, thickened skull, and mental deficiency. Less common features include "bird-headed" facies; loss of subcutaneous fat; photodermatitis; anhidrosis; normal pressure hydrocephalus; peripheral neuropathy, and extrapyramidal, pyramidal, and cerebellar signs (428).

On neuropathological examination (179, 302), the brain is consistently small, and leptomeninges are diffusely thickened. The optic nerves are atrophic. Blood vessels at the base of the brain show no abnormality. When the brain is cut, there is often a gritty texture correlating with the extensive calcification (Fig. 8.24A), especially in the basal ganglia (Fig. 8.24B). Coronal sections show a moderately dilated ventricular system, with an atrophic cortical mantle and reduced white matter. The cerebellum is also atrophic.

Microscopic examination confirms the extensively fibrosed leptomeninges. The cortex shows prominent perivascular and extravascular mineralization, which stains positively for calcium and iron. One report describes a prominent lipofuscin accumu-

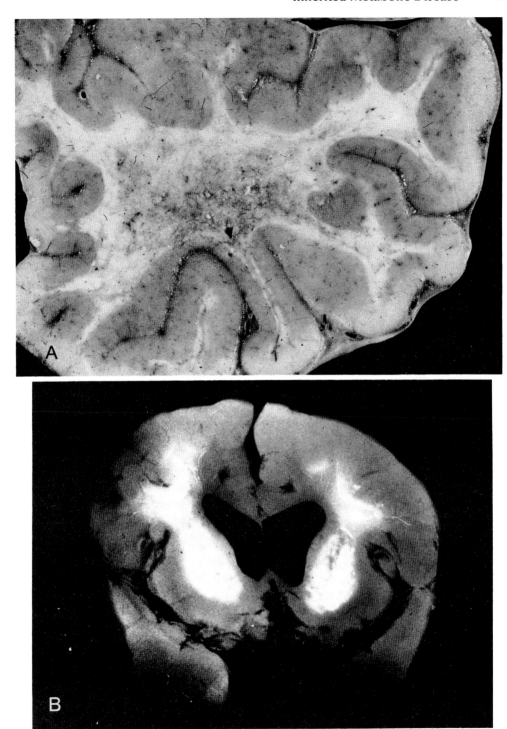

Figure 8.24. Frontal coronal section from Cockayne's disease. (*A*) Patchy demyelination and focal calcification. (*B*) Brain exposed to roentgenography showing extensive calcification in caudate, putamen, and centrum ovale.

lation within the cytoplasm of neurons (428). In the white matter, there is patchy demyelination with preservation of islands of perivascular myelin (Fig. 8.25A). The arcuate fibers are not spared. Soffer et al. (428) described the proliferation of large,

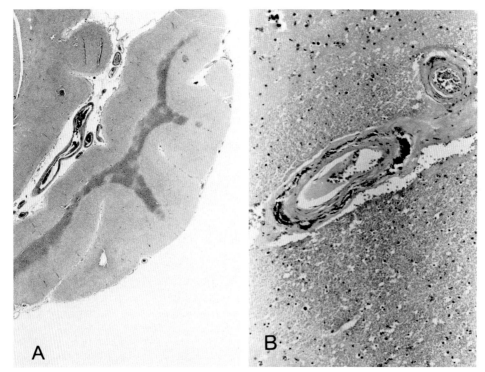

Figure 8.25. Cockayne's disease. (*A*) Focal myelin loss evident in the temporal white matter. LFB. (Original magnification ×1.5.) (*B*) Vascular calcification prominent throughout the brain parenchyma. H & E. (Original magnification ×100.)

bizarre astrocytes involving both grey and white matter. In the basal ganglia, especially in the putamen, basophilic calcospherites of various sizes can be found mainly in the walls of capillaries and arteries. Axonal spheroids in caudate nuclei, internal capsule, and substantia nigra have been described. In the cerebellum, there is a diffuse paucity of Purkinje and granule cells with proliferation of Bergmann astroglia. Golgi preparations of cerebellar cortex are normal except for single Purkinje cells, which lack secondary and tertiary branches and have a large, sunflower-like density, presumably representing a tangle of dendritic branches (428). Peripheral nerves have segmental demyelination (386).

The major neuropathological findings are micrencephaly, patchy demyelination (tigroid), and cerebral calcification. Because of variations from case to case, some authors have stressed the calcifying vasculopathy, and others the tigroid demyelination. In fact, Seitelberger, in 1970 (413),

included Cockayne's syndrome as a type of Pelizaeus-Merzbacher disease because of the pattern of demyelination; however, this does not appear to be justified on the basis of the many other abnormalities in Cockayne's syndrome.

The pathogenesis of Cockayne's syndrome is unknown. Some of the changes in the brain suggest an acceleration of the aging process (428). Using cultured skin fibroblasts from patients with Cockayne's syndrome, Schmickel et al. (401) showed decreased colony-forming ability after ultraviolet irradiation in vitro, but the fibroblasts have a normal rate of ultraviolet-induced, unscheduled deoxyribonucleic acid (DNA) synthesis, one measure of the repair of DNA. However, there has been no further clarification in this area, and a true understanding of the pathogenesis of the disease process remains unknown.

Sudanophilic Leukodystrophies

Although the term sudanophilic leukodystrophy (SLD) could be used very broadly to include all those leukodystrophies with orthochromatically staining neutral lipid in which metachromasia cannot be demonstrated, it now has a more restricted meaning. We are applying it to leukodystrophies that cannot be classified as inflammatory demyelinating disease, those without metachromatic substances, and those without other distinguishing diagnostic features. The "pure" form, simple type is described below, and the "pure" form, pigmented type and the "combined" forms described by Peiffer (346) are discussed under "Other Leukodystrophies."

Even cases with the "pure" form, simple type have different clinical features. Some have occurred in the perinatal period with markedly deficient CNS myelination and death early in life (395). Patients dying later in infancy have histological evidence of demyelination with sudanophilic lipid-laden macrophages (325). Juvenile (101) and adult (18) cases have occurred with severe CNS demyelination and large periventricular cavities. Although the demyelination is usually widespread, being most marked in cerebrum, some cases have had atypical distribution of demyelinating lesions. Histologically, there is evidence of demyelination with axonal loss usually in proportion to myelin damage. Foamy macrophages with sudanophilic birefringent material are seen in frozen sections. Reactive astrocytes and fibrillary gliosis are variable but may be quite pronounced.

Neurochemical studies have been performed on cerebral tissues of patients with several different types of "pure" SLD (482). Slight quantitative differences in several constituents have been found, but in general the changes in white matter reflect two morphological features: myelin loss—decreased levels of cerebroside, sulfatide, sphingomyelin, and free cholesterol—and sudanophilic material—increased amounts of cholesterol ester.

Ramsey et al. (371) also found greatly elevated levels of free fatty acid in a case of perinatal SLD. They believed this elevation was the chemical basis of sudanophilia in that case. The cholesterol ester in many cases is probably produced only as a byproduct of myelin degradation. Evidence for this comes from another case of perinatal SLD in which cholesterol esters were

moderately elevated (7.8% dry weight), but cholesteryl ester hydrolase activity was normal (372). However, Yates et al. (513) described a case of SLD in an adult with levels of cholesterol ester in degenerated white matter so high (33.6% of dry weight) that they considered it to be a metabolic abnormality with storage of cholesterol esters. Therefore, this case is an example of the disorders that will be removed from the SLD category and reclassified when specific biochemical abnormalities are recognized.

Other Leukodystrophies

In the miscellaneous category are a number of rare but characteristic diseases as well as others that are rare, incompletely described, and difficult to categorize (346). Those in the latter group will not be further mentioned.

Dermatoleukodystrophy with neuroaxonal spheroids (284) has been described in two Japanese siblings. The skin changes are those of ichthyosis. The neuropathologic findings are irregular loss of myelin, astrogliosis, sudanophilic-filled macrophages, and axonal spheroids containing granular material that ultrastructurally resembles ceroid lipofuscin.

SLD with meningeal angiomatosis (197) is a disease consisting of a noncalcifying meningeal angiomatosis and a SLD.

The pigmented glial cell type of leukodystrophy consists of diffuse demyelination characterized by yellow-black or green-black granules in astrocytes and macrophages, the nature of which has not been determined (346).

Polycystic lipomembranous osteodysplasia with sclerosing leukoencephalopathy (membranous lipodystrophy) is a disease that occurs in adults and is associated with cysts in the bones of the extremities and diffuse brain demyelination. The demyelination is maximal in the frontotemporal lobes with preservation of subcortical arcuate fibers and conspicuous astrogliosis (432).

OTHER METABOLIC DISEASES

A wide spectrum of metabolic disorders affects the nervous system to varying degrees by a variety of mechanisms. For example, in Fabry's disease, Menkes disease, and homocystinuria, the vasculature can be altered sufficiently to initiate thrombosis and cerebral infarction. In other diseases, liver dysfunction may cause encephalopathy. In still others, there may be profound mental retardation without sufficient pathological changes to explain the neurologic dysfunction adequately. To represent some of these uncommon metabolic diseases that may present to the neurologic consultant, the following metabolic encephalopathies will be discussed: amino acid, hyperammonemia, metabolic acidosis, hypoglycemia, copper, and Lesch-Nyhan.

Encephalopathies Associated with Disorders of Amino Acid Metabolism

Although disorders of amino acid metabolism are rare, they are important because they can cause severe, potentially treatable, disturbances of neurologic development (382). These disorders are associated with specific enzyme defects that result in accumulation of specific amino acids. Accompanying the aminoacidopathy, there may be systemic acidosis, hypoglycemia, or hyperammonemia. Because these secondary abnormalities may predominate, they are discussed under separate headings. Some of the aminoacidopathies, for example, maple syrup urine disease (MSUD) and nonketotic hyperglycinemia, present in the neonatal period with seizures, hypotonia, lethargy, and intermittent coma. Others, such as phenylketonuria, may be associated with minor signs in the neonatal period but failure to develop intellectually.

Rosenberg and Scriver (382) gave a detailed list of 48 clinical syndromes in which there is a specific catabolic enzyme defect. At least 23 of the syndromes are associated with mental retardation. An additional 20 disorders are associated with a primary defect in renal membrane transport of amino acids, and several of these are associated with mental retardation. In homocystinuria, still another group of aminoacidopathies, vascular abnormalities, predominate. Mass neonatal screening is used for three main disorders: phenylketonuria, hypothyroidism, and galactosemia. Three other main disorders must be diagnosed clinically on the basis of symptom-sign complexes: MSUD, hyperammonemia, and glycine encephalopathy.

Neuropathological descriptions of the aminoacidopathies have been largely confined to conventional histology, with few EM or Golgi impregnation studies available in the literature. In general, neonates who die with aminoacidopathy have vacuolation (spongiosus) of areas undergoing myelination. In older children, there is diminution in the amount of myelin. Five aminoacidopathies will be discussed here: MSUD, phenylketonuria, hyperglycinemia, homocystinuria, and Hartnup disease. For complete documentation of disorders of amino acid metabolism, see Stanbury et al. (439).

MAPLE SYRUP URINE DISEASE (MSUD)

MSUD is an autosomal recessive, neonatal, neurologic disorder associated with elevated plasma levels of branched-chain essential amino acids such as leucine, isoleucine, and valine, and their ketoacids. Isoleucine gives the maple syrup odor to the urine. Leukocytes of patients with MSUD transaminate the branched-chain amino acids but do not decarboxylate the resulting ketoacids, showing the site of abnormality to be at the point of oxidative decarboxylation (94). An infant with MSUD appears to be normal at birth but within the first week may feed poorly, vomit, be lethargic, and have seizures. The maple syrup odor to the urine may be detected within the 1st week of life. Death is usually due to an infection, although hypoglycemic episodes may also occur (422).

Morphological changes in infants dying in the early stages of disease consist of vacuolation in the areas that are undergoing myelination. A reduction of oligodendroglia with preservation of axons has been noted together with astrogliosis (86). Vacuolation without evident lack of myelination is present in lateral lemniscus, brachium conjunctivum cerebelli, and medial longitudinal fasciculus. Tracts that appear incompletely myelinated include the spinocerebellar, olivospinal, tectospinal, pyramidal, and the brachium pontine. In general, there is no evidence of myelin breakdown such as sudanophilic debris or lipid-filled macrophages (494). The grey matter, peripheral nerves, and dorsal root ganglia show no significant change (422).

Menkes et al. (293) reported that the phospholipid, cholesterol, cerebroside, and sulphatide contents of such brain samples are within normal limits (494). The deleterious effects of ketoacids are primarily due to the leucine ketoacid (α-ketoisocaproic acid), which inhibits myelination in cultures of cerebellum (421).

PHENYLKETONURIA

Phenylketonuria is characterized chemically by the excretion of large amounts of phenylpyruvic acid, clinically by mental retardation, seizures, and impaired hair pigmentation, and genetically by autosomal recessive inheritance. It is the most common aminoaciduria (1:12,500 live births) (7). The biochemical abnormality is impaired hydroxylation of phenylalanine to tyrosine based on a defective enzyme (phenylalanine hydroxylase) (213) and, in some cases, a deficiency of a cofactor (tetrahydrobiopterin) (314). The success of dietary therapy (37) has prompted a newborn screening program (178) that is now in general use.

Nine subtypes of phenylketonuria have been described (480). Since tetrahydrobiopterin is the coenzyme of phenylalanine hydroxylase, tyrosine-3 hydroxylase and tryptophan 5-hydroxylase, biopterin deficiency causes not only hyperphenylalanemia but also impaired biosynthesis of

the neurotransmitters, dopamine and serotonin (Fig. 8.26) (314).

In morphological descriptions of untreated phenylketonuria (14, 269), both grey and white matter changes are noted. Minor architectural abnormalities of cortex are described, such as lobar disproportion and gyral convolutional irregularities. There is one report (82) of ulegyria, presumably secondary to an ischemic insult. The major changes are in white matter, where vacuolation is seen in the CNS of children and demyelination and astrogliosis in the CNS of adults. Vacuolation consistently involves the central white matter of cerebrum and cerebellum, optic tracts, and fornix. Demyelination follows the same pattern with a tendency for preservation of arcuate fibers. Intense astrogliosis and sudanophilic and PAS-positive macrophages are also evident. One ultrastructural study (344) describes membrane-bound, parallel lamellar inclusions believed to be within oligodendrocytes. Lipids and proteolipids associated with myelin are decreased (10, 365).

The pathogenetic relationship between mental retardation and morphological and biochemical alterations is not clear. Several suggestions have been made (10): metabolites acting as toxins to brain, inhibition of inhibitory neurotransmitters (γ-aminobutyric acid), impaired synthesis of serotonin, impaired transport of essential amino acids into brain cells, impaired synthesis of struc-

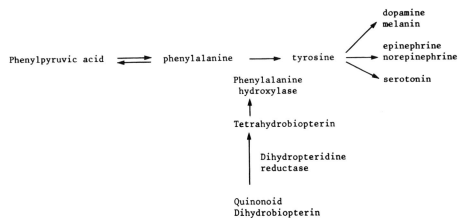

Figure 8.26. Outline of phenylalanine metabolism. In classic phenylketonuria the deficient enzyme is phenylalanine hydroxylase; however, defective cofactor may also produce hyperphenylalanemia.

tural proteolipids, chronic insufficiency of glutamine, or inhibition of brain pyruvate kinase. In general, it is agreed that elevated levels of phenylalanine could alter the biochemical milieu sufficiently to arrest differentiation of the CNS and result in retardation of neuronal development. Once maturation is complete, elevated levels of phenylalanine should not affect intellectual capacity (294).

HYPERGLYCINEMIA

Two types of hyperglycinemia are recognized: ketotic and nonketotic. In ketotic hyperglycinemia, there is a primary block in the catabolism of several organic acids, such as methylmalonic, propionic, and isovaleric acids and isoleucine (417), with a secondary defect in the metabolism of glycine. Neonates with ketotic hyperglycinemia have a severe metabolic acidosis, often with neutropenia, anemia, and thrombocytopenia. Only nonketotic hyperglycinemia is due to a primary defect of glycine metabolism. This type has severe neurologic deterioration with intractable seizures, spasticity, severe mental retardation, and early death (353). Since glycine is a major inhibitory neurotransmitter, the neurological manifestations have been attributed to an exaggerated postsynaptic inhibitory effect (426).

In both types of hyperglycinemia there is vacuolation and loss of myelin in the CNS similar to what has also been described in other aminoacidopathies, such as phenylketonuria, MSUD, tyrosinemia, methionine malabsorption syndrome, and hyperbetaalanemia (417). Ultrastructurally, the myelin vacuoles result from intraperiod splitting (9). Using immunoperoxidase methods, the walls of the vacuoles stain for myelin basic protein, suggesting that the vacuoles originate in compact myelin and not from the adaxonal portion of the sheath or from glial processes (9).

HOMOCYSTINURIA

Homocystinuria is the second most common inborn error of amino acid metabolism. It is an autosomal recessive inherited deficiency of cystothionine β-synthase in which there is elevated plasma methionine and homocystine and urinary excretion of

the homocystine. The clinical features are mental retardation, ectopia lentis, skeletal disproportion, osteoporosis, livedo reticularis over the limbs, and vascular thromboses (305).

Ischemic necrosis is the most dramatic neuropathological abnormality resulting from degeneration of the arterial muscularis and internal elastica in association with thrombosis. The pathogenesis of the vascular occlusion is not known, although enhanced platelet adhesiveness and homocystine accumulation in vessel walls have been suggested (352).

HARTNUP DISEASE

Hartnup disease is an autosomal recessive disorder associated with diminished renal tubular reabsorption and diminished intestinal transport of amino acids often presenting in late childhood or adolescence. Clinical signs are variable and may be intermittent but include a pellagra-like rash, episodes of cerebellar ataxia, dementia, and spasticity. Neuropathological examination shows cortical atrophy and severe neuronal loss especially pronounced in visual cortex and cerebellum (471).

Encephalopathy Associated with Hyperammonemia

The breakdown of amino acids results in the formation of ammonia (416), which is probably toxic to the nervous system, especially in infants. The cause of this toxicity is not clear. Encephalopathies occur mainly in the neonatal period as soon as milk feeding starts, but also may present in early childhood and adolescence. The characteristics are vomiting, lethargy, and seizures in neonates and feeding problems, episodic vomiting, and altered consciousness in infants. Ammonia is normally eliminated by a series of enzymes constituting the urea cycle. Individuals with enzymatic deficiencies at each step of the cycle have been described (385) (Table 8.7). Among the deficiencies, lack of ornithine transcarbamylase and argininosuccinase are most frequent. Hyperammonemia can also be associated with other hereditary disorders not related to a specific urea cycle enzyme (385).

Table 8.7
Urea Cycle Disorders[a]

Enzyme defect	Reaction catalyzed[b]
1. Carbamyl phosphate synthetase	Ammonia + bicarbonate + 2ATP → carbamyl phosphate + 2ADP + Pi
2. Ornithine transcarbamylase	Carbamyl phosphate + ornithine → citrulline + Pi
3. Argininosuccinic acid synthetase	Citrulline + aspartate + ATP → argininosuccinic acid + AMP + pyrophosphate
4. Argininosuccinase	Argininosuccinic acid → arginine + fumaric acid
5. Arginase	Arginine + water → urea + ornithine

[a] From L. P. Rowland (385).
[b] ADP, adenosine diphosphate; AMP, adenosine monophosphate; ATP, adenosine triphosphate.

The most consistent neuropathological change in encephalopathies with hyperammonemia is prominent, Alzheimer type II astrogliosis, which has been reported in ornithine transcarbamylase (60), argininosuccinase (31), and carbamyl-phosphate synthetase deficiencies (129). Although Alzheimer type II cells are very common in the brains of infants dying of other causes, the consistency and prominence of such cells in infants with hyperammonemia are probably significant. The liver in these cases is usually normal.

Other neuropathologic abnormalities have also been described. The etiology of these pathological changes is unknown, but hypoxic-ischemic insults may be contributory. Abnormalities varying from extensive neuronal loss and astrogliosis to foci of frank necrosis with maximum involvement of cerebral cortex, centrum ovale, and basal ganglia have been described (60). In addition, brains with vacuolation of white matter, delayed myelin formation without myelin breakdown, linear calcification in subpial areas of cerebrum and brain stem, as well as spongiosus, astrogliosis, and capillary proliferation maximum in the lateral thalamus, red nucleus, and inferior colliculi have been documented (31, 88, 430). Evaluation of these neuropathological findings is hindered by the difficulties of distinguishing hypoxic from metabolic effects. However, Solitare et al. (430) make a point of suggesting a primary disturbance of myelin formation on the basis of a deficiency of myelin breakdown products and absence of astrogliosis.

Table 8.8
Metabolic Acidosis Disorders

Organic acidurias
  Isovaleric acidemia
  Propionic acidemia
  Methylmalonic acidemia
  Ketotic hyperglycinemia

Congenital lactic acidosis
  Pyruvate carboxylase
  Pyruvate decarboxylase
  Fructose 1-6 diphosphate

Subacute necrotizing encephalopathy

Others
  Oculocerebrorenal syndrome
  Maple sugar urine disease
  Glycogen storage disease
  Renal tubular acidosis

Encephalopathy Associated with Metabolic Acidosis

The clinical findings associated with metabolic acidosis include hyperventilation and signs of neurological dysfunction, such as hypotonia, seizures, and impaired consciousness. There are three main groups of metabolic acidosis disorders (Table 8.8).

ORGANIC ACIDURIA

Organic aciduria is the designation of a group of metabolic disorders occurring in infants who often have prominent neurological signs and may show effects on their developing nervous systems. The main organic acidurias are isovaleric acidemia, propionic acidemia, methylmalonic acidemia, and ketotic hyperglycinemia. The catabolic enzyme sequence of each amino acid comprises several organic acids. Thus, for each aminoacidopathy there are five to ten related organic acidopathies.

The approximately 20 recognized aminoacidopathies are easily identified by relatively simple chemical procedures (e.g., paper or thin-layer chromatography). Specific identification of the approximately 100 potential organic acidopathies requires more sophisticated analytical procedures (e.g., gas chromatography, mass spectrometry). In organic acidurias, Shuman et al. (417) described marked myelin vacuolation and diminution of the amount of myelin, possibly occurring to the greatest degree in tracts actively myelinating at the time of illness. Impaired myelination may be due to disturbance in the synthesis of fatty acids or myelin protein caused by an amino acid imbalance.

CONGENITAL LACTIC ACIDOSIS

Congenital lactic acidosis can be caused by one of several different enzymatic deficiencies that produce both metabolic acidosis and increased lactic acid. The enzymatic defects that have been associated with congenital lactic acidosis are absence of pyruvate carboxylase, pyruvate decarboxylase, and fructose-1,6-diphosphatase (6). The neuropathological abnormalities described in congenital lactic acidosis include vacuolation and diminution of myelin (475), symmetrical subependymal cysts in the walls of the lateral and fourth ventricles (250), necrosis of globus pallidus, and hemorrhagic lesions (419). These abnormalities are similar to those described in patients with various aminoacidurias. The periventricular cystic change and the hemorrhagic lesions suggest a pathogenetic relationship to subacute necrotizing encephalomyelopathy.

SUBACUTE NECROTIZING ENCEPHALOMYELOPATHY (LEIGH'S DISEASE)

Subacute necrotizing encephalomyelopathy (SNEM) is an autosomal recessive disease characteristically occurring in infancy with a heterogeneous clinical picture. SNEM can affect older children and adults,

but it is most frequent in infancy (219). In the infant, the most common clinical abnormalities, which are sometimes intermittent, include psychomotor retardation, blindness, high-pitched crying, abnormal ocular movements, lethargy, vomiting, respiratory irregularities, and reduced nerve conduction velocities. Although acidosis with elevated blood lactate and pyruvate is usually present (especially during episodes of exacerbation), a definitive diagnosis can be established only when the characteristic morphological abnormalities are found, or when a sibling with the disease has been autopsied. In urine, serum, and CSF, Pincus et al. (359) have consistently found an inhibitor of the enzyme that transforms thiamine pyrophosphate to thiamine triphosphate. They feel the presence of this inhibitor is diagnostically useful.

The combination of morphological abnormalities in the CNS involves characteristic neuroanatomical localizations. The earliest change is a vacuolation of the neuropil followed by capillary proliferation, astrogliosis, and the appearance of histiocytes. Demyelination with relative preservation of neurons and axons helps distinguish these lesions from those that are hypoxic or ischemic in origin. The individual lesions involve both grey and white matter and tend to be patchy but are usually symmetrical in distribution. Microcysts and a spongy state are frequently present in the brain stem. The commonly involved sites are midbrain (periaqueductal grey matter and substantia nigra), pons and medulla (tegmentum and cranial nerve nuclei in the floor of the fourth ventricle, inferior olivary nuclei), cerebellum (dentate nuclei and cerebellar connections), basal ganglia and thalamus sparing of mammillary bodies) spinal cord (posterior columns and pyramidal tracts), optic nerves, posterior nerve roots, and peripheral nerves (301, 307, 359). There is also a report of a child with SNEM in whom skeletal muscle showed ragged-red fibers. By EM, enlarged mitochondria containing whorled cristae and electron-dense crystalloid inclusions are demonstrated, suggesting generalized abnormality of mitochondrial functions (91).

Several biochemical abnormalities have been documented, suggesting that more than one abnormality may be involved.

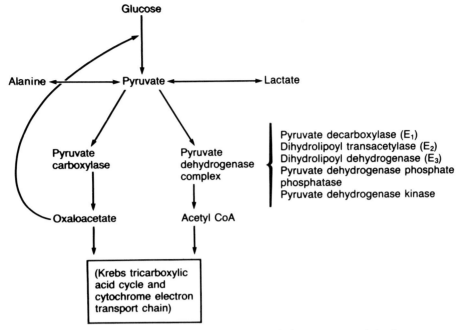

Figure 8.27. Deficiencies of pyruvate carboxylase and the pyruvate dehydrogenase complex sometimes reported in subacute necrotizing encephalomyelopathy.

Low levels of thiamine triphosphate have been demonstrated in areas of the brain that are most often involved pathologically (358). A nondialyzable inhibitor of the enzyme that catalyzes the formation of thiamine triphosphate from thiamine pyrophosphate has been found in brain and in 64 of 511 urine specimens. There have been no false negatives but 6.4% false positives (359).

Elevated levels of pyruvic and lactic acids in serum and increased excretion of alanine suggest an abnormality of pyruvate metabolism (Fig. 8.27). Pyruvate carboxylase deficiency has been reported in two cases with SNEM as well as in cases where the pathology has not been characteristic of SNEM (21). Defective activation of the dehydrogenase complex in SNEM has been correlated with the pathological abnormalities of SNEM. Five enzymes are involved in the conversion of pyruvate to acetyl coenzyme A, and abnormalities of several of these have been associated with SNEM (108).

Elevated levels of endorphin in cerebrospinal fluid during life and in brain tissue postmortem have been reported in a 23-month-old child (51). Morphological abnormalities were characteristic of SNEM. It remains to be determined whether increased synthesis or impaired endorphin metabolism is a characteristic feature of SNEM.

Deficient cytochrome C oxidase in muscle tissue was described in a 6-yr-old girl whose brain had the typical lesions of SNEM (501).

LOWE'S SYNDROME

Lowe's syndrome is an X-linked recessive disorder associated with congenital cataracts, severe mental retardation, hypotonia, and kidney disease (metabolic acidosis, aminoaciduria, proteinuria, and hypophosphatemic rickets). The exact metabolic defect remains unknown (1). Morphological abnormalities have not been consistent, ranging from descriptions of poor myelination to generalized cortical atrophy (381).

Encephalopathies Associated with Hypoglycemia

Hypoglycemia is clinically important because brain damage can be avoided if the condition is recognized early. The usually accepted critical levels of blood glucose are 20 mg/100 ml for low birth weight babies, 30 mg/100 ml for term babies less than 72 h old, and 40 mg/100 ml for older babies (308). The effects of hypoglycemia on the brain are similar to those of hypoxia, with necrosis of neurons in cerebral cortex, Ammon's horn, striatum, and cerebellum (15). Neonatal exposure to hypoglycemia may produce neuronal damage that is later expressed as mental retardation or seizures.

Among the genetic metabolic diseases causing hypoglycemia are type 1 glycogenosis (von Gierke's disease), hereditary fructose intolerance, hereditary fructose-1,6-diphosphate deficiency, glycogen synthetase deficiency, and galactosemia.

GALACTOSEMIA

In galactosemia, galactose-1-phosphate uridyl transferase is deficient, resulting in toxic effects on cellular metabolism due either to galactose or to galactitol. In the neonatal period, there is vomiting, diarrhea, hepatomegaly, and jaundice. By age 1 or 2 months, psychomotor retardation and cataracts can be identified.

There are at least two cases in which a neuropathologic description is available. The brain of an 8-yr-old child with mental retardation had micrencephaly, astrogliosis of white matter, and Purkinje- and granular-cell loss associated with astrogliosis. Large neurons contained lipofuscin (87). In a report on the brain of a 25-yr-old patient (180), there was micrencephaly, demyelination, and astrogliosis together with extensive cerebral and cerebellar neuronal cell loss. Lipofuscin was present in the globus pallidus and substantia nigra. Neuroaxonal spheroids were identified, especially in the thalamus. Related to the liver cirrhosis and hepatic failure associated with the galactosemia was extensive Alzheimer type II astrocytic change.

Disorders of Copper Metabolism

MENKES DISEASE (KINKY-HAIR SYNDROME)

In 1962, Menkes et al. (292) described an X-linked recessive disorder with growth retardation, peculiar hair (colorless and fria-

ble), and focal cerebral and cerebellar degeneration. In the neonatal period, hypothermia, poor feeding, seizures, and impaired weight gain are noted. Microscopically, there is pili torti (twisted hair) and trichorrhexis nodosa (fracture of the hair shaft at regular intervals). Low serum levels of copper and ceruloplasmin and low copper concentrations in liver were found by Danks et al. (95), who demonstrated a defect in intestinal absorption of copper (98). The defect involved a disturbance of intracellular transport in the mucosal cell or through the serosal aspect of the cell membrane.

The neuropathological abnormalities affect vessels, cortex, and white matter. Arteries are distorted, and the vessel wall is thickened. Abnormalities of elastin may be due to dysfunction of the copper-dependent lysyl oxidase, which is important in elastin cross-linking. The elastica shows extensive beading, fragmentation, and splitting with prominent, intimal hyperplasia (97).

Aguilar et al. (11) reported cystic degeneration of grey and white matter, especially in the temporal lobes. Others (502) described widespread nerve cell loss and gliosis, principally involving cerebral and cerebellar cortex and thalamus. Depopulation of stellate cells (neocortex, layer IV) and granule cells of the cerebellum is prominent. Golgi impregnations (367, 502) demonstrate alterations in size, branching pattern, and shape of dendrites, in addition to decreased spine density. Purkinje-cell dendrites tend to be very thick or dilated with many side branches (cactus-like). Axonal torpedos also occur. At the fine structural level, somatic spines are identified, some of which are unattached to any presynaptic element (194). Although Vagn-Hansen et al. (484) suggest that Menkes disease is a leukodystrophy, others disagree (502). They state that changes in the white matter are consistent with axonal degeneration secondary to neuronal cell death.

WILSON'S DISEASE

Wilson's disease is an autosomal recessive disorder due to a derangement in copper metabolism, resulting in heavy depositions of copper in liver (cirrhosis), cornea (Kayser-Fleischer rings), kidneys (impaired tubular absorption and transport), and CNS. Laboratory tests show low serum copper concentrations, decreased ceruloplasmin levels, and increased urinary copper excretion (106).

Neurologic findings are usually not apparent until adolescence. In the rapidly evolving form (Wilsonian or lenticular), there is spasticity, rigidity, dysarthria, dysphagia, and painful spasms. In the slowly evolving disease (Strümpell-Westphal disease or pseudosclerosis) flapping tremor of one arm may be the first sign before the characteristic, more generalized muscular rigidity develops. As the disease advances, there is slowed movement, rigidity, irregular tremor, and eventually extrapyramidal symptoms that incapacitate the patient.

Neuropathological findings (361) vary depending on the rate of progression of the disease. In the rapidly progressive fatal form, there is cavitation of the lenticular nuclei, and, in the more chronic form, the caudate and putamen may be shrunken and have light-brown discoloration. The histological findings are maximal in the putamen and consist of neuronal loss affecting large cells and small cells. Fibrillary astrogliosis is extensive, and macrophages containing lipid and hemosiderin are scattered throughout the tissue. Mononuclear Alzheimer type II astrocytes are abundant, and large multinucleate cells (Alzheimer type I astrocytes) have also been described. Cells approximately 15 μm in diameter with yellow-brown cytoplasmic granules stain heavily for copper and are thought to be a variant of Alzheimer type II astrocytes. Later, similar changes are present in the caudate, globus pallidus, and substantia nigra. In the globus pallidus, myelin is frequently diminished, and both Alzheimer type II astrocytes and Opalski cells are present. Opalski cells are up to 35 μm in diameter with a small central nucleus and slightly foamy cytoplasm. Their origin is not clear; some observers feel they may be degenerating neurons, some that they are derived from astrocytes, and others that they are phagocytes. There is usually less severe involvement of thalamus, brain stem, cerebellum, and cerebrum. In the cortex (frontal lobes), there may be focal spongy demyelination; widespread myelin loss has also been described (361).

Lesch-Nyhan Syndrome

The Lesch-Nyhan syndrome is an X-linked, recessive disease characterized by choreoathetosis, which is usually evident by one year of age, mental retardation, spasticity and compulsive self-mutilation. A deficiency in hypoxanthine guanine phosphoribosyltransferase is present, associated with systemic accumulation of uric acid. Therefore, patients are subject to all of the clinical features of gout including arthritis, urate nephropathy and tophi.

Neuropathological studies have shown no significant morphological abnormalities (300), suggesting that the striking neurological findings are entirely due to biochemical alterations. Lloyd et al. (256) showed that the neurochemical abnormalities are not restricted to low levels of hypoxanthine-guanine phosphoribosyl transferase. Using postmortem dissection of specific anatomical regions, they found evidence for a general deficit in dopamine-neuron content with normal norepinephrine- and serotonin-neuron content. In caudate nucleus, putamen, and nucleus accumbens septi (dopamine terminals), there are low dopamine and homovanillic acid levels and low dopadecarboxylase and tyrosine-hydroxylase activities. In substantia nigra, the dopamine levels are normal. They also found that in γ-aminobutyric acid (GABA) neurons L-glutamic acid carboxylase activities are normal, and in acetylcholine neurons choline acetyltransferase activity is low in putamen but not in globus pallidus.

Such alterations of the balance among GABA, dopamine, and acetylcholine neurons may account for the symptoms of extrapyramidal and behavioral dysfunction in the Lesch-Nyhan syndrome. The lack of morphologic abnormalities in the brain suggests that the neurotransmitter and associated enzyme losses are due to functional abnormalities rather than to cell loss.

CLINICAL FEATURES OF METABOLIC ERRORS

Although we are not discussing clinical signs and symptoms in detail, to make relevant clinicopathological correlations in metabolic diseases it is necessary to have an overall view of clinical signs and symptoms in these disorders (5). Because head size and ocular findings are of particular interest to the neuropathologist, these are specifically commented on below, and the other pertinent clinical features useful in diagnosis are summarized (Table 8.9).

For the different periods of childhood, neonatal refers to the 1st month of life, early infantile from 1 to 12 months, early childhood or late infantile from 1 to 4 yr, juvenile or late childhood from 5 to 12 yr, and adolescent from 13 to 19 yr.

Although the most incapacitating aspect of most of these metabolic diseases is related to the involvement of the brain, many have systemic manifestations that assist in clinical diagnosis.

Normally, brain weight increases rapidly during gestation and in the 1st yr of life. Since skull growth follows that of the brain, head circumference is a useful measurement of brain growth. In the 1st yr of life, normal head circumference increases from 34 to 46 cm and the brain weight from 335 to 950 g. In the 2nd yr, the circumference increases to 48 cm, and the brain weight increases to 1064 g. A head circumference smaller than three standard deviations below normal indicates microcephaly and one greater than three standard deviations above normal megacephaly. In neonates, Cockayne's syndrome is probably the only disorder of metabolic origin in which there is microcephaly. However, after 6 months of age, the failure of head circumference to increase, often associated with increased thickness of the skull, is very common in metabolic disorders. Megacephaly is associated with Alexander's, Canavan's, and Tay-Sachs diseases. In Alexander's and Canavan's diseases, the megacephaly occurs early in the course of the disease, but in Tay-Sachs disease it is a late occurrence.

The ocular features of metabolic disease are related to involvement of cornea, lens, retinal sensory epithelium (rods, cones, and pigmentary layer), retinal ganglion cells, optic nerves, optic pathways (geniculocalcarine tracts), and ocular movement centers (gaze palsies and nystagmus). Corneal opacities frequently occur in Hurler's syndrome and Fabry's disease. Cataracts are present in cerebrotendinous xanthomatosis, galactosemia, Lowe's syndrome, and Zellweger's syndrome. Lens dislocation occurs in homocystinuria. Retinitis pigmentosa is frequently associated with Jansky-Bielschowsky disease, Batten-Spielmeyer-Vogt disease, Bassen-Kornzweig syndrome, Refsum's syndrome, and Cockayne's syndrome. Neuronal storage in retinal ganglion cells produces a pale fundus with a red macula where choroidal vessels are visible (i.e., a cherry red spot). Macular cherry red spots are found in Tay-Sachs disease, Sandhoff disease, early infantile G_{M1} gangliosidosis, Niemann-Pick disease, and mucolipidosis type I. Although frequent in end stage disease, optic atrophy is uncommon as an early manifestation of this group of disorders; however, it is present in Leigh's disease, Canavan's disease, late onset lipidoses, and ALD. Ocular motor palsies have been described in Leigh's disease and infantile Gaucher's disease, supranuclear palsy in juvenile Niemann-Pick disease, jerk nystagmus in Leigh's disease, and pendular nystagmus in Pelizaeus-Merzbacher disease.

DIAGNOSIS

The diagnosis of metabolic disorders depends on biochemical analysis of excretion products in the urine, enzyme assay of leukocytes or microscopy of blood, bone marrow, or urine sediment. In some situations, tissue biopsies are necessary, but these are a small proportion of the total number of metabolic cases. Since metabolic disorders affect few children, each disorder is rare, and few neuropathologists, neurologists, or pediatricians will be familiar with the whole range of diagnostic possibilities. The procedures that are used to establish a diagnosis are lysosomal enzyme assays and examination of blood, bone marrow, urine, and biopsy tissue.

Blood and Bone Marrow

The presence of abnormal inclusions and vacuoles in neutrophilic leukocytes, lymphocytes, plasmacytes, and monocytes in the circulating blood and bone marrow may be important in establishing a diagnosis of sphingolipidosis, mucopolysaccharidosis, mucolipidosis, and lipofuscinosis. Atypical vacuolated lymphocytes are a common finding in storage diseases and may indicate that foamy histiocytes will be identified in the bone marrow. Patients with

Table 8.9
Major Clinical Manifestations of Some Metabolic Diseases

Disease and age at presentation	Psychomotor retardation/dementia	Bilateral pyramidal signs	Seizures	Cerebellar ataxia	Extrapyramidal signs[a]	Blindness[b]	Deafness	Peripheral neuropathy	Facial dysmorphism	Significant bone and/or joint abnormalities	Hepatosplenomegaly	Other major organ involvements[c]	Vacuolated cells (blood or bone marrow)
Gaucher													
Type 1 (adult)	+										+		+
Type 2 (early infantile)	+	+									+		+
Type 3 (juvenile)	+	+	+	+							+		+
Niemann-Pick													
A (early infantile)	+	+	+			+					+		+
B (late infantile)	+										+		+
C (late infantile)	+	+			+						+		+
D (late infantile)	+	+	+								+		+
Fabry's (adolescent)	+	+										K, S	+
Farber's (early infantile)	+									+		S	
G_{M1}													
Type 1 (neonatal)	+	+	+				+		+	+	+		+
Type 2 (late infantile)	+	+	+	+		+			+	+	+		+
G_{M2}													
Tay-Sachs (early infantile)	+	+	+			+							
Sandhoff (late infantile)	+	+	+			+					+		+
Neuronal ceroid lipofuscinosis													
Haltia-Santavuori (early infantile)	+			+		+							
Jansky-Bielschowsky (late infantile)	+	+	+	+	+	+							+
Batten-Spielmeyer-Vogt (juvenile)	+	+	+	+	+	+							+
Kufs' (adult)	+												
Cerebrotendinous xanthomatosis (juvenile)	+	+		+		+				+		L	+

Table 8.9—Continued

Disease and age at presentation	Psychomotor retardation/dementia	Bilateral pyramidal signs	Seizures	Cerebellar ataxia	Extrapyramidal signs[a]	Blindness[b]	Deafness	Peripheral neuropathy	Facial dysmorphism	Significant bone and/or joint abnormalities	Hepatosplenomegaly	Other major organ involvements[c]	Vacuolated cells (blood or bone marrow)
Refsum's (adolescent)				+		+		+					
Mucopolysaccharidoses													
Hurler (MPS I-H) (late infantile)	+	+				+	+		+	+	+	H, S	+
Scheie (MPS I-S) (juvenile)						+			+	+		S	+
Hunter (late infantile)	+						+		+	+	+	S	+
Sanfilippo (late infantile)	+	+					+		+	+	+	S	+
Morquio (late infantile)							+		+	+			
Maroteaux-Lamy (late infantile)						+			+	+			
Sly (late infantile)	+								+	+	+		+
Mucolipidoses													
I cherry red spot myoclonus syndrome (juvenile)						+							+
I dysmorphic syndrome (early infantile, juvenile)	+		+	+		+	+		+	+	+	S	+
II (neonatal)	+								+	+	+	S	+
III (late infantile)	+	+				+			+	+		H	+
IV (early infantile)	+	+				+			+				+
Fucosidosis (late infantile)	+	+							+	+	+	GB, S	+
Mannosidosis (late infantile)	+	+					+		+	+	+	S	+
Glycogenosis													
Type 2—Pompe's (early infantile)	+										+	H, M	+

Table 8.9—Continued

Disease and age at presentation	Psychomotor retardation/dementia	Bilateral pyramidal signs	Seizures	Cerebellar ataxia	Extrapyramidal signs[a]	Blindness[b]	Deafness	Peripheral neuropathy	Facial dysmorphism	Significant bone and/or joint abnormalities	Hepatosplenomegaly	Other major organ involvements[c]	Vacuolated cells (blood or bone marrow)
Metachromatic leukodystrophy													
Type 1 (late infantile)	+			+		+		+				GB	
Type 2 (juvenile)	+	+	+	+				+					
Type 3 (adult)	+	+			+								
Type 4 (early infantile)	+	+	+					+	+	+	+		
Krabbe's (early infantile)	+	+	+	+		+		+					
Adrenoleukodystrophy (classical juvenile)	+	+	+	+		+						A, S	
Alexander's (early infantile)	+	+	+										
Canavan's (early infantile)	+	+	+		+	+							
Pelizaeus-Merzbacher's (classical juvenile)	+	+		+	+								
Cockayne's (late infantile)	+	+		+	+	+	+	+	+	+		S	
Homocystinuria (juvenile)	+	+				+				+		S	
Hartnup (late infantile)	+	+	+	+									
Subacute necrotizing encephalomyelopathy (early infantile)	+	+				+		+				S	
Menkes (neonatal)	+		+										
Wilson's (adolescent)	+	+			+						+	S	
Lesch-Nyhan (early infantile)	+	+			+					+		S, K	

[a] Tremor, rigidity or choreoathetosis.
[b] Cherry red spot, corneal opacity or cataracts.
[c] A, adrenal; GB, gallbladder; H, heart; K, kidney; M, muscle; S, skin and/or hair.

mucopolysaccharidosis have atypical lymphocytes but do not have foam cells in the marrow. The foam cell is a lipid-laden histiocyte with droplets that are faintly sudanophilic and PAS-positive. In a small number of instances, these histiocytes have diagnositic features: Gaucher's cell with "crumpled silk" cytoplasm and juvenile Niemann-Pick disease with sea-blue histiocytes (in Giemsa or Wright's stains). EM of circulating lymphocytes is particularly valuable in establishing a diagnosis of ceroid lipofuscinosis (408).

Urine

In general, light microscopy of urinary sediment is useful only in metachromatic leukodystrophy where intracellular deposits of the material staining yellow-brown with toluidine blue stain are characteristic. Biochemical analysis of urine is of particular importance in the diagnosis of amino acid disorders, organic acidurias, mucopolysaccharidoses, and mucolipidoses.

Lysosomal Enzyme Assays

The identification of lysosomal enzyme defects utilizes complicated techniques that require careful controls and should be carried out only in specialized laboratories with experienced personnel. Before the tissue or fluid is taken, the preferred sample and its subsequent handling must be ascertained from personnel of the laboratory that will be processing and interpreting it. Lysosomal enzymes can be assayed in serum, plasma, leukocytes, urine, tears, skin, conjunctiva, muscle, liver, and amniotic fluid. Most enzyme assays can be performed on leukocytes, although for carrier detection, cultured fibroblasts may be preferred (234, 383).

Examination of Biopsied Tissue

Failure to establish a diagnosis by clinical, biochemical, or radiological data may necessitate histological examination of biopsied adrenal gland (ALD), hair (Menkes disease), rectum, appendix, liver, brain, muscle, sural nerve, skin, or conjunctiva. Brain biopsy (268) including both grey and white matter is required to make a definitive diagnosis of Alexander's disease

and Canavan's disease, although computerized tomographic scans may suggest the diagnosis (241). Muscle biopsy is useful in Pompe's disease. A sural nerve biopsy may be of help in the diagnosis of MLD. Krabbe's disease, ALD, and Refsum's syndrome.

Since biopsy of the skin or conjunctiva poses no risk to the patient, it is the tissue diagnostic procedure of choice. In ceroid lipofuscinosis, for which there is no enzymatic assay, skin or conjunctiva biopsy is especially valuable. Although neurons are not present, the ubiquitous character of the storage phenomena results in abnormal inclusions in several different cell elements: unmyelinated or myelinated axons, Schwann cells, fibroblasts, endothelial cells, exocrine sweat glands, bulbs of hair follicles, and histiocytes. A conjunctival biopsy is also a simple procedure that allows examination of the same cell types as the skin, except for the sweat glands, hair follicles, and myelinated axons.

Skin and conjunctiva biopsies have demonstrated abnormal inclusions in many of the lysosomal storage diseases, including lipidoses without clinically evident visceral involvement such as G_{M2}-gangliosidosis (278, 424, 511). Such biopsies of heterozygotes for the mutant genes causing the metabolic disorder have not shown any abnormality except Fabry's disease (249), where conjunctiva of the female carrier shows ultrastructural abnormalities.

Morphologic studies of cultured fibroblasts have not been as valuable as chemical studies because of artifacts induced by cell culture. In I-cell disease, cultured fibroblasts show filling of the cytoplasm by numerous pleomorphic, electron-dense inclusions that differ a great deal from the membrane-bound vacuoles in the fibroblasts and other cells of the skin or conjunctiva seen in biopsies (244).

At present, most metabolic disorders that affect the nervous system cannot be adequately treated, except for some of the oligosaccharidoses and aminoacidurias and, to a limited degree, Wilson's and Menkes diseases. Enzyme replacement is being investigated as a method of therapy (47, 48), but, to be successful, the normal enzyme probably must be introduced into the nervous system at an early age before neurons are already damaged. In many disorders, this would have to be before birth.

Because treatment is so limited, prevention becomes an important aim. The clinical identification of the heterozygote in autosomal recessive disease and of the female carrier in X-linked recessive disease is not possible in many metabolic disorders (298). However, the heterozygote sometimes has enzyme levels intermediate between those of the normal and the homozygote.

If two individuals with a recessive trait marry, the risk of having children affected by the specific disease is 25% for each pregnancy. If one child in the family is affected, or if two known or suspected heterozygotes marry and pregnancy occurs, then amniocentesis should be considered. It should be done by the 14th week of gestation and appropriate biochemical assays performed on the cells cultured from the amniotic fluid. The amniotic-fluid cells are of fetal origin and derived mainly from fetal skin and amnion. Although the main purpose of amniocentesis is to provide cells for appropriate lysosomal enzyme analysis, cells can also be examined for ultrastructural features.

Ornoy et al. (343) found that cultured skin fibroblasts are not reliable for morphological diagnosis because EM changes in affected fibroblasts cannot be distinguished from those in fibroblasts of heterozygotes and normal patients. In contrast, only cultured amniotic-fluid cells from affected individuals show characteristic changes, suggesting that EM examination of these cells is useful, but biochemical confirmation should always be sought if possible. If the fetus is affected, then the parents may elect to terminate the pregnancy.

For example, it is possible to prevent almost all Tay-Sachs disease. It is found only in Ashkenazic Jews and, therefore, a limited number of individuals can be screened by a reliable, well standardized blood test (260). When heterozygotes are identified, parents can be advised about the risks of having affected children.

Pathological examination of aborted fetuses provides an extension of the spectrum of involvement in metabolic disease and, in several instances, storage products have been well documented in gestations less than 20 weeks. Examination of dorsal root ganglia has been particularly fruitful in illustrating storage products (92).

CONCLUSION

Although the categorization of metabolic diseases is in flux, the classification in this chapter provides a framework to which other nosological entities can be added. We fully expect that the pathogenesis of many disorders will be altered and other disorders added to this "metabolic" category, which encompasses such a wide spectrum of disease processes.

ACKNOWLEDGMENTS

This chapter was prepared with the help of the Department of Medical Publications, The Hospital for Sick Children.

References

1. Abbassi V, Lowe CU, Calcagno PL. Oculo-cerebro-renal syndrome. *Am J Dis Child* 115:145–168, 1968.
2. Adachi M, Wallace BJ, Schneck L: Fine structure of central nervous system in early infantile Gaucher's disease. *Arch Pathol* 83:513–526, 1967.
3. Adachi M, Torri J, Schneck L, et al: Electron microscopic and enzyme histochemical studies of the cerebellum and spongy degeneration (van Bogaert and Bertrand type). *Acta Neuropathol (Berl)* 20:22–31, 1972.
4. Adachi M, Schneck L, Cara J, et al: Spongy degeneration of the central nervous system (van Bogaert and Bertrand type; Canavan's disease). *Hum Pathol* 4:331–347, 1973.
5. Adams RD, Lyon G: *Neurology of Hereditary Metabolic Diseases of Children.* Toronto, McGraw-Hill, 1982, p 1.
6. Adams RD, Lyon G: *Neurology of Hereditary Metabolic Diseases of Children.* Toronto, McGraw-Hill, 1982, p 82.
7. Adams RD, Lyon G: *Neurology of Hereditary Metabolic Diseases of Children.* Toronto, McGraw-Hill, 1982, p 177.
8. Adornato BT, O'Brien JS, Lampert PW, et al: Cerebral spongy degeneration of infancy: a biochemical and ultrastructural study of affected twins. *Neurology* 22:202–210, 1972.
9. Agamanolis DP, Potter JL, Herrick MK, et al: The neuropathology of glycine encephalopathy: a report of five cases with immunohistochemical and ultrastructural observations. *Neurology* 32:975–985, 1982.
10. Agrawal HC, Davison AN: Myelination and amino acid imbalance in the developing brain. In Himwich WA (ed): *Biochemistry of the Developing Brain.* New York, Dekker, 1973, vol 1, p 143.
11. Aguilar MJ, Chadwick DL, Okuyama K, et al: Kinky hair disease. I. Clinical and pathological features. *J Neuropathol Exp Neurol* 25:507–522, 1966.
12. Aleu FP, Terry RD, Zellweger H: Electron microscopy of two cerebral biopsies in gargoylism. *J Neuropathol Exp Neurol* 24:304–317, 1965.
13. Alexander WS: Progressive fibrinoid degeneration of fibrillary astrocytes associated with mental retardation in a hydrocephalic infant. *Brain* 72:373–381, 1949.
14. Alvord EC Jr, Stevenson LD, Vogel FS, et al: Neuropathological findings in phenyl-pyruvic oligophrenia (phenylketonuria). *J Neuropathol Exp Neurol* 9:298–310, 1950.
15. Anderson JM, Milner RDG, Strich SJ: Effects of neonatal hypoglycaemia on the nervous system: a patholog-

ical study. *J Neurol Neurosurg Pyschiatry* 30:295–310, 1967.

16. Andrews JM, Sorenson V, Cancilla PA, et al: Late infantile neurovisceral storage disease with curvilinear bodies. *Neurology* 21:207–217, 1971.

17. Anzil AP, Blinzinger K, Mehraein P, et al: Cytoplasmic inclusions in a child affected with Krabbe's disease (globoid leucodystrophy) and in the rabbit injected with galactocerebrosides. *J Neuropathol Exp Neurol* 31:370–388, 1972.

18. Anzil AP, Gessaga E: Late-life cavitating dystrophy of the cerebral and cerebellar white matter: a form of sudanophil leucodystrophy. *Eur Neurol* 7:79–94, 1972.

19. Arsénio-Nunes ML, Goutières F: An ultramicroscopic study of the skin in the diagnosis of the infantile and late infantile types of ceroid-lipofuscinosis. *J Neurol Neurosurg Psychiatry* 38:994–999, 1975.

20. Arsenio-Nunes ML, Goutières F, Aicardi JK: An ultramicroscopic study of skin and conjunctival biopsies in chronic neurological disorders of childhood. *Ann Neurol* 9:163–173, 1981.

21. Atkin BM, Buist NRM, Utter MF, et al: Pyruvate carboxylase deficiency and lactic acidosis in a retarded child without Leigh's disease. *Pediatr Res* 13:109–116, 1979.

22. Aula P, Autio S, Raivio KO, et al: Salla disease: a new lysosomal storage disorder. *Arch Neurol* 36:88–94, 1979.

23. Austin JH: Metachromatic form of diffuse cerebral sclerosis. I. Diagnosis during life by urine sediment examination. *Neurology* 7:415–426, 1957.

24. Austin J: Metachromatic sulphatides in cerebral white matter and kidney. *Proc Soc Exp Biol Med* 100:361–364, 1959.

25. Austin J, Armstrong D, Fouch S, et al: Metachromatic leukodystrophy (MLD). VIII. MLD in adults; diagnosis and pathogenesis. *Arch Neurol* 18:225–240, 1968.

26. Austin JH: Studies in metachromatic leukodystrophy. XII. Multiple sulfatase deficiency. *Arch Neurol* 28:258–264, 1973.

27. Bach G, Friedman R, Weissmann B, et al: The defect in the Hurler and Scheie syndromes: deficiency of α-L-iduronidase. *Proc Natl Acad Sci USA* 69:2048–2051, 1972.

28. Bale PM, Clifton-Bligh P, Benjamin BNP, et al: Pathology of Tangier disease. *J Clin Pathol* 24:609–616, 1971.

29. Banker BQ, Miller JQ, Crocker AC: The cerebral pathology of infantile Gaucher's disease. In Aronson SM, Volk BW (eds): *Cerebral Sphingolipidoses. A Symposium on Tay-Sachs' Disease and Allied Disorders.* New York, Academic Press, 1962, p 73.

30. Baumann RJ, Markesbery WR: Juvenile amaurotic idiocy (neuronal ceroid lipofuscinosis) and lymphocyte fingerprint profiles. *Ann Neurol* 4:531–536, 1978.

31. Baumgartner R, Scheidegger S, Stalder G, et al: Arginin-bernsteinsäure-Krankheit des Neugeborenen mit letalem Verlauf (Neonatal death due to argininosuccinic aciduria). *Helv Paediat Acta* 23:77–106, 1968.

32. Becker LE, Armstrong JB, Meloff KL: A large head in a 2-year-old boy. *J Pediatr* 91:499–502, 1977.

33. Benke PJ, Reyes PF, Parker JC Jr: New form of adrenoleukodystrophy. *Hum Genet* 58:204–208, 1981.

34. Berard M, Toga M, Bernard R, et al: Pathological findings in one case of neuronal and mesenchymal storage disease: its relationship to lipidoses and to mucopolysaccharidoses. *Pathol Eur* 3:172–183, 1968.

35. Berman ER, Livni N, Shapira E, et al: Congenital corneal clouding with abnormal systemic storage bodies. A new variant of mucolipidosis. *J Pediatr* 84:519–526, 1974.

36. Besley GTN, Hoogeboom AJM, Hoogeveen A, et al: Somatic cell hybridisation studies showing different gene mutations in Niemann-Pick variants. *Hum Genet* 54:409–412, 1980.

37. Bickel H, Gerrard J, Hickmans EM: Influence of phenylalanine intake on phenylketonuria. *Lancet* 2:812–813, 1953.

38. Besson JAO: A diagnostic pointer to adult metachromatic leucodystrophy. *Br J Psychiatry* 137:186–187, 1980.

39. Blaw ME: Melanodermic type leukodystrophy (adrenoleukodystrophy). In Vinken PJ, Bruyn GW (eds): *Leucodystrophies and Poliodystrophies. Handbook of Clinical Neurology.* Amsterdam, North-Holland, 1970, vol 10, p 128.

40. Boehme DH, Cottrell JC, Leonberg SC, et al: A dominant form of neuronal ceroid-lipofuscinosis. *Brain* 94:745–760, 1971.

41. Bootsma D, Galjaard H: Heterogeneity in genetic diseases studied in cultured cells. In Hommes FA ed: *Models for the Study of Inborn Errors of Metabolism.* Amsterdam, Elsevier, 1979, p 241.

42. Bourre JM, Jacque C, Nguyen-Legros J, et al: Pelizaeus-Merzbacher disease: biochemical analysis of isolated myelin (electron-microscopy; protein, lipid and unsubstituted fatty acids analysis). *Eur Neurol* 17:317–326, 1978.

43. Bourre JM,, Bornhofen JH, Araoz CA, et al: Pelizaeus-Merzbacher disease: brain lipid and fatty acid composition. *J Neurochem* 30:719–727, 1978.

44. Brady RO, Kanfer JN, Mock MB, et al: The metabolism of sphingomyelin. II. Evidence of an enzymatic deficiency in Niemann-Pick disease. *Proc Natl Acad Sci USA* 55:366–369, 1966.

45. Brady RO, Kanfer JN, Shapiro D: Metabolism of glucocerebrosides. II. Evidence of an enzymatic deficiency in Gaucher's disease. *Biochem Biophys Res Commun* 18:221–225, 1965.

46. Brady RO: Glucosyl ceramide lipidosis: Gaucher's disease. In Stanbury JB, Wyngaarden JB, Fredrickson DS (eds): *The Metabolic Basis of Inherited Disease*, ed 4. New York, McGraw-Hill, 1978, p 731.

47. Brady RO, Barranger JA: Therapeutic strategies for lipid storage diseases. *Trends Neurosci* 4:265–267, 1981.

48. Brady RO: Inherited metabolic storage disorders. *Annu Rev Neurosci* 5:33–56, 1982.

49. Brain WR, Greenfield JG: Late infantile metachromatic leuco-encephalopathy, with primary degeneration of the interfascicular oligodendroglia. *Brain* 73:291–317, 1950.

50. Brandt IK, DeLuca VA Jr: Type III glycogenosis: a family with an unusual distribution of the enzyme lesion. *Am J Med* 40:779–784, 1966.

51. Brandt NJ, Terenius L, Jacobsen BB, et al: Hyperendorphin syndrome in a child with necrotizing encephalomyelopathy. *N Engl J Med* 303:914–916, 1980.

52. Brante G: Gargoylism: a mucopolysaccharidosis. *Scand J Clin Lab Invest* 4:43–46, 1952.

53. Breen L, Morris HH, Alperin JB, et al: Juvenile Niemann-Pick disease with vertical supranuclear ophthalmoplegia: two case reports and review of the literature. *Arch Neurol* 38:388–390, 1981.

54. Brett EM, Ellis RB, Haas L, et al: Late onset G$_{M2}$-gangliosidosis: clinical, pathological, and biochemical studies on 8 patients. *Arch Dis Chld* 48:775–785, 1973.

55. Brown FR III, Shimizu H, McDonald JM, et al: Auditory evoked brainstem response and high-performance liquid chromatography sulfatide assay as early indices of metachromatic leukodystrophy. *Neurology* 31:980–985, 1981.

56. Brown FR III, McAdams AJ, Cummins JW, et al: Cerebro-hepato-renal (Zellweger) syndrome and neonatal adrenoleukodystrophy: similarities in phenotype and accumulation of very long chain fatty acids. *Johns Hopkins Med J* 151:344–351, 1982.

57. Brownstein S, Carpenter S, Polomeno RC, et al: Sandhoff's disease (G$_{M2}$ gangliosidosis type 2): histopathology and ultrastructure of the eye. *Arch Ophthalmol* 98:1089–1097, 1980.

58. Brunberg JA, McCormick WF, Schochet SS Jr: Type III glycogenosis: an adult with diffuse weakness and muscle wasting. *Arch Neurol* 25:171–178, 1971.

59. Brunngraber EG, Witting LA, Haberland C, et al: Glycoproteins in Tay-Sachs disease: isolation and carbohy-

drate composition of glycopeptides. *Brain Res* 38:151–162, 1972.

60. Bruton CJ, Corsellis JAN, Russell A: Hereditary hyperammonaemia. *Brain* 93:423–434, 1970.

61. Byrd JC III, Powers JM: Wolman's disease: ultrastructural evidence of lipid accumulation in central and peripheral nervous systems. *Acta Neuropathol (Berl)* 45:37–42, 1979.

62. Cable WJL, Dvorak AM, Osage JE, et al: Fabry disease: significance of ultrastructural localization of lipid inclusions in dermal nerves. *Neurology* 32:347–353, 1982.

63. Cable WJL, Kolodny EH, Adams RD: Fabry disease: impaired autonomic function. *Neurology* 32:498–502, 1982.

64. Callahan JW, Khalil M, Philippart M: Sphingomyelinases in human tissues. II. Absence of a specific enzyme from liver and brain of Niemann-Pick disease, type C. *Pediatr Res* 9:908–913, 1975.

65. Cammermeyer J: Neuropathological changes in hereditary neuropathies: manifestation of the syndrome heredopathia atactica polyneuritiformis in the presence of interstitial hypertrophic polyneuropathy. *J Neuropathol Exp Neurol* 15:340–361, 1956.

66. Canavan MM: Schilder's encephalitis periaxialis diffusa: report of a case in a child aged sixteen and one-half months. *Arch Neurol Psychiatry* 25:299–308, 1931.

67. Cantz M, Gehler J, Spranger J: Mucolipidosis I: increased sialic acid content and deficiency of an α-N-acetylneuraminidase in cultured fibroblasts. *Biochem Biophys Res Commun* 74:732–738, 1977.

68. Cardiff RD: A histochemical and electron microscopic study of skeletal muscle in a case of Pompe's disease (glycogenosis II). *Pediatrics* 37:249–259, 1966.

69. Carpenter S, Karpati G, Andermann F: Specific involvement of muscle, nerve, and skin in late infantile and juvenile amaurotic idiocy. *Neurology* 22:170–186, 1972.

70. Carroll M, Dance N, Masson PK, et al: Human mannosidosis—the enzymic defect. *Biochem Biophys Res Commun* 49:579–583, 1972.

71. Chang PL, Davidson RG: Complementation of arylsulfatase A in somatic hybrids of metachromatic leukodystrophy and multiple sulfatase deficiency disorder fibroblasts. *Proc Natl Acad Sci USA* 77:6166–6170, 1980.

72. Chilcote RR, Miller M, Dawson G, et al: Foamy histiocytes in the CSF of a patient with infantile Niemann-Pick disease. *Am J Dis Child* 135:76–77, 1981.

73. Chou SM, Thompson HG: Electron microscopy of storage cytosomes in Kufs' disease. *Arch Neurol* 23:489–501, 1970.

74. Christomanou H: Niemann-Pick disease, type C: evidence for the deficiency of an activating factor stimulating sphingomyelin and glucocerebroside degradation. *Hoppe-Seyler Z Physiol Chem* 361:1489–1502, 1980.

75. Clark JR, Miller RG, Vidgoff JM: Juvenile-onset metachromatic leukodystrophy: biochemical and electrophysiologic studies. *Neurology* 29:346–353, 1979.

76. Cockayne EA: Dwarfism with retinal atrophy and deafness. *Arch Dis Child* 11:1–8, 1936.

77. Collier J, Greenfield JG: The encephalitis periaxialis of Schilder: a clinical and pathological study with an account of two cases, one of which was diagnosed during life. *Brain* 47:489–519, 1924.

78. Constantopoulos G, McComb RD, Dekaban AS: Neurochemistry of the mucopolysaccharidoses: brain glycosaminoglycans in normals and four types of mucopolysaccharidoses. *J Neurochem* 26:901–908, 1976.

79. Conzelmann E, Sandhoff K: AB variant of infantile G_{M2} gangliosidosis: deficiency of a factor necessary for stimulation of hexosaminidase A-catalyzed degradation of ganglioside G_{M2} and glycolipid G_{A2}. *Proc Natl Acad Sci USA* 75:3979–3983, 1978.

80. Conzelmann E, Sandhoff K, Nehrkorn H, et al: Purification, biochemical and immunological characterisation of hexosaminidase A from variant AB of infantile G_{M2} gangliosidosis. *Eur J Biochem* 84:27–33, 1978.

81. Cornog JL, Jr, Gonatas NK, Feierman JR: Effects of

intracerebral injection of ouabain on the fine structure of rat cerebral cortex. *Am J Pathol* 51:573–590, 1967.

82. Coulson WF, Bray PF: An association of phenylketonuria with ulegyria. *Dis Nerv Syst* 30:129–132, 1969.

83. Crandall BF, Philippart M, Brown WJ, et al: Review article: mucolipidosis IV. *Am J Med Genet* 12:301–308, 1982.

84. Crocker AC, Farber S: Niemann-Pick disease; a review of eighteen patients. *Medicine (Baltimore)* 37:1–95, 1958.

85. Crocker AC: The cerebral defect in Tay-Sachs disease and Niemann-Pick disease. *J Neurochem* 7:69–80, 1961.

86. Crome L, Dutton G, Ross CF: Maple syrup urine disease. *J Pathol Bacteriol* 81:379–384, 1961.

87. Crome L: A case of galactosaemia with the pathological and neuropathological findings. *Arch Dis Child* 37:415–421, 1962.

88. Crome L, France NE: The pathological findings in a case of argininosuccinic aciduria. *J Ment Defic Res* 15:266–270, 1971.

89. Crome L, Hanefeld F, Patrick D, et al: Late onset globoid cell leukodystrophy. *Brain* 96:841–848, 1973.

90. Crome L, Stern J: Inborn lysosomal enzyme deficiencies. In Blackwood W, Corsellis JAN (eds): *Greenfield's Neuropathology*, ed 3. London, Edward Arnold, 1976, p 500.

91. Crosby TW, Chou SM: "Ragged-red" fibers in Leigh's disease. *Neurology* 24:49–54, 1974.

92. Cutz E, Lowden JA, Conen PE: Ultrastructural demonstration of neuronal storage in fetal Tay-Sachs disease. *J Neurol Sci* 21:197–202, 1974.

93. D'Agostino AN, Sayre GP, Hayles AB: Krabbe's disease: globoid cell type of leukodystrophy. *Arch Neurol* 8:82–96, 1963.

94. Dancis J, Hutzler J, Levitz M: The diagnosis of maple syrup urine disease (branched-chain ketoaciduria) by the in vitro study of the peripheral leukocyte. *Pediatrics* 32:234–237, 1963.

95. Danks DM, Campbell PE, Cartwright E, et al: The Sanfilippo syndrome: clinical, biochemical, radiological, haematological and pathological features of nine cases. *Aust Paediatr J* 8:174–186, 1972.

96. Danks DM, Stevens BJ, Campbell PE, et al: Menkes' kinky-hair syndrome. *Lancet* 1:1100–1102, 1972.

97. Danks DM, Campbell PE, Stevens BJ, et al: Menkes's kinky hair syndrome: an inherited defect in copper absorption with widespread effects. *Pediatrics* 50:188–201, 1972.

98. Danks DM, Cartwright E, Stevens BJ, et al: Menkes' kinky hair disease: further definition of the defect in copper transport. *Science* 179:1140–1142, 1973.

99. Dawson RMC: Phosphoinositides of nervous tissue. *Biochem J* 98:19P, 1966.

100. Dehkharghani F, Sarnat HB, Brewster MA, et al: Congenital muscle fiber-type disproportion in Krabbe's leukodystrophy. *Arch Neurol* 38:585–587, 1981.

101. Deisenhammer E, Jellinger K: Höhlenbildende Neutralfett-Leukodystrophie mit Schubverlauf. *Neuropaediatrie* 7:111–121, 1976.

102. Dekaban AS, Patton VM: Hurler's and Sanfilippo's variants of mucopolysaccharidosis: cerebral pathology and lipid chemistry. *Arch Pathol* 91:434–443, 1971.

103. Dekaban AS, Constantopoulos G, Herman MM, et al: Mucopolysaccharidosis type V (Scheie syndrome): a postmortem study by multidisciplinary techniques with emphasis on the brain. *Arch Pathol Lab Med* 100:237–245, 1976.

104. Dekaban AS, Constantopoulos G: Mucopolysaccharidosis types I, II, IIIA and V: pathological and biochemical abnormalities in the neural and mesenchymal elements of the brain. *Acta Neuropathol (Berl)* 39:1–7, 1977.

105. DeMyer W: Megalencephaly in children: clinical syndromes, genetic patterns, and differential diagnosis from other causes of megalocephaly. *Neurology* 22:634–643, 1972.

106. Denny-Brown D: Hepatolenticular degeneration (Wilson's disease): two different components. *N Engl J Med* 270:1149–1156, 1964.

107. Desnick RJ, Sweeley CC: Fabry's disease: α-galactosidase A deficiency. In Stanbury JB, Wyngaarden JB, Fredrickson DS, et al (eds): *The Metabolic Basis of Inherited Disease*, ed 5. New York, McGraw-Hill, 1983, p 906.

108. Devivo DC, Haymond MW, Obert KA, et al: Defective activation of the pyruvate dehydrogenase complex in subacute necrotizing encephalomyelopathy (Leigh disease). *Ann Neurol* 6:483–494, 1979.

109. DiMauro S, Stern LZ, Mehler M, et al: Adult-onset acid maltase deficiency: a postmortem study. *Muscle Nerve* 1:27–36, 1978.

110. DiMauro S, Hartlage PL: Fatal infantile form of muscle phosphorylase deficiency. *Neurology* 28:1124–1129, 1978.

111. Dische MR, Porro RS: The cardiac lesions in Bassen-Kornzweig syndrome: report of a case, with autopsy findings. *Am J Med* 49:568–571, 1970.

112. Djaldetti M, Fishman P, Bessler H: The surface ultrastructure of Gaucher cells. *Am J Clin Pathol* 71:146–150, 1979.

113. Dolman CL, Chang E: Visceral lesions in amaurotic familial idiocy with curvilinear bodies. *Arch Pathol* 94:425–430, 1972.

114. Dolman CL, MacLeod PM, Chang E: Skin punch biopsies and lymphocytes in the diagnosis of lipidoses. *Can J Neurol Sci* 2:67–73, 1975.

115. Dolman CL, Chang E, Duke RJ: Pathologic findings in Sandhoff disease. *Arch Pathol* 96:272–275, 1973.

116. Dolman CL, McLeod PM, Chang EC: Lymphocytes and urine in ceroid lipofuscinosis. *Arch Pathol Lab Med* 104:487–490, 1980.

117. Dorfman A, Lorincz AE: Occurrence of urinary acid mucopolysaccharides in the Hurler syndrome. *Proc Natl Acad Sci USA* 43:443–446, 1957.

118. Dorfman A, Matalon R: The mucopolysaccharidoses (a review). *Proc Natl Acad Sci USA* 73:630–637, 1976.

119. Dowson JH: Neuronal lipofuscin accumulation in ageing and Alzheimer dementia: a pathogenic mechanism? *Br J Psychiatry* 140:142–148, 1982.

120. Dreborg S, Erikson A, Hagberg B: Gaucher disease—Norrbottnian type. I. General clinical description. *Eur J Pediatr* 133:107–118, 1980.

121. Duffy PE, Kornfeld M, Suzuki K: Neurovisceral storage disease with curvilinear bodies. *J Neuropathol Exp Neurol* 27:351–370, 1968.

122. Dulaney JT, Moser HW: Farber disease (lipogranulomatosis). In Glew RH, Peters SP (eds): *Practical Enzymology of the Sphingolipidoses: Laboratory and Research Methods in Biology and Medicine*. New York, Alan R. Liss, 1977, vol 1, p 283.

123. Dulaney JT, Moser HW: Metachromatic leukodystrophy. In Glew RH, Peters SP (eds): *Practical Enzymology of the Sphingolipidoses: Laboratory and Research Methods in Biology and Medicine*. New York, Alan R. Liss, 1977, vol 1, p 137.

124. Dunn HG, Lake BD, Dolman CL, et al: The neuropathy of Krabbe's infantile cerebral sclerosis (globoid cell leucodystrophy). *Brain* 92:329–344, 1969.

125. Dunn HG, Dolman CL, Farrell DF, et al: Krabbe's leukodystrophy without globoid cells. *Neurology* 26:1035–1041, 1976.

126. Durand D, Gatti R, Cavalieri S, et al: Sialidosis (mucolipidosis I). *Helv Paediatr Acta* 32:391–400, 1977.

127. Durand P, Borrone C, Della Cella G, et al: Fucosidosis. *Lancet* 1:1198, 1968.

128. Ebato H, Abe T, Yamakawa T, et al: Characterization of the cytoplasmic inclusion bodies of the spleens from patients with adult form Gaucher's disease. *J Biochem (Tokyo)* 88:1765–1772, 1980.

129. Ebels EJ: Neuropathological observations in a patient with carbamylphosphate-synthetase deficiency and in two sibs. *Arch Dis Child* 47:47–51, 1972.

130. Eeg-Olofsson O, Kristensson K, Sourander P, et al: Tay-Sachs disease: a generalized metabolic disorder. *Acta Paediatr Scand* 55:546–562, 1966.

131. Elfenbein IB: Dystonic juvenile idiocy without amau- rosis. A new syndrome: light and electron microscopic observations of cerebrum. *Johns Hopkins Med J* 123:205–221, 1968.

132. Engel AG, Gomez MR, Seybold ME, et al: The spectrum and diagnosis of acid maltase deficiency. *Neurology* 23:95–106, 1973.

133. Engel WK, Dorman JD, Levy RI, et al: Neuropathy in Tangier disease α-lipoprotein deficiency manifesting as familial recurrent neuropathy and intestinal lipid storage. *Arch Neurol* 17:1–9, 1967.

134. Escourolle R, Berger B, Poirier J: Biopsie cérébrale d'un cas de mucopolysaccharidose H.S. (oligophrénie polydystrophique ou maladie de Sanfilippo): étude histochimique et ultrastructurale. *Presse Med* 74:2869–2874, 1966.

135. Espinas OE, Faris AA: Acute infantile Gaucher's disease in identical twins: an account of clinical and neuropathologic observations. *Neurology* 19:133–140, 1969.

136. Eto Y, Meier C, Herschkowitz NN: Chemical compositions of brain and myelin in two patients with multiple sulphatase deficiency (a variant form of metachromatic leukodystrophy). *J Neurochem* 27:1071–1076, 1976.

137. Faraggiana T, Churg J, Grishman E, et al: Light- and electron-miroscopic histochemistry of Fabry's disease. *Am J Pathol* 103:247–262, 1981.

138. Farber S: A lipid metabolic disorder—disseminated "lipogranulomatosis"—a syndrome with similarity to, and important difference from Niemann-Pick and Hand-Schüller-Christian disease. *Am J Dis Child* 84:499–500, 1952.

139. Farrell DF, Ochs U: G_{M1} gangliosidosis: phenotypic variation in a single family. *Ann Neurol* 9:225–231, 1981.

140. Farrell DF, Sumi SM: Skin punch biopsy in the diagnosis of juvenile neuronal ceroid-lipofuscinosis: a comparison of leukocyte peroxidase assay. *Arch Neurol* 34:39–44, 1977.

141. Fensom AH, Benson PF, Neville BRG, et al: Prenatal diagnosis of Farber's disease. *Lancet* 2:990–992, 1979.

142. Ferrans VJ, Fredrickson DS: The pathology of Tangier diseases: a light end electron microscopic study. *Am J Pathol* 78:101–158, 1975.

143. Ferrer I, Arbizu T, Peña J, et al: A Golgi and ultrastructural study of a dominant form of Kufs' disease. *J Neurol* 222:183–190, 1980.

144. Fine DIM, Barron KD, Hirano A: Central nervous system lipidosis in an adult with atrophy of the cerebellar granular layer: a case report. *J Neuropathol Exp Neurol* 19:355–369, 1960.

145. Fratantoni JC, Hall CW, Neufeld EF: The defect in Hurler's and Hunter's syndromes: faulty degradation of mucopolysaccharide. *Proc Natl Acad Sci USA* 60:699–706, 1968.

146. Fratantoni JC, Hall CW, Neufeld EF: Hurler and Hunter syndromes: mutual correction of the defect in cultured fibroblasts. *Science* 162:570–572, 1968.

147. Fredrickson DS, Sloan HR: Glucosyl ceramide lipidoses: Gaucher's disease. In Stanbury JB, Wyngaarden JB, Fredrickson DS (eds): *The Metabolic Basis of Inherited Disease*, ed 3. New York, McGraw-Hill, 1972, p 730.

148. Fredrickson DS, Sloan HR: Sphingomyelin lipidoses: Niemann-Pick disease. In Stanbury JB, Wyngaarden JB, Fredrickson DS, (eds): *The Metabolic Basis of Inherited Disease*, ed. 3. New York, McGraw-Hill, 1972, p 783.

149. French JH, Brotz M, Poser CM: Lipid composition of the brain in infantile Gaucher's disease. *Neurology* 19:81–86, 1969.

150. Fukuhara N, Suzuki M, Fujita N, et al: Fabry's disease on the mechanism of the peripheral nerve involvement. *Acta Neuropathol (Berl)* 33:9–21, 1975.

151. Gadbois P, Moreau J, Laberge C: La maladie de Morquio dans la province de Québec. *Union Med Can* 102:602–607, 1973.

152. Gadoth N, O'Croinin P, Butler IJ: Bone marrow in the Batten-Vogt syndrome. *J Neurol Sci* 25:197–203, 1975.

153. Gal AE, Brady RO, Barranger JA, et al: The diagnosis

of type A and type B Niemann-Pick disease and detection of carriers using leukocytes and a chromogenic analogue of sphingomyelin. *Clin Chim Acta* 104:129–132, 1980.

154. Gambetti P., DiMauro S, Baker L: Nervous system in Pompe's disease: ultrastructure and biochemistry. *J Neuropathol Exp Neurol* 30:412–430, 1971.

155. Garret R, Ames RP: Alexander disease: case report with electron microscopical studies and review of the literature. *Arch Pathol* 98:379–385, 1974.

156. Gatti R, Borrone C, Trias X, et al: Genetic heterogeneity in fucosidosis. *Lancet* 2:1024, 1973.

157. Gaucher PCE: De l'Épithélioma Primitif de la Rate: Hypertrophie Idiopathique de la Rate sans Leucémie. Doctoral thesis, Paris, 1882.

158. Ghatak NR, Fleming DF, Hinman A: Neuropathology of Sanfilippo syndrome. *Ann Neurol* 2:161–166, 1977.

159. Ghatak NR, Nochlin D, Peris M, et al: Morphology and distribution of cytoplasmic inclusions in adrenoleukodystrophy. *J Neurol Sci* 50:391–398, 1981.

160. Gilbert EF, Dawson G, Zu Rhein GM, et al: I-cell disease, mucolipidosis II: pathological, histochemical, ultrastructural and biochemical observations in four cases. *Z Kinderheilk* 114:259–292, 1973.

161. Gilbert EF, Varakis J, Opitz JM, et al: Generalized gangliosidosis type II (juvenile GM_1 gangliosidosis): a pathological, histochemical and ultrastructural study. *Z Kinderheilk* 120:151–180, 1975.

162. Gilles FH, Deuel RK: Neuronal cytoplasmic globules in the brain in Morquio's syndrome. *Arch Neurol* 25:393–403, 1971.

163. Glees P, Hasan M: Lipofuscin in neuronal aging and diseases. *Norm Pathol Anat (Stuttg)* 32:1–68, 1976.

164. Goebel HH, Argyrakis A, Shimokawa K, et al: Adult metachromatic leukodystrophy. IV. Ultrastructural studies on the central and peripheral nervous system. *Eur Neurol* 19:294–307, 1980.

165. Goebel HH, Koppang N: Retinal ultrastructure in certain lysosomal disorders. In Zimmerman HM (ed): *Progress in Neuropathology.* New York, Raven Press, 1979, vol 4, p 141.

166. Goldberg MF, Duke JR: Ocular histopathology in Hunter's syndrome: systemic mucopolysaccharidosis type II. *Arch Ophthalmol* 77:503–512, 1967.

167. Goldberg MF, Scott CI, McKusick VA: Hydrocephalus and papilledema in the Maroteaux-Lamy syndrome (mucopolysaccharidosis type VI). *Am J Ophthalmol* 69:969–975, 1970.

168. Goldman JE, Yamanaka T, Rapin I, et al: The AB-variant of G_{M2}-gangliosidosis. Clinical, biochemical, and pathological studies of 2 patients. *Acta Neuropathol (Berl)* 52:189–202, 1980.

169. Gonatas NK, Terry RD, Winkler R, et al: A case of juvenile lipidosis: the significance of electron microscopic and biochemical observations of a cerebral biopsy. *J Neuropathol Exp Neurol* 22:557–580, 1963.

170. Gonatas NK, Gonatas J: Ultrastructural and biochemical observations on a case of systemic late infantile lipidosis and its relationship to Tay-Sachs disease and gargoylism. *J Neuropathol Exp Neurol* 24:318–340, 1965.

171. Gonatas NK, Gambetti P, Baird H: A second type of late infantile amaurotic idiocy with multilamellar cytosomes. *J Neuropathol Exp Neurol* 27:371–389, 1968.

172. Gravel RA, Lowden JA, Callahan JW, et al: Infantile sialidosis: a phenocopy of type 1 G_{M1} gangliosidosis distinguished by genetic complementation and urinary oligosaccharides. *Am J Hum Genet* 31:669–679, 1979.

173. Grégoire A, Périer O, Dustin P Jr: Metachromatic leukodystrophy, an electron microscopic study. *J Neuropathol Exp Neurol* 25:617–636, 1966.

174. Griffin JW, Goren E, Schaumburg H, et al: Adrenomyeloneuropathy: a probable variant of adrenoleukodystrophy. I. Clinical and endocrinologic aspects. *Neurology* 27:1107–1113, 1977.

175. Grossman H, Dorst JP: The mucopolysaccharidoses and mucolipidoses. In Kaufman HJ (ed): *Progress in Pediatric Radiology.* Basel, Switzerland, Karger, 1973, vol 4, p 495.

176. Grunnet ML, Spilsbury PR: The central nervous system in Fabry's disease: an ultrastructural study. *Arch Neurol* 28:231–234, 1973.

177. Gumbinas M, Larsen M, Liu HM: Peripheral neuropathy in classic Niemann-Pick disease: ultrastructure of nerves and skeletal muscles. *Neurology* 25:107–113, 1975.

178. Guthrie R, Susi A: A simple phenylalanine method for detecting phenylketonuria in large populations of newborn infants. *Pediatrics* 32:338–343, 1963.

179. Guzzetta F: Cockayne-Neill-Dingwall syndrome. In Vinken PJ, Bruyn GW (eds): *Neuroretinal Degenerations, Handbook of Clinical Neurology.* Amsterdam, North-Holland, 1972, vol 13, p 431.

180. Haberland C, Perou M, Brunngraber EG, et al: The neuropathology of galactosemia: a histopathological and biochemical study. *J Neuropathol Exp Neurol* 30:431–447, 1971.

181. Haberland C, Brunngraber E, Witting L, et al: Juvenile metachromatic leucodystrophy: case report with clinical, histopathological, ultrastructural and biochemical observations. *Acta Neuropathol (Berl)* 26:93–106, 1973.

182. Hadfield MG, Mamunes P, David RB: The pathology of Sandhoff's disease. *J Pathol* 123:137–144, 1977.

183. Hadfield MG, Ghatak NR, Nakoneczna I, et al: Pathologic findings in mucopolysaccharidosis type IIIB (Sanfilippo's syndrome B). *Arch Neurol* 37:645–650, 1980.

184. Hagberg B: The clinical diagnosis of Krabbe's infantile leucodystrophy. *Acta Paediatr Scand* 52:213, 1963.

185. Hahn AF, Gordon BA, Gilbert JJ, et al: The AB-variant of metachromatic leukodystrophy (postulated activator protein deficiency): light and electron microscopic findings in a sural nerve biopsy. *Acta Neuropathol (Berl)* 55:281–287, 1981.

186. Hall CW, Cantz M, Neufeld EF: A β-glucuronidase deficiency mucopolysaccharidosis: studies in cultured fibroblasts. *Arch Biochem Biophys* 155:32–38, 1973.

187. Hall CW, Liebaers I, Di Natale P, et al. Enzymic diagnosis of the genetic mucopolysaccharide storage disorders. *Methods Enzymol* 50:439–456, 1978.

188. Haltia M, Rapola J, Santavuori P, et al: Infantile type of so-called neuronal ceroid-lipofuscinosis. Part 2. Morphological and biochemical studies. *J Neurol Sci* 18:269–285, 1973.

189. Haltia T, Palo J, Haltia M, et al: Juvenile metachromatic leukodystrophy: clinical, biochemical and neuropathologic studies in nine new cases. *Arch Neurol* 37:42–46, 1980.

190. Haust MD, Landing BH: Histochemical studies in Hurler's disease: a new method for localization of acid mucopolysaccharide, and an analysis of lead acetate "fixation". *J Histochem Cytochem* 9:79–86, 1961.

191. Herndon RM, Rubinstein LJ: Leucodystrophy with Rosenthal fibers (Alexander's disease): a histochemical and electron microscopic study (abstr). *Neurology* 18:300, 1968.

192. Hers HG: Inborn lysosomal disease. *Gastroenterology* 48:625–633, 1965.

193. Hickman S, Neufeld EF: A hypothesis for I-cell disease: defective hydrolases that do not enter lysosomes. *Biochem Biophys Res Commun* 49:992–999, 1972.

194. Hirano A, Llena JF, French JH, et al: Fine structure of the cerebellar cortex in Menkes kinky-hair disease: X-chromosome-linked copper malabsorption. *Arch Neurol* 34:52–56, 1977.

195. Hoeg JM, Demosky SJ Jr, Brewer HB Jr: Characterization of neutral and acid ester hydrolase in Wolman's disease. *Biochim Biophys Acta* 711:59–65, 1982.

196. Hogan GR, Richardson EP Jr: Spongy degeneration of the nervous system (Canavan's disease): report of a case in an Irish-American family. *Pediatrics* 35:284–294, 1965.

197. Hooft C, Deloore G, van Bogaert L, et al: Sudanophilic leucodystrophy with meningeal angiomatosis in two brothers: infantile form of diffuse sclerosis with meningeal angiomatosis. *J Neurol Sci* 2:30–51, 1965.

198. Horoupian DS, Ross RT: Pigment variant of neuronal ceroid-lipofuscinosis (Kufs' disease). *Can J Neurol Sci* 4:67–75, 1977.

199. Horoupian DS, Yang SS: Paired helical filaments in neurovisceral lipidosis (juvenile dystonic lipidosis). *Ann Neurol* 4:404–411, 1978.

200. Horoupian DS, Kress Y, Yen SH, et al: Nickel-induced changes and reappraisal of Rosenthal fibers in focal CNS lesions. *J Neuropathol Exp Neurol* 41:664–675, 1982.

201. Horrocks LA, Van Rollins M, Yates AJ: Lipid changes in the ageing brain. In Davison AN, Thompson RNS (eds): *The Molecular Basis of Neuropathology.* London, Edward Arnold, 1981, p 601.

202. Howard RO, Albert DM: Ocular manifestations of subacute necrotizing encephalomyelopathy (Leigh's disease). *Am J Ophthalmol* 74:386–393, 1972.

203. Howell RR, Williams JC: The glycogen storage disease. In Stanbury JB, Wyngaarden JB, Fredrickson DS, et al (eds): *The Metabolic Basis of Inherited Disease*, ed 5. New York, McGraw-Hill, 1983, p 141.

204. Hueck W: Pigmentstudien. *Beitr Pathol Anat* 54:68–232, 1912.

205. Hug G: Pre- and postnatal pathology, enzyme treatment, and unresolved issues in five lysosomal disorders. *Pharmacol Rev* 30:565–591, 1978.

206. Itoh T, Li Y-T, Li S-C, et al: Isolation and characterization of a novel monosialosylpentahexosyl ceramide from Tay-Sachs brain. *J Biol Chem* 256:165–169, 1981.

207. Iwamori M, Nagai Y: Ganglioside-composition of brain in Tay-Sachs disease: increased amounts of GD2 and N-acetyl-beta-D-galactosaminyl GD1a ganglioside. *J Neurochem* 32:767–777, 1979.

208. Jatzkewitz H, Sandhoff K: On a biochemically special form of infantile amaurotic idiocy. *Biochim Biophys Acta* 70:354–356, 1963.

209. Jatzkewitz H: Zwei Typen von Cerebrosid-schwefelsäureestern als sog. Prälipoide und Speichersubstanzen bei der Leukodystrophie, Typ Scholz (metachromatische Form der diffusen Sklerose). *Hoppe-Seylers Z Physiol Chem* 311:279–282, 1958.

210. Jeanloz RW: The nomenclature of mucopolysaccharides. *Arthritis Rheum* 3:233–237, 1960.

211. Jellinger K, Seitelberger F: Juvenile form of spongy degeneration of the CNS. *Acta Neuropathol (Berl)* 13:276–281, 1969.

212. Jensen OA: Mucopolysaccharidosis type III (Sanfilippo's syndrome): histochemical examination of the eyes and brain with a survey of the literature. *Acta Pathol Microbiol Scand [A]* 79:257–273, 1971.

213. Jervis GA: Phenylpyruvic oligophrenia deficiency of phenylalanine-oxidizing system. *Proc Soc Exp Biol Med* 82:514–515, 1953.

214. Jervis GA, Degenerative encephalopathy of childhood (cortical degeneration, cerebellar atrophy, cholesterinosis of basal ganglia). *J Neuropathol Exp Neurol* 16:308–320, 1957.

215. Johnson WG: The clinical spectrum of hexosaminidase deficiency diseases. *Neurology* 31:1453–1456, 1981.

216. Jolly RD: The pathology of the central nervous system in pseudolipidosis of Angus calves. *J Pathol* 103:113–121, 1971.

217. Joosten E, Hoes M, Gabreëls-Festen A, et al: Electron microscopic investigation of inclusion material in a case of adult metachromatic leukodystrophy; observations on kidney biopsy, peripheral nerve and cerebral white matter. *Acta Neuropathol (Berl)* 33:165–171, 1975.

218. Kaback MM, Sloan HR, Sonneborn M, et al: G$_{m1}$-gangliosidosis type I: in utero detection and fetal manifestations. *J Pediatr* 82:1037–1041, 1973.

219. Kalimo H, Lundberg PO, Olsson Y: Familial subacute necrotizing encephalomyelopathy of the adult form (adult Leigh syndrome). *Ann Neurol* 6:200–206, 1979.

220. Kamoshita S, Aron AM, Suzuki K, et al: Infantile Niemann-Pick disease: a chemical study with isolation and characterization of membranous cytoplasmic bodies and myelin. *Am J Dis Child* 117:379–394, 1969.

221. Karpati G, Carpenter S, Eisen AA, et al: Multiple peripheral nerve entrapments: an unusual phenotypical variant of the Hunter syndrome (mucopolysaccharidosis II) in a family. *Arch Neurol* 31:418–422, 1974.

222. Karpati G, Carpenter S, Wolfe LS, et al: Juvenile dystonic lipidosis: an unusual form of neurovisceral storage disease. *Neurology* 27:32–42, 1977.

223. Kelly TE, Thomas GH, Taylor HA Jr, et al: Mucolipidosis III (pseudo-Hurler polydystrophy): clinical and laboratory studies in a series of 12 patients. *Johns Hopkins Med J* 137:156–175, 1975.

224. Kelly TE, Graetz G: Isolated acid neuraminidase deficiency: a distinct lysosomal storage disease. *Am J Med Genet* 1:31–46, 1977.

225. Kelly TE, Bartoshesky L, Harris DJ, et al: Mucolipidosis I (acid neuraminidase deficiency): three cases and delineation of the variability of the phenotype. *Am J Dis Child* 135:703–708, 1981.

226. Kennedy JF: Chemical and biochemical aspects of the glycosaminoglycans and proteoglycans in health and disease. *Adv Clin Chem* 18:1–101, 1976.

227. Kenyon KR, Maumenee IH, Green WR, et al: Mucolipidosis IV: histopathology of conjunctiva, cornea, and skin. *Arch Ophthalmol* 97:1106–1111, 1979.

228. Kidd M: An electronmicroscopical study of a case of atypical cerebral lipidosis. *Acta Neuropathol (Berl)* 9:70–78, 1967.

229. Kjellman B, Gamstorp I, Brun A, et al: Mannosidosis: a clinical and histopathologic study. *J Pediatr* 75:366–373, 1969.

230. Klenk E. Über die Natur der Phosphatide der Milz bei der Niemann-Pickschen Krankheit. *Z Physiol Chem* 229:151–156, 1934.

231. Klintworth GK, Vogel FS: Macular corneal dystrophy: an inherited acid mucopolysaccharide storage disease of the corneal fibroblast. *Am J Pathol* 45:565–586, 1964.

232. Kohn G, Livni N, Ornoy A, et al: Prenatal diagnosis of mucolipidosis IV by electron microscopy. *J Pediatr* 90:62–66, 1977.

233. Kolodny EH, Hass WK, Lane B, et al: Refsum's syndrome: report of a case including electron microscopic studies of the liver. *Arch Neurol* 12:583–596, 1965.

234. Kolodny EH, Cable JWL: Inborn errors of metabolism. *Ann Neurol* 11:221–232, 1982.

235. Kolodny EH, Moser HW: Sulfatide lipidosis: metachromatic leukodystrophy. In Stanbury JB, Wyngaarden JB, Fredrickson DS, et al (eds): *The Metabolic Basis of Inherited Disease*, ed 5. New York, McGraw-Hill, 1983, p 881.

236. Koneff H: Beitrage zur Kenntnis der Nervenzellen der peripheren Ganglien. Mit Holzschnitten im text. *Mitt Naturforsch Gesselsch Bern* 1143–1168, 1886–1887 (13–44).

237. Koto A, Horwitz AL, Suzuki K, et al: The Morquio syndrome: neuropathology and biochemistry. *Ann Neurol* 4:26–36, 1978.

238. Krabbe K: A new familial, infantile form of diffuse brain-sclerosis. *Brain* 39:74–114, 1916.

239. Kraus-Ruppert R, Sommer H: The late form of metachromatic leukodystrophy. II. Ultrastructural correlations with morphological and neurochemical findings. *J Neurol Sci* 17:383–387, 1972.

240. Kristensson K, Rayner S, Sourander P: Visceral involvement in juvenile amaurotic idiocy. *Acta Neuropathol (Berl)* 4:421–424, 1965.

241. Lane B, Carroll BA, Pedley TA: Computerized cranial tomography in cerebral diseases of white matter. *Neurology* 28:534–544, 1978.

242. Lee RE, Peters SP, Glew RH: Gaucher's disease: clinical, morphologic, and pathogenetic considerations. *Pathol*

Annu 12(Part 2):309–339, 1977.

243. Lehner T, Adams CWM: Lipid histochemistry of Fabry's disease. *J. Pathol Bacteriol* 95:411–415, 1968.

244. Leroy JG, DeMars RI, Opitz JM: I-cell disease. *Birth Defects* 5(4):174–189, 1969.

245. Levine S, Hoenig EM: Astrocytic gliosis of vascular adventitia and arachnoid membrane in infantile Gaucher's disease. *J Neuropathol Exp Neurol* 31:147–154, 1972.

246. Levy LA, Lewis JC, Sumner TE: Ultrastructures of Reilly bodies (metachromatic granules) in the Maroteaux-Lamy syndrome (mucopolysaccharidosis VI): a histochemical study. *Am J Clin Pathol* 73:416–422, 1980.

247. Li S-C, Hirabayashi Y, Li Y-T: A protein activator for the enzymic hydrolysis of G_{M2} ganglioside. *J Biol Chem* 256:6234–6240, 1981.

248. Libert J, Van Hoof F, Toussaint D, et al: Ocular findings in metachromatic leukodystrophy: an electron microscopic and enzyme study in different clinical and genetic variants. *Arch Ophthalmol* 97:1495–1504, 1979.

249. Libert J, Tondeur M, Van Hoof F: The use of conjunctival biopsy and enzyme analysis in tears for the diagnosis of homozygotes and heterozygotes with Fabry disease. *Birth Defects* 12(3):221–239, 1976.

250. Lie SO, Löken AC, Strömme JH, et al: Fatal congenital lactic acidosis in two siblings. I. Clinical and pathological findings. *Acta Paediatr Scand* 60:129–137, 1971.

251. Liebaers I, Neufeld EF: Iduronate sulfatase activity in serum, lymphocytes, and fibroblasts—simplified diagnosis of the Hunter syndrome. *Pediatr Res* 10:733–736, 1976.

252. Lillie RD, Ashburn LL, Sebrell WH, et al: Histogenesis and repair of the hepatic cirrhosis in rats produced on low protein diets and preventable with choline. *Public Health Rep* 57:502–508, 1942.

253. Lin HJ, Lie Ken Jie MSF, Ho FCS: Accumulation of glyceryl ether lipids in Wolman's disease. *J Lipid Res* 17:53–56, 1976.

254. Liss L: Etiology of uncommon distribution of anoxic lesions (abstr). *J Neuropathol Exp Neurol* 37:649, 1978.

255. Livni N, Merin S: Mucolipidosis IV: ultrastructural diagnosis of a recently defined genetic disorder. *Arch Pathol Lab Med* 102:600–604, 1978.

256. Lloyd KG, Hornykiewicz O, Davidson L, et al: Biochemical evidence of dysfunction of brain neurotransmitters in the Lesch-Nyhan syndrome. *N Engl J Med* 305:1106–1111, 1981.

257. Loeb H, Tondeur M, Jonniaux G, et al: Biochemical and ultrastructural studies in a case of mucopolysaccharidosis "F" (fucosidosis). *Helv Paediatr Acta* 24:519–537, 1969.

258. Lowden JA, Cutz E, Conen PE, et al: Prenatal diagnosis of G_{M1}-gangliosidosis. *N Engl J Med* 288:225–228, 1973.

259. de Léon GA, Kaback MM, Elfenbein IB, et al: Juvenile dystonic lipidosis. *Johns Hopkins Med J* 125:62–77, 1969.

260. Lowden JA, Zuker S, Wilensky AJ, et al: Screening for carriers of Tay-Sachs disease: a community project. *Can Med Assoc J* 111:229–233, 1974.

261. Lowden JA, O'Brien JS: Sialidosis: a review of human neuraminidase deficiency. *Am J Hum Genet* 31:1–18, 1979.

262. Lowden JA, Callahan JW, Gravel RA, et al: Type 2 GM_1 gangliosidosis with long survival and neuronal ceroid lipofuscinosis. *Neurology* 31:719–724, 1981.

263. Löwenberg K, Hill TS: Diffuse sclerosis with preserved myelin islands. *Arch Neurol Psychiatry* 29:1232–1245, 1933.

264. Luijten JAFM, Straks W, Blikkendaal-Lieftinck LF, et al: Metachromatic leukodystrophy: a comparative study of the ultrastructural findings in the peripheral nervous system of three cases: one of the late infantile, one of the juvenile and one of the adult form of the disease. *Neuropaediatrie* 9:338–350, 1978.

265. Lynn R, Terry RD: Lipid histochemistry and electron microscopy in adult Niemann-Pick disease. *Am J Med* 37:987–994, 1964.

266. Lyons JC, Scheithauer BW, Ginsburg WW: Gaucher's disease and glioblastoma multiforme in two siblings: a clinicopathologic study. *J Neuropathol Exp Neurol* 41:45–53, 1982.

267. MacBrinn M, Okada S, Woollacott M, et al: Beta-galactosidase deficiency in the Hurler syndrome. *N Engl J Med* 281:338–343, 1969.

268. MacGregor DL, Humphrey RP, Armstrong DL, et al: Brain biopsies for neurodegenerative disease in children. *J Pediatr* 92:903–905, 1978.

269. Malamud N: Neuropathology of phenylketonuria. *J Neuropathol Exp Neurol* 25:254–268, 1966.

270. Mancall EL, Aponte GE, Berry RG: Pompe's disease (diffuse glycogenosis) with neuronal storage. *J Neuropathol Exp Neurol* 24:85–96, 1965.

271. Manz HJ, Schuelein M, McCullough DC, et al: New phenotypic variant of adrenoleukodystrophy: pathologic, ultrastructural, and biochemical study in two brothers. *J Neurol Sci* 45:245–260, 1980.

272. Markesbery WR, Shield LK, Egel RT, et al: Late-infantile neuronal ceroid-lipofuscinosis: an ultrastructural study of lymphocyte inclusions. *Arch Neurol* 33:630–635, 1976.

273. Maroteaux P, Levêque B, Marie J, et al: Une nouvelle dysostose avec elimination urinaire de chondroitine-sulfate B. *Presse Med* 71:1849–1852, 1963.

274. Maroteaux P, Lamy M: La pseudo-polydystrophie de Hurler. *Presse Med* 74:2889–2892, 1966.

275. Martin JJ, Joris C: The sciatic nerve in juvenile metachromatic leucodystrophy: a quantitative evaluation. *Acta Neurol Belg* 73:175–191, 1973.

276. Martin JJ, Barsy Th de, Van Hoof F, et al: Pompe's disease: an inborn lysosomal disorder with storage of glycogen: a study of brain and striated muscle. *Acta Neuropathol (Berl)* 23:229–244, 1973.

277. Martin JJ, Leroy JG, Farriaux JP, et al: I-cell disease (mucolipidosis II): a report on its pathology. *Acta Neuropathol (Berl)* 33:285–305, 1975.

278. Martin JJ, Ceuterick C: Morphological study of skin bipopsy specimens: a contribution to the diagnosis of metabolic disorders with involvement of the nervous system. *J Neurol Neurosurg Psychiatry* 41:232–248, 1978.

279. Martin JJ, Ceuterick C, Van Dessel G, et al: Two cases of mucopolysaccharidosis type III (Sanfilippo). An anatomopathological study. *Acta Neuropathol (Berl)* 46:185–190, 1979.

280. Martin JJ, Ceuterick C, Libert J: Skin and conjunctival nerve biopsies in adrenoleukodystrophy and its variants. *Ann Neurol* 8:291–295, 1980.

281. Martin JJ, Leroy JG, Ceuterick C, et al: Fetal Krabbe leukodystrophy. A morphologic study of two cases. *Acta Neuropathol (Berl)* 53:87–91, 1981.

282. Matalon R, Dorfman A: The structure of acid mucopolysaccharides produced by Hurler fibroblasts in tissue culture. *Proc Natl Acad Sci USA* 60:179–185, 1968.

283. Matalon R, Dorfman A: Hurler's syndrome, and α-L-iduronidase deficiency. *Biochem Biophys Res Commun* 47:959–964, 1972.

284. Matsuyama H, Watanabe I, Mihm MC, et al: Dermatoleukodystrophy with neuroaxonal spheroids. *Arch Neurol* 35:329–336, 1978.

285. McArdle B: Myopathy due to a defect in muscle glycogen breakdown. *Clin Sci* 10:13–35, 1951.

286. McKusick VA, Howell RR, Hussels IE, et al: Allelism, non-allelism, and genetic compounds among the mucopolysaccharidoses. *Lancet* 1:993–996, 1972.

287. McKusick VA, Neufeld EF: The mucopolysaccharide storage diseases. In Stanbury JB, Wyngaarden JB, Fredrickson DS, et al (eds): *The Metabolic Basis of Inherited Disease*, ed 5. New York, McGraw-Hill, 1983, p 751.

288. McKusick VA: *Heritable Disorders of Connective Tissue*, ed 4. St Louis, Mosby, 1972.

289. McMaster KR, Powers JM, Hennigar GR Jr, et al: Nervous system involvement in type IV glycogenosis.

Arch Pathol Lab Med 103:105–111, 1979.

290. Meier C, Bischoff A: Sequence of morphological alterations in the nervous system of metachromatic leucodystrophy. Light and electronmicroscopic observations in the central and peripheral nervous system in a prenatally diagnosed foetus of 22 weeks. *Acta Neuropathol (Berl)* 36:369–379, 1976.

291. Meier C, Wiesmann U, Herschkowitz N, et al: Morphological observations in the nervous system of prenatal mucopolysaccharidosis II (M. Hunter). *Acta Neuropathol (Berl)* 48:139–143, 1979.

292. Menkes JH, Alter M, Steigleder GK, et al: A sex-linked recessive disorder with retardation of growth, peculiar hair, and focal cerebral and cerebellar degeneration. *Pediatrics* 29:764–779, 1962.

293. Menkes JH, Philippart M, Fiol RE: Cerebral lipids in maple syrup disease. *J Pediatr* 66:584–594, 1965.

294. Menkes JH: The pathogenesis of mental retardation in phenylketonuria and other inborn errors of amino acid metabolism. *Pediatrics* 39:297–308, 1967.

295. Menkes JH, Schimschock JR, Swanson PD: Cerebrotendinous xanthomatosis: the storage of cholestanol within the nervous system. *Arch Neurol* 19:47–53, 1968.

296. Menkes JH, O'Brien JS, Okada S, et al: Juvenile G_{M2} gangliosidosis: biochemical and ultrastructural studies on a new variant of Tay-Sachs disease. *Arch Neurol* 25:14–22, 1971.

297. Migeon BR, Moser HW, Moser AB, et al: Adrenoleukodystrophy: evidence for X linkage, inactivation, and selection favoring the mutant allele in heterozygous cells. *Proc Natl Acad Sci USA* 78:5066–5070, 1981.

298. Milunsky A, Littlefield JW, Kanfer JN, et al: Prenatal genetic diagnosis. *N Engl J Med* 283:1370–1381, 1441–1447, 1498–1504, 1970.

299. Miyatake T, Suzuki K: Globoid cell leukodystrophy: additional deficiency of psychosine galactosidase. *Biochem Biophys Res Commun* 48:538–543, 1972.

300. Mizuno T, Endoh H, Konishi Y, et al: An autopsy case of the Lesch-Nyhan syndrome: normal HGPRT activity in liver and xanthine calculi in various tissues. *Neuropaediatrie* 7:351–355, 1976.

301. Montpetit VJA, Andermann F, Carpenter S, et al: Subacute necrotizing encephalomyelopathy: a review and a study of two families. *Brain* 94:1–30, 1971.

302. Moossy J: The neuropathology of Cockayne's syndrome. *J Neuropathol Exp Neurol* 26:654–660, 1967.

303. Morquio L: Sur une forme de dystrophie osseuse familiale. *Bull Soc Pediatr Paris* 27:145–152, 1929.

304. Moser HW, Moser AB, Kawamura N, et al: Adrenoleukodystrophy: studies of the phenotype, genetics and biochemistry. *Johns Hopkins Med J* 147:217–224, 1980.

305. Mudd SH, Levy HL: Disorders of transsulfuration. In Stanbury JB, Wyngaarden JB, Fredrickson DS, et al (eds): *The Metabolic Basis of Inherited Disease*. ed 5. New York, McGraw-Hill, 1983, p 522.

306. Nagashima K, Kikuchi F, Suzuki Y, et al: Retinal amacrine cell involvement in Tay-Sachs disease. *Acta Neuropathol (Berl)* 53:333–336, 1981.

307. Namiki H: Subacute necrotizing encephalomyelopathy: case report with special emphasis on associated pathology of peripheral nervous system. *Arch Neurol* 12:98–107, 1965.

308. Neligan G: Hypoglycaemia in infancy and childhood. *J Clin Pathol* 22(Suppl 2):51–56, 1969.

309. Neufeld EF: The biochemical basis for mucopolysaccharidoses and mucolipidoses. *Prog Med Genet* 10:81–101, 1974.

310. Neufeld EF, Cantz MJ: Corrective factors for inborn errors of mucopolysaccharide metabolism. *Ann NY Acad Sci* 179:580–587, 1971.

311. Neville BGR, Lake BD, Stephens R, et al: A neurovisceral storage disease with vertical supranuclear ophthalmoplegia, and its relationship to Niemann-Pick disease: a report of nine patients. *Brain* 96:97–120, 1973.

312. Ng Ying Kin NMK, Wolfe LS: Oligosaccharides accu-

mulating in the liver from a patient with G_{M2}-gangliosidosis variant O (Sandhoff-Jatzkewitz disease). *Biochem Biophys Res Commun* 59:837–844, 1974.

313. Ng Ying Kin NMK, Palo J, Haltia M, et al: High levels of brain dolichols in neuronal ceroid-lipofuscinosis and senescence. *J Neurochem* 40:1465–1473, 1983.

314. Niederwieser A, Curtius HC, Wang M, et al: Atypical phenylketonuria with defective biopterin metabolism. Monotherapy with tetrahydrobiopterin or sepiapterin, screening and study of biosynthesis in man. *Eur J Pediatr* 138:110–112, 1982.

315. Niemann A: Ein unbekanntes Krankheitsbild. *Jb Kinderheilk* 79:1–10, 1914.

316. Nilsson O, Månsson JE, Håkansson G, et al: The occurrence of psychosine and other glycolipids in spleen and liver from the three major types of Gaucher's disease. *Biochim Biophys Acta* 712:453–463, 1982.

317. Nishimura RN, Barranger JA: Neurologic complications of Gaucher's disease, type 3. *Arch Neurol* 37:92–93, 1980.

318. Nitowsky HM, Grunfeld A: Lysosomal α-glucosidase in type II glycogenosis; activity in leukocytes and cell cultures in relation to genotype. *J Lab Clin Med* 69:472–484, 1967.

319. Noonan SM, Desousa J, Riddle JM: Lymphocyte ultrastructure in two cases of neuronal ceroid-lipofuscinosis. *Neurology* 28:472–477, 1978.

320. Nordén NE, Öckerman PA: Urinary mannose in mannosidosis. *J Pediatr* 82:686–688, 1973.

321. Norman MG: Leukodystrophy: diffuse cerebral sclerosis or Schilder's disease revisited. *Perspect Pediatr Pathol* 2:61–100, 1975.

322. Norman RM, Urich H, Lloyd OC: The neuropathology of infantile Gaucher's disease. *J Pathol Bacteriol* 72:121–131, 1956.

323. Norman RM, Urich H, Tingey AH: Metachromatic leuco-encephalopathy: a form of lipidosis. *Brain* 83:369–380, 1960.

324. Norman RM, Oppenheimer DR, Tingey AH: Histological and chemical findings in Krabbe's leucodystrophy. *J Neurol Neurosurg Psychiatry* 24:223–232, 1961.

325. Norman RM, Tingey AH: Sudanophil leukodystrophy and Pelizaeus-Merzbacher disease. In Folch-Pi J (ed): *Brain Lipids, Lipoproteins and Leucodystrophies*. Amsterdam, Elsevier, 1963, p 169.

326. Norman RM, Tingey AH: Sudanophil leucodystrophy and Pelizaeus-Merzbacher disease. In Folch-Pi J, Bauer H (eds): *Brain Lipids and Lipoproteins and the Leucodystrophies*. Amsterdam, Elsevier, 1963, p 169.

327. Norman RM, Forrester RM, Tingey AH: The juvenile form of Niemann-Pick disease. *Arch Dis Child* 42:91–96, 1967.

328. O'Brien JS, Stern MB, Landing BH, et al: Generalized gangliosidosis—an inborn error of ganglioside metabolism? *Am J Dis Child* 109:338–346, 1965.

329. O'Brien J: Generalized gangliosidosis. *J Pediatr* 75:167–186, 1969.

330. O'Brien JS: Ganglioside storage diseases. *Hum Genet* 3:39–98, 1972.

331. O'Brien JS, Ho MW, Veath ML, et al: Juvenile GM_1 gangliosidosis: clinical, pathological, chemical and enzymatic studies. *Clin Genet* 3:411–434, 1972.

332. O'Brien JS: Neuraminidase deficiency in the cherry red spot-myoclonus syndrome. *Biochem Biophys Res Commun* 79:1136–1141, 1977.

333. O'Brien JS: Suggestions for a nomenclature for the G_{M2} gangliosidoses making certain (possibly unwarrantable) assumptions. *Am J Hum Gent* 30:672–675, 1978.

334. Öckerman PA: A generalised storage disorder resembling Hurler's syndrome. *Lancet* 2:239–241, 1967.

335. Öckerman PA: Mannosidosis: isolation of oligosaccharide storage material from brain. *J Pediatr* 75:360–365, 1969.

336. Ogino T, Osuka T, Yokoi S: Atypical GM_1 ganglioside accumulation in a case of juvenile amaurotic idiocy. *Clin Chim Acta* 78:9–16, 1977.

337. Ohkura T, Yamashita K, Kobata A: Urinary oligosaccharides of G_{M1}-gangliosidosis: structures of oligosaccharides excreted in the urine of type 1 but not in the urine of type 2 patients. *J Biol Chem* 256:8485–8490, 1981.

338. Ohnishi A, Dyck PJ: Loss of small peripheral sensory neurons in Fabry disease: histologic and morphometric evaluation of cutaneous nerves, spinal ganglia, and posterior columns. *Arch Neurol* 31:120–127, 1974.

339. Okada S, McCrea M, O'Brien JS: Sandhoff's disease (GM_2 gangliosidosis *type 2*): clinical, chemical, and enzyme studies in five patients. *Pediatr Res* 6:606–615, 1972.

340. O'Neill B, Butler AB, Young E, et al: Adult-onset GM_2 gangliosidosis: seizures, dementia, and normal pressure hydrocephalus associated with glycolipid storage in the brain and arachnoid granulation. *Neurology* 28:1117–1123, 1978.

341. O'Neill BP, Marmion LC, Feringa ER: The adrenoleukomyeloneuropathy complex: expression in four generations. *Neurology* 31:151–156, 1981.

342. Oppenheimer DR, Norman RM, Tingey AH, et al: Histological and chemical findings in juvenile Niemann-Pick disease. *J Neurol Sci* 5:575–588, 1967.

343. Ornoy A, Sekeles E, Cohen R, et al: Electron microscopy of cultured skin fibroblasts and amniotic fluid cells in the diagnosis of hereditary storage diseases. *Monogr Hum Genet* 10:32–39, 1978.

344. Oteruelo FT: "PKU bodies": characteristic inclusions in the brain in phenylketonuria. *Acta Neuropathol (Berl)* 36:295–305, 1976.

345. Pearse AGE: *Histochemistry, Theoretical and Applied*, ed 3. London, Churchill, 1968, Vols 1 and 2.

346. Peiffer J: The pure leucodystrophic forms of orthochromatic leucodystrophies (simple type, pigment type). In Vinken PJH, Bruyn GW (eds): *Leucodystrophies and Poliodystrophies, Handbook of Clinical Neurology*. Amsterdam, North-Holland, 1970, vol 10, p 105.

347. Pellissier JF, Hassoun J, Gambarelli PA, et al: Maladie de Niemann-Pick type "C" de Crocker: étude ultrastructurale d'un cas. *Acta Neuropathol (Berl)* 34:65–76, 1976.

348. Pellissier JF, Barsy Th de, Faugere MC, et al: Type III glycogenosis with multicore structures. *Muscle Nerve* 2:124–132, 1979.

349. Pellissier JF, Van Hoof F, Bourdet-Bonerandi D, et al: Morphological and biochemical changes in muscle and peripheral nerve in Fabry's disease. *Muscle Nerve* 4:381–387, 1981.

350. Pennock CA, Barnes IC: The mucopolysaccharidoses. *J Med Genet* 13:169–181, 1976.

351. Percy AK, Kaback MM, Herndon RM: Metachromatic leukodystrophy: comparison of early- and late-onset forms. *Neurology* 27:933–941, 1977.

352. Perry TL: Unsolved problems in homocystinuria. In Nyhan WL (ed): *Amino Acid Metabolism and Genetic Variation*. New York, McGraw-Hill, 1967, p 279.

353. Perry TL, Urquhart N, MacLean J, et al: Nonketotic hyperglycemia: glycine accumulation due to absence of glycine cleavage in brain. *N Engl J Med* 292:1269–1273, 1975.

354. Peterson L, Nelson A, Parkin J: Mucopolysaccharidosis type VII. A morphologic, cytochemical, and ultrastructural study of the blood and bone marrow (abstr). *Lab Invest* 44:5P, 1981.

355. Phillippart M, Martin L, Martin JJ, et al. Niemann-Pick disease: morphologic and biochemical studies in the visceral form with late central nervous system involvement (Crocker's group C). *Arch Neurol* 20:227–238, 1969.

356. Pick L: Der Morbus Gaucher und die ihm ähnlichen Erkrankungen (Die Lipoidzellige Splenohepatomegalie Typus Niemann und die diabetische Lipoidzellenhypoplasie der Milz). *Ergeb Inn Med Kinderheilkd* 29:519–627, 1926.

357. Pilz H, Müller D: Studies on adult metachromatic leukodystrophy. Part 2. Biochemical aspects of adult cases of metachromatic leukodystrophy. *J Neurol Sci* 9:585–595, 1969.

358. Pincus JH, Cooper JR, Piros K, et al: Specificity of the urine inhibitor test for Leigh's disease. *Neurology* 24:885–890, 1974.

359. Pincus JH, Solitare GB, Cooper JR: Thiamine triphosphate levels and histopathology. Correlation in Leigh disease. *Arch Neurol* 33:759–763, 1976.

360. Poduslo SE, Miller K, Jang Y: Biochemical studies of the late infantile form of metachromatic leukodystrophy. *Acta Neuropathol (Berl)* 57:13–22, 1982.

361. Popoff N, Budzilovich G, Goodgold A, et al: Hepatocerebral degeneration: its occurrence in the presence and in the absence of abnormal copper metabolism. *Neurology* 15:919–930, 1965.

362. Powell H, Tindall R, Schultz P, et al: Adrenoleukodystrophy: electron microscopic findings. *Arch Neurol* 32:250–260, 1975.

363. Powers JM, Schaumberg HH: Adreno-leukodystrophy (sex-linked Schilder's disease). A pathogenetic hypothesis based on ultrastructural lesions in adrenal cortex, peripheral nerve and testis. *Am J Pathol* 76:481–500, 1974.

364. Powers JM, Schaumburg HH: The testis in adrenoleukodystrophy. *Am J Pathol* 102:90–98, 1981.

365. Prensky AL, Carr S, Moser HW: Development of myelin in inherited disorders of amino acid metabolism: a biochemical investigation. *Arch Neurol* 19:552–558, 1968.

366. Probst A, Ulrich J, Heitz PU, et al: Adrenomyeloneuropathy, a protracted, pseudosystematic variant of adrenoleukodystrophy. *Acta Neuropathol (Berl)* 49:105–115, 1980.

367. Purpura DP, Hirano A, French JH: Polydendritic Purkinje cells in X-chromosome linked copper malabsorption: a Golgi study. *Brain Res* 117:125–129, 1976.

368. Purpura DP, Suzuki K: Distortion of neuronal geometry and formation of aberrant synapses in neuronal storage disease. *Brain Res* 116:1–21, 1976.

369. Quigley HA, Kenyon KR: Ultrastructural and histochemical studies of a newly recognized form of systemic mucopolysaccharidosis (Maroteaux-Lamy syndrome, mild phenotype). *Am J Ophthalmol* 77:809–818, 1974.

370. Rahman AN, Lindenberg R: The neuropathology of hereditary dystopic lipidosis. *Arch Neurol* 9:373–385, 1963.

371. Ramsey RB, Sarnat HB, Adelman LS: Lipid analysis of perinatal sudanophilic leukodystrophy. *Am J Dis Child* 127:294–295, 1974.

372. Ramsey RB, Banik NL, Ramsey ML, et al: Neurochemical findings in a perinatal sudanophilic leukodystrophy rich in steryl ester. *J Neurol Sci* 30:95–111, 1976.

373. Rao BG, Spence MW: Niemann-Pick disease type D: lipid analyses and studies on sphingomyelinases. *Ann Neurol* 1:385–392, 1977.

374. Rapin I, Suzuki K, Suzuki K, et al: Adult (chronic) G_{M2} gangliosidosis: atypical spinocerebellar degeneration in a Jewish sibship. *Arch Neurol* 33:120–130, 1976.

375. Rapin I, Goldfischer S, Katzman R, et al: The cherry-red spot-myoclonus syndrome. *Ann Neurol* 3:234–242, 1978.

376. Raynaud EJ, Escourolle R, Baumann N, et al: Metachromatic leukodystrophy: ultrastructural and enzymatic study of a case of variant O form. *Arch Neurol* 32:834–838, 1975.

377. Refsum S: Heredopathia atactica polyneuritiformis phytanic-acid storage disease, Refsum's disease: a biochemically well-defined disease with a specific dietary treatment. *Arch Neurol* 38:605–606, 1981.

378. Renlund M, Aula P, Raivio KO, et al: Salla disease: a new lysosomal storage disorder with disturbed sialic acid metabolism. *Neurology* 33:57–66, 1983.

379. Résibois-Grégoire A: Electron microscopic studies of metachromatic leucodystrophy. II. Compound nature of the inclusions. *Acta Neuropathol (Berl)* 9:244–253, 1967.

380. Résibois A: Electron microscopic studies of metachromatic leucodystrophy. IV. Liver and kidney alterations. *Pathol Eur* 6:278–298, 1971.

381. Richards W, Donnell GN, Wilson WA, et al: The oculo-cerebro-renal syndrome of Lowe. *Am J Dis Child* 109:185–203, 1965.

382. Rosenberg LE, Scriver CR: Disorders of amino acid metabolism. In Bondy PK, Rosenberg LE (eds): *Metabolic Control and Disease*, ed 8. Philadelphia, Saunders, 1980, p 583.

383. Rosenberg RN: Biochemical genetics of neurologic disease. *N Engl J Med* 305:1181–1193, 1981.

384. Rowland LP, Lovelace RE, Schotland DL, et al: The clinical diagnosis of McArdle's disease: identification of another family with deficiency of muscle phosphorylase. *Neurology* 16:93–100, 1966.

385. Rowland LP: Hyperammonemia, congenital. In Vinken PJ, Bruyn CW (eds): *Neurogenetic Directory, Handbook of Clinical Neurology*. Amsterdam, North-Holland, 1981, vol 42, p 560.

386. Roy S, Srivastava RN, Gupta PC, et al: Ultrastructure of peripheral nerve in Cockayne's syndrome. *Acta Neuropathol (Berl)* 24:345–349, 1973.

387. Russo LS Jr, Aron A, Anderson PJ: Alexander's disease: a report and reappraisal. *Neurology* 26:607–614, 1976.

388. Rutsaert J, Menu R, Résibois A: Ultrastructure of sulfatide storage in normal and sulfatase-deficient fibroblasts *in vitro*. *Lab Invest* 29:527–535, 1973.

389. Salen G, Shefer S, Cheng FW, et al: Cholic acid biosynthesis: the enzymatic defect in cerebrotendinous xanthomatosis. *J Clin Invest* 63:38–44, 1979.

390. Sanchez JE, Lopez VF: Sex-linked sudanophilic leukodystrophy with adrenocortical atrophy (so-called Schilder's disease). *Neurology* 26:261–269, 1976.

391. Sandhoff K, Andreae U, Jatzkewitz H: Deficient hexoaminidase activity in an exceptional case of Tay-Sachs disease with additional storage of kidney globoside in visceral organs. *Life Sci* 7:283–288, 1968.

392. Sandhoff K, Christomanou H: Biochemistry and genetics of gangliosidosis. *Hum Genet* 50:107–143, 1979.

393. Santavuori P, Haltia M, Rapola J, et al: Infantile type of so-called neuronal ceroid-lipofuscinosis. Part 1. A clinical study of 15 patients. *J Neurol Sci* 18:257–267, 1973.

394. Santavuori P, Haltia M, Rapola J: Infantile type of so-called neuronal ceroid-lipofuscinosis. *Dev Med Child Neurol* 16:644–653, 1974.

395. Sarnat HB, Adelman LS: Perinatal sudanophilic leukodystrophy. *Am J Dis Child* 125:281–285, 1973.

396. Schärer K, Marty A, Muhlethaler JP: Chronic congenital lactic acidosis: a fatal case with hyperphosphotemia and hyperlipemia. *Helv Paediat Acta* 23:107–127, 1968.

397. Schaumburg HH, Powers JM, Raine CS, et al: Adrenoleukodystrophy: a clinical and pathological study of 17 cases. *Arch Neurol* 32:577–591, 1975.

398. Schaumburg HH, Powers JM, Raine CS, et al: Adrenomyeloneuropathy: a probable variant of adrenoleukodystrophy. II. General pathologic, neuropathologic, and biochemical aspects. *Neurology* 27:1114–1119, 1977.

399. Schimschock JR, Alvord EC Jr, Swanson PD: Cerebrotendinous xanthomatosis. Clinical and pathological studies. *Arch Neurol* 18:688–698, 1968.

400. Schlaepfer WW, Prensky AL: Quantitative and qualitative study of sural nerve biopsies in Krabbe's disease. *Acta Neuropathol (Berl)* 20:55–66, 1972.

401. Schmickel RD, Chu EHY, Trosko J: The definition of a cellular defect in two patients with Cockayne syndrome (abstr). *Pediatr Res* 9:317, 1975.

402. Schmitt HP, Berlet H, Volk B: Peripheral intraaxonal storage in Tay-Sachs' disease (G_{M2}-gangliosidosis type 1). *J Neurol Sci* 44:115–124, 1979.

403. Schmoeckel C, Hohlfed M: A specific ultrastructural marker for disseminated lipogranulomatosis (Farber). *Arch Dermatol Res* 266:187–196, 1979.

404. Schneck L: The clinical aspects of Tay-Sachs' disease. In Volk BW (ed): *Tay-Sachs Disease*. New York, Grune & Stratton, 1964, p 16.

405. Schneck L, Adachi M, Volk BW: Congenital failure of

406. Schochet SS, McCormick WF, Powell GF: Krabbe's disease. A light and electron microscopic study. *Acta Neurpathol (Berl)* 36:153–160, 1976.

407. Schotland DL, Spiro D, Rowland LP, et al: Ultrastructural studies of muscle in McArdle's disease. *J Neuropathol Exp Neurol* 24:629–644, 1965.

408. Schwendemann G: Lymphocyte inclusions in the juvenile type of generalized ceroid-lipofuscinosis: an electron microscopic study. *Acta Neuropathol (Berl)* 36:327–338, 1976.

409. Scully RE, Galdabini JJ, McNeely BU: Case records of the Massachusetts General Hospital: case 18-1979. *N Engl J Med* 300:1037–1045, 1979.

410. Seitelberger F: Histochemistry and classification of the Pelizaeus-Merzbacher disease. In Cumings JN (ed): *Cerebral Lipidoses: A Symposium*. Oxford, Blackwell Scientific Publications, 1957, p 92.

411. Seitelberger F, Simma A: On the pigment variant of amaurotic idiocy. In Aronson SM, Volk BW (eds): *Cerebral Sphingolipidoses. A Symposium on Tay-Sachs' Disease and Allied Disorders*. New York, Academic Press, 1962, p 29.

412. Seitelberger F, Jacob H, Schnabel R: The myoclonic variant of cerebral lipidosis. In Aronson SM, Volk BW (eds): *Inborn Disorders of Sphingolipid Metabolism*. Oxford, Pergamon Press, 1967, p 43.

413. Seitelberger F: Pelizaeus-Merzbacher disease. In Vinken PJ, Bruyn GW (eds): *Leucodystrophies and Poliodystrophies, Handbook of Clinical Neurology*. Amsterdam, North-Holland, 1970, vol. 10, p 150.

414. Seitelberger F: Pelizaeus-Merzbacher disease. In Vinken PJ, Bruyn GW (eds): *Neurogenetic Directory Part 1. Handbook of Clinical Neurology*. Amsterdam, North-Holland, 1981, vol 42, p 502.

415. Sherwin RM, Berthrong M: Alexander's disease with sudanophilic leukodystrophy. *Arch Pathol* 89:321–328, 1970.

416. Shih VE: Congenital hyperammonemic syndromes. *Clin Perinatol* 3:3–11, 1976.

417. Shuman RM, Leech RW, Scott CR: The neuropathology of the nonketotic and ketotic hyperglycinemias: three cases. *Neurology* 28:139–146, 1978.

418. Siakotos AN, Armstrong O: Age pigment, a biochemical indicator of intracellular ageing. In Ordy JM, Brizzee KR (eds): *Neurobiology of Ageing*. New York, Plenum Press, 1975, p 369.

419. Sidbury JB Jr, Smith EK, Harlan W: An inborn error of short-chain fatty acid metabolism: the odor-of-sweaty-feet syndrome. *J Pediatr* 70:8–15, 1967.

420. Siemerling E, Creutzfeld HG: Bronzekrankheit und Sklerosierende Encephalomyelitis. *Arch Psychiatr Nervenkr* 68:217–244, 1923.

421. Silberberg DH: Maple syrup urine disease metabolites studied in cerebellum cultures. *J Neurochem* 16:1141–1146, 1969.

422. Silberman J, Dancis J, Feigin I: Neuropathological observations in maple syrup urine disease: branched-chain ketoaciduria. *Arch Neurol* 5:351–363, 1961.

423. Singh I, Moser HW, Moser AB, et al: Adrenoleukodystrophy: impaired oxidation of long chain fatty acids in cultured skin fibroblasts and adrenal cortex. *Biochem Biophys Res Commun* 102:1223–1229, 1981.

424. Sipe JC, O'Brien JS: Ultrastructure of skin biopsy specimens in lysosomal storage diseases: common sources of error in diagnosis. *Clin Genet* 15:118–125, 1979.

425. Sly WS, Quinton BA, McAlister WH, et al: Beta glucuronidase deficiency: report of clinical, radiologic, and biochemical features of a new mucopolysaccharidosis. *J Pediatr* 82:249–257, 1973.

426. Snyder SH: Fifth Gaddum Memorial Lecture, University of Bristol, September 1974. The glycine synaptic receptor in the mammalian central nervous system. *Br J Pharmacol* 53:473–484, 1975.

myelination: Pelizaeus-Merzbacher disease? *Neurology* 21:817–824, 1971.

427. Sobrevilla LA, Goodman ML, Kane CA: Demyelinating central nervous system disease, macular atrophy and acanthocytosis (Bassen-Kornzweig syndrome). *Am J Med* 37:821–828, 1964.

428. Soffer D, Grotsky HW, Rapin I, et al: Cockayne syndrome: unusual neuropathological findings and review of the literature. *Ann Neurol* 6:340–348, 1979.

429. Soffer D, Yamanaka T, Wenger DA, et al: Central nervous system involvement in adult-onset Gaucher's disease. *Acta Neuropathol (Berl)* 49:1–6, 1980.

430. Solitare GB, Shih VE, Nelligan DJ, et al: Argininosuccinic aciduria: clinical, biochemical, anatomical and neuropathological observations. *J Ment Defic Res* 13:153–170, 1969.

431. Solt LC, Jimenez C, Becker L, et al: A study of Rosenthal fibres in five cases of Alexander's disease (abstr). *J Neuropathol Exp Neurol* 38:342, 1979.

432. Sourander P, Järvi O, Hakola P, et al: Neuropathological aspects of polycystic lipomembranous osteodysplasia with sclerosing leukoencephalopathy (membranous lipodystrophy). In Yonezawa T (ed): *International Symposium on the Leucodystrophy and Allied Diseases.* Kyoto, September 19–20, 1981. The Japanese Society of Neuropathology, "Neuropathology" Suppl 1, n.d.

433. Søvik O, Lie SO, Fluge G, et al: Fucosidosis: severe phenotype with survival to adult age. *Eur J Pediatr* 135:211–216, 1980.

434. Spranger J, Wiedemann HR, Tolksdorf M, et al: Lipomucopolysaccharidose. Eine neue Speicherkrankheit. *Z Kinderheilk* 103:285–306, 1968.

435. Spranger JW, Wiedemann HR: The genetic mucolipidoses: diagnosis and differential diagnosis. *Humangenetik* 9:113–139, 1970.

436. Spranger J: The systemic mucopolysaccharidoses. *Ergeb Inn Med Kinderheilk* 32:165–265, 1972.

437. Spranger J, Gehler J, Cantz M: Mucolipidosis I—a sialidosis. *Am J Med Genet* 1:21–29, 1977.

438. Stam FC: Concept, classification, and nosology of the leucodystrophies: an historical introductory review. In Vinken PJ, Bruyn GW (eds): *Leucodystrophies and Poliodystrophies, Handbook of Clinical Neurology.* Amsterdam, North-Holland, 1970, vol 10, p 1.

439. Stanbury JB, Wyngaarden JB, Fredrickson DS, et al (eds): *The Metabolic Basis of Inherited Disease. Part 3: Disorders of Amino Acid Metabolism,* ed 5. New York, McGraw-Hill, 1983, p 231.

440. Steinman L, Tharp BR, Dorfman LJ, et al: Peripheral neuropathy in the cherry-red spot-myoclonus syndrome (sialidosis type I). *Ann Neurol* 7:450–456, 1980.

441. Stevenson RE, Howell RR, McKusick VA, et al: The iduronidase-deficient mucopolysaccharidoses: clinical and roentgenographic features. *Pediatrics* 57:111–122, 1976.

442. Strecker G, Herlant-Peers M-C, Fournet B, et al: Structure of seven oligosaccharides excreted in the urine of a patient with Sandhoff's disease (GM₂ gangliosidosis-variant O). *Eur J Biochem* 81:165–171, 1977.

443. Strecker G: Oligosaccharides in lysosomal storage diseases. In Callahan JW, Lowden JA (eds): *Lysosomes and Lysosomal Storage Diseases.* New York, Raven Press, 1981, p 95.

444. Stumpf D, Neuwelt E, Austin J, et al: Metachromatic leukodystrophy (MLD). X. Immunological studies of the abnormal sulfatase A. *Arch Neurol* 25:427–431, 1971.

445. Sudo M: Brain glycolipids in infantile Gaucher's disease. *J Neurochem* 29:379–381, 1977.

446. Sugita M, Dulaney JT, Moser HW: Ceramidase deficiency in Farber's disease (lipogranulomatosis). *Science* 178:1100–1102, 1972.

447. Sung JH, Hayano M, Desnick RJ: Mannosidosis: pathology of the nervous system. *J Neuropathol Exp Neurol* 30:807–820, 1977.

448. Sung JH: Autonomic neurons affected by lipid storage in the spinal cord in Fabry's disease: distribution of autonomic neurons in the sacral cord. *J Neuropathol Exp Neurol* 38:87–98, 1979.

449. Suzuki K: Ganglioside patterns of normal and pathological brains. In Aronson SM, Volk BW (eds): *Inborn Disorders of Sphingolipid Metabolism.* Oxford, Pergamon Press, 1967, p 215.

450. Suzuki K: Peripheral nerve lesion spongy degeneration of the central nervous system. *Acta Neuropathol (Berl)* 10:95–98, 1968.

451. Suzuki K, Suzuki K, Chen GC: Morphological histochemical and biochemical studies on a case of systemic late infantile lipidosis (generalized gangliosidosis). *J Neuropathol Exp Neurol* 27:15–38, 1968.

452. Suzuki K, Suzuki K, Chen GC: Isolation and chemical characterization of metachromatic granules from a brain with metachromatic leukodystrophy. *J Neuropathol Exp Neurol* 26:537–550, 1967.

453. Suzuki K, Johnson AB, Marquet E, et al: A case of juvenile lipidosis: electron microscopic, histochemical and biochemical studies. *Acta Neuropathol (Berl)* 11:122–139, 1968.

454. Suzuki K, Suzuki K, Kamoshita S: Chemical pathology of G_{M1}-gangliosidosis (generalized gangliosidosis). *J Neuropathol Exp Neurol* 28:25–73, 1969.

455. Suzuki K: Ultrastructural study of experimental globoid cells. *Lab Invest* 23:612–619, 1970.

456. Suzuki K, Suzuki K, Rapin I, et al: Juvenile G_{M2}-gangliosidosis: clinical variant of Tay-Sachs disease or a new disease. *Neurology* 20:190–204, 1970.

457. Suzuki K, Tanaka H, Suzuki K: Studies on the pathogenesis of Krabbe's leukodystrophy: cellular reaction of the brain to exogenous galactosylsphingosine, monogalactosyl diglyceride, and lactosyl ceramide. In Volk BW (ed): *Current Trends in Sphingolipidoses and Allied Diseases.* New York, Plenum Press, 1976, p 99.

458. Suzuki K, Suzuki Y: Galactosylceramide lipidosis: globoid cell leukodystrophy (Krabbe's disease). In Stanbury JB, Wyngaarden JB, Fredrickson DS, et al (eds): *The Metabolic Basis of Inherited Disease,* ed 5. New York, McGraw-Hill, 1983, p 857.

459. Suzuki Y, Suzuki K: Krabbe's globoid cell leukodystrophy: deficiency of galactocerebrosidase in serum, leukocytes and fibroblasts. *Science* 171:73–75, 1971.

460. Suzuki Y, Jacob JC, Suzuki K, et al: G_{M2}-gangliosidosis with total hexosaminidase deficiency. *Neurology* 21:313–328, 1971.

461. Suzuki Y, Nakamura N, Shimada Y, et al: Macular cherry-red spots and β-galactosidase deficiency in an adult: an autopsy case with progressive cerebellar ataxia, myoclonus, thrombocytopathy, and accumulation of polysaccharide in liver. *Arch Neurol* 34:157–161, 1977.

462. Suzuki Y, Nakamura N, Fukuoka K: G_{M1}-gangliosidosis: accumulation of ganglioside G_{M1} in cultured skin fibroblasts and correlation with clinical types. *Hum Genet* 43:127–131, 1978.

463. Svennerholm L: Lipidoses. In Dawson RMC, Rhodes DN (eds): *Metabolism and Physiological Significance of Lipids.* New York, John Wiley & Sons, 1964, p 553.

464. Svennerholm L: The patterns of gangliosides in mental and neurological disorders. *Biochem J* 98:20P, 1966.

465. Svennerholm L, Håkansson G, Vanier MT: Chemical pathology of Krabbe's disease. IV. Studies of galactosylceramide and lactosylceramide β-galactosidases in brain, white blood and amniotic fluid cells. *Acta Paediatr Scand* 64:649–656, 1975.

466. Svennerholm L: The chemical structure of normal human brain and Tay-Sachs gangliosides. *Biochem Biophys Res Commun* 9:436–441, 1962.

467. Swanson PD, Sumi SM, Stahl WL: Subcellular distribution of cerebral cholestanol in cerebrotendinous xanthomatosis (abstr). *Clin Res* 18:188, 1970.

468. Swift TR, McDonald TF: Peripheral nerve involvement in Hunter syndrome (mucopolysaccharidosis II). *Arch Neurol* 33:845–846, 1976.

469. Tabira T, Goto I, Kuroiwa Y, et al: Neuropathological and biochemical studies in Fabry's disease. *Acta Neuropathol (Berl)* 30:345–354, 1974.

470. Tagliavini F, Pietrini V, Pilleri G, et al: Adult metachro-

matic leucodystrophy: clinicopathological report of two familial cases with slow course. *Neuropathol Appl Neurobiol* 5:233–243, 1979.

471. Tahmoush AJ, Alpers DH, Feigin RD, et al: Hartnup disease. *Arch Neurol* 33:797–807, 1976.

472. Takashima S, Matsui A, Fujii Y, et al: Clinicopathological differences between juvenile and late infantile metachromatic leukodystrophy. *Brain Dev* 3:365–374, 1981.

473. Tanaka J, Garcia JH, Max SR, et al: Cerebral sponginess and GM₃ gangliosidosis: ultrastructure and probable pathogenesis. *J Neuropathol Exp Neurol* 34:249–262, 1975.

474. Taori GM, Iyer GV, Mokashi S, et al: Sanfilippo syndrome (mucopolysaccharidosis-III). *J Neurol Sci* 17:323–345, 1972.

475. Tarui S, Okuno G, Ikura Y, et al: Phosphofructokinase deficiency in skeletal muscle: a new type of glycogenosis. *Biochem Biophys Res Commun* 19:517–523, 1965.

476. Tatematsu M, Imaida K, Ito N, et al: Sandhoff disease. *Acta Pathol (Jpn)* 31:503–512, 1981.

477. Taubold RD, Siakotos AN, Perkins EG: Studies on chemical nature of lipofuscin (age pigment) isolated from normal human brain. *Lipids* 10:383–390, 1975.

478. Tellez-Nagel I, Rapin L, Iwamoto T, et al: Mucolipidosis IV: clinical, ultrastructural, histochemical, and chemical studies of a case, including a brain biopsy. *Arch Neurol* 33:828–835, 1976.

479. Terry RD, Weiss M: Studies in Tay-Sachs disease. II. Ultrastructure of the cerebrum. *J Neuropathol Exp Neurol* 22:18–55, 1963.

480. Tourian A, Sidbury JB: Phenylketonuria and hyperphenylalaninemia. In Stanbury JB, Wyngaarden JB, Fredrickson DS, et al: (eds): *The Metabolic Basis of Inherited Disease*, ed 5. New York, McGraw-Hill, 1983, p 270.

481. Tsay GC, Dawson G: Oligosaccharide storage in brains from patients with fucosidosis, G_{M1} gangliosidosis and G_{M2}-gangliosidosis (Sandhoff's disease). *J Neurochem* 27:733–740, 1976.

482. Tsuchiya Y, Numabe T, Yokoi S: Neuropathological and neurochemical studies of three cases of sudanophilic leucodystrophy. *Acta Neuropathol (Berl)* 16:353–366, 1970.

483. Tsuji S, Sano T, Argia T, et al: Increased synthesis of hexacosanoic acid (C26:0) by cultured skin fibroblasts from patients with adrenoleukodystrophy (ALD) and adrenomyeloneuropathy (AMN). *J Biochem* 90:1233–1236, 1981.

484. Vagn-Hansen PL, Reske-Nielsen E, Lou HC: Menkes' disease—a new leucodystrophy (?): a clinical and neuropathological review together with a new case. *Acta Neuropathol (Berl)* 25:103–119, 1973.

485. Van Bogaert L, Scherer HJ, Epstein E: Une forme cérébrale de la cholestérinose généralisée: type particulier de lipidose à cholestérine. Paris, Masson, 1937.

486. Van Bogaert L, Bertrand I: Sur une idiotie familiale avec dégénérescence spongieuse du névraxe (note préliminaire). *Acta Neurol Psychiatr Belg* 49:572–587, 1949.

487. Van Hoof F, Hers HG: L'ultrastructure des cellules hépatiques dans la maladie de Hürler (gargoylisme). *C R Acad Sci (Paris)* 259:1281–1283, 1964.

488. Van Hoof F, Hers HG: The abnormalities of lysosomal enzymes in mucopolysaccharidoses. *Eur J Biochem* 7:34–44, 1968.

489. Van Hoof F, Hers HG: Mucopolysaccharidosis by absence of α-fucosidase. *Lancet* 1:1198, 1968.

490. Vanier MT, Svennerholm L: Chemical pathology of Krabbe's disease. I. Lipid composition and fatty acid patterns of phosphoglycerides in brain. *Acta Paediatr Scand* 63:494–500, 1974.

491. Vietor KW, Havesteen B, Harms D, et al: Ethanolaminosis: a newly recognized generalized storage disease with cardiomegaly, cerebral dysfunction and early death. *Eur J Pediatr* 126:61–75, 1977.

492. Volk BW: Pathologic anatomy. In Volk BW (ed): *Tay-*

Sachs Disease. New York, Grune & Stratton, 1964, p 36.

493. Von Sallmann L, Gelderman AH, Laster L: Ocular histopathologic changes in a case of a-beta-lipoproteinemia (Bassen-Kornzweig syndrome). *Doc Ophthalmol* 26:451–460, 1969.

494. Voyce MA, Montgomery JN, Crome L, et al: Maple syrup urine disease. *J Ment Defic Res* 11:231–238, 1967.

495. Walkley SU, Blakemore WF, Purpura DP: Alterations in neuron morphology in feline mannosidosis. *Acta Neuropathol (Berl)* 53:75–79, 1981.

496. Wallace BJ, Kaplan D, Adachi M, et al: Mucopolysaccharidosis type III: Morphologic and biochemical studies of two siblings with Sanfilippo syndrome. *Arch Pathol* 82:462–473, 1966.

497. Walsh PJ: Adrenoleukodystrophy: report of two cases with relapsing and remitting courses. *Arch Neurol* 37:448–450, 1980.

498. Weismann U, Neufeld EF: Scheie and Hurler syndromes: apparent identity of the biochemical defect. *Science* 169:72–74, 1970.

499. Wenger DA, Kudoh T, Sattler M: et al: Niemann-Pick disease type B: prenatal diagnosis and enzymatic and chemical studies on fetal brain and liver. *Am J Hum Genet* 33:337–344, 1981.

500. Wherrett JR, Rewcastle NB: Adult neurovisceral lipidosis (abstr). *Clin Res* 17:665, 1969.

501. Willems JL, Monnens LAH, Trijbels JMF, et al: Leigh's encephalomyelopathy in a patient with cytochrome c oxidase deficiency in muscle tissue. *Pediatrics* 60:850–857, 1977.

502. Williams RS, Marshal PC, Lott IT, et al: The cellular pathology of Menkes steely hair syndrome. *Neurology* 28:575–583, 1976.

503. Williams RS, Lott IT, Ferrante RJ, et al: The cellular pathology of neuronal ceroid-lipofuscinosis: a Golgi-electronmicroscopic study. *Arch Neurol* 34:298–305, 1977.

504. Williams RS, Ferrante RJ, Caviness VS Jr: The isolated human cortex: a golgi analysis of Krabbe's disease. *Arch Neurol* 36:134–139, 1979.

505. Willner JP, Grabowski GA, Gordon RE, et al: Chronic GM₂ gangliosidosis masquerading as atypical Friedreich ataxia: clinical, morphologic, and biochemical studies of nine cases. *Neurology* 31:787–798, 1981.

506. Wilson D, Melnik E, Sly W, et al: Neonatal beta-glucuronidase-deficiency mucopolysaccharidosis (MPS VII): autopsy findings (abstr). *J Neuropathol Exp Neurol* 41:344, 1982.

507. Witting C, Müller KM, Kresse H, et al: Morphological and biochemical findings in a case of mucopolysaccharidosis type III A (Sanfilippo's disease type A). *Beitr Pathol* 154:324–338, 1975.

508. Wolfe LS, Ng Ying Kin NMK, Baker RR, et al: Identification of retinoyl complexes as the autofluorescent component of the neuronal storage material in Batten disease. *Science* 195:1360–1362, 1977.

509. Wolfe LS, Ng Ying Kin NMK, Palo J, et al: Dolichols in brain and urinary sediment in neuronal ceroid lipofuscinosis. *Neurology* 33:103–106, 1983.

510. Yajima K, Fletcher TF, Suzuki K: Sub-plasmalemmal linear density: a common structure in globoid cells and mesenchymal cells. *Acta Neuropathol (Berl)* 39:195–200, 1977.

511. Yamano T, Shimada M, Okada S, et al: Electron microscopic examination of skin and conjunctival biopsy specimens in neuronal storage diseases. *Brain Dev* 1(1):16–25, 1979.

512. Yamashita K, Ohkura T, Okada S, et al: Urinary oligosaccharides of G_{M1}-gangliosidosis: different excretion patterns of oligosaccharides in the urine of type 1 and type 2 subgroups. *J Biol Chem* 256:4789–4798, 1981.

513. Yates AJ, Wyatt RH, Kishimoto Y, et al: A leukodystrophy accumulating large amounts of cholesterol ester. *J Neurochem Pathol* 1:103–123, 1983.

514. Zeman W, Hoffman J: Juvenile and late forms of amaurotic idiocy in one family. *J Neurol Neurosurg Psychiatry*

25:352–362, 1962.

515. Zeman W, Donahue S: Fine structure of the lipid bodies in juvenile amaurotic idiocy. *Acta Neuropathol (Berl)* 3:144–149, 1963.

516. Zeman W, Demyer W, Falls HF: Pelizaeus-Merzbacher disease: a study in nosology. *J Neuropathol Exp Neurol* 23:334–354, 1964.

517. Zeman W, Donahue S, Dyken P, et al: The neuronal ceroid-lipofuscinoses (Batten-Vogt syndrome). In Vinken PJ, Bruyn GW (eds): *Handbook of Clinical Neurology.* Amsterdam, North-Holland, 1970, vol 10, p 588.

518. Zeman W: *Presidential address*: studies in the neuronal ceroid-lipofuscinoses. *J Neuropathol Exp Neurol* 33:1–12, 1974.

CHAPTER 9

Exogenous Toxic-Metabolic Diseases Including Vitamin Deficiency

SYDNEY S. SCHOCHET, Jr., M.D.

INTOXICATIONS

Introduction

People are exposed daily to an ever expanding array of toxic compounds. Many of these affect the nervous system either selectively or in association with involvement of other organ systems. Appreciation of the importance of neurotoxicity is reflected by the appearance in recent years of journals and monographs devoted exclusively to this aspect of toxicology. In this brief chapter, discussion is limited to selected exogenous toxins that are relatively common and/or known to produce morphologically demonstrable central nervous system lesions.

Hypoxia and Toxic Gases

CLASSIFICATION

Several intoxication states share in common deficient delivery and/or utilization of oxygen and substrate. The hypoxic effects of such intoxications are particularly apparent in the heart and brain. The latter normally receives about 15% of the cardiac output, consumes about 20% of the blood oxygen, and metabolizes about 10–20% of the blood glucose. The oxygen and substrate deficiencies have been variously classified. The following is a simplified but useful version.

1. Anoxic or hypoxic hypoxia results from the absence or insufficiency of inhaled oxygen. This may be due to impaired ventilatory activity or insufficient oxygen in inhaled gases, e.g., anesthetic accidents. It may also result from pulmonary disorders that prevent absorption of oxygen, e.g., pulmonary edema.
2. Anemic hypoxia results from a decrease in oxygen transport due to either anemia or a reduced capacity of the hemoglobin to transport oxygen, e.g., carbon monoxide poisoning.
3. Stagnant hypoxia results from reduction or cessation of blood flow due to reduced cardiac output or impaired local perfusion. The cerebral lesions seen with stagnant hypoxia actually reflect the combined effects of inadequate oxygen supply, inadequate glucose supply, and the accumulation of catabolites such as lactic acid.
4. Histotoxic hypoxia results from cellular intoxications that render the cells incapable of utilizing oxygen and substrate, e.g., cyanide intoxication which poisons the respiratory enzymes.
5. Oxyachrestic hypoxia results from hypoglycemia in which oxygen is not utilized because of the substrate deficiency.

CARBON MONOXIDE

Carbon monoxide is a colorless, odorless gas that is produced by the incomplete combustion of various fuels. The toxic effects result predominantly from impaired transport of oxygen. Hemoglobin combines reversibly with carbon monoxide but has about a 250-fold greater affinity for carbon monoxide than for oxygen. In addition, the carbon monoxide causes the oxygen that is bound to hemoglobin to be released less easily to other tissues. Therefore a given degree of carboxyhemoglobinemia produces more severe tissue hypoxia than a comparable degree of anemia. Still further toxic effects may result from the interaction of carbon monoxide with other hemoproteins such as myoglobin, cytochrome oxidase, cytochrome P_{450}, catalases, and peroxidases. The magnitude of the toxicity from the combination with these other hemoproteins remains unknown.

The clinical manifestations of acute carbon monoxide intoxication can be correlated with the concentration of carboxyhemoglobin (percent saturation) in the blood. Thus they are influenced by both the duration of exposure and the concentration of carbon monoxide in the environment. Symptoms are referable to the tissues with the greatest oxygen demands, i.e., brain and heart. In general, a previously healthy individual will experience severe headache and dizziness with 20–30% saturation; impaired vision, hearing, and mental function at 40–50% saturation; coma and convulsions at 50–60% saturation; and cardiorespiratory failure and death when over 70% saturation. The toxicity may be markedly potentiated by preexisting cardiovascular disease. Many of the immediate acute deaths are the result of myocardial dysfunction.

Although carboxyhemoglobin has a distinctive bright red color, acutely intoxicated patients may appear flushed, pallid, or even cyanotic while still alive. The classical "cherry-red" color of skin, blood, and viscera is observed more often as a post mortem phenomenon. The skin may show extensive blister or bullae formation. Petechial hemorrhages, retinal hemorrhages, and pulmonary edema also have been observed. Brains from individuals dying within a few hours of the carbon monoxide intoxication generally show congestion and edema, an abnormal color, and rare petechial hemorrhages (Fig. 9.1). The "cherry red" color of the fresh brain may become less apparent with prolonged formalin fixation. Brains from individuals dying 1–7 days after intoxication commonly show more extensive petechial hemorrhages (30). Pallidal necrosis is classically associated with delayed deaths from carbon monoxide intoxication. Grossly discernible foci of pallidal necrosis are encountered most often in individuals who survive for 6 or more days following the intoxication (30, 58). Microscopic foci of necrosis and/or petechial hemorrhages may be seen sooner. Lapresle and Fardeau (58) observed pallidal necrosis in 16 of 22 patients who survived for 1–139 days following intoxication. Rarely, the lesion is unilateral; more often, the lesions are merely asymmetrical, and bilateral lesions can be demonstrated in multiple planes of section. The necrosis most often involves the inner segment of the pallidum but may extend laterally into the outer segment or dorsally into the internal capsule (Fig. 9.2). It must be emphasized that while characteristic of delayed death from carbon monoxide, the pallidal necrosis is not unique to this condition and has been seen in a wide variety of intoxications and anoxic states (14). The pathogenesis of the pallidal necrosis has been the subject of much debate over the years. Many authors regard pallidal necrosis as a manifestation of impaired circulation through the pallidal branches of the anterior choroidal arteries. Hemorrhagic and necrotic lesions of the cerebral cortex and Ammon's horn are also commonly encountered. Lapresle and Fardeau (58) found foci of cortical necrosis in 12 of their 22 cases and varying degrees of hippocampal injury in 10 of 20 cases. The cerebellum may show loss of Purkinje cells and loss of cells from the internal granular cell layer.

Lesions of the white matter are encountered equally as often and in association with grey matter lesions in individuals with delayed death from carbon monoxide intoxication. Four categories of white matter lesions have been delineated; however, there is much overlap among these groups

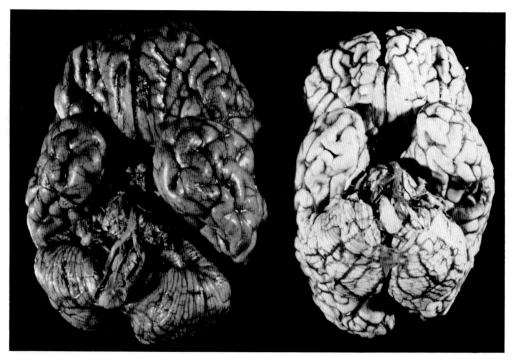

Figure 9.1. Acute carbon monoxide poisoning. Compare with control brain on right.

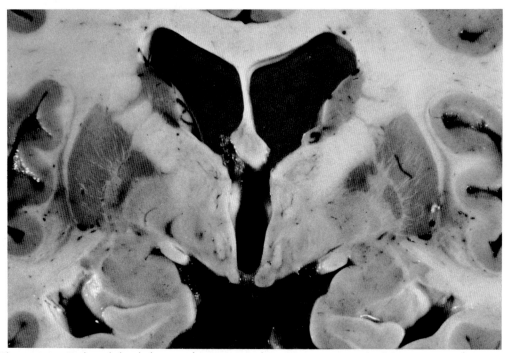

Figure 9.2. Delayed death from carbon monoxide poisoning. Note the bilateral pallidal necrosis.

(58). The first category consists of multiple small necrotic foci in the centrum semiovale (Fig. 9.3) and interhemispheric commissures. These small necrotic lesions are found predominantly in the anterior deep central white matter and anterior portion

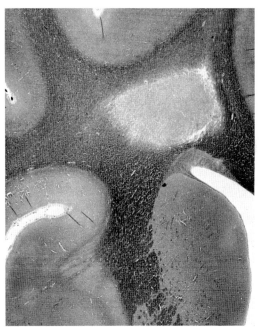

Figure 9.3. Macrophotograph showing white matter demyelination and necrosis secondary to carbon monoxide poisoning. Trichrome. (Original magnification ×2.)

of the corpus callosum. The necrotic foci are centered about small blood vessels that contain swollen endothelial cells with vesicular nuclei. Some of the endothelial cells may even contain mitotic figures. The second category of lesions consists of extensive, confluent areas of necrosis. These necrotic zones may extend from the frontal to the occipital poles within the deep periventricular white matter and throughout the corpus callosum. The lesions are sharply demarcated and tend to spare the arcuate fibers. Histologically, the lesions show extensive axonal destruction and contain numerous lipid-laden macrophages. The third category of lesions consists of demyelination with relative preservation of axons in the deep periventricular white matter. The lesions may be small and discrete, extensive, or even confluent. Arcuate fibers tend to be spared. This third category is the type that is seen most often in patients with delayed deterioration or the so-called biphasic myelinopathy of Grinker. The fourth category consists of very small necrotic foci limited to the hemispheric white matter. The last category seems merely to be a restricted earlier form of the first cat-

egory. As with the gray matter lesions, identical white matter lesions can be seen in other anoxic or hypoxic states. However, in the case of carbon monoxide poisoning, direct toxic effects on the white matter may be contributory to the development of the lesions. In a careful experimental study of carbon monoxide poisoning in primates, Ginsberg et al. (35) found closer correlation between the size of the white matter lesions and the degree of metabolic acidosis and systolic hypotension than the extent of hypoxia per se.

NITROUS OXIDE

Nitrous oxide has long been used as an anesthetic agent. Accidents with this and other inhalation anesthetics may lead to hypoxic hypoxia with pallidal necrosis and white matter lesions. These are morphologically quite similar to those seen following carbon monoxide intoxication. Recently, much attention has been focused on a myeloneuropathy that has been encountered in individuals, most often dental personnel, who have had prolonged exposure to nitrous oxide (59). Although histopathological studies in man are lacking, the clinical manifestations are similar to subacute combined degeneration. The nitrous oxide is thought to produce the myeloneuropathy by inactivating vitamin B_{12}. Experimental studies with this agent have produced degeneration of the spinal cord involving both myelin sheaths and axons.

CYANIDES

The toxicity of cyanides results from the reversible but strong bonding between the cyanide ion and the iron in cytochrome oxidase. This leads to rapid inhibition of cellular respiration throughout the body. Cyanides are thus considered histotoxic or cytotoxic agents.

In acute intoxication, death rapidly ensues, with respiratory arrest preceded by convulsions. Brains from such individuals show, at most, edema and occasional small subarachnoid hemorrhages. With more delayed deaths, the brains may show petechial hemorrhages and necrotic foci in the white matter, loss of Purkinje cells, and necrotic foci in the basal ganglia, both the putamena and pallida. Recently, bilateral pallidal necrosis, presumed to be the result of subacute cyanide intoxication, has been reported in a patient treated for 14 days with sodium nitroprusside for uncontrolled hypertension (47). The unexpected accumulation of cyanide to toxic levels was attributed to impaired liver function.

Experimental cyanide intoxication in rats has produced extensive white matter lesions that involve predominantly the corpus callosum. The callosal lesions are more extensive toward the splenium and are surrounded by a peripheral rim of intact white matter. The myelin loss is considered to be secondary to axonal degeneration, and the distribution of the lesions is determined by vascular perfusion (45). Evidence linking chronic cyanide intoxication with optic nerve and tract degeneration in man has been reported but is not well documented.

Cyanide intoxication also may result from degradation of cyanogenic glucosides. Acute cyanide intoxication has been reported following the ingestion of amygdalin in the form of laetrile. In one such case, an 11-month-old child died 71 hours after the drug ingestion (12). Autopsy disclosed small necrotic lesions in the putamena, focal hemorrhages in the internal granular layer of the cerebellum, and degeneration of Purkinje cells. Chronic consumption of foodstuffs containing cyanogenic glucosides has been implicated in causing an ataxic neuropathy in Nigeria.

HYDROGEN SULFIDE

Intoxication with hydrogen sulfide is a rare event encountered most often among miners and sewer workers. Low concentrations of this toxic gas are readily detected by its characteristic "rotten-egg" odor. Unfortunately, higher, potentially lethal concentrations of this gas rapidly produce olfactory paralysis and may go undetected. Hydrogen sulfide in sufficiently high concentrations can cause almost instantaneous respiratory arrest.

Individuals who have been poisoned by this compound may display a distinctive gray-green skin color and have hemorrhagic pulmonary edema. The cerebral gray matter, both cortex and basal ganglia, may show a distinctive greenish-purple discoloration (2). The white matter and intravascular blood retain a more nearly normal appearance. The greenish-purple color is rapidly lost upon formalin fixation. The chemical composition of this distinctively colored compound is unknown. It is thought not to be sulfhemoglobin or sulfmethemoglobin, compounds which impart a greenish-gray color to putrefying tissue.

Alcohols

ETHANOL

General

Ethanol has many effects upon the central nervous system, some of which fall into the purview of the neuropathologist. It is well known that alcoholism potentiates infections and precipitates traumatic injuries to the nervous system. Acute ethanol intoxication has been claimed to increase the risk of both aneurysmal and primary subarachnoid hemorrhage (43). Alcoholism is an important cause of peripheral neuropathy. Although these various effects are of concern to the neuropathologist, they are largely outside the domain of this chapter. Some of the direct and indirect toxic effects will be considered here, while the Wernicke-Korsakoff syndrome will be treated later among the deficiency states.

Acute intoxication with large quantities of alcohol can lead to death from central cardiorespiratory paralysis. Blood levels over 450–500 mg/dl are generally considered as potentially lethal. Nevertheless, there is considerable individual variation, and numerous patients have survived even higher levels. This has been attributed to the increased CNS tolerance encountered in alcoholics. Children are often considered more susceptible than adults to this intoxication. Here, too, individual cases surviving exceptionally high blood levels have been reported. Fatalities from acute intoxication are often the result of ingesting alcohol along with other drugs. Examination of the brain following death from acute intoxication usually reveals little more than cerebral edema.

Patients with chronic alcoholism may show cerebral atrophy. The frequency, severity, and relation of this finding to the alcoholism remains controversial. At one extreme is the position taken by Courville (23), who regarded chronic alcoholism as "the most common cause of cerebral cortical atrophy in the fifth and sixth decades of life." Although this conclusion would be disputed by many, other workers had found at least a mild degree of cortical atrophy or ventricular enlargement in one-fourth to one-half of their autopsied cases. More recently, use of computerized tomography has confirmed ventricular enlargement and cerebral atrophy (17) in alcoholic patients, even in the absence of significant hepatic disease.

A wide variety of histological changes in the cerebral cortex, including loss of small pyramidal cells and swelling, pycnosis, and "pigmentary atrophy" of remaining neurons, have been described in alcoholic patients (23). Most of these changes are now regarded as nonspecific or even artifactual. Other histopathological alterations are associated with Wernicke's encephalopathy, cerebellar degeneration, Marchiafava-Bignami disease, and central pontine myelinolysis.

Alcoholic Cerebellar Degeneration

Degeneration and atrophy of the superior vermis and adjacent portions of the superior surface of the cerebellar hemispheres occur commonly in individuals with chronic alcoholism (115). This form of cerebellar degeneration may be encountered as an isolated lesion or in conjunction with other alcohol-related lesions such as Wernicke's encephalopathy. The clinical manifestations of the cerebellar degeneration evolve slowly over a period of months or years and include truncal instability, leg ataxia, and a wide-based stance and gait.

Grossly, the folia of the rostral vermis and, to a lesser extent, the folia of the anterosuperior aspect of the cerebellar hemispheres are atrophic and separated by widened interfolial sulci. The atrophy is most readily demonstrated by a sagittal section through the vermis (Fig. 9.4). The cerebellar vermal atrophy can be demonstrated antemortem by the use of computerized tomography (52).

Histological studies have shown the folial crests to be more severely affected than the depths of the interfolial sulci. This is in contrast to the pattern of alteration resulting from hypoxia. In the more severely affected areas, there is loss of Purkinje cells, patchy loss of granular cells, and atrophy of the molecular layer. In addition,

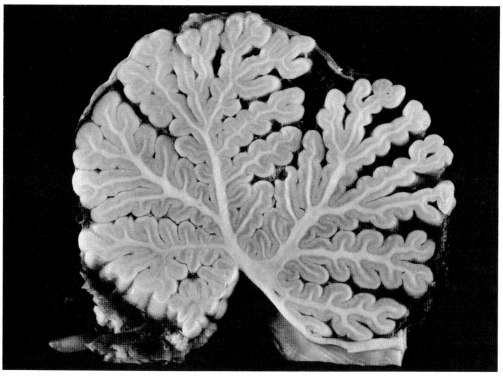

Figure 9.4.   Cerebellar vermal atrophy in a patient with chronic alcoholism.

there is gliosis with proliferation of Bergmann glia. The white matter remains relatively unaffected. Opinion varies as to whether the granular cells or the Purkinje cells are damaged initially in this condition. The acute and subacute stages of this degeneration have not been well documented morphologically.

Alcoholic cerebellar degeneration generally has been attributed to direct toxic effects of alcohol or nutritional deficiencies, especially thiamine deficiency. More recently, experimental studies have suggested that electrolyte imbalances, specifically excessively rapid or overcorrection of hyponatremia, may be responsible for this lesion as well as for central pontine myelinolysis (48). Some authors feel that a similar but generally milder cerebellar atrophy can occur independent of alcoholism as an age related phenomenon.

Marchiafava-Bignami Disease

Marchiafava-Bignami disease is a rare, predominantly demyelinative disorder that was originally described in poorly nourished Italian males who were addicted to the chronic consumption of crude red wine. Subsequently, the disorder was described in other populations with different preferences in alcoholic beverages (51, 98). Although most cases have occurred in individuals with alcoholism, a few have been reported in poorly nourished individuals who abstained from alcohol (60). In several instances Marchiafava-Bignami disease has been found in association with Wernicke's encephalopathy (51), and in at least one case, there was concurrent central pontine myelinolysis (33).

Grossly the lesion appears as a discolored or even partially cystic demyelinated region in the corpus callosum. Involvement is generally maximal in the genu and body of the corpus callosum. Characteristically the lesion spares thin layers of myelinated fibers along both the dorsal and ventral surfaces of the corpus callosum. In some cases, similar lesions have been seen in the optic chiasm, anterior commissure, centrum semiovale, and middle cerebellar peduncles. The lesions tend to be bilaterally symmetrical and spare gray matter. Similarities between the gross appearance of the lesions in Marchiafava-Bignami disease and experimental cyanide intoxication have been emphasized.

Microscopically the lesions display predominantly demyelination with relative sparing of axis cylinders. Oligodendrocytes are markedly reduced in number while lipid-laden macrophages are abundant. Astrocytes generally show only mild reactive changes; however, these may be prominent in the more destructive cases with cyst formation. Vessels in and about these lesions may show proliferation and hyalinization of their walls.

Central Pontine Myelinolysis

Central pontine myelinolysis is an uncommon demyelinative condition that affects predominantly the basis pontis. This disorder was first described in detail by Adams et al. in 1959 (1). Three of the four patients suffered from chronic alcoholism, and all had serious malnutrition. Although most of the cases reported subsequently have occurred in adults with alcoholism or malnutrition, the spectrum of underlying background disorders has been expanded, and even childhood cases have been reported (120). Because of the diverse circumstances in which the disorder has occurred, etiological factors other than alcohol and nutritional deficiencies had to be considered. In recent years, the role of electrolyte imbalances, especially the excessively rapid correction or overcorrection of hyponatremia has received much support from review of clinical material and experimental studies (49, 73).

The explanation for the preferential involvement of the ventral pons and the precise pathogenesis of the demyelination remain unsettled. Some authors have attributed the selective pontine involvement to the detrimental effect of edema in the anatomic grid within the pons formed by the longitudinal and transverse myelinated fibers with interposed gray matter (70). It has been postulated that the edema results from osmotic opening of the blood-brain barrier or from osmotic vascular injury (73).

The clinical manifestations of central pontine myelinolysis are determined in part by the size of the lesion. In many cases, the lesions are too small to be clinically manifest. In other cases, signs and symptoms attributable to the pontine lesions are obscured by coma from the underlying disease. In only a small proportion of cases do the findings of quadriparesis, pseudobulbar palsy, and pseudocoma permit the clinical diagnosis of central pontine myelinolysis. Formerly the diagnosis was usually made at autopsy. More recently, the diagnosis has been established antemortem by the use of computerized tomography (109).

Grossly the typical lesion of central pontine myelinolysis appears as a discolored, finely granular demyelinated area in the basis pontis (Fig. 9.5). In some instances, the demyelination can be seen only in stained sections. The demyelinated lesions vary from a few millimeters in diameter to extensive lesions that involve almost the entire cross-sectional area of the basis pontis. Generally there is at least a thin rim of intact myelin at the periphery of the brain stem (Fig. 9.6). The demyelination is maximal in the middle and rostral portions of the pons. Rarely, the lesions extend rostrally into the midbrain while caudally, the lesions generally stop at the pontomedullary junction. Only in rare instances has the medulla been involved.

Histologically, central pontine myelinolysis is characterized by demyelination with relative preservation of axis cylinders and neurons (Fig. 9.7). The more acute lesions contain numerous lipid-laden macrophages but minimal or no perivascular inflammatory cell infiltrates. Oligodendrocytes are markedly reduced in number or even absent. Occasionally, foci of necrosis may be present in the center of the more severe lesions. These may be surrounded by reactive axons. Astrocytes in and about the demyelinated lesions may undergo hypertrophy and hyperplasia. Rarely, some of the astrocytes may contain arrested mitotic figures. Occasionally, Alzheimer type II astrocytes may be seen in the demyelinated portion of the basis pontis and in the overlying pontine tegmentum.

In some cases of central pontine myelinolysis, especially more severe cases, the pontine lesions are accompanied by extrapontine demyelinative lesions. These have been encountered in the striatum, internal

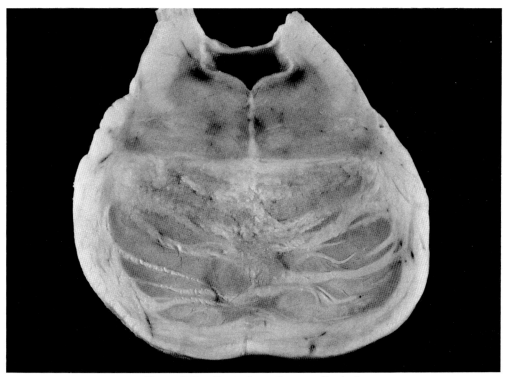

Figure 9.5. Central pontine myelinolysis.

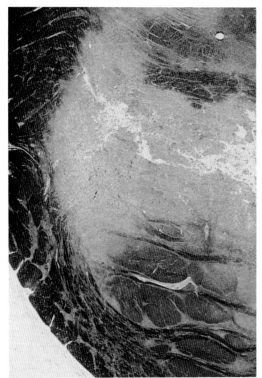

Figure 9.6. Central pontine myelinolysis, hemisection of pons. Note the central demyelination with preservation of peripheral rim of myelin. Luxol fast blue. (Original magnification ×4.)

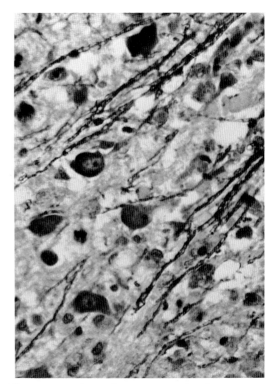

Figure 9.7. Central pontine myelinolysis. Note the preservation of neurons despite loss of myelin. Luxol fast blue. (Original magnification ×450.)

and external capsules, white matter of cerebellar folia, thalami, and lateral geniculate bodies (37, 109, 120). In common with the pons, these areas have bundles of myelinated fibers surrounded by gray matter.

Fetal Alcohol Syndrome

The so-called fetal alcohol syndrome is thought to result from the adverse effects of chronic maternal alcoholism on the fetus. The extent of maternal alcohol consumption and the critical stages in gestation for the development of this disorder are not yet known. Furthermore, it is uncertain as to whether the alcohol itself, a catabolite of the alcohol, or an associated nutritional deficiency is actually responsible for the teratogenic effects. The syndrome is common and is regarded as one of the leading causes of birth defects associated with mental retardation (54). A wide spectrum of abnormalities have been observed in these infants. Clarren (21) has grouped the abnormalities in four cate-

gories: pre- and postnatal growth retardation; a characteristic facial appearance; central nervous system dysfunction and malformations; and variable major and minor malformations of other organs. The facial anomalies include short palpebral fissures, short nose, thinned upper lip vermilion, hypoplastic philtrum, and flattened maxilla. The nervous system dysfunction includes mental retardation, irritability, tremulousness, seizures, hypotonicity, and cerebellar dysfunction.

Despite the frequency with which this syndrome is diagnosed clinically, the number of neuropathological studies are relatively limited. Nevertheless, a wide spectrum of malformations have been reported. The most consistent neuropathological lesions have been microcephaly, reduction in cerebral white matter, enlargement of the ventricular system, cerebellar hypoplasia, and neuroglial heterotopias. The neuroglial heterotopias may be periventricular and project into the cavities of the ventricular system, or they may be in the leptomeninges. Peiffer et al. (81) studied brains from three fetal and three childhood cases. They found a wide spectrum of lesions, ranging from mild dysplasias to severe malformations, including syringomyelia, the Dandy-Walker malformation, porencephaly, agenesis of the corpus callosum, and hydranencephaly. Anencephaly, meningomyelocele, and a lumbosacral lipoma also have been reported. Of particular interest is a 4-year-old girl with this syndrome who died as the result of an accident. She was found to have a small brain with reduced cerebral white matter, ventricular dilatation, and neuronal heterotopias along the lateral ventricular surfaces. This case may provide a more accurate description of the neuropathological lesions in the numerous milder cases of fetal alcohol syndrome who otherwise would have survived (21).

METHANOL

The toxicity of methanol was not fully appreciated until the end of the first quarter of the 20th century. When originally produced from destructive distillation of wood, "wood alcohol" contained so many unpleasant smelling and tasting contaminants that little thought was given to human consumption. After production methods improved, methanol was included in alcoholic beverages, cosmetics, and medicinals. The toxicity was generally accepted only after a group of Hamburg dock-workers were poisoned with pure methanol in 1923. Methanol intoxication has continued to occur, most often as the result of consumption of adulterated "moonshine" (Bennett et al. reported an "outbreak" of 323 such cases (7)) or from the ingestion of various methanol-containing fluids not intended for oral consumption. It has been estimated that about 6% of blindness in American troops during World War II was due to methanol intoxication.

There is marked variation in individual susceptibility to ingested methanol. Blindness has followed ingestion of as little as 4 ml of pure methanol, and Bennett et al. (7) reported death from drinking no more than 15 ml of adulterated whiskey containing 40% methanol. Conversely, the same authors recorded survival following consumption of a pint of the same adulterated whis-

key. The usual lethal dose is in the range of 100–250 ml. Severe intoxication also can result from topical application or inhalation of methanol vapors.

Methanol itself produces central nervous system depression. However, the more serious sequelae are produced by the catabolites of this alcohol. Methanol is slowly oxidized by hepatic alcohol dehydrogenase to formaldehyde, which is about 30 times more toxic than methanol, and to formic acid, which is also more toxic than the original methanol. Formic acid and formates, which block cellular respiration, contribute to the development of the associated metabolic acidosis.

Because of the frequent occurrence of blindness in methanol intoxication, the ocular pathology has been investigated extensively but with conflicting findings. Older reports emphasized degeneration of the retinal ganglion cells and photoreceptors. In more recent investigations, optic disc edema and retrolaminar demyelination and necrosis have been the principal findings (101). Experimental studies in primates have suggested that the ocular toxicity is due to the formation of formates which inhibit cellular respiration (68). This in turn blocks axoplasmic transport at the nerve head and leads to optic disc swelling. The retrolaminar optic nerve localization has been attributed to high regional concentrations of the formates in a watershed area between cerebral and optic nerve circulations (101).

Neuropathological changes include cerebral edema and, when death is delayed, necrosis of the lateral aspects of the putamena and the claustra (Fig. 9.8). Initially, the lesions in the putamen are hemorrhagic while those in the claustrum and intervening external capsule tend to be more ischemic. Later, the necrotic areas can undergo cystic transformation. Orthner (76) originally described this distinctive pattern of putamenal necrosis in autopsies on 41 of 124 fatal cases. More recently, the putamenal necrosis has been demonstrated antemortem by the use of computerized tomography (64). Some patients with especially prolonged survival following severe methanol intoxication will show, in addition, extensive necrosis of cerebral and cerebellar white matter. This too has been

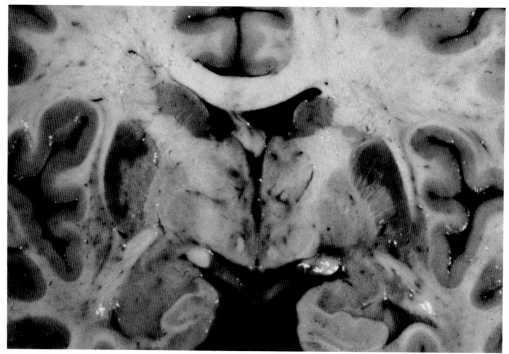

Figure 9.8. Delayed death from methanol intoxication. Note the bilateral early putamenal necrosis.

demonstrated antemortem by computerized tomography (64). The pathogenesis of the putamenal lesions remains unclear. Sharpe et al. (101) have suggested that cerebral white matter lesions, as well as the retrolaminar demyelination of the optic nerves, represent histotoxic myelinoclastic damage caused by formates.

ETHYLENE GLYCOL

Ethylene glycol is a dihydroxy alcohol that is widely used as a solvent and component of certain antifreezes and coolants. Intoxication with ethylene glycol is encountered most often when it is consumed as an ill-advised substitute for ethanol or is used as a vehicle for suicide. The minimum lethal dose is estimated to be in excess of 100 ml. Ethylene glycol is progressively oxidized, in part by alcohol dehydrogenase, to a series of toxic compounds including glycoaldehyde, glycolic acid, and glyoxylic acid. A small proportion is oxidized eventually to oxalic acid.

The clinical manifestations of ethylene glycol intoxication can be divided into three fairly distinct stages. These are central nervous system dysfunction with severe metabolic acidosis, cardiopulmonary failure, and acute renal failure (80). The initial cerebral manifestations, including drowsiness, stupor, and coma, coincide with the period of maximal aldehyde formation. The intoxicated patients may be thought to be "drunk" but lack the expected odor of alcohol. A wide variety of neurological complications, including altered consciousness, meningismus, ocular abnormalities, cranial nerve dysfunction, seizures, and movement disorders, have been tabulated by Berger and Ayyar (8). The acidosis has been attributed to the formation of oxalic acid; however, this seems unlikely since only a small proportion of the ethylene glycol is oxidized to this compound. However, the oxalic acid is responsible for the hypocalcemia and crystalluria seen with this intoxication.

Gross examination of brains from fatal cases reveals cerebral edema, meningeal congestion and, occasionally, petechial hemorrhages. Microscopically, acute inflammatory cell infiltrates may be seen in the meninges and about intraparenchymal blood vessels. Crystalline deposits of calcium oxalate may be seen in and about vessels in the meninges, neural parenchyma, and choroid plexus. These crystals are better demonstrated when the tissue is examined with polarized light (Fig. 9.9). Although previously implicated, the crystals probably do not contribute directly to the coma.

Drugs and Diagnostic Agents

DIPHENYLHYDANTOIN

Loss of Purkinje cells and gliosis of the cerebellar cortex have been observed in patients with seizure disorders who have been treated with diphenylhydantoin for prolonged periods. The relation of these findings to the diphenylhydantoin therapy is difficult to interpret since loss of Purkinje cells may result from hypoxia during seizures or from preexisting brain damage. Furthermore, it has been claimed that loss of Purkinje cells may occur in patients with epilepsy apart from the effects of generalized hypoxia. This conclusion was based on a study of cerebellar biopsy specimens (97). Nevertheless, the rare reports of Purkinje

cell degeneration in patients with few or no seizures support the view that diphenylhydantoin itself can act as a neurotoxin. Ghatak et al. (34) observed cerebellar atrophy, total loss of Purkinje cells throughout the entire cerebellum, and mild loss of granule cells in a patient who had only rare seizures. Similarly, Rapport and Shaw (92) observed loss of Purkinje cells in another patient without seizures. However, evaluation of this report is complicated by the presence of tuberculous meningitis which was treated with isoniazide. Experimental studies have yielded conflicting results.

Administration of anticonvulsants, including diphenylhydantoin to pregnant women, has been implicated in the production of various congenital anomalies, i.e., the so-called fetal hydantoin syndrome. The spectrum of nervous system malformations described in such individuals includes hydrocephalus, microcephaly, and neural tube defects. In other cases the lesions are much more subtle. Mallow et al. (66) studied a case in whom the brain was grossly normal but microscopically showed

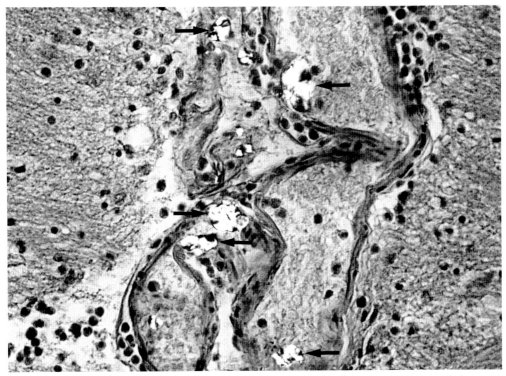

Figure 9.9.   Ethylene glycol poisoning. Note the birefringent calcium oxalate crystals (*arrows*) in the vessel walls and the perivascular inflammatory cell infiltrates. Hematoxylin & eosin. Photographed with polarized light. (Original magnification ×400.)

diffuse cerebral gliosis, malformation of the dentate nucleus, neuronal heterotopias, and dendritic cacti on the Purkinje cells. The effects of maternal infections and possible prenatal exposure to other teratogens must be considered before directly attributing these fetal anomalies to maternal use of anticonvulsants.

HEXACHLOROPHENE

Hexachlorophene is a chlorinated bisphenol that is commonly employed as a topical germicide. Some of the drug is absorbed through the skin; however, adults and older children rarely suffer any ill effects from the topical use of this agent on intact skin. Increased absorption with neurotoxicity manifested by tremulousness, seizures, lethargy, and coma have been observed following application of this compound to mucous membranes, diseased skin, and burns. Neurotoxicity has been encountered most frequently in low birthweight premature infants who were bathed with hexachlorophene (88, 103). These infants are especially susceptible because of the increased permeability of their skin and the decreased capacity of their liver to detoxify and excrete the drug. Spongy degeneration of white matter was found in infants weighing less than 1400 g who were repeatedly bathed with a hexachlorophene emulsion. The spongy degeneration was most pronounced in the brain stem, especially the medullary reticular formation, the medial longitudinal fasciculus, the medial lemniscus, and the superior cerebellar peduncle. Ultrastructural study showed the spongy degeneration to result from intramyelinic edema (88).

Rare fatalities have resulted from accidental or intentional oral ingestion of hexachlorophene. Martinez et al (69) reported a 7-year-old boy who had been given approximately 45 ml of a 3% hexachlorophene emulsion. Neuropathologic studies disclosed severe cerebral swelling and spongy degeneration of white matter due to intramyelinic edema. In addition, there was necrosis of the optic nerves, chiasm, and tracts.

Intramyelinic edema has been produced in laboratory animals experimentally intoxicated with hexachlorophene. In addition, these animals show vacuolation of peripheral nerve myelin, degeneration of retinal photoreceptor cells, and degeneration of axons within the optic nerves. The precise mechanism by which hexachlorophene exerts its toxic effect on the lipid-rich membranes of the myelin sheath and photoreceptor cells remains unsettled.

ANTIBIOTICS AND ANTIVIRAL AGENTS

When administered in high dosages for prolonged periods of time, chloramphenicol had been observed to produce a peripheral polyneuropathy and an optic neuropathy. These complications are rare now that the drug is used for shorter periods of time. Pathological finding included loss of retinal ganglion cells with atrophy, gliosis, and fibrosis of the corresponding portions of the optic nerves.

Gentamicin is an aminoglycoside antibiotic used in the treatment of infections due to various gram-negative organisms. Transient neurotoxicity manifested by ototoxicity, encephalopathy, psychosis, and neuromuscular blockade has been observed clinically. Microscopically, multiple necrotic foci were encountered in the mesencephalon and pons of a patient treated with intrathecal gentamicin for pseudomonas meningitis (117). The individual lesions consisted of axonal swellings, some of which were calcified, surrounded by a sparsely cellular zone of spongiosis. This spongiosis was due to loss of axis cylinders, oligodendrocytes, and astrocytes. Similar lesions were reproduced experimentally in rabbits by intrathecal administration of high doses of the antibiotic (117).

Other antimicrobial agents such as isoniazid, dapsone, metronidazole, and nitrofurantoin are well known but rare causes of peripheral neuropathy in man. Experimentally, isoniazid has been observed to produce intramyelinic edema in the central nervous system of ducklings (56) and dogs (10). Comparable lesions have not been encountered in man.

At the present time, there is considerable optimism regarding the efficacy of vidarabine (adenine arabinoside) in the treatment of herpes simplex encephalitis and disseminated varicella-zoster infections. Most of the complications of therapy with this drug have been related to the large volume fluid needed to administer this agent intravenously. In addition, several authors have described movement disorders, dysarthria, confusion, and coma which they attributed to direct neurotoxicity of this drug (72, 112). Neuropathologic studies are limited but have shown widespread central chromatolysis and acute degeneration of neurons (112). The changes were most severe in the brain stem. We have observed similar changes in pontine neurons from a patient who was treated for herpes simplex encephalitis (Fig. 9.10A and B). The metabolic basis for this neurotoxicity is unclear.

ANTINEOPLASTIC AGENTS

A variety of clinically manifested neurological complications have been encountered in the course of systemic or intrathecal chemotherapy with various antineoplastic agents (36). Of particular interest at the present time are those associated with methotrexate, a widely used folic acid antagonist. The systemic toxic effects of this drug on the bone marrow, gastrointestinal tract, liver, reproductive organs, and fetal tissues have long been known. More recently, neurotoxicity has been observed under various circumstances. Acute or subacute chemical meningitis, meningoencephalitis, and even transverse myelitis have occurred shortly after intrathecal administration of methotrexate. The meningitis may be accompanied by cerebrospinal fluid pleocytosis, but further histopathological features are unknown. Examination of the spinal cords from patients with transverse myelitis following intrathecal methotrexate have shown either no abnormalities, or demyelination of spinal cord nerve roots and small regions of superficial spinal white matter. At least one case of an acute encephalomyelopathy has followed repeated intrathecal methotrexate administration. Neuropathological studies on this patient disclosed multiple sharply circumscribed areas of partial necrosis and gliosis. The affected areas were largely confined to the external surfaces of the brain and spinal cord adjacent to the subarachnoid space. In the spinal cord, the root entry zones were especially severely affected. No lesions were encountered in the deep white matter of the brain or spinal cord or in the periventricular regions (104).

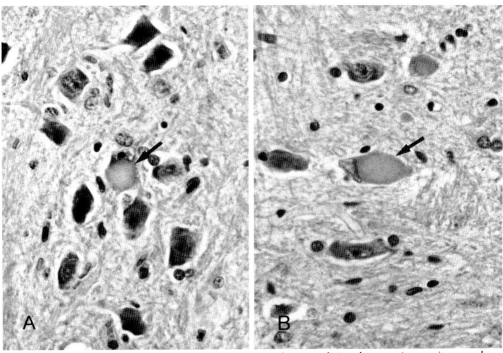

Figure 9.10. (A and B). Pontine neurons showing chromatolytic changes (arrows) secondary to vidarabine toxicity. H&E. (Original magnification ×400.)

Rarely, the acute onset of neurological deficits has been recorded following intravenous administration of methotrexate. Transient hemiplegia and focal seizures have been observed in patients being treated with high dose intravenous methotrexate followed by citrovorum factor "rescue." Intracarotid infusion of high dose methotrexate has on at least one occasion resulted in the production of multiple hemorrhagic infarcts with fibrinoid necrosis and thrombosis of small vessels (36).

Of great concern have been the delayed encephalopathies which most often follow a combination of high-dose, long-term systemic and/or intrathecal methotrexate therapy and cranial irradiation in children with leukemia (26, 90, 91, 95). The clinical manifestations usually appear insidiously and include confusion, mental deterioration, ataxia, seizures and, eventually, stupor or coma (36). Neuropathological studies have disclosed several patterns of injury. The best known of these lesions has been designated as disseminated necrotizing leukoencephalopathy by Rubinstein et al. (95) and as subacute encephalopathy by Price and Jamieson (91). The lesions consist of multiple discrete or confluent foci of coagulative necrosis scattered throughout the white matter (Fig. 9.11). Some of the lesions may be surrounded by a border of petechial hemorrhages. In the more severely affected cases, the lesions may be roughly symmetrical and especially prominent within the central white matter of the cerebral hemispheres. Microscopically, the lesions are characterized by coagulative necrosis, demyelination, spongiosus, gliosis, and mineralization of reactive axonal swellings and cellular debris (Fig. 9.12). Lipid-laden macrophages may be abundant, but inflammatory cells are conspicuously sparse. Vascular changes are present in some but not all of the cases. Price and Birdwell (90) reported another series of children with leukemia who had a noninflammatory mineralizing angiopathy. The

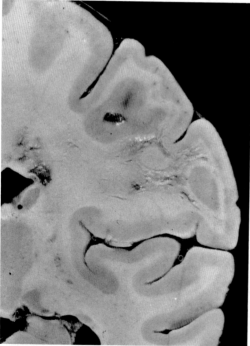

Figure 9.11. Necrotizing encephalomyelopathy secondary to synergistic effects of methotrexate and radiation. Note the demyelinated and necrotic white matter lesions in this patient who had received intrathecal methotrexate and cranial radiation for leukemia.

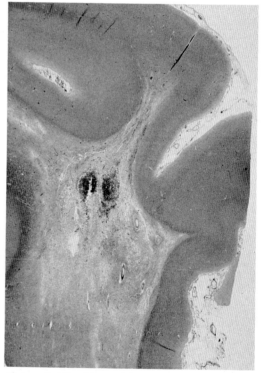

Figure 9.12. Necrotizing encephalomyelopathy secondary to synergistic effects of methotrexate and radiation. Note the demyelination, necrosis, and mineral deposits in the white matter. H&E. (Original magnification ×3.5.)

vascular alterations were most severe in the lenticular nuclei. Parenchymal necrosis and mineralization were variable. Although the authors attributed the microangiopathy to irradiation, all of the affected cases had been given methotrexate. Crosley et al. (26) emphasized the frequent occurrence (65%) of cerebral atrophy, both in children treated with intrathecal methotrexate alone and in combination with radiation therapy. These authors also described a necrotizing vasculitis in some of their cases. Additional mild cases of encephalopathy have been detected by computerized tomography of asymptomatic children with leukemia who had received intrathecal methotrexate and cranial irradiation (86). The abnormalities demonstrated by the computerized tomography included ventricular dilatation, enlargement of the subarachnoid space, areas of decreased attenuation, and intracerebral calcification.

Lesions similar to those of disseminated necrotizing leukoencephalopathy but with a more pronounced periventricular distribution have been encountered in patients given intraventricular methotrexate without radiation. Obstruction of the normal cerebrospinal fluid pathways is regarded as an essential factor in the development of the lesions under these circumstances. Focal intraparenchymal lesions have also occurred when intraventricular catheters were misplaced delivering the drug directly into the neural parenchyma (77).

The Vinca alkaloids, vincristine and vinblastine, are mitotic spindle inhibitors that are used as antineoplastic agents. Both are neurotoxic. A peripheral neuropathy is usually the dose-limiting factor when vincristine is employed. Vincristine neuropathy is manifested initially by suppression of the Achilles tendon reflex. This is followed by paresthesias, distal motor weakness, and cranial nerve palsies. Constipation and colicky abdominal pain reflect involvement of the autonomic nervous system. Vincristine binds to microtubule protein and, according to some authors, disrupts fast axonal transport. Histological studies on peripheral nerves from patients and experimental animals with this neuropathy have shown predominantly axonal degeneration. Inappropriate antidiuretic hormone secretion and seizures have been reported occasionally,

but the central nervous system is generally spared from the neurotoxic effects of the drug by the blood-brain barrier.

On a few occasions, the vincristine has been inadvertently administered intrathecally (105). This has been following by ascending paralysis, sensory deficits, respiratory failure, and death 3–14 days later. Examination of the spinal cord has disclosed swollen motor neurons with dispersed Nissl granules and aggregates of neurofilaments. One case also contained prominent eosinophilic crystals (Fig. 9.13) which were thought to be derived from reaggregration of microtubule proteins.

Cytosine arabinoside, or Ara-C, is a pyrimidine analog that inhibits DNA synthesis. This antineoplastic agent is commonly used in the therapy of myelocytic leukemia. Few neurotoxic reactions have been reported when used systemically; however, manifestations ranging from meningismus to paraplegia have been observed following intrathecal administration. Pathological

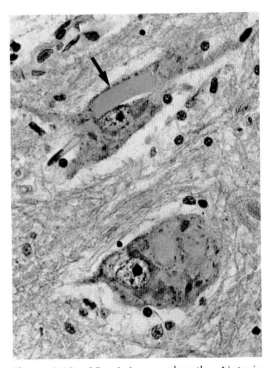

Figure 9.13. Vincristine myelopathy. Note in eosinophilic intracytoplasmic inclusion (*arrow*) and aggregates of filaments (lower neuron) in anterior horn motor neurons from a patient who had received intrathecal vincristine. H&E. (Original magnification ×800.)

studies on a patient who died 6 months after the onset of paraparesis induced by Ara-C showed loss of myelin, microvacuolation, and axonal degeneration in the spinal cord (13). Mild cases of encephalopathy, similar to those associated with methotrexate and radiation, have been detected by computerized tomography of asymptomatic children with leukemia who had received intrathecal cytosine arabinoside and cranial irradiation (86).

Cerebellar cortical degeneration also has been observed following high-dose systemic cytosine arabinoside therapy (119). Clinical manifestations began within a week of administration of the drug and included ataxia, dysarthria, and nystagmus. Postmortem examination disclosed patchy degeneration of the cerebellar cortex involving primarily Purkinje cells and the molecular layer.

Another pyrimidine analog that inhibits DNA synthesis is 5-Fluorouracil. This agent is often used in the treatment of various gastrointestinal, breast, and ovarian carcinomas. Neurotoxicity is relatively uncommon and consists mainly of a cerebellar syndrome that is often reversible. Pathological studies have shown loss of neurons from the Purkinje cell layer, internal granular cell layer, dentate nuclei, and inferior olivary nuclei (93). 5-Fluorouracil itself is relatively nontoxic to the nervous system. It has been suggested that the neurotoxic manifestations result from inhibition of the Krebs cycle by catabolites of the drug including fluoroacetate and fluorocitrate.

Nitrogen mustard (mechlorethamine) is the prototype of the so-called "alkylating" antineoplastic agents. Reports of neurotoxicity are rare when the drug has been given intravenously in conventional doses. One patient with Hodgkin's disease was reported to have developed hemiplegia and coma after two intravenous doses of nitrogen mustard. Examination of the brain, 4 years later, disclosed only focal areas of neuronal loss and gliosis (9). More severe reactions with seizures, coma, and death within 12 hours have been reported following intraarterial infusion of nitrogen mustard. Histological studies on one such case that we personally examined revealed an extensive area of edema and necrosis in the white matter. Similar adverse reactions with hemiplegia have followed "isolation perfusion" with phenylalanine mustard.

Cyclophosphamide is another alkylating agent that is commonly employed both as an antineoplastic agent and as an immunosuppresive agent. Neurotoxicity in man is unusual; however, hemorrhagic and necrotizing choroid plexitis has been produced in rats with high doses of this compound.

Doxorubicin (Adriamycin) and daunorubicin are members of another class of antineoplastic agents, the anthracyclines. These drugs are relatively new but widely employed in the treatment of a variety of neoplasms. In addition to the usual toxic effects of antineoplastic agents, serious cardiotoxicity has been observed. Clinical neurotoxicity has not yet been described in man but remains a concern. Administration of adriamycin to rats has been reported to produce progressive ataxia affecting predominantly the hind limbs. Pathological studies (20) have demonstrated alterations in the peripheral nervous system. Spinal, paravertebral, and trigeminal ganglia showed neuronal necrosis and proliferation of nerve sheath cells. This was preceded, in dorsal root ganglia, by an increase in the number of neurofilaments and mitochondria. Somewhat similar neuronal changes have been observed in cardiac ganglion cells of children treated with daunorubicin for leukemia.

BCNU (1,3-bis(2-chloroethyl)-1-nitrosourea) is a nitrosourea compound that is used in the chemotherapy of various cerebral neoplasms. Systemic therapy is complicated by bone marrow suppression and pulmonary fibrosis but usually minimal neurotoxicity. However, high dose systemic BCNU has been reported to produce a necrotizing encephalomyelopathy (15). Currently the drug is also being administered intraarterially for regional perfusion of cerebral neoplasms. Although comparable lesions have not been reported in patients, intracarotid administration of BCNU in dogs has resulted in the production of a hemorrhagic encephalitis with necrotizing arteriolitis (75).

Cis-platin (cis-diamine dichloroplatinum II) is one of several platinum compounds that is being used in the therapy of various malignancies, usually in advanced stages of the disease. Neurotoxicity in the form of cranial nerve dysfunction (deafness and optic neuritis) and distal polyneuropathies have been reported. Morphological studies are limited and difficult to evaluate because of underlying disease and concurrent use of other neurotoxic antineoplastic agents. Walsh et al. (116) reported the neuropathological findings with a 3½-year-old girl who had been given cisplatin and doxorubicin for a sacrococcygeal teratoma. They observed swelling of the optic nerve head, loss of axons from dorsal spinal roots, and demyelination and gliosis in the dorsal columns of the spinal cord.

METRIZAMIDE

Metrizamide is currently employed extensively for diagnostic neuroradiologic studies. Seizures and encephalopathy are well-recognized complications following the use of this contrast agent. These effects are thought to result from inhibition of hexokinase. Morphological changes consisting predominantly of inflammatory cell infiltrates have been observed in animal studies. Auer et al. (4) have reported perivascular mononuclear inflammatory cell infiltrates, including numerous plasmacytoid cells, in a patient who died 11 days after intraventricular instillation of metrizamide. The infiltrates were most marked within 3 mm of the ventricular surface. The authors attributed these changes to the metrizamide and considered them comparable to those previously observed in laboratory animals.

Industrial Solvents

Methyl *n*-butylketone and *n*-hexane have been employed extensively as organic solvents. These two hexacarbons and their common catabolite, 2,5-hexanedione, are capable of producing a morphologically distinctive form of "dying-back" peripheral neuropathy. These so-called "hexacarbon induced giant axonal neuropathies" are characterized by the formation of focal enlargements on axons prior to degeneration of the more distal segments of the affected nerves. The enlargements are situated proximal to nodes of Ranvier and are filled with accumulations of neurofilaments. Similar axonal enlargements have been encountered following acrylamide monomer

and carbon disulfide intoxications, in hereditary giant axonal neuropathy, and in a neuropathy thought to be associated with vitamin B_{12} malabsorption (50, 99, 106). The formation of the axonal enlargements is thought to result from partial impairment of the centrifugal transport of neurofilaments at the nodes of Ranvier (96). In the case of the hexacarbon-induced giant axonal neuropathies, the impaired transport has been attributed to a localized block in glycolysis (96) or linkage between 2,5-hexanedione and amino groups on the neurofilaments (38).

These hexacarbon-induced neuropathies are regarded as forms of central-peripheral distal axonopathies (106). This terminology emphasizes the fact that the distal axonal segments in both the central and peripheral nervous systems are similarly affected. Long fiber tracts in the central nervous system that are especially vulnerable include the fasciculus gracilis, the corticospinal tracts, and the spinocerebellar tracts. Although less extensively studied, the distal segments of these central pathways contain axonal enlargements that are distended with neurofilaments similar to those in the peripheral nerves (106).

Carbon tetrachloride is commonly employed as a solvent and has been used in certain types of fire extinguishers. This compound is neurotoxic as well as hepatotoxic and nephrotoxic. Relatively few reports document the morphological changes in the human nervous system. Multiple small hemorrhages ranging from 0.1 to 0.5 cm have been encountered in the pons, middle cerebellar peduncles, and cerebellum. Microscopically these lesions display perivenular demyelination and necrosis accompanied by extravasation of erythrocytes. This apparently resulted from necrosis of the vessel walls. The lesions were sufficiently large to be grossly apparent in the patient reported by Luse and Wood (62). More recent studies of experimental carbon tetrachloride intoxication in laboratory animals have emphasized an increase in the number of astrocytes and an enlargement of astrocytic nuclei. These glial changes may be secondary to the hepatic toxicity since they do not appear until several weeks after the onset of hepatic necrosis.

Trichloroethylene is another chlorinated hydrocarbon that has been employed extensively as a solvent. It has also been used as an inhalation anesthetic and at one time was used in the treatment of trigeminal neuralgia. The compound is neurotoxic with prominent involvement of the optic, facial, and especially trigeminal nerves. One postmortem study described both demyelination and axonal degeneration in the trigeminal root and nerves (16). The corresponding brain stem nuclei showed severe loss of neurons and degenerative changes in the remaining neurons.

Metal Intoxications

A wide variety of metals, in sufficient concentration and appropriate form, are known to be toxic to man. Most of these adversely affect multiple systems of the body, including the nervous system. Space will permit only brief consideration of selected metals, with emphasis on central nervous system toxicity.

ALUMINUM

The neurotoxicity of aluminum is highly controversial. This abundant element has long been regarded as nontoxic for man. There is now evidence that this may not always be the case. Various aluminum compounds applied directly onto or injected into the cerebral cortex of certain laboratory animals produce seizures and a type of neurofibrillary degeneration. Ultrastructural studies have shown that these experimentally induced neurofibrillary tangles are composed of skeins of smooth filaments 10 nm in diameter. These are quite different from the paired helical filaments that comprise the naturally occurring Alzheimer neurofibrillary tangles in man. Nevertheless, Crapper and colleagues (24) have reported significantly elevated aluminum content in muliple samples of brain from patients with Alzheimer's disease. They correlated neurofibrillary tangle formation with a regional content of aluminum in excess of 4 μg/g dry weight. These findings have not been accepted by all workers, and some relate the increased aluminum content merely to advancing age (63, 67). Furthermore, experimental aluminum intoxication has not resulted in the formation of other histological manifestations of Alzheimer's disease such as granulovacuolar degeneration and senile plaques.

Aluminum has been implicated more convincingly in the development of at least some cases of the so-called dialysis encephalopathy syndrome. This potentially lethal disorder is characterized by dyspraxia, asterixis, convulsions, and dementia. It has been encountered most often in individuals who have undergone chronic hemodialysis for renal failure. Use of oral medications containing aluminum compounds and a high aluminum content in the dialysate contribute to the development of this disorder. Although the brain aluminum content may be elevated to levels even greater than reported in Alzheimer's disease, neurofibrillary tangles have not been detected.

ARSENIC

Arsenic intoxication is now encountered most often as the result of occupational exposure or following ingestion with homicidal or suicidal intent. In the past, a number of cases resulted from consumption of illicit liquor contaminated with arsenic and from the therapeutic use of arsenical compounds.

Peripheral neuropathy is a well-known and often disabling sequela of both acute and chronic arsenical intoxication. Arsenic is thought to exert its deleterious effects by binding to sulfhydryl groups on lipoic acid and thus interfering with pyruvate metabolism. The histopathological changes encountered in peripheral nerve biopsy specimens have been interpreted as predominantly axonal degeneration with secondary segmental demyelination (108).

Encephalopathy also has been observed with both acute and chronic arsenic intoxication. However, few recent reports discuss the morphological features accompanying this clinical manifestation. Older reports described edema and petechial hemorrhages in the corpus callosum, periventricular white matter, internal capsule, and brain stem following arsphenamine therapy. It is not clear whether these lesions resulted from the arsenic intoxication or a hypersensitivity reaction.

CADMIUM

Cadmium, in low concentrations and usually in association with zinc, is widespread throughout our environment. Acute cadmium intoxication is variously manifested by vomiting and abdominal cramps or dyspnea and pulmonary edema, depending upon the mode of exposure. Emphysema and renal dysfunction with proteinuria are among the major manifestations of subacute and chronic intoxication. Chronic exposure to excess cadmium in drinking water in Japan produced a syndrome that was further characterized by severe bone pain. Neurotoxicity manifested by anosmia has been recognized in industrial workers who were exposed to cadmium for many years (61). Although human neuropathological studies are sparse, a number of experimental studies in laboratory animals appear to be relevant. Administration of cadmium to newborn mice induced hemorrhages, edema, and foci of neuronal necrosis throughout much of the immature brain. The changes were progressively less severe in older animals; however, the olfactory bulbs were among the structures still affected in the more mature animals. The neuronal damage was considered secondary to vascular injury (118). Acute hemorrhagic lesions in sensory and trigeminal ganglia have been produced by parenteral administration of cadmium to older animals. Again capillary damage was considered the initial event in the development of these ganglionic lesions. In addition, direct neurotoxicity has been suggested by in vitro tissue culture studies. Organotypic cultures of sensory ganglia displayed intraneuronal aggregates of glycogen granules, lipid droplets, and neurofilamentous whorls when exposed to cadmium compounds (110).

LEAD

Lead poisoning has afflicted man since antiquity. Although many occupational, domestic, and environmental sources have been eliminated or reduced, unacceptably high blood levels are still present in large numbers of children, especially among lower socioeconomic groups. Lead can enter the body through the gastrointestinal and respiratory tracts and, when in organic compounds, through the skin. Many systems of the body, including the hematopoietic, genitourinary, and nervous systems, are affected adversely by an excessive lead burden.

Lead neurotoxicity may be manifested as an encephalopathy, a neuropathy, or both. Lead encephalopathy is now relatively rare and is encountered predominantly in young children who chew objects coated with lead paint. In adults, chronic poisoning is now most often manifested as a motor neuropathy. In the past, when lead intoxication was more prevalent, encephalopathy was more often seen in adults (19). Most cases of lead encephalopathy in adults and teenagers are now the result of consumption of contaminated "moonshine" whiskey, of occupational exposure to tetraethyl lead, or of "sniffing" leaded gasoline (111).

Children with lead encephalopathy typically display excessive irritability, convulsions, ataxia, and an altered state of consciousness ranging from drowsiness to coma. The brains from these cases are often swollen with flattened gyri and compressed ventricles (83). Uncal and tonsillar herniations may be present. The histopathologic changes include congestion, petechial hemorrhages, and foci of necrosis. A variety of vascular changes have been described. Capillaries may be obliterated or unusually prominent as the result of dilatation and proliferation. Some may be surrounded by a PAS-positive proteinaceous exudate. Clasen et al. (22) have emphasized the diagnostic significance of small PAS-positive globules located within the perivascular astrocytes. Similar globular deposits with variable staining characteristics had been described previously by other authors. Diffuse astrocytic proliferation in both gray and white matter has been reported even in the absence of capillary changes (83).

Many authors have attributed the encephalopathy, predominantly if not exclusively, to vascular injury. Pentschew and Garro (85) were able to produce an experimental model of lead encephalopathy in suckling rats by feeding lead carbonate to the nursing mothers. The suckling rats developed edema, discoloration, and petechial hemorrhages in their cerebellum. Lesser degrees of edema, capillary proliferation and dilatation, and abnormal vascular permeability were evident in the cerebrum and spinal cord. Pentschew and Garro (85) regarded the changes as a manifestation of a "dysoric encephalopathy" and focused attention on abnormal vascular permeability.

Subsequent ultrastructural and isotope studies using this and similar models confirmed the endothelial damage and abnormal capillary permeability. Press (89) emphasized the selective vulnerability of the developing vascular bed in the immature cerebellum and stressed the sensitivity of the endothelial bud or angioblast in this model. Some authors feel that the vascular changes have been overemphasized and that other neurotoxic effects of lead have been inadequately investigated (19). Following intracerebral implantation of lead acetate in rats, Hirano and Kochen (44) observed the formation of intracytoplasmic and intranuclear inclusions in astrocytes. These astrocytic inclusions resembled the intranuclear inclusions in renal tubular epithelium of lead intoxicated patients and animals.

Lead peripheral neuropathy, now the more common manifestation of lead neurotoxicity in the adult, is a remarkably pure motor neuropathy that often is most severe in the radial nerves. Recent histopathological studies on patients with this disorder are exceedingly sparse. Behse and Carlsen (6) mentioned sural nerves from eight men who had 1–8 years of occupational exposure to lead but no overt signs or symptoms of neuropathy. The sural nerves merely showed a slightly increased incidence of paranodal demyelination and an increased incidence of degeneration among the un-myelinated fibers. By contrast, numerous studies of experimental lead neuropathy have been reported. Fullerton (31) described segmental demyelination in teased nerve preparations from guinea pigs after lead intoxication for up to 2 years. An ultrastructural study on chronic lead neuropathy in rats was performed by Lampert and Schochet (57), who found endoneurial edema, degenerating Schwann cells and segmental demyelination. Occasional fibers showed remyelination and even "onion bulb" formations. Only rare axons appeared to be degenerating. More recent studies by Powell et al. (87) have suggested that the Schwann cell damage is due to a direct toxic effect of lead rather than being secondary to the endoneurial edema. Intranuclear inclusions in Schwann cells developed early in the course of the disease while endoneurial edema did not appear until the neuropathy was already established.

MANGANESE

The neurotoxicity of manganese has been studied most extensively in Chilian miners who have had chronic exposure to manganese dioxide. The clinical manifestations include transient psychiatric disturbances (so-called "manganese madness"), headaches, and parkinsonian-like extrapyramidal dysfunction. The latter manifestations persist even after exposure has been terminated and much of the manganese has been cleared from the body. The limited pathological studies have been summarized by Barbeau et al. (5). Collectively the reports document lesions predominantly in the pallidum and subthalamic nucleus and to a lesser extent in the caudate and putamen. The substantia nigra was involved in only one patient. Experimental chronic manganese intoxication in monkeys, produced by intramuscular injection of a manganese dioxide suspension, resulted in lesions that were most severe in the subthalamic nucleus and pallidum. These lesions displayed neuronal loss and gliosis (84).

MERCURY

The toxicity of mercury has been recognized since antiquity. All forms of the element—metallic, inorganic compounds, and organic compounds—are potential sources of human intoxication. Inorganic and elemental mercury poisoning have become relatively uncommon since the risk of occupational exposure has been reduced and the medicinal use of mercury and mercury compounds has been sharply curtailed. Acute poisoning from inorganic mercury compounds is manifested predominantly by gastrointestinal tract and renal tubular injury. Pulmonary damage occurs when the acute intoxication is caused by inhalation of metallic mercury vapors. Neurotoxicity is a prominent manifestation of chronic inorganic mercury poisoning. The initial symptoms often consist of bizarre behavioral changes called "erethism." Other common manifestations include intention tremor and movement disorders. Occasionally, patients have peripheral neuropathy. Peripheral neuropathy was also one of the major manifestations of acrodynia or "pink disease." This disorder was thought to result from chronic mercury poisoning in infants and young children. The mercury was acquired most often from teething powders and antihelminthic agents.

There are relatively few reports of the neuropathological inorganic mercury poisoning in man. Some of the older accounts reported no histopathological abnormalities. Davis et al. (28) described the morphological findings in two women who had used a laxative containing calomel (mercurous chloride) for many years. The brains showed cerebellar atrophy with loss of internal granular layer cells and, possibly, some Purkinje cells.

Organic mercury compounds have been responsible for major outbreaks of poisoning in recent years. Large numbers of Japanese individuals living in the Minamata Bay and Niigata districts developed chronic organic mercury intoxication from fish contaminated by methylmercury (102). Other large outbreaks have resulted from the consumption of grain treated with an organic mercury fungicide. The clinical manifestations are dominated by constriction of visual fields, paresthesias, ataxia, dysarthria, and impaired hearing. Neuropathological studies have shown cerebral atrophy most pronounced along the anterior portions of the calcarine fissures and, to a lesser extent, in the pre- and postcentral gyri. In these areas, there was neuronal loss, especially from the outer cortical layers, and gliosis. Cerebellar atrophy was encountered almost as frequently as the atrophy of the calcarine cortex. Microscopically, there was loss of neurons from the internal granular cell layers, proliferation of Bergmann glia, and mild loss of Purkinje cells. Cavanagh (19) has suggested that the lesions caused by organic and inorganic mercury are essentially the same. The apparent differences may simply reflect variations in the rate of entry of the compounds into the nervous system.

THALLIUM

Thallium compounds have long been recognized to be highly toxic. They are now employed primarily as components of certain pesticides used for insect and rodent control. In the past, some thallium compounds were used medically for the control of night sweats from tuberculosis and as depilatory agents. Oral ingestion of thallium compounds produces a wide spectrum of toxic manifestations, including neuro-

toxicity. Massive acute intoxication is characterized initially by gastrointestinal manifestations, including nausea, vomiting, diarrhea, and abdominal pain. This may be followed by cardiac and pulmonary involvement, altered states of consciousness, and limb pain. Initially the limb pain involves the legs predominantly and is localized about the joints with distal paresthesias. Later a predominantly sensory neuropathy and muscular wasting develop. Neuropathy may be the initial manifestation from milder intoxication. Behavioral changes, convulsions, and movement disorders also have been reported, especially in cases of chronic intoxication. Death in at least some cases results from myocardial necrosis. Alopecia is the most widely recognized manifestation of thallium intoxication but does not become evident for several weeks and, even then, does not occur in all patients.

Some reports have described rather varied neuropathological changes, including edema, congestion, neuronal loss, chromatolysis neuronal vacuolization, and degeneration of the posterior columns of the spinal cord (19). Recently Davis et al. (27) studied a patient who died about 9 days after ingestion of 5–10 g of thallium nitrate. They found no histopathological abnormalities in the brain and only questionable chromatolysis of scattered neurons in the anterior horns of the spinal cord. Nevertheless, the cerebral gray matter contained some of the highest concentrations of thallium in the body.

Peripheral nerves from patients and experimental animals have been studied extensively. Most reports have emphasized axonal degeneration, which may be preceded or accompanied by vacuolation of mitochondria (27, 106). Involvement of the autonomic nervous system has been implicated in the development of the alopecia and cardiac dysfunction.

DEFICIENCIES

Vitamin Deficiencies

GENERAL

Nutritional deficiencies, especially certain vitamin deficiencies, are responsible for an important group of neurological disorders. Nutritional deficiency from inadequate food supply is widespread in certain underdeveloped nations and afflicts smaller, less fortunate segments of the population in other countries. In the highly developed nations of Europe and in the United States, many cases of vitamin deficiency are associated with alcoholism. Alcohol is substituted for other dietary items, impairs the absorption of various vitamins and, due to the carbohydrate load, imposes additional needs for certain vitamins such as thiamine. Occasionally, vitamin deficiency is encountered among food faddists, in individuals with gastrointestinal diseases that impair the absorption of vitamins, and in individuals on medications that impede the utilization of vitamins.

THIAMINE DEFICIENCY

Thiamine deficiency is responsible for causing several neurological disorders, including the Wernicke-Korsakoff syndrome and certain nutritional polyneuropathies. Although the Wernicke-Korsakoff syndrome is encountered most often in patients suffering from chronic alcoholism, it is clearly due to the associated thiamine deficiency rather than direct toxic effects of the alcohol. This was evident even from the cases originally reported by Wernicke in 1881. Two of his three patients were alcoholics; the third was a young woman who developed pyloric stenosis from ingestion of sulfuric acid. Over the years at least a small number of cases of Wernicke's encephalopathy has been reported in association with a wide variety of conditions other than alcoholism. Included among these are uremia, chronic hemodialysis, neoplasms of the gastrointestinal tract, prolonged intravenous therapy, and gastric plication for obesity (39, 71, 78).

Abnormalities of ocular motility including gaze paralysis, nystagmus, ataxia, and mental confusion are regarded as the clinical hallmarks of Wernicke's encephalopathy. Retrograde amnesia and an impaired ability to acquire new information are considered the essential clinical features of Korsakoff's psychosis. The latter disorder usually occurs along with Wernicke's encephalopathy in alcoholic patients. Rarely, however, Korsakoff's psychosis may occur independently, even in nonalcoholic individuals, as the result of other diencephalic lesions.

Morphological evidence of Wernicke's encephalopathy has been encountered in 1.7–2.7% of consecutive cases in at least three large autopsy series (25, 42, 113). The pathological features vary with the stage and severity of the disease process. Patients who die in the acute stages may have lesions in the mammillary bodies, hypothalamus, periventricular region of the thalamus, about the aqueduct, and beneath the floor of the fourth ventricle. The mammillary bodies, especially the medial nuclei are the most frequently affected structures and are involved in virtually all cases (Fig. 9.14). Involvement of the other locations is less constant (113). The mammillary bodies and other affected areas typically display a gray-to-brown discoloration. A narrow band of tissue immediately adjacent to the ventricular system and about the aqueduct generally remains unaffected. Occasionally the lesions contain petechial hemorrhages. Only rarely are the hemorrhages large and conspicuous. Even among acute cases, pathological changes may not be discernible grossly. For example, Harper (42) recorded no grossly recognizable changes in the mammillary bodies in 5 of 10 acute

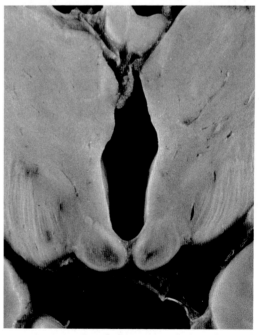

Figure 9.14. Wernicke's encephalopathy. Diffusely discolored, focally necrotic mammillary bodies.

cases. Patients with more chronic or previously treated disease may have only mildly discolored and mildly atrophic mammillary bodies. Under these circumstances, lesions in periventricular and periaqueductal regions may be very inconspicuous.

The histopathological findings also vary with the stage and severity of the disease. Acute lesions display edema, necrosis, demyelination, and some loss of neurons (Fig. 9.15). Vessels are abnormally prominent due to swelling and hyperplasia of the endothelial cells (Fig. 9.16). Lipid-laden macrophages may be present in the enlarged perivascular spaces. When petechial hemorrhages are present, extravasated erythrocytes and hemosiderin-laden macrophages may be seen. The astrocytes may be enlarged and abnormally conspicuous. Rarely, unusually prominent, chromatolytic appearing neurons may be encountered in the mammillary bodies. This striking neuronal change was found in 7 of 92 cases reported by Peña (82). In the chronic stages of the disease and in treated cases, the affected regions may show little more than mild loss of neurons and gliosis.

Victor (113) regarded lesions in the medial dorsal nuclei of the thalamus as the morphological substrate of the Korsakoff component of the Wernicke-Korsakoff syndrome. Support for this interpretation is derived from cases of Korsakoff psychosis associated with hemorrhages and neoplasms in this particular anatomic location. More recently, however, Mair et al. (65) studied two patients with the Wernicke-Korsakoff syndrome and found lesions in the mammillary bodies and midline region of the thalamus but not the medial dorsal nuclei. For that reason, they questioned the specificity of the association between the medial dorsal nuclei and Korsakoff's psychosis.

Thiamine deficiency also produces peripheral neuropathies, beriberi neuropathy, and probably most cases of so-called "alcoholic" neuropathy. In contrast to some of the older reports, a recent study of beriberi neuropathy in nonalcoholic patients revealed predominantly axonal degeneration (74). Similarly, most histopathological

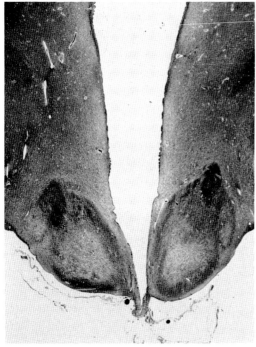

Figure 9.15. Wernicke's encephalopathy. Note the demyelination of the mammillary bodies. Trichrome. (Original magnification ×5.)

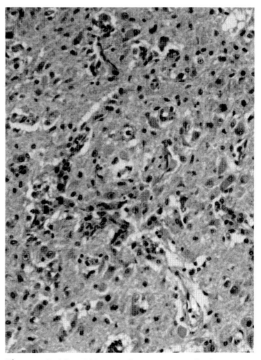

Figure 9.16. Wernicke's encephalopathy showing endothelial proliferation, lipid-laden macrophages, and reactive astrocytes in a mammillary body. Trichrome. (Original magnification ×175.)

studies on specimens from patients with alcoholic neuropathy have disclosed axonal degeneration. Segmental demyelination, when present, may be secondary to the axonal changes.

Thiamine in the form of thiamine pyrophosphate is an essential cofactor for certain enzyme systems such as the pyruvate dehydrogenase complex, ketoglutarate dehydrogenase, and transketolase. However, the neurochemical basis for the selective distribution of lesions in Wernicke's encephalopathy has not been fully elucidated. The mammillary bodies which are almost invariably affected in Wernicke's encephalopathy have the highest regional activity of transketolase in the normal human brain (29). Experimental studies have shown that thiamine deficiency produces a widespread reduction in cerebral glucose utilization. The decline in glucose utilization is more rapid in many of the structures that are known to develop lesions in patients with the Wernicke-Korsakoff syndrome (40). Blass and Gibson (11) have attributed the relatively infrequent development of the Wernicke-Korsakoff syndrome among alcoholics to genetically determined differences in the binding of thiamine by transketolase. They found that transketolase in fibroblasts from patients with the Wernicke-Korsakoff syndrome bound thiamine less avidly than transketolase in fibroblasts from controls. Since this defect persisted in multiple generations of cultured fibroblasts, the authors interpreted the binding abnormality as genetically determined. This finding has been correlated with the observation that Wernicke-Korsakoff syndrome occurs most often among individuals of European extraction.

NIACIN DEFICIENCY

Pellagra, characterized by the triad of dermatitis, diarrhea, and dementia, has long been recognized in various parts of the world among poverty-stricken people who used corn as a major part of their diet. During the early part of the 20th century, the disease was endemic in the southern part of the United States. After many attempts to identify a toxin in spoiled corn or an infectious agent, Goldberger showed that the disease was due to a dietary deficiency and could be prevented with additional protein. Later Elvehjem and associates showed that niacin would prevent experimental pellagra (100). It is now known that dietary deficiency of the vitamin itself or of tryptophan, an amino acid precursor of niacin, can lead to pellagra. The disease has now become very rare largely as the result of enriching common foods, such as bread, with niacin. Most recent cases have been encountered in patients with alcoholism and are often clinically atypical, e.g. without associated skin lesions (46).

The neuropathological changes classically associated with niacin deficiency consist of neuronal enlargement, nuclear displacement, and loss of Nissl granules. These alterations resemble chromatolysis following axonal disruption. The changes are most pronounced among the large neurons in the cerebral cortex and basal ganglia, in various brain stem nuclei, in the cerebellar roof nuclei, and among the anterior horn motor neurons of the spinal cord. Typically unaffected are neurons in Ammon's horn, hypoglossal neurons, and Purkinje cells. In addition, some cases have been reported to show degeneration of the posterior columns and corticospinal tracts. Vacuolation of myelin and tissue spongiosus is less severe than in patients with myelopathy secondary to vitamin B_{12} deficiency. Peripheral neuropathy has also been observed in niacin deficiency.

Experimental pyridoxine deficiency in monkeys reproduces the neuronal changes classically associated with human niacin deficiency (114). Furthermore, the neurological deficits in some patients with pellagra persist despite niacin therapy. For these reasons, it has been suggested that the neurological deficits in patients with pellagra may actually be due to an associated pyridoxine deficiency.

B_{12} DEFICIENCY

Man cannot synthesize vitamin B_{12} and must obtain this essential vitamin from dietary sources, principally meats and dairy products. Prior to absorption from the ileum, the vitamin is bound to intrinsic factor, a glycoprotein produced by gastric parietal cells. Human vitamin B_{12} deficiency results most often from inadequate production of intrinsic factor. An immunologically mediated atrophic gastritis is responsible for the failure of intrinsic factor production in patients with pernicious anemia. Rarely, inadequate intrinsic factor production is associated with gastric neoplasms or following gastrectomy. Vitamin B_{12} deficiency can also result from diseases that impede absorption of the vitamin from the small intestine. These include various malabsorption syndromes, intestinal tuberculosis, regional enteritis, and lymphomas. Still other cases have resulted from competitive uptake of the vitamin by fish tapeworm infestation or bacterial overgrowth in blind loops and diverticula of the small intestine (78).

Vitamin B_{12} is currently known to be a coenzyme for only two reactions in man, conversion of L-methylmalonyl-CoA to succinyl-CoA and methylation of homocysteine to methionine. The deficiency has profound effects on the hematopoietic system, epithelial surfaces, and the nervous system. The biochemical basis for the deleterious effects of this vitamin deficiency upon the nervous system remains to be elucidated.

Grossly discernible alterations are evident only with long-standing severe disease. Under these circumstances, the spinal cord may be mildly shrunken with discolored translucent posterior and lateral columns. Microscopically, confluent patchy lesions displaying varying degrees of demyelination, spongiosus, and gliosis are found in the posterior and lateral columns (Fig. 9.17). In the most severe cases, the anterior columns also may be involved. Conversely, lesions may be confined to the posterior columns in milder cases. The lesions are typically most severe in the lower cervical and thoracic spinal cord segments but may extend rostrally to the medulla.

The earliest lesions recognizable by light microscopy consist of vacuolar distension of myelin sheaths (79). Fibers with the greatest diameter are affected predominantly. The pathological changes begin in small foci that later coalesce to become

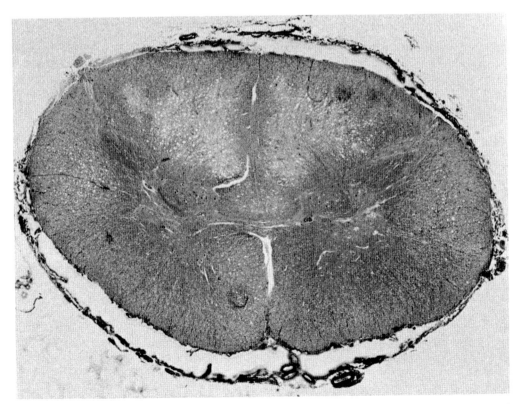

Figure 9.17. Myelopathy associated with vitamin B_{12} deficiency. Note the status spongiosus in the dorsal, lateral, and ventral columns. Luxol fast blue. (Original magnification ×9.)

large patchy lesions. The vacuolation in the myelin imparts a characteristic spongy appearance to the affected white matter (Fig. 9.18). Demyelination ensues and lipid-laden macrophages become scattered throughout the spongy lesions. At least some of the axons are eventually destroyed and undergo Wallerian degeneration. Although an astrocytic response is not marked initially, dense gliosis can be seen in long-standing cases with extensive destruction. The degree of gliosis appears to correlate more closely with the duration of the disease than therapy.

Occasionally, somewhat similar appearing spongy mixed demyelination and destructive lesions may be seen in the cerebral white matter. These lesions have been designated as Lichtheim plaques. Very rarely, the lesions may involve the optic nerves affecting, in particular, the papillomacular bundles. Vitamin B_{12} deficiency induced experimentally in rhesus monkeys has produced neuropathological changes that are similar to those in man except for the more

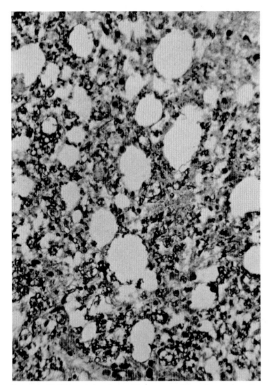

Figure 9.18. Myelopathy associated with vitamin B_{12} deficiency. Luxol fast blue. (Original magnification ×250.)

severe involvement of the visual pathways (3).

The frequency and nature of peripheral nerve involvement in vitamin B_{12} deficiency is controversial. Although Pallis and Lewis (78) regard peripheral neuropathy as the most common neurological complication of this vitamin deficiency, other authors find this manifestation uncommon. Although some of the earlier studies emphasized a reduction in the number of large myelin sheaths suggesting segmental demyelination, more recent reports (53) have described predominantly axonal degeneration. In one report of B_{12} deficiency associated with malabsorption, the peripheral nerve changes were those of a giant axonal neuropathy (99).

VITAMIN E DEFICIENCY

Experimental vitamin E deficiency has been studied extensively in various laboratory animals. In the rat, deficiency of this vitamin consistently produces a slowly evolving ataxia and hind limb paralysis. The most conspicuous neuropathological alterations in these animals consist of demyelination of the dorsal funiculi of the spinal cord and the presence of dystrophic axons in the medulla. The so-called "dystrophic axons" are terminal or preterminal spherical to fusiform enlargements that may be many times larger than the axons from which they are derived. Most of the dystrophic axons are homogeneous or granular in appearance although some may be vacuolated or appear as spiked balls. They can be seen with hematoxylin and eosin but are better demonstrated with trichrome and silver stains. Ultrastructural studies have shown the dystrophic axons to contain strikingly pleomorphic accumulations of filaments, membranes, tubules, altered mitochondria, and osmiophilic granular material (55).

In recent years, a number of reports have appeared suggesting that prolonged severe deficiency of vitamin E also may adversely affect the human nervous system. These reports have been based largely on neuropathological observations in individuals who have had diseases that impair absorption and transport of this fat-soluble vitamin. Dystrophic axons are characteristically abundant in certain degenerative neurological disorders and increase nonspecifically in number with aging. However, Sung et al. (107) have found dystrophic axons in large numbers, disproportionate to age, in the gracile nuclei of children and young adults with biliary atresia or cystic fibrosis (Fig. 9.19). Furthermore, the dystrophic axons were more numerous in those patients who had not received supplemental vitamin E. In two other large series of patients with cystic fibrosis, demyelination of the fasciculus gracilis was found in 11 and 19% of the cases (18, 32).

In relatively few instances have clinical manifestations been correlated with these neuropathological alterations and/or low serum levels of vitamin E. Rosenblum et al. (94) described a progressive neurological syndrome in six children with chronic cholestatic liver disease. Serum vitamin E levels were low in all patients. Neuropathological studies were performed on two of the patients. These showed dystrophic axons, demyelination of the posterior columns of the spinal cord, and loss of large

myelinated fibers from peripheral nerves. Patients with abetalipoproteinemia also have peripheral neuropathy, spinocerebellar manifestations, and low serum vitamin E levels; however, neuropathologic studies are limited. Recently, Harding et al. (41) reported two adults with chronic fat malabsorption who developed progressive neurological disorders resembling spinocerebellar degeneration. Serum vitamin E was undetectable, and one adult showed clinical improvement with vitamin E therapy. Until more correlative long-term studies are available, the role of vitamin E deficiency in the pathogenesis of human neurological disease will remain controversial.

ACKNOWLEDGMENTS

The author wants to thank Ms. Linda Kent Tomago for typing the manuscript and Ms. Sally Anderson for preparing illustrations.

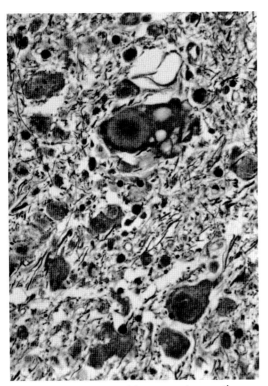

Figure 9.19. Dystrophic axons in gracile nucleus from a child with mucoviscidosis. Bodian silver. (Original magnification ×420.)

References

1. Adams RD, Victor M, Mancall EL: Central pontine myelinolysis: A hitherto undescribed disease occurring in alcoholics and malnourished patients. *Arch Neurol Psychiatry* 81:154, 1959.
2. Adelson L, Sunshine I: Fatal hydrogen sulfide intoxication. *Arch Pathol* 81:375, 1966.
3. Agamanolis DP, Chester EM, Victor M, Kark JA, Hines JD, Harris JW: Neuropathology of experimental vitamin B$_{12}$ deficiency in monkeys. *Neurology* 26:905, 1976.
4. Auer RN, Fox AJ, Kaufmann JCE: The histologic effect of intraventricular injection of metrizamide. *Arch Neurol* 39:60, 1982.
5. Barbeau A, Inoué N, Cloutier T: Role of manganese in dystonia. In: Eldridge R, Fahn S (eds): *Dystonia. Advances in Neurology.* New York, Raven Press, 1976, pp 339–351.
6. Behse F, Carlsen F: Histology and ultrastructure of alterations in neuropathy. *Muscle Nerve* 1:368, 1978.
7. Bennett IL Jr, Carey FH, Mitchell GL Jr, Cooper MN: Acute methyl alcohol poisoning: a review based on experiences in an outbreak of 323 cases. *Medicine* 32:431, 1953.
8. Berger JR, Ayyar DR: Neurological complications of ethylene glycol intoxication. Report of a case. *Arch Neurol* 38:724, 1981.
9. Bethlenfalvay NC, Bergin JJ: Severe cerebral toxicity after intravenous nitrogen mustard therapy. *Cancer* 29:366, 1972.
10. Blakemore WF, Palmer AC, Noel PRB: Ultrastructural changes in isoniazid-induced brain oedema in the dog. *J Neurocytol* 1:263, 1972.
11. Blass JP, Gibson GE: Abnormality of a thiamine-requiring enzyme in patients with Wernicke-Korsakoff syndrome. *N Engl J Med* 297:1367, 1977.
12. Braico KT, Humbert JR, Terplan KL, Lehotay JM: Laetrile intoxication. Report of a fatal case. *N Engl J Med* 300:238, 1979.
13. Breuer AC, Pitman SW, Dawson DM, Schoene WC: Paraparesis following intrathecal cytosine arabinoside. *Cancer* 40:2817, 1977.
14. Brucher JM: Neuropathological problems posed by car-

bon monoxide poisoning and anoxia. *Prog Brain Res* 24:75, 1967.

15. Burger PC, Kamenar E, Schold SC, Fay JW, Phillips GL, Herzig GP: Encephalomyelopathy following high-dose BCNU therapy. *Cancer* 48:1318, 1981.

16. Buxton PH, Hayward M: Polyneuritis cranialis associated with industrial trichloroethylene poisoning. *J Neurol Neurosurg Psychiatr* 30:511, 1967.

17. Carlen PL, Wilkinson DA, Wortzman G, Holgate R, Cordingley J, Lee MA, Huzar L, Moddel G, Singh R, Kiraly L, Rankin JG: Cerebral atrophy and functional deficits in alcoholics without clinically apparent liver disease. *Neurology* 31:377, 1981.

18. Cavalier SJ, Gambetti P: Dystrophic axons and spinal cord demyelination in cystic fibrosis. *Neurology* 31:714, 1981.

19. Cavanagh JB: Metallic toxicity and the nervous system. In: Smith, WT, Cavanagh JB: *Recent Advances in Neuropathology.* Edinburgh, Churchill Livingstone, 1979, ch 10, pp 247–275.

20. Cho E-S: Toxic effects of adriamycin on the ganglia of the peripheral nervous system: a neuropathological study. *J Neuropathol Exp Neurol* 36:907, 1977.

21. Clarren SK: Recognition of fetal alcohol syndrome. *JAMA* 245:2436, 1981.

22. Clasen RA, Hartman JF, Starr AJ, Coogan PS, Pandolfi S, Laing I, Becker R, Hass GM: Electron microscopic and chemical studies of the vascular changes and edema of lead encephalopathy. A comparative study of the human and experimental disease. *Am J Pathol* 74:215, 1974.

23. Courville CB: *Effects of Alcohol on the Nervous System of Man.* Los Angeles, San Lucas Press, 1966, ed 2.

24. Crapper DR, Krishnan SS, Quittkat S: Aluminum, neurofibrillary degeneration and Alzheimer's disease. *Brain* 99:67, 1976.

25. Cravioto H, Korein J, Silberman J: Wernicke's encephalopathy: a clinical and pathological study of 28 autopsied cases. *Arch Neurol* 4:510, 1961.

26. Crosley CJ, Rorke LB, Evans A, Nigro M: Central nervous system lesions in childhood leukemia. *Neurology* 28:678, 1978.

27. Davis LE, Standefer JC, Kornfeld M, Abercrombe DM, Butler C: Acute thallium poisoning: toxicological and morphological studies of the nervous system. *Ann Neurol* 10:38, 1981.

28. Davis LE, Wands JR, Weiss SA, Price DL, Girling EF: Central nervous system intoxication from mercurous chloride laxatives. Quantitative, histochemical, and ultrastructural studies. *Arch Neurol* 30:428, 1974.

29. Dreyfus PM: The regional distribution of transketolase in the normal and the thiamine-deficient nervous system. *J Neuropathol Exp Neurol* 24:119, 1965.

30. Finck PA: Exposure to carbon monoxide: review of the literature and 567 autopsies. *Milit Med* 131:1513, 1966.

31. Fullerton PM: Chronic peripheral neuropathy produced by lead poisoning in guinea-pigs. *J Neuropathol Exp Neurol* 25:214, 1966.

32. Geller A, Gilles F, Schwachman H: Degeneration of fasciculus gracilis in cystic fibrosis. *Neurology* 27:185, 1977.

33. Ghatak NR, Hadfield MG, Rosenblum WI: Association of central pontine myelinolysis and Marchiafava-Bignami disease. *Neurology* 28:1295, 1978.

34. Ghatak NR, Santoso RA, McKinney WM: Cerebellar degeneration following long-term phenytoin therapy. *Neurology* 26:818, 1976.

35. Ginsberg MD, Myers RE, McDonagh BF: Experimental carbon monoxide encephalopathy in the primate. II. Clinical aspects, neuropathology and physiologic correlation. *Arch Neurol* 30:209, 1974.

36. Goldberg ID, Bloomer WD, Dawson DM: Nervous system toxic effects of cancer therapy. *JAMA* 247:1437, 1982.

37. Goldman JE, Horoupian DS: Demyelination of the lateral geniculate nucleus in central pontine myelinolysis. *Ann Neurol* 9:185, 1981.

38. Graham DG, Shaw BB, Richards RG, Wolfram JW: An hypothesis for the molecular pathogenesis of hexane neuropathy. *J Neuropathol Exp Neurol* 39:356, 1980.

39. Haid RW, Gutmann L, Crosby TW: Wernicke-Korsakoff encephalopathy after gastric plication. *JAMA* 247:2566, 1982.

40. Hakim AM, Pappius HM: The effect of thiamine deficiency on local cerebral glucose utilization. *Ann Neurol* 9:334, 1981.

41. Harding AE, Muller DPR, Thomas PK, Willison HJ: Spinocerebellar degeneration secondary to chronic intestinal malabsorption: a vitamin E deficiency syndrome. *Ann Neurol* 12:419, 1982.

42. Harper C: Wernicke's encephalopathy: a more common disease than realized. A neuropathological study of 51 cases. *J Neurol Neurosurg Psychiatr* 42:226, 1979.

43. Hillbom M, Kaste M: Alcohol intoxication: a risk factor for primary subarachnoid hemorrhage. *Neurology* 32:706, 1982.

44. Hirano A, Kochen JA: Further observations on the effects of lead implantation in rat brains. *Acta Neuropathol* 34:87, 1976.

45. Hirano A, Levine S, Zimmerman HM: Experimental cyanide encephalopathy: electron microscopic observations of early lesions in white matter. *J Neuropathol Exp Neurol* 26:200, 1967.

46. Ishii N, Nishihara Y: Pellagra among chronic alcoholics: clinical and pathological study of 20 necropsy cases. *J Neurol Neurosurg Psychiatr* 44:209, 1981.

47. Kim YH, Foo M, Terry RD: Cyanide encephalopathy following therapy with sodium nitroprusside. *Arch Pathol Lab Med* 106:392, 1982.

48. Kleinschmidt-DeMasters BK, Norenberg MD: Cerebellar degeneration in the rat following rapid correction of hyponatremia. *Ann Neurol* 10:561, 1981.

49. Kleinschmidt-DeMasters BK, Norenberg MD: Neuropathologic observations in electrolyte-induced myelinolysis in the rat. *J Neuropathol Exp Neurol* 41:67, 1982.

50. Koch T, Schultz P, Williams R, Lambert P: Giant axonal neuropathy: a childhood disorder of microfilaments. *Ann Neurol* 1:438, 1977.

51. Koeppen AH, Barron KD: Marchiafava-Bignami disease. *Neurology* 28:290, 1978.

52. Koller WC, Glatt SL, Perlik S, Huckman MS, Fox JH: Cerebellar atrophy demonstrated by computed tomography. *Neurology* 31:405, 1981.

53. Kosik KS, Mullins TF, Bradley WG, Tempelis LD, Cretella AJ: Coma and axonal degeneration in vitamin B12 deficiency. *Arch Neurol* 37:590, 1980.

54. Krous HF: Fetal alcohol syndrome: a dilemma of maternal alcoholism. *Pathol Annu* 16 (1):295, 1981.

55. Lampert PW: A comparative electron microscopic study of reactive, degenerating, regenerating and dystrophic axons. *J Neuropathol Exp Neurol* 26:345, 1967.

56. Lampert PW, Schochet SS Jr: Electron microscopic observations on experimental spongy degeneration of the cerebellar white matter. *J Neuropathol Exp Neurol* 27:210, 1968.

57. Lampert PW, Schochet SS Jr: Demyelination and remyelination in lead neuropathy: Electron microscopic studies. *J Neuropathol Exp Neurol* 27:527, 1968.

58. Lapresle J, Fardeau M: The central nervous system and carbon monoxide poisoning. II. Anatomical study of brain lesions following intoxication with carbon monoxide (22 cases). *Prog Brain Res* 24:31, 1967.

59. Layzer RB: Myeloneuropathy after prolonged exposure to nitrous oxide. *Lancet* 2:1227, 1978.

60. Leong ASY: Marchiafava-Bignami disease in a non-alcoholic Indian male. *Pathology* 11:241, 1979.

61. Louria DB, Joselow MM, Browder AA: The human toxicity of certain trace elements. *Ann Intern Med* 76:307, 1972.

62. Luse SA, Wood WG: The brain in fatal carbon tetrachloride poisoning. *Arch Neurol* 17:304, 1967.

63. McDermott JR, Smith AI, Iqbal K, Wisniewski HM: Brain aluminum in aging and Alzheimer disease. *Neurology* 29:809, 1979.

64. McLean DR, Jacobs H, Mielke BW: Methanol poisoning: a clinical and pathological study. *Ann Neurol* 8:161, 1980.

65. Mair WGP, Warrington EK, Weiskrantz L: Memory disorder in Korsakoff psychosis: a neuropathological and neuropsychological investigation of two cases. *Brain* 102:749, 1979.

66. Mallow DW, Herrick MK, Gathman G: Fetal exposure to anticonvulsant drugs. Detailed pathological study of a case. *Arch Pathol Lab Med* 104:214, 1980.

67. Markesbery WR, Ehmann WD, Hossain TIM, Alauddin M, Goodin DT: Instrumental neutron activation analysis of brain aluminum in Alzheimer disease and aging. *Ann Neurol* 10:511, 1981.

68. Martin-Amat G, McMartin KE, Hayreh SS, Hayreh MS, Tephly TR: Methanol poisoning: ocular toxicity produced by formate. *Toxicol Appl Pharmacol* 45:201, 1978.

69. Martinez AJ, Boehm R, Hadfield MG: Acute hexachlorophene encephalopathy: clinico-neuropathological correlation. *Acta Neuropathol* 28:93, 1974.

70. Messert B, Orrison WW, Hawkins MJ, Quaglieri CE: Central pontine myelinolysis: considerations on etiology, diagnosis, and treatment. *Neurology* 29:147, 1979.

71. Meyers CC, Schochet SS Jr, McCormick WF: Wernicke's encephalopathy in infancy: development during parenteral nutrition. *Acta Neuropathol* 43:267, 1978.

72. Nadel AM: Vidarabine therapy for herpes simplex encephalitis: the development of an unusual tremor during treatment. *Arch Neurol* 38:384, 1981.

73. Norenberg MD, Leslie KO, Robertson AS: Association between rise in serum sodium and central pontine myelinolysis. *Ann Neurol* 11:128, 1982.

74. Ohnishi A, Tsuji S, Igisu H, Murai Y, Goto I, Kuroiwa Y, Tsujihata M, Takamori M: Beriberi neuropathy: morphometric study of sural nerve. *J Neurol Sci* 45:177, 1980.

75. Omojola MF, Fox AJ, Auer RN, Viñuela FV: Hemorrhagic encephalitis produced by selective non-occlusive intracarotid BCNU injection in dogs. *J Neurosurg* 57:791, 1982.

76. Orthner H: Neuartige Hirnbefunde bei Methyl-Alkohol-Vergiftung. *Zentralbl. Allg. Pathol.* 85:11, 1949.

77. Packer RJ, Zimmerman RA, Rosenstock J, Rorke LB, Norris DG, Berman PH: Focal encephalopathy following methotrexate therapy: administration via a misplaced intraventricular catheter. *Arch Neurol* 38:450, 1981.

78. Pallis CA, Lewis PD: *The Neurology of Gastrointestinal Disease*. London, W B Saunders, 1974.

79. Pant SS, Asbury AK, Richardson EP Jr: The myelopathy of pernicious anemia. A neuropathological reappraisal. *Acta Neurol Scand Suppl* 44(35):1, 1968.

80. Parry MF, Wallach D: Ethylene glycol poisoning. *Am J Med* 57:143, 1974.

81. Peiffer J, Majewski F, Fischbach H, Bierch JR, Volk B: Alcohol embryo- and fetopathy. *J Neurol Sci* 41:125, 1979.

82. Peña CE: Wernicke's encephalopathy: report of seven cases with severe nerve cell changes in the mamillary bodies. *Am J Clin Pathol* 51:603, 1969.

83. Pentschew A: Morphology and morphogenesis of lead encephalopathy. *Acta Neuropathol* 5:133, 1965.

84. Pentschew A, Ebner FF, Kovatch RM: Experimental manganese encephalopathy in monkeys: a preliminary report. *J Neuropathol Exp Neurol* 22:488, 1963.

85. Pentschew A, Garro F: Lead encephalo-myelopathy of the suckling rat and its implications on the porphyrinopathic nervous diseases: with special reference to the permeability disorders of the nervous system's capillaries. *Acta Neuropathol* 6:266, 1966.

86. Peylan-Ramu N, Poplack DG, Pizzo PA, Adornato BT, Dichiro G: Abnormal CT scans of the brain in asymptomatic children with acute lymphocytic leukemia after prophylactic treatment of the central nervous system with radiation and intrathecal chemotherapy. *N Engl J Med* 298:815, 1978.

87. Powell HC, Myers RR, Lampert PW: Changes in schwann cells and vessels in lead neuropathy. *Am J Pathol* 109:193, 1982.

88. Powell H, Swarner O, Gluck L, Lampert P: Hexachlorophene myelinopathy in premature infants. *J Pediatr* 82:976, 1973.

89. Press MF: Lead encephalopathy in neontal Long-Evans rats: morphologic studies. *J Neuropathol Exp Neurol* 36:169, 1977.

90. Price RA, Birdwell DA: The central nervous system in childhood leukemia. III. Mineralizing microangiopathy and dystrophic calcification. *Cancer* 42:717, 1978.

91. Price RA, Jamieson PA: The central nervous system in childhood leukemia. II. Subacute leukoencephalopathy. *Cancer* 35:306, 1975.

92. Rappport RL, Shaw CM: Phenytoin-related cerebellar degeneration without seizures. *Ann Neurol* 2:437, 1977.

93. Riehl JL, Brown WJ: Acute cerebellar syndrome secondary to 5-fluorouracil therapy. *Neurology* 14:961, 1964.

94. Rosenblum JL, Keating JP, Prensky AL, Nelson JS: A progressive neurologic syndrome in children with chronic liver disease. *N Engl J Med* 304:503, 1981.

95. Rubinstein LJ, Herman MM, Long TF, Wilbur JR: Disseminated necrotizing leukoencephalopathy: a complication of treated central nervous system leukemia and lymphoma. *Cancer* 35:291, 1975.

96. Sabri MI, Spencer PS: Toxic distal axonopathy: biochemical studies and hypothetical mechanisms. In: Experimental and Clinical Neurotoxicology, Spencer PS, Schumberg HH, Baltimore, Williams & Wilkins, 1980, ch 14, pp 206–219.

97. Salcman M, Defendini R, Correll J, Gilman S: Neuropathological changes in cerebellar biopsies of epileptic patients. *Ann Neurol* 3:10, 1978.

98. Sato Y, Tabira T, Tateishi J: Marchiafava-Bignami disease, striatal degeneration and other neurological complications of chronic alcoholism in a Japanese. *Acta Neuropathol* 53:15, 1981.

99. Schochet SS Jr, Chesson AL Jr: Giant axonal neuropathy: possibly secondary to vitamin B12 malabsorption. *Acta Neuropathol* 40:79, 1977.

100. Sebrell WH Jr: History of pellagra. *Fed Proc* 40:1520, 1981.

101. Sharpe JA, Hostovsky M, Bilbao JM, Rewcastle NB: Methanol optic neuropathy. A histopathological study. *Neurology* 32:1093, 1982.

102. Shiraki H: Neuropathological aspects of organic mercury intoxication, including minamata disease. In: *Handbook of Clinical Neurology*, Vinken PJ, Bruyn GW (eds): Amsterdam, North-Holland, 1979, vol 36, ch 5, pp 83–145.

103. Shuman RM, Leech RW, Alvord EC Jr: Neurotoxicity of hexachlorphene in humans. II. A clinicopathological study of 46 premature infants. *Arch Neurol* 32:320, 1975.

104. Skullerud K, Halvorsen K: Encephalomyelopathy following intrathecal methotrexate treatment in a child with acute leukemia. *Cancer* 42:1211, 1978.

105. Slyter H, Liwnicz B, Herrick MK, Mason R: Fatal myeloencephalopathy caused by intrathecal vincristine. *Neurology* 30:867, 1980.

106. Spencer PS, Schaumburg HH: Central-peripheral distal axonopathy—The pathology of drying-back polyneuropathies. In: *Progress in Neuropathology*, Zimmerman HM (ed): New York, Grune & Stratton, 1977, vol 3, ch 9, pp 253–295.

107. Sung JH, Park SH, Mastri A, Warwick WJ: Axonal dystrophy in the gracile nucleus in congenital biliary atresia and cystic fibrosis (mucoviscidosis): beneficial effect of vitamin E therapy. *J Neuropathol Exp Neurol* 39:584, 1980.

108. Telerman-Toppet N, Flament-Durand J, Khoubesserian P, Couck AM, Lambelin D, Cöers C: Encephalomyeloneuropathy in acute arsenic poisoning: an ultrastructural study of the sural nerve. *Clin Neuropathol* 1:47, 1982.

109. Thompson DS, Hutton JT, Stears JC, Sung JH, Norenberg MD: Computerized tomography in the diagnosis of central and extrapontine myelinolysis. *Arch Neurol* 38:243, 1981.

110. Tischner KH, Schröder JM: The effects of cadmium chloride on organotypic cultures of rat sensory ganglia: a light and electron microscopic study. *J Neurol Sci*

16:383, 1972.

111. Valpey R, Sumi SM, Copass MK, Goble GJ: Acute and chronic progressive encephalopathy due to gasoline sniffing. *Neurology* 28:507, 1978.

112. Van Etta L, Brown J, Mastri A, Wilson T: Fatal vidarabine toxicity in a patient with normal renal function. *JAMA* 246:1703, 1981.

113. Victor M: The Wernicke-Korsakoff syndrome. In: Vinken PJ, Bruyn GW: (eds): *Handbook of Clinical Neurology.* Amsterdam, North-Holland, 1976, vol 28, Ch 9, pp 243-270.

114. Victor M, Adams RD: The neuropathology of experimental vitamin B_6 deficiency in monkeys. *Am J Clin Nutr* 4:346, 1956.

115. Victor M, Adams RD, Mancall EL: A restricted form of cerebellar cortical degeneration occurring in alcoholic patients. *Arch Neurol* 1:579, 1959.

116. Walsh TJ, Clark AW, Parhad IM, Green WR: Neurotoxic effects of cisplatin therapy. *Arch Neurol* 39:719, 1982.

117. Watanabe I, Hodges GR, Dworzack DL, Kepes JJ, Duesing GF: Neurotoxicity of intrathecal gentamicin: a case report and experimental study. *Ann Neurol* 4:564, 1978.

118. Webster WS, Valois AA: The toxic effects of cadmium on the neonatal mouse CNS. *J Neuropathol Exp Neurol* 40:247, 1981.

119. Winkelman MD, Hines JH: Cerebellar cortical degeneration caused by high-dose systemic therapy with cytosine arabinoside. *Ann Neurol* 12:77, 1982.

120. Wright DG, Laureno R, Victor M: Pontine and extrapontine myelinolysis. *Brain* 102:361, 1979.

CHAPTER 10

Central Nervous System Manifestations of Systemic Disease

MICHAEL D. NORENBERG, M.D.
JOCELYN B. GREGORIOS, M.D.

INTRODUCTION

The immense complexity of the nervous system along with its great metabolic demands renders it extremely dependent on the integrity of other organs for the provision of oxygen, nutrients, and hormones, the maintenance of proper electrolyte and pH status, and the elimination of potential toxins. It is therefore not surprising that one of the earliest and most dramatic manifestations of organ system failure is a central nervous system derangement.

Clinically, patients often present with a generalized disorder of the nervous system. There is often a decline in sensorium with stupor, coma, and frequently, myoclonus. When the metabolic insult is acute, it is often associated with generalized seizures and severe neurological derangements. However, with chronic insults, the brain demonstrates a remarkable capacity to call forth a number of compensatory mechanisms that result in little to no clinical change (for review of clinical aspects, see Plum and Posner (441), and Griggs and Satran (229)).

Symptoms may occasionally be focal. This is usually explained by the presence of a subclinical anatomical lesion which in the setting of a superimposed metabolic insult results in focal symptoms.

From a morphological point of view the changes are often minimal and unremarkable, suggesting that in most instances one is dealing principally with a biochemical derangement rather than an anatomical one. This perhaps explains why clinically these processes are often reversible. It is only when the metabolic insult has been excessive and prolonged that anatomical changes occur, thus accounting for the permanent clinical deficits that some of these patients display.

ANOXIC-ISCHEMIC ENCEPHALOPATHY AND RELATED DISORDERS

General Considerations

The brain is a metabolically very active organ, accounting for approximately 20% of the body's oxygen utilization. Additionally, because there are no significant stores of oxygen in brain and since the brain's metabolism is almost exclusively oxidative, as much as 15% of the cardiac output (55 ml/100 g/min) goes to the brain to meet that incessant demand. The principal function of oxygen is to provide high energy phosphates (ATP and phosphocreatine) for transmembrane ion transport, for axoplasmic transport of organelles and nutrients, for the manufacture of neurotransmitters, and for the synthesis of cellular

403

constituents required for the maintenance of tissue integrity (521).

Failure to provide sufficient oxygen to the tissues (anoxia) represents the commonest form of metabolic encephalopathy. Because of the brain's great and constant requirement for oxygen it is very vulnerable to any curtailment in this supply. Oxygen lack will lead to a cessation of oxidative phosphorylation and energy failure, eventually resulting in the disruption of cellular function and ultimately, destruction of cellular structure.

Cerebral oxygen deficiency is dramatically displayed in clinical settings. A decrease in arterial oxygen tension (PaO_2) to 40–50 mm Hg leads to impaired cognitive function. Levels of PaO_2 below 30 mm Hg for 10 sec lead to loss of consciousness and for 20 sec to loss of spontaneous electrical activity. Total circulatory arrest in man for 10–15 sec such as following a Stokes-Adams attack will result in loss of consciousness (471).

Anoxia is observed in a wide variety of clinical conditions where insufficient oxygen reaches blood (anoxic anoxia), such as following drowning, choking, anesthetic accidents, high altitude exposure; where there is insufficient oxygen content in blood (anemic anoxia) as in anemia, carbon monoxide poisoning, and with the formation of methemoglobin; and where certain poisons interfere with the utilization of oxygen (histotoxic anoxia), such as in cyanide intoxication. Most commonly, however, it is seen in conditions resulting in decreased cerebral blood perfusion (stagnant anoxia), such as following a cardiac arrest, hypotension, and increased intracranial pressure, a phenomenon referred to as global cerebral ischemia. The critical value of cerebral blood flow necessary to prevent brain injury is about 15 ml/100 g/min.

Pure anoxic injuries, however, are rare in humans, inasmuch as anoxia invariably induces cardiac failure very quickly (255, 557), thus adding a component of ischemia to the cerebral injury. It is likely that the cardiac status following anoxia is the critical factor in the brain's response to anoxic injury (503). Ischemia is considerably less well tolerated by tissues than uncomplicated anoxia, since in addition to deprivation of oxygen (and nutrients) there is also a failure to remove metabolic wastes that may be toxic (see below). Moreover, the brain manifests a remarkable resistance to pure anoxia (43, 384). Most probably it is only when anoxia is combined with perfusion failure that significant clinical and morphological derangements occur. Thus, despite a PaO_2 of 21 mm Hg, as long as perfusion pressure can be maintained, high energy phosphate levels are not significantly depressed, and lesions do not occur (147, 201, 216). Accordingly, most anoxic processes are better termed as anoxic-ischemic encephalopathy.

Mechanisms of Anoxic-Ischemic Injury

While cerebral protective mechanisms against hypoxic injury exist (e.g., increase in cerebral blood flow and more efficient extraction of oxygen) (147), this protection is however limited. When the anoxia occurs in sufficient duration and intensity there is an abrupt drop in the levels of high energy phosphates (521). Complete cerebral ischemia for 1 min results in a 50% fall in ATP, and after 2 min ATP becomes virtually undetectable. This energy failure and the inability of the cell to perform ATP-requiring functions appear to be the principal mechanism responsible for injury and damage to nervous tissue (461). In general, as long as high energy levels are maintained the potential for recovery is present. (For review of energy metabolism in anoxic-ischemic states see Siesjö (521) and Duffy and Plum (147).)

Not all of the problems associated with hypoxia, however, can be explained simply by energy failure (522). With a PaO_2 of 30 mm Hg there is a significant impairment in the level of consciousness, yet there is no substantial fall in high energy phosphates (147). Recent studies have suggested that abnormalities in neurotransmitters may be responsible for this early neurological deterioration. Depression in the synthesis of catecholamines has been described (126). Hypoxia initiates a perturbation in the tricarboxylic acid intermediates that subsequently affects the level of the neurotransmitter amino acids glutamate, aspartate, and GABA (57, 148). It is possible that these amino acids, particularly glutamic acid, may additionally cause destructive changes (66). Acetylcholine synthesis has also been shown to be depressed (211). Related to abnormalities in neurotransmitter metabolism is the elevation of cyclic AMP (303). It would seem that the early phase of brain failure following anoxia-ischemia is probably due to derangements in neurotransmitter metabolism rather than to structural anatomical changes. This phase appears to be fully reversible.

The precise mechanisms by which anoxia-ischemia and associated energy failure bring about irreversible tissue injury to the CNS have not been completely elucidated as yet. A number of events, however, have been identified, some of which may have a deleterious effect on the nervous system. These include the development of edema, increase in lactic acid, free fatty acids, generation of free radicals, increase in extracellular potassium and ammonia, abnormalities in calcium flux, and reperfusion problems. This currently represents an important area of investigation because of the potential for reversal by pharmacological means. Detailed reviews of these factors are provided in articles by Siesjö (522), Plum (439), and Raichle (452).

EDEMA

Among the most significant and earliest sequelae of hypoxia-ischemia is the development of edema. Its harmful effect stems from the elevation of intracranial pressure as well as its interference in the diffusion of nutrients and disturbance in gaseous exchange (70). Edema is initially cytotoxic (intracellular) (507), as brain swelling occurs before there is endothelial injury (199, 201). With the eventual development of endothelial injury there is a disturbance of the blood-brain barrier, and the edema becomes vasogenic (extracellular) (42, 329, 409).

Several factors appear to be operative in the development of cytotoxic edema: (a) Energy failure will lead to impaired ion homeostasis resulting in an excessive amount of intracellular water and sodium ions (236, 264). (b) Anoxia-ischemia is associated with elevation in extracellular K^+ concentration (249) and a K^+-stimulated Cl-transport system has been described in astrocytes leading to increased transport of fluid into these cells (70). (c) Increased osmolality (from either tissue breakdown or release of osmols from tissue stores) has been found in anoxic-ischemic brain which will osmotically draw fluid into the brain (358). (d) The increase in free fatty acids (see below) may also be responsible for edema (101).

The disturbance in the permeability properties of the blood-brain barrier leading to the vasogenic component of edema appears to be particularly related to the presence of hypercapnia (42) and perhaps more importantly to overall tissue necrosis (432), rather than to a specific vascular pathology. It is only observed at least 4–6 h following an anoxic insult.

LACTIC ACID

In recent years the potential toxic role of lactic acid has been extensively investigated. When oxygen tension falls below 50 mm Hg there is an increase in the glycolytic rate, leading to lactate formation through the activation of phosphofructokinase (41). Myers (382, 383), developing on the earlier views of Lindenberg (325) and Ames and Gurian (12), postulated that lactate and/or its associated acidosis may have a deleterious effect on both neurons and glia, an observation which has received substantial experimental support (217, 282, 450, 519). Although the mechanism by which lactate causes injury has not been established, the potential harmful effects of lactate are demonstrated when brain glucose and glycogen stores (required for lactate synthesis) are raised. Thus, when experimental animals are pretreated with glucose and then subsequently exposed to an anoxic-ischemic injury, they develop increased brain lactate, do poorly clinically, and have more extensive lesions pathologically than control nonpretreated animals.

FATTY ACIDS AND FREE RADICALS

Following anoxia the levels of free fatty acids are increased (51, 349), possibly due to the calcium activation of phospholipases. These fatty acids appear to be harmful especially to mitochondria and may inhibit Na-K ATPase (8, 101). The elevation of the polyunsaturated fatty acid, arachidonic acid, and the subsequent formation of prostaglandins and leukotrienes appear to produce a number of injurious effects, dealing principally with altered hemodynamics, abnormalities in platelet aggregation, and the generation of free radicals (350). The reported beneficial effects of indomethacin in anoxic-ischemic encephalopathy (206) may perhaps be mediated by inhibition of cyclooxygenase which is required for the synthesis of prostaglandins.

The role of free radicals has also been explored in recent years (181, 187, 305). As noted above, some of the problems associated with elevated arachidonic acid may be through the generation of free radicals (192). Free radicals appear to cause damage by injuring cell membranes through the peroxidation of phospholipids. Perhaps the reported beneficial effects of barbiturates (257, 630) may partially be explained by their action as free radical scavengers (130).

CALCIUM, POTASSIUM, AND AMMONIA

Abnormalities in calcium flux have been described (237) and have been given great emphasis by Siesjö (522). During anoxia calcium shifts from the extracellular space into the cytosol followed by an additional release from intracellular storage sites. Such increase in intracellular calcium may trigger a chain of reactions culminating in cell death. In part this may be mediated by the activation of phospholipase leading to the release of free fatty acids. Additionally, the entry of calcium into mitochondria may be the first phase in the process of irreversible neuronal injury (197, 522). Calcium may also stimulate the activity of protease (165), as well as produce deleterious effects on microtubules and myelin (494, 496).

Following anoxia there is an elevation of the extracellular potassium ion concentration (249). This may lead to an increased vascular resistance with a subsequent fall in cerebral blood flow (47). In addition, such increase may serve as the principal trigger in the astroglial swelling so commonly seen initially following anoxia (71, 249). This swelling may also impair cerebral blood flow (33). The rise in extracellular potassium may also result in seizures (427).

Following anoxia-ischemia there is also a rise in brain ammonia (331), a substance which is neurotoxic, causing seizures and coma and which may additionally have vasoactive actions (see liver disease section).

NO-REFLOW AND REPERFUSION ABNORMALITIES

The concept of no-reflow phenomenon was proposed whereby the brain became incapable of being completely reperfused after a period of total cerebral ischemia (13, 262). Thus, the anoxic-ischemic episode initiated a chain of events that appeared to preclude the restoration of tissue viability by preventing in some manner the reestablishment of circulation. Indeed, it has been shown that if recirculation can be reestablished, even after 60 min of ischemia, some functional recovery can be achieved (262).

There has been considerable controversy over the existence and mechanism involved in recirculation failure (321). Originally it was felt that recirculation failure was due to blockage of the vascular lumen secondary to swelling of endothelial cells and astroglia. Others have later proposed that abnormalities in red blood cell aggregation and increased blood viscosity might be more important (173, 261).

Some have seriously questioned whether the phenomenon of no-reflow is clinically relevant (546). Typically it is observed only after a 20–30 min period of total ischemia, and by then, irreversible tissue damage has already occurred, so that the lack of reperfusion may actually be of no real material significance.

Although controversial (see below), it appears that the reestablishment of circulation (after a critical period of anoxia-ischemia), which will allow a suboptimal degree of metabolic activity to occur, may be associated with a greater degree of tissue damage than if reperfusion was not allowed to occur (33, 262, 283). Similarly, greater tissue damage is found if the ischemia has not been complete (522) as compared to complete ischemia. These paradoxical findings have been explained by several mechanisms. Indeed, many of the aforementioned mechanisms possibly involved in anoxic-ischemic injury occur only during the reperfusion period. Following the restoration of circulation the presence of oxygen may initiate the formation of free radicals, which subsequently may cause tissue injury (305). Similarly, the formation of prostaglandins is increased only during recirculation (their synthesis requires oxygen) and not during the ischemic period (207). The K^+-stimulated Cl-transport into astrocytes resulting in glial swelling also requires the presence of oxygen (248). Furthermore, the formation of edema (either cytotoxic or vasogenic) necessitates fluid which can only be derived from plasma (636). Perhaps most importantly, the reestablishment of circulation provides glucose which when metabolized to lactic acid may contribute to the development of cerebral injury.

The relevance of these observations in man, however, is uncertain, since the period of complete ischemia in the experimental studies was 20–60 min, while total ischemia for more than 4 min in man is rarely tolerated (441). Moreover, the studies involving reversibility following 60 min of ischemia showed improvement of metabolic and electrophysiologic parameters only. Clinical recovery was not described. Additionally, the animals had received barbiturates, which may have had a protective effect. Lastly, studies by Steen et al. (546) have strongly disputed the claim that incomplete ischemia results in a worse outcome than complete ischemia.

Morphology

As noted by Steegmann (545) and Moossy (374) the morphology of cerebral anoxia ischemia is highly variable and unpredictable possibly as a result of the interaction of a number of complex factors. Such factors as the severity and duration of anoxia-ischemia, nutritional state, circulatory status, level of intracranial pressure, history of previous injury that perhaps sensitizes the brain to ischemic injury (295), the presence of incomplete ischemia and reinstitution of circulation, body temperature, drugs, hypercapnia, and acidosis may all interact in ways that result in a variety of morphological patterns. Additionally, the phenomenon of "maturation" as delineated by Klatzo (295) has to be considered, in that a variable period of time may be required following an anoxic-ischemic insult for morphological changes to occur.

REGIONAL AND CELLULAR VULNERABILITIES

The entire brain is not uniformly involved following an anoxic-ischemic insult. Certain areas of the brain seem to be preferentially involved. Thus, grey matter is more vulnerable than white matter. In grey matter the boundary (watershed) zones between arterial circulations are particularly involved, a phenomenon first described by Meyer (369), emphasized in man by Zülch and Behrend (642) and by Romanul and Abramowicz (472), and reproduced experimentally by Brierley et al. (81). As these zones are the last to be perfused they are also the most vulnerable to a fall in perfusion pressure.

Neurons are the elements most sensitive to anoxia-ischemia. The earliest histopathological changes consist of isolated neuronal necrosis. In general, small neurons tend to be more sensitive than larger ones. With greater severity of injury total tissue necrosis follows (infarction). The hippocampus, especially the pyramidal cells of Sommer's sector (h1 segment) (Fig. 10.1) and the end-plate region, the cerebral cortex particularly lamina III, V, and VI, the cerebellum notably the Purkinje cells (Fig. 10.2), as well as the caudate and putamen are highly sensitive to anoxia-ischemia. Lesser degree of sensitivity to anoxia is observed in the globus pallidus, thalamus, hemispheric white matter, brain stem, and spinal cord.

Variable sensitivity is observed even among neurons in the same area. In the cerebellum the Purkinje cells are more sensitive as compared to granule cells, which in turn are more sensitive than Golgi II neurons (505). In the hippocampus the h2 segment (resistant sector) is usually spared together with the granule cells (fascia dentata).

Some have attempted to describe patterns, depending on whether anoxia or ischemia was the predominant insult. Thus Scholz (505) believed that ischemia was the responsible factor for injuries to the cerebral cortex, striatum, thalamus, hippocampus, and cerebellar cortex, whereas when anoxia was the offending agent, the globus pallidus, subthalamic nucleus, and dentate nucleus showed more severe damage. As

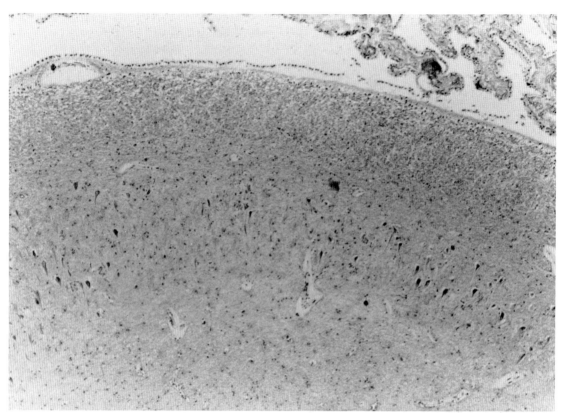

Figure 10.1. Section taken from Sommer's sector of Ammon's horn (hippocampus). This area is extremely vulnerable to anoxia and shows prominent neuronal shrinkage, neuronal loss, and diffuse gliosis. Bodian stain. (Original magnification ×40.)

noted previously pure anoxic insults are rare, and in the majority of instances both anoxia and ischemia appear to be involved. Moreover, such characteristic topographical responses to uncomplicated anoxia or uncomplicated ischemia as described by Scholz (505) have not been observed (80).

The rationale for the regional or selective vulnerability of anoxic-ischemic injury remains controversial. The vascular theory originally suggested by Spielmeyer (541), whereby the pattern is dependent on the degree of vascularity or the proximity of vessels to parenchymal structures, may account for some of the lesions (especially the watershed lesions) but not all. Thus laminar necrosis of the cortex cannot be explained on the basis of local circulatory derangements, as adjacent structures are supplied by the same vessels. The pattern of necrosis in the cerebellum similarly cannot be accounted for by circulatory factors.

Another proposed mechanism suggests that individual neuronal characteristics may account for such differential responses (pathoclisis of Vogt and Vogt) (601). Biochemical differences in various types of neurons have indeed been described (188, 287), as well as differences in oxygen requirements (550), perhaps accounting for the sensitivity or resistance to anoxic-ischemic injury. It is likely that combinations of both circulatory and local biochemical differences explain the differential response of nervous tissue to anoxia-ischemia. Recently, issues such as recirculation and nutritional status have been invoked to explain some of these morphologic patterns (381, 383).

In addition to regional sensitivities, different nervous tissue cells respond variably to anoxia so that neurons, astrocytes, oligodendrocytes, and endothelial cells show greater sensitivity in decreasing order (197, 272). Some feel that oligodendrocytes are more vulnerable than astrocytes (250).

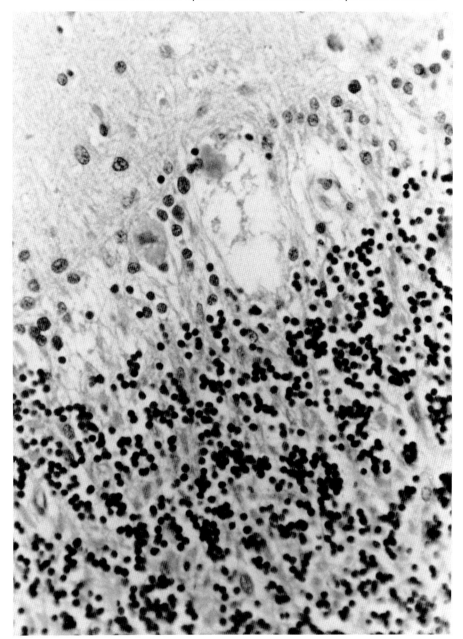

Figure 10.2. Cerebellar changes in early anoxia consisting of eosinophilia and disintegration of Purkinje cells with spongiform change of the Purkinje cell layer (lamina dissecans). Hemotoxylin and eosin (H&E) stain. (Original magnification ×400.)

FINDINGS IN MAN

The gross appearance of anoxic-ischemic encephalopathy consists of more or less symmetrical areas of injury involving the aforementioned sites. The brain is swollen (although not invariably so) and soft, while the grey matter may be pale or dusky. As the lesion gradually evolves, areas of cavitation in a laminar pattern may be observed in the cerebral cortex, particularly in the vascular boundary zones (600) as well as in the parietooccipital cortex (198) (Figs. 10.3–10.5). The terms laminar or pseudolaminar necrosis are commonly used to describe this state. Pseudolaminar necrosis

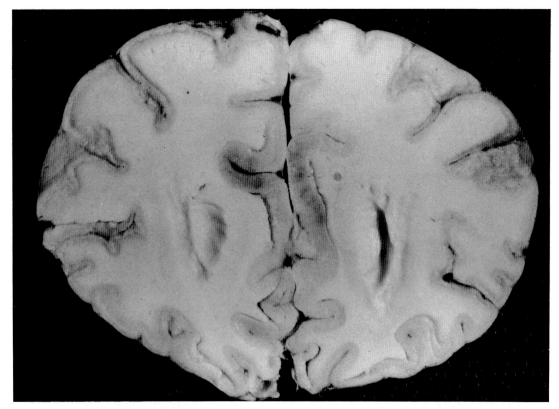

Figure 10.3. Coronal section through frontal lobes from a patient who died 3 weeks after cardiac arrest. Note the greyish discoloration and shrinkage of the cortex, causing a laminar cavitation at the junction of grey and white matter.

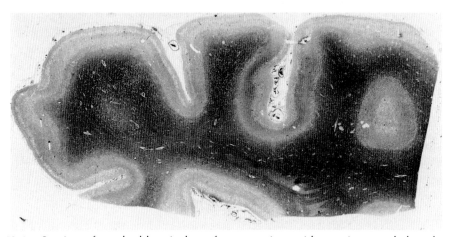

Figure 10.4. Section of cerebral hemisphere from a patient with anoxic encephalopathy. Pseudolaminar necrosis is indicated by pallor in layers 3 and 5. Note the more severe involvement of sulcal cortex. Luxol-fast blue/H&E. (Original magnification ×5.)

implies the involvement of more than one lamina, which is the usual case. In the cortex the sulcal depths are especially affected (629) (Fig. 10.4).

The light microscopic changes in man are not fundamentally different from infarcts as described in detail elsewhere in this text. During the first several hours,

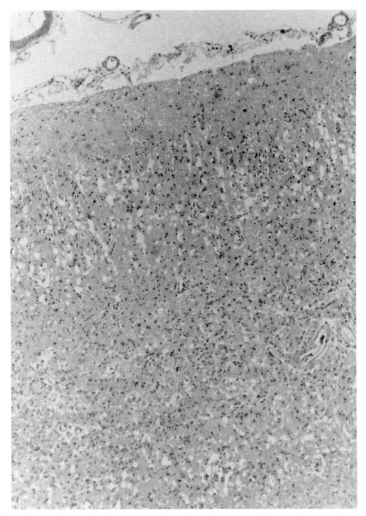

Figure 10.5. Section of cerebral cortex showing the spongiform change in a pseudolaminar pattern, predominantly involving layers 2, 3, and 5. Vacuolation is present in a pericellular distribution as well as within the neuropil. H&E. (Original magnification ×40.)

there may be some sponginess of the neuropil (dendritic and astrocytic swelling), some change in the tinctorial properties of neurons and glia, and neurons may be swollen or shrunken (Fig. 10.6). These changes may be difficult to distinguish from common artifacts. After about 6–8 h, the eosinophilic (ischemic or homogenizing) change heralds the unequivocal and irreversible neuronal damage associated with anoxia-ischemia. The neurons are shrunken with loss of Nissl substance and possess intensely eosinophilic cytoplasm and pyknotic, frequently triangular nuclei (Fig. 10.6). Over the next few days there is gradual dissolution of the cell with its eventual

disappearance. Over the succeeding days there is endothelial nuclear swelling, endothelial hyperplasia, microglial reaction (especially rod forms), infiltration of neutrophils (depending on presence of recirculation), and other glial responses similarly seen in infarcts (Fig. 10.7).

EXPERIMENTAL FINDINGS

Under carefully controlled experimental conditions of *complete* cerebral ischemia for up to 20–30 min and without reperfusion (reversible phase) the principal changes are predominantly that of disturbance of ion and water homeostasis, resulting in hydropic changes (33, 197, 272, 280) occurring

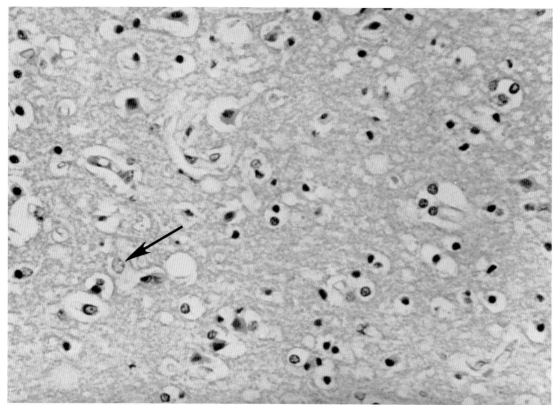

Figure 10.6. Cerebral cortex showing early anoxic encephalopathic changes, characterized by neuronal necrosis and spongiform change (perineuronal, periglial, perivascular, and within the neuropil). Occasional astroglial nuclear swelling is noted resembling an Alzheimer type II astrocyte (*arrow*) H&E. (Original magnification ×250.)

in a more or less uniform distribution (272). The initial alteration appears to be the swelling of astrocytes (66, 196, 330), with similar changes in neurons shortly thereafter especially in postsynaptic dendrites (196). There is swelling of smooth endoplasmic reticulum, rough endoplasmic reticulum, and mitochondria, as well as an increased lucency of the cytosol. Breakup of ribosomal rosettes into individual particles has been described (33) in keeping with deranged protein synthesis (299). Minor microtubular changes have also been observed during this early phase, possibly the result of intracellular calcium accumulation. Subtle changes in the chromatin of both astrocytes and neurons and nucleolar condensation are found, which perhaps may be related to elevation in lactate (273). Chromatin clumping was seen as early as 1½ min following ischemia.

Although the principal concern regarding the morphologic changes following anoxia-ischemia has been focused on neurons, recent studies have emphasized the role of astroglial cells, which appear to be the first cells to respond to anoxia-ischemia. Mention has been made of their capacity to quickly swell. Diemer and Klinken (138), Petito and Babiak (431), and Garcia et al. (202) have additionally described reactive changes in these cells. They appear to be increased in number quite early and manifest enlarged, pleomorphic mitochondria as well as a greater abundance of rough endoplasmic reticulum. In view of current concepts of astroglial functions these changes may reflect an attempt by these cells to restore the deranged extracellular milieu (increased K^+, ammonia, lactate, amino acids) brought about by the anoxic-ischemic injury.

Although more resistant to anoxia-ischemia, endothelial changes do occur. Early on there is enhanced pinocytosis (33, 430) but no significant disturbance in the permea-

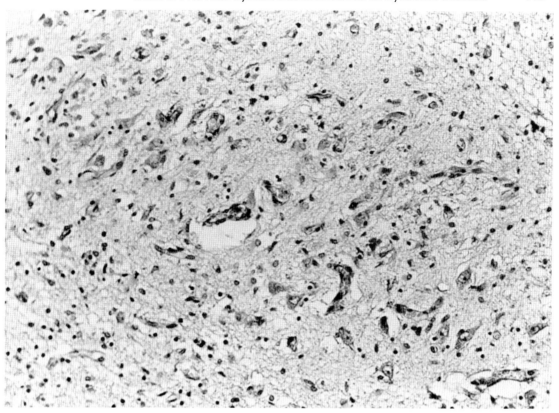

Figure 10.7. Anoxic encephalopathy of 1 week duration. Note the significant capillary proliferation with prominent endothelial nuclei. H&E. (Original magnification ×100.)

bility properties of the blood-brain barrier (433). This appears to be a functional change perhaps involved in the provision of nutrients to the brain (91, 430). With more extensive injury, endothelial cell necrosis is observed, at which time a gross breakdown of the blood-brain barrier occurs.

With longer periods of complete cerebral ischemia (irreversible phase) and without reperfusion there is a greater degree of swelling of all cell processes, and most importantly, mitochondria become swollen and their cristae are broken (33). In the "Levine" model (unilateral carotid clamping and nitrogen exposure) Brown and Brierley (84) observed that neuronal mitochondrial swelling (microvacuolization) was the first change occurring as early as 5–10 min following anoxia-ischemia. The subsequent presence of flocculent densities within mitochondria appear to signify the onset of irreversible cellular injury (200).

With the reestablishment of circulation after a prolonged period of complete cerebral ischemia, even more severe destructive changes are observed in a heterogeneous and haphazard distribution (215, 273). Neurons become markedly shrunken, electron-dense (dark neurons), and have few identifiable subcellular structures. These shrunken neurons are often surrounded by swollen astroglial processes, and there seems to be a reciprocal relationship between the degree of neuronal shrinkage and glial swelling. Brierley (79) believed that this reciprocal pattern was due to the compression of neurons by swollen glial cells. Recent studies by Kalimo et al. (283) indicate, however, that this finding is reflective of recirculation, as glial swelling can only occur in the presence of some oxygen.

Respirator Brain

The designation "respirator brain" has been applied to the brain of patients who suffered severe global anoxic-ischemic episodes and were clinically comatose, without cephalic reflexes, usually with isoelectric electroencephalograms, and with radiographic evidence of a severe reduction or absence of cerebral blood flow as a result of increased intracranial pressure. The brains are swollen, congested, dusky, friable, and remain soft despite adequate fixation (376, 607). There is usually transtentorial and tonsillar herniation with or without Duret hemorrhages. The ventricular lining sloughs off easily, and fragments of macerated cerebellum may occasionally be found alongside the spinal cord. The pituitary gland is often necrotic, and the sagittal and transverse venous sinuses may be clotted. It requires 12 to 24 h following anoxia-ischemia to develop these changes (315, 425). The nature and duration of the offending process, extent of residual cerebral blood flow, and degree of acidosis influence the extent of neuropathological change.

The histopathological features, while variable, are similar to those of anoxia-ischemia, except for the absence of inflammation and lack of reactive glial or vascular changes. Neurons may show eosinophilic change, or the cytoplasm may be pale and ghost-like. Nuclear changes vary from extreme pallor to pyknosis. Glial cells show similar alterations. Blood vessels are often congested, and the endothelial cells show blurring of cytoplasmic detail and nuclear pallor.

The mechanism for the "respirator brain" is felt to represent in vivo autolysis that was allowed to occur as a result of the patient being maintained on a mechanical respirator following an anoxic-ischemic episode. It should not be construed that the respirator in itself was in some fashion responsible for these pathological changes (197, 425).

Postanoxic Encephalopathy

Following an anoxic episode severe enough to produce coma, patients may recover in 24–48 h but after a period of 4–14 d occasionally will again undergo severe neurological deterioration (213, 442). At autopsy, changes are confined to the white matter, although cerebral cortical and pallidal lesions have sometimes been described (Fig. 10.8). The mechanism for this delayed postanoxic state is unclear. The lesions are to a varying degree demyelinative and ne-

crotic. Early lesions are located in a perivascular location. The mechanisms involved appear to be a combination of prolonged but lesser degrees of hypoxia and depressed blood perfusion perhaps with added hypocapnia (213, 383, 405). Kamijyo et al. (284) and Garcia and Conger (198) noted that with long-standing fluctuation in blood pressure, white matter necrosis became prominent. The reason for such sensitivity of the white matter to blood pressure fluctuations is not known, but Okeda et al. (405) showed an unusual degree of vasodilation in white matter as opposed to grey matter following anoxia.

Carbon Monoxide Intoxication

Carbon monoxide (CO) has 250 times the affinity of oxygen for hemoglobin, thus reducing the oxygen-carrying capacity of blood. When approximately two-thirds of hemoglobin is converted to carboxyhemoglobin, death ensues. CO also may interact with cytochrome oxidase, perhaps adding a histotoxic component to the anoxia.

The pathologic changes in brain in acute lethal cases are minimal. The brain may present a pink-red color due to the presence of carboxyhemoglobin. In addition, slight congestion and petechial hemorrhages may be evident. In longer surviving cases the changes are similar, if not identical, with that already described for anoxia-ischemia. For unexplained reasons, the globus pallidus is commonly affected (Fig. 10.9), perhaps more so than in anoxia-ischemia, suggesting a specific cytotoxic effect of CO for the pallidum.

A delayed encephalopathy similar to that seen with anoxia-ischemia may occur (Grinker's myelinopathy). As in anoxia-ischemia, the hemispherical white matter bears the brunt of the pathological changes resulting in symmetrical diffuse damage.

Symmetrical white matter lesions have been produced in monkeys following exposure to CO (214). The authors felt that in some manner the combination of hypotension and metabolic acidosis led to that pattern of injury.

Hypoglycemia

The brain has a high metabolic rate and is very much dependent upon a constant supply of glucose for normal activity. The

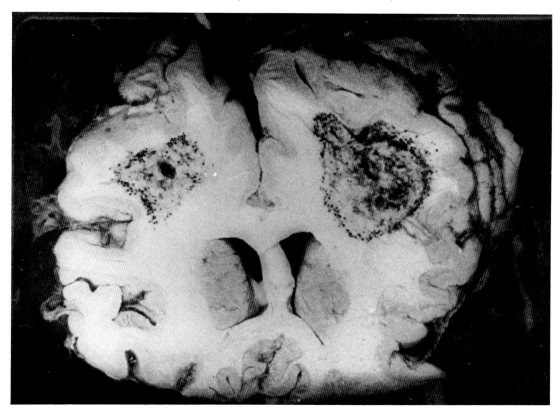

Figure 10.8. Postanoxic leukoencephalopathy. Coronal section of the brain shows symmetrical areas of necrosis in white matter. The presence of petechial hemorrhages within the necrotic zone is not usually found. (Courtesy of Myron D. Ginsberg, M.D.)

brain's respiratory quotient of 1 indicates that glucose is the predominant substrate in energy metabolism. Circulating glucose enters the brain by facilitated diffusion or via saturable passive carrier-mediated mechanisms (40). Once glucose reaches the cellular compartment, it is metabolized almost exclusively by glycolytic and oxidative pathways (38). Cerebral stores of glucose and glycogen are sufficient to maintain an overall rate of energy consumption in man for only a few minutes (39).

The brain may utilize exogenous substrates in certain circumstances, such as starvation, when ketone bodies are generated. The use of ketone bodies as alternative sources of energy by the fasting adult may explain the occasional poor correlation between blood glucose levels and the severity of symptoms in hypoglycemia. On the other hand, neonates and children are less capable of maintaining a normal glucose level when deprived of calories even during

short periods of fasting (413). One factor that probably contributes to the high glucose requirement of young children is their relatively larger ratio between brain mass and total body mass. In addition, children have less gluconeogenic potential and are less able to mobilize an adequate supply of gluconeogenic substrates.

Insulin-induced hypoglycemia has been the most extensively used experimental model for studying the effects of low glucose level on brain function. Various workers have reported conflicting results regarding the effect of insulin on CNS metabolism. Strang and Bachelard (548) found a 60% increase in glucose-6-phosphate and a 50% increase in glycogen but no change in glucose, glutamate, or lactate levels following administration of insulin to rats. Mellerup and Rafaelsen (363) induced a 25% increase in brain glycogen following direct application of insulin by intracisternal route. Nelson et al. (387) showed increased brain

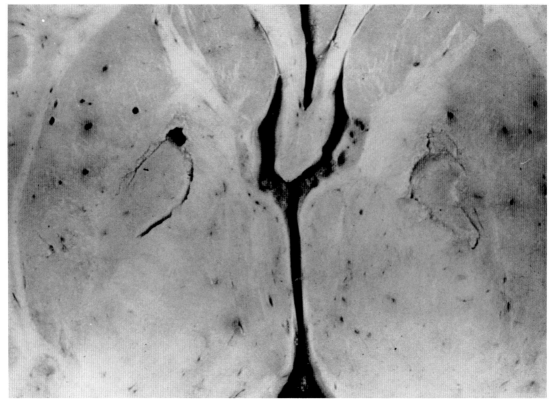

Figure 10.9. Section of the basal ganglia showing symmetrical destruction and necrosis of the pallidum. The patient survived 5 days after carbon monoxide intoxication. (Courtesy of Lowell W. Lapham, M.D.)

glucose and glycogen levels after insulin and glucose were administered systemically to alloxan-diabetic mice. In contrast, Tews et al. (564) reported a reduction of glucose and to a lesser extent, of glycogen, lactic acid, glutamic acid, and glutamine in brain of hypoglycemic dogs.

Other biochemical derangements have been identified in insulin-induced hypoglycemia. A rise in brain ammonia level in dogs was felt to contribute significantly to the development of seizures (564). Geiger (208) suggested that hypoglycemic symptoms may be due to the accumulation of toxic breakdown products of endogenous noncarbohydrate substrates. Other workers (167) maintain that development of neural dysfunction is due to alteration of glucose-dependent metabolic processes rather than to interference in energy metabolism and is associated with a decrease in DNA and protein content as well as decreased rate of formation of sulfatides and cerebrosides.

Mild hypoglycemia has been shown to cause a significant decrease in the rate of acetylcholine turnover (211), although the energy required directly for neurotransmitter function is only about 1% of that produced in the brain as a whole (37).

CLINICAL FEATURES

Cerebral dysfunction develops when arterial blood concentration of glucose falls below 40 mg/100 ml in infants, children, and adults, and below 30 mg/100 ml in full-term and premature neonates (521). Hypoglycemic episodes may occur during primary hyperinsulinism (e.g., with islet cell adenoma), during functional hyperinsulinism (i.e., with reactive hypoglycemia in prediabetics, following gastrointestinal surgery or with overt peptic disease), and in diabetic patients following insulin therapy. The condition may also be seen in association with adrenal insufficiency, hypothyroidism, hypopituitarism, hepatic disease, and liver enzyme deficiency (glucose 6-phosphatase, liver phosphorylase, glycogen synthetase, amylo-1,6-glucosidase), and prematurity.

Hypoglycemia affects cerebral cortical function first and later involves brain stem functions. The clinical picture is variable and may consist of headache, confusion, irritability, incoordination, and lethargy leading to stupor, convulsion, and coma. The latter is usually accompanied by a decrease in oxygen consumption. If prolonged and frequent, hypoglycemic episodes may result in permanent CNS dysfunction.

Seizures are the most frequent presenting signs at any age, but are especially common in children under the age of 1 yr (153). Convulsions are believed to be possibly due to impairment of membrane integrity and instability of ion gradient resulting from derangement of certain metabolic functions and insufficiency of energy reserves (615). The role of increased brain ammonia level has been suggested (564).

Ketotic hypoglycemia, the most common form of hypoglycemia in young children, is characterized by episodes of irritability, apathy, convulsion or coma, usually occurring after prolonged fasting. It is associated with the presence of acetone in urine and decreased hyperglycemic response to glucagon.

NEUROPATHOLOGIC ALTERATIONS

Grossly, brain swelling is usually slight or absent. Some cases surviving less than 12 h may show vascular congestion and marked brain edema with uncal and/or tonsillar herniation, without focal changes (467). Microscopic alterations may be mild and are generally similar to anoxic-ischemic changes observed following circulatory arrest, arterial hypotension (81), and status epilepticus (368). The earliest neuronal alterations are manifested by microvacuolation in the perikaryon and proximal parts of axons and dendrites. Neurons become eosinophilic, shrunken, and show pyknotic hyperchromatic nuclei. The changes are seen earlier in small neurons and later become most prominent in the 3rd, 5th, and 6th layers of the cerebral cortex in a pseudolaminar distribution. They are most extensive in the temporal lobes with involvement of the Ammon's horn, especially in

Sommer's sector. In contrast to anoxia-ischemia, degenerative changes in Purkinje cells are often absent or generally less severe when present (314).

Diffuse destructive changes with associated ventricular dilatation are seen following survival for months or years. The lesions are generally most severe in cerebral cortex and hippocampus with relative preservation of parahippocampal gyrus. The cerebral cortex shows pseudolaminar necrosis involving the middle cortical layers with relative sparing of the subpial and deeper laminae. The caudate nucleus and putamen are severely affected, and the small neurons are especially involved. The globus pallidus is relatively spared. There is variable involvement of the thalamus and less severe affection of the cerebellum. Minor changes are seen in brain stem nuclei and spinal cord (279, 314, 343). There is often widespread gliosis in the subpial zone and in the cerebral and cerebellar white matter. Parenchymal petechial and perivascular hemorrhages of varying ages and distribution and gliotic microcavitation have also been observed occasionally (44). A case of chronic, irreversible hypoglycemic coma caused by sulfonylurea was recently reported, with only minor structural alterations at gross and microscopic levels (279).

Infants dying from hypoglycemia do not exhibit the same pattern of "selective vulnerability" as shown in adults. Examination of neonates who died following untreated and verified hypoglycemia has shown diffuse acute nerve cell degeneration throughout the CNS. No selective laminar cortical involvement was observed (14).

Induction of hypoglycemia in monkeys (82, 83) resulted in ischemic cell change within the cerebral cortex in all animals. The changes were confined to the 3rd, 5th, and 6th layers and were more numerous within sulcal cortex than over the gyral crest. Involvement of the hippocampus, striatum, and cerebellum was only occasionally noted. The earliest neuronal alteration was microvacuolation of neuronal perikaryon, especially of larger pyramidal neurons, which was discernible as early as 15 min after induction of hypoglycemia. Ischemic eosinophilic change within neurons occurred after 30 min. Agardh et al. (7) and Kalimo et al. (281) studied perfused brains of rats with insulin-induced hypo-glycemia and described two types of nerve cell injury. Type I injury, considered irre-versible, was characterized by shrunken, angulated, darkly stained neurons with nu-clear condensation and perineuronal vacu-olated astrocytic processes. Small neurons in cortical layer 3 were mainly affected. Ultrastructural alterations consisted of condensed nuclei, compact ribosomes, di-lated RER cisterns, contracted mitochon-dria, and swollen perineuronal astrocytic processes. Type II injury, felt to be revers-ible, was characterized by cytoplasmic swelling, subplasmalemmal clearing and vacuolation, and mainly involved larger neurons in layers 5 and 6. Electron micro-scopic studies showed reorganization and reduction of RER cisterns, disintegration of ribosomes, contraction of mitochondria, and formation of membranous whorls. No nuclear alteration was noted.

HYPOGLYCEMIC NEUROPATHY

A rare complication of hypoglycemia consists of peripheral neuropathy due to an insulin-secreting tumor. This illness, which clinically resembles motor neuron disease, usually develops over a period of 6–72 months, although it sometimes has a more rapid onset. The symptoms improve follow-ing correction of hypoglycemia. Pathologic changes in man (573) as well as in animals (625) consist of degeneration of anterior horn and posterior root ganglion cells. In rabbits, the lesion appears to be in anterior horn cells (378). Conduction times are of-ten abnormal, suggesting that peripheral nerves themselves may also be involved. Evidence of primary damage to peripheral nerve in hypoglycemia is equivocal. Danta (122) postulates that the peripheral neu-ropathy is due to axonal reaction from de-generating nerve cell bodies.

DISORDERS OF TEMPERATURE REGULATION

Hypothermia

Hypothermia is defined as a core tem-perature of 35°C. It is usually seen after environmental exposure often in the alco-holic patient (465). It may occur in associ-ation with hypopituitarism, hypothyroid-ism, hypoadrenalism, Wernicke's disease,

and other conditions (465). It is occasion-ally induced in certain surgical procedures. It may present clinically with incoordina-tion, apathy, and confusion. When severe, the patient may be obtunded or comatose (365).

The morphological changes associated with hypothermia have not been clearly defined. A postmortem study of 43 cases of hypothermia did not describe CNS lesions (347). Some reports have described white matter edema, neuronal swelling, and as-trocytic proliferation (65, 544), although this has been denied by others (563). Some pathological changes possibly could be sec-ondary to circulatory failure arising from arrhythmias complicating hypothermia rather than hypothermia per se (55). It is likely that the encephalopathic state asso-ciated with hypothermia is the result of decreased cerebral metabolism without any morphological counterpart (154).

Hyperthermia

Neurological features are often the first clinical manifestation of hyperthermia. In-crease in body temperature over 41°C is usually associated with severe neurological symptoms, including an alteration in the level of consciousness, profound mental changes, and seizures (360, 513). Temper-ature over 42°C may be fatal.

Hyperthermia is usually seen following strenuous physical activity in hot and hu-mid environmental conditions (513). The elderly may be affected when exposed to hot weather, especially when they do not have access to water. Cases of hyperthermia have also been associated with infections, fever therapy, and malignant hyperther-mia. The latter occurs with the administra-tion of certain anesthetics and appears to have a genetic predisposition (388).

If the patient dies early minimal patho-logical changes are found. If the patient survives for a few days the brain often shows diffuse swelling with petechial hem-orrhages widely distributed but particularly around the third and fourth ventricles (224, 344, 513). Subarachnoid and subdural hem-orrhages have also been described. Degen-erative neuronal changes (swelling and shrinkage) are found throughout the brain but especially in the cerebellum where the Purkinje cells are often lost associated with a proliferation of Bergmann glial cells (224, 344). The vermis is as equally involved as the hemispheres. The upper layers of the cerebral cortex are more affected than the lower. The striatum, thalamus, and the pallidum show changes similar to the cortex but are less severe.

The pathogenesis of the cerebral changes is not clear. Many of these patients have associated cardiovascular collapse, fluid and electrolyte derangements, particularly hypernatremia, renal and hepatic failure, and disseminated intravascular coagulation. The hemorrhagic changes could possibly be secondary to the hypernatremia and/or the disseminated intravascular coagulation. To what extent the direct physical effect of excessive heat (i.e., denaturation of enzymes, etc.) may result in destructive injury to nervous tissue is not known (513). In general, the changes in brain have a strong resemblance to that of anoxia-ischemia (238). Since many of these patients have associated cardiovascular failure it is likely that many if not most of the pathological findings may be on the basis of perfusion failure. Additionally, hyperthermia is associated with an increase in the cerebral metabolic rate, which may thus result in a state of relative oxygen deficiency (48, 513).

DISORDERS OF ACID-BASE BALANCE

The pH of brain and CSF remains remarkably constant, despite substantial changes in arterial pH (variations from 6.8 through 7.6) (24, 288). The mechanism largely responsible for the maintenance of pH values in the nervous system is mediated via the protective effect of the blood-brain barrier (415) through its limitation of the entry of H^+ and HCO_3^- (24), by the generation or loss of HCO_3^- (444), and the generation or loss of organic acids (26, 520). As in other metabolic encephalopathies these adaptive changes require a certain period of time to efficiently develop. Thus, abrupt pH alterations give rise to marked neurological symptoms such as seizures and coma (26), while chronically developing ones may be relatively asymptomatic.

There is no significant barrier to CO_2 because of its high permeability so that most of the neurological consequences of acid-base disturbances are principally due to alteration in serum CO_2 tension (respiratory acidosis and alkalosis). Accordingly, there is a fairly good correlation between the degree of pH derangement in blood during respiratory disorders and clinical findings, whereas metabolically induced acid-base disorders tend to correlate poorly with plasma pH levels (24, 445).

Respiratory Acidosis

Patients with pulmonary disease often manifest a wide ranging set of neurological signs and symptoms. These include headache, personality changes, memory disturbance, somnolence, lethargy, weakness, depression, irritability, confusion, delirium, papilledema and increased cerebrospinal fluid pressure, extensor plantar reflexes, asterixis, myoclonus, seizures, and coma (113, 411). Various pulmonary disorders may be responsible for these findings. By far, the most common cause is chronic obstructive pulmonary disease secondary to emphysema and chronic bronchitis. They may be seen with kyphoscoliosis, infection, obesity, myxedema, chest trauma, the use of CNS depressant drugs, and aspiration (370).

While a number of abnormalities such as anoxia, acidosis, polycythemia, and cor pulmonale which are associated with pulmonary disease may contribute to the symptomatology, it appears that the principal factor in the development of pulmonary encephalopathy is hypercapnia. It is the factor that best correlates with the symptomatology of these individuals (441, 518).

CO_2 has profound and complex effects on the central nervous system. It has depressant and anesthetic properties (CO_2 narcosis) (626). It also causes marked vessel dilatation as well as increased cerebral blood flow (60, 290). As these effects are partly independent of the associated acidosis it would appear that most of the problem is CO_2 itself.

The principal mechanism whereby the CNS adapts to respiratory acidosis is through the generation and secretion of HCO_3^- by the choroid plexus into the CSF (24). This process can be blocked by acetazolamide (288), and accordingly HCO_3^- secretion into the CSF would appear to be a carbonic anhydrase-mediated function. There is also enhanced formation of HCO_3 in the brain parenchyma which apparently does not necessitate the mediation of carbonic anhydrase (24).

A number of adaptive biochemical alterations have been identified in the brain of hypercapneic animals. There is a decrease in the level of metabolic acids, including lactate, pyruvate, α-ketoglutarate, malate, citrate, aspartate, and glutamate (183, 289, 493). In addition, there is an increase in ammonia, glutamine, and GABA (183, 289, 587, 616).

The rise in ammonia may be helpful, as the alkaline ammonia partly neutralizes the acidity. It is of interest that many of the clinical features, including the EEG of patients with pulmonary encephalopathy, tend to mimic that of hepatic coma. Possibly the elevation in ammonia in both conditions may be a common factor. The elevation in ammonia and GABA as well as the fall in glutamate may contribute to the symptomatology, as these substances have potent neurophysiological properties.

The gross pathological findings of hypercapnia in man are usually unremarkable, except for duskiness of the brain which is a reflection of the increased blood content as a result of the vascular dilatation caused by CO_2. In severe cases there also may be edema, flattening of the convolutions, and evidence of uncal and tonsillar herniation (113, 527). To what extent some of these changes are due strictly to hypercapnia or to certain complications such as seizures, vascular collapse, and anoxia is uncertain.

In experimental animals there is an increase in the water content of the brain particularly within the white matter (43), probably as a result of a breakdown of the blood-brain barrier and increased capillary permeability (120, 275). The swelling appears to be predominantly within astrocytes (43, 357). However, the CO_2 levels required to impair the blood-brain barrier in animals are excessive and are rarely seen in humans. Studies by Paljärvi and coworkers (414) showed that with CO_2 tensions of 150 mm Hg astroglial swelling occurred while neurons remained normal. At levels of 300 mm Hg, neuronal changes were observed consisting of coarse chromatin clumping, mild mitochondrial swelling, dispersion of polysomes, stripping of ribosomes from the rough endoplasmic reticulum, and dilatation of the endoplasmic reticulum cisternae. These changes were generally mild and reversible.

Respiratory Alkalosis

Respiratory alkalosis (hypocapnia) may be seen with asthma, cirrhosis, salicylate intoxication, hypoxia, sepsis, and certain brain lesions (24). A modest degree of respiratory alkalosis may result in paresthesias and dizziness (24), while a more severe degree of respiratory alkalosis (pH 7.52–7.65), especially when associated with hypoxia, may result in asterixis, myoclonus, coma, seizures, and death (292).

Hypocapnia usually results in decreased cerebral blood flow (60), but this fall is rarely to such a degree that it results in frank ischemic changes. The principal compensation for a respiratory alkalosis is a fall in HCO_3^- (26). In addition, there is a rise in CSF lactate (440), as well as an increase in brain lactate, pyruvate, glutamate, and tricarboxylic acid intermediates (26, 520). Such changes in the levels of organic acids ameliorate the existing alkalosis. No significant morphological changes have been described in respiratory alkalosis.

Metabolic Acidosis

Metabolic acidosis may be seen with diabetes mellitus, renal insufficiency, toxicity with methanol and ethylene glycol, and inborn errors of metabolism (332). Thus far, very little investigation has been done on the effect of metabolic acidosis on the central nervous system (24). Severe metabolic acidosis results in minor and inconsistent change on brain pH (24). The paucity of CNS effects is probably due to the inability of the hydrogen ion to adequately penetrate the blood-brain barrier. Metabolic acidosis does have a significant depressant effect on the cardiovascular system, so that some of the neurological effects may be largely due to ischemia from the cardiac failure rather than a primary effect of pH derangement on the brain. Additionally, some of the conditions giving rise to acidosis have effects on the nervous system independent of the effect of pH.

The brain's adaptive response to metabolic acidosis is to increase formation of HCO_3^- as well as to elevate ammonia (247).

LACTIC ACIDOSIS

A special form of metabolic acidosis occurs with rises in lactic acid. Lactic acid appears to have a detrimental effect on the nervous system, and a detailed discussion of this subject is included in the section on anoxic-ischemic encephalopathy. Lactic acidosis may be seen following hypoxia, cardiac failure, renal disease, shock, the use of phenformin, ethanol ingestion, anemia, leukemia, liver disease, diabetes mellitus, and nonketotic hyperglycemic coma (332). Whether or not the neurological effects are directly due to increased lactate is uncertain.

A number of probably heterogeneous congenital conditions characterized by severe mental retardation, hypotonia, and choreoathetosis appear to be associated with serum elevations in lactic acid. Most of these cases have depicted small brains, mild ventricular dilatation, spongy degeneration of the hemispherical and cerebellar white matter, with either marked demyelination or undermyelination and the presence of subependymal cysts (324, 487).

Metabolic Alkalosis

Metabolic alkalosis results in very minor neurological deficits. It may be seen with liver disease, gastric suction, and bicarbonate ingestion (332). There is an increase in brain lactate and pyruvate and relatively little change in brain pH (24).

DISORDERS OF SERUM ELECTROLYTES

Sodium

HYPONATREMIA

Hyponatremia is a very common clinical condition (24, 29, 127), which almost always is due to dilution but may occur in the presence or absence of depletion of total body sodium. As such this state can be viewed as water intoxication.

Hyponatremia may occur acutely such as following the intake of hypotonic fluids (bladder irrigation, intravenous solutions, beer drinking, and excessive water ingestion as in psychogenic polydipsia). It may

also occur chronically, the most common cause being the syndrome of inappropriate antidiuretic hormone secretion. It may also be seen in cirrhosis, renal failure, and congestive heart failure.

Central nervous system symptoms are often the first and most prominent feature of hyponatremia (24). Patients may present with weakness, twitching, myoclonus, asterixis, confusion, delirium, and psychosis (619). It may also present as a life-threatening condition with stupor, coma, and generalized seizures (177). In general, symptoms do not occur until the sodium falls to 120–125 meq/l. Symptoms, however, are more dependent on the rate of development of hyponatremia than on absolute sodium levels (27, 177). Thus the acute reduction of serum sodium to 120–125 meq/l may result in severe symptoms, whereas if the hyponatremia evolves slowly to even as low as 110 meq/l the patient may remain relatively asymptomatic. Similar findings can also be obtained experimentally. Rabbits rendered hyponatremic within a 2- or 3-h period develop seizures with a high incidence of mortality, whereas when the same level is achieved over a period of 3–5 days the animals frequently demonstrate no clinical symptoms (27).

The effects of hyponatremia on the brain can perhaps be more properly understood by noting the unique ability of the brain to respond to hypoosmotic stress. In the setting of hyponatremia the brain becomes swollen and edematous (142, 482, 613). However, the amount of water actually present in brain is less than predicted on the basis of simple osmotic equilibrium (482). Thus, the brain adapts in some manner to prevent an excessive accumulation of fluid, thereby mitigating the effects of increased intracranial pressure. The mechanisms by which the brain accomplishes this phenomenon are through the loss of osmotically active particles, principally potassium, as well as sodium, glucose, and a number of amino acids, including alanine and glutamate (21, 140, 482, 568). Another mechanism by which the brain limits the water content is by diminishing extracellular water by increasing bulk flow into the cerebral spinal fluid (204, 364). These adaptive mechanisms require time (1–3 d). Rabbits with acute hyponatremia show a 17%

increase in water content, whereas chronically it only increases by 7% (27). Thus, the longer time the brain has to apply these mechanisms, the less the volumetric effects and accordingly the less severe degree of clinical symptoms.

The precise cause of the neurological disorder in hyponatremia is still unclear. Some have argued for increased intracranial pressure from the increased water content as the responsible mechanism (21, 482). Others have proposed that the loss of intracellular potassium may be the important factor (140). In addition, some of the alterations in amino acids may change the excitability of the brain, as some of them are putative neurotransmitters (21, 24). Abnormalities in cerebral metabolic rate have not been found (205), and the levels of ATP are unaltered (21).

The principal morphologic effect on the brain in hyponatremia is the presence of edema (142, 614). The edema is intracellular (cytotoxic), and the blood-brain barrier remains intact (482). In experimental animals the accumulation of fluid is principally in astrocytes (614). A mild form of Alzheimer type II alteration in astrocytes has also been observed (399).

With regards to changes observed in humans there have been relatively few reports. All have shown swollen brains and evidence of increased intracranial pressure (241, 458). One case appeared to be normal (327). That patient, however, had received very rapid treatment, and it is probable that the lethal consequences of edema had already occurred prior to therapy.

Central Pontine Myelinolysis

Originally described by Adams and colleagues (5), central pontine myelinolysis is a demyelinative disorder affecting the pontine base principally, although other regions of the nervous system may be involved, particularly the thalamus, striatum, lateral geniculate, and the grey-white junctions of the cerebral and cerebellar cortices (220, 222, 627). This disorder invariably occurs in a hospital setting usually in patients who are malnourished, alcoholic, and often have a chronic underlying illness, frequently liver disease, and often have derangements in serum electrolytes. Clinically, it may present with quadriparesis,

hyperreflexia, extensor plantar responses, and evidence of bulbar involvement. It not uncommonly presents as an incidental finding at autopsy.

The condition occurs as a symmetrical process involving the pontine base, only rarely affecting the tegmentum (Fig. 10.10). The lesion is most extensive at the level of the fifth cranial nerve and gradually tapers rostrally and caudally. The lesion may have a triangular, diamond, or butterfly shape. Early on, the lesion presents without any distinctive gross features, although after 1–2 weeks it is often greyish and granular. Older severe areas may display frank cavitation, although this is a rare event. The paramount gross features are its central location in the pontine base, its symmetry, and the preservation of the most ventral portions of the pons.

Microscopically, it has the usual features of a primary demyelinative disease. There is destruction of myelin, loss of oligodendrocytes, mild reactive astrocytosis, presence of reactive astrocytes, and macrophages containing sudanophilic lipids. Neuronal cell bodies and axis cylinders are preserved, although in severe cases there may be frank neuronal necrosis. Axonal spheroids are commonly observed (499). Early on, there may be prominence of capillaries with endothelial nuclear swelling (Fig. 10.11). Inflammatory changes are not seen. The corticospinal tracts are the structures usually least affected in the pontine base. Electron microscopy has disclosed the presence of intramyelin edema (446).

Of the various potential etiologic factors, electrolyte disturbances, especially hyponatremia, have been most commonly identified (92, 367). Recent studies, however, appear to implicate a rapid rise in serum sodium, usually from hyponatremic levels as a key factor in the pathogenesis of this disorder (300, 311, 400). Demyelination has been induced experimentally by rapid correction of hyponatremia (Fig. 10.12). This appears to be especially so when the preceding hyponatremia is of long-standing duration (399). How such sodium fluxes bring about demyelinative lesions in such precise loci of the nervous system is not known, although speculations have been proposed (396). It is believed that the rich admixture of grey and white matter in the

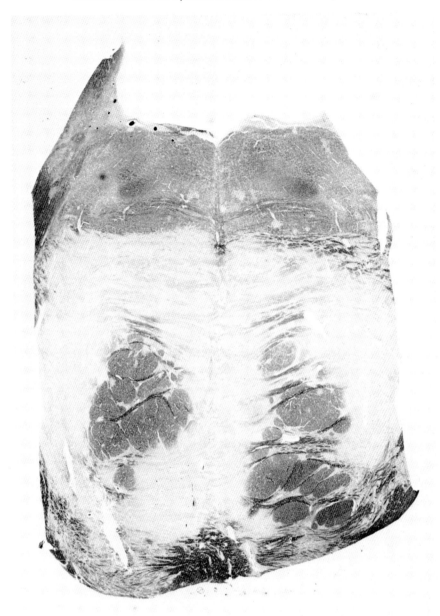

Figure 10.10.   LFB-PAS stain of pons showing central pontine myelinolysis. Note the symmetrical demyelination of basis pontis with minimal involvement of the adjacent tegmentum. There is sparing of ventral pons as well as the corticospinal tracts.

pontine base may explain the predisposition of that site to demyelinative lesions.

HYPERNATREMIA

Hypernatremia generally results from insufficient fluid intake. It is thus seen in the incapacitated patient who does not receive adequate water. It may also be seen in individuals with hypothalamic damage who have impairment in thirst mechanisms, as well as impaired release of antidiuretic hormone (essential hypernatremia) (233, 437, 543). It may rarely be seen following excessive sodium bicarbonate administration for the treatment of cardiopulmonary arrest and metabolic acidosis,

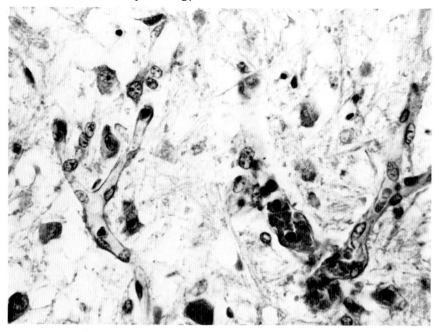

Figure 10.11.   Light micrograph of pons in early central pontine myelinolysis showing diffuse pallor of neuropil (demyelination), preservation of neuronal cell bodies, and prominent capillaries with endothelial nuclear swelling. H&E. (Original magnification ×300.)

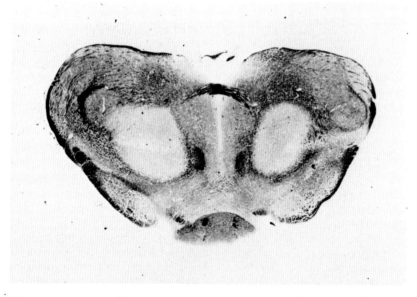

Figure 10.12.   Cross-section of the brain stem-thalamic junction in the rat following rapid correction of hyponatremia. Note the bilateral, symmetrical, well-circumscribed zones of pallor indicating the presence of demyelination. Luxol-fast-blue stain. (From B. K. Kleinschmidt-DeMasters and M. D. Norenberg: *Science* 211:1068, 1981 ©AAAS.)

from malfunctioning dialysis equipment, therapeutic abortion, and improper preparation of infant formula (443). Chronic hypernatremia may be seen with excessive intestinal losses from osmotic laxatives, renal losses, nephrogenic diabetes insipidus, burns, excessive insensible losses (fever, tachypnea), and the use of steroids.

The symptoms of hypernatremia, as in other electrolytes disorders, are principally neurological, with the presence of an altered sensorium, decrease in spontaneous activity, lethargy, ataxia, stupor, and coma (443, 556). Seizures have occasionally been described but are probably the result of overly rapid hydration of hypernatremic patients (171, 555). As in other metabolic encephalopathies neurological manifestations tend to correlate with the speed with which changes occur. Symptoms may develop with serum sodium levels of 150 meq/ l, although most symptomatic patients have values greater than 160 meq/l. Levels over 180 meq/l are frequently lethal (441).

Hypernatremia, as in other hyperosmolar states, may produce symptoms by causing an osmotic diuresis, thereby decreasing the cerebral blood volume and diminishing cerebral blood flow. An increase in blood viscosity may also interfere with cerebral circulation. It is believed, however, that the principal effect of hypernatremia is simply that of a brain dehydration as a result of osmotic forces.

As in hyponatremia, the brain has adaptive responses that with ample time appear to prevent excessive water shifts. The principal mechanism for the retention of brain volume and prevention of water loss is by the generation of osmotically active particles. These appear to be in part due to an increase in sodium and chloride (21) and in organic solutes including amino acids (glutamate, glutamine, aspartate, glycine, GABA), lactate, glucose, tricarboxylic acid intermediates, and ammonia (178, 333, 443, 568, 569). The increased brain osmolality cannot, however, be accounted for by all of these described metabolites, and thus a significant number of still unidentified substances appear to be responsible for the maintenance of osmotic equilibrium with plasma (idiogenic osmoles) (28).

The precise mechanism for the production of symptoms is not clear. While a decrease in energy metabolism has been identified, ATP levels appear to be intact (443). The rise in ammonia, glutamate, and GABA, all of which have neurophysiological effects, may in some fashion contribute to the symptomatology. A hemorrhagic encephalopathy occurs with severe hypernatremia, and this may likewise contribute to the development of symptoms.

Our principal knowledge of the pathological effects of hypernatremia in man was obtained from a nursery disaster in which improper infant formula was administered to infants (171). At autopsy the infants showed venous and capillary congestion, subarachnoid hemorrhage, intracerebral hemorrhage, cortical venous thrombosis, and venous infarcts. Several cases in adults have similarly shown widespread cerebral hemorrhages (95, 633). It is believed that hemorrhages are secondary to mechanical trauma as the result of brain shrinkage. Maccauley and Watson (341), however, described no anatomical lesions in some patients.

Similar hemorrhagic findings have been reproduced in experimental animals (170, 539). Additionally, disruption of the blood-brain barrier has been observed (143).

Cerebral edema may develop in hypernatremic patients in whom hypernatremia has been rapidly corrected. This complication appears to be more common in children (169).

Calcium

HYPOCALCEMIA

The level of CSF calcium is normally kept within a narrow range (2–3 mg/dl) (24). This relative constancy is seen, despite wide variations in plasma calcium. Calcium has a number of important functions in the nervous system. It has an effect on the excitability properties of cell membranes, probably by stabilizing in some manner the cell membrane and maintaining selective membrane permeability (243). Calcium is also involved in the release and uptake of neurotransmitters (46, 268, 457), in axoplasmic transport (235), and in the modulation of cyclic nucleotides (168, 514).

Hypocalcemia is defined as a total serum level of less than 9 mg/dl. Florid signs, however, are usually not seen until the calcium levels fall to 6–7 mg/dl (470). Hypocalcemia is most commonly seen in association with renal disease. It is also seen in hypoparathyroidism, vitamin D deficiency, pancreatitis, and malnutrition.

The clinical manifestations of hypocalcemia can be divided into those that affect the peripheral nervous system such as paresthesias, laryngeal stridor, and carpopedal spasms, and central nervous system manifestations which include hyperexcitability, psychosis, seizures, delirium, stupor, and rarely coma (125, 186). Parkinsonism and choreoathetosis have also been described (298, 525). Rarely, the patient may present only with dementia (469, 452). Increased intracranial pressure has been described, although the mechanism is not known (125). Associated with these clinical features are abnormal EEG patterns (125).

Pathological changes in brain, when present, are limited to calcification of the basal ganglia, particularly the pallidum, as well as the dentate nucleus of the cerebellum (see next section). The reason for the calcification is unclear.

Except for the extrapyramidal findings, which may be caused by the basal ganglia calcification, there is no adequate morphologic basis for the bulk of the clinical symptoms. It appears, therefore, that clinical derangements are due chiefly to biochemical defects rather than to any specific anatomical abnormalities.

Fahr's Disease

A relatively minor degree of basophilic granular deposition is a very common incidental postmortem finding in the pallidum and to a lesser extent in the dentate nucleus and hippocampus, especially in the elderly. The material consists of an admixture of calcium, iron, and other metals embedded in a PAS-positive, mucopolysaccharide matrix (Fig. 10.13). In some patients there may be an extraordinary degree of mineralization to the extent of visibility on routine skull films. This condition, which may be familial, is sometimes referred to as Fahr's disease, although as documented by Löwenthal and Bruyn (337), Fahr neither was the first to describe it nor was his description particularly thorough. Patients may be asymptomatic or have a history of seizures, mental deterioration, psychosis, parkinsonism, and cerebellar symptoms.

In this more severe form of the disorder,

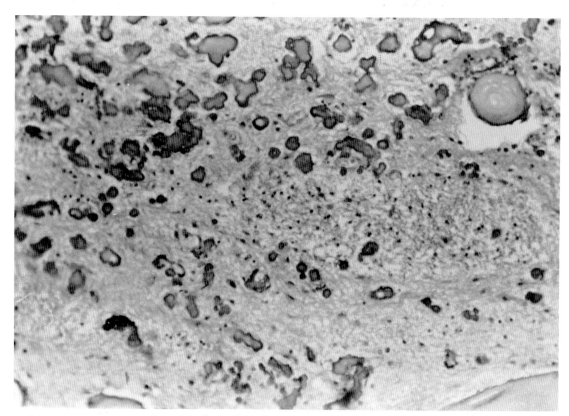

Figure 10.13. Section from basal ganglia of a patient with Fahr's disease. Note the extensive calcification in blood vessel walls as well as in the parenchyma. H&E. (Original magnification × 20.)

the mineralization is additionally seen in the striatum, sulcal depths of the cerebral cortex, and other sites as well. The mineralization is primarily localized to small and medium sized blood vessels. There is often no parenchymal reaction, although in some cases there is a varying degree of neuronal degeneration and gliosis. It seems likely that the presence or absence of symptoms relate to the degree of parenchymal damage.

In about 70–80% of patients, this disorder results from hypoparathyroidism and related disturbances in calcium and phosphate metabolism (337). In some patients, however, no such metabolic alterations have been identified, so that the cause of mineral deposition in these patients is still obscure.

Infantile cases of mineralization similar to Fahr's disease have been described with associated microcephaly and demyelinization (274).

HYPERCALCEMIA

Hypercalcemia is seen with hyperparathyroidism, a variety of neoplastic disorders, vitamin D intoxication, sarcoid, milk-alkali syndrome, and dialysis accidents (502). Elevation in serum calcium may result in lethargy, confusion, delirium, psychosis, stupor, and coma (125, 318). Seizures may occur but are uncommon (108). Patients may display an abnormal electroencephalographic pattern. Although rare cases of intracranial calcifications have been described (337), to date no consistent neuropathological features have been attributed to hypercalcemia (118, 243).

Magnesium

HYPOMAGNESEMIA

Magnesium is an essential component of a large number of metabolically important enzymes (9, 150). It is also involved in axoplasmic transport, the synthesis and release of neurotransmitters, and in cyclic AMP metabolism (517).

Hypomagnesemia is usually seen in individuals with poor dietary intake as well as in individuals with malabsorption, chronic alcoholism, prolonged parenteral nutrition, and hypoparathyroidism. Hypomagnesemia is associated with weakness,

tremor, personality changes, psychotic behavior, vertigo, nystagmus, ataxia, and seizures (150). The electroencephalogram often shows a diffuse hyperexcitability (150).

No specific histopathological changes have been described in humans other than a rare case of focal cerebral vessel calcification (585). Studies in experimental animals have shown vasculitis (336) and degenerative changes in Purkinje cells (49, 63). A decrease in the number of Gomoripositive glia has been described (542). The significance of this observation is unclear.

HYPERMAGNESEMIA

Elevation in serum magnesium is usually seen in patients with renal disease who have been treated with magnesium-containing antacids and occasionally following its use for sedative purposes (150). Patients may manifest respiratory depression, weakness, hyporeflexia, dysarthria, and ataxia (175). Excess magnesium may suppress the release of neurotransmitters and antagonizes the effect of calcium (375). However, since magnesium also depresses cardiovascular function (375), some of the clinical findings attributed to hypermagnesemia may be on the basis of a reduction in cerebral blood flow. No histopathological changes have thus far been described in hypermagnesemia.

Hypophosphatemia

Phosphate is the major intracellular anion (301). It is essential for the integrity of cells, required for synthetic and catabolic processes, required for the formation of ATP, and is involved in the delivery of oxygen by regulating the level of 2,3-diphosphoglycerate in the red blood cell. Hypophosphatemia is seen in many clinical conditions but especially in association with hyperalimentation, alcohol withdrawal, the use of phosphate binders, and in the presence of respiratory alkalosis.

Hypophosphatemia is very commonly found (normal values 2.7–4.5 mg/dl), but its symptoms are not usually seen until levels fall below 1 mg/dl (229). Symptoms consist of irritability, apprehension, muscular weakness, numbness, paresthesias, dysarthria, confusion, obtundation, seizures, and coma (180, 301).

The mechanism involved in the production of neurological symptoms is not clear. It is believed that an important factor may be related to the reduction in red blood cell 2,3-diphosphoglycerate and adenosinetriphosphate (323). There is an increased red blood cell affinity for oxygen, resulting in a decreased availability of oxygen for tissues. Patients who have associated respiratory alkalosis, commonly associated with hypophosphatemia, are particularly vulnerable, since they already have a decrease in cerebral blood flow (229). Morphological changes have thus far not been described in patients with hypophosphatemia.

RENAL DISEASE

Uremic Encephalopathy

Among the early clinical manifestations in patients with renal failure are a number of neurological abnormalities (18, 581, 582). The clinical features are usually generalized and include disorientation, drowsiness, and insomnia, extending all the way to stupor and coma. Occasionally the patient may present with frank psychosis. Other abnormalities include a slurring of speech, gait imbalance, tremor, twitching, myoclonus, asterixis, and rarely, chorea and ballismus. Seizures, if they occur, are usually a late manifestation. There is often a fluctuation of symptoms from day to day and even from hour to hour. The more rapid the development of uremia, the more pronounced are the clinical changes.

Symptoms correlate poorly with any single laboratory abnormality, although the BUN is often a useful index of severity of the disorder. The correlation of BUN to clinical symptoms is influenced by the rate of development of the renal failure. Thus, when the disorder is acute the BUN may only be as high as 40–50 mg/dl, and the patient may be severely encephalopathic; yet, when renal disease is chronic the elevation of BUN may be over 200 mg/dl, and there may still be relatively little in the way of neurological deficit.

PATHOGENESIS

While a large number of biochemical abnormalities in blood and brain have been described in human and experimental uremia, to date the precise biochemical defect is not known. The fact that CNS manifestations of uremia are reversed by dialysis indicates that low molecular compounds are responsible for the syndrome, but the precise nature of these elusive compounds remains to be identified (54, 386).

Although the rise in BUN often mirrors the severity of the uremic state, urea itself is not responsible for the features of uremia (366). Abnormalities in blood sodium, potassium, pH, calcium, chloride, phosphate, and osmolalities have been described, but none of these clearly correlates with the uremic state (24). Certain organic acids (508) and phenolic acids (218) are elevated in sera and have the capacity of inhibiting a number of enzymes in brain concerned with respiration, anaerobic glycolysis, and transamination, as well as have effects on nucleotidase and glutamic acid decarboxylase. Inhibition of Na-K ATPase has also been shown in uremic rats (372).

Considerable interest has recently focused on the pathogenetic role of parathyroid hormone (PTH). PTH levels in serum are increased, so that it has been suggested that PTH might perhaps be the uremic CNS toxin (36, 355). There is an elevation of calcium in brain, presumably secondary to the elevation in PTH (23). In keeping with this view, some clinical improvement with hypoparathyroidectomy has been reported (355).

Brain tissue obtained at autopsy has disclosed an increase in serotonin and a decrease in dopamine (271, 516). Elevation in free plasma tryptophan, the serotonin precursor, has been described (516, 552). Alterations in neurotransmitter metabolism may yet turn out to be of great importance. Other abnormalities include a decrease in glucose and oxygen utilization, although it is not clear whether these are primary or secondary phenomena (61, 489). Experimental uremia does not result in brain energy failure (586). Permeability changes of the blood-brain barrier have been described in experimental uremia, but edema was not observed (25, 176, 179).

In sum, it may be said that despite a large number of potential toxins and abnormalities that have been identified in blood and brain to date, there is no clear cut explanation for the uremic state.

PATHOLOGY

An abundant early literature regarding a large number of morphologic alterations in patients dying with uremia has been reviewed by Knutson and Baker (302) and Olsen (406). These abnormalities have included meningeal fibrosis, a variety of glial changes, edema, vascular degeneration, focal and diffuse degeneration of neurons, and focal demyelination. Although many alterations have been noted, no consistent pattern has been identified.

The detailed studies by Olsen are especially noteworthy. He examined 104 uremic brains and described neuronal changes in many areas. In general, the changes were more severe in chronic forms of uremia. Small infarcts were commonly identified and attributed to hypertension. A few brains showed hemorrhages, presumably also on the basis of hypertension. Acute granule cell necrosis of the cerebellum was found in 60% of cases, as compared to only 8% of the control group. This cerebellar change is a relatively common nonspecific abnormality that is a terminal event of unknown significance. Also described were demyelination and focal necrosis, which were probably related to the associated vascular pathology. In summary, Olsen concluded that the neuropathologic changes were nonspecific and inconsistent, an opinion which the authors fully share.

The major difficulty in defining the pathological changes in uremia stems from the fact that these patients often have other coexisting diseases and abnormalities, such as hypertension, infections, seizures, diabetes, and lupus erythematosis which complicate the interpretation. Furthermore, a number of other associated problems to be discussed below may confuse the picture. In a study of eight severely uremic patients, no clear-cut histological abnormalities were observed (94). It appears that the uremic state itself is unassociated with any histopathological alterations and that most, if not all, of the various pathological changes described in patients with renal disease can be attributed to complicating features of the uremic state or may be agonal and/or artifactual. Experimental studies in rats made acutely uremic have shown no histopathological alterations by light microscopy (179). By electron microscopy, minor endothelial and astrocytic changes were observed (588), but these are difficult to interpret as the animals were not fixed by perfusion.

Complications Associated with Dialysis

DISEQUILIBRIUM SYNDROME

The disequilibrium syndrome refers to the occurrence of headache, nausea, vomiting, muscle cramps, agitation, delirium, obtundation, muscle twitching, disorientation, tremors and most importantly, generalized seizures and coma in a setting of a rapid dialysis usually early in the phase of a dialysis program (429, 473). It appears to be more common in children. Typically the symptoms are seen towards the end of a dialysis run, although sometimes they occur 8–24 h after dialysis. The symptoms are usually self-limiting, but when the delirium appears it may persist for several days.

This syndrome has been attributed to the development of cerebral edema, as there is an increase in intracranial pressure (231, 604). The edema originally was felt to be secondary to the retention of urea in brain, thus creating an osmotic gradient between brain and blood resulting in a shift of water into brain. Subsequent studies have shown that the increased osmolarity of the brain could not be attributed solely to urea; instead, studies by Arieff and coworkers (25) have indicated that an as yet unidentified solute(s) appears to be generated in brain during uremia ("idiogenic osmoles"), and these solutes appear to be responsible for the development of edema and increased pressure. As yet, no pathological studies have been described in individuals with this syndrome.

DIALYSIS ENCEPHALOPATHY (DIALYSIS DEMENTIA)

A progressive and ultimately fatal syndrome has been described in patients who have been on renal dialysis for at least 2 yr, with most of the patients having been on hemodialysis for 4 yr (10, 94, 342, 403). There is initially an insidious alteration in behavior and memory, which subsequently progresses to dementia, myoclonus, seizures, and death. A characteristic dysarthria (dyspraxia) may herald this syndrome. Unlike uremic encephalopathy, the neurologic symptoms are not modified by biochemical improvement of the uremic state. The syndrome typically occurs during the later phases of the hemodialysis run. Early in the course the symptoms clear in the ensuing 4–12 h. Eventually, however, the remissions cease. Within 6 months after the onset of symptoms, patients become incapable of communicating verbally. A characteristic EEG has been identified consisting of diffuse, multifocal slow (delta) waves interrupted by bilaterally synchronous, high voltage complexes. Late in the course of this disorder, the syndrome cannot be reversed by renal transplantation; however, early on it may be reversible (524, 551). Most patients have died within 18 months of the diagnosis.

The pathogenesis of this condition appears to be related to an accumulation of aluminum in blood and particularly in brain (11, 359, 621). Aluminum is derived from the frequent use of phosphate-binding alumina gels and from the water used in the dialysis bath, especially the latter. The syndrome has been described in nondialyzed patients, who, however, did receive aluminum gels orally (184, 456). How this accumulation of aluminum brings about the syndrome has not been defined. Subtle alterations in the blood-brain barrier have been described (252), although cerebral edema is not a component of this syndrome. It should be noted that the pathogenetic role of aluminum is not universally accepted; the deposition of aluminum in brain may be simply an epiphenomenon secondary to the increase in parathyroid hormone (29).

Pathological descriptions of this condition have differed from the comment of no neuropathological finding to a variety of nonspecific alterations (94, 96, 136, 149, 483, 610). Sabouraud et al. (483) described neuronal loss, accumulation of lipofuscin pigment, neurofibrillary degeneration, especially in the motor cortex, red nucleus, and the dentate, and olivary nuclei. In one study (94), neuronal changes were identified consisting of slight nuclear hyperchromaticity, cytoplasmic shrinkage, increase in lipofuscin pigment, no obvious neuronal loss, a slight increase in microglia with rod forms, a slight Alzheimer type II change, and a slight sponginess of the neuropil. These findings were principally observed in the cerebral cortex. The microglial changes appeared to be the earliest morphological change. Similar changes, however, were observed in a comparable group of dialyzed

patients who did not have this syndrome. The changes observed in the dialyzed patients were not found in a comparable group of uremic but nondialyzed patients. There was no evidence of inflammation, and no neurofibrillary tangles were found as might have been expected since in experimental animals aluminum produces these tangles (296). Nor was there any evidence of significant atrophy, although some CT scan studies have suggested a slight atrophy (417). In sum, it would appear that the neuropathological changes in dialysis dementia are relatively minor compared to the severity of the syndrome and are mostly nonspecific.

SUBDURAL HEMATOMA

Subdural hematomas have been a complication of hemodialysis (320, 559). These are believed to be the result of anticoagulation and clotting difficulties associated with renal failure rather than due to the dialysis procedure itself.

Complications of Renal Transplantation

Patients with renal transplants are highly susceptible to a number of opportunistic infections. The immunosuppression that is attendant with transplantation is responsible for many of these infections. Fungal infections are common, with *Aspergillus* and *Candida* accounting for the majority of fungal infections, while *Histoplasma* accounted for the rest (468). Other opportunistic infections have included toxoplasmosis (576), cytomegalovirus infection (498), and nocardia (468). Measles encephalitis has also been described (6). Progressive multifocal leukoencephalopathy, usually occurring in a setting of immunodeficiency, has also been identified (317, 348).

The occurrence of primary CNS lymphomas has been noted in patients with renal transplantation. Typically they tend to occur within 5–46 months following transplantation (259, 501). The high incidence of lymphomas has usually been ascribed to the presence of a chronic antigenic stimulation provided by the transplant, which results in immunoblast proliferation with possible neoplastic transformation. The relatively high incidence of these tumors within brain has been attributed to the privileged immunologic conditions present in the brain, perhaps secondary to the lack of lymphatics and the presence of the blood-brain barrier, all of which would protect the neoplasm from an immunologic attack. In addition, the patient's capacity for immunologically responding to these tumors might be impaired by the associated immunosuppression.

Central pontine myelinolysis has been described in association with renal transplantation (499). This complication has only been observed in a minority of patients and might perhaps be more related to associated electrolyte disturbances than to the transplant itself (see above).

LIVER DISEASE

Hepatic Encephalopathy

Patients with liver disease may develop a neurological syndrome commonly referred to as hepatic encephalopathy, hepatic coma, or portal-systemic encephalopathy. The clinical picture is characterized by a fall of intellect, personality changes, impairment in the level of consciousness, asterixis, and characteristic electroencephalographic changes. This syndrome may develop in a wide variety of liver disorders but is most commonly seen with alcoholic cirrhosis.

ETIOLOGY AND PATHOGENESIS

The precise etiology and pathogenesis of hepatic encephalopathy is not known. The most favored view is that toxic substances elaborated by the gut are not detoxified by the liver, either because of the presence of shunts or because of inability of the injured liver to detoxify these substances. The principal issue to date has been which of the relatively large number of candidates may be the responsible factor. It is likely that several factors acting synergistically may give rise to the neurological deficit, a concept strongly championed by Zieve (637).

Possibly the most important toxin and certainly the one which has received the greatest attention is ammonia. Strong arguments in support of an important role of ammonia has been adequately marshaled by Conn and Lieberthal (112). They showed that while the correlation between blood ammonia and clinical symptoms has not always been perfect, it has been fairly good. Reasonable explanations have been offered by these authors to account for those occasional episodes where the correlation did not appear to be as good as it could have been. Further support for the etiological role of ammonia is that any condition that results in an elevation of blood ammonia tends to aggravate hepatic encephalopathy (administration of ammonium salts and resins, hypokalemia, elevation of blood urea, gastrointestinal bleeding, and ingestion of a high protein diet) (123, 606). Importantly, almost all of the therapeutic maneuvers currently employed in the therapy of hepatic coma are aimed towards the reduction of blood ammonia levels (77). Also, infants with congenital urea cycle defects which result in hyperammonemia have shown histopathological changes similar to that seen in hepatic encephalopathy (91, 97, 319, 322, 353, 412, 538). Lastly, a wide variety of experimental situations which produce an elevation of brain or blood ammonia results in a histopathology identical to that seen in hepatic encephalopathy in man (see Norenberg (395) for review).

Ammonia is clearly neurotoxic (251). In animals, high doses result in seizures, while lower doses cause coma. It is still unclear how ammonia exerts its toxic effect in man and animals. It was earlier suggested that ammonia may initiate bioenergetic failure through the mechanism by which the brain detoxifies ammonia (58). Ammonia is detoxified by the formation of glutamine following the pathway shown below:

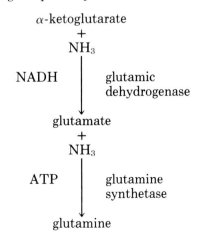

α-ketoglutarate
+
NH_3

NADH $\quad$ glutamic dehydrogenase

glutamate
+
NH_3

ATP $\quad$ glutamine synthetase

glutamine

The detoxification of ammonia consumes ATP, NADH, and α-ketoglutarate, so that it seemed that bioenergetic failure was a reasonable proposition. More recent studies by Hindfelt and Siesjö (253) and Hawkins and coworkers (239), however, have failed to identify bioenergetic failure at least in acute ammonia encephalopathy. Yet, the possibility that bioenergetic failure may be confined to a small but crucial compartment in brain has not been precluded. This is particularly important since ammonia metabolism is a compartmentalized process (56), and the best evidence to date suggests that that compartment is the astrocyte (394, 398).

Ammonia has potent electrophysiological effects. It depolarizes the cell membrane and causes hyperexcitability by blocking postsynaptic inhibition (340, 451). Additionally, ammonia may lead to abnormalities in acetylcholine metabolism (74, 419, 583). Ammonia may also affect the levels of GABA and glutamate (62, 254), substances that are putative neurotransmitters. A variety of other abnormalities induced by ammonia has been described, including effects on the activity of ATPase (491), carbonic anhydrase (380), alterations in the blood-brain barrier (312), and loss of vascular autoregulation (294) (for review of these and other mechanisms see Norenberg (395)).

Next to ammonia, the false neurotransmitter hypothesis and its modifications have received the greatest amount of contemporary interest. It was proposed that gut-derived catecholamine byproducts of bacterial decarboxylation (octopamine, phenylethanolamine, and perhaps others) are circulated around the liver and enter the brain to displace normal neurotransmitters. Serum levels of octopamine have appeared to correlate well with the level of encephalopathy (307, 345). The status of false neurotransmitters is currently uncertain, since the intraventricular injection of very high doses of octopamine to rats has so far been without clinical effect (638). Furthermore, the experimental reduction of norepinephrine and dopamine, substances which presumably are displaced by the false neurotransmitters, did not cause significant alterations in the level of consciousness in animals (352).

A modification of the false neurotransmitter hypothesis has been proposed by Soeters and Fischer (535). They observed a characteristic pattern in the amino acids found in plasma typified by elevation in the levels of aromatic amino acids (phenylalanine, tyrosine) and a depression in the levels of branched-chain amino acids (valine, leucine, isoleucine). The imbalance in the ratio of these amino acids leads to an increased entry of the aromatic amino acids into brain, resulting in an altered neurotransmitter status chiefly by raising serotonin levels. The elevation in brain glutamine (by ammonia) simply aids in the transport of these aromatic amino acids by acting as a coupling agent (269).

Other potential toxins have been proposed, but their evidence is not nearly as strong as for ammonia. Some of these include short chain fatty acids (637), α-ketoglutaramate (591), mercaptans (637), false neurotransmitters (174), and GABA (488).

PATHOLOGY

The only consistent histopathological change observed in patients dying from portal-systemic encephalopathy has been a change in grey matter astrocytes referred to as the Alzheimer type II change (protoplasmic astrocytosis). While the association of astroglial changes to acquired liver disease was made earlier by Scherer (492), it was the classical and detailed studies of Adams and Foley (4) that clearly emphasized the characteristic astroglial changes associated with liver disease.

The Alzheimer type II astrocyte as observed in hematoxylin-eosin preparations is characterized by an enlarged, vacuolated nucleus with chromatin margination and often a prominent nucleolus (Fig. 10.14). The astrocytes show little visible cytoplasm, which frequently contains excessive lipofuscin pigment. Intranuclear inclusions consisting of glycogen may be observed particularly in chronic cases (594) (Fig. 10.14C), and occasionally some glycogen may also be found in the cytoplasm as well (267).

These astroglial changes are found throughout the grey matter of brain and are only minimally observed or even absent in the white matter. In the cerebral cortex they are best noted in the deeper layers.

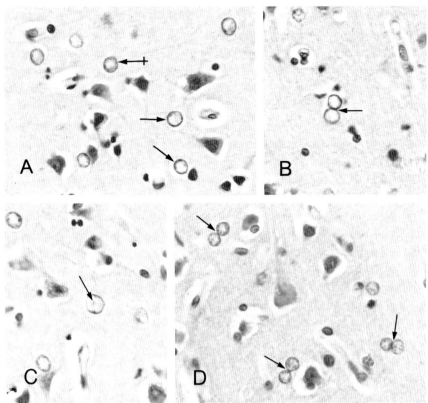

Figure 10.14. (A) Alzheimer type II astrocytes from a patient with hepatic encephalopathy are characterized by enlarged vacuolated nuclei with margination of chromatin (arrows). A comparably less involved astrocyte is indicated by cross-arrow. (B) Astroglial hyperplasia is manifested by the presence of paired nuclei (arrow). (C) PAS-positive intranuclear inclusion in an Alzheimer II astrocyte (arrow). (D) Section from cerebral cortex of a patient with hepatorenal syndrome. Note that the characteristic vacuolization of Alzheimer type II cells is not fully developed, although astroglial proliferation is represented by the presence of three paired nuclear forms (arrows). (From *Adv in Cell Neurobiol* 2:303, 1981, Academic Press (395).)

They are also prominent in the striatum, globus pallidus, thalamus, substantia nigra, inferior olives, dentate nucleus, and the Bergmann cells of the cerebellum. The brain stem and spinal cord show a lesser degree of this change. Alzheimer type II cells are not observed in the pyramidal layer of the hippocampus and yet may be conspicuous in the adjacent subiculum. The reasons for these topographical differences are not known. For unexplained reasons Alzheimer type II cells tend not to be conspicuous in patients with hepatorenal syndrome (Fig. 10.14D).

In the cerebral cortex, striatum, and thalamus, the astrocyte has a rounded outline. However, in the pallidum, substantia nigra, inferior olives, and dentate nucleus of the cerebellum, the astrocyte is highly lobulated (Fig. 10.15). Whether this morphological variation represents distinct and separate responses to liver injury or whether it merely reflects local anatomical differences is not known. It is likely that the latter view is correct and that there is probably no significant differences between the rounded, "naked glial nuclei" as observed in cortex and the more lobulated forms as originally described in the pallidum by Von Hosslin and Alzheimer (602).

Another characteristic astrocyte response to liver disease is the apparent increase in the number of these cells. Typically, astroglial nuclei are clustered in pairs, triplets, and even quadruplets (Fig. 10.14B). Adams and Foley (4) indicated an approximate two-fold increase in these cells. The conspicuous lack of mitotic fig-

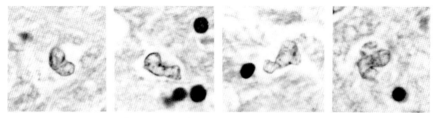

Figure 10.15.   Representative forms of Alzheimer type II astrocytes from globus pallidus in hepatic encephalopathy showing varying degrees of nuclear lobulation and irregularity. H&E. (Original magnification ×600.) (From *Adv Cell Neurobiol* 2:303, 1981, Academic Press (395).)

ures, however, was and continues to be a puzzling aspect of this astroglial response. Lapham (310) found that some astrocytes possessed tetraploid amounts of DNA and thus considered the possibility of amitotic division as an explanation for the apparent increase in the number of astroglial cells. A study by Brun et al. (90) also showed an increase in the number of astrocytes, but they observed no increase in the total number of glial cells.

Experimental studies concerned with the issue of astroglial proliferation have been performed. Norenberg (393) and Taylor et al. (561) noted an apparent proliferation of astroglial cells in their models of hepatic encephalopathy. Again, mitotic figures were not observed. Diemer (137) has extensively studied the problem of quantitation and noted an increased number of Alzheimer type II cells. Similar to the observations of Brun et al. (90) in man, he also was not able to find an increase in the total number of glial cells. He concluded that a true proliferation of astrocytes in hepatic encephalopathy probably does not occur but rather that cells not originally recognized as astrocytes are subsequently interpreted as astrocytes once they develop the typical Alzheimer type II appearance. In any event, while the issue of glial proliferation remains controversial, the apparent proliferation is indeed one of the most characteristic features of the histopathology of human hepatic encephalopathy.

Electron microscopic studies of hepatic encephalopathy in man have been few. Martinez (354) observed that the astrocyte cytoplasm was swollen and contained membrane-bound vacuoles. Minor mitochondrial changes and an apparent increase in the lipofuscin pigment were observed. Foncin and Nicolaidis (185) demonstrated en-

larged, irregular nuclei with coarse chromatin. The cytoplasm was increased in size and was associated with an increase in ribosomes and glycogen.

There is a fairly good correlation between the clinical severity of hepatic encephalopathy and the extent of these astroglial changes (4, 395). Since hepatic encephalopathy may be clinically reversible, one suspects that these astroglial changes may also be reversible. However, a definitive statement on this aspect in man cannot be made at this time. This issue has been studied experimentally by Diemer and Laursen (139) and by Norenberg (395) who have shown that it is a reversible process at least in experimental settings.

Experimental Studies

A large number of experimental studies have been performed to assess the astroglial response to liver disease. These have been recently summarized (395). Most of these studies were designed to either injure the liver or to elevate the blood and/or brain ammonia content. With a few exceptions, all studies have resulted in the formation of cells resembling the Alzheimer type II change seen in man.

Electron microscopic studies by Zamora et al. (634), Norenberg and Lapham (397), and Norenberg (393) showed similar findings. These consisted of hypertrophic cytoplasmic changes, including a proliferation of mitochondria and rough endoplasmic reticulum (Fig. 10.16). These changes occurred early in the phase of this disorder. As the clinical state worsened, the cytoplasmic features appeared degenerative and were characterized by hydropic degeneration, presence of membrane-bound vacuoles, degenerated mitochondria, and swollen Golgi and endoplasmic reticulum (Fig.

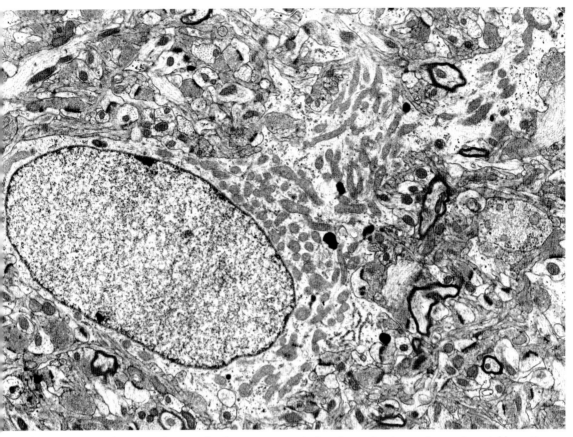

Figure 10.16. Electron micrograph of an astrocyte during the early phase of experimental hepatic encephalopathy. Note the enlarged cytoplasmic compartment with an abundant number of mitochondria. (Original magnification ×10,000.) (From *Lab Invest* 36:618, 1977 (394).)

10.17). These degenerative changes occurring terminally were the electron microscopic counterpart of the Alzheimer type II cell as seen by light microscopy. Significant nuclear alterations were not observed. This is in keeping with the observations of Cavanagh and Kyu (100) and Norenberg and Lapham (397) that the nuclear swelling observed by light microscopy is in part an artifactual change.

It was tentatively concluded that the initial hypertrophic astroglial appearance reflected heightened metabolic activity perhaps for ammonia detoxification. This appears plausible, since glutamine synthetase, the principal enzyme involved in ammonia detoxification, is exclusively found in astrocytes (398). Eventually, perhaps due to energy failure, degenerative changes develop. Thus, impaired astroglial function (water, electrolyte, pH, neurotransmitter regula-

tion) (see Scheffeniels et al. (504) for review) leads to an encephalopathic state.

Fulminant Hepatic Failure

Following acute toxic or viral injuries to the liver, patients may develop an explosive syndrome characterized by the rapid development of delirium, coma, and seizures. Alzheimer type II changes tend not to be very striking, although they are present. Perhaps the short duration of the condition may be responsible for the paucity of astroglial changes, or perhaps the marked severity of the condition alters the ability of the astrocyte to assume this characteristic morphology. Instead, the predominant change is that of cerebral edema (566, 611, 620). The edema appears to be of the cytotoxic type (98). As indicated previously, excessive serum ammonia may cause vasoparalysis resulting in vasodilatation, and

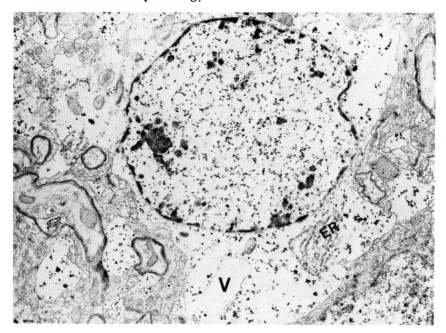

Figure 10.17. Electron micrograph of an astrocyte at the terminal phase of experimental hepatic encephalopathy. Note the cytoplasmic swelling, prominent lamellae of endoplasmic reticulum (*ER*), scattered glycogen granules, and large membrane-bound vacuole (*V*). (Original magnification ×10,000.) (From *J Neuropathol Exp Neurol* 33:423, 1974 (397).)

edema. Additionally, there are often diffuse neuronal changes of an ischemic nature. Whether these neuronal changes are due to the excessive effect of a toxin or represent secondary complications such as hypoglycemia, anoxia, or seizures has not been determined.

Acquired Hepatocerebral Degeneration

Patients suffering from repeated bouts of hepatic encephalopathy may develop a syndrome consisting of dementia, tremor, dysarthria, ataxia, and choreoathetosis (172, 515, 594). Histopathologically the lesions are found predominantly in the cerebral cortex, striatum, and subthalamus, although other parts may be affected. The lesions are characterized by neuronal loss, spongiform changes in the neuropil, and the presence of Alzheimer types I and II astrocytes. Opalsky cells are rarely seen. Astrocytes often possess prominent intranuclear inclusions consisting of glycogen. In the cerebral cortex the changes are best seen in the gyral crests. In severe cases the white matter may also be affected.

These morphological changes have generally been viewed as the sequelae of a progressive metabolic disorder which initially was characterized by the Alzheimer type II change. With progressive insults more severe anatomical changes occur that eventually result in progressive neurological deficits. It is also possible that these patients may have incurred additional metabolic injury (e.g., electrolyte disturbance, anoxia, etc.) that combined with the underlying hepatic encephalopathic state resulted in destructive anatomical changes.

Waggoner et al. (603) and Victor et al. (594) have pointed out the similarity of these cases to those of Wilson's disease, suggesting that a significant component of the neuropathology of Wilson's disease was secondary to liver disease rather than the direct effect of copper on the central nervous system.

"Shunt" Myelopathy

Patients with long-standing portocaval shunts may develop a progressive myelopathy characterized by degenerative and demyelinative changes in the white matter columns of the spinal cord, especially the lateral columns (316, 416, 639, 641). Some patients have not had shunts but instead had severe cirrhosis. The cause of this uncommon disorder is unclear. Whether this condition falls within the spectrum of acquired hepatocerebral degeneration or is due to an additional nutritional or toxic insult not known.

Reye's Syndrome

Reye's syndrome (RS) comprises an acute form of encephalopathy associated with fatty degeneration of the viscera, particularly the liver. It predominantly affects children whose age group ranges from 6 weeks to 16 yr (420). Simultaneous occurrence in siblings has been reported (623). The majority of cases present with a viral or viral-like illness prior to the clinical onset of encephalopathy and hepatocellular dysfunction. Symptoms are characterized by persistent vomiting, anorexia, hyperventilation, and a variable degree of CNS disturbance, which ranges from lethargy and delirium to stupor and coma. Many patients die from the complications of cerebral edema. Surviving patients usually manifest neurologic sequelae, including a variable degree of learning disability, mental retardation, hypotonia, choreoathetosis, and spastic quadriplegia (124). It appears that the degree of neuropsychologic impairment is related to the severity of the initial symptoms and age of onset, with fewer and less severe residua in children who have been affected at an older age.

METABOLIC ABNORMALITIES

Patients with RS usually have increased levels of BUN, SGOT and SGPT, prolonged prothrombin time, and hypoglycemia (266). Bilirubin is rarely increased beyond 3 m$_f$ 'dl, despite massive liver injury and abnormal liver function tests (420).

The most characteristic and consistent abnormality in RS is hyperammonemia. Although a direct relationship between serial changes in blood ammonia levels and clinical severity of the disease has not been consistently shown, the initial level of ammonia is felt to be directly related to the progression and severity of the symptoms (112).

A significant increase in plasma lactate levels has been reported to correlate with the clinical stage of the disease (574), suggesting that lactic acidemia may also be an important factor in this disorder. Such an elevation, however, is not consistently seen in all patients, has not been prominent in the mild and early stages, and may occur only as a late event (115). An elevation of serum-free fatty acids also has been observed (86).

PATHOLOGY

The gross neuropathologic alterations in RS are relatively constant, albeit nonspecific, and consist chiefly of cerebral edema with or without evidence of herniation and vascular congestion. The light microscopic findings are likewise nonspecific and consist mainly of congestion and edema (102). Neuronal eosinophilic degeneration may be seen in the cerebral cortex, Purkinje cell layer, visual cortex, hippocampus, basal ganglia, periaqueductal grey matter, and brain stem nuclei (68). Microglial and astrocytic hyperplasia may be present (119). These changes are felt to be at least in part secondary to hypoxic-anoxic damage. Cytoplasmic inclusion bodies in Purkinje cells, similar to those seen in rabies, were reported in one patient with RS, with negative viral studies and without previous history of animal contact (58). No evidence of inflammation has been described, although satellitosis and neuronophagia are sometimes noted in severe cases (68). Alzheimer type II cells are neither frequent nor characteristic.

By electron microscopy, mitochondrial abnormalities similar to those seen within hepatocytes are noted chiefly within neurons (102, 421, 422). These changes consist of mitochondrial swelling, rarefaction, pleomorphism, and matrix expansion. Disaggregation of neuronal ribosomes, dilatation of endoplasmic reticulum, and a variable increase in number of residual dense bodies are seen within the electron-dense cytoplasm. Cerebral edema, believed to be cytotoxic in nature, is characterized by an accumulation of fluid within myelin lamellae and by swelling of astrocytes and satellite cells. Such changes occur especially in the acute stage of the disease and are reversible. Astrocytic swelling is reportedly reduced after cerebral decompression and treatment by exchange transfusion (421). The recovery period is characterized by the presence of normal mitochondria, reactive astrocytes containing lipid droplets and myelin debris, a variable increase in microglial cells, and enlarged oligodendrocytes (422). Wallerian-type changes and regeneration of myelin sheath are also noted. The ultrastructural morphology of cerebral microvasculature is generally preserved (134), although lysosomal dense bodies containing lipid have been described in pericytes (102).

ETIOLOGIC FACTORS

It appears from the numerous clinical and experimental studies that RS may be due to an interaction of various agent(s) capable of inducing a distinct neurologic entity. Some of these include viruses, toxins, and possible inborn errors of metabolism (112).

Epidemiologic studies have shown serologic evidence of recent infection with influenza B virus in affected patients (256). Influenza A, parainfluenza, adenovirus, vaccinia, and varicella zoster viruses have also been implicated (326).

Clinical and morphological features similar to RS have been reported in patients who die of salicylate intoxication and were attributed to the hepatocellular damage induced by the drug (631). However, not all patients exposed to drug overdose are affected, and marked hyperammonemia is not as prominent with salicylate-induced hepatotoxicity as it is with RS, so that the drug is felt to be merely an "innocent bystander" (112). The validity of studies concerning possible relationship between salicylate toxicity and RS has been critically reviewed (121).

Food contamination by aflatoxin, a metabolic product of *Aspergillus flavus*, has been implicated in the pathogenesis of RS. It causes an illness in children that is indistinguishable from RS (67). Reye's syndrome-like symptoms and metabolic alterations in brain and liver have been induced experimentally when monkeys were given toxic amounts of aflatoxin B (69).

Hypoglycin A, a toxic product of the akee fruit, induces Jamaican vomiting sickness, a condition which is clinically very similar to RS. The active component of hypoglycin A is believed to be its 4-pentenoic acid moiety which when injected intraperitoneally into rats caused RS-like clinical symptoms and morphologic changes in liver. No neuropathologic alterations were reported (219). Goldstein (223) isolated capillaries from rat brain and reported that palmitate-induced potassium uptake by endothelial cells in the brain was completely blocked by 4-pentenoic acid. He suggested that impaired regulation of active cation transport and the consequent inability to maintain water and electrolyte homeostasis might contribute to the formation of brain edema in RS.

PATHOGENETIC MECHANISMS

Hyperammonemia in RS is believed to be due to mitochondrial injury causing a deficiency of carbamylphosphate synthetase and ornithine transcarbamylase (OTC), thereby resulting in impaired liver synthesis of urea (99, 89, 129). Thaler et al. (565) have suggested that the syndrome might represent one of a spectrum of heritable defects in the conversion of ammonia to urea, which then becomes manifest following exposure to various agents including viruses, drugs, and toxins.

Hyperammonemia exerts a toxic effect on the nervous system (see liver disease section). Experimentally, it causes vasoparalysis (293) which might be a key mechanism for the increased intracranial pressure seen in RS patients. In agreement with this view are the studies of Giannotta et al. (210) showing enhancement of cerebral cortex on computerized tomography following injection of contrast material, suggesting the presence of cerebral vasodilatation and increased blood volume. The intramyelinic edema induced following infusion of ammonia to calves (104), which is similar to that seen in RS, further supports the toxic role of ammonia. Lastly, it should be noted that the pathologic changes in RS are similar, if not identical, to those of fulminant hepatic failure. This suggests, at least in part, that the CNS abnormalities may be secondary to severe acute liver disease rather than representing a direct effect on the CNS by the agent(s) causing liver injury.

Short chain fatty acids may play a role in RS. Brown et al. (87) presented clinical and experimental data implicating excessive vomiting as a possible factor in the fatty acidemia by inducing lipolysis, mobilization of fat from body stores, and subsequent accumulation of lipid in certain tissues. Brown and Madge (86) felt that increased fatty acid levels might aggravate the disturbance of mitochondrial metabolism by shifting the normal intracellular metabolic pathways towards an anaerobic cycle. In keeping with the potential toxic role of fatty acids, Ansevin (15) reported that the addition of RS-serum impaired cell respiration, stimulated ATPase activity, and decreased the rate of phosphorylation in isolated rat brain mitochondria. Such alterations in brain mitochondrial function were blocked by preincubating and binding RS-serum with fatty acid-free albumin, which eluted the fatty acids from the test serum.

Intravenous infusion of the short chain fatty acid, sodium octanoate, in rabbits caused significant increase in intracranial pressure, hyperammonemia, lactic acidemia, and clinical features similar to RS (598). Pathologic changes consisted mainly of swelling and pleomorphism of hepatic mitochondria and less consistent swelling of astrocytic processes in brain (597).

Despite these studies that support the role of fatty acids in the pathogenesis of RS, serum-free acid level has not been correlated with the severity of coma, cerebral edema, or extent of neuropathologic alteration in RS (129).

A synergistic effect of aspirin, influenza infection, and ammonia in arginine-deficient rats with clinical and morphological features of RS has been demonstrated (133). Similarly, RS-like features have been induced by treating animals with encephalomyocarditis virus and a variety of chemical agents such as salicylate, pentachlorophenol, and butylated hydroxytoluene (265). These experiments have been performed based on the hypothesis that RS results from a synergistic interaction between environmental, dietary or chemical agents, and viral infection. Schubert et al. (506) maintain that the associated prodrome of viral or viral-like infections acts by sensitizing the host to some ingested toxin. Conversely, Mullen (379) believes that potentially toxic foreign compounds or their biotransformation products (i.e., aflatoxin and hypoglycin A) may be capable of altering the biochemical and immunologic status of the body, thereby making it more susceptible to viral infections.

ENDOCRINE DISORDERS

Disorders of the Pancreas

DIABETES MELLITUS

Cerebral Dysfunction

Diabetes mellitus has a great propensity of causing neurologic complications. Metabolic derangements leading to ketoacidosis, intracellular dehydration, and hyperosmolarity have been responsible for CNS depression, coma, and death in many cases. Prior to the discovery of insulin, 63.8% of diabetic patients died in coma, while 17.5% died of cardiorenal vascular disease (278). With the advent of insulin therapy, there has been a decreased frequency of death from ketoacidotic coma. Associated abnormalities of small and large vessels have accounted for an increased death rate from cardiorenal vascular disorders, as well as an increased incidence of cerebrovascular disease (203). Uremia and worsening chronic renal failure secondary to diabetic nephropathy also cause significant neurologic dysfunction (for further details, see section on renal disease). Other diabetic complications have been related to infection and disorders of peripheral and autonomic nervous system.

Cerebrovascular Disease. Clinical and epidemiological studies have established that diabetic patients have a significantly higher incidence of cerebrovascular disease as well as nonfatal or subclinical infarction, compared to the normal population (31). Hypertension and generalized atherosclerosis occur at an earlier age and with greater severity in diabetics (313). Autopsy studies (35) show a high proportion of atherosclerosis and cerebral infarcts, predominantly in maturity-onset diabetes, as well as a lower survival of diabetic patients with stroke. The Framingham study indicates a six-fold increased risk of atherothrombotic cerebral infarction in diabetic patients with hypertension, even with only modest evidence of impaired glucose tolerance (285). Increased platelet aggregation has, likewise, been observed in diabetic patients (111) and may constitute a risk factor in progressive atherosclerosis and thromboembolic phenomena in diabetes.

Aronson (32) reported an increased incidence of ischemic encephalomalacia in diabetic patients, particularly in the older age group and especially when associated with hypertension. Major cerebral artery occlusion and fatal hemispheric infarcts are only slightly higher, while infratentorial lesions are far more frequent in diabetic than in nondiabetic patients. There is a threefold or greater increase in the rate of infarction within the pontine base, thalamus, and basal ganglia. These lesions consist usually of lacunar infarcts and are rarely fatal.

Massive fatal cerebral hemorrhage, on the other hand, occurs less frequently in an older population of hypertensive diabetic patients, compared to nondiabetic groups (32). This low frequency is probably related to a lower incidence of disseminated fibrinoid necrosis of parenchymatous arterioles and arteries, regarded as precursors of cerebral hemorrhage. Diabetes mellitus may induce structural changes in small arterial walls which may serve as a protective barrier against hypertensive arteriolar necrosis and subsequent cerebral hemorrhage.

The greater activity and generally poor outcome of ischemic strokes are believed to be related to high glucose levels resulting in increased lactate production in brain (35, 439, 450). Glucose administration prior to induction of bilateral forebrain ischemia in rats has caused severe morphologic damage and more extensive infarction throughout the neocortical layers as well as in the striatum, hippocampus, and cerebellum. Brain lactate levels above 16 mmol/kg appear to contribute to cerebral ischemic infarction by causing neuronal death, as well as astrocytic and endothelial injury, and resulting in greater destruction of parenchyma (see section on anoxia-ischemia).

Diabetic Coma. The exact pathogenetic mechanism involved in CNS depression leading to stupor, coma, and death in diabetic ketoacidosis is still controversial. Earlier workers (291) implicated β-hydroxybutyric acid and acetoacetate as the of-

fending anions, causing acidosis, decreased oxygen consumption, and subsequent coma. However, recent studies have indicated that the depth of stupor in uncontrolled diabetes may be more related to the severity and duration of osmotic disequilibrium between blood and brain, rather than to the degree of ketoacidosis (19). Marked dehydration and hyperosmolarity could result in hemoconcentration, increased blood viscosity, decreased blood flow, and decreased oxygen consumption, leading to suppression of aerobic metabolism and irreversible coma (632).

Disseminated intravascular coagulation has also been observed in patients with diabetic ketoacidotic coma (572) and has been precipitated by infection and hypovolemia (52). Abnormal coagulation state and diminished fibrinolytic activity have been observed in a prospective study of patients with uncomplicated diabetic ketoacidotic coma (424). Disseminated intravascular coagulation is more readily induced in alloxan-treated rats, suggesting the metabolic role of diabetes in this coagulation disorder (16).

Cerebral Edema. The initial favorable response to treatment of diabetic ketoacidosis is occasionally followed by sudden rapid deterioration associated with elevated intracranial pressure, coma, and death. The occurrence of fatal acute cerebral edema complicating the treatment of diabetic coma was initially reported by Dillon et al. (141) and later reappraised by Young and Bradley (632). As a rule, the condition occurs in an otherwise healthy, young diabetic following rapid improvement of blood glucose levels and plasma electrolyte concentration with insulin and intravenous therapy. A sudden drop of glucose following insulin therapy is believed to be the cause of cerebral edema. Tornheim (575) measured the brain water content in streptozotocin diabetic rats following fluid and insulin therapy and found preferential accumulation of edema fluid in cerebral cortex as early as 1 h after the initiation of therapy, increasing in magnitude after 5 h, and later also involving the white matter.

The occurrence of cerebral edema following correction of diabetic ketoacidosis has been related to a disturbance of the glucuronate or sorbitol pathway in brain cells. A significant increase of sorbitol, fructose, and the enzymes that catalyze their formation is found in brain, spinal cord, and peripheral nerve of alloxan and streptozotocin diabetic rats (194). Sorbitol crosses membranes slowly, and its accumulation within the tissue is associated with increased water content due to its osmotic effect (449). Clements et al. (107) have postulated that hypertonicity of plasma might counteract and minimize the effect of increased fructose and sorbitol synthesis during hyperglycemia. However, rapid lowering of blood glucose concentration and plasma osmolality by insulin and hypotonic fluids induces a sudden shift of water into the brain, resulting in cerebral edema (448).

An alternate theory has been proposed by Arieff and Kleeman (22), implicating idiogenic osmols in the pathogenesis of cerebral edema. They reported that abrupt lowering of plasma osmolality after sustained hyperglycemia in rabbits caused an osmotic gradient between blood and brain, forcing fluid into the brain. They maintained that the cerebral cortex adapted to extracellular hyperosmolality mainly by accumulation of undetermined solutes (idiogenic osmols), rather than through loss of water or increase in concentration of electrolytes, lactate, amino acids, or other glucose metabolites. Insulin was felt to enhance the transport of electrolytes into the CNS and aid in the uptake of osmotically active particles by brain tissue, thereby causing an increase in water content and volume of the brain. Cerebral edema, however, did not occur until plasma glucose level had fallen to at least 250 mg%.

Hyperosmolar, Hyperglycemic, Nonketotic Coma. Hyperosmolar, hyperglycemic, nonketotic diabetic coma (HHNC) may occur in middle-aged or older patients with recent onset of diabetes, in the absence of significant acidosis or ketonemia. Although accounting for only 10% of hospital admissions for diabetic coma, this condition has been described in up to 90% of autopsied patients with diabetic coma (562). The majority of cases are precipitated by infection or drugs that complicate diabetic control such as thiazides, adrenocorticosteroids, or diphenylhydantoin (449). Almost all patients are clinically dehydrated, while a third are febrile and in

shock upon hospital admission. Hallmarks of the disease include severe hyperglycemia (frequently greater than 1000 mg/dl), severe glycosuria without significant acetonuria, and normal serum ketone levels. The serum hyperosmolality is due to increased Na^+ content from osmotic diuresis, as well as due to hyperglycemia itself.

Neurologic dysfunction has been related to serum hyperosmolality, intracellular dehydration, or abnormal electrolyte distribution (large deficits of Na^+ and K^+) and alteration of respiratory enzyme activity in CNS tissue (234). Arieff and Carroll (20) maintain that hyperglycemia contributes to the development of coma only when there is a resultant elevation of plasma osmolality. Other workers (163) suggest that total body sodium deficit, rather than hyperosmolality itself, plays a critical role in producing neurologic dysfunction by causing a disturbance in cellular membrane potential.

In contrast to diabetic ketoacidosis, focal neurologic deficits are common in HHNC. Focal seizures occur in about 20% of patients with diabetic nonketotic hyperglycemia and comprise the chief clinical manifestation in 6% (182). These usually affect patients in the 5th decade or older and do not cause severe depression of consciousness. Focal seizures are felt to be due to activation of small, previously silent foci of cerebral ischemia by hyperglycemia and hyperosmolality (589). Venna and Sabin (590) reported three patients in whom recurrent focal motor seizures occurred as the initial manifestation of HHNC. They implicated focal cortical venous sludging or thrombosis induced by hyperglycemia, hyperosmolality, and/or dehydration because of the parasaggital localization of the postural seizures in two patients. However, pathologic study of patients with unequivocal HHNC has failed to reveal any significant abnormality (418).

Diabetic Encephalopathy. Reports of primary brain parenchymal involvement by diabetes have been very meager and are difficult to evaluate because of the concomitant vascular damage, hyperosmolarity, acidosis, and shock so frequently associated with the condition. Most clinicians regard the cerebral manifestations in diabetes to be due to cerebrovascular disease. Warren et al. (612) maintain that there are no changes distinctive of diabetes other than occasional abnormal glycogen deposits in ganglion cells. However, morphologic changes have been described in some patients who have had no focal cerebrovascular abnormality. The use of the term "diabetic encephalopathy" is perhaps justified in the few reported cases where ganglion cell abnormalities in long-term diabetics were felt to represent a primary metabolic disorder. Such a term is possibly best regarded on a morphologic basis rather than as a specific clinical entity, since most of the cases reported do not show good clinicopathological correlation.

Reske-Nielsen and Lundbaek (462) reported diffuse degeneration of ganglion cells and nerve fibers in cerebral hemispheres, cerebellum, and brain stem of three patients who had diabetes for 24–30 yr. Subpial gliosis, thickened axis cylinders in white matter, slight diffuse astrocytosis, and oligodendroglial hyperplasia were also described. Degenerative changes and loss of Purkinje cells were noted in the cerebellum. The changes were felt to be due partly to ischemic angiopathy and partly to a primary metabolic derangement in the ganglion cells.

In 1965, Reske-Nielsen et al. (464) studied the neuropathologic changes in 16 juvenile diabetics who died of diabetic angiopathy. They found diffuse degeneration of brain tissue with symmetrical pseudocalcinosis and atrophy of the dentate nucleus of the cerebellum. The ganglion cell abnormality consisted of an accumulation of PAS-positive and lipid-laden cytoplasmic granules (? lipofuscin). Demyelination of cranial nerves, cerebral vascular angiopathy, and fibrosis of the leptomeninges were also described. The changes seemed more severe than would be expected from alterations caused by angiopathy alone. The degenerative lesions were therefore thought to be of dual etiology—either due to ischemia or secondary to a primary metabolic abnormality of the brain parenchyma. There was a poor correlation of the brain pathology with hypertension, uremia, or hyperglycemic episodes.

Diffuse degeneration of cortical neurons, loss of Purkinje cells, Bergmann gliosis, edema of cerebellar granular cell layer, and degeneration of melanin-containing neurons were described by Olsson et al. (408) in nine diabetic patients. These were, however, felt to be similar to those seen in anoxia and ischemia.

Thickening of cerebral cortical capillary basement membrane has been observed by electron microscopy in diabetic patients (277), in streptozotocin diabetic rats (377), and in spontaneously diabetic hamsters (339). The capillary basement membrane thickening is thought to be associated with an increased permeability of the blood-brain barrier, allowing for increased transport of substances that may be potentially harmful to the neural parenchyma. In diabetic patients, an enhanced release of growth hormone during dopamine infusion has been reported (335), indicating a possible abnormality in blood-brain barrier. It is conceivable that the primary ganglion cell abnormalities observed in the so-called "diabetic encephalopathy" may be related to this microangiopathy and increased vascular permeability.

Dysfunction of Spinal Cord, Cranial, Autonomic, and Peripheral Nerves

Myeloradiculoneuropathy. Diabetes mellitus has been associated with loss of deep tendon reflexes, disturbance in proprioceptive sensation, paresthesias, and weakness. These are attributed to the secondary effects of diabetes on spinal cord, nerve roots, and peripheral nerves and may be pathologically related to arteriosclerotic involvement of their respective nutrient vessels.

Routine spinal cord examination in 200 consecutive autopsies (530) revealed occult lesions in 40% of diabetic patients, which consisted of degeneration of spinal tracts, particularly of the posterior columns and microinfarcts. Diffuse, symmetrical degeneration of ganglion cells associated with PAS-positive and lipid-containing granules has been described in anterior and posterior horns (463), as well as in dorsal root ganglia (408). Demyelination and swelling or focal loss of axons were more pronounced in posterior roots than in posterior columns (144, 463), suggesting that the posterior column involvement is probably secondary to Wallerian degeneration. Vascular changes were mild or absent in spinal cord but more pronounced in peripheral nerves. Intimal proliferation and narrowing of the lumen of the anterior spinal artery were noted in a few cases. There was PAS-stained hyalinization of intraneural and perineural arteries. Capillary thickening has been noted only in juvenile diabetes. Neuronal dropout and microinfarcts in spinal cord were reported to have greater frequency and occur at an earlier age in diabetic patients compared to age-matched nondiabetic controls (500). There is no evidence that myelopathy increases with the duration of the illness or correlates with the clinical symptoms of peripheral neuropathy (529).

The precise pathological change in diabetic neuropathy has been in dispute. Segmental demyelination was felt to be the initial and basic pathologic lesion. Electron microscopy of affected nerves show variable internodal lengths of myelinated fibers, myelin breakdown at the nodes of Ranvier, segmental demyelination and remyelination, and Schwann cell proliferation (105, 567). Combined axonal and myelin loss suggestive of Wallerian degeneration and regeneration is less frequent and seen mostly in elderly diabetic patients.

Primary axonal degeneration, especially of unmyelinated and small myelinated fibers, however, has also been reported in early diabetes (64). This is characterized by disintegration of neurofilaments, a corresponding increase in tubular and vesicular elements of the endoplasmic reticulum, accumulation of axoplasmic organelles, and hyperplasia or reduplication of the basement membrane surrounding the Schwann cell. Pathologic changes in motor endplates, characterized by reduction or shrinkage of the terminal arborization and diffuse thickening of preterminal nerve fibers, have been observed in some patients, even in the absence of obvious symptoms of peripheral neuropathy. However, most recent studies appear to indicate that nerve fiber loss secondary to distal axonal neuropathy is the predominant feature of diabetic polyneuropathy (85).

Autonomic Neuropathy. Disorders of autonomic nervous system function associated with diabetes can lead to diverse clinical manifestations. Symptoms may include pupillary abnormalities, impaired pilomotor, vasomotor and sweat gland reflexes (189), gastrointestinal symptoms (155), orthostatic hypotension, and tachycardia, bladder dysfunction, and impotence (156).

Reports on the pathology associated with autonomic dysfunction are variable. Dolman (144) found no significant changes in the lumbar sympathetic chain of diabetic patients with autonomic dysfunction. Berge et al. (53) reported no demonstrable abnormality in mucosal, muscular, vascular, or neural components of the gastrointestinal tract in symptomatic patients. On the other hand, Appenzeller and Richardson (17) found variable stages of degeneration in ganglion cells of the paravertebral sympathetic chains associated with the presence of intracytoplasmic PAS-positive eosinophilic refractile material. The final stage of degeneration was characterized by disappearance of the cell with formation of a "gliocytic" capsule. "Giant" sympathetic neurons and dendritic degeneration of postganglionic neurons have been noted (242).

Axonal degeneration and segmental demyelination in preganglionic communicating rami to the thoracic sympathetic trunk, as well as neurolysis, cytoplasmic vacuolation, and degenerative changes were seen in paravertebral and prevertebral ganglia of patients with autonomic dysfunction (407). These changes were related to marked thickening of the nutrient vessels of both communicating rami and ganglia.

Cranial Neuropathy. Cranial nerves, especially the 3rd and 6th nerves, may be affected in diabetic neuropathy causing external ophthalmoplegia (640). The symptoms are usually abrupt in onset, occurring in patients with poorly controlled long-standing diabetes. The pupil is usually spared, and recovery usually occurs within a few weeks to 9 months.

A combination of various factors such as neuropathy, atherosclerosis, and microangiopathy may play a role in the etiology of diabetic ophthalmoplegia. Dreyfus et al. (146) studied a patient who died with diabetic ophthalmoplegia and found fusiform enlargement of the retroorbital part of the oculomotor nerve, with focal destruction of myelin sheath and axis cylinders in the central portion of the nerve trunk. There was Wallerian degeneration of the distal segment and axonal reaction in the oculomotor nerve nucleus. Although no occluded artery or vein was found, the lesion was believed to be compatible with incomplete ischemic neuropathy. Selective sparing of the peripheral subepineural fibers was felt to be responsible for the retention of the pupilloconstrictor and accommodation fibers of the nerve.

Asbury et al. (34) studied an 88-yr-old diabetic patient with recent and remote oculomotor palsy and showed a circumscribed demyelinating lesion in the intracavernous portion of the 3rd nerve, with relative sparing of the axons, paucity of Wallerian degeneration distally, and absence of central chromatolysis in the cell bodies within the third nerve nuclei. Due to widespread arteriolar disease and the absence of recognizable compressive mechanisms, they implicated ischemia as the basis for the demyelination, although no vessel near the lesion was found to be occluded.

Optic nerve involvement may also occur and may be secondary to toxic-metabolic change (528) or due to ischemic microangiopathy and vascular occlusion of the nutrient vessels (371). Capillary abnormalities in the superficial disc area, similar to those seen in diabetic retinopathy, have also been described (628).

Several mechanisms have been proposed to explain the occurrence of nerve dysfunction in diabetes mellitus. One of the most popular concepts implicates ischemia of peripheral nerves secondary to atherosclerosis (509). Thickening of the basement membrane in endoneurial capillaries can increase blood-brain barrier permeability and affect local metabolite exchange, possibly causing nerve damage (596). Polyneuropathy is also believed to be the result of a disturbance in Schwann cell metabolism leading to breakdown of myelin (567) and an increase in phospholipids (64). Accumulation of sorbitol has been reported which could result in altered cellular integrity, loss of Schwann cells, and segmental demyelination (195). A decrease in nerve myoinositol with deficient myelin synthesis and repair as well as a reduction in myoinositol-related sodium-potassium ATPase activity have also been described (85, 624).

Infection in Diabetes

Diabetic patients account for up to 80% of all reported cases of rhinoorbitocerebral infections by *Mucor* (*Rhizopus*) species (3,286). Mucormyocosis is most often associated with diabetic ketoacidosis. The infection usually begins in the nose and spreads by direct extension to the paranasal sinuses, orbit, cribriform plate, meninges, and brain. The pathology includes invasion of blood vessel wall by the nonseptal fungal hyphae with consequent thrombotic vascular occlusion and infarction of neural parenchyma. The close relationship between uncontrolled diabetic ketoacidosis and mucormycosis is explained by the fact that the *Mucor* species have an active ketone reductase system, grow best in a glucose-rich medium, and have their peak metabolic activity at a low pH level (286). Abrahamson et al. (3) noted that acute alloxan-induced ketotic diabetes in rats and mice permitted invasive growth of preinstilled *Mucor* organisms, while infusional hyperglycemia and nonketotic diabetes did not, implicating acidosis in the pathogenesis of this condition.

PANCREATIC INSUFFICIENCY

Pancreatic Encephalopathy

Patients with acute pancreatitis may develop electrolyte derangements, hypocalcemia, hypoglycemia, hyperosmolality, diabetes mellitus, liver disease, hypotension, and hemorrhagic shock, all of which may induce considerable neurologic dysfunction. Nevertheless, a neurologic syndrome apparently independent of these metabolic alterations has been ascribed to the pancreatic disease itself. Pancreatic encephalopathy has been characterized by acute delirium, hallucinations, convulsive seizures, and multifocal neurologic signs occurring usually between the 2nd and 5th day after the onset of acute pancreatitis (510).

The first comprehensive pathological description of pancreatic encephalopathy is credited to Rothermich and Von Haam (475) who examined five patients with acute hemorrhagic pancreatitis and/or chronic interstitial pancreatitis. The neuropathologic findings were characterized by focal areas of capillary hemorrhage, perivascular edema, and reactive gliosis. The petechial hemorrhages which were most numerous in patients who died of acute pancreatitis were most frequently observed in the basal ganglia and periventricular regions and were only occasionally seen in cortex and white matter. Necrosis and hyalinization of capillary vessel wall as well as subependymal gliosis were also present.

Delarue et al. (128) described areas of cerebral infarction with diffuse demyelination, macrophage reaction, and petechial hemorrhages in the cortex, thalamus, and brain stem. Vogel (598) noted patchy loss of myelin in contiguous portions of grey and white matter, often in a perivascular distribution, with very little neuronal alteration and no inflammation. The perivascular distribution of the lesions, with greater frequency in the more highly vascularized grey matter, suggested that circulating pancreatic enzymes may induce necrosis of cerebral fat and destruction of surrounding myelin sheaths. Embolization of fat particles from bone marrow and other extrapancreatic sites has also been implicated (338).

Vogel (597) has shown that lipase is capable of destroying myelin and may play a role in pancreatic encephalopathy. Pathologic lesions similar to those seen in humans were produced following intracerebral and intravascular injection of purified lipase in rabbits. Loss of stainable myelin in peripheral nerves and in spinal nerve roots were also noted following incubation of segments of spinal cord with lipolytic enzymes, but not with trypsin or chymotrypsin.

Pancreatitis and Central Pontine Myelinolysis

Acute and chronic pancreatitis have been occasionally associated with central pontine myelinolysis (CPM) (512, 599). Vogel felt that lipolytic enzymes released by the damaged pancreas may have been responsible for the demyelination. Since electrolyte abnormalities appear to be important in the development of CPM the pontine demyelination in pancreatitis is probably more closely related to the electrolyte imbalance which is often seen in pancreatic disease (see electrolyte section).

Neuroaxonal Dystrophy and Cystic Fibrosis of Pancreas

Precocious occurrence of neuroaxonal dystrophy has been reported in about two-thirds of patients with cystic fibrosis of the pancreas (361, 553). This occurs in as early as the first decade, increasing progressively with the severity and duration of the clinical course. Axonal spheroids in the sensory nuclei of spinal cord and the gracile and cuneate nuclei are usually accompanied by considerable nerve cell loss and astrogliosis. Bilateral degeneration of fasciculus gracilis in thoracic and cervical segments of the cord has also been described in patients dying with cystic fibrosis (209). Such spinal cord changes are less common and do not necessarily correlate with the presence of dystrophic axons in the gracile and cuneate nuclei. These dystrophic axonal changes have been attributed to vitamin E deficiency (554).

Disorders of Thyroid Gland

BIOCHEMICAL CONSIDERATIONS

The principal thyroid hormones, thyroxine and triiodothyronine, can increase brain excitability, enhance the capacity of the brain to support maximal electroshock seizures, and shorten postictal depression by altering brain electrolyte distribution within the cell (571). There is experimental evidence that extracellular Na^+ is decreased, while intracellular Na^+ is increased in brain during hyperthyroidism (570). Noradrenaline synthesis and/or turnover is also increased (161, 549). Increased noradrenaline plasma level during stimulation of sympathetic flow in hyperthyroidism following removal of CNS control in pithed rats may reflect an increase in neurotransmitter release and a reduction in sympathetic tone (385). Hyperthyroid patients have decreased levels of CSF homovanillic acid, which is a major end product of dopamine breakdown (297), suggesting an alteration in dopamine metabolism.

A decrease in thyroid hormone, on the other hand, results in impaired cyclic adenosine monophosphate accumulation possibly due to a decrease in the density of β-adrenoreceptors in cortical membranes (230). Behavioral syndromes reflecting activation of central serotonergic receptors are much less intense in hypothyroid compared to euthyroid animals (584), implying a state of serotonergic hypoactivity. The latter is believed to be relevant in the etiology of mental retardation occurring in neonatal and juvenile hypothyroidism. Thyroid deficiency also leads to transitory decrease in concentration of glutamic acid, glutamine, and GABA, and permanent depression in levels of aspartic acid and taurine in brain (453). Reduction of both cholesterol and glycolipids is felt to be responsible for the failure of myelin formation in hypothyroidism (131, 423). Neonatal thyroidectomy causes a marked decrease in the activity of certain membrane-bound enzymes which may diminish the formation of the structural membrane components of the CNS during early stages of brain maturation (45, 423).

HYPERTHYROIDISM

Hyperthyroidism is characterized clinically by irritability, insomnia, hyperreflexia, tremors, chorea, seizures, and psychiatric manifestations. No specific morphological abnormalities have been observed in humans. Most of the symptoms have been explained on biochemical and functional grounds alone.

Hyperthyroid Chorea

Hyperthyroid chorea is a distinct clinical entity seen in 2% of patients with hyperthyroidism (334). Choreiform movements are characterized by brief, rapid, incoordinated jerks of the face, limbs, or trunk, and are much less common than the hyperthyroid tremors associated with increased sympathetic tone (555). Morphologic alterations in the brain are lacking. The reversibility of the symptoms following treatment with dopamine antagonists implies a functional rather than a structural striatal defect (297). The symptoms are likewise believed to be related to hypersensitivity of dopamine receptor sites rather than to increased catecholamine production (227).

Hyperthyroid Optic Neuropathy

Optic neuropathy may occur in hyperthyroid patients. The major manifestation, impairment of visual acuity, may be accompanied by papilledema, restriction of ocular motility, or proptosis (579). The cause is thought to be either a mechanical compression of optic nerve by the enlarged extraocular muscles of patients with exophthalmos or a neurotoxic effect of thyroid hormone on the optic nerve.

Acute Thyrotoxic "Encephalomyopathy"

The syndrome of acute thyrotoxic "encephalomyopathy" was described by Waldenstrom (605) who reported six patients in addition to 35 cases in the literature. The syndrome is characterized by acute bulbar manifestations with paralysis of pharyngeal muscles and dysphagia. Paralysis of vocal cords and palate and, rarely, paralysis of 7th and 12th cranial nerves may also be present. Associated signs include choreiform movements, aphasia, apraxia, confusion, and psychosis. Coma may occur, suggesting a cerebral origin of the dysfunction. Pathologic alterations in the brain are lacking. The muscle changes consist of varying degrees of fatty infiltration and muscle fiber atrophy with nonspecific focal myofibrillar degeneration, mitochondrial hypertrophy, and focal dilatation of the transverse tubular system (159).

Parkinsonism and Thyrotoxicosis

The coexistence of Parkinsonism and thyrotoxicosis has been reported and reviewed by Bartels and Rohart (50). Although there is no concrete evidence for any direct relationship between the two conditions, some therapeutic improvement has been reported with the use of ^{131}I in some cases of Parkinsonism.

Myasthenia Gravis and Thyrotoxicosis

A close association between myasthenia gravis and hyperthyroidism, particularly Graves disease, is well known (484). Muscle atrophy and lymphorrhages occur in both conditions, probably because of a common autoimmune mechanism (526). Thyroid antibodies are present in 24% of patients with myasthenia, strongly suggesting related autoimmunity (454). However, there is no evidence that thyroid disorder causes myasthenia gravis or vice-versa, so that the frequent occurrence of both conditions in the same patient is probably related to a genetic predisposition to an autoimmune disease (227).

HYPOTHYROIDISM

Hypothyroidism presents itself in a variety of clinical syndromes, depending upon the severity of hormonal deficiency and the age at which the dysfunction becomes manifest. Severe neonatal thyroid deficiency results in cretinism, while a later onset or less severe dysfunction causes myxedema.

Cretinism

Administration of thyroxine in neonatal rats causes increased growth and development of apical dendritic spines, aberrant hippocampal mossy fibers, early differentiation in cerebellar molecular and internal granular layers, terminal decrease in granule cells, basket cells, and astrocytes, and an overall increase in brain weight (45, 389, 390). On the other hand, induction of hypothyroidism causes impairment of growth of apical dendritic spines, impaired development of cell processes and perikaryon of cortical neurons, and retarded myelination of axons.

Hypothyroidism in children is characterized by apathy, hypomotility, retarded mental and motor development, deafness, and a combination of pyramidal and extrapyramidal signs. Deafness, sometimes associated with tinnitus and vertigo, is common in endemic acquired cretinism and is felt to be due to lesions in the inner ear, nervous tract, or central cochlear components (135). Demonstrable changes in the brain include cerebral hypoplasia, decreased brain weight, and vascular abnormalities (152). Maldevelopment of hypothalamus has been reported (558).

Myxedema

The neurologic dysfunction in adult hypothyroidism may range from mild paresthesia and sensory disturbance to hyporeflexia, slowness of thought, memory loss, delusions, hallucinations, paranoia, lethargy, and coma (391). Unsteadiness of gait and ataxia are commonly attributed to involvement of cerebellum and its connections. Price and Netsky (447) reported focal degeneration of cerebellar cortex with accumulation of glycogen-containing granular bodies ("neural myxedema bodies") in

two patients with myxedema. However, a concomitant history of alcohol abuse in both cases lends some doubt on the significance of such findings. No other pathology has been ascribed to hypothyroidism.

Myxedema coma occurs in less than 1% of hypothyroid patients. It is usually seen in long-standing, severe, undiagnosed cases and particularly affects elderly women (555). The syndrome is often associated with hypothermia in the absence of shivering and with depressed respirations. The associated hypercapnia may be of special importance. Seizures commonly occur and have been reported in 20–25% of patients (164). Some neurologic signs of myxedema have been ascribed to interstitial accumulation of fluid in the nervous system or to changes in cerebral hemodynamics (410, 490). A role of magnesium in the production of myxedema coma has also been postulated (560).

Hypothyroid Neuropathy

Limb paresthesias occur in approximately 80% of patients with hypothyroidism (391). The symptoms usually present as a mononeuropathy associated with compression of median nerve (carpal tunnel syndrome). The changes are probably related to increased amounts of acid mucopolysaccharides in the perineurium and endoneurium as well as in surrounding connective tissue. In addition, Nickel et al. (392) described segmental demyelination, axonal degeneration, metachromasia, and fibrosis of the lateral femoral cutaneous nerve in association with myxedema neuropathy.

Peripheral polyneuropathy has also been documented. Biopsy findings of sural nerves in such cases are consistent with segmental demyelination and remyelination, as well as focal axonal degeneration (151). Electron microscopic studies show increased glycogen accumulation in Schwann cell cytoplasm and axis cylinders, as well as lipid droplets, some abnormal mitochondria, and lamellar bodies.

Disorders of Adrenal and Pituitary Glands

ADDISON'S DISEASE

Adrenocortical insufficiency (Addison's disease) not uncommonly presents as a chronic insidious disorder secondary to destruction of adrenal cortical tissue. It may be caused by tuberculosis, syphilis, tumor metastasis, and fungal infections. Neuropsychiatric disturbances range from nervousness, irritability and depression to disorientation, memory deficit, personality changes, delirium, and coma (106). Some of these symptoms may be associated with evidence of hypoglycemia (109). Neuropathologic findings are rarely reported and consist chiefly of generalized cerebral edema probably resulting from disturbed water metabolism (270). Walsh (609) has also implicated thrombosis of the intracranial dural sinuses as a contributary factor.

Addisonian patients may also present with paresthesias and flaccid paralysis. The latter is usually ascending, bilaterally symmetrical, and related to decrease of neurotransmitter excitability from electrolyte disturbance, especially of potassium (351). Spastic paraplegia has been described associated with patchy degeneration of spinal cord (428). Polyradiculoneuropathy, characterized by segmental peripheral nerve demyelination and a mononuclear inflammatory reaction, has also been reported (1).

ADRENOLEUKODYSTROPHY AND ADRENOMYELONEUROPATHY

These related syndromes, associated but not directly caused by adrenal atrophy, are discussed in Chapter 8.

CUSHING'S DISEASE

Cushing's disease manifests with hypercortisolism secondary to inappropriate ACTH secretion or hypothalamic stimulation of pituitary function by bilateral adrenocortical hyperplasia. Increasing knowledge of neurotransmitter regulation of corticotrophin-releasing hormone/ACTH release has led to the hypothesis that Cushing's disease may represent a functional disorder of CNS regulation of ACTH release (166). Krieger et al. (306) have reported successful treatment of Cushing's disease by a neurotropic drug, cyproheptadine, which has antiserotonergic, anticholinergic, and antidopaminergic effects. Similar results have been obtained following administration of bromocriptine, a dopamine antagonist (308). The normalization of growth hormone response to hypo-

glycemia following bromocriptine administration to patients with Cushing's disease (308) suggests some relationship to altered dopamine metabolism, although a direct effect of excess glucocorticoid on the hypothalamus cannot be excluded. Depression, the most common psychiatric manifestation in patients with Cushing's disease (583), is felt to be a sequel of neurotransmitter disturbance in the hypothalamic-pituitary-adrenal axis (212).

Despite numerous studies on the physiopathology of Cushing's disease, neuropathologic changes in brain parenchyma itself have been only infrequently reported. Hypertensive encephalopathy (162), intracranial hemorrhage (346), and cerebrovascular stroke (438) have been related to the frequent occurrence of hypertension in Cushing's syndrome. Internal hydrocephalus, cerebral cortical and cerebellar atrophy have been reported (373). Specific studies in the hypothalamus have failed to reveal any significant morphologic abnormality (536).

HYPOPITUITARISM

Hypopituitarism may result from intrinsic pituitary gland disease damaging the secretory cells, from hypothalamic disease damaging the hypophysiotropic area, or from extrasellar structural disease impinging on the hypothalamic-pituitary endocrine unit. Complications of hypopituitarism may therefore be related to the causative lesion (i.e., visual field defect from pituitary tumor) or may be secondary to pituitary failure itself. Patients with hypopituitarism are prone to certain metabolic or endocrine crises due to water intoxication, hypoglycemia, or disturbance of temperature regulation and may also exhibit inordinate sensitivity to CNS depressants (2). Reports on the morphologic alterations in CNS induced by pituitary failure are nil.

REMOTE EFFECTS OF CARCINOMA

Several distinct neurologic disorders have been recognized as complications of malignancy in the absence of CNS metastasis. The major categories include cerebellar cortical degeneration, encephalomyelitis, peripheral neuropathy, and neuromuscular disorders. Progressive multifocal leukoencephalopathy is a well-recognized entity which occurs predominantly with lymphoreticular malignancies. Other complications may be secondary to opportunistic infections in the face of impaired immune response, to abnormal hemorrhagic or thromboembolic tendency, or to the effects of radiation and chemotherapy.

Cerebellar Degeneration

It is estimated that at least 50% of patients with acquired progressive subacute cerebellar degeneration have an underlying malignancy (244). Conversely, symptomatic cerebellar degeneration is seen in 16% of patients with carcinoma, being second in frequency to paraneoplastic neuropathy which occurs in 22% of cases (497). The most common associated neoplasm is lung cancer followed by those in the ovary, breast, and uterus (75). Clinical manifestations often occur prior to the discovery of the underlying tumor, although they may initially appear months after tumor resection. Ataxia and dysarthria are the most common symptoms followed by nystagmus, dysphagia, and dementia. There may also be associated cranial nerve dysfunction, motor weakness, sensory disturbance, and abnormal deep tendon reflexes.

Unlike alcoholic cerebellar degeneration where changes are mostly restricted to the superior vermis, paraneoplastic cerebellar degeneration consists of a diffuse loss of Purkinje cells without specific involvement of neo- or paleocerebellum. The greatest degree of neuronal loss is seen with ovarian carcinoma (497). This may be accompanied by a less conspicuous loss of granule cells with slight atrophy and gliosis of the molecular layer. The cerebellar white matter may show evidence of secondary degeneration. The deep cerebellar nuclei are only rarely involved (547). There may be associated degeneration of spinocerebellar tracts with less severe damage of the posterior columns (75). Perivascular lymphocytic infiltration and microglial nodules may be found to a variable degree (76). Occasional cases have associated demyelination of the globus pallidus and Parkinsonian features (75), Wernicke's type of degenerative changes in the mamillary bodies and mesencephalic tectum (592), or loss of motor neurons in brain stem and spinal cord (246). The variable course and lack of cor-

relation between tumor size and occurrence of cerebellar degeneration makes the simple toxic effect of tumor an unlikely factor. It has been suggested that the changes seen in cerebellar degeneration may be due to the flare-up of a viral infection or to carcinoma-induced nutritional or metabolic imbalance (593). Antibodies to Purkinje cells have been documented in patients with carcinomatous cerebellar degeneration, suggesting that the pathogenetic mechanism may be immune-mediated (228).

Encephalomyelitis

Perivascular cellular infiltrates typically but not exclusively affecting the grey matter of brain, brain stem, cerebellar nuclei, spinal cord, posterior nerve roots, and ganglia are commonly observed in patients with carcinoma. They are usually associated with oat cell carcinoma of the lung but may also be seen with adenocarcinoma of uterus and breast (116). Occasional cases have been reported with Hodgkin's disease (608). Patients may be asymptomatic, with neuropathologic changes discovered incidentally on postmortem examination. Symptoms, if present, may vary depending on the CNS area involved and may precede, accompany, or follow the discovery of the associated malignancy. The course of this disorder may last between 2 and 24 months. Progressive mental symptoms such as selective impairment of recent memory, confusion, hallucination, and disorientation occur with limbic encephalitis. Vertigo, ataxia, nystagmus, and bulbar palsy (brain stem involvement), muscle wasting and weakness with or without fasciculation (spinal cord involvement) or sensory neuropathy (posterior root and ganglion involvement) are also observed.

The neuropathologic features resemble those of a viral infection and consist principally of perivascular lymphocytic infiltration, microglial nodule formation, and a variable degree of neuronal degeneration and gliosis (245). Wallerian degeneration of nerve tracts arising from damaged neurons may be seen. There is no strict correlation between the intensity of lymphocytic infiltration and the severity of neuronal loss or gliosis.

In so-called limbic encephalitis, the inflammatory reaction is most severe in the medial temporal lobe, amygdaloid nucleus, hypothalamus, and hippocampus, usually extending into the subiculum and parahippocampal gyrus (14). Although generally associated with lung carcinoma, limbic encephalitis may occasionally occur in the absence of malignancy (309).

The changes in brain stem encephalitis are most severe in the medulla where grey matter structures along the floor of the 4th ventricle, cranial nerve nuclei, and inferior olives are predominantly affected. The lesions may also involve the pontine base and tegmentum and are sometimes associated with degeneration of olivocerebellar tracts. Occasionally, the midbrain may be specifically involved (460). In the spinal cord, the grey matter (especially the anterior horn) is most severely affected and is associated with degeneration of pyramidal and spinocerebellar tracts. The inflammatory reaction not infrequently extends into the peripheral nerve roots and dorsal root ganglia with formation of residual nodules of Nageotte (635).

Although specific areas may be singly and predominantly affected, it is not uncommon to find involvement of the whole CNS constituting an encephalomyeloganglioradiculitis, sometimes in association with subacute cerebellar degeneration and peripheral neuropathy (145, 232, 593). The concurrence of these lesions suggests a common or related pathogenetic mechanism linking these various paraneoplastic syndromes.

The exact pathogenesis of the perivascular infiltrates is still unclear. They were initially felt to represent a secondary reaction to degenerating nervous tissue (76). A viral etiology was later proposed (246, 481) and is presently the accepted view to account for the inflammatory nature of the lesion. However, supporting evidence by direct studies and viral cultures is lacking. The alternative view is that it may represent altered host immune response either due to infection or to autoimmunity (481) or that it may be secondary to some neurotoxic or neuroirritative factors from the neoplasm (145). None of these hypotheses has been satisfactorily proven.

Necrotizing Myelopathy

Patients with visceral carcinoma (lung, breast, kidney) sometimes develop a progressive necrotizing myelopathy in the absence of metastasis within the spinal cord, meninges, or epidural space (466, 622). The neurologic disorder may occur prior to or after the onset of malignancy. It may also manifest in the absence of tumor recurrence. The etiology and pathogenesis of this disorder is unclear, although some workers believe that the changes may have been related to an organ-specific toxic factor elaborated by the neoplasm (466). A prevailing theory is that the syndrome may be related to direct viral invasion or represents an allergic response to viral, bacterial, or toxic agents (258, 328, 643, 651, 653).

The illness is characterized by a sudden onset of ascending sensory loss followed by progressive flaccid paralysis which may change into spasticity within a week or two (328, 643, 648). The initial loss of deep tendon reflexes is later followed by hyperreflexia, clonus, positive Babinski sign, and loss of bowel and bladder control. The cerebrospinal fluid may show normal to very high protein levels. Pleocytosis, when present, is usually transient and consists initially of polymorphonuclear leukocytes which are later replaced by mononuclear cells (648, 655).

The duration of the illness may be acute or subacute (258, 649, 651). In acute cases, the loss of spinal cord function is usually complete within several days to a couple of weeks. Subacute cases generally have a more gradual course without any remission, reaching the greatest degree of neurologic impairment within 8 weeks to 6 months.

The pathologic process usually extends through several segments of the spinal cord and is most frequently seen at the thoracic and lumbosacral levels (258, 651, 655). The affected cord may be swollen during the initial phase or shrunken in the later stages (651). The lesion is generally not confined to a particular vascular distribution (258, 654). The white matter is more involved than the grey (258, 648). In some cases, there is a predominant involvement of the anterolateral columns, while in others, the posterior columns are more severely affected (466).

Microscopically, the morphologic alteration is characterized by patchy areas of nonspecific necrosis involving white more than grey matter, associated with swelling of myelin sheaths, Wallerian degeneration, and reactive gliosis (466, 649). Fragmentation and loss of axis cylinders are accompanied by degeneration and loss of myelin (466, 643). Inflammatory reaction, if present, is minimal, consisting of perivenular collections of histiocytes and macrophages (258, 655). Perivascular cuffing by lymphocytes and plasma cells occurs rarely (258, 466). Focal leptomeningeal thickening may be present. Meningeal inflammation is usually absent, although some cases may show a variable degree of inflammatory cell infiltration (648). Minor vascular abnormalities characterized by endothelial hyperplasia, thrombosis, vasculitis, fibrinoid necrosis, or adventitial fibrosis of the walls of intramedullary or meningeal vessels may be seen inconstantly (258, 466, 649). These changes are felt to be part of the overall necrotizing process rather than having a primary pathogenetic significance (258).

A clinically and morphologically similar syndrome exists in the absence of carcinoma. In these cases, no specific vascular etiology can be found, and the exact pathogenetic mechanism is obscure (328).

The illness may occur at any age but is generally more common in the 3rd and 4th decades of life (328, 648). Some patients may be in good health prior to the onset of symptoms (643, 648). In others, the neurologic disorder may be preceded by an upper respiratory infection, minor systemic disease, or a history of exposure to a variety of toxins or physical agents (643, 648, 655). Some patients die within 2 weeks to 3 months from the onset of symptoms because of respiratory failure, especially when the cervical cord segments are involved (655). Others succumb at a later date from the effects of bedsores or urinary infection (651, 654). However, a number of patients may survive the episode and may either remain incapacitated or gradually recover from their neurologic dysfunction (328).

Carcinomatous Neuromyopathy

Peripheral neuropathy is the most frequently recognized paraneoplastic syndrome, sometimes occurring in combination with subacute cerebellar cortical degeneration. It is most often associated with carcinoma of the lung (especially the oat-cell variant) and ovary, followed by stomach, prostate, breast, colon, cervix, and uterus in descending order (466). Neurological symptoms may occur long before or after malignancy is discovered (117). The patients may present with either a purely sensory neuropathy or a subacute or chronic distal sensorimotor polyneuropathy. There is no definite correlation between the degree of peripheral nerve involvement and the extent and course of malignancy (650).

Sensory neuropathy has a generally subacute course characterized by loss of all modalities of sensation (especially joint and position sense) associated with relatively intact motor function (117, 260). Pain and paresthesia initially affect distal extremities, progressing proximally and accompanied by unsteady gait, sensory ataxia, and pseudoathetosis. CSF protein is usually high (>100 mg/dl) with normal or increased cell count (260). The pathology primarily consists of variable degeneration and loss of neurons in the dorsal root ganglia (260, 644). This is generally accompanied by secondary degeneration and gliosis of the posterior columns, atrophy of posterior roots, and secondary degeneration of peripheral nerves. There is relative preservation of anterolateral columns and various cell groups in the anterior and posterior horns (117). Inflammatory cellular response and neuronophagia, if present, are usually confined to the dorsal root ganglia with little extension into the nerve roots (260). However, in some cases there may be associated encephalomyelitic changes in the limbic areas, brain stem, and spinal cord parenchyma.

Subacute or chronic distal sensorimotor polyneuropathy with loss of tendon reflexes frequently overlaps with a myopathic syndrome characterized by weakness and wasting of proximal extremities (646, 650). It is often difficult clinically to determine whether the symptoms are primarily due to disease of motor neurons, peripheral nerves, or muscle, or a combination of the three (245). The polyneuropathy is characterized histologically by combined axonal and myelin degeneration and is felt to be secondary to degeneration of neurons, spinal sensory ganglia, and spinal cord. Some patients with carcinomatous sensorimotor dysfunction show evidence of vasculitis of epineural vessels in addition to active nerve fiber degeneration (276). Associated perivascular inflammation (brain stem encephalitis) in two reported autopsied cases suggests a somewhat related pathogenetic mechanism involving these entities (276). Muscle biopsy of affected areas shows focal nonspecific myofiber necrosis in the absence of inflammation.

Carcinoma and Muscle Disease

Polymyositis or dermatomyositis occurring in the older age group (>40) has a very high incidence of associated malignancy (477). The inflammatory disorder usually occurs independently of the neoplasm and often appears before the diagnosis of malignancy is made. There is no predilection for any particular tumor and no correlation between the course of muscle disorder and the treatment or extent of malignancy (477, 645). Clinically, the patients present with a rapid evolution of proximal muscle weakness associated with increased serum enzyme levels (creatine phosphokinase, lactic dehydrogenase), high erythrocyte sedimentation rate, and characteristic fibrillations and myopathic action potentials on electromyography (647). Pathologic features consist of a perivascular or interstitial chronic inflammatory reaction with necrosis and regeneration of muscle fibers (477, 647).

Certain neoplastic conditions have been associated with defects in neuromuscular transmission. About 33% of patients with thymoma have myasthenia gravis (477), while 10% of myasthenic patients have thymoma (476). Histologic changes are usually nonspecific. In some cases, scattered degenerating fibers and lymphocytic infiltrates (lymphorrhages), either in perivenous location or adjacent to the necrotic fibers, are seen, superficially resembling polymyositis (480). Abnormal arborization of nerve terminals, simplification of the postsynaptic region, and decrease in nerve terminal area have been described (485). The primary fault is felt to be either a reduction in amount of ACh/quantum or diminished postsynaptic sensitivity (157). Immune complexes (IgG, C3) have been demonstrated in postsynaptic membrane and degenerating junctional folds, supporting the theory that a destructive autoimmune reaction in postsynaptic membrane may be an important pathogenetic factor (160).

Eaton-Lambert syndrome is a myasthenic disorder associated with a high frequency of intrathoracic tumors, especially oat cell carcinoma of the lung, developing 3 months to 2 yr after the diagnosis of muscle disease (652). Cases likewise have been reported of cerebellar degeneration and Eaton-Lambert syndrome in association with bronchogenic carcinoma (486). There is no consistent histologic abnormality, and end-plate sensitivity to ACh is normal. The defect is felt to be presynaptic and due to impaired release of ACh from the nerve terminals (158).

Infections

Infection of the CNS by fungi and gram-negative rods are more common in cancer patients than in the general population (103). Almost one-third of all cases of meningitis are secondary to fungal infections, particularly *Cryptococcus neoformans*. The most common bacterial agent in patients with malignancy is *Listeria monocytogenes* (22%), which is responsible for less than 1% of bacterial meningitis in the general population. *Diplococcus pneumoniae* accounts for 14% of bacterial meningitis. Brain abscesses, although less common than meningitis, occur with greater frequency in the cancer population and are most frequent in patients with leukemia. In lymphoma patients, the type of infection depends upon the degree of WBC depression. With WBC counts greater than 2700/cu mm, *Cryptococcus*, *Listeria*, and *D. pneumoniae* are the predominant organisms involved. *Proteus* infections occur when WBC count is less than 2700/cu mm. The incidence of herpes zoster-varicella infection ranges from 0.06–13.4% (221, 537). The latter is particularly seen in patients with Hodgkin's disease and most frequently involves the thoracic cord. Infections with multiple organisms may occur (618). The propensity of these infectious processes to affect patients with malignancy is generally felt to be due to immunologic deficiency related to the neoplasm or to therapy.

Several cases of "measles inclusion body encephalitis" have been reported following treatment of acute lymphocytic leukemia (540). Usually occurring while patients are in clinical remission, the symptoms develop about 2–5 months after uncomplicated measles and generally prove fatal within a couple of weeks. The measles antibody titer is usually increased but may be normal. Pathologic findings include parenchymal necrosis and eosinophilic nuclear and cytoplasmic inclusions in neurons and glial cells, predominantly in cortex and basal ganglia. Nucleocapsids of paramyxoviruses are seen with electron microscopy.

CNS toxoplasmosis is most frequently associated with Hodgkin's lymphoma and acute leukemias but has also been described with melanoma and ovarian carcinoma (99, 595). The majority of patients have had malignancy for more than a year and have received radiation and/or chemotherapy (531, 595). They may manifest clinically with symptoms of diffuse encephalopathy, meningoencephalitis, or cerebral mass lesions and may often have simultaneous infection with cytomegalovirus and herpes (479). Pathologic features vary from acute focal encephalomyelitis to massive necrosis of brain parenchyma with involvement of grey and white matter and usually accompanied by acute vasculitis, thrombosis, perivascular cuffing by mononuclear cells, collection of macrophages, and reactive astrocytosis. Toxoplasma occurring as pseudocysts or as free organisms may be seen within the necrotic areas.

Progressive Multifocal Leukoencephalopathy

Progressive multifocal leukoencephalopathy is a subacute demyelinative disorder sometimes found in association with lymphoproliferative disorders and carcinomas. It results from a papovavirus infection in an immunocompromised host. For further discussion see Chapter 14.

Hemorrhage and Thrombosis

Intracerebral hemorrhage is a well-known complication of acute myelogenous and acute lymphocytic leukemia (190, 435). Fatal parenchymal hemorrhage correlates best with blastic crisis and is seen frequently in patients with WBC counts ranging from 50,000 to 300,000/cu mm or more (434). Its relationship with thrombocytopenia is less well-defined, except in cases where the leukocyte count is less than 50,000/cu mm. Leukocytosis with consequent leukostasis and increased blood vis-

cosity is believed to be a major pathogenetic mechanism in this disorder. Loss of integrity of the vascular endothelium secondary to vasodilatation and increased vascular permeability have also been suggested as contributing factors.

Nontraumatic subdural hematoma and spontaneous subarachnoid hemorrhage, on the other hand, are felt to be more directly related to low platelet levels than to leukocytosis (434), although the degree of thrombocytopenia is claimed not to correlate with the neurologic status of the patients (436). Venous obstruction by tumor cells as well as a coagulation defect secondary to disseminated intravascular coagulation has also been described (193).

An increased incidence of cerebral infarction has been reported in patients with systemic cancer (459). Collins et al. (110) found cerebrovascular disease in 10% of 1459 autopsied patients with cancer. Twelve of these patients showed multifocal acute and subacute hemorrhagic or pale infarcts secondary to disseminated intravascular coagulation. Ten patients had leukemia or lymphoma, while two had breast carcinoma.

Thrombosis of major venous channels including the dural sinuses has also been reported, particularly in patients with acute leukemia, less frequently with cancer of lung and breast (523), and occasionally with occult malignancy (534). Although sagittal sinus thrombosis more commonly occurs as a metastatic complication, non-metastatic occlusion has been noted and is believed to be possibly due to either local injury to the sinus or to a hypercoagulable state that is so often seen with systemic malignancy (426).

Miscellaneous Conditions

A chronic form of Wernicke's encephalopathy characterized by petechiae, neuronal depletion, loss of myelinated fibers, and gliosis in mamillary bodies, periaqueductal region, and areas adjacent to 3rd and 4th ventricles has been described in three patients with tumors of hematopoietic and lymphoid system (132). An association between ALS and a variety of malignant neoplasms, most commonly adenocarcinoma, has been noted by some investigators (402). In 50% of their cases the motor neuron disease occurred prior to the diagnosis of carcinoma. Granulomatous angiitis, characterized by segmental vasculitis, focal obliteration of small vessels, and infiltration by histiocytes, multinucleated cells, and chronic inflammatory cells has been observed in several patients with Hodgkin's lymphoma (226). The concurrent presence of lymphoma, herpes zoster, and granulomatous angiitis has led to the speculation that the latter may be related to viral infection in an immunocompromised host, although no infectious agent has been identified (474).

Complications of Therapy

Parenchymal foci of necrosis with predilection for white matter, vascular proliferation, and atypical astrogliosis are not uncommonly observed in patients who have received radiation therapy for primary or metastatic tumors in brain. Vascular injury is generally felt to be the important factor in causing parenchymal damage. In monkeys, delayed radiation necrosis induces a selective vulnerability of white matter, beginning as areas of demyelination and progressing into actual necrosis with axonal degeneration (240). This is associated with vasculitis, aneurysmal formation, telangiectasia, and endothelial hyperplasia. Hypertrophy of oligodendroglial cells with cytoplasmic glycogen accumulation is described as one of the earliest manifestations of parenchymal injury. Experimental studies on spinal cord of Wistar rats exposed to radiation show lamellated myelin balls in paranodal regions associated with Wallerian degeneration throughout white matter, most numerous in the ventral half and in superficial portions of the dorsal columns. Widening and variable lengths of nodal gap become more prominent 2 months after radiation and are felt to be unrelated to the axonal degeneration (356).

Subacute disseminated necrotizing leukoencephalopathy has been described in patients who have been treated with combined intrathecal antimetabolite chemotherapy (particularly methotrexate) and radiation for leukemia/lymphoma (478) or following ventriculocisternal administration of methotrexate for posterior fossa tumors (401). Similar necrotizing lesions have been reported predominantly in basis pontis (78). Such lesions consist of discrete foci of coagulation necrosis randomly scattered in subcortical and deep white matter in the absence of inflammatory cellular response and with relative paucity of macrophage reaction. Demyelination and axonal damage with conspicuous axonal swelling and astrocytic response are present. Axonal swelling is a constant early feature representing a disturbance in functional metabolism of the axoplasm. This is believed to be related to inhibition of DNA synthesis with subsequent effect on neuronal protein synthesis and metabolism of axoplasm by the antimetabolite. Pyknosis, karyorrhexis, and eventual loss of oligodendroglial cells with edema and spongiosis of adjacent parenchyma are also noted. No intranuclear inclusions are seen. There is usually no correlation between the extent of white matter damage and the dosage of methotrexate or radiation. The changes are different from cerebral radionecrosis because of the usual lack of conspicuous vascular fibrinoid necrosis, endothelial hyperplasia, and fibrin extravasation in neural parenchyma.

Mixed sensorimotor peripheral neuropathy is the most common manifestation of vincristine toxicity, although cranial nerve dysfunction (involving oculomotor, trigeminal, abducens, and facial nerves) and autonomic dysfunction have also been reported (617). Peripheral nerve damage consists of primary axonal degeneration rather than segmental demyelination both in clinical as well as in experimental studies (72, 73, 225). Vincristine also has been reported to result in neuroaxonal dystrophy with formation of axonal spheroids in brain stem and upper cervical cord (362). Axonal damage is thought to be secondary to disruption of neurotubules with consequent impairment of axoplasmic transport mechanisms (495, 511). Neurofibrillary degeneration, proliferation of neurofilaments, and loss of neurotubules have been seen in electron microscopic studies of neuron cultures and mouse spinal ganglia (93, 511).

A syndrome of transient, reversible cerebellar, vestibular and pyramidal tract dysfunction has been observed in 2–7% of patients receiving intensive high dose courses of 5-fluorouracil (304). The patients present with ataxia, gross dysmetria, slurred speech, and coarse nystagmus which may be difficult to differentiate clinically from carcinomatous cerebellar degeneration. Neuropathologic changes consist of acute neuronal changes in olivary and dentate nuclei and dropout of cerebellar granule cells. The cause of cerebellar toxicity is unknown. Experimental studies in cats have suggested that its major catabolite, α-fluoro-β-alanine is further degraded to form fluoroacetate and fluorocitrate, which are potent inhibitors of the Krebs cycle (304).

L-asparaginase, an enzyme used for the treatment of acute lymphoblastic leukemia, has been known to cause marked cerebral dysfunction characterized by lethargy, somnolence, and confusion, usually beginning within a day or so of therapy and clearing rapidly after the end of treatment (617). Less commonly, a delayed form of organic brain syndrome resembling delirium tremens or Korsakoff's psychosis has also been observed about 1 week after therapy, often lasting for several weeks. The acute form of encephalopathy is probably related to L-aspartic acid intoxication or to increased ammonia liberated by the enzymatic action of L-asparaginase on its substrates, L-asparagine and L-glutamine (404). The delayed organic syndrome is felt to be due to defective protein synthesis resulting from L-asparagine deficiency. Although no definite pathology has been described in brain, abnormal clotting, decreased plasminogen, and elevated fibrin degradation products have been noted in patients receiving asparaginase therapy (455).

Seizures, coma, progressive cerebral dysfunction, and death have occasionally been observed in association with intracarotid and regional nitrogen mustard perfusion (30). Examination of the brain has revealed only focal areas of gliosis with neuronal loss (59). Occasional cases of myelopathy have also been reported following treatment with cytosine arabinoside (78). The lesion, possibly due to direct toxic effect of the drug, affects white matter of the spinal cord and consists of microvacuolation, fat-laden macrophages, axonal swelling, loss of myelin, and minimal fibrillary gliosis.

ACKNOWLEDGMENTS

The authors are grateful to Drs. Robert C. Griggs and Richard Satran for allowing us to review their manuscript on clinical aspects of metabolic encephalopathy, to Mrs. Linda Williams for her meticulous preparation of the text, and to Dr. Luz-Oliva B. Norenberg for her tireless review of the manuscript.

References

1. Abbas DJ, et al: Polyradiculoneuropathy in Addison's disease. Case report and review of literature. *Neurology (Minneap)* 27:494, 1977.
2. Abboud CF, Laws ER Jr: Clinical endocrinological approach to hypothalamic-pituitary disease. *J. Neurosurg* 51:271, 1979.
3. Abrahamson E, et al: Rhinocerebral phycomycosis in association with diabetic ketoacidosis. *Ann Intern Med* 66:735, 1967.
4. Adams RD, Foley JM: The neurological disorder associated with liver disease. *Res Publ Assoc Res Nerv Ment Dis Proc* 32:198, 1953.
5. Adams RD, et al: Central pontine myelinolysis: a hitherto undescribed disease occurring in alcoholic and malnourished patients. *Arch Neurol Psychiatry* 81:154, 1959.
6. Agamanolis DP, et al: Immunosuppressive measles encephalitis in a patient with a renal transplant. *Arch Neurol* 36:686, 1979.
7. Agardh CD, et al: Hypoglycemic brain injury. I. Metabolic and light microscopic findings in rat cerebral cortex during profound insulin-induced hypoglycemia and in the recovery period following glucose administration. *Acta Neuropathol (Berl)* 50:31, 1980.
8. Ahmed K, Thomas BS: The effects of long chain fatty acids on sodium plus potassium ion-stimulated adenosine triphosphatase in rat brain. *J Biol Chem* 246:103, 1971.
9. Aikawa JK: The relationship of magnesium to disease in domestic animals and humans. Springfield, IL, Charles C Thomas, 1971, pp 10–36.
10. Alfrey AC, et al: Syndrome of dyspraxia and multifocal seizures associated with chronic hemodialysis. *Trans Am Soc Artif Organs* 18:257, 1972.
11. Alfrey AC, et al: The dialysis encephalopathy syndrome: possible aluminum intoxication. *N Engl J Med* 294:184, 1976.
12. Ames A III, Gurian BS: Effects of glucose and oxygen deprivation on function of isolated mammalian retina. *J Neurophysiol* 26:617, 1963.
13. Ames A III, et al: Cerebral ischemia. II. The no-reflow phenomenon. *Am J Pathol* 52:437, 1968.
14. Anderson JM, et al: Pathological changes in the nervous system in severe neonatal hypoglycemia. *Lancet:* 1:372, 1966.
15. Ansevin CF: Reye syndrome: serum-induced alterations in brain mitochondrial function are blocked by fatty-acid-free albumin. *Neurology* 30:160, 1980.
16. Antoniades HN, et al: Effects of nutritional, endocrine and metabolic state on the development of intravascular coagulation induced by human serum preparations with procoagulant activity. *Thromb Diath Haemorrh* 29:33, 1973.
17. Appenzeller O, Richardson EP: Sympathetic chain in patients with diabetic and alcoholic neuropathy. *Neurology (Minneap)* 16:1205, 1966.
18. Arieff AI: Neurological complications of uremia. In Brenner BM, Rector FC, (eds) *The Kidney.* Philadelphia, WB Saunders, 1981.
19. Arieff AI, Carroll HJ: Nonketotic hyperosmolar coma with hyperglycemia: clinical features, pathophysiology, renal function, acid-base balance, plasma CSF equilibria and the effects of therapy in 37 cases. *Medicine (Baltimore)* 51:73, 1972.
20. Arieff AI, Carroll HJ: Cerebral edema and depression of

sensorium in nonketotic hyperosmolar coma. *Diabetes* 23:525, 1974.

21. Arieff AI, Guisado R: Effects on the central nervous system of hypernatremic and hyponatremic states. *Kidney Int* 10:104, 1976.

22. Arieff AI, Kleeman CR: Cerebral edema in diabetic comas. II. Effects of hyperosmolality, hyperglycemia and insulin in diabetic rabbits. *J Clin Endocrinol Metab* 38:1057, 1974.

23. Arieff AI, Massry S: Calcium metabolism of brain in acute renal failure. *J Clin Invest* 53:387, 1974.

24. Arieff AI, Schmidt RW: Fluid and electrolyte disorders of the central nervous system. In Maxwell MH, Kleeman CR (eds): *Clinical Disorders of Fluid and Electrolyte Metabolism*, ed 3. New York, McGraw-Hill, 1980, pp 1409–1480.

25. Arieff AI, et al: Brain water and electrolyte metabolism in uremia: effects of slow and rapid hemodialysis. *Kidney Int* 4:77, 1973.

26. Arieff AI, et al: Intracellular pH of brain: alterations in acute respiratory acidosis and alkalosis. *Am J Physiol* 230:804, 1976.

27. Arieff AI, et al: Neurological manifestations and morbidity of hyponatremia: correlation with brain water and electrolytes. *Medicine* 55:121, 1976.

28. Arieff AI, et al: The pathophysiology of hyperosmolar states. In Andreoli TE, Grantham JJ, Rector FC (eds): *Disturbances in Body Fluid Osmolality*. Bethesda, MD, American Physiological Society, 1977, pp 227–250.

29. Arieff AI, et al: Dementia, renal failure, and brain aluminum. *Ann Intern Med* 90:741, 1979.

30. Ariel IM: Intra-arterial chemotherapy for metastatic cancer to the brain. *Am J Surg* 102: 647, 1961.

31. Aronson SM: Some ecologic features of cerebral vascular disease. *Patologos.* 7:147, 1969.

32. Aronson SM: Intracranial vascular lesions in patients with diabetes mellitus. *J Neuropathol Exp Neurol* 32:183, 1973.

33. Arsénio-Nunez ML, et al: Ultrastructural and histochemical investigation of the cerebral cortex of cat during and after complete ischemia. *Acta Neuropathol* 26:329, 1973.

34. Asbury AK, et al: Oculomotor palsy in diabetes mellitus: a clinicopathological study. *Brain* 93:555, 1970.

35. Asplund K, et al: The natural history of stroke in diabetic patients. *Acta Med Scand* 207:417, 1980.

36. Avram MM, et al: Uremic syndrome in man: new evidence for parathormone as a multisystem neurotoxin. *Clin Nephrol* 11:59, 1979.

37. Bachelard HS: Energy utilized by neurotransmitters. In Ingvar DH, Lassen NA (eds): *Brain Work.* Copenhagen, Munksgaard, 1975, p 79.

38. Bachelard HS: Carbohydrate and energy metabolism of the central nervous system: biochemical approach. In Vinken PJ, Bruyn GW (eds): *Handbook of Clinical Neurology.* Amsterdam, North Holland, 1976, vol 27, p 1.

39. Bachelard H: Cerebral metabolism and hypoglycemia. In Marks V, Clifford RF (eds): *Hypoglycemia*, ed 2. Oxford, England, Blackwell Scientific Publications, 1981, pp 51–65.

40. Bachelard HS, et al: The transport of glucose into the brain of rat in vivo. *Proc R Soc Lond [Biol]* 183:71, 1973.

41. Bachelard HS, et al: Mechanisms activating glycolysis in the brain in arterial hypoxia. *J Neurochem* 22:395, 1974.

42. Bakay L, Bendixen HH: Central nervous system vulnerability in hypoxaemic states. Isotope uptake studies. In Schade JP, McMenemey WH (eds): *Selective Vulnerability of the Brain in Hypoxaemia.* Philadelphia, FA Davis, 1963.

43. Bakay L, Lee JC: The effect of acute hypoxia and hypercapnia on the ultrastructure of the central nervous system. *Brain* 91:697, 1968.

44. Baker AB, Lufkin NH: Cerebral lesions in hypoglycemia. *Arch Pathol* 23:190, 1937.

45. Balazs R, et al: Effect of thyroid hormone on the bio-

chemical maturation of rat brain: postnatal cell formation. *Brain Res* 25:555, 1971.

46. Baldessarini RJ, Kopin IJ: The effect of drugs on the release of norepinephrine-^{3}H from central nervous system tissues by electrical stimulation in vitro. *J Pharmacol Exp Ther* 156:31, 1967.

47. Baldy-Moulinier M: Cerebral blood flow and membrane ionic pump. *Eur Neurol* 6:107, 1971/72.

48. Banet M: Fever and survival in the rat. The effect of enhancing the cold defense response. *Experientia* 37:985, 1981.

49. Barron GP, et al: Histological manifestations of a magnesium deficiency in the rat and rabbit. *Proc Soc Exp Biol* 70:220, 1949.

50. Bartels EC, Rohart RR: The relationship of hyperthyroidism and Parkinsonism. *AMA Arch Intern Med* 101:562, 1958.

51. Bazán NG Jr: Effects of ischemic and electroconvulsive shock on free fatty acid pool in the brain. *Biochim Biophys Acta* 218:1, 1970.

52. Beck RL: Disseminated intravascular coagulation and related syndromes: etiology, pathophysiology, diagnosis and management. *Am J Hematol* 5:265, 1978.

53. Berge KG, et al: The intestinal tract in diabetic diarrhoae: a pathologic study. *Diabetes* 5:289, 1956.

54. Bergström J, et al: Uremic middle molecules exist and are biologically active. *Clin Nephrol* 11:229, 1979.

55. Bering EA: Effects of profound hypothermia and circulatory arrest on cerebral oxygen metabolism and cerebrospinal fluid electrolyte composition in dogs. *J Neurosurg* 39:199, 1974.

56. Berl S, Clarke DD: Compartmentation of amino acid metabolism. In Lajtha A (ed): *Handbook of Neurochemistry.* New York, Plenum Press, 1969, vol 2, pp 447–472.

57. Berntman L, Siesjo BK: Cerebral metabolic and circulatory changes induced by hypoxia in starved rats. *J Neurochem* 31:1265, 1978.

58. Bessman SP, Bessman AN: The cerebral and peripheral uptake of ammonia in liver disease with an hypothesis for the mechanism of hepatic coma. *J Clin Invest* 34:622, 1955.

59. Bethlenfalvay NC, Bergin JJ: Severe cerebral toxicity after intravenous nitrogen mustard therapy. *Cancer* 29:366, 1972.

60. Betz E: Cerebral blood flow: its measurement and regulation. *Physiol Rev* 52:595, 1970.

61. Bianchi Porro G, Maiolo AT: Cerebral ammonia metabolism in uremia. *Life Sci* 9:43, 1970.

62. Biebuyck JF, et al: Neurochemistry of hepatic coma: alterations in putative transmitter amino acids. In Williams R, Murray-Lyon IM (eds): *Artificial Liver Support.* London, Pitman, 1974, pp 51–60.

63. Bird FH: Mg deficiency in chick. I. Clinical and neuropathologic findings. *J Nutr* 39:13, 1949.

64. Bischoff A: Ultrastructural pathology of peripheral nervous system in early diabetes. *Adv Metab Disord Suppl* 2:441, 1973.

65. Björk VO, Hultquist G: Brain damage in children after deep hypothermia for open heart surgery. *Thorax* 15:284, 1960.

66. Bosley TM, et al: Effects of anoxia on the stimulated release of amino acid neurotransmitters in the cerebellum in vitro. *J Neurochem* 40:189, 1983.

67. Bourgeois CH, et al: Udorn encephalopathy: fatal cerebral edema and fatty degeneration of the viscera in Thai children. *J Med Assoc Thai* 52:553, 1969.

68. Bourgeois C, et al: Encephalopathy and fatty degeneration of the viscera: a clinicopathologic analysis of 40 cases. *Am J Clin Pathol* 56:558, 1971.

69. Bourgeois CH, et al: Acute aflatoxin B toxicity in the macaque and its similarities to Reye's syndrome. *Lab Invest* 24:206, 1971.

70. Bourke RS, et al: Chloride transport in mammalian astroglia. In Schoffeniels E, Franck G, Hertz L, Tower DB (eds): *Dynamic Properties of Glia Cells.* Oxford, England, Pergamon Press, 1978.

71. Bourke RS, et al: Biology of glial swelling in experimental edema. *Adv Neurol* 28:99, 1980.
72. Bradley WG: Neuropathy of vincristine in the guinea pig. An electrophysiological and pathological study. *J Neurol Sci* 10:133, 1970.
73. Bradley WG: Neuropathy of vincristine in man. *J Neurol Sci* 10:107, 1970.
74. Braganca BM, et al: Effects of inhibitors of glutamine synthesis on the inhibition of acetylcholine synthesis in brain slices by ammonium ions. *Biochim Biophys Acta* 10:83, 1953.
75. Brain L, Wilkinson M: Subacute cerebellar degeneration associated with neoplasms. *Brain* 88:465, 1965.
76. Brain WR, et al: Subacute cortical cerebellar degeneration and its relation to carcinoma. *J Neurol Neurosurg Psychiatry* 14:59, 1951.
77. Breen J, Schenker S: Hepatic coma: present concepts of pathogenesis and therapy. *Prog Liver Dis* 4:301–322, 1972.
78. Breuer AC, et al: Paraparesis following intrathecal cytosine arabinoside: a case report with neuropathologic findings. *Cancer* 40:2817, 1977.
79. Brierley JB: Pathology of cerebral ischemia. In McDowell FH, Brennan RW (eds): *Cerebral Vascular Diseases, VIII Princeton Conference*. New York, Grune & Stratton, 1973, pp 59–75.
80. Brierley JB, Cooper JE: Cerebral complications of hypotensive anaesthesia in a healthy adult. *J Neurol Neurosurg Psychiatry* 25:24, 1962.
81. Brierley JB, et al: Brain damage in the Rhesus monkey resulting from profound arterial hypotension. I. Its nature, distribution and general physiological correlates. *Brain Res* 13:68, 1969.
82. Brierley JB, et al: The nature and time course of the neuronal alterations resulting from oligaemia and hypoglycaemia in the brain of *Macaca Mulatta*. *Brain Res* 25:483, 1971.
83. Brierley JB, et al: The neuropathology of insulin-induced hypoglycemia in a primate (M. Mulatta). Topography and cellular nature. *Clin Dev Med* 39/40:225, 1971.
84. Brown AW, Brierley JB: The earliest alterations in rat neurones and astrocytes after anoxia-ischemia. *Acta Neuropathol* 23:9, 1973.
85. Brown MJ, Asbury AK: Diabetic neuropathy. *Ann. Neurol.* 15:2, 1983.
86. Brown RE, Madge GE: Fatty acids and metabolic disturbances in Reye's syndrome. *Arch. Pathol.* 94:475, 1972.
87. Brown, RE, et al: Observations on the pathogenesis of Reye's syndrome. *South Med J* 64:942, 1971.
88. Brown RE: The biochemistry of Reye's syndrome. *CRC Crit Rev Clin Lab Sci* 17:247, 1982.
89. Brown T, et al: Transiently reduced activity of carbamyl phosphate synthetase and ornithine transcarbamylase in liver of children with Reye's syndrome. *N Engl J Med* 294:861, 1976.
90. Brun A, et al: Brain protein in hepatic encephalopathy. *Acta Neurol Scand* 55:213, 1977.
91. Bruton CJ, et al: Hereditary hyperammonaemia. *Brain* 93:423, 1970.
92. Burcar PJ, et al: Hyponatremia and central pontine myelinolysis. *Neurology (Minneap)* 27:223, 1977.
93. Burdman JA: Note of the selective toxicity of vincristine sulfate on chick-embryo sensory ganglia in tissue culture. *J Natl Cancer Inst* 37:331, 1966.
94. Burks JS, et al: A fatal encephalopathy in chronic hemodialysis patients. *Lancet* 1:764, 1976.
95. Cameron JM Dagan AD: Association of brain damage with therapeutic abortion induced by amniotic-fluid replacement: report of two cases. *Br Med J* 1:1010, 1966.
96. Cameron KR, et al: Isolation of a foamy virus from patient with dialysis encephalopathy. *Lancet* 2:796, 1978.
97. Campbell AGM, et al: Ornithine transcarbamylase deficiency: a cause of lethal neonatal hyperammonemia in males. *N Engl J Med* 288:1, 1973.
98. Canalese J, et al: Controlled clinical trial of dexamethasone and mannitol for cerebral edema of fulminant hepatic failure. *Gut* 23:625, 1982.
99. Carey R, et al: Toxoplasmosis: clinical experiences in a cancer hospital. *Am J Med* 54:30, 1973.
100. Cavanagh JB, Kyu MH: Type II Alzheimer change experimentally produced in astrocytes in the rat. *J Neurol Sci* 12:63, 1971.
101. Chan PH, Fishman RA: Brain edema: induction in cortical slices by polyunsaturated fatty acids. *Science* 201:358, 1978.
102. Chang LW, et al: Reye syndrome: light and electron microscopic studies. *Arch Pathol* 96:127, 1973.
103. Chernik NL, et al: Central nervous system infections in patients with cancer. *Medicine* 52:563, 1973.
104. Cho DY, Leipold HW: Experimental spongy degeneration in calves. *Acta Neuropathol* 39:115, 1977.
105. Chopra JJ, et al: The pathogenesis of sural nerve changes in diabetes mellitus. *Brain* 92:391, 1969.
106. Cleghorn RA: Adrenal cortical insufficiency: psychological and neurological observations. *Can Med Assoc J* 65:449, 1951.
107. Clements RS Jr, et al: Acute cerebral edema during treatment of hyperglycemia: an experimental model. *Lancet* 2:384, 1968.
108. Cogan MG, et al: Central nervous system manifestations of hyperparathyroidism. *Am J Med* 65:963, 1978.
109. Cohen SI, Marks IM: Prolonged organic psychosis with recovery in Addison's disease. *J Neurol Neurosurg Psychiatry* 24:366, 1961.
110. Collins, et al: Neurologic manifestations of intravascular coagulation in patients with cancer. *Neurology* 25:795, 1975.
111. Colwell JA, et al: Altered platelet function in diabetes mellitus. *Diabetes* 25(Suppl 2):826, 1976.
112. Conn HO, Lieberthal ML: *The Hepatic Coma Syndromes and Lactulose*. Baltimore, Williams & Wilkins, 1979.
113. Conn HO, et al: Pulmonary emphysema simulating brain tumor. *Am J Med* 22:524, 1957.
114. Corsellis JAN, et al: Limbic encephalitis and its association with carcinoma. *Brain* 91:481, 1968.
115. Crocker JFS: Reye's syndrome. *Semin Liver Dis* 2:340, 1982.
116. Croft PB, Wilkinson M: The incidence of carcinomatous neuromyopathy in patients with various types of carcinoma. *Brain* 88:427, 1965.
117. Croft PB, et al: Sensory neuropathy with bronchial carcinoma: a study of four cases showing serological abnormalities. *Brain* 88:501, 1965.
118. Crome L, Sylvester PE: A case of severe hypercalcemia of infancy with an account of the neuropathological findings. *Arch. Dis. Child.* 35:620, 1960.
119. Cullity GJ, Kakulas BA: Encephalopathy and fatty degeneration of the viscera: an evaluation. *Brain* 93:77, 1970.
120. Cutler RWP, Barlow CF: The effect of hypercapnia on brain permeability to protein. *Arch. Neurol.* 14:54, 1966.
121. Daniels SR, et al: Scientific uncertainties in the studies of salicylate use and Reye's syndrome. *JAMA* 249:1311, 1983.
122. Danta G: Clinical features of peripheral neuropathy associated with hypoglycemia. In Camerrini-Davalos A, Cole HS (eds): *Vascular and Neurological Changes in Early Diabetes*. New York, Academic Press, 1973, p 465.
123. Davidson CS, Gabuzda GJ: Hepatic coma. In Schiff L (ed): *Diseases of the Liver*, ed 4. Philadelphia, Lippincott, 1975, pp 466–499.
124. Davidson PW, et al: Neurological and intellectual sequelae of Reye's syndrome: a preliminary report. In Pollack JD (ed): *Reye's Syndrome*. New York, Grune & Stratton, 1975, pp 55–60.
125. Davis FA, Schauf CL: Neurological manifestations of calcium imbalance. In Vinken PJ, Bruyn GW (eds): *Handbook of Clinical Neurology*. Amsterdam, North Holland, 1976, vol 28.
126. Davis JN, et al: The effect of hypoxia on brain neurotransmitter systems. In Fahn S, Davis JN, Rowland LP

(eds): *Cerebral Hypoxia and its Consequences.* New York, Raven Press, 1979, pp 219–223.

127. Defronzo RA, Thier SO: Pathophysiologic approach to hyponatremia. *Arch Intern Med* 140:897, 1980.

128. Delarue J, et al: Encephalopathie subaigue secondaire à une pancreatite necrosante hemorragique. *Arch. Anat. Pathol. (Paris)* 13:45, 1965.

129. Delong GR, Glick TH: Encephalopathy of Reye's syndrome: a review of pathogenetic hypotheses. *Pediatrics* 69:53, 1982.

130. Demopoulos HB, et al: Antioxidant effects of barbiturates in model membranes undergoing free radical damage. *Acta. Neurol. Scand. (Suppl)* 64:7.12, 1977.

131. Deraveglia IF, et al: Hormonal regulation of brain development. V. Effect of neonatal thyroidectomy on lipid changes in cerebral cortex and cerebellum of developing rats. *Brain Res.* 43:181, 1972.

132. Dereuck JL, et al: Wernicke's encephalopathy in patients with tumors of the lymphoid-hemopoietic systems. *Arch. Neurol.* 37:338, 1980.

133. Deshmukh DR, et al: Interactions of aspirin and other potential etiologic factors in an animal model of Reye syndrome. *Proc. Natl. Acad. Sci.* USA 79:7557, 1982.

134. Devivo DC, et al: Intensive supportive approach to the treatment of Reye's syndrome. In Pollack JD (ed): *Reye's Syndrome.* New York, Grune & Stratton, 1975, pp 315–327.

135. Devoz JA: Deafness in hypothyroidism. *J Laryngol* 77:390, 1963.

136. Dewberry FL, et al: The dialysis dementia syndrome: report of fourteen cases and review of the literature. *ASAIO J* 3:102, 1980.

137. Diemer NH: Glial and neuronal changes in experimental hepatic encephalopathy. A quantitative morphological investigation. *Acta Neurol. Scand. Suppl.* 58:1, 1978.

138. Diemer NH, Klinken L: Astrocyte mitoses and Alzheimer type I and II astrocytes in anoxic encephalopathy. *Neuropathol. Appl. Neurobiol.* 2:313, 1976.

139. Diemer NH, Laursen H: Glial cell reactions in rats with hyperammonemia induced by urease or portocaval anastomosis. *Acta Neurol. Scand.* 55:425, 1977.

140. Dila CF, Pappius HM: Cerebral water and electrolytes: an experimental model of inappropriate secretion of antidiuretic hormone. *Arch. Neurol.* 26:85, 1972.

141. Dillon ES, et al: Cerebral lesions in uncomplicated fatal diabetic acidosis. *Am. J. Med. Sci.* 192:360, 1936.

142. Dodge PR, et al: Studies in experimental water intoxication. *Arch. Neurol.* 3:513, 1960.

143. Dodge PR, et al: Influence of hypertonicity of the body fluids on the blood-brain barrier. *Trans. Am Neurol. Assoc.* 86:12, 1961.

144. Dolman CL: The morbid anatomy of diabetic neuropathy. *Neurology (Minneap.)* 13:135, 1963.

145. Dorfman LJ, Forno LS: Paraneoplastic encephalomyelitis. *Acta Neurol Scand* 48:556, 1972.

146. Dreyfus PM, et al: Diabetic ophthalmoplegia. *Arch Neurol Psychiatry (Chic)* 77:337, 1957.

147. Duffy TE, Plum F: Seizures, coma and major metabolic encephalopathies. In Siegel GJ, Albers RW, Agranoff BW, Katzman R (eds): *Basic Neurochemistry,* ed 3. Boston, Little, Brown, 1981, pp 693–718.

148. Duffy TE, et al: Cerebral carbohydrate metabolism during acute hypoxia and recovery. *J. Neurochem* 19:959, 1972.

149. Dunea G, et al: Role of aluminum in dialysis dementia. *Ann. Intern Med.* 88:502, 1978.

150. Durlach J: Neurological manifestations of magnesium imbalance. In Vinken PJ, Bruyn GW (eds): *Handbook of Clinical Neurology.* Amsterdam, North-Holland, 1976, vol 28, p 545.

151. Dyck PJ, Lambert EH: Polyneuropathy associated with hypothyroidism. *J. Neuropathol. Exp. Neurol.* 29:631, 1970.

152. Eayrs JT: Influence of the thyroid on the central nervous system. *Br Med. Bull.* 16:122, 1960.

153. Ehrlich RM: Hypoglycemia in infancy and childhood.

Arch. Dis. Child. 46:716, 1971.

154. Ehrmantraut WR, et al: Cerebral hemodynamics and metabolism in accidental hypothermia. *Arch. Intern. Med.* 99:57, 1957.

155. Ellenberg M: Diabetic enteropathy. *Am. J. Gastroenterol* 40:269, 1961.

156. Ellenberg M: Diabetic neurogenic vesical dysfunction. *Arch. Intern Med.* 117:348, 1966.

157. Elmqvist D: Neuromuscular transmission with special reference to myasthenia gravis. *Acta. Physiol. Scand.* 64(Suppl 249):1, 1965.

158. Elmqvist D, Lambert E: Neuromuscular transmission in the patient with the myasthenic syndrome sometimes associated with bronchogenic carcinoma. *Mayo Clin Proc* 43:689, 1968.

159. Engel AG: Electron microscopic observations in thyrotoxic and corticosteroid myopathies. *Mayo Clin Proc* 41:785, 1966.

160. Engel AG, et al: Immune complexes (IgG and C₃) at the motor end-plate in myasthenia gravis. Ultrastructural and light microscopic localization and electrophysiologic correlation. *Mayo Clin Proc* 52:267, 1977.

161. Engstrom G, et al: Thyroxine and brain catecholamines: increased transmitter synthesis and increased receptor sensitivity. *Brain Res.* 77:471, 1974.

162. Ernest I, Ekman H: Adrenalectomy in Cushing's disease. *Acta Endocrinol* 69(Suppl 160):1, 1972.

163. Espinas DE, Poser CM: Blood hyperosmolality and neurologic deficit. *Arch. Neurol. (Chic.)* 20:182, 1969.

164. Evans EC: Neurologic complications of myxedema: convulsions. *Ann. Intern Med.* 52:434, 1960.

165. Farber JL: The role of calcium in cell injury. *Life Sci.* 29:1289, 1981.

166. Fehm HL, Voigt KH: Pathophysiology of Cushing's disease. *Pathobiol Ann* 9:225–255, 1979.

167. Ferrendelli JA, Chang MM: Brain metabolism during hypoglycemia. Effect of insulin on regional central nervous system glucose and energy reserves in mice. *Arch. Neurol. (Chic.)* 28:173, 1973.

168. Ferrendelli JA, et al: Influence of divalent cations regulations of cyclic GMP and cyclic AMP levels in brain tissue. *J. Neurochem.* 26:741, 1976.

169. Finberg L: Hypernatremic (hypertonic) dehydration in infants. *N Engl J Med* 289:196, 1973.

170. Finberg L, et al: Pathogenesis of lesions in the nervous system in hypernatremic states. II. Experimental studies of gross anatomic changes and alteration of chemical composition of the tissues. *Pediatrics* 23:46, 1959.

171. Finberg L, et al: Mass accident salt poisoning in infancy. *JAMA* 184:187, 1963.

172. Finlayson MH, Superville B: Distribution of cerebral lesions in acquired hepatocerebral degeneration. *Brain* 104:79, 1982.

173. Fischer EG, et al: Reassessment of cerebral capillary changes in acute global ischemia and their relationship to the "no-reflow phenomenon." *Stroke* 8:36, 1977.

174. Fischer JE, Baldessarini RJ: Pathogenesis and therapy of hepatic coma. *Prog Liver Dis* 5:363–397, 1976.

175. Fishman RA: Neurological aspects of magnesium metabolism. *Arch. Neurol.* 12:562, 1965.

176. Fishman RA: Permeability changes in experimental uremic encephalopathy. *Arch. Intern. Med.* 126:835, 1970.

177. Fishman RA: Neurological manifestations of hyponatremia. In Vinken PJ, Bruyn GW (eds): *Handbook of Clinical Neurology,* Part II. Amsterdam, North-Holland, 1976, vol 28, pp 495–505.

178. Fishman RA, Chan PH: Changes in ammonia and amino acid metabolism induced by hyperosmolality in vivo and in vitro. *Trans. Am. Neurol. Assoc.* 101:1, 1976.

179. Fishman RA, Raskin NH: Experimental uremic encephalopathy: permeability and electrolyte metabolism of brain and other tissues. *Arch Neurol* 17:10, 1967.

180. Fitzgerald F: Clinical hypophosphatemia. *Ann Rev Med* 29:177, 1978.

181. Flamm ES, et al: Free radicals in cerebral ischemia.

Stroke 9:445, 1978.

182. Flugel KA: Metabolically induced focal seizures: hyperosmolar nonketoacidotic hyperglycemia. *Schweiz Arch Neurol Neurochir Psychiatr* 120:3, 1977.

183. Folbergrova J, et al: The effect of hypercapnic acidosis upon some glycolytic and level cycle associated intermediates in the rat brain. *J. Neurochem.* 19:2507, 1972.

184. Foley CM, et al: Encephalopathy in infants and children with chronic renal disease. *Arch. Neurol.* 38:656, 1981.

185. Foncin J-F, Nicolaidis S: Encephalopathie portocave: contribution a la pathologie ultrastructurale de la glie chez l'homme. *Rev. Neurol.* 123:81, 1970.

186. Fonseca OA, Calverley JR: Neurological manifestations of hypoparathyroidism. *Arch. Intern. Med.* 120:202, 1967.

187. Fridovich I: Hypoxia and oxygen toxicity. *Adv. Neurol.* 26:255, 1979.

188. Friede RL: The histochemical architecture of the Ammons horn as related to its selective vulnerability. *Acta. Neuropathol* 6:1, 1966.

189. Friedman SA, et al: Vasomotor tone in diabetic neuropathy. *Ann. Intern. Med.* 77:353, 1972.

190. Fritz RD, et al: The association of fatal intracranial hemorrhage and "blastic crisis" in patients with acute leukemia. *N. Engl. J. Med.* 261:59, 1959.

191. Fujimoto T, et al: Pathophysiologic aspects of ischemic edema. In Pappius HM, Feindel W (eds): *Dynamics of Brain Edema.* New York, Springer-Verlag, 1976, pp 171–180.

192. Furlow TW, Hallenbeck JM: Indomethacin prevents impaired perfusion of the dog's brain after global ischemia. *Stroke* 9:591, 1978.

193. Furui T, et al: Subdural hematoma associated with disseminated intravascular coagulation in patients with advanced cancer. *J Neurosurg* 58:398, 1983.

194. Gabbay KH: The sorbitol pathway and the complications of diabetes. *N Engl J Med.* 288:831, 1973.

195. Gabbay KH, O'Sullivan JB: The sorbitol pathway: enzyme localization and content in normal and diabetic nerve and cord. *Diabetes* 17:239, 1968.

196. Garcia JH: Reversibility of regional cerebral ischemia. In McDowell FH, Brennan RW (eds): *Cerebral Vascular Diseases, VIII Princeton Conference.* New York, Grune & Stratton, 1973, pp 133–143.

197. Garcia JH: Ischemic injuries of the brain. *Arch. Pathol. Lab. Med.* 107:157, 1983.

198. Garcia JH, Conger KA: Ischemic brain injuries: structural and biochemical effects. In Grenvik A, Safar P (eds): *Brain Failure and Resuscitation.* New York, Churchill Livingstone, 1981, pp 35–54.

199. Garcia JH, et al: Ultrastructure of the microvasculature in cerebral infarction. *Acta. Neuropathol (Berl.)* 18:273, 1971.

200. Garcia JH, et al: Cerebral ischemia: the early structural changes and correlation of these with known metabolic and dynamic abnormalities. In Whisnant JP, Sandok BA (eds): *Cerebral Vascular Diseases, IX Princeton Conference.* New York, Grune & Stratton, 1975, pp 313–325.

201. Garcia JH, et al: Fine structure and biochemistry of brain edema in regional cerebral ischemia. In Price TR, Nelson E (eds): *Cerebral Vascular Diseases, XI Princeton Conference.* New York, Grune & Stratton, 1979, pp 169–189.

202. Garcia JH, et al: Postischemic brain edema: quantitation and evolution. *Adv Neurol* 28:147–169, 1980.

203. Garcia MJ, et al: Morbidity and mortality in diabetes in the Framingham population. *Diabetes* 23:105, 1974.

204. Gardiner RM: Potassium transfer from brain to blood during sustained hyponatraemia in the calf. *J. Physiol. (Lond.)* 306:463, 1980.

205. Gardiner RM, Wilkinson AG: Potassium transfer from brain to blood during sustained hyponatraemia in the newborn calf. *Experientia* 36:990, 1980.

206. Gaudet RJ, Levine L: Transient cerebral ischemia and brain prostaglandins. *Biochem. Biophys. Res. Commun.* 86:893, 1979.

207. Gaudet RJ, et al: Accumulation of arachidonic acid metabolites in gerbil brain during reperfusion after bilateral carotid artery occlusion. *J. Neurochem.* 35:653, 1980.

208. Geiger A: Correlation of brain metabolism and function by the use of a brain perfusion method in situ. *Physiol. Rev.* 38:1, 1958.

209. Geller A, et al: Degeneration of fasciculus gracilis in cystic fibrosis. *Neurology* 27:185, 1977.

210. Giannotta SL, et al: Computerized tomography in Reye's syndrome: evidence for pathological cerebral vasodilatation. *Neurosurgery* 2:201, 1978.

211. Gibson GE, Blass JP: Impaired synthesis of acetylcholine accompanying mild hypoxia and hypoglycemia. *J. Neurochem.* 27:37, 1976.

212. Gifford S, Gunderson IG: Cushing's disease as a psychosomatic disorder. *Medicine* 49:397, 1970.

213. Ginsberg MD: Delayed neurological deterioration following hypoxia. In Davis JN, Rowland LP (eds): *Cerebral Hypoxia and its Consequences.* New York, Raven Press, 1979, pp 21–44.

214. Ginsberg MD, Myers RE: Experimental carbon monoxide encephalopathy in the primate. I. Physiologic and metabolic aspects. *Arch Neurol* 30:202, 1974.

215. Ginsberg MD, et al: Diffuse cerebral ischemia in the cat. I. Local blood flow during severe ischemia and recirculation. *Ann Neurol* 3:482, 1978.

216. Ginsberg MD, et al: Diffuse cerebral ischemia in the cat. III. Neuropathologic sequelae of severe ischemia. *Ann. Neurol.* 5:350, 1979.

217. Ginsberg MD, et al: Deleterious effect of glucose pretreatment on recovery from diffuse cerebral ischemia in the cat. I. Local cerebral blood flow and glucose utilization. *Stroke* 11:347, 1980.

218. Glaser GH: Brain dysfunction in uremia. *Res. Publ. Assoc. Res. Nerv. Ment. Dis.* 53:173, 1974.

219. Glasgow AM, Chase HP: Production of the features of Reye's syndrome in rats with 4-pentenoic acid. *Pediatr. Res.* 9:133, 1975.

220. Goebel HH, Herman-Ben Zur P: Central pontine myelinolysis. In Vinken PJ, Bruyn GW (eds): *Handbook of Clinical Neurology.* Amsterdam, North Holland, 1976, vol 28, pp 285–316.

221. Goffinet DR, et al: Herpes zoster-varicella infections and lymphoma. *Ann. Intern. Med.* 76:235, 1973.

222. Goldman JE, Horoupian DS: Demyelination of the lateral geniculate nucleus in central pontine myelinolysis. *Ann. Neurol.* 9:185, 1981.

223. Goldstein GW: Cerebral edema: role of fatty acid metabolism of brain capillaries. *N Engl. J. Med.* 296:632, 1977.

224. Gore I, Isaacson NH: The pathology of hyperpyrexia: observations at autopsy in 17 cases of fever therapy. *Am J Pathol* 25:1029, 1949.

225. Gottschalk PG, et al: Vinca alkaloid neuropathy: nerve biopsy studies in rats and in man. *Neurology (Minneap)* 18:875, 1968.

226. Greco FA, et al: Hodgkin's disease and granulomatous angiitis of the central nervous system. *Cancer* 38:2027, 1976.

227. Greene R: The thyroid gland: its relationship to neurology. In Vinken PJ, Bruyn GW (eds): *Handbook of Clinical Neurology.* Amsterdam, North Holland, 1976, vol 27, ch11.

228. Greenlee JE, Brashear HR: Antibodies to cerebellar Purkinje cells in patients with paraneoplastic cerebellar degeneration and ovarian carcinoma. *Ann. Neurol.* 14:609, 1983.

229. Griggs RC, Satran R: Metabolic encephalopathy. In Rosenberg RN (ed): *Clinical Neurosciences.* New York, Churchill Livingstone, 1983, vol 1, pp 645–677.

230. Gross G, et al: Decreased number of β-adrenoreceptors in cerebral cortex of hypothyroid rats. *Eur. J. Pharmacol.* 61:191, 1980.

231. Hagstam KE, et al: Mannitol infusion in regular haemodialysis treatment for chronic renal insufficiency. *Scand. J. Urol. Nephrol.* 3:257, 1969.

232. Halperin JJ, et al: Paraneoplastic encephalomyelitis and

neuropathy. *Arch. Neurol.* 38:773, 1981.

233. Halter JB, et al: Selective osmoreceptor dysfunction in the syndrome of chronic hypernatremia. *J. Clin. Endocrinol. Metab.* 44:609, 1977.

234. Hamberger A, Lovtrup S: The effect of brain dehydration on the activity of respiratory enzymes in isolated neurons, neuroglial cells and in brain mitochondria. *J. Neurochem.* 11:687, 1964.

235. Hammerschlag R, et al: Mechanism of axonal transport: a proposed role for calcium ions. *Science* 188:273, 1975.

236. Hansen AJ: Extracellular ion concentrations in cerebral ischemia. In Zenther T (ed): *The Application of Ionselective Microelectrodes.* New York, Elsevier/North-Holland, 1981, pp 239–254.

237. Harris RJ, et al: Changes in extracellular calcium activity in cerebral ischaemia. *J Cereb Blood Flow Metabol* 1:203, 1981.

238. Hartman FW: Lesions of the brain following fever therapy: etiology and pathogenesis. *J. Am Med. Assoc.* 109:2116, 1937.

239. Hawkins RA, et al: The acute action of ammonia on rat brain metabolism in vivo. *Biochem. J.* 134:1001, 1973.

240. Haymaker W, et al: Delayed radiation effects in the brains of monkeys exposed to X- and gamma rays. *J. Neuropathol. Exp. Neurol.* 27:50, 1968.

241. Helwig FC, et al: Water intoxication: report of a fatal human case with clinical, pathological and experimental studies. *JAMA* 104:1569, 1935.

242. Hensley GT, Soergel KH: Neuropathologic findings in diabetic diarrhea. *Arch. Pathol.* 85:587, 1968.

243. Henson RA: The neurological aspects of hypercalcemia: with special reference to primary hyperparathyroidism. *J. Coll. Physicians Lond.* 1:41, 1966.

244. Henson RA: Nonmetastatic neurological manifestations of malignant disease. In Williams D (ed): *Modern Trends in Neurology.* New York, Appleton-Century-Crofts, 1970, vol 5.

245. Henson RA, Urich H: *Cancer and the Nervous System: The Neurological Manifestations of Systemic Disease.* Boston, Blackwell Scientific, 1982.

246. Henson RA, et al: Encephalomyelitis with carcinoma. *Brain* 88:449, 1965.

247. Herrera L, Kazemi H: CSF bicarbonate regulation in metabolic acidosis: role of HCO_3^- formation in CNS. *J Appl Physiol* 49:778, Nov 1980.

248. Hertz L: Energy metabolism of glial cells. In Schoffeniels E, Franck G, Hertz L, Tower DB (eds): *Dynamic Properties of Glia Cells.* Oxford, England, Pergamon Press, 1978, pp. 121–132.

249. Hertz L: Features of astrocyte function apparently involved in the response of the central nervous system to ischemia-hypoxia. *J Cereb Blood Flow Metabol* 1:143, 1981.

250. Hicks SP: Vascular pathophysiology and acute and chronic oxygen deprivation. In Minckler J (ed): *Pathology of the Nervous System.* New York, McGraw-Hill, 1968, pp 341–350.

251. Hindfelt B: On mechanisms in hyperammonemic coma—with particular reference to hepatic encephalopathy. *Ann. NY Acad. Sci.* 252:116, 1975.

252. Hindfelt B, Olsson J-E: Soluble brain proteins in dialysis encephalopathy. *Acta. Neuropathol* 50:241, 1980.

253. Hindfelt B, Siesjö BK: Cerebral effects of acute ammonia intoxication. II. The effect upon energy metabolism. *Scand. J. Clin. Lab. Invest.* 28:365, 1971.

254. Hindfelt B, et al: Effect of acute ammonia intoxication on cerebral metabolism in rats. *J. Clin. Invest.* 59:386, 1977.

255. Hirsch H, et al: Über die Erholung des gehirns nach kompletter Ischämie Hypothermie. *Pflugers Arch.* 265:314, 1957.

256. Hochberg FH, et al: Influenza type-B related encephalopathy: the 1971 outbreak of Reye syndrome in Chicago. *JAMA* 231:817, 1975.

257. Hoff JT, et al: Barbiturate protection from cerebral infarction in primates. *Stroke* 6:28, 1975.

258. Hoffman HL: Acute necrotic myelopathy. *Brain* 78:377, 1955.

259. Hoover R, Fraumeni JF Jr: Risk of cancer in renal-transplant recipients. *Lancet* 2:55, 1973.

260. Horwich MS, et al: Subacute sensory neuropathy: a remote effect of carcinoma. *Ann Neurol* 2:7, 1977.

261. Hossmann K-A, Hossmann V: Coagulopathy following experimental cerebral ischemia. *Stroke* 8:249, 1977.

262. Hossmann K-A, Kleihues P: Reversibility of ischemic brain damage. *Arch. Neurol.* 29:375, 1973.

263. Hossmann K-A, Sato K: Recovery of neuronal function after prolonged cerebral ischemia. *Science* 168:375, 1970.

264. Hossmann K-A, Schuier FJ: Metabolic cytotoxic type of brain edema following middle cerebral artery occlusion in cats. In Price TR, Nelson E (eds): *Cerebrovascular Diseases.* New York, Raven Press, 1979, pp 141–165.

265. Hug G, et al: Reye's syndrome simulacra in liver of mice after treatment with chemical agents and encephalo-myocarditis virus. *Lab. Invest.* 45:89, 1981.

266. Huttenlocher PR, Trauner DA: Reye's syndrome. In Vinken PJ, Bruyn GW (eds): *Handbook of Clinical Neurology.* Amsterdam, North Holland, 1977, vol 29, pp 331–344.

267. Inose T, et al: A histochemical study of hepatocerebral degeneration in liver disease (glycogen findings). *Arch. Psychiatr Nervenkr.* 200:505, 1960.

268. Iversen LC, et al: The effect of stimulation of inhibitory pathways on the release of endogenous gamma-amino-butyric acid from the cat cerebral cortex. *Br. J. Pharmacol* 38:452, 1970.

269. James JH, et al: Hyperammonaemia, plasma amino acid imbalance, and blood-brain amino acid transport: a unified theory of portal-systemic encephalopathy. *Lancet.* 2:772, 1979.

270. Jefferson A: A clinical correlation between encephalopathy and papilloedema in Addison's disease. *J Neurol Neurosurg Psychiatry* 19:21, 1956.

271. Jellinger K, Riederer P: Brain monoamines in metabolic (endotoxic) coma. A preliminary biochemical study in human postmortem material. *J Neurol Transm* 41:275, 1977.

272. Jenkins LW, et al: Complete cerebral ischemia. An ultrastructural study. *Acta. Neuropathol.* 48:113, 1979.

273. Jenkins LW, et al: The role of postischemic recirculation in the development of ischemic neuronal injury following complete cerebral ischemia. *Acta. Neuropathol.* 55:205, 1981.

274. Jervis GA: Microcephaly with extensive calcium deposits and demyelination. *J. Neuropathol. Exp Neurol.* 13:318, 1954.

275. Johansson B, Nilsson B: The pathophysiology of the blood-brain barrier dysfunction induced by severe hypercapnia and by epileptic brain activity. *Acta Neuropathol.* 38:153, 1977.

276. Johnson PC, et al: Paraneoplastic vasculitis of nerve: a remote effect of cancer. *Ann. Neurol.* 5:437, 1979.

277. Johnson PC, et al: Thickened cerebral cortical capillary basement membranes in diabetes. *Arch. Pathol. Lab. Med.* 106:214, 1982.

278. Joslin EP, et al: *The Treatment of Diabetes Mellitus,* ed 10. Philadelphia, Lea & Febiger, 1959, pp 492–493.

279. Kalimo H, Olsson Y: Effects of severe hypoglycemia on the human brain. *Acta Neurol. Scand.* 62:345, 1980.

280. Kalimo H, et al: The ultrastructure of "brain death." II. Electron microscopy of feline cortex after complete ischemia. *Virchows Arch [B Cell Pathol]* 25:207, 1977.

281. Kalimo H, et al: Hypoglycemic brain injury. VI. Electron microscopic findings in rat cerebral cortical neurons during profound insulin-induced hypoglycemia and in the recovery period following glucose administration. *Acta Neuropathol (Berl)* 50:43, 1980.

282. Kalimo H, et al: Brain lactic acidosis and ischemic cell damage. II. Histopathology. *J Cereb Blood Flow Metabol* 1:313, 1981.

283. Kalimo H, et al: Structural changes in brain tissue under hypoxic-ischemic conditions. *J. Cereb. Blood Flow Met-*

abol. 2(Suppl 1):S19, 1982.

284. Kamijyo Y, et al: Temporary MCA occlusion: a model of hemorrhagic and subcortical infarction. *J. Neuropathol. Exp. Neurol.* 36:338, 1977.

285. Kannel WB: Current status of epidemiology of brain infarction associated with occlusive arterial disease. *Stroke* 2:259, 1971.

286. Kasper LH, et al: Bilateral rhinocerebral phycomycosis. *Ann. Neurol.* 6:131, 1979.

287. Kato T, Lowry OH: Enzymes of energy-converting systems in individual mammalian nerve cell bodies. *J. Neurochem.* 20:151, 1973.

288. Katzman R, Pappius HM: *Brain Electrolytes and Fluid Metabolism.* Baltimore, Williams & Wilkins, 1973.

289. Kazemi H, et al: Brain organic buffers in respiratory acidosis and alkalosis. *J. Appl. Physiol.* 34:478, 1973.

290. Kety SS, Schmidt CF: The effect of altered arterial tensions of carbon dioxide and oxygen on cerebral blood flow and oxygen consumption of normal young men. *J. Clin. Invest.* 27:484, 1948.

291. Kety SS, et al: Blood flow and oxygen consumption of human brain in diabetic ketoacidosis and coma. *J Clin Invest* 27:500, 1948.

292. Kilburn KH: Shock, seizures and coma with alkalosis during mechanical ventilation. *Ann Intern Med* 65:977, 1966.

293. Kindt GW, et al: Intracranial pressure in Reye syndrome: monitoring and control. *JAMA* 231:822, 1975.

294. Kindt FW, et al: Blood/brain barrier and brain edema in ammonia intoxication. *Lancet* 1:201, 1977.

295. Klatzo I: Cerebral oedema and ischemia. In Smith TW, Cavanagh JB (eds): *Recent Advances in Neuropathology.* Edinburgh, Churchill Livingstone, 1979, vol 1, pp 27–39.

296. Klatzo I, et al: Experimental production of neurofibrillary degeneration. I. Light microscopic observations. *J. Neuropathol Exp. Neurol.* 24:187, 1965.

297. Klawans HL, et al: Observations on the dopaminergic nature of hyperthyroid chorea. In Barbeau A, Chase RN, Paulson GW (eds): *Advances in Neurology.* New York, Raven Press, 1973, vol 1, pp 543–549.

298. Klawans HL, et al: Calcification of the basal ganglia as a cause of levodopa resistant Parkinsonism. *Neurology* 26:221, 1976.

299. Kleihues P, et al: Protein synthesis in the cat brain after prolonged cerebral ischemia. *Brain Res.* 35:409, 1971.

300. Kleinschmidt-Demasters BK, Norenberg MD: Neuropathologic observations in electrolyte-induced myelinolysis in the rat. *J. Neuropathol Exp. Neurol.* 41:67, 1982.

301. Knochel JP: The pathophysiology and clinical characteristics of severe hypophosphatemia. *Arch. Intern Med.* 137:203, 1977.

302. Knutson J, Baker AB: The central nervous system in uremia: clinicopathologic study. *Arch Neurol* 54:130, 1945.

303. Kobayashi M, et al: Concentrations of energy metabolites and cyclic nucleotides during and after bilateral ischemia in the gerbil cerebral cortex. *J. Neurochem* 29:53, 1977.

304. Koenig H, Patel A: Biochemical basis of the acute cerebellar syndrome in 5-fluorouracil chemotherapy. *Trans Am Neurol Assoc* 94:290, 1969.

305. Kogure K, et al: Involvement of lipid peroxidation in postischemic brain damage. *Neurology* 29:546, 1979.

306. Krieger DT, et al: Cyproheptadine-induced remission of Cushing's disease. *N. Engl. J. Med.* 293:893, 1975.

307. Lam KC, et al: Role of false neurotransmitter, octopamine, in the pathogenesis of hepatic and renal encephalopathy. *Scand. J. Gastroenterol.* 8:465, 1973.

308. Lamberts SWJ, et al: The role of dopaminergic depletion in the pathogenesis of Cushing's disease and the possible consequences for medical therapy. *Clin. Endocrinol* 7:185, 1977.

309. Langston JW, et al: Encephalomyeloneuritis in the absence of cancer. *Neurology* 25:633, 1975.

310. Lapham LW: Cytologic and cytochemical studies of neuroglia. I. A study of the problem of amitosis in reactive protoplasmic astrocytes. *Am. J. Pathol.* 41:1, 1962.

311. Laureno R: Central pontine myelinolysis following rapid correction of hyponatremia. *Ann. Neurol.* 13:232, 1983.

312. Laursen H, Westergaard E: Enhanced permeability to horseradish peroxidase across cerebral vessels in the rat after portocaval anastomosis. *Neuropathol Appl. Neurobiol.* 3:29, 1977.

313. Lavy S, et al: Hypertension and diabetes as risk factors in stroke patients. *Stroke* 4:751, 1973.

314. Lawrence RD, et al: The pathological changes in the brain in fatal hypoglycemia. *Q J Med* 11:181, 1942.

315. Leestma JE, et al: Temporal correlates in brain death: EEG and clinical relationships to the respirator brain. *Arch Neurol* 41:147, 1984.

316. Lefer LG, Vogel FS: Encephalomyelopathy with hepatic cirrhosis following portosystemic venous shunts. *Arch. Pathol.* 93:91, 1972.

317. Legrain M, et al: Leucoencephalopathie multifocale progressive apres transplantation rénale. *J. Neurol. Sci.* 23:49, 1974.

318. Lehrer GM, Levitt MF: Neuropsychiatric presentation of hypercalcemia. *J. Mount Sinai Hosp.* 27:10, 1960.

319. Leibowitz J, et al: Citrullinemia. *Virchows Arch. A. Pathol Anat. Histol.* 377:249, 1978.

320. Leonard A, Shapiro FL: Subdural hematoma in regularly hemodialyzed patients. *Ann. Intern. Med.* 82:650, 1975.

321. Levy DE, et al: Ischemic brain damage in the gerbil in the absence of "no-reflow." *J. Neurol. Neurosurg. Psychiatry* 38:1197, 1975.

322. Lewis PD, Miller AL: Argininosuccinic aciduria: case report with neuropathological findings. *Brain* 93:413, 1970.

323. Lichtman MA, et al: Reduced red cell glycolysis 2,3-diphosphoglycerate and adenosine triphosphate concentration and increased hemoglobin oxygen affinity caused by hypophosphatemia. *Ann. Intern. Med.* 74:562, 1971.

324. Lie SO, et al: Fatal congenital acidosis in two siblings. I. Clinical and pathological findings. *Acta. Paediatr. Scand.* 60:129, 1971.

325. Lindenberg R: Morphotropic and morphostatic necrobiosis: investigations on nerve cells of the brain. *Am. J. Pathol.* 32:1147, 1956.

326. Linnemann CC, et al: Association of Reye's syndrome with viral infection. *Lancet* 1:179, 1974.

327. Lipsmeyer E, Ackerman GL: Irreversible brain damage after water intoxication. *JAMA* 196:286, 1966.

328. Lipton H, Teasdall R: Acute transverse myelopathy in adults. *Arch Neurol (Chic)* 28:252, 1973.

329. Little JR: Microvascular alterations and edema in focal cerebral ischemia. In Pappius H, Feindel W (eds): *Dynamic Aspects of Cerebral Edema.* New York, Springer-Verlag, 1976, pp 236–243.

330. Little JR: Morphological changes in acute focal ischemia: response to osmotherapy. *Adv. Neurol.* 28:443, 1980

331. Ljunggren B, et al: Cerebral metabolic state following complete compression ischemia. *Brain Res.* 73:291, 1974.

332. Lockman LA: Neurological aspects of acid-base metabolism. In Vinken PJ, Bruyn GW (eds): *Handbook of Clinical Neurology.* Amsterdam, North-Holland, 1976, vol 28, pp 507–525.

333. Lockwood AH: Adaptation to hyperosmolality in the rat. *Brain Res.* 200:216, 1980.

334. Logothetis J: Neurologic and muscular manifestation of hyperthyroidism. *Arch. Neurol.* 5:533, 1961.

335. Lorenzi M, et al: Increased growth hormone response to dopamine infusion in insulin dependent diabetic subjects: indication of possible blood-brain barrier abnormality. *J. Clin. Invest.* 65:146, 1980.

336. Lowenhaupt E, et al: Basic histologic lesions of magnesium deficiency in the rat. *Arch. Pathol.* 49:427, 1950.

337. Löwenthal A, Bruyn GW: Calcification of the striopallidaldentate system. In Vinken PJ, Bruyn GW (eds): *Handbook of Clinical Neurology.* Amsterdam, North Holland, 1968, vol 6, pp 703–725.

338. Lukash WM: Complications of acute pancreatitis. *Am J Gastroenterol* 49:120, 1968.

339. Luse SA, et al: Cerebral abnormalities in diabetes mellitus: an ultrastructural study of the brain in early-onset diabetes mellitus in the Chinese hamster. *Diabetologia* 6:192, 1970.

340. Lux HD, et al: The action of ammonium on post-synaptic inhibition of cat spinal motoneurons. *Exp. Brain. Res.* 11:431, 1970.

341. Maccaulay D, Watson M: Hypernatremia in infants as a cause of brain damage. *Arch. Dis. Child.* 42:485, 1967.

342. Mahurkar SD, et al: Dialysis dementia. *Lancet* 1:1412, 1973.

343. Malamud N: Fatalities resulting from treatment with subshock doses of insulin. *Am. J. Psychiatry* 105:373, 1948.

344. Malamud N, et al: Heatstroke: a clinico-pathologic study of 125 fatal cases. *Milit. Surg.* 99:397, 1946.

345. Manghani KK, et al: Urinary and serum octopamine in patients with portal-systemic encephalopathy. *Lancet.* 2:943, 1975.

346. Mannix H, Glenn F: Hypertension in Cushing's syndrome. *J. Am Med. Assoc.* 180:225, 1962.

347. Mant AK: Autopsy diagnosis of accidental hypothermia. *J. Forensic Med.* 16:126, 1969.

348. Manz JH, et al: Progressive multifocal leucoencephalopathy after renal transplantation. *Ann. Intern. Med.* 75:77, 1971.

349. Marion J, Wolfe L: Origin of the arachidonic acid released post-mortem in rat forebrain. *Biochim Biophys Acta* 574:25, 1979.

350. Markelonis J, Garbus J: Alterations of intracellular oxidative metabolism as stimuli evoking prostaglandin biosynthesis. A review of prostaglandins in cell injury and a hypothesis. *Prostaglandins* 10:1087, 1975.

351. Marks LJ, Feit E: Flaccid quadriplegia, hyperkalemia and Addison's disease. *Arch Intern Med* 91:56, 1953.

352. Marshall JP, et al: Biochemistry of hepatic coma in alcohol-induced liver disease and other types of hepatic dysfunction. In Majchrowicz E, Noble EP (eds): *Biochemistry and Pharmacology of Ethanol.* New York, Plenum Press, 1979, vol 1, pp 479–502.

353. Martin J-J, Schlote W: Central nervous system lesions in disorders of amino acid metabolism. A neuropathologic study. *J. Neurol. Sci.* 15:49, 1972.

354. Martinez A: Electron microscopy in human hepatic encephalopathy. *Acta. Neuropathol* 11:82, 1968.

355. Massry SG, Goldstein DA: The search for uremic toxin(s) "X":"X" = PTH. *Clin. Nephrol.* 11:181, 1979.

356. Mastaglia FL, et al: Effects of X-radiation on the spinal cord: an experimental study of the morphological changes in central nerve fibers. *Brain* 99:101, 1976.

357. Matakas F, et al: The effect of prolonged experimental hypercapnia on the brain. *Acta Neuropathol* 41:207, 1978.

358. Matsuoka Y, Hossmann K-A: Brain tissue osmolality after middle cerebral artery occlusion in cats. *Exp. Neurol.* 77:599, 1982.

359. McDermott JR, et al: Brain-aluminum concentration in dialysis encephalopathy. *Lancet* 1:901, 1978.

360. Mehta AC, Baker RN: Persistent neurologic deficits in heat stroke. *Neurology* 20:336, 1970.

361. Mei Liu H: Reactive neuroaxonal dystrophy in children. *Acta Neuropathol* 42:237, 1978.

362. Mei Liu H, et al: Neuroaxonal dystrophy of the brain in patients receiving antineoplastic chemotherapy. *Acta Neuropathol (Berl.)* 37:207, 1977.

363. Mellerup ET, Rafaelsen OJ: Brain glycogen after intracisternal insulin injection. *J. Neurochem.* 16:777, 1969.

364. Melton JE, Nattie EE: Brain and CSF water and ions during dilutional and isosmotic hyponatremia in the rat. *Am. J. Physiol.* 244:R724, 1983.

365. Meriwether WD, Goodman RM: Severe accidental hypothermia with survival after rapid rewarming. *Am. J. Med.* 53:505, 1972.

366. Merrill JP, et al: Observations on the role of urea in uremia. *Am. J. Med.* 14:519, 1953.

367. Messert B, et al: Central pontine myelinolysis: considerations on etiology, diagnosis and treatment. *Neurology*

368. *(Minneap.)* 29:147, 1979.

368. Meyer A, et al: Unusually severe lesions in the brain following status epilepticus. *J. Neurol. Neurosurg. Psychiatry* 18:24, 1955.

369. Meyer JE: Über die Lokalisation frühkindlicher Hirnschäden in arteriellen Grenzgebieten. *Arch. Psychiatr Nervenkr* 190:328, 1953.

370. Miller A, et al: The neurologic syndrome due to marked hypercapnia, with papilledema. *Am. J. Med.* 33:309, 1962.

371. Miller GR, Smith JL: Ischemic optic neuropathy. *Am. J. Ophthalmol* 62:103, 1966.

372. Minkoff L, et al: Inhibition of brain sodium-potassium ATPase in uremic rats. *J Lab Clin Med* 80:71, 1972.

373. Momose KJ, et al: High incidence of cortical atrophy of the cerebral and cerebellar hemispheres in Cushing's disease. *Radiology* 99:341, 1971.

374. Moossy J: Validation of ischemic stroke models. In Price TR, Nelson E (eds): *Cerebrovascular Diseases. XI Princeton Conference.* New York, Raven Press, 1979, pp 3–10.

375. Mordes JP, Wacker WE: Excess magnesium. *Pharmacol. Rev.* 29:273, 1977.

376. Moseley JI, et al: Respirator brain: report of a survey and review of current concepts. *Arch. Pathol. Lab. Med.* 100:61, 1976.

377. Mukai N, et al: Cerebral lesion in rats with streptozotocin induced diabetes. *Acta Neuropathol.* 51:79, 1980.

378. Mulder DW: Hyperinsulin neuronopathy. *Neurology* 6:627, 1956.

379. Mullen PW: Immunopharmacological considerations in Reye's syndrome: a possible xenobiotic initiated disorder? *Biochem. Pharmacol.* 27:145, 1978.

380. Muntwyler E, et al: Kidney glutaminase and carbonic anhydrase activities and renal electrolyte excretion in rats. *Am. J. Physiol.* 184:83, 1956.

381. Myers RE: Anoxic brain pathology and blood glucose. *Neurology* 26:345, 1976.

382. Myers RE: Lactic acid accumulation as cause of brain edema and cerebral necrosis resulting from oxygen deprivation. In Korobkin R, Guilleminault C (eds): *Advances in Perinatal Neurology.* New York, SP Medical and Scientific Books, 1979, vol 1, pp 85–114.

383. Myers RE: A unitary theory of causation of anoxic and hypoxic brain pathology. In Fahn S, Davis JN, Rowland LP (eds): *Cerebral Hypoxia and its Consequences.* New York, Raven Press, 1979, pp 195–213.

384. Myers RE, et al: Failure of marked hypoxia with maintained blood pressure to produce brain injury in cats (abstr.) *J Neuropathol Exp Neurol* 39:378, 1980.

385. Nagel-Hiemke M, et al: Influence of hypo- and hyperthyroidism on plasma catecholamines in pithed rats. *Arch Pharmacol* 317:159, 1981.

386. Navarro J, et al: Are middle molecules responsible for toxic phenomena in chronic renal failure? *Nephron* 32:301, 1982.

387. Nelson SR, et al: Control of glycogen levels in brain. *J. Neurochem.* 15:1271, 1968.

388. Nelson TE, Flewellen EH: The malignant hyperthermia syndrome. *N Engl. J. Med.* 309:416, 1983.

389. Nicholson JLM, Altman J: The effects of early hypo- and hyperthyroidism on the development of rat cerebellar cortex. I. Cell proliferation and differentiation. *Brain Res.* 44:13, 1972.

390. Nicholson JL, Altman J: The effects of early hypo- and hyperthyroidism on the development of the cerebellar cortex. II. Synaptogenesis in the molecular layer. *Brain Res.* 44:25, 1972.

391. Nickel SN, Frame B: Neurologic manifestations of myxedema. *Neurology (Minneap.)* 8:511, 1958.

392. Nickel SN, et al: Myxedema neuropathy and myopathy: a clinical and pathologic study. *Neurology (Minneap)* 11:125, 1961.

393. Norenberg MD: A light and electron microscopic study of experimental portal-systemic (ammonia) encephalopathy. *Lab. Invest.* 36:618, 1977.

394. Norenberg MD: The distribution of glutamine synthetase in the rat central nervous system. *J. Histochem Cytochem* 27:756, 1979.

395. Norenberg MD: The astrocyte in liver disease. In Fedoroff S, Hertz L (eds): *Advances in Cellular Neurobiology.* New York, Academic Press, 1981, vol 2, pp 303–352.

396. Norenberg MD: A hypothesis of osmotic endothelial injury. A pathogenetic mechanism in central pontine myelinolysis. *Arch Neurol* 40:66, 1983.

397. Norenberg MD, Lapham LW: The astrocyte response in experimental portal-systemic encephalopathy: an electron microscope study. *J Neuropathol Exp Neurol* 33:422, 1974.

398. Norenberg MD, Martinez-Herenandez A: Fine structural localization of glutamine synthetase in astrocytes of rat brain. *Brain Res.* 161:303, 1979.

399. Norenberg MD, Pappendick RE: Chronicity of hyponatremia as a factor in experimental myelinolysis. *Ann. Neurol* 15:544, 1984.

400. Norenberg MD, et al: Association between rise in serum sodium and central pontine myelinolysis. *Ann. Neurol.* 11:128, 1982.

401. Norrell H, et al: Leukoencephalopathy following administration of methotrexate into the cerebrospinal fluid in the treatment of brain tumors. *Cancer* 33:923, 1974.

402. Norris FH, Engel WK: Carcinomatous amyotrophic lateral sclerosis. In Brain L, Norris F (eds): *The Remote Effects of Cancer on the Nervous System.* New York, Grune & Stratton, 1965, ch 2, pp 24–34.

403. O'Hare JA, et al: Dialysis encephalopathy: clinical, electroencephalographic and interventional aspects. *Medicine* 62:129, 1983.

404. Ohnuma T, et al: Biochemical and pharmacological studies with asparaginase in man. *Cancer Res* 30:2297, 1970.

405. Okeda R, et al: Comparative study on pathogenesis of selective cerebral lesions in carbon monoxide poisoning and nitrogen hypoxia in cats. *Acta Neuropathol* 56:265, 1982.

406. Olsen S: The brain in uremia. *Acta Psychiatr Scand.* 36(Suppl 156):1, 1961.

407. Olsson Y, Sourander P: Changes in the sympathetic nervous system in diabetes mellitus: a preliminary report. *J Neuro. Visc. Relat.* (*Wien*) 31:86, 1968.

408. Olsson Y, et al: Pathoanatomical study of the central and peripheral nervous systems in diabetes of early onset and long duration. *Pathol Eur* 3:62, 1968.

409. Olsson Y, et al: The blood-brain barrier to protein tracers in focal cerebral ischemia and infarction caused by occlusion of the middle cerebral artery. *Acta Neuropathol* 18:89, 1971.

410. Oppenheimer JH, Surks MI: Biochemical basis of thyroid hormone action. In Litwack I (ed): *Biochemical Action of Hormones.* New York, Academic Press, 1975, pp 128–148.

411. Ortiz Vazquez J: Neurological manifestations of chronic respiratory diseases. In Vinken PJ, Bruyn GW (eds): *Handbook of Clinical Neurology.* Amsterdam, Elsevier/North Holland, 1979, vol 38, pp 285–307.

412. Packman S, et al: Severe hyperammonemia in a newborn infant with methylmalonyl-CoA mutase deficiency. *J Pediatr* 92:769, 1978.

413. Pagliara AS, et al: Hypoglycemia in infancy and childhood. *J Pediatr* 82:365, 1973.

414. Paljärvi L, et al: The brain in extreme respiratory acidosis. A light- and electron-microscopic study in the rat. *Acta Neuropathol* (*Berl*) 58:87, 1982.

415. Pannier JL, et al: Effect of non-respiratory alkalosis on brain tissue and cerebral blood flow in rats with damaged blood-brain barrier. *Stroke* 9:354, 1978.

416. Pant SS, et al: Spastic paraparesis following portocaval shunts. *Neurology* 18:134, 1968.

417. Papageorgiu C, et al: A comparative study of brain atrophy by computerized tomography in chronic renal failure and chronic hemodialysis. *Acta Neurol Scand* 66:378, 1982.

418. Park BE, et al: Nonketotic hyperglycemic hyperosmolar coma. Report of neurosurgical cases with a review of mechanism and treatment. *J Neurosurg* 44:409, 1976.

419. Parker TH, et al: The effect of acute and subacute ammonia intoxication in regional cerebral acetylcholine levels in rats. *Biochem Med* 18:235, 1977.

420. Partin JC: Reye's syndrome (encephalopathy and fatty liver): diagnosis and treatment. *Gastroenterology* 69:511, 1975.

421. Partin JC, et al: Brain ultrastructure in Reye's syndrome (encephalopathy and fatty infiltration of the viscera). *J Neuropathol Exp Neurol* 34:425, 1975.

422. Partin JC, et al: Brain ultrastructure in Reye's disease. II. Acute injury and recovery processes in three children. *J Neuropathol Exp Neurol* 37:796, 1978.

423. Pasquini JM, et al: Neonatal hypothyroidism and early undernutrition in the rat: defective maturation of structural membrane components in the central nervous system. *Neurochem Res* 6:979, 1981.

424. Patton RC: Haemostatic changes in diabetic coma. *Diabetologia* 21:172, 1981.

425. Pearson J, et al: Brain death. II. Neuropathological correlation with the radioisotopic bolus technique for evaluation of critical deficit of cerebral blood flow. *Ann Neurol* 2:206, 1977.

426. Peck SD, Reiquam CW: Disseminated intravascular coagulation in cancer patients: supportive evidence. *Cancer* 31:1114, 1973.

427. Pedley TA: The pathophysiology of focal epilepsy: neurophysiological considerations. *Ann. Neurol.* 3:2, 1978.

428. Penman RWB: Addison's disease in association with spastic paraplegia. *Br Med J* 1:402, 1960.

429. Peterson H, Swanson AG: Acute encephalopathy occurring during hemodialysis. *Arch Intern Med* 113:877, 1964.

430. Petito CK: Early and late mechanisms of increased vascular permeability following experimental cerebral infarction. *J Neuropathol Exp Neurol* 38:222, 1979.

431. Petito CK, Babiak T: Early proliferative changes in astrocytes in postischemic noninfarcted rat brain. *Ann Neurol* 11:510, 1982.

432. Petito CK, et al: Ischemic brain edema requires tissue necrosis. *Ann Neurol* 8:91, 1980.

433. Petito CK, et al: Edema and vascular permeability in cerebral ischemia. *J Neuropathol Exp Neurol* 41:423, 1982.

434. Phair JP, et al: The central nervous system in leukemia. *Ann Intern Med* 61:863, 1964.

435. Pierce MI: Neurologic complications of acute leukemia in children. *Pediatr Clin North Am* 9:425, 1962.

436. Pitner SE, Johnson WW: Chronic subdural hematomata in childhood acute leukemia. *Cancer* 32:185, 1973.

437. Pleasure D, Goldberg M: Neurogenic hypernatremia. *Arch Neurol* 15:78, 1966.

438. Plotz M, et al: The natural history of Cushing's syndrome. *Am J Med* 13:597, 1952.

439. Plum F: What causes infarction in ischemic brain? *Neurology* 33:222, 1983.

440. Plum F, Posner JB: Blood and cerebrospinal fluid lactate during hyperventilation. *Am J Physiol* 212:864, 1967.

441. Plum F, Posner JB: *The Diagnosis of Stupor and Coma,* ed 3. Philadelphia, FA Davis, 1980.

442. Plum F, et al: Delayed neurological deterioration after anoxia. *Arch Intern Med* 110:18, 1962.

443. Pollock AS, Arieff AI: Abnormalities of cell volume regulation and their functional consequences. *Am J Physiol* 239:F195, 1980.

444. Pontén U: Consecutive acid-base changes in blood, brain tissue and cerebrospinal fluid during respiratory acidosis and baseosis. *Acta Neurol Scand* 42:455, 1966.

445. Posner JB, et al: Acid-base balance in cerebrospinal fluid. *Arch Neurol* 12:479, 1965.

446. Powers JM, McKeever PE: Central pontine myelinolysis: an ultrastructural and elemental study. *J Neurol Sci* 29:65, 1976.

447. Price TR, Netsky MG: Myxedema and ataxia: cerebellar alterations and "neural myxedema bodies" *Neurology*

(*Minneap*) 16:957, 1966.

448. Prockop, LD: Hyperglycemia, polyol accumulation and increased intracranial pressure. *Arch Neurol (Chic)* 25:126, 1971.

449. Prockop LD: Hyperglycemia: effects on the nervous system. In Vinken PS, Bruyn GW (eds): *Handbook of Clinical Neurology*, Amsterdam, North Holland, 1976, vol 27.

450. Pulsinelli WA, et al: Moderate hyperglycemia augments ischemic brain damage: A neuropathologic study in the rat. *Neurology* 32:1239, 1982.

451. Raabe W, Gummit RJ: Disinhibition in cat motor cortex by ammonia. *J Neurophysiol* 38:347, 1975.

452. Raichle ME: The pathophysiology of brain ischemia. *Ann Neurol* 13:2, 1983.

453. Ramirez de Guglielmo AE, Gomez CJ: Influence of neonatal hypothyroidism on amino acids in developing rat brain. *J Neurochem* 13:1017, 1966.

454. Ramsay ID: *Thyroid Disease and Muscle Dysfunction*. London, Heinemann, 1974.

455. Ramsay MKC, et al: The effect of L-asparaginase on plasma coagulation factors in acute lymphoblastic leukemia. *Cancer* 40:1398, 1977.

456. Randall ME: Aluminum toxicity in an infant not on dialysis. *Lancet* 1:1327, 1983.

457. Randic M, Padjec A: Effect of calcium ions on the release of acetylcholine from the cerebral cortex. *Nature* 215:990, 1967.

458. Raskind M: Psychosis, polydipsia, and water intoxication: report of a fatal case. *Arch Gen Psychiatry* 30:112, 1974.

459. Reagan TJ, Okazaki H: The thrombotic syndrome associated with carcinoma: a clinical and neuropathologic study. *Arch Neurol* 31:390, 1974.

460. Reddy RV, Vakili ST: Midbrain encephalitis as a remote effect of a malignant neoplasm. *Arch Neurol* 38:781, 1981.

461. Rehncrona S, Siesjo BK: Metabolic and physiologic changes in acute brain failure. In Grenvik A, Safar P (eds): *Brain Failure and Resuscitation*. New York, Churchill Livingstone, 1981, pp 11–33.

462. Reske-Nielsen E, Lundbaek K: Diabetic encephalopathy: diffuse and focal lesions of the brain in long-term diabetics. *Acta Neurol Scand* 39(Suppl 4):273, 1963.

463. Reske-Nielsen E, Lundbaek K: Pathological changes in the central and peripheral nervous system of young long-term diabetics. II. The spinal cord and peripheral nerves. *Diabetologia* 4:34, 1968.

464. Reske-Nielsen E, et al: Pathological changes in the central and peripheral nervous system of young long-term diabetics. I. Diabetic encephalopathy. *Diabetologia* 1:233, 1965.

465. Reuler JB: Hypothermia: pathophysiology, clinical settings and management. *Ann Intern Med* 89:519, 1978.

466. Richardson EP Jr: Neurologic effects of cancer. In Holland JF, Frei E (eds): *Cancer Medicine*. Philadelphia, Lea & Febiger, 1973, pp 1057–1067.

467. Richardson JC, et al: Encephalopathies of anoxia and hypoglycemia. *Arch Neurol* 1:178, 1959.

468. Rifkind D, et al: Systemic fungal infections complicating renal transplantation and immunosuppressive therapy: clinical microbiologic, neurologic and pathologic features. *Am J Med* 43:28, 1967.

469. Robinson KC, et al: Idiopathic hypoparathyroidism presenting as dementia. *Br Med J* 2:1203, 1954.

470. Robinson PK: The clinical effects of hypocalcemia on the nervous system. *J R Coll Physicians* 1:36, 1966.

471. Robson JG: The physiology and pathology of acute hypoxia. *Br J Anaesth* 36:536, 1964.

472. Romanul FCA, Abramowicz A: Changes in brain and pial vessels in arterial border zones: a study of 13 cases. *Arch Neurol* 11:40, 1964.

473. Rosen SM, et al: Haemodialysis disequilibrium. *Br Med J* 2:672, 1964.

474. Rosenblum WI, Hadfield MG: Granulomatous angiitis of the nervous system in cases of herpes zoster and lymphosarcoma. *Neurology* 22:348, 1972.

475. Rothermich NO, Von Haam E: Pancreatic encephalopathy. *J Clin Endocrinol* 1:872, 1941.

476. Rowland LP: Myasthenia gravis. In Goldensohn ES, Appel SH (eds): *Scientific Approaches to Clinical Neurology*. Philadelphia, Lea & Febiger, 1977, ch 89, pp 1518–1554.

477. Rowland LP, Schotland DL: Neoplasms and muscle disease. In Brain L, Norris F (eds): *The Remote Effects of Cancer on the Nervous System*. New York, Grune & Stratton, 1965, pp 67–80.

478. Rubinstein LS, et al: Disseminated necrotizing leukoencephalopathy: a complication of treated central nervous system leukemia and lymphoma. *Cancer* 35:291, 1975.

479. Ruskin J, Remington JS: Toxoplasmosis in the compromised host. *Ann Intern Med* 84:193, 1976.

480. Russell DS: Histological changes in the striped muscles in myasthenia gravis. *J Pathol Bacteriol* 65:279, 1953.

481. Russell DS: Encephalomyelitis and carcinomatous neuropathy. In Van Bogaert L, Radermecker J, Hozay J, Lowenthal A (eds): *The Encephalitides*. Amsterdam, Elsevier, 1961, pp 131–135.

482. Rymer MM, Fishman RA: Protective adaptation of brain to water intoxication. *Arch Neurol* 28:49, 1973.

483. Sabouraud O, et al: L'encéphalopathie myoclonique progressive des dialyses (E.M.P.D): étude clinique, électroencephalographique et neuropathologique. Discussion pathogénique. *Rev Neurol* 134:575, 1978.

484. Sahay BM, et al: Relation between myasthenia gravis and thyroid disease. *Br Med J* 1:762, 1965.

485. Santa T, et al: Histometric study of neuromuscular junction ultrastructure. I. Myasthenia gravis. *Neurology* 22:71, 1972.

486. Satoyoshi E, et al: Subacute cerebellar degeneration and Eaton-Lambert syndrome with bronchogenic carcinoma. A case report. *Neurology* 23:764, 1973.

487. Saudubray JM, et al: Neonatal congenital lactic acidosis with pyruvate carboxylase deficiency in two siblings. *Acta Paediatr Scand* 65:717, 1976.

488. Schafer DF, Jones EA: Potential neural mechanisms in the pathogenesis of hepatic encephalopathy. *Prog Liver Dis* 7:615, 1982.

489. Scheinberg P: Effects of uremia on cerebral blood flow and metabolism. *Neurology* 4:101, 1954.

490. Scheinberg P, et al: Correlative observations on cerebral metabolism and cardiac output in myxoedema. *J Clin Invest* 29:1139, 1950.

491. Schenker S, et al: Studies on the intracerebral toxicity of ammonia. *J Clin Invest* 46:838, 1967.

492. Scherer H-J: Zur Frage der Beziehungen zwischen Leberund Gehirnveränderungen. *Virchows Arch Pathol Anat* 288:333, 1933.

493. Schindler U, Betz E: Influence of severe hypercapnia upon cerebral cortical metabolism, CSF electrolyte concentrations and EEG in the cat. *Bull. Physiopathol Respir (Nancy)* 12:277, 1976.

494. Schlaepfer WW: Experimental alterations of neurofilaments and neurotubules by calcium and other ions. *Exp Cell Res* 67:73, 1971.

495. Schlaepfer WW: Vincristine-induced axonal alterations in rat peripheral nerve. *J Neuropathol Exp Neurol* 30:488, 1971.

496. Schlaepfer WW: Vesicular disruption of myelin simulated by exposure of nerve to calcium ionophore. *Nature* 265:734, 1977.

497. Schmid AH, Riede UN: A morphometric study of the cerebellar cortex from patients with carcinoma: a contribution on quantitative aspects in carcinotoxic cerebellar atrophy. *Acta Neuropathol.* 28:343, 1974.

498. Schneck SA: Neuropathological features of human organ transplantation. I. Probable cytomegalovirus infection. *J Neuropathol Exp Neurol* 24:415, 1965.

499. Schneck SA: Neuropathological features of human organ transplantation. II. Central pontine myelinolysis and neuroaxonal dystrophy. *J Neuropathol Exp Neurol* 25:18, 1966.

500. Schneck SA: Diabetes and the nervous system. *Acta*

Diabetol Lat 6:713, 1969.

501. Schneck SA, Penn I: De novo brain tumors in renal transplant recipients. *Lancet* 1:983, 1971.

502. Schneider AB, Sherwood LM: Calcium homeostasis and the pathogenesis and management of hypercalcemic disorders. *Metabolism* 23:975, 1974.

503. Schneider M: Survival and revival of the brain in anoxia and ischemia. In Guastaut H, Meyer JS (eds): *Cerebral Anoxia and the Electroencephalogram.* Springfield, IL, Charles C Thomas, 1961, pp 134–143.

504. Schoffeniels E, Franck G, Hertz L, Tower DB (eds): *Dynamic Properties of Glia Cells.* Oxford, England, Pergamon Press, 1978.

505. Scholz W: Selective neuronal necrosis and its topistic patterns in hypoxemia and oligemia. *J Neuropathol Exp Neurol* 12:249, 1953.

506. Schubert WK, et al: Encephalopathy and fatty liver (Reye's syndrome). *Prog Liver Dis* 4:489–510, 1972.

507. Schuier FJ, Hossmann K-A: Experimental brain infarcts in cats. II. Ischemic brain edema. *Stroke* 11:593, 1980.

508. Seligson H, Seligson D: N-methyl-2-pyridone-5-carboxylic acid and N-methyl-2-pyridone-5-formamido acetic acid isolated from dialysis fluids of uremic patients. *Clin Chim Acta* 12:137, 1965.

509. Seneviratna KN, Peires DA: The effect of ischaemia on the excitability of sensory nerves in diabetes mellitus. *J Neurol Neurosurg Psychiatry* 31:348, 1968.

510. Sharf B, Bental E: Pancreatic encephalopathy. *J Neurol Neurosurg Psychiatry* 34:357, 1971.

511. Shelanski ML, Wisniewski H: Neurofibrillary degeneration induced by vincristine therapy. *Arch Neurol* 20:199, 1969.

512. Sherins RJ, Verity MA: Central pontine myelinolysis associated with acute hemorrhagic pancreatitis. *J Neurol Neurosurg Psychiatry* 31:583, 1968.

513. Shibolet S, et al: Heat stroke: a review. *Aviat Space Environ Med* 47:280, 1976.

514. Shimizu H, et al: Cyclic 3′5′-monophosphate formation in brain slices: stimulation by batrachotoxin, ouabain, veratridine and potassium ions. *Molec Pharmacol* 6:184, 1970.

515. Shiraki H, Oda M: Neuropathology of hepatocerebral disease with emphasis on comparative studies. In Minckler J (ed): *Pathology of the Nervous System.* New York, McGraw-Hill, 1968, vol 1, pp 1089–1103.

516. Siassi F, et al: Plasma tryptophan levels and brain serotonin metabolism in chronically uremic rats. *J Nutr* 107:840, 1977.

517. Siegel GJ, Albers RW, Agranoff BW, Katzman R (eds): *Basic Neurochemistry*, ed 3. Boston, Little, Brown, 1981.

518. Sieker HO, Hickam JB: Carbon dioxide intoxication. *Medicine* 35:389, 1956.

519. Siemkowicz E, Hansen AJ: Clinical restitution following cerebral ischemia in hypo-, normo-, and hyperglycemic rats. *Acta Neurol Scand* 58:1, 1978.

520. Siesjö BK: Metabolic control of intracellular pH. *Scand J Clin Lab Invest* 32:97, 1973.

521. Siesjö BK: *Brain Energy Metabolism.* New York, Wiley, 1978, pp 453–526.

522. Siesjö BK: Cell damage in the brain: a speculative synthesis. *J Cereb Blood Flow Metabol* 1:155, 1981.

523. Sigsbee B, et al: Nonmetastatic superior sagittal sinus thrombosis complicating systemic cancer. *Neurology* 29:139, 1979.

524. Silke B, et al: Dialysis dementia and renal transplantation. *Dial Transplant* 7:486, 1978.

525. Simpson JA: The neurological manifestations of idiopathic hypoparathyroidism. *Brain* 75:76, 1952.

526. Simpson JA: Myasthenia gravis and myasthenic syndromes. In Walton JN (ed): *Disorders of Voluntary Muscle.* London, Churchill, 1969, pp 336–368.

527. Simpson T: Acute respiratory infections in emphysema. *Br Med J* 1:297, 1954.

528. Skillern PG, Lockhart G: Optic neuritis and uncontrolled diabetes mellitus in 14 patients. *Ann Intern Med* 51:468, 1959.

529. Slager UT: Diabetic myelopathy. *Arch Pathol Lab Med* 102:467, 1978.

530. Slager UT, Webb AT: Pathologic findings in the spinal cord. *Arch Pathol* 96:388, 1973.

531. Slavick HE, Lipman IJ: Brainstem toxoplasmosis complicating Hodgkin's disease. *Arch Neurol* 34:636, 1977.

532. Slyter H: Idiopathic hypoparathyroidism presenting as dementia. *Neurology* 29:393, 1979.

533. Smith CK, et al: Psychiatric disturbance in endocrinologic disease. *Psychosom Med* 34:69, 1972.

534. Smith W, et al: Sagittal sinus thrombosis and occult malignancy. *J Neurol Neurosurg Psychiatry* 46:187, 1983.

535. Soeters PB, Fischer JE: Insulin, glucagon, amino acid imbalance, and hepatic encephalopathy. *Lancet* 2:880, 1976.

536. Soffer LJ, et al: Cushing's syndrome: a study of fifty patients. *Am J Med* 30:129, 1961.

537. Sokal JE, Firat D: Varicella-zoster infection in Hodgkin's disease. *Am J Med* 39:452, 1965.

538. Solitare GB, et al: Argininosuccinic aciduria: clinical, biochemical, anatomical and neuropathological observations. *J Ment Defic Res* 13:153, 1969.

539. Sotos JF, et al: Studies in experimental hypertonicity. *Pediatrics* 26:925, 1960.

540. Spalke G, Eschenbach C: Infantile cortical measles inclusion body encephalitis during combined treatment of acute lymphoblastic leukemia. *J Neurol* 220:269, 1979.

541. Spielmeyer W: *Histopathologie des Nervensystems.* Berlin, Springer Verlag, 1922.

542. Srebro F, Stachura J: Gomori-positive glia in magnesium-deficient rats. *Acta Neuropathol* 21:256, 1972.

543. Sridhar CB, et al: Syndrome of hypernatremia hypodipsia and partial diabetes insipidus. A new interpretation. *J Clin Endocrinol Metab* 38:890, 1974.

544. Steegmann AT: The influence of hypothermia on the brain. In Minckler J (ed): *Pathology of the Nervous System.* New York, McGraw-Hill, 1968, vol 1, pp 948–967.

545. Steegmann AT: Neuropathology of cardiac arrest. In Minckler J (ed): *Pathology of the Nervous System.* New York, McGraw-Hill, 1968, vol 1, pp 1005–1029.

546. Steen PA, et al: Incomplete versus complete cerebral ischemia: improved outcome with a minimal blood flow. *Ann Neurol* 6:389, 1979.

547. Steven MM, et al: Cerebellar cortical degeneration with ovarian carcinoma. *Postgrad Med J* 58:47, 1982.

548. Strang RHC, Bachelard HS: Effect of insulin on levels and turnover of intermediates of brain carbohydrate metabolism in vivo. *J Neurochem.* 18:1799, 1971.

549. Stromborn U, et al: Hyperthyroidism: specifically increased response to central NA (α) receptor stimulation and generally increased monoamine turnover in brain. *J Neural Transm* 41:73, 1977.

550. Subramanyam R, et al: A model for regional cerebral oxygen distribution during continuous inhalation of $^{15}O_2$, $C^{15}O$, and $C^{15}O_2$. *J Nucl Med* 19:48, 1978.

551. Sullivan PA, et al: Dialysis dementia: recovery after transplantation. *Br Med J* 2:740, 1977.

552. Sullivan PA, et al: Cerebral transmitter precursors and metabolites in advanced renal disease. *J Neurol Neurosurg Psychiatry* 41:581, 1978.

553. Sung JH: Neuroaxonal dystrophy in mucoviscidosis. *J Neuropathol Exp Neurol* 25:341, 1966.

554. Sung JH, et al: Axonal dystrophy in the gracile nucleus in congenital biliary atresia and cystic fibrosis (mucoviscidosis): beneficial effect of vitamin E therapy. *J Neuropathol Exp Neurol* 39:584, 1980.

555. Swanson JW, Kelly JJ Jr: Neurologic aspects of thyroid dysfunction. *Mayo Clin Proc* 56:504, 1981.

556. Swanson PD: Neurological manifestations of hypernatremia. In Vinken PJ, Bruyn GW (eds): *Handbook of Clinical Neurology.* Amsterdam, North Holland, 1976, vol 28, pp 443–461.

557. Sylvester JT, et al: Hypoxia and CO-hypoxia in dogs: hemodynamics, carotid reflexes, and catecholamines.

Am J Physiol 218:H22, 1979.

558. Szanto L, et al: Interrelations of thyroid and mesencephalic activity. *Acta Microbiol Acad Sci Hung* 27:235, 1970.

559. Talalla A, et al: Subdural hematoma associated with long-term hemodialysis for chronic renal disease. *JAMA* 212:1847, 1970.

560. Tapley DF: Magnesium balance in myxedematous patients treated with triiodothyronine: preliminary note. *Bull Johns Hopkins Hosp* 96:274, 1955.

561. Taylor P, et al: Quantitative changes in astrocytes after portocaval shunting. *Arch Pathol Lab Med* 103:82, 1979.

562. Tchertkoff V, et al: Hyperosmolar nonketotic diabetic coma: vascular complications. *J Am Geriat Soc* 22:462, 1974.

563. Tempel GE, Musacchia XJ: The hypothermic hamster brain: its water and electrolyte content and perfusion. *Cryobiology* 18:585, 1981.

564. Tews JK, et al: Chemical changes in the brain during insulin hypoglycemia and recovery. *J Neurochem* 12:679, 1965.

565. Thaler MM, et al: Reye's syndrome due to a novel protein-tolerant variant of ornithine-transcarbamylase deficiency. *Lancet* 2:438, 1974.

566. Thölen H: Hirnödem. Eine Todesursache beim endogenen Leberkoma. *Klin. Wochenschr.* 50:296, 1972.

567. Thomas PK, Lascelles RG: The pathology of diabetic neuropathy. *Q J Med* 35:489, 1966.

568. Thurston JH, et al: Effects of salt and water loading on carbohydrate and energy metabolism and levels of selected amino acids in the brain of young mice. *J Neurochem* 24:953, 1975.

569. Thurston JH, et al: Taurine: a role in osmotic regulation of mammalian brain and possible clinical significance. *Life Sci* 26:1561, 1980.

570. Timiras PS, Woodbury DM: Effect of thyroid activity on brain function and brain electrolyte distribution in rats. *Endocrinology* 58:181, 1956.

571. Timiras PS, et al: Effects of thyroxine on brain function and electrolyte distribution in intact and adrenalectomized rats. *J Pharmacol Exp Ther* 115:154, 1955.

572. Timperley WR, et al: Cerebral intravascular coagulation in diabetic ketoacidosis. *Lancet* 1:952, 1974.

573. Tom MI, Richardson JC: Hypoglycaemia from islet cell tumour of pancreas with amyotrophy and cerebrospinal nerve cell changes: a case report. *J Neuropathol Exp Neurol* 10:57, 1951.

574. Tonsgard JH, et al: Lactic acidemia in Reye's syndrome. *Pediatrics* 69:64, 1982.

575. Tornheim PA: Regional localization of cerebral edema following fluid and insulin therapy in streptozotocin-diabetic rats. *Diabetes* 30:762, 1981.

576. Townsend JJ, et al: Acquired toxoplasmosis: a neglected cause of treatable nervous system disease. *Arch Neurol* 32:335, 1975.

577. Trauner DA: Pathologic changes in a rabbit model of Reye's syndrome. *Pediatr Res* 16:950, 1982.

578. Trauner DA, Adams H: Intracranial pressure elevations during octonoate infusion in rabbits: an experimental model of Reye's syndrome. *Pediatr Res* 15:1097, 1981.

579. Trobe JD, et al: Dysthyroid optic neuropathy: clinical profile and rationale for management. *Arch Ophthalmol* 96:1199, 1978.

580. Turel AP, et al: Reye's syndrome and cerebellar intracytoplasmic inclusion bodies. *Arch Neurol* 32:624, 1975.

581. Tyler HR: Neurologic disorders in renal failure. *Am J Med* 44:734, 1968.

582. Tyler HR: Neurologic disorders seen in renal failure. In Vinken PJ, Bruyn GW (eds): *Handbook of Clinical Neurology.* Amsterdam, North Holland, 1976, vol 27, pp 321–348.

583. Ulshafer TR: The measurement of changes in acetylcholine level (ACh) in rat brain following ammonium ion intoxication and its possible bearing on the problem of hepatic coma. *J Lab Clin Med* 52:718, 1958.

584. Vaccari A: Decreased central serotonin function in hy-

585. Vainsel M, et al: Tetany due to hypomagnesaemia with secondary hypocalcemia. *Arch Dis Child* 45:254, 1970.

586. Van Den Noort S, et al: Brain metabolism in experimental uremia. *Arch Intern Med* 126:831, 1970.

587. Van Leuven F, et al: Influence of PCO_2 on amino acids in the brain of the rat. *Arch. Int. Physiol. Biochim.* 82:419, 1973.

588. Várkonyi T, et al: Die feinstrukturellen Veranderungen des nucleus caudatus bei der experimentellen uramischen encephalopathie. *Beitr Pathol* 140:110, 1969.

589. Vastola EF, et al: Activation of epileptogenic foci by hyperosmolarity. *Neurology* 17:520, 1967.

590. Venna N, Sabin TD: Tonic focal seizures in nonketotic hyperglycemia of diabetes mellitus. *Arch Neurol* 38:512, 1981.

591. Vergara F, et al: α-Ketoglutaramate: increased concentrations in the cerebrospinal fluid of patients in hepatic coma. *Science* 183:81, 1974.

592. Verhaart WJC: Grey matter degeneration of the central nervous system in carcinosis. *Acta Neuropathol* 1:107, 1961.

593. Vick N, et al: Carcinomatous cerebellar degeneration, encephalomyelitis and sensory neuropathy (radiculitis). *Neurology* 19:425, 1969.

594. Victor M, et al: The acquired (non-Wilsonian) type of chronic hepatocerebral degeneration. *Medicine* 44:345, 1965.

595. Vietzke W, et al: Toxoplasmosis complicating malignancy—experience at the National Cancer Institute. *Cancer* 21:816, 1968.

596. Vital C, et al: Les neuropathies peripheriques du diabeti sucré. *J Neurol Sci* 18:381, 1973.

597. Vogel FS: Demyelination induced in living rabbits by means of a lipolytic enzyme preparation. *J Exp Med* 93:297, 1951.

598. Vogel FS: Cerebral demyelination and focal visceral lesions in a case of acute hemorrhagic pancreatitis. *AMA Arch Pathol* 52:355, 1951.

599. Vogel FS: Conundrum of central pontine myelinolysis. *Pathol Annu* 13:29, 1978.

600. Vogel FS: The morphological consequences of cerebral hypoxia. In Fahn S, Doors JN, Rowland LP (eds): *Cerebral Hypoxia and its Consequences.* New York, Raven Press, 1979, pp 147–154.

601. Vogt C, Vogt O: Erkrankungen der grosshirnrinde im lichte der Topistick Pathoklise und Pathoarchitektonik. *J Psychol Neurol* 28:1, 1922.

602. Von Hösslin C, Alzheimer A: Ein Beitrag zur Klinik und pathologischen Anatomie der Westphal-Strümpellschen Pseudosklerose. *Z Neurol Psychiatr* 8:183, 1912.

603. Waggoner RW, et al: Wilson's disease in the light of cerebral changes following ordinary acquired liver disorders. *J Nerv Ment Dis* 96:410, 1942.

604. Wakim KG: The pathophysiology of the dialysis disequilibrium syndrome. *Mayo Clin Proc* 44:406, 1969.

605. Waldenstrom J: Acute thyrotoxic encephalo- or myopathy, its cause and treatment. *Acta Med Scand* 121:251, 1945.

606. Walker CO, Schenker S: Pathogenesis of hepatic encephalopathy with special reference to the role of ammonia. *Am J Clin Nutr* 23:619, 1970.

607. Walker AE, et al: The neuropathological findings in irreversible coma. *J Neuropathol Exp Neurol* 34:295, 1975.

608. Walton JN, et al: Subacute "poliomyelitis" and Hodgkin's disease. *J Neurol Sci* 6:435, 1968.

609. Walsh FB: Papilledema associated with increased intracranial pressure in Addison's disease. *Arch Ophthalmol* 47:86, 1952.

610. Ward MK, et al: Dialysis encephalopathy syndrome. *Proc Eur Dial Transplant Assoc* 13:348, 1976.

611. Ware AJ, et al: Cerebral edema: a major complication of massive hepatic necrosis. *Gastroenterology* 61:877, 1971.

612. Warren S, et al: *The Pathology of Diabetes Mellitus,* ed 4. Philadelphia, Lea & Febiger, 1966.

pothyroidism. *Eur J Pharmacol* 82:93, 1982.

613. Wasterlain CG, Posner JB: Cerebral edema in water intoxication. I. Clinical and chemical observations. *Arch Neurol* 19:71, 1968.

614. Wasterlain CG, Torack RM: Cerebral edema in water intoxication. II. An ultrastructural study. *Arch Neurol* 19:79, 1968.

615. Watkins JC: Metabolic derangements and other causative factors in toxic convulsions. *Biochem J* 106:4P, 1968.

616. Wayne J, et al: Metabolism of glutamic acid and related amino acids in the brain studied with ^{14}C-labeled glucose, butyric acid and glutamic acid in hypercapnic rats. *J Neurochem* 29:469, 1977.

617. Weiss HD, et al: Neurotoxicity of commonly used antineoplastic agents. *N Engl J Med* 291:75, 127, 1974.

618. Weitzman S, et al: Case report: simultaneous fungal and viral infection of the central nervous system. *Am J Med Sci* 276:127, 1978.

619. Welti W: Delirium with low serum sodium. *Arch Neurol Psychiatry* 76:559, 1956.

620. Williams R: Hepatic encephalopathy. *J R Coll Physicians* 8:63, 1973.

621. Wills MR, Savory J: Aluminum poisoning: dialysis encephalopathy, osteomalacia, and anaemia. *Lancet* 2:29, 1983.

622. Wilson JWL, et al: Necrotizing myelopathy associated with renal cell carcinoma. *Urology* 21:390, 1983.

623. Wilson R, et al: Reye's syndrome in three siblings: association with type A influenza infection. *Am J Dis Child* 134:1032, 1980.

624. Winegrad AL, Greene DA: Diabetic polyneuropathy: the importance of insulin deficiency-hyperglycemia and alterations in myoinositol metabolism in its pathogenesis. *N Engl J Med* 295:1416, 1976.

625. Winkelman NW, Moore MT: Neurohistopathologic changes with metrazol and insulin shock therapy: an experimental study on the cat. *Arch Neurol Psychiatry* 43:1108, 1940.

626. Woodbury DB, Karler T: The role of carbon dioxide in the nervous system. *Anaesthesiology* 21:686, 1960.

627. Wright DG, et al: Pontine and extrapontine myelinolysis. *Brain* 102:361, 1979.

628. Yanko L, et al: Optic nerve involvement in diabetes. *Acta Ophthalmol* 50:556, 1972.

629. Yanzer RC, Friede RL: Perisulcal infarcts: lesions caused by hypotension during increased intracranial pressure. *Ann Neurol* 6:399, 1979.

630. Yatsu FM, et al: Experimental brain ischemia: protection from irreversible damage with a rapid-acting barbiturate (methohexital). *Stroke* 3:726, 1972.

631. You K: Salicylate and mitochondrial injury in Reye's syndrome. *Science* 221:163, 1983.

632. Young E, Bradley RF: Cerebral edema with irreversible coma in severe diabetic ketoacidosis. *N Engl J Med* 276:665, 1967.

633. Young RSK, Truax BT: Hypernatremic hemorrhagic encephalopathy. *Ann Neurol* 5:588, 1979.

634. Zamora AJ, et al: Ultrastructural responses of the astrocytes to portocaval anastomosis in the rat. *J Neurol Sci* 18:25, 1973.

635. Zangemeister WH, et al: Carcinomatous encephalomyelopathy in conjunction with encephalomyeloradiculitis. *J Neurol* 218:63, 1978.

636. Zaren HA, et al: Experimental ischemic brain swelling. *J Neurochem* 32:227, 1970.

637. Zieve L: Pathogenesis of hepatic coma. *Arch Intern Med* 118:211, 1966.

638. Zieve L, Olsen RL: Can hepatic coma be caused by a reduction of brain noradrenaline or dopamine? *Gut* 18:688, 1977.

639. Zieve L, et al: Shunt encephalomyelopathy: II. Occurrence of permanent myelopathy. *Ann Intern Med* 53:53, 1960.

640. Zorilla E, Kozak GP: Ophthalmoplegia in diabetes mellitus. *Ann Intern Med* 67:968, 1967.

641. Zucker G, et al: Myelopathy associated with cirrhosis of liver and portocaval shunt: *NY State J Med* 74:402, 1974.

642. Zülch KJ, Behrend RCH: The pathogenesis and topography of anoxia, hypoxia and ischemia of the brain in man. In Gastaut H, Meyer JS (eds): *Cerebral Anoxia and the Electroencephalogram.* Springfield, IL, Charles C Thomas, 1961, pp 144–163.

Additional References

643. Altrocchi PH: Acute transverse myelopathy. *Arch Neurol* 9:111, 1963.

644. Bruyn GW: Carcinomatous polyneuropathy. In Vinken PJ, Bruyn BW (eds): *Handbook of Clinical Neurology.* Amsterdam, North Holland, 1979, vol 38, ch 28, pp 679–693.

645. Croft P: Neuromuscular syndromes associated with malignant disease. *Br J Hosp Med* 17:356, 1977.

646. Denny-Brown D: Primary sensory neuropathy with muscular changes associated with carcinoma. *J Neurol Neurosurg Psychiatry* 11:73, 1947.

647. DeVere R, Bradley WG: Polymyositis: its presentation, morbidity and mortality. *Brain* 98:637, 1975.

648. Folliss AGH, Netski MG: Progressive necrotic myelopathy. In Vinken PJ, Bruyn GW (eds): *Handbook of Clinical Neurology.* Amsterdam, North Holland, 1970, vol 9, ch 16, pp 452–468.

649. Greenfield JG, Turner JWA: Acute and subacute necrotic myelitis. *Brain* 62:227, 1939.

650. Henson RA, et al: Carcinomatous neuropathy and myopathy: a clinical and pathological study. *Brain* 77:82, 1954.

651. Jaffe D, Freeman W: Spinal necrosis and softening of obscure origin: necrotic myelitis versus myelomalacia. Review of literature and clinico-pathologic case studies. *Arch Neurol Psychiatry* 49:683, 1943.

652. Lambert EH, Rooke ED: Myasthenic state and lung cancer. In Lord Brain, Morris F (eds): *The Remote Effects of Cancer on the Nervous System.* New York, Grune & Stratton, 1965, ch 8, pp 67–80.

653. Margolis G, et al: Contrast medium injury to the spinal cord produced by aortography: pathologic anatomy of the experimental lesion. *J Neurosurg* 13:349, 1956.

654. Moersch FP, Kernohan JW: Progressive necrosis of the spinal cord. *Arch Neurol Psychiatry* 31:504, 1934.

655. Veron JR, et al: Acute necrotic myelopathy. *Eur Neurol* 11:83, 1974.

CHAPTER 11

Demyelinating Diseases

CEDRIC S. RAINE, Ph.D, D.Sc.

INTRODUCTION

It is probably safe to assume that in 1854, when Virchow (147) first described myelin in the central nervous system (CNS), he was unaware that this fatty substance would later become the most characteristic membrane of nervous tissue, a membrane unique morphologically, biochemically, immunologically, and physiologically, and one which would form the common denominator in the classification of important groups of human conditions, the acquired demyelinating and the hereditary dysmyelinating diseases. The following paragraphs emanate from the pen of one acquainted more with experimental demyelination than with clinical neuropathology, and, inasmuch as the understanding of this unique membrane is central to the present subject, the reader might anticipate a reappraisal with a fundamental flavor.

The demyelinating diseases are a heterogeneous group epitomized by multiple sclerosis, the most common member of the group and the archtype and yardstick with which all other primary diseases of myelin are measured. Indeed, in all teachings on this group, multiple sclerosis must be kept as the frame of reference. The component diseases (*vide infra*) are linked by an acquired infectious etiology (either proven or suspected), white matter lesions or "plaques" possessing a prominent perivenous inflammatory response and at least some evidence for an autoimmune pathogenesis, and within the lesions, a selective loss of myelin with relative sparing of axons.

Clinically, the demyelinating diseases have a broad base of manifestations ranging from acute to chronic, monophasic to polyphasic, benign to fatal, and within each subcategory, variation is legend. Diagnosis is often difficult. For some members, no specific diagnostic test exists, and final diagnosis is made either after a process of elimination or retrospectively at autopsy. In general, the demyelinating diseases afflict young adults, and the most common forms have long-term disabling effects giving the group important socioeconomic ramifications. For a fuller understanding of the clinical breadth and scope of these conditions, the reader is referred to the texts of Hallpike et al. (53), McAlpine et al. (76), and Vinken and Bruyn (146).

DEFINITION

Demyelination refers to the removal of apparently normal myelin from axons of the central and peripheral nervous systems (CNS and PNS), usually against a background of perivenular infiltration by small lymphocytes, plasma cells, and large mononuclear cells. This is the hallmark lesion of the demyelinating diseases which have an acquired (usually viral) etiology. Some texts refer to the process of demyelination as "primary" or "secondary demyelination," a confusing nomenclature since the adjectives, though illustrative, are redundant. "Secondary demyelination" is an archaic term used to describe the loss of myelin which follows parenchymal (including axonal) destruction in a wide spectrum of neuropathologic states. It is most frequently applied to Wallerian degeneration in the PNS, where, for example, after traumatic insult, the segment of nerve distal to the injury undergoes axonal depletion and, secondarily, loss of myelin. To apply the term "demyelination" to the latter phenomenon is therefore a contradiction of terms since axons no longer exist. "Myelinoclasis," a term used in some classic texts (e.g., *Greenfield's Neuropathology*), was introduced and strongly recommended by Poser (89), who states that this nomenclature was "chosen over the more traditional term 'demyelinating' in order to emphasize the difference between these diseases and the dysmyelinating diseases" (90). The reason for the demise of the term myelinoclasis is also (like "secondary demyelination") probably related to its redundancy. "Demyelination" is a term carefully avoided by most authors in references to the hereditary dysmyelinating diseases (metachromatic leukodystrophy, Krabbe's disease, adrenoleukodystrophy, etc.) on account of the extensive, early axonal destruction and the hereditary-metabolic etiology. Therefore, there is no need to distinguish it from the type of myelin loss encountered in the latter group. It is interesting to note that in texts published as recently as 1982 (121), "demyelination" is still being applied to some hereditary dysmyelinating conditions like adrenoleukodystrophy, which is also referred to as "Schilder's disease" (121).

Thus, there is currently a consensus among neuropathologists that "demyelination" should be a term reserved for the multiple sclerosis group of conditions. In the words of Adams and Sidman (5), "it serves no useful purpose" to apply the term to disorders of nervous tissue merely because they are located in the white matter. Nevertheless, it is pertinent to point out that myelin loss (N.B., "myelin loss," not "demyelination"), is a common sequela of a multitude of conditions, many of which initially affect other elements of white matter, such as blood vessels, glia, and axons. Therefore, although the major component of white matter, myelin is frequently damaged secondarily by neoplasia, trauma, infarct, necrosis, abscess, edema, anoxia, and hemorrhage in addition to degeneration of overlying cortex (Alzheimer's disease) or the small subcortical cerebral arteries (Binswanger's disease). It will become apparent in the forthcoming pages that with the com-

bination of routine and contemporary morphologic techniques, there is ample justification for the dogmatic application of this definition.

THE TARGET—WHITE MATTER

No human disease can match the specificity of the destruction which distinguishes from other conditions the demyelinating diseases where a single, sequestered membrane becomes the target of a complex, probably immunologic, attack. This profound proclamation on the pathologic uniqueness of multiple sclerosis is predated by many early workers on multiple sclerosis like Dawson (31), who noted in 1916 that "The pathologic anatomy of disseminated sclerosis bears no analogy to any other known pathological process in the body. We know e.g., of no process in other organs in which the relative integrity of the specific functioning parenchymatous tissue is associated with the enormous increase of the interstitial tissue occurring in definite circumscribed areas." As was pointed out in an earlier chapter in this volume (Chapter 2), myelin is elaborated in the CNS by the oligodendrocyte and in the PNS by the Schwann cell. Biochemically, it stands apart from other membranes both in its possessing unique proteins and its unusually high percentage (70%) of lipids. Among the 30% of the membrane made up of protein, one component in particular, myelin basic protein, has characteristic properties which render the sheath highly susceptible to immunologic attack. An 18,000 molecular weight, 170 amino acid molecule, myelin basic protein is cross-reactive and highly encephalitogenic when inoculated into most species (38). Even short sequences of this molecule are encephalitogenic, and it has been demonstrated that different polypeptides along the molecule influence cell-mediated and antibody-mediated immunity to the membrane.

In normal white matter, myelin is the major structural element, and related to its biochemistry, a wide variety of lipid stains exist which clearly differentiate white from grey matter. While such general stains are of little value for detailed examination, they are most useful for demonstrating widespread or diffuse myelin loss which show up as paler areas of staining. A routine hematoxylin and eosin (H&E) preparation gives little information on the integrity of myelin except to delineate white from grey matter and to show cell nuclei. Axis cylinder (axon) stains are useful for determining the density of nerve fibers for comparison with diseased areas. The differential astroglial and oligodendroglial cell stains of Cajal and Hortega (respectively), together with the Hortega microglial and the Holzer glial fibrillary stains (among others), afford the neuropathologist a comprehensive (albeit laborious) armamentarium of techniques for the analysis of white matter. However, due to preparative artifacts, none of the above gives reliable insight into myelin integrity.

In recent years, the light microscope analysis of the demyelinating diseases has been augmented significantly by the application of 1-μm epoxy sections from blocks prepared for ultrastructural study. These preparations can be stained with a variety of reagents, the most popular applied being toluidine blue/borax. Blocks up to 0.25 $\times$ 0.5 inch are possible; therefore, orientation and topography are preserved. With such preparations, myelinated fibers stand out in transverse sections as dense rings (due to their osmiophilia) and axons, as pale staining profiles in which mitochondria and filamentous elements can be discerned (Fig. 11.1). Astrocytes are identifiable by their elliptical or irregular nuclei which always display a perimeter of denser chromatin and sometimes one or two nucleoli. The cellular boundaries are often difficult to determine since the cytoplasm stains in a pale fashion. Oligodendrocytes are easy to distinguish since they possess nuclei which are more rounded and made up of clumped heterochromatin. The cytoplasm is usually a narrow perinuclear rim which stains moderately densely. Resting microglial cells in normal white matter are difficult to find, but cells with elongated densely staining nuclei can be detected which might correspond to microglia. Debris-laden macrophages, ciliated ependyma around the ventricles, and blood vessels with the occasional fibroblast, macrophage, or pericyte within the Virchow-Robin space, complete the light microscope image.

Ultrastructurally, white matter is made up of densely packed, electron-dense, lipid-rich (osmiophilic) myelin sheaths surrounding pale-staining axons (Fig. 11.2). Each sheath has the characteristic spiral lamellar pattern (88, 108, and Chapter 2). The sheath of one fiber is often contiguous with and separated from its neighbor by a single myelin period (10.6 nm, approximately). Groups of unmyelinated axons are sometimes seen. Nerve fibers often lie in groups separated by fibrous astrocytic septae and interfascicular oligodendrocytes. Blood vessels in normal white matter display little or no space between the closely apposed basal laminae of the endothelial cells and the glia limitans (the potential Virchow-Robin space), except for that occupied by an occasional pericyte, macrophage, smooth muscle cell, fibroblast, or collagen pocket.

CLASSIFICATION

As more sophisticated diagnostic criteria evolve, some component members of the demyelinating diseases are being removed from the list, in particular those conditions now categorized as hereditary dysmyelinating or storage diseases, the leukodystrophies. Nevertheless, it is still probably impossible to classify the demyelinating diseases to the satisfaction of all neuropathologists, since inconsistencies in definitive criteria abound. For example, the lack of a prominent inflammatory component in progressive multifocal leukoencephalopathy and the absence of a viral etiology and inflammation in diphtheritic neuropathy compel us to exercise some flexibility.

With the above provisos in mind, the following list outlines the demyelinating diseases as of this date:

1. Chronic multiple sclerosis
2. Variants of multiple sclerosis
   a. Acute multiple sclerosis
   b. Neuromyelitis optica
   c. Concentric sclerosis
3. Acute disseminated encephalomyelitis
   a. Postinfectious encephalomyelitis
   b. Postvaccinal encephalomyelitis
4. Acute hemorrhagic leukoencephalopathy
5. Progressive multifocal leukoencephalopathy
6. Idiopathic polyneuritis
7. Diphtheritic neuropathy

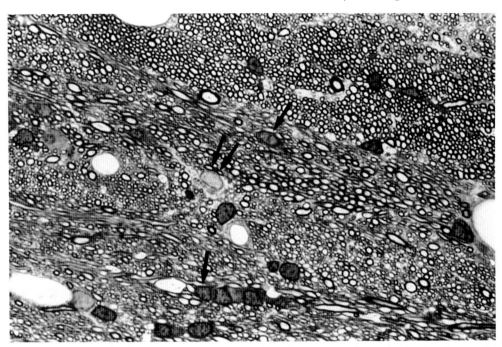

Figure 11.1. Normal white matter. Paraventricular white matter from the brain of a rat shows myelinated central nervous system (CNS) fibers cut longitudinally (*below*) and transversely (*above*). Note the rounded, densely staining oligodendroglia which are arranged below in interfascicular rows (*single arrows*). An astrocyte is seen near the center (*double arrow*). Toluidine blue-stained, 1-μm epoxy section. (Original magnification ×400.)

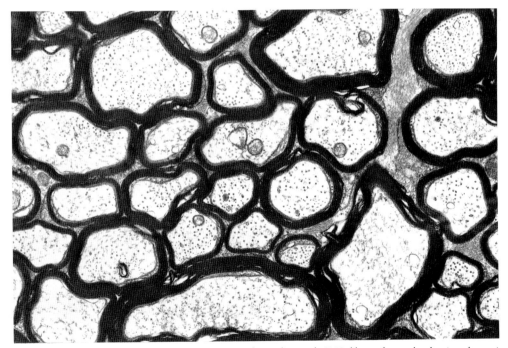

Figure 11.2. Normal white matter. A group of myelinated CNS fibers from the brain of a guinea pig is shown. Note the multilamellar myelin sheaths which often abut, the lack of an extensive extracellular space, and the intervening processes from fibrous astroglia. (Original magnification ×15,000.)

Chronic Multiple Sclerosis

History

Multiple sclerosis has become recognized as one of the most common causes of chronic neurological disability in young adults and has been estimated to account for one of every thousand in the adult deaths around the world.

The chronology and nationality of the first reports on multiple sclerosis have been debated for many years. Credit for the first clinical investigation of multiple sclerosis appears to go to Frerichs in 1849 (44), and it is generally agreed that multiple sclerosis as a pathological entity was not recognized until the latter half of the 19th century (32), before which it was often concealed among the medley of spinal paraplegias. Popular opinion holds that the correlative clinical and pathologic parameters of multiple sclerosis were not firmly established prior to the publication of the lectures of the great French neurologist, Charcot in 1868 (22), who is "given credit for the first clinical description of multiple sclerosis as well as the first pathologic delineation" (32). Incidentally, the latter historical review of multiple sclerosis by Dejong is a well-documented account of some of the earliest case histories and other details on multiple sclerosis as a clinical entity. Charcot (22, 23) described several cases of what would be classed today as typical chronic progressive multiple sclerosis. In retrospect, it is interesting to note that most of the early descriptions of multiple sclerosis tend to be of the chronic progressive type, rather than the relapsing and remitting form. Whether this was real or a reflection of the prevailing clinical analysis remains unknown. However, in Charcot's dissertations on the subject, he named the condition "sclérose en plaques" (23). He also recognized other forms affecting the spinal cord which he termed "paraplégie par degeneration grise des cordons de la moelle" in which he noted the specific disease process as "sclérose en taches" or "sclérose en îles" (hardness in spots or islands), and that these sclerotic areas appeared to grow at the expense of adjacent normal white matter. Following Charcot's pioneer contributions to the symptomatology and pathology of multiple sclerosis came the analysis of its ocular manifestations by Uhthoff in 1889 (144). Despite the emphasis by Marie in 1884 (74) on the role of an infectious agent in its etiology, by the end of the nineteenth century, multiple sclerosis was considered to be due to an inborn error in myelin metabolism, a view which changed early in the twentieth century as the autoallergic concept emerged.

While it is recognized that Charcot's perceptive analysis gave multiple sclerosis its present standing, his were certainly not the first descriptions of the disease. Indeed, one report has appeared in recent years which describes the clinical history of a 53-yr-old woman, St. Ludwina of Schiedam (Holland), who died in 1433 after a 37-yr history interpreted by Medaer (79) as chronic multiple sclerosis. However, the history is rather incomplete, and the diagnosis, though ostensibly credible, might well be an overinterpretation. The first seriously considered, reported case of multiple sclerosis was a grandson of George III of Great Britain, and a cousin of Queen Victoria who had a 25-yr history of neurological deficits which were considered cumulatively to be an excellent example of chronic (progressive) multiple sclerosis (32).

Charcot and many contemporary authorities regard 1835 and the description of Cruveilhier (27) as the beginning of the clinicopathologic history of multiple sclerosis. This view was also supported in 1869 by Charcot's students, Bourneville and Guerard (16). Cruveilhier's accounts mainly covered diseases of the spinal cord in which he described and illustrated very convincingly what might well have been the spinal cord manifestations of chronic multiple sclerosis. However, in the face of yet another report originally dated 1835, credit for the first clinical description and account of the pathology of spinal cord lesions in multiple sclerosis might equally go to a Scot, R. Carswell (20). As mentioned above, the first diagnosis of multiple sclerosis in the living subject is attributed to Frerichs of Göttingen in 1849 (44), where it was classified as a type of "spinal sclerosis." The first autopsy-proven case of disseminated or "insular" sclerosis in England was presented by Moxon (84) in 1873. In researching the literature on this subject, one is impressed by the initial prominence of the French neurologists who retained Charcot's terminology, sclérose en plaques (disseminées), and then the domination of the field by the German school. Among the earliest references to the term "multiple sclerosis" appears to come from the latter. Schüle in 1870 (127), a few years after Charcot's lectures, refers to "multiple sklerose" as a term in common usage at that time. Interestingly, Dejong (32) attributes the term multiple "cerebral" sclerosis to a report by Hammond in the United States in 1871. Towards the end of the nineteenth century and in the early twentieth, the British school emerged, together with its preferred terminology, "disseminated sclerosis," a term believed to have its roots in an article by Seguin et al. (129), an American, who is also given the credit for the first New World report on the subject in 1878. However, Dejong (32) also quotes a report on what appears to be multiple sclerosis given by Morris in Philadelphia in 1867.

It is highly unlikely that the above, brief synopsis of the history of multiple sclerosis will be the last word. It is also apparent that even the earliest reports on the subject detected great variation in disease presentation. For fuller coverage on the history of multiple sclerosis, the reader is referred to the erudite accounts by Dawson (31), Dejong (32), and Poser (90).

Clinical Parameters

While the individual components which comprise the diagnostic, clinical tableau of multiple sclerosis have long been delineated, their sequence and severity of presentation from case to case are subject to great variation (53, 76, 122, and 135). It is fair to say that no two patients with multiple sclerosis are alike, and consequently, there is contention as to what constitutes the stereotypic clinical history. Basically, the clinician seeks CNS lesions which are defined by the time-honored adage as being "separated in time and space." It is a disease known by its affinity to strike in the prime of life (between 18 and 40 yr of age) and which demonstrates a greater incidence among females.

Multiple sclerosis typically presents with symptoms and signs (usually visual or sensory) which remit and relapse over 30 or more years and in itself is rarely fatal. With each exacerbation, new signs may appear or old signs may worsen (or both), and with each remission, some residual deficit is detectable. Therefore, although the pattern is one of a chronic relapsing disorder, there is a progressive downhill trend with time. The disease is not always debilitating, and of the 75% of subjects surviving after 25 yr of affliction, two-thirds of these (i.e., 50% of the total) lead useful lives (135). Many clinicians will debate what constitutes the typical case history in multiple sclerosis and will advocate that a chronic, progressive course is more common. Perusal of the literature does little to clarify the issue because of the innate variation from case to case and perhaps from one geographic area to another.

As a final point before presenting the major accepted clinical manifestations, it should be pointed out that the diagnosis of multiple sclerosis is fraught with difficulties, is sometimes reached only by a process of elimination, and in any large population of patients, one can anticipate an incorrect diagnosis in about 5–10% of cases. Confusion, for example, often arises from spinal cord or brain stem tumors or some of the systemic degenerative states. While these problems are gradually diminishing as diagnostic tests become more sophisticated (e.g., CT and NMR technology), be wary of the study on multiple sclerosis which reports that in 90% (or higher) of examined patients, a specific response to some immunologic factor or structural entity is claimed. In addition to the innate percentage of misdiagnoses, many such studies, e.g., on antibody titers, are conducted by nonclinicians or on referred cases where the diagnosis might not have been rigorously checked.

In general, the primary manifestations of chronic progressive and chronic relapsing multiple sclerosis do not vary greatly. Evidence for an insidious disease (apathy, depression, fatigue, loss of weight, muscle pains) can often be uncovered prior to the first neurological manifestations. Among the first signs in about 50% of all definite multiple sclerosis cases are limb weakness, numbness or tingling (paresthesias) in one or more limbs, the extremities, or around the trunk. There is often discordance between signs and symptoms summarized by Adams and Victor (6) who mention that "it is a common aphorism that the patient with multiple sclerosis presents with symptoms in one leg and signs (bilateral Babinski) in both." Another common initial sign is a short-lived episode of retrobulbar neuritis affecting one or both eyes. Many of these patients will display papillitis (swelling of the optic nerve head) which depends upon the proximity of the demyelinated plaque to the nerve head. There is considerable debate as to whether optic neuritis in a significant percentage of cases constitutes a separate disease or subclass of multiple sclerosis, but in about 40% of cases, the disease progresses to multiple sclerosis (10).

Cerebellar signs form a less common group of early presenting features, and in some patients are manifested by nystagmus, cerebellar ataxia, scanning speech, rhythmic movements of the upper extremities, intention tremors, and lack of coordination. The occurrence of nystagmus, scanning speech, and intention tremor constitutes "Charcot's triad," which is held by some to be almost pathognomonic of multiple sclerosis. While sometimes included among the early clinical manifestations of multiple sclerosis, many clinicians contend that Charcot's triad does not usually become apparent until at least some signs are well established. Among the remaining manifestations classed as "initial" are unsteadiness, brain stem dysfunction (diplopia, vertigo, vomiting), bladder dysfunction, and Lhermitte's sign, tingling of the upper torso after flexion or extension of the neck. The latter is believed to be related to mechanical deformation of the spinal cord which evokes impulses in demyelinated sensory fibers. Less commonly, hemiplegia, trigeminal neuralgia, facial paralysis, deafness, or seizures, in various combinations, may present initially.

Psychologic disturbances are frequently observed and may present as an inappropriate euphoric state, attributed by Adams and Victor (6) probably to extensive white matter lesions in the frontal lobes, or in a much higher percentage of patients, as depression and irritability.

As diagnosis becomes established, a more regular group of clinical syndromes develop either progressively or in a remitting fashion. The majority of patients display a mixed or generalized type of disease involving optic nerves, brain stem, cerebellum, and spinal cord. About one-third will exhibit a spinal form, about 5% will display a cerebellar or pontobulbar-cerebellar form, and a similar percentage will have an amaurotic form. Adams and Victor (6) estimate that at least 80% of their own clinical material was comprised of cerebrospinal and spinal forms of the disease. Other clinical accounts are given by Hallpike et al. (53), McAlpine et al. (76), and Poser (90).

Precipitating Factors

The onset and clinical worsenings (exacerbations) of multiple sclerosis can sometimes be linked to recent, antecedent events—these come under the general heading of precipitating factors. Prime among these are infection, trauma, and pregnancy. For example, it is common knowledge that upper respiratory tract infections (influenza, etc.) might elicit an exacerbation, and it is claimed in the case of trauma that the site of the injury may share a relationship with the site of the initial symptoms. The first documented causal relationship between "exposure to cold and damp, trauma, mental stress, and antecedent infections" appears to come from Leyden in 1863, quoted by Brain in 1930 (17), and supports the so-called "exogenous" (as opposed to "developmental") etiology of the disease—so hotly contested at the turn of the twentieth century. Abrupt elevation of body temperature (the hot bath test), first noted by Uhthoff in 1889 (144), is well known for its ability to precipitate an exacerbation.

Neuropathology

Macroscopic Examination. In the majority of cases, the multiple sclerosis brain displays no outward abnormalities. On rare occasions, a mild degree of cortical atrophy with widening of the sulci can be seen. The brain weight is usually within normal limits. The optic nerves are frequently atrophic and display grey zones from which myelin has been depleted. The optic chiasm can be similarly affected. Gross examination of the brain stem some-

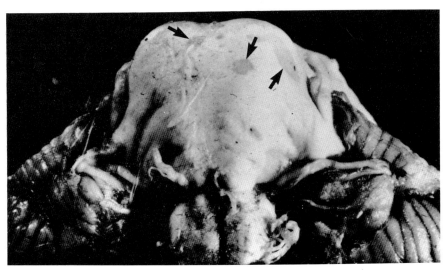

Figure 11.3. Chronic multiple sclerosis—gross specimen. The pons is inverted and rests upon the cerebellum with the medulla in the foreground. Note the many, small, grey demyelinated lesions (*arrows*) which have broken through to the surface from deeper layers. (Courtesy of Dr. S. Aronson.)

times reveals grey (demyelinated) patches on the surface of the basis pontis (Fig. 11.3), the roof and floor of the fourth ventricle, the cerebellar peduncles, and the surface of the medulla where lesions have either developed superficially or broken through from deeper levels. Similarly, the spinal cord might be atrophic and show completely disseminated, grey, firm, depressed surface patches along its entire length. There is no predilection for any one level or tract. Sometimes, the proximal segments of cranial nerves and spinal nerve roots display greyness or atrophy, presumably due to the loss of CNS myelin in these areas or to the presence of an adjacent lesion in the CNS proper. The PNS is macroscopically normal.

Coronal section of the brain reveals large lesions (plaques) which vary in appearance, texture, size, shape, number, and topography (Figs. 11.4–11.6). Variations in appearance and texture reflect the age and activity of the lesions. Pink, soft lesions indicate areas of recent activity, while older lesions are grey, sometimes rather translucent (hyaline, glossy), gelatinous, and firm to the touch. They are difficult to section thinly, since they have the consistency of soft rubber and shrink away from more normal white matter upon contact with air. Lesions in the spinal cord and optic nerve

are usually very firm and have a brittle texture. Sometimes, areas of old hemispheric lesions may have a chalky appearance due to the large number of lipid-laden macrophages. Lesions vary in size from less than a millimeter to several centimeters across (e.g., the entire margin of a lateral ventricle). Plaques may unite and arborize throughout the white matter, presumably along the vasculature. Therefore, a small circular lesion centered on a vessel might well be connected elsewhere to larger plaques (Figs. 11.8 and 11.38), and as such constitute a "Dawson's finger" (31). With regard to shape, plaques can be cup-shaped (ventricular wall), spherical, elliptical, angular, or striated. Some cases of multiple sclerosis will display large confluent lesions almost on a scale comparable to the leukodystrophies; others may display cavitary changes (Figs. 11.6*B* and 11.7), while in others, only a few are found, one or two of which may have occurred in strategic (clinically detectable) locations, e.g., the brain stem.

The location of multiple sclerosis lesions usually defies clinical and anatomical explanation, and it is frequently found that the degree of involvement revealed at autopsy exceeds by far that indicated by the clinical history. Indeed, multiple sclerosis has frequently been diagnosed only at au-

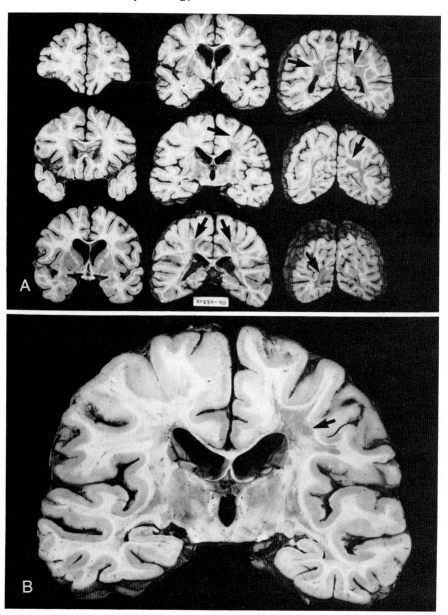

Figure 11.4. (A) Chronic multiple sclerosis. A series of coronal slices from the frontal (*upper left*) to the occipital lobes (*lower right*) demonstrates the involvement of white matter, in particular periventricular zones, in the disease process. Some lesions are indicated at the *arrows*. (Courtesy of Dr. W. Schoene.) (B) The central section from (A) shows the common involvement of the area between the angle of the lateral ventricle and the caudate nucleus (*arrow*)—the so-called Wetter-winkel zone. Elsewhere, other white matter lesions are apparent. (Courtesy of Dr. Schoene.)

topsy in the total absence of a clinical history, so-called "benign multiple sclerosis." Just as no area of predilection can be identified with certainty in multiple sclerosis (some neuropathologists may debate this point on the basis of the frequent occurrence of paraventricular involvement), no

area of sparing exists. The entire central neuraxis is vulnerable, and in the vast majority of cases, the cerebrum is involved. The heaviest concentration of paraventricular plaques appears to occur in relationship to subependymal vasculature. One commonly involved area (sometimes over-

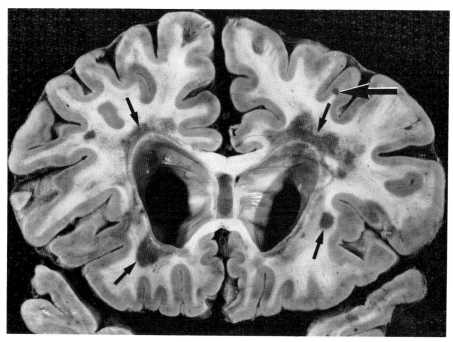

Figure 11.5. Chronic multiple sclerosis. The disseminated distribution of old, intensely sclerotic plaques is evident (*arrows*). Note the predilection for periventricular areas and the small lesion in the gyrus to the upper right (*large arrow*) which involves both grey and white matter.

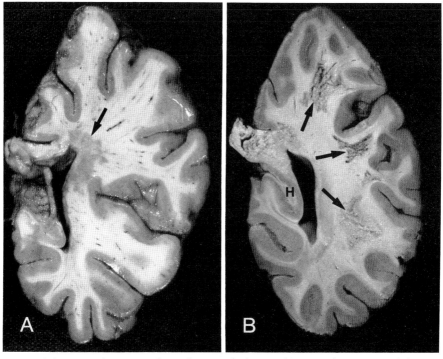

Figure 11.6. (*A*) Coronal section through a single hemisphere in the region of the ventricular trigone shows a single large demyelinated lesion at the angle of the lateral ventricle (*arrow*). This lesion is less chronic than those depicted in Figure 11.5. (*B*) A hemispheric section more rostral to (*A*) (note the posterior hippocampus at *H*) contains several large white matter lesions (*arrows*) which show cystic degeneration.

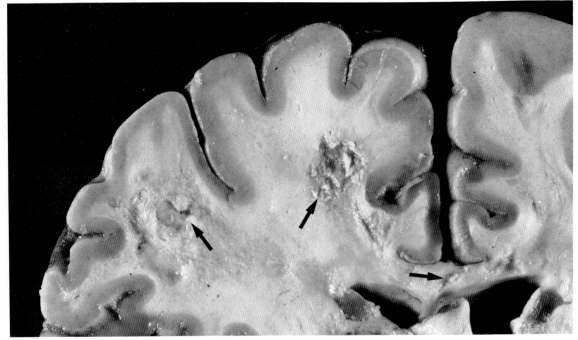

Figure 11.7. Chronic multiple sclerosis. Close-up of a coronal brain slice with several large cystic lesions (*arrows*). (Courtesy of Dr. J. Powers.)

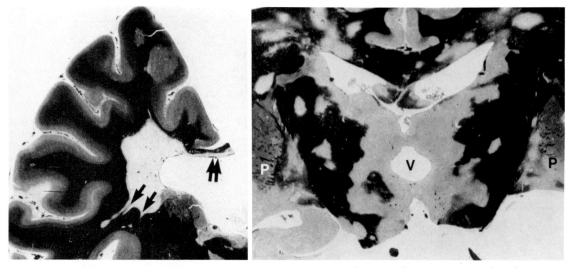

Figure 11.8. (*Left*) A myelin-stained preparation depicts a chronic silent periventricular plaque (note the sharply demarcated edge) from which several Dawson's fingers radiate—sleeves of demyelination which follow blood vessels (*arrows, left*). The plaque also continues subependymally along the corpus callosum (*double arrows, right*). (From C. E. Lumsden (73).)

Figure 11.9. (*Right*) Note the symmetrical, extensive involvement of the white matter around the third ventricle (*V*) at the level of the mass intermedia. Scattered old plaques are seen elsewhere in this myelin preparation. The putamen (*P*) is shown to the *left* and *right*.

emphasized since no plaque-related region can be classed as pathognomonic in multiple sclerosis) is the angle between the cau-

date nucleus and the corpus callosum—the so-called "Wetterwinkel" or "storm center" of Steiner (133) (Figs. 11.4*B*, 11.5, and

11.8). Smaller lesions commonly occur in the white matter at the tips of gyri where they may spill over into grey matter (subcortical grey matter also contains myelinated nerve fibers) (Figs. 11.5 and 11.11). Plaques may also be found in the striatum, pallidum, and thalamus. Lesions also occur around the margins of the third ventricle (Fig. 11.9) and hypothalamic pathways.

Moving caudally, plaques will often be revealed in the cerebellar peduncles and white matter of the folia (Fig. 11.10), deeper regions in the vicinity of the dentate nucleus, and the roof and floor of the fourth ventricle. The brain stem is a common area of involvement, with discrete lesions being found around the aqueduct of Sylvius and around the margin of the basis pontis. Similar lesions often extend down into the medulla and upper cervical spinal cord. Brain stem lesions can sometimes be correlated with recent clinical activity in that patients who become comatose or suffer respiratory arrest may display active inflammatory lesions in this location.

Optic nerve, chiasm, and tract lesions might be deeply or superficially located, focal or extensive and might traverse the entire nerve for considerable lengths (Figs. 11.12–11.16). There are suggestions that they are related initially to the pial vasculature, and a similar relationship has been noted in the spinal cord. Sometimes where regions of grey matter containing myelinated fibers are overlaid by pial vessels,

small demyelinated lesions can also be found. Spinal cord lesions demonstrate no regularity in their topography and disregard anatomical and functional boundaries (Fig. 11.17). Cervical cord is more likely to be involved than lower levels. It is not unusual to find an entire cross-section of spinal cord completely devoid of myelin and severely atrophic. In most cases of multiple sclerosis, evidence of spinal cord involvement can be found, and in the so-called spinal form of the disease, spinal cord lesions may predominate.

Microscopic Examination. To the neuropathologist writing the microscopic description of multiple sclerosis plaques in the 1980s, it is almost embarrassing to have to admit that relatively little new has been added to the analyses of pioneer investigators like Dawson (31). For example, it might be difficult, except for more sophisticated illustrative methods, to improve on the 1911 abstract of Bruce and Dawson, quoted in Dawson's 1916 monograph (31), which states "The plaques in disseminated sclerosis, wherever they are situated, are distributed evidently without any relation to nerve tracts. Their character and appearance suggest a gradual infiltration from some central source into the surrounding neighbouring tissues. In the cord their tendency is to pass inwards from the meninges in a more or less wedge-shaped form, their relationship to blood vessels being often difficult or impossible to trace except

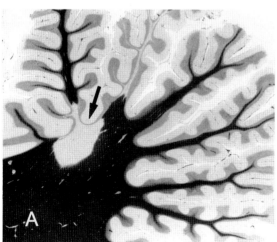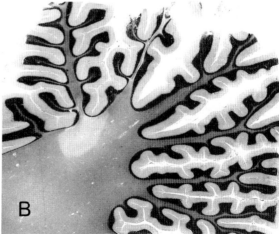

Figure 11.10. (*A*) In this myelin (Heidenhain) preparation of the cerebellum, a small chronic plaque lies at the base of a folium (*arrow*). (*B*) The same plaque shows as a diffusely stained area in a parallel H&E preparation.

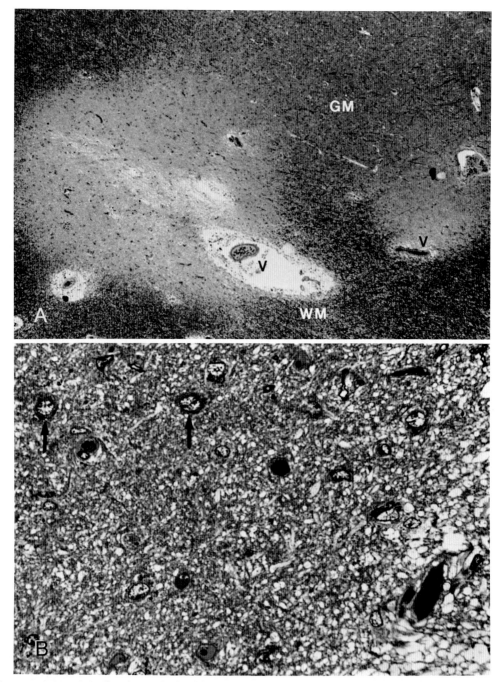

Figure 11.11. (A) Chronic multiple sclerosis. Two small plaques, centered on vessels (V), lie at the tip of a gyrus and involve both white matter (WM) and grey matter (GM). Toluidine blue stained, 1-µm epoxy section. (Original magnification ×160.) (B) Detail from A. Note the demyelinated gliotic white matter below, which extends upwards into grey matter containing neurons (arrows). (Original magnification ×640.)

in the earlier stages. The cerebrum and cerebellum are better adapted to give an idea as to their mode of formation because of the independence of the arterial and venous paths. Within the cerebrum the veins pass towards the walls of the ventri-

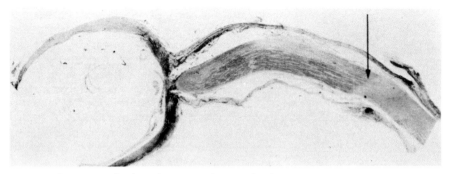

Figure 11.12. Chronic multiple sclerosis. A longitudinal section of optic nerve attached to the optic globe is stained for myelin and reveals a diffuse loss of myelin which traverses the entire nerve at the *arrow*. (From C. E. Lumsden (73).)

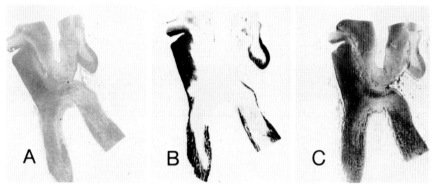

Figure 11.13. A series of sections across the optic chiasm shows the general picture in *A*, an H&E preparation; widespread loss of myelin in *B*, a Heidenhain preparation; and axonal sparing in *C*, a Bodian preparation. (Courtesy of Dr. R. D. Terry.)

cles and the choroid plexus towards the veins of Galen, and have in this way a distribution altogether different from that of the arteries. The same is true of the cerebellum. A study of a series of sections shows that the plaques are deposited in relation to the distribution of the veins and to the walls of the ventricles. An examination of sections of the cerebral hemispheres strongly suggests that the infiltration is along the lymphatic channels (*sic*) surrounding the veins. Similar conclusions are suggested by study of the sections of the pons, cerebellum, and medulla." Thus, with this verbatum 1911 synopsis in mind, the reader may experience an element of *déjà vu* in the forthcoming paragraphs.

Recognizing that within each group, further subdivision can be made, the lesions of chronic (progressive or relapsing) multiple sclerosis fall into three categories:

a. Chronic, inactive plaques
b. Chronic, active plaques
c. Shadow plaques.

Chronic, Inactive Plaques. In general, inactive (burnt-out) lesions correlate clinically with long-term (20–30 yr), stable disease and are sometimes revealed at autopsy in patients without any previous history of multiple sclerosis. The most common locations are paraventricular, the optic nerves and chiasm, and the spinal cord. Myelin stains will reveal demyelinated areas sharply demarcated from the adjacent myelinated white matter, imparting upon them a punched-out appearance (49). It is an established fact in multiple sclerosis lesions that sharpness of contour equates with chronicity (Figs. 11.5, 11.8, 11.9, and 11.11). Furthermore, staining of parallel sections from the same brain will reveal

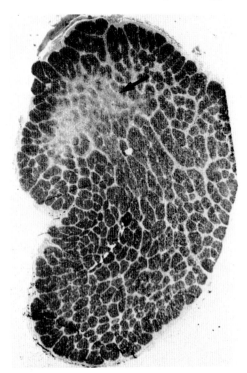

Figure 11.14. A transverse section of an optic nerve shows an area of diffuse demyelination (*arrow*). Toluidine blue-stained, 1-μm epoxy section. (Original magnification ×15.)

that the areas of myelin loss in myelin preparations can be matched by areas of fibrillary gliosis (Fig. 11.18).

Axon stains will disclose a moderate decrease in the density of axons toward the periphery of the plaque, but deeper areas will be more depleted. This progressive dropout of axons with time and distance from more normal areas has been recognized for many years. A feature noted as long ago as 1871 by Schüle (128) is the observation that the surviving axons within the lesion display marked shrinkage. Axonal shrinkage subsequent to demyelination has been documented in many subsequent studies in both the CNS and PNS, most recently by Prineas and Connell (96) and Raine (107). A paucity of Wallerian degeneration is apparent, an observation made by Charcot himself, although some axons may display periodic dilatations or beading. Rarely are all axons lost, and even in the deepest (oldest) regions of the largest lesions, scattered axons can be found—for example, beneath the ependymal plate in

the wall of the lateral ventricle. From a series of 125 cerebral plaques, Greenfield and King (48) noted "severe loss of axons" (i.e., a reduction of one-fifth–one-seventh of the normal number) in only 10% of the total. However, the only real exception to the rule of relative sparing of axons is the occasional brain which displays cystic lesions where parenchymal elements are replaced by a glial mesh (Figs. 11.6*B* and 11.7). Such cystic degeneration is presumed to result from particularly severe inflammatory changes during early stages of plaque formation.

The loss of myelin from a fiber is abrupt at the lesion edge (Fig. 11.19) and is visu-

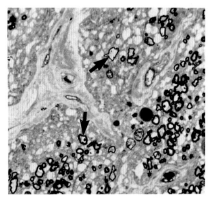

Figure 11.15. Detail from the lesion in Figure 11.14. Gliosis, naked axons, and thinly remyelinated fibers (*arrows*) are apparent. (Original magnification ×640.)

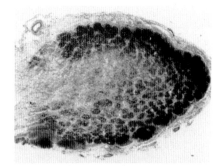

Figure 11.16. The optic nerve from another case of chronic multiple sclerosis (same magnification as Fig. 11.14) displays severe atrophy and a large area of demyelination. Toluidine blue-stained, 1-μm epoxy section. (Original magnification ×15.)

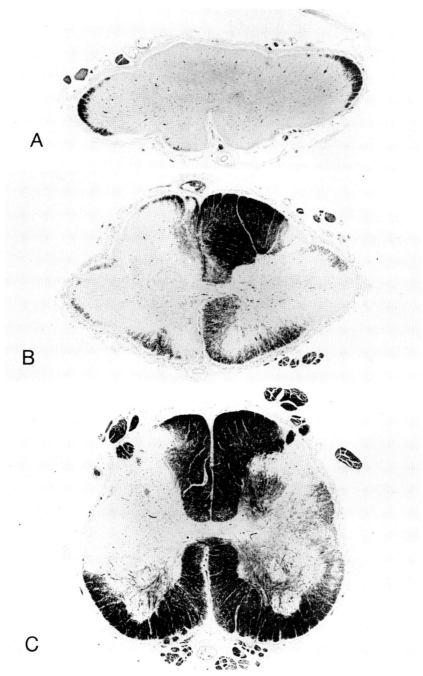

Figure 11.17. Chronic multiple sclerosis. Three different levels of spinal cord (*A*, cervical/thoracic; *B*, midthoracic; *C*, lumbar) demonstrate variation in the degree of involvement. Note the almost total loss of myelin in *A* where axons were well preserved—see Figure 11.22–11.24, the large lesions in *B*, and the disseminated involvement in *C*.

alized as a myelinated segment becoming naked and continuing into the lesion as a demyelinated fiber (Fig. 11.20). Frequently, even in silent lesions, foamy macrophages can be seen, presumably engaged in smoldering disease activity (Fig. 11.21).

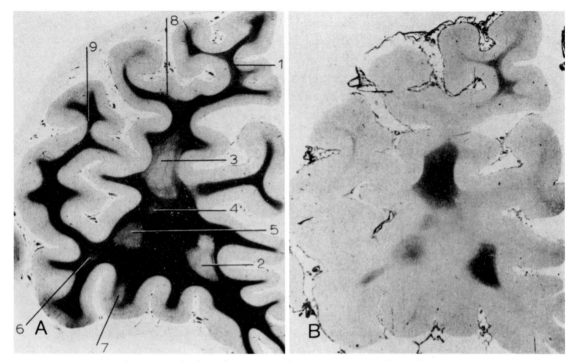

Figure 11.18. Chronic multiple sclerosis. Myelin-stained (*A*) and gliofibril (Holzer)-stained (*B*) adjacent sections show numbered plaques of different degrees of demyelination and of different ages, as judged by fibrillary gliosis. (From C. E. Lumsden (73).)

As a result of loss of parenchymal elements and intense gliosis, considerable atrophy of affected regions is not uncommon. This might be manifested by a shrunken appearance of a paraventricular plaque, hydrocephalus *ex vacuo*, or severe atrophy of the optic nerves and spinal cord. Particularly in the spinal cord, the atrophy can be regional, with proximal and distal segments more or less of normal dimensions (Fig. 11.17). These observations support Charcot's claim of a lack of Wallerian degeneration in tracts, and, despite the atrophy, the degree of axonal sparing is often remarkable (Figs. 11.22–11.24). Similar appearances are seen in inactive lesions in the optic nerve (Figs. 11.18 and 11.19). Sometimes, membrane specializations are encountered between naked axons and the investing, scarring fibrous astroglial cells (105).

Histologically, most inactive lesions have a rather acellular appearance, consisting of a fibrillary astroglial feltwork which is responsible for the sclerosis, color, and tex-ture of the tissue (Figs. 11.25 and 11.26). Microscopically, this appears as a diffuse mesh of twig-like processes emanating from large, hypertropic cell bodies which may sometimes be multinucleated (Fig. 11.27). The fibrous astroglial processes stain positively with appropriate reagents, and by electron microscopy are seen to contain compact bundles of 9-nm filaments (Fig. 11.24). Hypertrophic astrocytes and their processes end abruptly at the plaque edge, from which they may also extend for a short distance into the normal appearing white matter (Figs. 11.28 and 11.29). Immunocytochemical studies have shown these cells, but not normal astrocytes, to bind IgG. However, this propensity is not specific for multiple sclerosis, and hypertrophic astrocytes in the vicinity of lesions from a number of CNS conditions display the same phenomenon (37, 99). To date, no specificity for this IgG binding has been attributed to nervous system components or to multiple sclerosis. Astrocytes and their foot processes in normal white matter may also

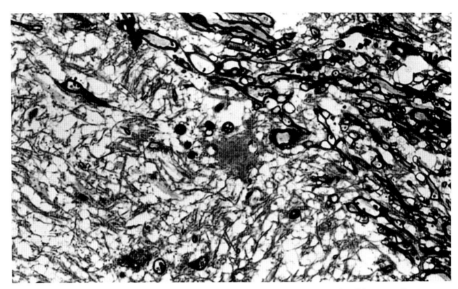

Figure 11.19. The edge of a chronic multiple sclerosis lesion is marked by an abrupt interphase between the completely demyelinated gliotic plaque (*lower left*) and the myelinated white matter (*upper right*). Toluidine blue-stained, 1-μm epoxy section. (Original magnification ×640.)

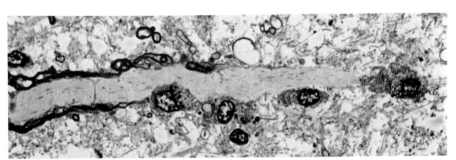

Figure 11.20. A myelinated CNS nerve fiber entering a plaque to the right has lost its sheath, and the naked segment is flanked by macrophages. Toluidine blue-stained, 1-μm epoxy section. (Original magnification ×1,000.)

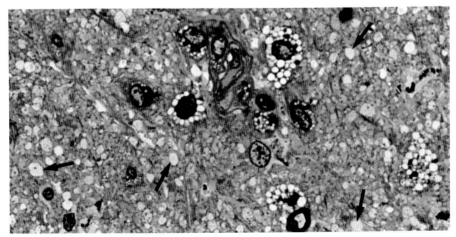

Figure 11.21. Within the center of a chronically demyelinated lesion (naked axons at *arrows*), foamy macrophages (microglia) encircle a small vessel (*upper center*) and are scattered throughout the parenchyma. Toluidine blue-stained, 1-μm epoxy section. (Original magnification ×1,000.)

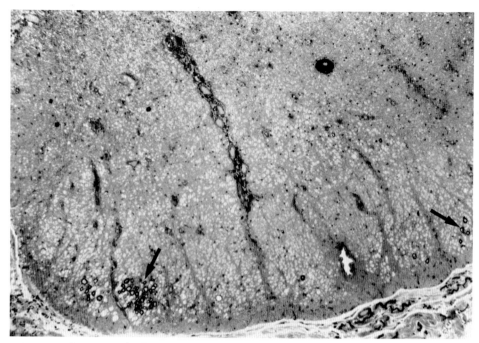

Figure 11.22.   Chronic multiple sclerosis—same case as Figure 11.17. A section of cervical cord shows almost total depletion of myelin and many small, pale profiles—naked axons at higher magnification (Fig. 11.23). Macrophages flank some blood vessels, and a few small groups of preserved myelinated axons (*arrows*) can be discerned. Toluidine blue-stained, 1-μm epoxy section. (Original magnification ×20.)

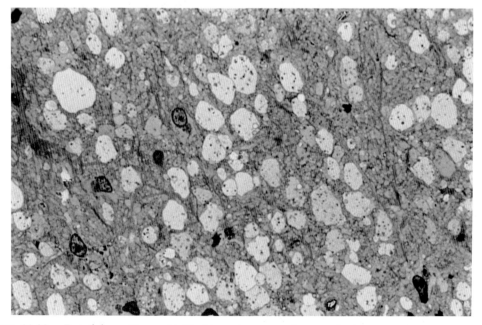

Figure 11.23.   Detail from Figure 11.22. Note the many, large naked axons which reside in an intensely gliotic matrix. No oligodendroglia can be seen, and the nuclei present belong to fibrous astrocytes. (Original magnification ×1,000.)

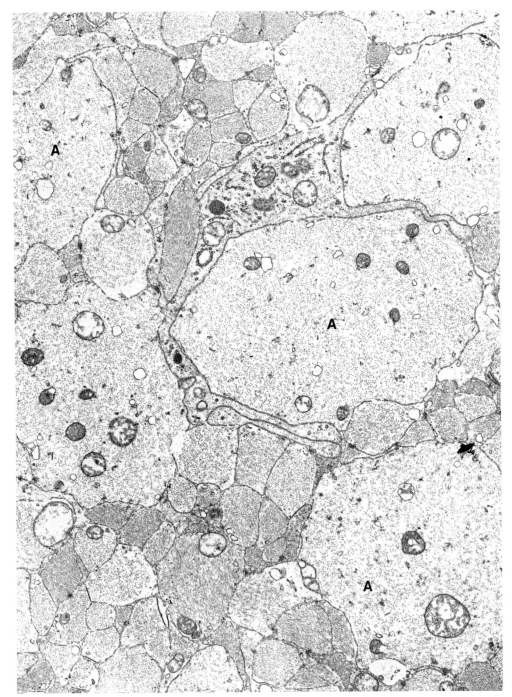

Figure 11.24.   Electron micrograph of the lesion shown in Figure 11.22. Naked axons (*A*) reside in a mosaic of processes from fibrous astroglial cells. These processes are filled with bundles of 9-nm gliofilaments. (Original magnification ×11,000.)

display hypertrophy and fibrosis in relationship to perivascular areas (glial sleeves, hyaline vessels), presumably a response to a previous vascular insult and perhaps in continuity with large lesion areas elsewhere. In the plaque itself, the degree of astroglial proliferation varies enormously from the dense mosaic one often sees in

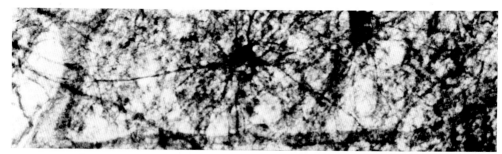

Figure 11.25. Chronic multiple sclerosis. A Cajal-stained preparation from a chronic plaque shows hypertrophic fibrillary astrocytes in abundance. (Original magnification ×1,000.)

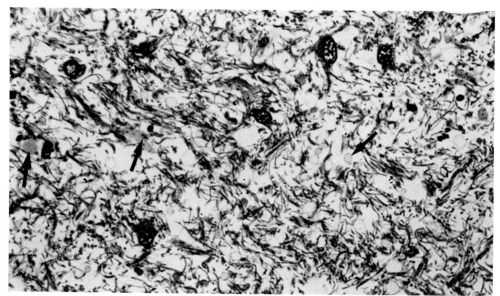

Figure 11.26. The center of a silent plaque is made up of a meshwork of fibrous astrocytes and their twig-like processes between which naked axons (*arrows*) can invariably be found. Toluidine blue-stained, 1-μm epoxy section. (Original magnification ×1,000.)

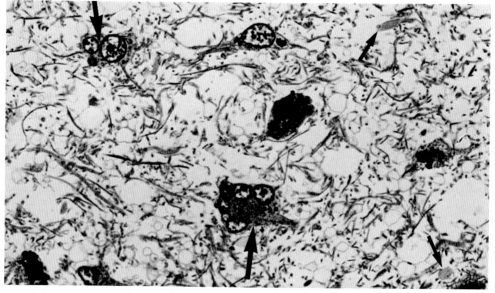

Figure 11.27. This area of a silent lesion contains multinucleated astrocytes (*large arrows*), fibrous astroglial processes, and a few naked axons (*arrows*). The densely staining material in some astroglial somata is lipofuscin. (Original magnification ×1,000.)

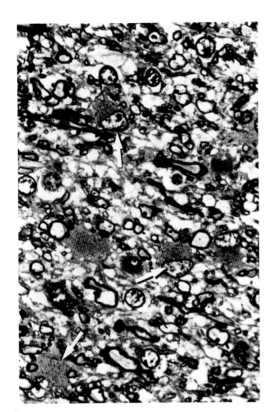

Figure 11.28. Chronic multiple sclerosis. The myelinated white matter adjacent to a chronic silent plaque contains an abundance of hypertrophic astrocytes (*arrows*). The rounded nuclei of several oligodendrocytes are also apparent. Toluidine blue-stained, 1-μm epoxy section. (Original magnification ×1,000.)

midbrain, optic nerve, and spinal cord lesions (Figs. 11.23 and 11.24) to the loose meshwork typical of cerebral lesions or to the sometimes regular, grid-like (reticular) arrangement encountered in the deepest regions of old lesions (Figs. 11.26 and 11.27). Not infrequently, these hypertrophic astrocytes contain lipid droplets and lipofuscin (Fig. 11.27).

The stroma of most chronic lesions contains a few sudanophilic, lipid-laden macrophages, fat granule cells, compound granular corpuscles, foamy cells, histiocytes, among other synonyms), which are randomly scattered throughout the parenchyma or exist in small collections around blood vessels (Figs. 11.21 and 11.30). These cells are regarded as being of hematogenous (monocytic) lineage and stain positively

with most lipid stains. Inflammatory cells are usually rare within silent lesions. An occasional plasma cell is encountered in an enlarged Virchow-Robin space, but small lymphocytes are difficult to find. An ultrastructural study of chronic multiple sclerosis lesions enumerated the infiltrating cell population and came to the conclusion that plasma cells are the most common element, and small lymphocytes are rare (101). Moreover, adjacent normal white matter also contained plasma cells and small lymphocytes, albeit in much lower numbers. Interestingly, immunocytochemical study of inflammatory events in chronic multiple sclerosis lesions, which employed monoclonal antibody technology (140), has more precisely delineated these

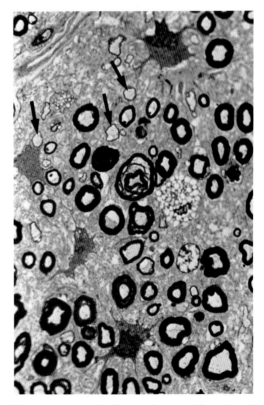

Figure 11.29. At the perimeter of a chronic plaque in the spinal cord, densely staining, spider-like astrocytes are present. A single foamy macrophage lies near the center of the field. A few remyelinated CNS fibers (*arrows*) can also be seen. Toluidine blue-stained, 1-μm epoxy section. (Original magnification ×1,000.)

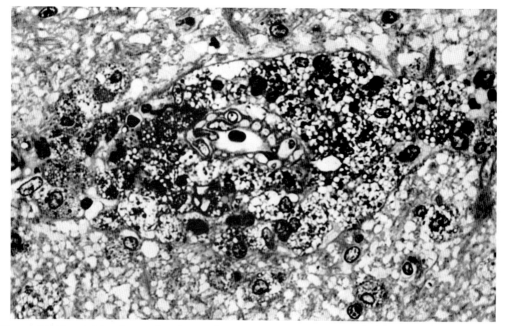

Figure 11.30. A blood vessel within a chronic plaque contains lipid-laden (foamy) macrophages within its Virchow-Robin space and within the adjacent parenchyma. Toluidine blue-stained, 1-µm epoxy section. (Original magnification ×1,000.)

cells and has shown a few helper and suppressor/cytotoxic T cells within the lesion and the normal white matter and many Ia-bearing cells (B cells and macrophages). Other components of inactive chronic multiple sclerosis lesions include corpora amylacea, fibroblasts, and deposits of collagen, the latter particularly within enlarged perivascular spaces (Fig. 11.31).

Oligodendrocytes have purposely been left to the end of this section. As has been known for years, oligodendroglial depletion is severe in lesions of multiple sclerosis. Their destruction has been regarded by some as primary in lesion formation—the so-called "oligodendrogliolysis" postulate of Lumsden (72), or secondary (117), while some authors speak of an initial hyperplasia of oligodendroglia leading to death (57, 58). Their role in plaque formation notwithstanding, oligodendroglia are absent from the centers of established chronic inactive lesions (Figs. 11.23 and 11.27). This correlates well with the reported absence of pseudocholinesterase activity, an enzyme reputedly associated with oligodendrocytes and of an acid lipase-esterase (1). Sometimes, toward the edge of the lesions and in

the adjacent white matter, a zone of oligodendrocytes with small round nuclei can be discerned. The white matter in close proximity to chronic lesions frequently contains oligodendrocytes among nerve fibers with thin myelin sheaths, appearances now interpreted as indicative of CNS remyelination (Figs. 11.29 and 11.32). Within chronic lesions in the spinal cord, myelination of CNS axons (presumably, previously demyelinated) by Schwann cells and PNS myelin has been documented on several occasions (46) (Fig. 11.33). Such a phenomenon is well-described in animal systems (115), and while initially an exciting observation in multiple sclerosis in view of therapeutic implications, large scale PNS myelination of CNS axons has yet to be linked with functional improvement.

Despite the existence of a few isolated reports, PNS involvement *per se* is unusual in multiple sclerosis, although proximal segments of spinal nerve roots, sometimes close to or in continuity with large silent lesions, may sometimes contain groups of demyelinated fibers in the CNS (glial) region of the root (Fig. 11.34) or remyelinated PNS fibers more distally (Fig. 11.35).

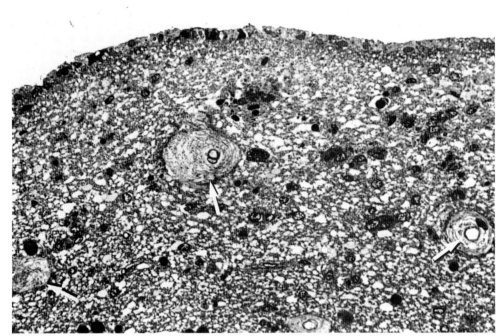

Figure 11.31. Beneath the ventricular surface (*above*) in the deepest layers of a chronic silent plaque, many blood vessels contain fibrotic changes (*arrows*). Elsewhere, intense fibrous astrogliosis is in evidence. Toluidine blue-stained, 1-μm epoxy section. (Original magnification ×400.)

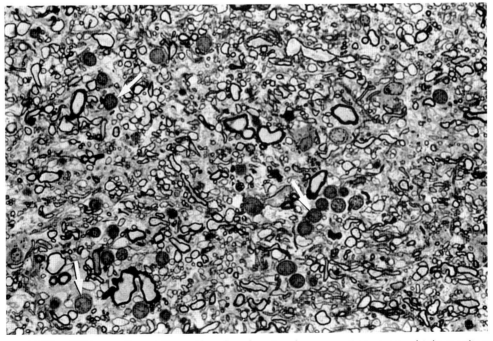

Figure 11.32. White matter at the edge of a chronic plaque contains many thinly myelinated (remyelinated) CNS fibers and an unusually large number of oligodendrocytes (*arrows*). Toluidine blue-stained, 1-μm epoxy section. (Original magnification ×640.)

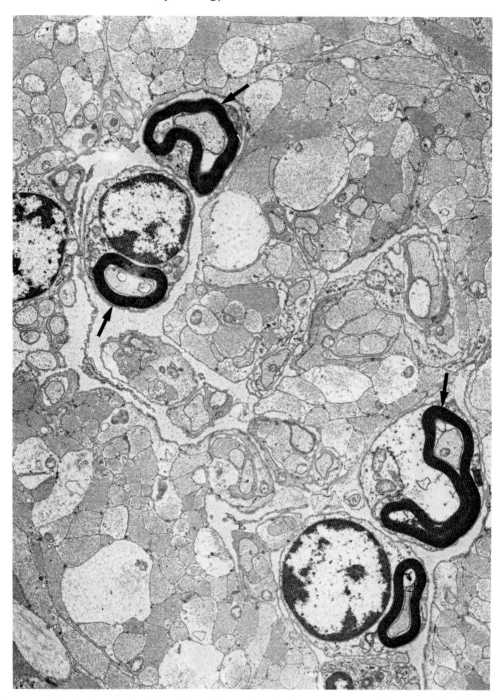

Figure 11.33. A chronically demyelinated spinal cord plaque contains Schwann cells which have elaborated peripheral nervous system (PNS) myelin around CNS axons (*arrows*). Elsewhere, a mosaic of fibrous astroglial processes and a few naked CNS axons can be seen. (Original magnification ×9,000.)

Chronic, Active Plaques. Precisely what constitutes an active chronic multiple sclerosis lesion is sometimes difficult to deter- mine and depends upon the technique applied. Frequently, for example, a large, ostensibly inactive lesion will contain at one

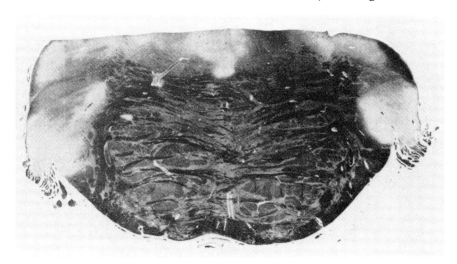

Figure 11.34. Chronic multiple sclerosis. A section of pons shows bilateral plaques at the trigeminal nerve root entry zones and diffuse plaques above. (From C. E. Lumsden (73).)

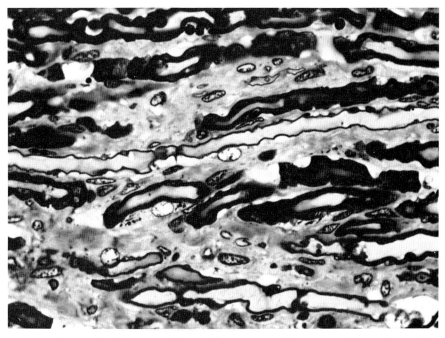

Figure 11.35. A longitudinal section of a spinal nerve root shows remyelinated PNS fibers among unaffected fibers. Toluidine blue-stained, 1-μm epoxy section. (Original magnification ×650.)

pole, a focus of florid disease activity. In other cases, patients who have succumbed to an intercurrent infection might display large, inactive lesions with massive perivascular infiltrates deep within the lesions. Other reports exist where lesion activity has been claimed on the basis of an increased level of hydrolytic enzymes, bound immunoglobulin, myelin basic protein depletion, or the presence of myelin degradation products. The above indices of lesion activity fail to satisfy entirely the classical definition of a chronic active multiple sclerosis lesion which in most circles is regarded as an established lesion along the edges of which is a broad zone of perivas-

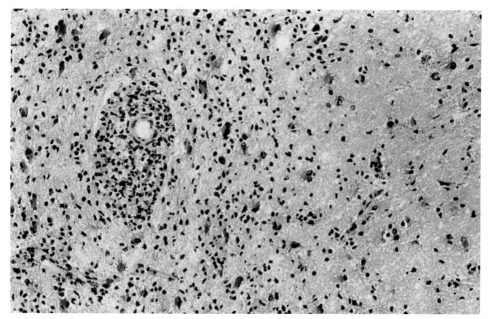

Figure 11.36. Chronic multiple sclerosis. The perimeter of an active chronic lesion displays extensive perivascular and parenchymal inflammation which tapers off as normal white matter is approached. H&E section. (Original magnification ×300.)

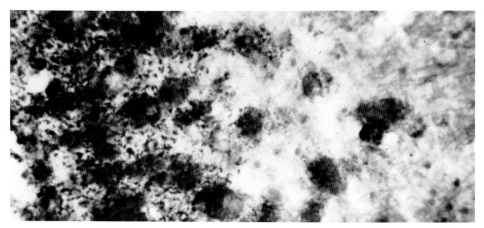

Figure 11.37. Oil red O-positive macrophages extend away from a perivascular exudate at the edge of a chronic active lesion. (Original magnification ×800.)

cular and parenchymal inflammation together with diffuse ongoing demyelination (as judged by stains showing myelin breakdown products) (Fig. 11.36). Macrophage activity manifested by PAS- or oil red O-positive material, glial hypertrophy, and hypercellularity, and some edema are also in evidence (Fig. 11.37). On gross examination, such a lesion would appear to have a pink or white tinge about its margins, corresponding to inflammation and macrophage activity, respectively. Frequently, the location of an active chronic multiple sclerosis lesion correlates with recent clinical history, e.g., brain stem lesions in cases of respiratory failure.

Chronic active lesions have a less well demarcated margin on myelin staining. Stains for neutral fat, lipofuscin, and myelin breakdown products are intensely positive, with the reactions extending considerable distances into the apparently normal

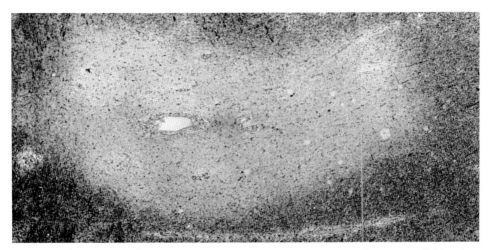

Figure 11.38. A Dawson's finger cut in transverse section is centered on a small blood vessel around which inflammatory cells can be seen. Toluidine blue-stained, 1-μm epoxy section. (Original magnification ×40.)

white matter. Similar small lesions can often be found centered on small veins within the white matter proper (Figs. 11.38 and 11.39). Presumably such small demyelinating foci will eventually coalesce to form larger lesions. The adjacent myelinated white matter is often hypercellular and contains proliferated oligodendrocytes (Fig. 11.40).

Foamy macrophages are invariably found throughout the normal white matter far away from lesions. Such a phenomenon might be representative of persistent low level activity or more likely, in the light of the reported presence of T cells (in particular, helper T cells) in normal white matter removed from active chronic multiple sclerosis plaques (140), antigen presentation. Ia antigens, a marker for macrophages and antigen-presenting cells, are sometimes observed on endothelial cells in multiple sclerosis (141).

Macrophages within active lesions contain recognizable myelin debris and participate in active demyelination (Fig. 11.41). The latter involves the encirclement of the fiber by the macrophage which then proceeds to phagocytose droplets of myelin as they are peeled away from the outer layers of the otherwise normal-appearing myelin sheath (Fig. 11.42). Eventually, naked axons reside in a parenchyma of macrophages, fibrous astrocytes, and rounded oligodendroglia. The mechanism of myelin

uptake is believed to involve IgG and the ingestion of myelin droplets into phagosomes within the macrophage by receptor-mediated endocytosis (36, 97). This mechanism has been postulated to involve the attachment of myelin (by ligands yet to be identified) to receptors on coated vesicles located at the surface of the macrophage and the uptake of the droplets into phagosomes within the cell. The subsequent stages in the structural degradation of myelin have been outlined elsewhere (65, 107). The end-products of myelin breakdown are lamellar inclusions (Fig. 11.42) which, on the basis of superficial resemblances to paramyxoviruses, have in the past been identified as viral and unique to multiple sclerosis, but their derivation from myelin and occurrence in several disorders is now well-documented. Histochemically, these inclusions are tertiary lysosomes. At the biochemical level, myelin breakdown has been expressed as the formation of esterified cholesterol from unesterified or free cholesterol, although some authors believe this to be a late event (1).

The involvement of proteolytic enzymes in the genesis of lesions has received careful scrutiny (1). Undoubtedly an integral component, whether or not enzyme activity plays a specific or primary role in demyelination remains speculative. The activity of hydrolytic enzymes in these regions is probably causally related to the reported

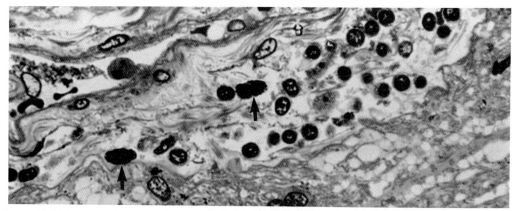

Figure 11.39. Detail from Figure 11.38, to show the nature of the perivascular cellular infiltrates. Small mononuclear cells and a few mast cells (*arrows*) are seen. (Original magnification ×820.)

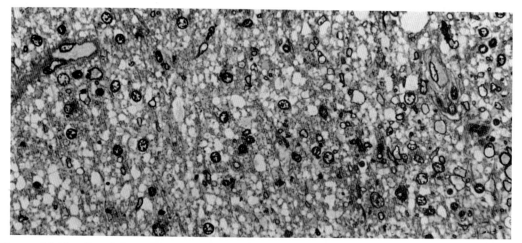

Figure 11.40. Detail from Figure 11.38, to show the margins of the lesion. A broad zone of hypercellularity lies to the left of the myelinated white matter (*right*). These cells have the features of oligodendrocytes. (Original magnification ×520.)

depletion of myelin basic protein and myelin-associated glycoprotein (59). Also of interest are suggestions that the proteinase activity by macrophages during autoimmune demyelination might be T cell or antibody-dependent (19). It has also been demonstrated in multiple sclerosis (104, 107), canine distemper encephalomyelitis (103), and during demyelination in vitro (109), that the astrocyte is capable of myelin phagocytosis. This activity might also be mediated via antibody/hydrolytic enzyme pathways.

While macrophage activity and demyelination probably represent the ultimate manifestations of the destructive process in multiple sclerosis, the hallmark, probably antecedent, event is the accumulation of inflammatory cells, best visualized as perivascular infiltrates around vessels along the interphase between the myelinated and demyelinated zones. The parenchyma is hypercellular throughout, due to infiltrating hematogenous cells and proliferating oligodendroglia (Fig. 11.41). Among the infiltrates, small mononuclear cells, presumably lymphocytes, are the most common elements (Fig. 11.43). Large PAS- or oil red O-positive mononuclear cells can be seen within the Virchow-Robin space, and the parenchyma and plasma cells are present but not prominent. The occasional mast

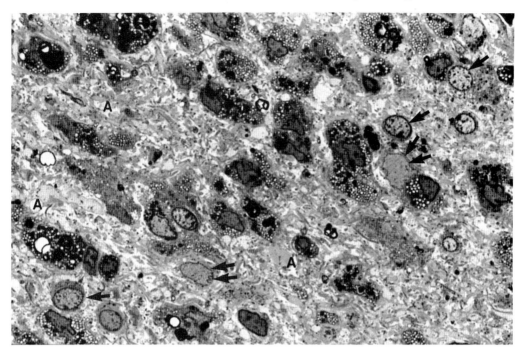

Figure 11.41. At the edge of a chronic active lesion sampled at biopsy, microglial cells containing recognizable myelin debris as well as lipid droplets are prominent. Surviving oligodendrocytes (*single arrows*), a few astrocytes (*double arrows*), and scattered demyelinated axons (A) are also in evidence. Toluidine blue-stained, 1-μm epoxy section. (Original magnification ×1,000.)

cell is seen towards the margins of perivascular infiltrates (Fig. 11.39), but polymorphonuclear leukocytes, hemorrhage, and fibrin deposition are not features of active chronic multiple sclerosis lesions.

Until recently, neuropathologists had to be satisfied with the above, largely descriptive categorization of infiltrating cell types in the active lesion in multiple sclerosis. With the aid of the Sternberger peroxidase-antiperoxidase technique and monoclonal antibodies, it has been possible to dissect with relative certainty the components of the immune system within the target tissue, the CNS (137, 140, 141). Within the center of active lesions, only a few T cells and many Ia-positive (macrophages and B cells) are present. At the lesion margin, there is concentration of helper T cells (T4$^+$), particularly in the parenchyma, and these cells spread for great distances into the adjacent normal appearing white matter. Suppressor/cytotoxic T cells (T8$^+$) are localized in perivascular locations, mainly at the lesion edge. Scattered Ia$^+$ macrophages are always found in normal white matter, some closely associated with helper T cells, a relationship perhaps reminiscent of antigen presentation. Lesion progression correlates with the presence of helper (T4$^+$) T cells, and myelin degradation is macrophage (Ia$^+$)-related. The ability to identify functionally the subunits of the immune system within a target tissue affords the neuropathologist a valuable new tool for conditions in which immunologic phenomena are implicated.

Throughout active lesions, astrocytic hypertrophy is common, particularly in the white matter adjacent to the lesion. Hypertrophic astrocytes extend for some distance into the surrounding white matter. These cells show binding of antihuman IgG, a feature perhaps related to active endocytosis of extravasated or locally produced immunoglobulin. Not infrequent in active lesions is a small amount of axonal degeneration and spheroids within the zone of ongoing demyelination (107).

The role of oligodendrocytes in the active

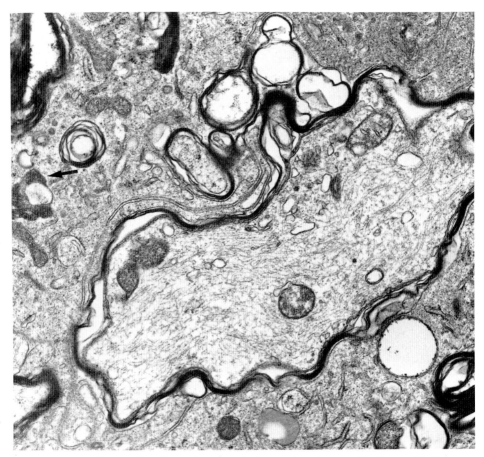

Figure 11.42. A myelinated fiber from the same lesion as that depicted in Figure 11.41 is invested by macrophage processes which have penetrated the outer layers of myelin and are engaged in its phagocytosis. Various stages of myelin breakdown are seen, including multilamellar inclusions (*arrow*), identified by some investigators as being of possible viral origin. (Original magnification ×22,000.)

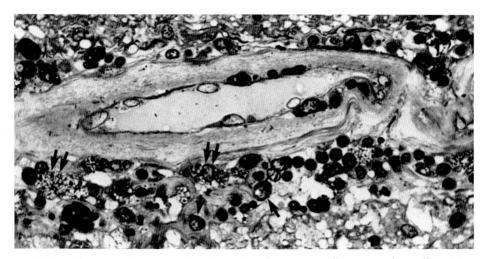

Figure 11.43. At the periphery of a chronic active plaque, a small perivascular cuff contains small lymphocytes, plasma cells (*single arrows*), and foamy macrophages (*double arrows*). Within the Virchow-Robin space, some fibrosis is also in evidence. Toluidine blue-stained, 1-μm epoxy section. (Original magnification ×640.)

chronic multiple sclerosis lesion has been enigmatic. While some can be identified positively on purely morphologic grounds by their proclivity to form interfascicular chains (1), on most occasions they are difficult to distinguish light microscopically from small lymphocytes. With the advent of monoclonal antibodies to T cells, antisera to oligodendroglial and myelin components, double-labeling techniques, and the resolution of the electron microscope, such pitfalls are now less problematical. Along the demyelinated edge of an active chronic multiple sclerosis lesion, there is pronounced hyperplasia of oligodendroglia (57, 58), an event reputed to denote the impending demise of oligodendrocytes in this region. However, it is now believed that these cells survive the initial demyelinative and inflammatory insults and that they proliferate and probably remain after the growth phase of the lesion has ceased. For example, in one chronically active lesion sampled at biopsy (117), it was seen that despite the presence of ongoing demyelination, inflammation, and macrophages containing recognizable myelin debris, surviving and proliferating oligodendroglia were common (Fig. 11.44). Indeed, in some regions around the lesion, remyelination was evident. These observations support the conclusion that the myelin sheath, and not the oligodendrocyte, is the primary target in this condition.

In addition to active inflammation around blood vessels, desease activity in multiple sclerosis has been attributed to generalized increased prominence of vessels where there is widening of the Virchow-Robin space or swelling of glial end-feet. Nevertheless, while such changes are now deemed artifactual, their consistent prominence may herald an innate, increased leakiness exaggerated by histologic processing. Sometimes, vessels surrounded by thick sleeves of fibrous astrocytes will contain rims of inflammatory cells confined to the Virchow-Robin space. A persistent problem in active multiple sclerosis lesions has been the chronology of the inflammatory events and that in the final analysis, many "recent" inflammatory cuffs might have been present for months. It is known from inflammatory demyelinating diseases in animals that perivascular cuffs can persist in the CNS long after disease progression has subsided.

A feature of active chronic multiple sclerosis lesions often overlooked is the presence of inflammation in the leptomeninges, more akin to acute multiple sclerosis and the acute disseminated encephalomyelitides. This brings to mind a common trap in chronic multiple sclerosis, which is to apply the term "acute" instead of "active" to growing lesions. Strictly speaking, an *acute* multiple sclerosis lesion is one from that rare, fatal form of multiple sclerosis, acute multiple sclerosis (*vide infra*). However, it is not unusual in chronic multiple sclerosis to find microscopic, active lesions centered on small vessels which have features of acute multiple sclerosis lesions. Whether or not these represent truly *acute* (i.e., initial, new) lesions or merely growing fingers from *active chronic* plaques must remain speculative.

Shadow Plaques. A unique lesion to multiple sclerosis, the shadow plaque has had a controversial history since its earliest description. Greenfield and Norman (49) point out that shadow plaques ("Markschattenherde" of the German school) were regarded by Alzheimer in 1910 and later by Zimmerman and Netsky (158), as plaques in the early stages of development. Dawson (31) questioned Alzheimer's interpretation and suggested that shadow plaques might "indicate a simple atrophy which results in a progressive reduction of the volume of the sheath without affecting the remaining myelin."

Shadow plaques are claimed to be most commonly seen in the spinal cord where they lie in isolated positions or adjacent to older lesions. They also occur on a larger scale in the cerebral hemispheres where they stain in myelin preparations as pale grey zones interposed between nonstaining plaque proper and densely staining white matter (Figs. 11.39 and 11.40). Often, they form satellitic areas on the posterior aspects of paraventricular lesions over the angles of the lateral ventricles and on demyelinated areas in the pons, medulla oblongata, and cerebellum.

Shadow plaques show up pale by H&E and myelin stains and contain diffusely distributed, thinly myelinated fibers. Today, the consensus is that they represent

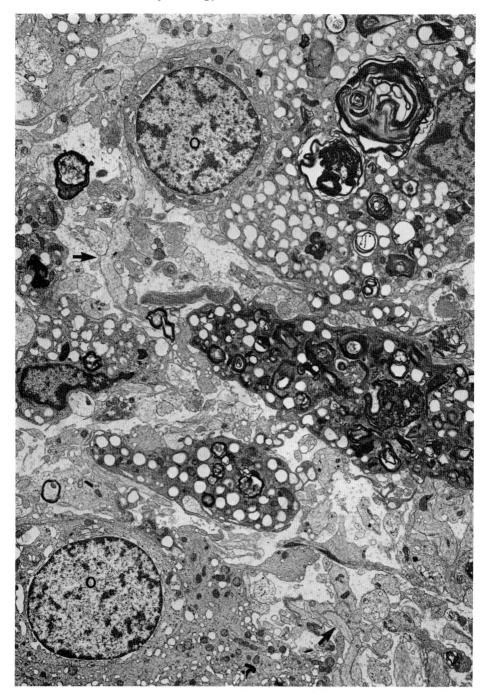

Figure 11.44. This electron micrograph is taken from the same chronic active lesion as that depicted in Figure 11.41. The area is almost totally demyelinated, and naked axons are present (*arrows*). Two surviving oligodendrocytes (*O*) lie among microglial cells containing myelin debris and lipid droplets. (Original magnification ×5,600.)

areas of CNS remyelination (Figs. 11.45 and 11.46). This conclusion is based on a preponderance of large diameter axons with thinner than normal myelin sheaths, attenuated sheaths containing aberrant collections of oligodendroglial cytoplasm, and a

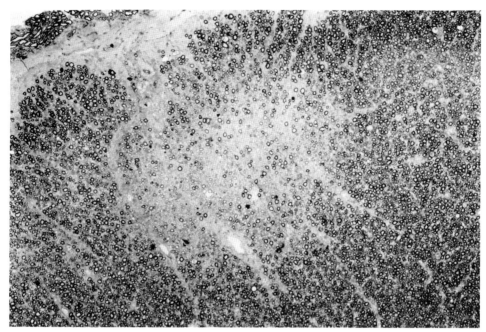

Figure 11.45. Chronic multiple sclerosis. A shadow plaque is seen within an interior column of the spinal cord. There is obvious myelin pallor but no evidence of ongoing disease activity. Toluidine blue-stained, 1-μm epoxy section. (Original magnification ×100.)

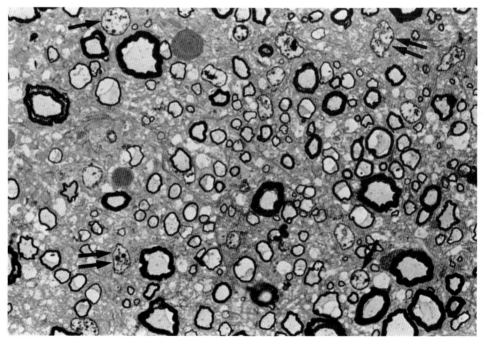

Figure 11.46. Detail from the lesion shown in Figure 11.45. Note the prominence of nerve fibers with relatively large diameter axons and thin myelin sheaths—the morphologic hallmarks of remyelination. A mild background gliosis is present, and a corpus amylaceum, a few oligodendrocytes (*single arrows*), and astrocytes (*double arrows*) can be discerned. (Original magnification ×1,000.)

modest increase in the number of oligodendrocytes (96, 107, 117). Evidence of previous damage can be found in the form of a moderate background gliosis, an abundance of nonspecific corpora amylacea, a few fibrotic blood vessels, and the occasional foamy macrophage. Inflammatory cells are absent, as are prominent fibrous astroglial and macrophage responses.

Earlier descriptions of shadow plaques may have included lesions in more active stages of evolution, since Marchi-positive material (myelin debris or "myelin-Abbau") and many macrophages are mentioned. Therefore, it is conceivable that active chronic multiple sclerosis lesions with a broad advancing edge of ongoing demyelination have in the past been interpreted as shadow plaques. The lesion illustrated by Zimmerman and Netsky (158, figure 65, loc. cit.) is highly reminiscent of the spinal cord lesion illustrated here (Figs. 11.45 and 11.46), albeit by a different technique. Anecdotally, Lumsden (73) refers to "an incidental remark in a paper by Bornstein et al. (1962) on remyelination in tissue cultures—that shadow plaques may indicate attempts at remyelination of plaques." Lumsden discounts the possibility and continues by saying that shadow plaques are most likely areas in which the demyelinating process did not reach completion and that "remyelination may be a possibility in the cat (Bunge et al., 1961), but it remains to be proved that it occurs in man." In 1969, Suzuki et al. (134) documented remyelination in multiple sclerosis, and it has since been confirmed on a number of occasions (93, 96, 107, 117). In animals, CNS remyelination is a well-proven phenomenon (106).

As a final note on remyelination, close examination of most chronic multiple sclerosis lesions will often reveal a circumferential narrow zone of remyelination, perhaps 0.5–1.0 mm across. Why such areas never progress to the dimensions of shadow plaques may be related to the degree of oligodendroglial depletion, the intensity of the gliotic response, or the duration and severity of preceding inflammatory events.

Pathologic Mechanisms

Towards the end of the nineteenth century, neuropathologists favored the notion that underlying the demyelinative process in multiple sclerosis was an inherited defect in the biochemistry of the sheath manifested during development. As we entered the twentieth century, opinions focused on the vascular component of the lesion and the involvement of diffusable "noxious" or "exogenous" factors. In Dawson's monograph (31) in 1916, the prevailing view was one in which there was a primary effect upon the glia, expressed as "an enlargement of the protoplasm and protoplasmic processes of the normally existing spider cell," i.e., astrocyte. (The reader should bear in mind that at the time Dawson's insightive analysis was compiled, our present day glial cell terminology did not exist, oligodendroglia had not been identified, and glia were believed to belong to a common syncytium.) Myelin degeneration was regarded as an event secondary to this glial overgrowth. Indeed, few neuropathologists will disagree that astroglial hypertrophy appears to be early and widespread in active multiple sclerosis and often precedes other abnormalities. Of course, whether this glial overgrowth reflects a response to an unseen, antecedent event (e.g., humoral factors) remains to be clarified. Therefore, what constitutes the initial event in lesion formation is open to question. McAlpine et al. (76) claim that based upon clinical data, the duration of the primary insult for a lesion is less than 1 week in the majority of cases and that maximal intensity is achieved within hours of the onset of an exacerbation. Given these constraints, Prineas (94) has pointed out that the lesions which become available for study are possibly not recently active but are indeed inactive and contain reactive and reparative changes only.

Regardless of the nature of the putative etiological factor in multiple sclerosis, in the face of an increasing literature on immunological anomalies, it is more than likely that immune-mediated events play a significant role in the expression of the ensuing disease. That these immunological vagaries and their fluctuations might herald pathogenetic events provides a convenient scaffold for discussion but must remain speculative. While the variation in clinical picture innate to multiple sclerosis renders correlation of findings from the various immunological parameters hazardous, the morphology of demyelinating lesions in multiple sclerosis is better appreciated when presented against the backcloth of the growing evidence for an immunogenic process. In this context and supporting the possibility of a generalized immunological abnormality in multiple sclerosis, a large number of works exist. The following two paragraphs, abstracted from the reviews of McFarlin and McFarland (78), Raine (107), and Traugott and Raine (135), represent but a few on this subject; these reviews should be consulted for actual references.

An elevated IgG level in the cerebrospinal fluid (CSF) is a common finding in a significant number of multiple sclerosis subjects, a feature suggestive of local antibody synthesis. Other studies reported IgM and oligoclonal IgG in the cerebrospinal fluid of subjects, indicative perhaps of some specificity in the cerebrospinal fluid antibody responses. Within the circulation, abnormalities in lymphocyte subpopulations and dynamics are well documented, some of which fluctuate with disease activity. Fluctuations in suppressor T cell activity and possible cross-reactivity between circulating human suppressor T cells and lamb oligodendrocytes in culture have been reported. In a later study, the latter was not confirmed in fresh frozen human CNS tissue (137). As has been the experience with most other immunological parameters, none of the above T cell phenomena has proven to be specific for multiple sclerosis. Circulating immune complexes in multiple sclerosis have been reported, and within the cerebrospinal fluid, immunological techniques have revealed myelin basic protein (MBP) or its fragments, phenomena thought not to be specific for multiple sclerosis but indicative of white matter damage.

Within the CNS proper, immunological events have been difficult to document at the structural level, but IgG has been demonstrated within plaques, particularly in reactive astrocytes. However, clear roles for either immunoglobulin or lymphocytes within the nervous system are lacking, although the recent study by Traugott *et al.* (140, 141) does impart some functional significance upon the presence of identified T cell subsets in lesions. Since functional expression of T cell subsets is still not fully understood, the assignment of function to the T cell subsets recognized by the presently available monoclonal antibodies must be viewed with caution. Sensitization against MBP has been a hotly debated issue for many years. Using T cell rosetting techniques, some works have been able to show an enhanced recognition of MBP by T cells in multiple sclerosis, but this response is not multiple sclerosis-specific. "Antibodies" against oligodendrocytes were described in multiple sclerosis but were later found to be nonspecific and related to binding to Fc receptors. The presence of circulating antimyelin factors in multiple sclerosis serum, first demonstrated on myelinated CNS cultures, has been confirmed repeatedly but appears to be unreleated to antibody (50).

Etiology and Epidemiology

From an etiologic standpoint, despite periodic flurries of excitement, no direct evidence for a causal agent exists in multiple sclerosis. Epidemiologic evidence indicates that the putative agent is contracted during the first 15 hr of life, after which a latent period occurs before the disease becomes manifest. The disease therefore is the end stage, or at best a late manifestation, of the disease mechanism, a stage which almost certainly involves immune mediation.

An infectious etiology in multiple sclerosis has been considered since Marie, in 1884 (74), noted an association between infections and the onset of clinical worsenings and stated that "the cause of insular sclerosis is intimately connected with infectious diseases" (87). On the basis of repeated reports of an abnormal immune response to measles virus (60, 104), measles has become the major candidate in the causation of multiple sclerosis. Paramyxovirus-like material was described in multiple sclerosis lesions in the early 1970s but was later found to be nonspecific for multiple sclerosis and probably represented degenerating nuclear chromatin (113). Several other infectious agents have been isolated from a variety of multiple sclerosis tissues, but none has been confirmed as being causally related (78). To date, unequivocal virus has not been observed within the CNS in this condition.

Laboratory testing of antigens of the major histocompatibility complex has revealed an association of certain HLA antigens and the ability to develop multiple sclerosis. Among whites in Europe, North America, and Australia, such an association occurs between multiple sclerosis and the combination of HLA-A3 and B7, and most frequent in these populations is a strong association with Dw2 and DRw2. These associations are not found in all populations where multiple sclerosis is endemic, and in Italy and Jordan the association is with DRw4, and in Japan, with DRw6 (78). Since the strongest immunogenetic link appears to be with the DRw region of the major histocompatibility complex, it has been postulated that there exists a relationship between susceptibility to multiple sclerosis and genetic control of immune regulation. Attempts have been made to demonstrate familial traits in the incidence of the disease, but from such studies, a haplotype or gene product shared by affected members but absent in healthy relatives has not been uncovered. Some concordance between monozygotic and dizygotic twins has been described. However, the current view is that it is unlikely that the increased incidence of multiple sclerosis in families or between twins is based solely on genetic influence (78).

Epidemiologic studies have documented without equivocation that definite high and low risk areas for multiple sclerosis exist and that the highest risk occurs in the northern hemisphere north of latitude 40°N. In general, prevalence increases with distance northwards. For example, in the United States, in New Orleans, Louisiana (30°N), the prevalence is 6 per 100,000; in Denver, Colorado (40°N), 38 per 100,000; and in Rochester, Minnesota, the highest prevalence area in the United States, 64 per 100,000. The highest prevalence in the world is found in the Orkney Islands (59°N), off the north coast of Scotland, where it is 317 per 100,000, but one must take into account that the total population is a little more than 60,000, and the statistics may be somewhat skewed. However, latitude alone does not always correlate with the incidence and prevalence of multiple sclerosis, since Japan (30–45°N) has about 4 per 100,000, and the form of multiple sclerosis which occurs there is of the neuromyelitis optica-type (*vide infra*).

The existence of high and low prevalence areas and the mass migrations which have occurred in the past few decades (e.g., from Europe to Israel and South Africa) have afforded epidemiologists fertile ground for the examination of susceptibility and age in multiple sclerosis. In brief, it has been found that persons migrating before the age of 15 from a high to a low risk zone (e.g., Ukraine to Israel) acquire the low risk of the new country. Persons migrating after the age of 15 from high to low risk areas, or *vice versa*, take with them the risk frequency of their country of origin. Thus, the evidence is consistent with a childhood exposure to a putative causative factor.

Variants of Multiple Sclerosis

In addition to the wide clinical and neuropathologic variability among patients with chronic multiple sclerosis, there exist at least three demyelinating conditions with features distinct enough to assign them separate identities. In the case of the first (acute multiple sclerosis), this can be justified on both clinical and neuropathologic grounds; in the second (neuromyelitis optica), on a purely clinical basis; and in the third (concentric sclerosis), the diagnosis can only be made at autopsy.

ACUTE MULTIPLE SCLEROSIS

Clinical Parameters

Difficult to distinguish from the acute disseminated encephalomyelitides (*vide infra*) except perhaps on the basis of an absence of a documentable antecedent infection, vaccination, or immunization, acute multiple sclerosis is a rare, invariably fatal form of multiple sclerosis. Reports exist which discuss long-lasting remissions and survival in acute multiple sclerosis, but such cases might be difficult to separate from chronic multiple sclerosis with a severe onset.

The usual clinical course is one of an acute or subacute neurological condition characterized by headache, vomiting, brain stem signs, and spinal cord and optic nerve involvement. The patient is often rendered stuporous or comatose or decerebrate with prominent cranial nerve or corticospinal abnormalities over a few weeks (6). Examination of the clinical history may reveal insidious signs (depression, lethargy) months prior to the neurologic deficits. Rarely, there may be one or two remissions. The course is commonly less than 10 months. Frequently, definitive diagnosis is made only at autopsy.

Neuropathology

Macroscopic Examination. The brain appears normal on gross examination and is within the normal weight range. Sectioning will usually reveal scattered, pink lesions of a uniform age within the white matter, with a distribution comparable to that of chronic multiple sclerosis and with some predilection for paraventricular zones. On occasion, it is difficult to detect some lesions grossly with certainty within the centrum semiovale, and, rarely, a few chronic lesions can be detected. Brainstem involvement is common, and lesions within the spinal cord and optic nerves are usually not evident grossly.

Microscopic Examination. Myelin stains will reveal areas of obvious pallor, although many of these may not have been apparent macroscopically (Fig. 11.47). Acute multiple sclerosis lesions have indistinct margins, where demyelinated zones blend gradually into densely myelinated areas (Fig. 11.48). H&E examination reveals the entire lesion to be intensely inflammatory (Fig. 11.49), with small mononuclear cells in perivascular locations and in the parenchyma (Figs. 11.50–11.52). Perivascular cuffing is not particularly concentrated towards the lesion edge but occurs throughout the lesion. Macrophages reside within the perivascular cuffs and the affected parenchyma. Lipid stains reveal an intense PAS- or oil red O-positive reaction, with some concentration towards the perimeter. Hypertrophic astrocytes permeate the lesion proper, the broad marginal (presumably actively demyelinating) zone, and taper off towards more normal white matter. Oligodendrocytes are difficult to identify because of the intense inflammatory activity, and axon staining will reveal a diffuse loss, more so than in active chronic multiple sclerosis.

Immunocytochemistry has revealed binding of immunoglobulin to hypertrophic astrocytes and occasional plasma cells (99), and the application of monoclonal antibodies to human T cells and their subsets has shown the body of the affected area to be packed with T cells (141). There is a predominance of helper T cells which tend to congregate at the lesion margin. Unlike chronic multiple sclerosis, T cell involvement ceases at the lesion edge, and none can be found in the adjacent white matter. Ia^+ macrophages are homogeneously densely distributed across the lesion, and then decrease once the edge is reached.

Ultrastructural examination of lesions from acute multiple sclerosis has confirmed ongoing demyelination by macrophages, but despite intensive search and the application of immunoperoxidase technology, evidence in support of previous claims of virus involvement has not been found (114).

Ferraro (40) was among the first neuropathologists to point out the striking similarity between acute multiple sclerosis and acute experimental autoimmune (allergic) encephalomyelitis (EAE), on which the bulk of the laboratory studies on multiple sclerosis-related research has been conducted.

NEUROMYELITIS OPTICA

History

Known also since 1894 as Devic's disease (33), neuromyelitis optica is a form of multiple sclerosis characterized by an acute onset of partial or complete blindness and signs of myelopathy. Credit for its recognition has actually been traced back to Albutt in 1870 (7), and although Devic did not publish extensively on the subject, it was his perception as to its individuality which inspired his students, most notably Gault, to research it further (25). Neuromyelitis optica is a relatively rare condition (300 or so cases are in the literature) among Western countries, but is more common in India and the Far East, particularly Japan. These geographic differences notwithstanding, neuromyelitis optica must still be regarded as a rare variant of multiple sclerosis.

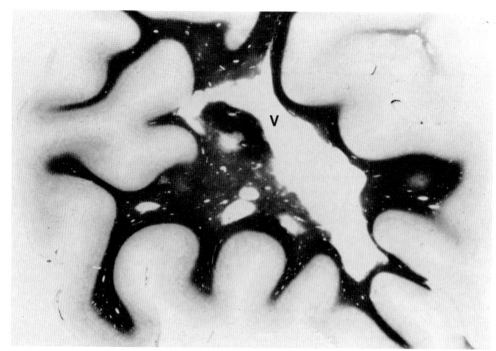

Figure 11.47. Acute multiple sclerosis. A section of an occipital lobe shows the ventricle (*V*) surrounded by a large area of demyelination. Elsewhere, diffusely demyelinated foci are scattered throughout the white matter. Note how most of the lesions have indistinct margins, indicative of ongoing demyelination, and a preferential distribution around small vessels. Heidenhain's myelin stain. (Courtesy of Dr. R. D. Terry.)

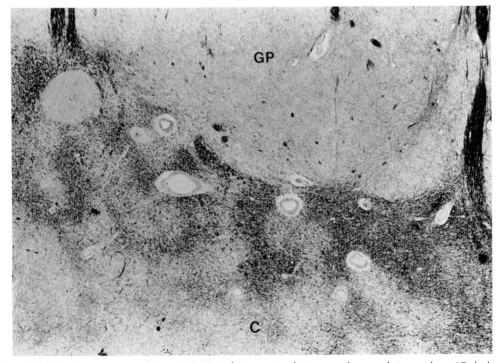

Figure 11.48. Same case as Figure 11.47. White matter between the caudate nucleus (*C, below*) and the globus pallidus (*GP, above*) shows rings of demyelination around perivascular inflammatory cuffs and a diffuse loss of myelin throughout. (Original magnification ×40.)

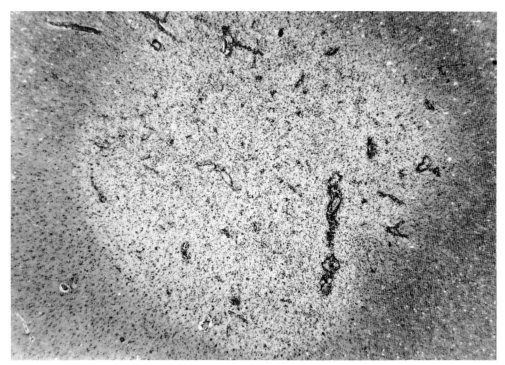

Figure 11.49.   Acute multiple sclerosis. A small lesion in the centrum semiovale is seen to be hypercellular and heavily infiltrated throughout, particularly around blood vessels. The lesion margin is relatively indistinct. H&E stain. (Original magnification ×80.)

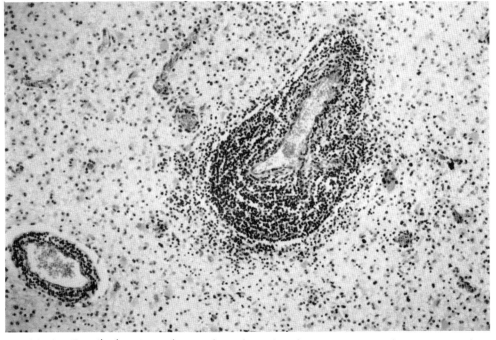

Figure 11.50.   Detail of perivascular exudates from the above case. Note the intense packing of small mononuclear cells in the Virchow-Robin spaces and adjacent CNS parenchyma. (Original magnification ×140.)

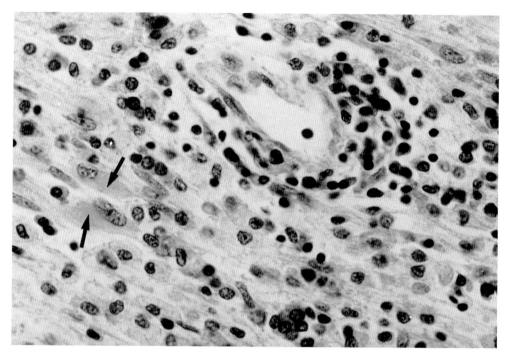

Figure 11.51. Higher magnification of the lesion in Figure 11.49. Note the predominance of infiltrating small mononuclear cells and the hypertrophic astrocytes (*arrows*). Foamy macrophages can be seen in the background. (Original magnification ×400.)

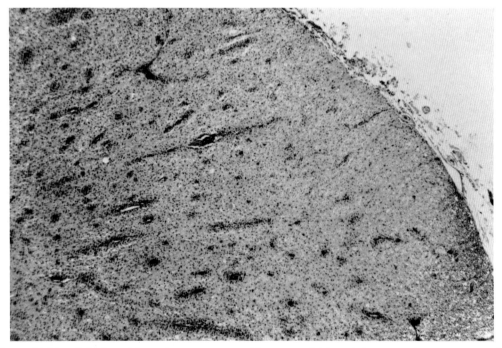

Figure 11.52. Spinal cord from the same case as Figure 11.47. Note the many radiating perivascular infiltrates accompanying the penetrating vessels, a few cells in the meninges, and the overall hypercellularity. (Original magnification ×50.) (Courtesy of Dr. R. D. Terry.)

Clinical Parameters

Like acute multiple sclerosis, neuromyelitis optica has features in common with acute disseminated encephalomyelitis (e.g., postinfectious encephalomyelitis), and indeed, a history of a recent viral infection precedes clinical onset in about one-third of cases. It often afflicts persons at the extremes of the age range associated with multiple sclerosis, i.e., under 10 and over 60 yr (121). Onset of disease is rapid, often with a decrease in visual acuity in one eye, which then progresses to total blindness as sight diminishes in the other eye over a period of a few hours. In some cases, the entire process may take a few months with intervening remissions. Bilateral blindness affects about 85% of patients. While the optic discs may sometimes be blurred and papilledema apparent, the most common visual sign is a central scotoma on one or both sides. Involvement of the extraocular muscles has been reported but is not common.

Spinal cord signs may occur initially in combination with the optic involvement or as a later development. The heralding signs of spinal cord disease are those of an acute transverse lesion. Progressive motor and sensory loss follows, usually until the patient is paraplegic. Bowel and bladder signs are also common. In about 20% of cases, the course is rapid and progresses to death with total blindness and respiratory failure in about 3 months. About 30% show a slow downhill course to death in a few years due to decubiti, pneumonia, or other complications. The remaining 50% survive with varying degrees of recovery. There is return of vision in some cases, but some residual weakness or paralysis of the extremities usually remains in evidence.

Neuropathology

All cases display severe involvement of the optic nerves, chiasm, and spinal cord. The optic nerves frequently display atrophic changes, and in some severe cases, there is necrosis of the spinal cord. Cystic changes are also seen in the optic nerves and chiasm. Other regions of the CNS may display a lesion distribution indistinguishable from chronic multiple sclerosis, although the extent of the involvement is considerably less. Histologically, perivascular demyelination or more commonly, total demyelination of entire segments of optic nerve and spinal cord, are common features. In more severe cases, inflammatory changes (both perivascular and diffusely parenchymal) are described, but meningeal infiltrates are not prominent. In some lesions, there is diffuse demyelination, while in others, they may be a total loss of all elements due to necrosis. In summary, the lesions of neuromyelitis optica have the features of multiple sclerosis, except for an increased severity in the optic nerves and spinal cord.

CONCENTRIC SCLEROSIS

History

In contrast to neuromyelitis optica which possesses distinctive clinical manifestations, concentric sclerosis (Balo's disease) is diagnosable only at autopsy and is a curious histologic variant of multiple sclerosis. Reviewed by Courville (26), this condition was originally termed encephalitis periaxialis scleroticans by Marburg in 1906, encephalitis periaxialis diffusa (Schilder), and encephalitis periaxialis concentrica by Balo (13). Concentric sclerosis is an exceedingly rare variant of multiple sclerosis, and the total number of reported typical cases amounts to less than two dozen. Another 14 reports exist on typical multiple sclerosis in which small regions of concentric sclerosis were found in addition to characteristic plaques.

Clinical Parameters

There is no singular feature which accounts for the unusual pathology typical of this form of multiple sclerosis (vide infra), and in general, the patient is not diagnosed during life as suffering from a demyelinating disease. Indeed, Courville (26) states that "a correct diagnosis of the disease has not been made ante mortem," and in only one case was a demyelinating disorder suspected. Retrospective clinical analysis has highlighted the following frequently occurring features in concentric sclerosis: acute onset; involvement of young individuals; early symptoms (like headaches) suggestive of a space-occupying lesion; marked motor symptoms in most of the cases or psychic syndromes in others; short survival period

(3–5 yr usually); absence of remissions and exacerbations; and death due to some intercurrent cause (26).

Neuropathology

Grossly, the brain contains areas of gray discoloration disseminated throughout the white matter ranging in size from a few millimeters to 3–4 cm (according to Balo, from the size of a lentil to a pigeon's egg). The lesions occur throughout the cerebral and cerebellar white matter, with sparing of gyri and arcuate fibers. Histologically, the lesions are distinctive and take the form of areas of white matter of varied shape, in which alternating bands of myelinated white matter are separated by almost equidistant zones of myelin depletion, but the usual bull's eye form is not as common as the literature might suggest (Fig. 11.53). This alternating pattern is reproduced in fibrillary glial and fat stains. Sometimes, the bands of demyelination are interlaced. Axonal preservation is apparent. Inflammation is usually not prominent, but can be seen on occasion (Fig. 11.54). The concentric lesions in their most rounded forms are sometimes centered on blood vessels.

The etiopathogenesis of concentric sclerosis still evades elucidation, but there is no reason to regard the disease as anything other than a variant of multiple sclerosis. The incidence of similar smaller, concentric lesions, sometimes satellitic to chronic plaques, in reports on clinically diagnosed multiple sclerosis underlines the concept that they are not the result of any particular etiologic factor. Furthermore, similar less well-defined lesions have been described adjacent to areas of focal softening and embolic infarctions, and claims exist that they have been produced after potassium cyanide intoxication (26).

The characteristic pattern of the CNS lesions has been debated for many years and remains unexplained. Neuropathologists have preferred the views that they are representative of waves of demyelination punctuated either by zones of disease quiescence or remyelination, or that they are due to an unusual vasculopathy. An old concept, promulgated by Hallervorden and Spatz (52), holds that the concentric lesion is the end product of a lecithinolytic exudate which "produces the physicochemical phenomenon generally known as 'Liesegang ring formation' as seen in nature (i.e. mosaics of plants)." Balo himself considered the etiology to be inflammatory, which smacks of a suspected infectious etiology (as in chronic multiple sclerosis), but precisely what underlies lesion formation must await clarification.

Acute Disseminated Encephalomyelitis

A collective term applied to a variety of severe, sometimes acutely fatal, infectious, inflammatory demyelinating diseases, acute disseminated encephalomyelitis has a history dating back to the early eighteenth century in association with smallpox infection (49), but the term did not appear in the medical literature until the late nineteenth century (155). The recognition that a separate family of diseases associated with a number of exanthems or vaccinations had a common inflammatory demyelinating pathology emanated from the work of Perdrau (87) and Greenfield and King (48). The term "disseminated vasculomyelinopathy" has also been applied on occasion to these conditions (90). It is known today that the member diseases share an almost identical pathology, consisting of multifocal, sometimes confluent, areas of inflammation which are usually exclusively perivenous and meningeal and accompanied by perivenous and subpial demyelination, and that the etiology probably resides in an allergic (perhaps autoimmune) response within the central (and sometimes, peripheral) nervous system (47, 83, 118, 145). In addition to cases which are clearly postinfectious and postvaccinal, some exist in which no precipitating factor has been traced—the so-called "spontaneous" or "idiopathic" acute disseminated encephalomyelitides.

POSTINFECTIOUS ENCEPHALOMYELITIS

Clinical Parameters

Post- or parainfectious encephalomyelitis embraces a number of neurological complications of some common acute infections which may be expressed as encephalitis, myelitis, or encephalomyelitis. The clinical parameters of the component members are

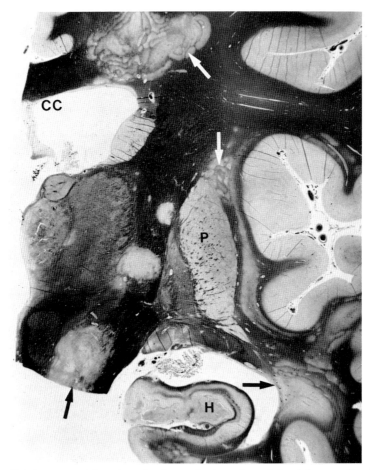

Figure 11.53. Balo's concentric sclerosis. A cerebral section stained for myelin shows multiple plaques of alternating demyelinated and myelinated layers giving an onion skin effect (*arrows*). These waves of demyelination appear to radiate from centers which at the microscopic level are related to blood vessels. *CC,* corpus callosum; *P,* putamen; *H,* hippocampus. (Courtesy of Dr. Y. Takei.)

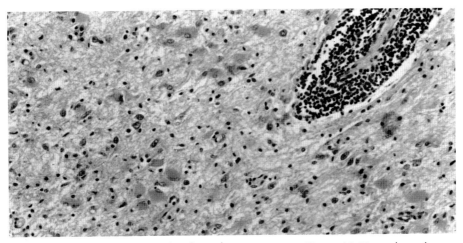

Figure 11.54. Low power H&E section from the same case as Figure 11.53, to show the occasional perivascular cuff within a demyelinated area and the many hypertrophic astrocytes. (Original magnification ×200.) (Courtesy of Dr. Takei.)

extensively reviewed by Miller and Evans (82) and Miller *et al.* (83). Postinfectious encephalomyelitis is associated most frequently with an antecedent infection by measles, varicella (chicken pox), and rubella (German measles), and less frequently, with influenza, mumps, streptococcal (scarlet fever), and pertussis infection. Disease incidence ranges from 1:5000 after rubella infection and 1:1000 (measles) to 1:800 for scarlet fever, although Miller *et al.* (83) point out that in pertussis, the incidence is undetermined but probably higher.

Neurological signs usually appear between 3 and 21 d after the rash. However, in some cases (parainfectious forms), the exanthem appears after the onset of symptoms. In 15–20%, the disease is fatal. In most patients, the disease is monophasic in that those who recover (particularly after a measles exanthem, the most common form), there is no relapse or recurrence of neurological signs. Persistent, residual (often psychiatric) signs are not uncommon (82). These diseases most frequently affect the 6–10 yr age group. The typical clinical features include headache and vomiting, followed by fever and stupor. Other signs include neck stiffness, strabismus, flaccid paraplegia, incontinence, drowsiness, absent abdominal and plantar or deep reflexes. Cases of myelitis have been reported as a sequela of infection—e.g., in 3% of cases after measles (83), mostly in children between 5–8 yr of age. Onset was acute and involved backache, retention of urine, and progressed in some cases to spastic paraplegia. In four cases, visual signs were apparent. In 20%, the myelitis was fatal in 1–17 d. In the majority of survivors, there was a return to full function, although some displayed persistent mild paraparesis. In a few instances (2% of measles cases), a nonfatal polyradiculitis is reported.

In mumps and streptococcal encephalomyelitis, while the above signs (which relate more to measles, varicella, and rubella cases) are present, the most common complication is that of a lymphocytic meningitis. In pertussis, a fulminating encephalopathy is the usual, if not the only, manifestation. In all instances of postinfectious encephalomyelitis, the only clinical features of definite prognostic significance are

coma and convulsions, both of which are of serious import (83).

Spinal fluid changes do not always occur but when present, usually take the form of a variable pleocytosis and moderate increase in protein.

Although circumstantial in most cases, a viral (or bacterial) etiology in these disorders is generally accepted. Direct evidence comes from the reported isolation of measles virus from cerebrospinal fluid cells, and from CNS tissue after cocultivation, as well as the presence of measles inclusion bodies in the CNS *in situ*. Mumps virus has been isolated from the cerebrospinal fluid in several cases (121).

Neuropathology

Macroscopic Examination. With minor differences only, the neuropathology of the postinfectious encephalomyelitides varies little. On gross examination, petechial hemorrhages may be visible on the surface of the brain and spinal cord. Brain weight is often increased and correlates with the presence of edema and swelling of the gyri. Coronal section reveals more congestion of blood vessels than one might expect, particularly in the white matter. Narrow grey zones can sometimes be traced around small venules in the white matter (Fig. 11.55) and the penetrating vessels of the spinal cord.

Microscopic Examination. The distinctive features of the CNS lesions in this condition are a vigorous inflammatory response with perivascular demyelination

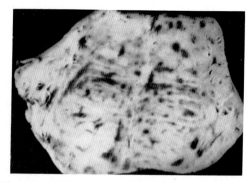

Figure 11.55. Acute disseminated encephalomyelitis: postmeasles encephalomyelitis. A gross specimen from the brain stem shows multiple punctate grey lesions. (Courtesy of Dr. H. M. Zimmerman.)

(Figs. 11.56–11.59). The extent of inflammation correlates with the duration of the disease. Longer survival is associated more with quiescent lesions, with a morphology similar to chronic multiple sclerosis. H&E stained sections reveal widespread involvement of white matter, with some predilection for the basis pontis. The prominent inflammatory response occurs around small- to medium-sized venules within the white matter (Figs. 11.56–11.59). The perivascular cuffing occurs around scattered vessels, and individual lesions range from

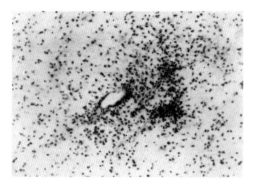

Figure 11.56. A Nissl preparation from the case depicted in Figure 11.55 shows perivascular and parenchymal infiltration by hematogenous cells. (Original magnification ×80.) (Courtesy of Dr. H. M. Zimmerman.)

0.1–1.0 mm in diameter. Small lesions often coalesce to form larger areas of involvement. Among the infiltrating cells, small lymphocytes are most prominent. Plasma cells are common, as are large mononuclear cells and occasional eosinophils and fat-laden macrophages (gitter cells). In more severe cases, polymorphonuclear leukocytes are prominent. Perivascular hemorrhages, though rare, may occur.

Around the perivascular cuffs, infiltrating cells may be scattered diffusely in the parenchyma, and each is associated with a narrow rim of demyelination. Adjacent rims of demyelination tend to fuse and produce lesions similar to multiple sclerosis. Within the narrow, almost uniform, sleeves of demyelination and in the adjacent parenchyma, hypertrophic astrocytes and fibrillary gliosis are apparent. Fat-laden microglial cells abut normal white matter around the lesions, a phenomenon termed "wall-formation" by Greenfield and King (48). As lesions become older, increasing numbers of macrophages are found in perivascular spaces, and inflammatory cells decrease in number. Also described in early lesions are spindle-shaped cells which become increasingly difficult to identify with age. Occasionally within the Virchow-Robin space, the lipid phagocytes contain mitotic figures in measles encephalitis and

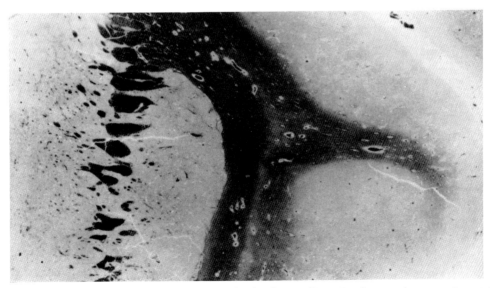

Figure 11.57. Postmeasles encephalitis. A Kultschitzky myelin-stained coronal preparation at the level of the internal capsule shows multiple foci of perivascular demyelination together with a diffuse loss of myelin. (Courtesy of Dr. H. M. Zimmerman.)

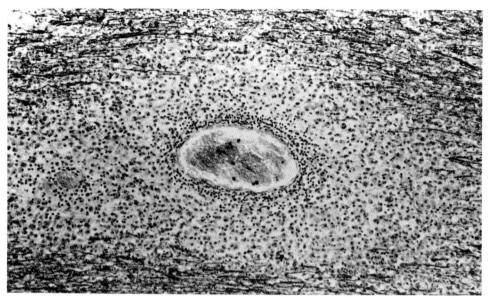

Figure 11.58. Postinfectious encephalomyelitis. A Luxol fast blue-stained section shows perivascular inflammation with associated demyelination. (Original magnification ×150.) (Courtesy of Dr. P. W. Lampert.)

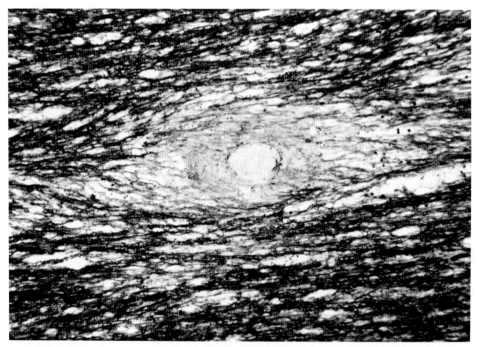

Figure 11.59. Postinfectious encephalomyelitis. A Heidenhain preparation shows loss of myelin around a perivascular cuff. (Original magnification ×160.)

cause some workers to refer to the condition as "microglial encephalitis" (121).

Around meningeal veins and vessels penetrating the spinal cord, inflammation is frequently apparent. Accompanying these are narrow zones of subpial demyelination and radiating sleeves of myelin loss, respectively (Fig. 11.60). Demyelination is also

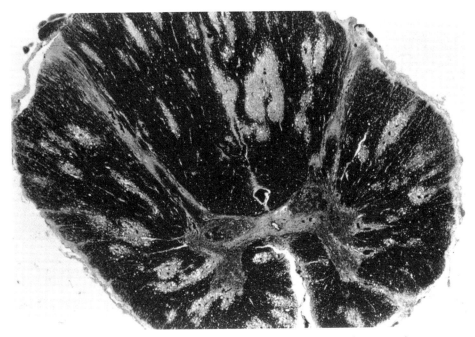

Figure 11.60. Postinfectious encephalomyelitis. A Kultschitzky myelin-stained preparation from the thoracic spinal cord displays multiple, radiating perivenular foci of demyelination. (Courtesy of Dr. A. Hirano.)

common along the walls of the lateral ventricles. In some cases of acute disseminated encephalomyelitis, viz. measles (2), viral inclusion bodies have been seen. Ependymal damage leading to aqueductal stenosis has been described in cases of mumps encephalitis. Some authors have attempted to classify lesion types further and relate the classification to clinical manifestations (15).

With regard to other changes, there is a moderate decrease in the number of axons in affected areas, and oligodendroglial hyperplasia has been reported. Involvement of grey matter is not unknown, and in such instances, perivenular inflammation and an intense microglial response are key features.

Pathogenesis

An area of intense debate, the genesis of the acute disseminated encephalomyelitis lesion has long been suspected of having an immunologic (allergic) basis. Selective infection and penetration of white matter endothelial cells have been implicated for the vascular damage which is believed to lead to the perivascular cuffing so typical

of this family of diseases. Attempts to demonstrate viral antigen in these areas have been generally unsuccessful, although a few cases have been reported where viral inclusions were described (2) and one where virus was isolated from brain tissue (81). Also, attempts to demonstrate specific sensitization to myelin components to support the concept of autosensitization to myelin or cross-reactivity with viral proteins have not been conclusive. However, on the basis of striking similarities between the member conditions and experimental autoimmune encephalomyelitis (EAE), most neuropathologists deem an immunologic attack upon CNS myelin to be the operative mechanism. Whether this demyelination is the result of a direct and specific attack or whether myelin and oligodendroglia are damaged due to a spillover of locally produced immunologic factors (e.g., lymphokines) hostile to CNS myelin, remains to be proven. Such a concept was considered originally by Perdrau in these conditions. Bystander destruction is a well-known phenomenon in immunology, where in the vicinity of a specific immune response between lymphocytes and antigen, uninvolved, local structures become victims and are lysed (123).

POSTVACCINAL ENCEPHALOMYELITIS

History

This group of iatrogenic conditions, nowadays exceedingly rare, represents diseases caused by vaccination against a number of conditions, most notably smallpox (vaccinia), typhoid-paratyphoid, and rabies. In the 1890s, a widespread "neuroparalytic accident" was reported among several thousand subjects following the use of Pasteur's antirabies vaccine. Postrabies immunization encephalomyelitis continued to be reported for many years (49) before it was found to be due to contamination of the inoculum by neural antigens (probably myelin) from the rabbit brain tissue in which it was cultivated (55). Encephalomyelitis occurred in about 1 in 750 inoculated with this vaccine, and in 20%, the condition was fatal. Subsequently, the vaccine was produced in duck embryo tissue. The characteristic pathological changes associated with the nervous complications of smallpox vaccination were first recognized by Turnbull and McIntosh (1926) in a report on seven cases of encephalitis following vaccination, although the condition had been recognized since 1860 (6). Incidence of the disease is about 1 in 4000 vaccinations. Smallpox vaccination has accounted for more than 200 deaths since reported in 1924 in Holland (121). Although no longer a major neurological condition, postrabies immunization encephalomyelitis has proven fatal in more than 400 cases since it was first described. More recently, Seitelberger *et al.* (130) reported a fatal encephalomyelitis in a patient who had received an inoculum containing, among other things, lyophilized calf brain cells as a treatment for progressive hemiparkinsonism. Following the termination of the treatment, about 18 months after the first injection, the patient developed severe CNS signs and died 7 weeks later.

Clinical Parameters

Postvaccinal or postimmunization encephalomyelitis presents as an acute monophasic syndrome with features more or less identical to postinfectious encephalomyelitis (headache, fever, stupor, etc.). In the majority of cases, the incubation period posttreatment varies from 8 to 14 days, with a decided predilection for the 10–12-d period. For example, in a study of 54 cases of postrabies immunization encephalomyelitis, Remlinger (118) reported that 10 presented with signs between days 7 and 10 after the first injection, 31 between days 11 and 14, and 13 between days 16 and 20.

Somewhat in contrast to the naturally occurring (i.e., postinfectious) forms, iatrogenic acute disseminated encephalomyelitis more frequently displays myelitic and radicular signs. Shiraki (132) reported 10 cases of fatal postrabies immunization encephalomyelitis which presented as two separate forms—an acute (survival time 16–47 d after the first injection) myelitic form with a preponderance of histologic changes in the spinal cord and brain stem, and a delayed (3–6 months), cerebral form, where the most pronounced changes occurred in the cerebral white matter.

Neuropathology

Macroscopic Examination. The brain resembles that of postinfectious encephalitis, with edema and swelling of the gyri and a slight increase in brain weight representing the major features. Petechial hemorrhages and increased vascular congestion are also common. Pink lesions are sometimes visible in periventricular locations, and many vessels, particularly in the spinal cord white matter, can be seen to have grey sleeves.

Microscopic Examination. Postvaccinal encephalomyelitis has a neuropathology very similar to that of acute multiple sclerosis, except that there is more subpial demyelination and meningeal infiltration. Lesions are intensely inflammatory and within the cerebral white matter, confluent and most extensive in periventricular regions. Some CNS necrosis has been reported. Grey matter inflammation, though minor in degree, is frequently seen. Perivascular cuffing is also prominent in the white matter immediately underlying the grey matter. In many cases, the most severe lesions are seen in the pons, medulla, and upper cervical cord. In some cases, optic nerve involvement occurs.

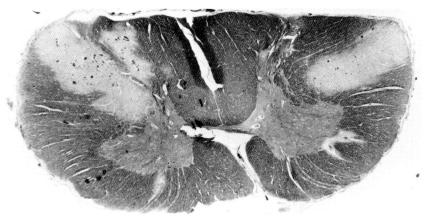

Figure 11.61. Acute disseminated encephalomyelitis: postrabies immunization encephalomyelitis. A myelin-stained section of cervical spinal cord shows several large radiating demyelinated plaques, some of which can be seen to be centered on blood vessels. (Courtesy of Dr. N. Peress.)

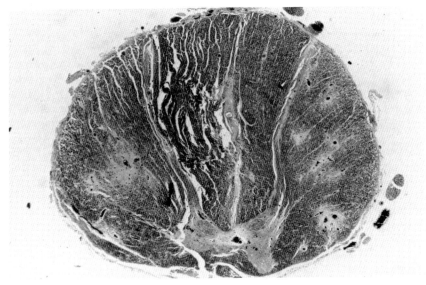

Figure 11.62. At the thoracic level, in the same case as Figure 11.61, the spinal cord contains multiple small perivenular foci of demyelination. (Courtesy of Dr. N. Peress.)

The inflammatory response, which is both perivascular and parenchymal, leads to large, coalescent lesions which show either total or diffuse loss of myelin around perivascular cuffs (Figs. 11.61–11.64). The lesion margins may be ill-defined, with a broad transition between the lesion proper and normal white matter. In the most protracted cases of postvaccinal or postimmunization encephalomyelitis, lesion margins are quite distinct (143).

Among the inflammatory cells, small mononuclear cells (lymphocytes) are the most common (Fig. 11.64). Plasma cells are also numerous, particularly in the Virchow-Robin space. Polymorphonuclear leukocytes are seen only very occasionally but are common where necrosis has occurred. Large mononuclear cells, sometimes in mitosis, are seen in the perivascular space. Perivascular and parenchymal macrophages laden with PAS-positive material occur throughout the lesion.

There is an intense microglial (rod cell) response within the area of damage. Hypertrophic astrocytes are scattered around the lesion margins and throughout the adjacent white matter. The area of demyelina-

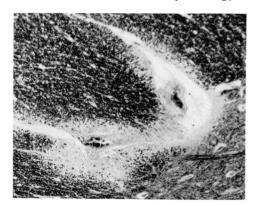

Figure 11.63. Detail of a perivenular lesion in the left dorsal horn, from the same case as Figure 11.61. (Courtesy of Dr. N. Peress.)

tion is mildly gliotic, and older lesions are very similar to those of chronic multiple sclerosis with some activity at the lesion margins.

In many cases, particularly after antirabies immunization, there is a distinct orientation of lesions to the subarachnoid space where inflammation is common. A broad zone of subpial demyelination sometimes circles the spinal cord and protrudes radially into the cord where penetrating vessels enter with their perivascular cuffs.

Pathogenesis

In many instances, it might be assumed that accidental infection of the CNS by virulent virus was causative. However, no definitive reports on the rescue of virus exist, and immunologic follow-up has been rare and negative in terms of a local reaction at the inoculation site and a circulating antibody response (132). Furthermore, the incidence of CNS complications after smallpox vaccination has been found to have no bearing on the source of the vaccine. While evidence of viral replication may be lacking, there remains the possibility that the virus causes the initial damage to the blood-brain barrier, thus exposing the usually sequestered CNS to components to the general circulation. Thereafter, a cascade of events culminating in an autoallergic (autoimmune) attack upon white matter (specifically, myelin) ensues. Evidence for such a sequence is stronger in the case of postrabies immunization encepha-

lomyelitis, in which it has been known for many years (3, 4, 55, 120) that the changes encountered in the human disease are related to the presence of myelin antigens within the inoculum. This aspect has been examined extensively in the EAE model (103, 152) in which a single subcutaneous inoculation of myelin antigens in an adjuvant leads in 2–3 weeks to an acute, fatal paralytic disease with an histology virtually identical to acute disseminated encephalomyelitis. However, while specific cell-mediated immunity to myelin antigens is well-documented in the experimental situation, the same is not the case in the human conditions.

Acute Hemorrhagic Leukoencephalopathy

History

Sometimes classed as a "leukoencephalitis," this condition (also known as Weston Hurst disease) is typified by severe damage to white matter vasculature which leads in most cases to varying degrees of CNS necrosis. For this reason, "leukoencephalopathy" is a more appropriate designation. This disease was separated from other forms of hemorrhagic encephalopathy by Hurst (56) in 1941 on the basis of a predilection for white matter involvement and the presence of inflammation and demyelination, although the latter might sometimes be obscured by hemorrhage and necrosis. Its relationship to the acute dissem-

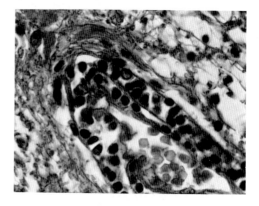

Figure 11.64. A demyelinated area from the same case as Figure 11.61 shows perivascular inflammation. (Original magnification ×200.) (Courtesy of Dr. N. Peress.)

inated encephalomyelitides was first noted by Russell (24), of which it is now considered to be an hyperacute form.

Clinical Parameters

Acute hemorrhagic leukoencephalopathy usually occurs in childhood (although many adult cases are known), more often in males than in females, and its onset can frequently be linked to an antecedent viral infection (e.g., influenza, chickenpox, or measles), urticarial rash, or vaccination. It is probably an hyperacute form of acute disseminated encephalomyelitis and is characterized by an abrupt onset of headache, fever, motor and sensory disturbances, and lethargy. These signs rapidly progress to stupor and coma. Within days, severe weakness develops, often with convulsions and paralysis of brain stem function (swallowing, breathing). In most instances, the disease has a fatal outcome in 1–6 d. It is difficult to diagnose during life, and claims of recovery after intensive corticosteroid therapy or massive cranial bony decompression might be equivocal in view of the lack of distinctive diagnostic criteria. Despite the hemorrhagic pathology, the cerebrospinal fluid is usually clear and similar to the picture in acute disseminated encephalomyelitis. In most cases, the cerebrospinal fluid is under increased pressure and has a white cell count of several hundred to over 1000, the majority of which are polymorphonuclear leukocytes. There is a corresponding increase in cerebrospinal fluid protein, but sugar and electrolytes are normal.

Neuropathology

Macroscopic Examination. The brain appears congested and swollen, and in hemiplegic cases, this may be more evident in one hemisphere. The sulci may contain a creamy exudate, but meninges are normal. Coronal section reveals widespread or localized involvement of white matter, ranging from small petechial hemorrhages to large confluent zones of hemorrhage and necrosis (liquefaction) (Figs. 11.65 and 11.66). Other areas may be swollen, grey, and faintly hemorrhagic (Fig.

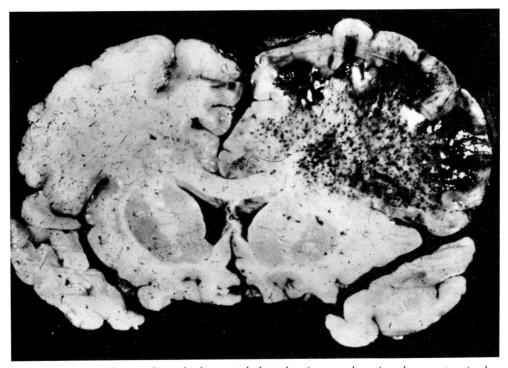

Figure 11.65. Acute hemorrhagic leukoencephalopathy. A coronal section shows extensive hemorrhage and swelling of the white matter of one hemisphere. Elsewhere, small hemorrhagic foci are apparent in the white matter. (Courtesy of Dr. R. D. Terry.)

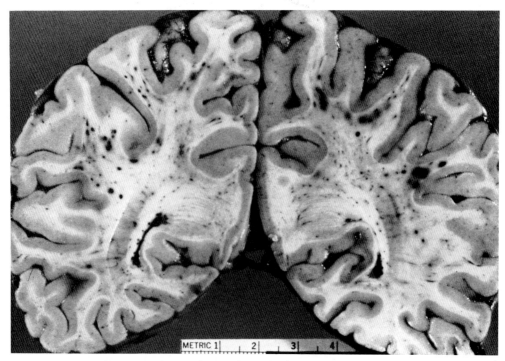

Figure 11.66.   Another case of acute hemorrhagic leukoencephalopathy shows, in a more rostral section, multiple small hemorrhagic foci disseminated throughout the white matter. (Courtesy of Dr. J. Garcia.)

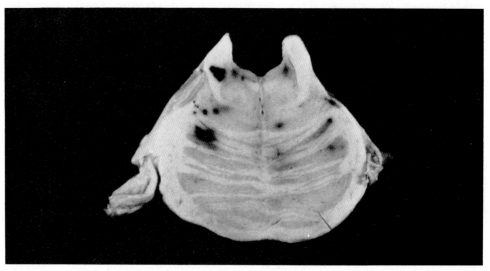

Figure 11.67.   In this case of acute hemorrhagic leukoencephalopathy, hemorrhagic lesions are seen in the pons. (Courtesy of Dr. G. R. W. Moore.)

11.67). Cerebral and cerebellar white matter and brain stem are equally vulnerable (Fig. 11.68). The basal ganglia, cerebral cortex, and spinal cord are usually spared.

Microscopic Examination. The key features of the lesions are partial vascular necrosis, fibrin deposition within Virchow-Robin spaces and narrow perivascular zones, perivascular edema, some necrosis of local CNS elements, multiple small, ring-

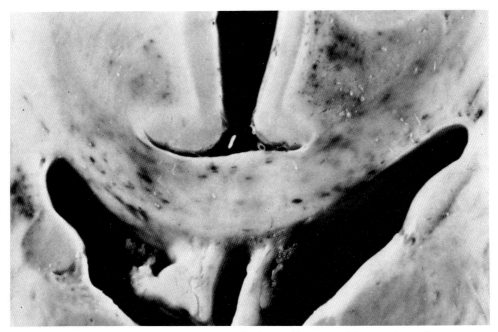

Figure 11.68. Same case as Figure 11.67. Multiple small grey and hemorrhagic lesions traverse the corpus callosum. (Courtesy of by Dr. G. R. W. Moore.)

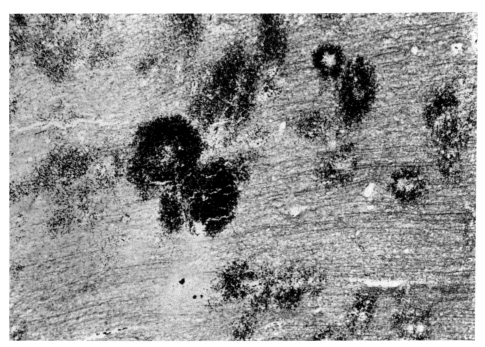

Figure 11.69. A low power view of a myelin stain from the case depicted in Figures 11.67 and 11.68 reveals punctate, ball-like hemorrhagic foci in the white matter. (Original magnification ×40.) (Courtesy of Dr. G. R. W. Moore and Dr. S. Chittal.)

shaped hemorrhages, hemosiderin-filled macrophages, and perivascular inflammation with demyelination (Figs. 11.69 and 11.70). The inflammation might be masked by tissue necrosis and hemorrhage, but close examination usually reveals scattered

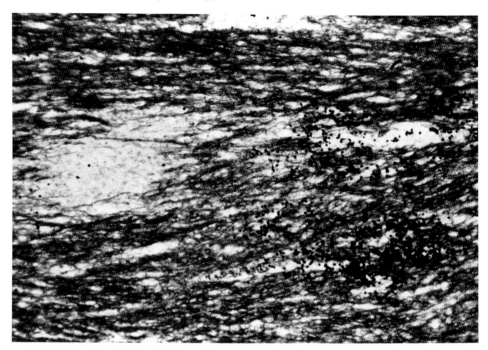

Figure 11.70. Higher magnification of a Heidenhain myelin-stained preparation reveals perivascular demyelination and erythrocytes (*right*) within the white matter parenchyma. Same case as Figures 11.67–11.69. (Original magnification ×160.)

small lymphocytes, large mononuclear cells, plasma cells, and an overriding number of polymorphonuclear leukocytes.

The above features immediately separate the condition from brain purpura, fat embolic encephalomalacia, herpes simplex encephalitis, and brain abscess. From case to case, there may be variation in the vascular reaction, depending upon survival time. Occasionally, the polymorphonuclear leukocyte response is an early event followed by the appearance of mononuclear cells. Some areas might display perivascular fibrin deposition and demyelination with little evidence of active inflammation. Mitosis is not uncommon among the many microglia and histiocytes (lipid-laden macrophages), but in general, the microglial response is less than that seen in acute disseminated encephalomyelitis. Other microscopic features include axonal degeneration and depletion, particularly in the immediate vicinity of fibrinoid deposits and hemorrhage, a mild astrogliosis, and some astrocytic and oligodendrocyte swelling. Ultrastructural examinations have likened the picture in acute hemorrhagic leukoencephalopathy to that occurring in EAE (75).

Pathogenesis

The astute observations of Russell (124) related this condition to the acute disseminated encephalomyelitides. It is generally considered that the condition reflects an hyperacute, anaphylactic-like reaction within the white matter. In support of this are the experimental data of Ferraro and Jervis (41) on anaphylaxis caused by systemic sensitization to egg albumin and the subsequent inoculation of the same antigen, and of Levine and Wenk (68) on hyperacute EAE caused by the addition of pertussis vaccine to an inoculum of CNS antigens. The prominence of polymorphonuclear leukocytes in lesions of acute hemorrhagic leukoencephalopathy is also consistent with an hyperacute reaction. However, the presence of lymphocytic infiltration in the white matter suggests either primary sensitization against myelin antigens or a tropism of the putative virus for white matter, with the myelin damage representing a secondary bystander event. These latter possibilities await clarification, but the early age of onset, the possible immaturity of the blood-brain barrier at the time of onset, and a history of allergic reactions appear to be key predisposing factors.

Progressive Multifocal Leukoencephalopathy

History

In many respects, this condition conforms poorly to the criteria laid down in the definition of the demyelinating diseases. It is included because it has a known infectious cause, a marked predilection for CNS white matter, and a remarkable sparing of axons. In future classifications, it may well be considered a neoplastic condition. In some of the most learned contemporary texts on the demyelinating diseases, progressive multifocal leukoencephalopathy is given brief mention only (6, 90, 121). Historically, this disease has been traced back to Hallervorden in 1930, quoted by Zu Rhein (160), who likened it to certain pleomorphic gliomas and dubbed it peculiar and unclassifiable. As a disease entity, progressive multifocal leukoencephalopathy was not recognized until 1958, when Aström *et al.* (12) coined the term and referred to it as an "hitherto unrecognized complication of chronic lymphatic leukemia and Hodgkin's disease." A viral etiology was first considered by Cavanagh *et al.* (21), a concept later strongly supported by Richardson (119). With the aid of electron microscopy, formaldehyde-fixed material, and a considerable amount of insight (tantamount to heresy for those who recall the occasion), Zu Rhein and Chou (161), at a meeting of the Association for Research in Nervous and Mental Diseases in 1964 (later published in 1968), described the ultrastructure of the intranuclear inclusions in the bizarre, pathognomonic oligodendrocytes as that consistent with a virus—a papovavirus. A few years later, as more sophisticated viral rescue techniques evolved, unequivocal papovavirus was indeed isolated from brain biopsy samples of several patients, and at least three serotypes were identified (153).

Clinical Parameters

Progressive multifocal leukoencephalopathy is a rare, fatal neurological disease of adults (male to female ratio, 3:2), usually between 40 and 60 yr of age, and has accounted for less than 100 deaths worldwide. Until 1964, it was a disease known principally to the neuropathologist. Neurologically, it develops most frequently against a background of lymphoproliferative disease, although it is also linked to nonlymphoproliferative diseases, like acute and chronic myelogenous leukemia and carcinomatosis and benign diseases of the reticuloendothelial system. An essential precipitating factor is aggressive immunosuppression (X-irradiation, cytotoxic agents, and/or adrenocorticosteroids), and it is widely held that during this period of immunodeficiency, there is recrudescence of a latent infection which is expressed in the CNS.

Clinically, cerebral signs predominate, and only rarely are cerebellar signs manifest. Motor, mental, and visual disturbances are the most common symptoms. Others include sensory deficits, incontinence, ataxia, and bulbar signs, and, in the terminal stages, paraparesis and coma. There is no increase in intracranial pressure. Typically, from insidious onset to death, the disease runs a 3- to 6-month course, but since the underlying disorder is relentlessly progressive, it is possible that the neurologic illness might be prevented from running its full natural course.

Neuropathology

Macroscopic Examination. Externally, the brain and leptomeninges appear normal. After sectioning, the brain reveals grey lesions mainly in the cerebral white matter, but in a few cases, the cerebellum, brain stem, and spinal cord are involved. Most common and characteristic are minute grey foci, often in clusters or chains oriented towards the cerebral subcortical white matter. Within gyri and deeper white matter, rounded, smooth grey lesions, from several millimeters to one or more centimeters in diameter, are frequently located (Fig. 11.71). These plaques are less discrete and less gliotic than multiple sclerosis lesions and lack a tendency to occur in paraventricular regions. Most prominent are large areas of nonhemorrhagic softening, sometimes occupying a major part of the white matter of one hemisphere, on a scale comparable to lesions seen in some of the leukodystrophies such as adrenoleukodys-

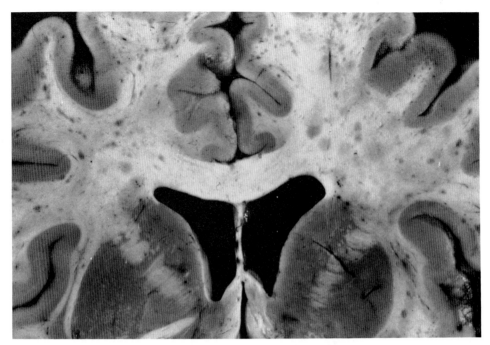

Figure 11.71. Progressive multifocal leukoencephalopathy. In this gross specimen, numerous small punctate lesions are scattered throughout the subcortical white matter. (Courtesy of Dr. D. S. Horoupian.)

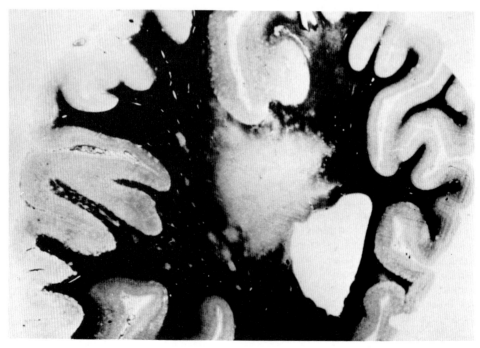

Figure 11.72. Another case of progressive multifocal leukoencephalopathy shows, in this myelin-stained preparation of an occipital lobe, a large area of demyelination with an irregular margin and several small puff-ball areas of myelin loss. (Courtesy of Dr. H. H. Schaumburg.)

trophy (110). Sometimes, cystic dehiscent and subcortical slit-like lesions (the end stages of tissue destruction) are encountered (160).

Microscopic Examination. The small (0.5–2.0 mm) grey lesions most easily seen in the subcortical white matter are believed to represent the early lesions in this condition. These areas are rounded, sometimes centered on vessels, and contain few normal oligodendrocytes, little myelin, preserved axons, gemistocytic astrocytes, and pleomorphic neuroglia. Oil red O-positive granules have been described in the gemistocytic astrocytes. In myelin stains, these lesions (plus many of the larger lesions) have a distinctive "puff-ball" appearance, with the demyelinated margin blending gradually into normal white matter, a feature distinguishing them from those of the multiple sclerosis group (Fig. 11.72). More striking, and indeed pathognomonic for progressive multifocal leukoencephalopathy, are the abnormal oligodendrocytes (type 1 cells) within the lesions (Figs. 11.73 and 11.74). Together with proliferated astrocytes and microglia, these cells lie towards the margin of the lesion and have nuclei up to 15 μm in diameter, thrice that of normal oligodendrocytic nuclei. These nuclei contain a variety of inclusion bodies, including Cowdry type A inclusions. Similar inclusions have been noted in nuclei of astrocytes and unidentified cells within lesions.

The large lesions are usually regarded as late lesion areas which have arisen by the coalescence of multiple early lesions. Along the "dense wall of glial proliferation" (12), abnormal oligodendrocytes predominate. Ultrastructurally, the nuclei of these cells have been shown to contain either rounded (icosahedral) virions, 30–40 nm in diameter, distributed randomly and in crystalline arrays (Figs. 11.76 and 11.77), or elongated virions, 0.1–0.7 μm in length. The virus inclusions appear almost exclusively to be associated with the abnormal oligodendrocytes (160). Also common in late lesions are giant astrocytes (type II cells), which might be multinucleated or have a single nucleus up to 60 μm across, containing profiles suggestive of multipolar mitosis (Fig. 11.75). These large lesions are devoid of myelin, but axons are relatively well preserved, although dehiscent lesions display varying degrees of axonal depletion. Glial macrophages (presumably astroglial) have been identified and contain a variety of cytoplasmic inclusions, as well as pleomorphic lamellar stacks similar to those described as terminal stages of myelin degradation (65).

Small lesions may be found microscopically in the grey matter and involve a reactive astrocytosis, proliferation of rod cells (microglia), some neuronal dropout, and axonal torpedoes. Along capillaries or between nerve cells in grey matter, type I and type II cells are found.

Notably absent from the pathologic tableau of progressive multifocal leukoencephalopathy is a conspicuous inflammatory component, a feature separating it from the multiple sclerosis family. Perivascular collections of small mononuclear cells have been seen in a few cases, but rarely are they a component of major areas of destruction. Whether they are related to the underlying lymphoproliferative disease or to ongoing destruction in the CNS remains to be evaluated.

Pathogenesis

Since an underlying disorder of the reticuloendothelial system and immunosuppression provides the most common backdrop for progressive multifocal leukoencephalopathy, it has been postulated that under these circumstances, a latent viral infection is activated. The agent then finds its way, unimpeded, to the CNS where it crosses the blood-brain barrier and apparently selectively infects oligodendroglia. In mixed cultures of astrocytes and oligodendrocytes, Shein (131) demonstrated selective destruction of oligodendrocytes by SV 40, one of the three papovaviruses linked to this disease. The selective infection of the myelinating cell has been causally linked to the slow depletion of myelin, with local glial cells providing the macrophage population. The absence of a florid inflammatory response is in keeping with such a sequence of events. Many appearances suggestive of neoplasia occur throughout affected areas, and these too may contribute to the inability of the region to support myelin. The relative hyporeactivity of the CNS tissue is probably related to the relentless progression of the condition and immunosuppression.

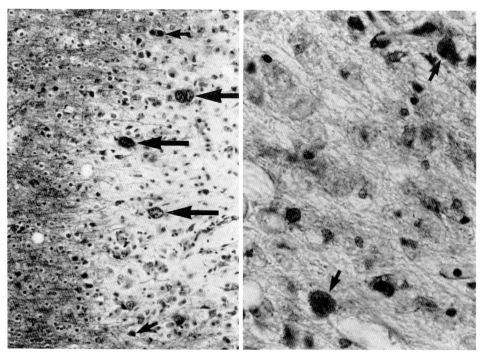

Figure 11.73. *(Left)* Progressive multifocal leukoencephalopathy. The edge of a small demyelinated lesion contains several type II cells (bizarre astrocytes, *large arrows*), and type I cells (atypical oligodendrocytes, *small arrows*). (Original magnification ×120.) (Courtesy of Dr. G. M. Zu Rhein.)
Figure 11.74. *(Right)* Higher magnification of an H&E preparation shows two atypical oligodendroglia *(arrows)* among more normal appearing glial cells. Note the difference in nuclear size. (Original magnification ×400.) (Courtesy of Dr. D. S. Horoupian.)

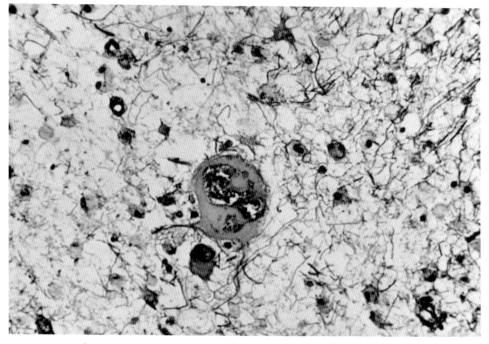

Figure 11.75. A bizarre astrocyte (type II cell) lies at the periphery of a small lesion. Note the peculiar form of the nucleus. (Original magnification ×500.) (Courtesy of Dr. H. H. Schaumburg.)

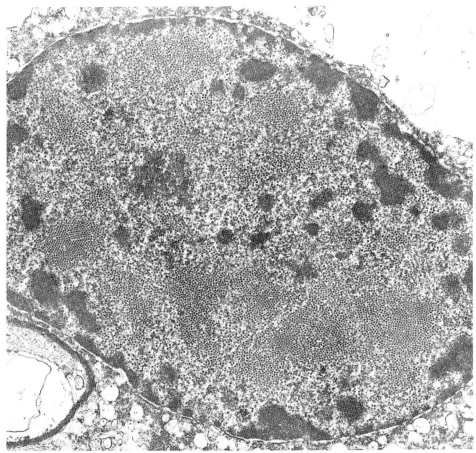

Figure 11.76. Progressive multifocal leukoencephalopathy. This electron micrograph shows the nucleus of an atypical oligodendrocyte containing paracrystalline collections of papovavirus virions. (Original magnification ×15,000.) (Courtesy of Dr. G. M. Zu Rhein.)

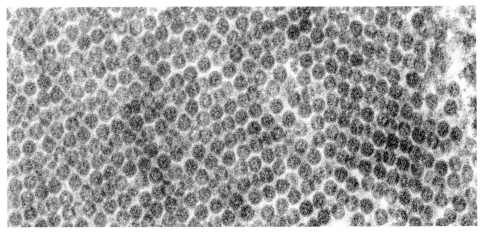

Figure 11.77. Higher magnification of the virions reveals a morphology typical of papovavirus (see text). (Original magnification ×92,000.) (Courtesy of Dr. G. M. Zu Rhein.)

Idiopathic Polyneuritis

History

Idiopathic polyneuritis covers a small group of acquired paralytic diseases of the PNS, usually of short duration, which are linked pathologically by the presence of endoneurial and perivascular infiltrates of hematogenous cells and demyelination. They account for approximately 40% of all adult polyneuropathies. In addition to the most common form, acute idiopathic polyneuritis (better known in North America as the Guillain-Barré syndrome, and in European circles as the Landry-Guillain-Barré syndrome), the term includes recurrent and chronic forms (11, 91, 92, 98). First delineated clinically by Landry in 1859 (67), and later reevaluated by Guillain et al. in 1916 (51), the Guillain-Barré syndrome lacked a generally accepted pathological basis for many years, even though Duménil in 1864 (34) had noted nerve fiber loss in the absence of spinal cord changes. In spite of this, it was held by many that the disease was a spinal cord disorder. The credit for the separation of the peripheral neuropathies from the amyotrophies of spinal cord goes to Leyden in 1880 (69). As more pathologic descriptions emerged, it gradually became evident that the nerve fiber damage was associated with myelin loss, axonal preservation, and endoneurial inflammation (54, 62). Recently reviewed by Prineas (95), "it is now well established that nerve damage in this disease is not a diffuse process but occurs in the form of discrete foci of inflammation scattered throughout the peripheral nervous system, especially in the major nerve plexuses, in the spinal nerves, and close to dorsal root ganglia."

Clinical Parameters

In its acute form, this is a severe paralytic illness of short duration that occurs typically 1–2 weeks after a banal respiratory infection. About half the patients have experienced an infectious bout (which may also be associated with certain well-defined viruses like measles, rubella, varicella zoster, and mumps), and in some, the infection may have been as subtle as low back pain. In a few, a recent vaccination (more often, revaccination) against agents like vaccinia are causal, and in others, the disease may surface after a surgical procedure, presumably a manifestation of surgical stress (9). The most prominent presenting feature of the neurologic syndrome is a rapid onset of flaccid, areflexic weakness which is often symmetrical. Weakness ranges from minimal paresis to total paralysis of all skeletal muscles, necessitating assisted ventilation. Sensory abnormalities occur but are usually less marked than motor signs. Approximately 50% of subjects have cranial nerve involvement, and autonomic abnormalities are seen. CNS findings occur in a small percentage of patients (35, 159). About 5% of patients succumb to the disease, although 20% might require ventilatory assistance. Only 60% display complete recovery. After about 1 week of symptoms, cerebrospinal fluid protein levels are elevated and often remain so after improvement. Transient oligoclonal bands have been described in the cerebrospinal fluid as well as increases in IgM in 25%, IgA in 35%, and IgG in 63% of patients (70). Usually less than 10 mononuclear cells/mm^3 are found in the cerebrospinal fluid.

In its chronic form, idiopathic neuritis may present as an insidiously progressive, stepwise progressive or a relapsing-remitting symmetrical sensorimotor neuropathy (98, 159). Weakness is the most common manifestation of the chronic form. This may be predominantly distal or involve both proximal and distal muscles. Respiratory muscles are involved in about 10% of patients, and cranial nerves in 10–25%. Sensory abnormalities are almost always found, and autonomic and CNS findings occur in up to 10%. Peak disability is from 3 weeks to 2 yr after onset, but is usually reached after 6–12 months. Cerebrospinal fluid proteins are elevated in 90% of patients, and protein levels higher than 100 mg% are quite common. A low grade pleocytosis is seen in 10% of patients, although the cerebrospinal fluid is usually acellular.

Neuropathology

Macroscopic Examination. Almost invariably, abnormalities of the PNS cannot be detected grossly. The CNS also appears normal.

Microscopic Examination. Affected regions of the PNS are focal, randomly scattered, and display edema, infiltration of the endoneurium by small mononuclear cells (lymphocytes), and macrophages

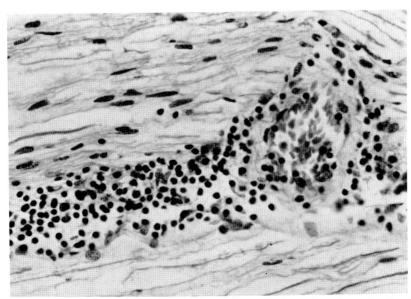

Figure 11.78. Landry-Guillain-Barré syndrome. A longitudinal section through a brachial plexus showing perivascular infiltration by mononuclear cells. Note the cigar-shaped Schwann cell nuclei. H&E stain. (Original magnification ×250.) (From Asbury AK: Hepatic neuropathy. In Dyck PJ, Thomas PK, Lambert EH (eds): *Peripheral Neuropathy*. Philadelphia, WB Saunders, 1975, pp 993–998.)

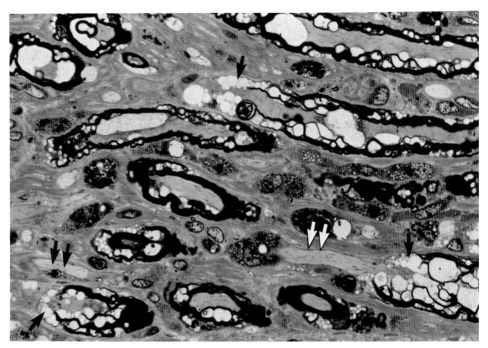

Figure 11.79. A longitudinal section through a spinal nerve root of another case of the Landry-Guillain-Barré syndrome reveals myelin vesiculation (*single arrows*), numerous segments of naked axons (*double arrows*), and many macrophages containing myelin debris. Toluidine blue-stained, 1-μm epoxy section. (Original magnification ×640.)

which tend to be concentrated in perivascular areas (Fig. 11.78). The selectivity of the disease process for the myelin sheath is quite remarkable (Fig. 11.79). The myelin damage is effected by macrophages which, sometimes together with small lymphocytes, enter the Schwann tube of the nerve fiber and phagocytose myelin (Figs. 11.80 and 11.81). During this process, the myelin sheath becomes attenuated and may show dissolution into vesicular arrays, similar to patterns described in autoimmune demyelination (102). Eventually, naked axons remain, invested only by a loose covering of Schwann cell cytoplasm. An infectious agent associated with areas of involvement has not been encountered.

With clinical recovery, PNS remyelination is observed. In severely affected areas of both acute and chronic lesions, some Wallerian degeneration is not unusual. In chronic relapsing cases, supernumerary Schwann cells, episodic demyelination, varying degrees of remyelination, and onion-bulb formation have been documented. The pattern of demyelination is almost indistinguishable from the laboratory analog of this condition, experimental autoimmune (allergic) neuritis (EAN), a demyelinating disease of the PNS induced by sensitization against PNS myelin or its proteins.

Pathogenesis

In the face of striking similarities between idiopathic polyneuritis and EAN, it is difficult to ignore the strong likelihood of autosensitization to PNS myelin in the human condition. The frequent association with an antecedent viral infection or vaccination might raise pathogenetic (as well as causal) questions reminiscent of multiple sclerosis, in which an alteration in the blood-tissue barrier might be effected by the agent. Presumably this might then lead to a cascade of immune-mediated events which are structurally expressed by the loss of myelin. Viral antibodies to members of the herpes family (cytomegalovirus and Epstein-Barr virus) might implicate these agents in the etiology in some cases (159). Cell-mediated immunity and humoral immunity to myelin antigens and circulating immune complexes have been documented in the Guillain-Barré syndrome. While apparently a secondary phenomenon, antibodies to myelin components appear to be important in the dissolution of myelin. This concept has been strengthened by experiments which showed that the local injection of Guillain-Barré serum into rat peripheral

nerve *in situ* induces focal demyelinated lesions (39, 126).

Diphtheritic Neuropathy

History

Included here on the basis of its infectious etiology, it is believed that diphtheritic neuropathy can be traced back to the time of the ancient Greeks, and in historical reviews on the subject, Fisher and Adams (42) and McDonald and Kocen (77) point out that the condition was documented in 1749 in Italy and France, and in 1771 in New York City. According to McDonald and Kocen (77), Bretonneau in 1826, and his pupil Trousseau in 1830 and 1835, were instrumental in the analysis of the clinical and pathological features of both the faucial and extrafaucial forms of the disease. The bacterial nature of the disease was established by Klebs in 1875 and by Loeffler in 1884, which led to the preparation of diphtheria toxin from cultures of *Corynebacterium diphtheriae* by Roux and Yersin in 1889 (77). Almost simultaneously in 1890, Brieger and Fraenkel (18) and Behring and Kitasato (14) published their findings on artificial immunity to the agent and therapy in this condition. Although more or less an eradicated or very rare disease in Western Europe and North America today, diphtheritic neuropathy is still common in many Third World countries. Key among the neuropathologic studies is the detailed study of Fisher and Adams (42). Except for an occasional case report and study on experimental demyelination, diphtheritic neuropathy has slid almost into obscurity.

Clinical Parameters

The principal varieties of diphtheria are faucial, laryngeal, and nasal, and present after an incubation period of 2 to 6 d. Signs consist of malaise, anorexia, irritability, headache, and generalized aching pains. The infected throat may show a greyish-white exudate, and local inflammation is common. This grey-membranous layer was given the name "la diphthérite" by Bretonneau in 1821 (77). In some cases, the signs lead to respiratory failure during the 1st week, and in the 2nd week, cardiac complications develop, often with a fatal outcome. The extrafaucial forms of diphtheria (skin,

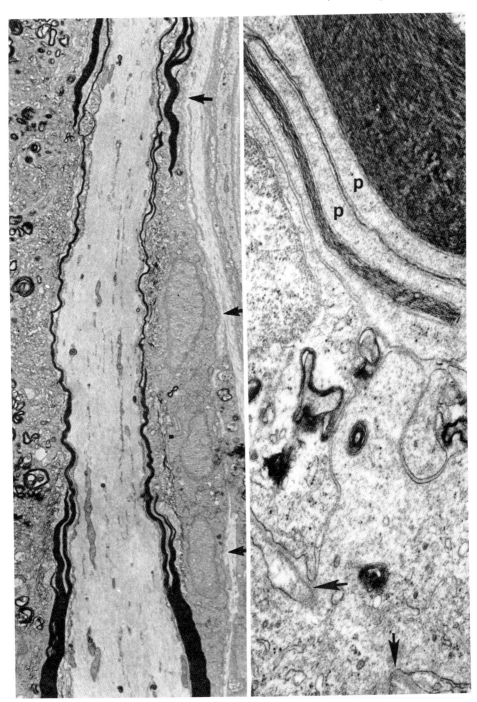

Figure 11.80. *(Left)* Landry-Guillain-Barré syndrome. In this acutely involved peripheral nerve, mononuclear cells, including lymphocytes and macrophages, have penetrated the basal lamina *(arrows)* of a PNS fiber. These cells are associated with severe disruption of a segment of myelin some distance from a node of Ranvier. (Original magnification ×27,000.) (From J. W. Prineas (92).)

Figure 11.81. *(Right)* A macrophage has extended a cytoplasmic process *(arrows)* through a gap in the basal lamina of a Schwann cell surrounding a myelinated PNS axon *(extreme upper right)*. The same cell process has further divided into finger-like processes *(p)* which are separating groups of myelin lamellae from the main sheath. Elsewhere, phagocytosed myelin debris can be seen. (Original magnification ×62,000.) (From J. W. Prineas (92).)

abrasions, umbilicus) lead to similar clinical complications. Early on, there are neurological signs which may be hard to diagnose (e.g., slight alteration in voice, transient reading difficulty) and may go unnoticed, while more definite signs (e.g., peripheral neuropathy) may develop months after the initial bout. Incidence rates vary from group to group. McDonald and Kocen (77) quote the figures of Paley and Truelove who reported in 1948 that 14.7% of their subjects displayed palatal paralysis; 5.7%, accommodation paralysis; 10.6%, peripheral neuropathy; 1.2%, paresis of extraocular muscles; and 0.4%, facial paralysis. Initial neurologic presentations stress a "nasal twang," attributable to a myositis of the palate secondary to local inflammation. Over the next few weeks, palatal and pharyngeal signs predominate, but a generalized peripheral neuropathy, typical of mixed sensory and motor type, does not make its appearance until the 8th to 12th week. Recovery varies with severity, and tendon reflexes are the last sign to return to normal.

Neuropathology

The dominant changes occur within the PNS, and the CNS appears almost not to be involved. Areas of particular vulnerability exist in the PNS, most notably within cranial nerve and spinal nerve ganglia and within the adjacent regions of dorsal, ventral, and mixed spinal nerve roots. The selectivity for ganglionic involvement was well documented experimentally by Waksman (148), where within 1 h postinjection of I^{131}-labeled diphtheria toxin, label was shown in dorsal root ganglia and spinal nerve roots. The outstanding feature of the lesion is the selective demyelination of isolated fibers, with a remarkable degree of axonal sparing. The demyelination is believed to commence paranodally and progress back towards the center of the internode. Myelin phagocytosis is carried out by the Schwann cell, which also shows some reactive changes, such as swelling. Minor axonal abnormalities have been described. Remyelination accompanies recovery, first documented experimentally by Webster et al. (151).

Of significant pathologic relevance is the repeated absence of mention of an inflammatory response within affected nerves. Indeed, accumulations of polymorphonuclear leukocytes, lymphocytes, plasma cells, or macrophages of hematogenous origin have not been reported. Although not described by Fisher and Adams (42), a meningeal reaction has been noted but was not considered to be of pathogenetic significance.

Pathogenesis

It is well known that diphtheria toxin is a potent inhibitor of protein synthesis, and Webster et al. (151) attributed the action of this exotoxin during demyelination to its specific affinity towards membrane systems. Following the release of the exotoxin by the bacterium, the blood-nerve barrier is apparently breached in areas where it is least patent (ganglia, nerve roots), and the toxin then exerts a direct lytic effect upon myelin. Some workers have claimed that the toxin blocks the synthesis of myelin proteolipid and basic protein, whereupon demyelination ensues. The demyelination has not been linked to an autoimmune mechanism.

ANIMAL MODELS

While no spontaneous animal equivalent exists for multiple sclerosis, models are available which are applicable to particular facets of the neuropathology of the condition and other members of the group. Chief among the dissimilarities have been the lack of a chronic, relapsing clinical course, and large, demyelinated plaques with a topography comparable to that of multiple sclerosis. Heaviest laboratory emphasis in recent years has been placed on the autoimmune aspect, although the virologic models of demyelination have been receiving increasing attention with the aid of some naturally occurring conditions.

Experimental Autoimmune Encephalomyelitis

This condition was first introduced in the 1930s as a model for postrabies immunization encephalomyelitis (120). It was subsequently recognized as having striking pathologic similarities to acute multiple sclerosis (40). In its commonest form, EAE is an acute, usually fatal, inflammatory disease of white matter induced in most laboratory species by a single subcutaneous inoculation of an emulsion containing white matter and complete Freund's adjuvant. EAE can also be actively induced with injections containing either purified central myelin, myelin basic protein, or encephalitogenic fragments of the myelin basic protein molecule. In support of EAE being a T-cell-mediated condition, the disease can be transferred passively to a naive recipient with T cells from an actively sensitized animal (with whole CNS tissue or myelin basic protein in complete Freund's adjuvant)—see reviews by Raine (103), Paterson (86), and Weigle (152). Passive transfer of EAE with serum has not been achieved.

Typically, animals sensitized for acute EAE display early signs 12–14 d postinoculation, consisting of abrupt weight loss, floppiness, tail droop, and hind limb paraparesis, signs which progress in about 48 h to quadriparesis and incontinence. Some species (e.g., rat) recover from this acute disease, but in the majority (rabbit, monkey, guinea pig), the condition has a fatal outcome. Neuropathologically, the CNS displays diffuse inflammation of the white matter. Periventricular foci of inflammation are common, diffuse infiltration of the meninges is typical, and there is severe involvement of the spinal cord. Demyelination is a regular component of the lesion and is usually manifested as a narrow rim of naked axons surrounding the perivascular cuffs of inflammatory cells made up of small lymphocytes, large mononuclear cells, and plasma cells (Figs. 11.82 and 11.83). More distinctive in acute EAE is a broad rim of subpial demyelination which underlies the meningeal infiltration, a change reminiscent of acute disseminated encephalomyelitis.

Ultrastructural studies have demonstrated that mononuclear cells leave the bloodstream, enter the CNS parenchyma, and invest myelinated fibers. One of the earliest structural changes in the myelin sheath is a transient uniform increase in the periodicity of the outer lamellae which then rapidly break down into vesicular masses. Cytoplasmic processes from macrophages undermine the outer layers of myelin and strip the sheath from the axon (Fig. 11.84). The process also appears to involve the attachment of myelin droplets to coated pits on the surface of macrophages and the uptake of the debris via a process reminiscent of receptor-mediated endocytosis (Fig. 11.85) (36). Oligodendrocytes survive the period of active demyelination, and in animals which recover, CNS remyelination invariably ensues. On occasion, there is involvement of the PNS in the proximal segments of the spinal nerve roots. Other features of EAE lesions include a mild hypertrophy of fibrillary astrocytes and some Wallerian degeneration (64, 65, 103, 106).

Acute EAE shares little in common with chronic multiple sclerosis (both clinically and pathologically), has some similarities to acute multiple sclerosis, and several features reminiscent of the acute disseminated encephalomyelitides. In some species, the neuropathology of acute EAE is similar to hyperacute EAE (e.g., mouse, monkey). EAE has been heavily explored from the therapeutic standpoint and can be successfully prevented, suppressed, and treated with a variety of compounds including myelin basic protein (107).

Hyperacute EAE is a form with a more severe clinical and pathologic outcome and is associated with the incorporation of pertussis vaccine into the induction protocol (68). Lesions are more destructive than regular acute EAE and contain polymorphonuclear leukocytes, fibrin and extravasated red cells, as well as the usual inflammatory components. The condition is highly reminiscent of acute hemorrhagic leukoencephalopathy, for which it provides a useful model.

Chronic relapsing EAE is a condition most frequently associated with inbred strain 13 guinea pigs (111), although it is also inducible in rats, mice, monkeys, and outbred strains of guinea pigs. The strain 13 model approximates, more closely than any other, the situation in multiple sclerosis. Animals are sensitized as juveniles and develop a delayed-onset EAE, which remits and relapses for up to 4 yr postinoculation. CNS lesions may be grossly visible and large (Fig. 11.86). A wide spectrum of lesion activity is seen, ranging from acutely demyelinating, chronic inactive (Fig. 11.87), chronic active (Fig. 11.88), and remyelinated lesions (Fig. 11.89). Axonal sparing is remarkable, and perivascular

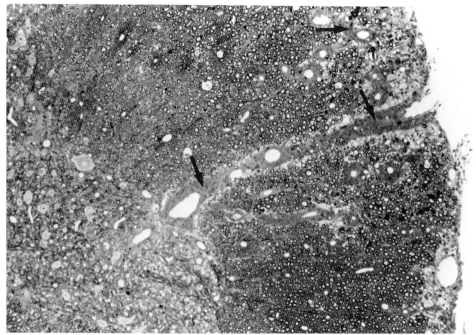

Figure 11.82. Experimental autoimmune (allergic) encephalomyelitis (EAE). A transverse section of the spinal cord of a guinea pig affected with EAE (caused by an injection of guinea pig spinal cord in adjuvant) shows meningeal and perivascular inflammation (*arrows*) with accompanying demyelination. Note the similarities between EAE and the acute disseminated encephalomyelitides (Figs. 11.60–11.62). Toluidine blue-stained, 1-μm epoxy section. (Original magnification ×100.)

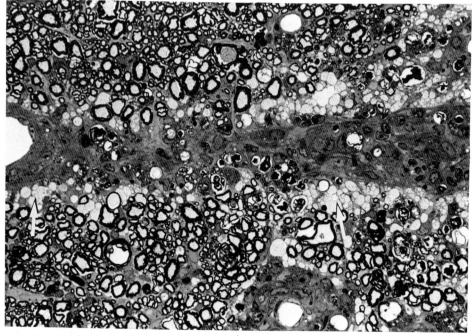

Figure 11.83. Higher magnification of Figure 11.82, to show the clear association between the demyelinated axons (*arrows*) and the perivascular infiltrates. (Original magnification ×400.)

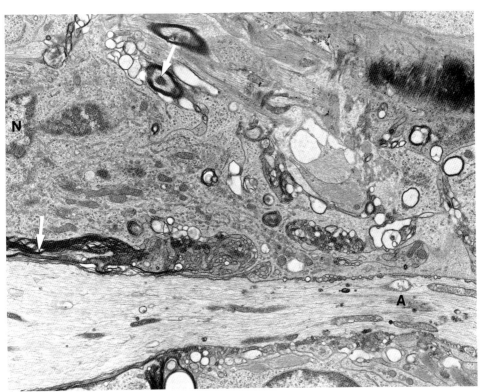

Figure 11.84. Acute EAE. An electron micrograph from the spinal cord of a rabbit with acute EAE shows processes from a macrophage (nucleus at *N*) encircling and lifting myelin from two nearby nerve fibers (*arrows*) by a process of vesiculation. The denuded segment of the lower axon (*A*) displays some decrease in diameter. (Original magnification ×9,000.)

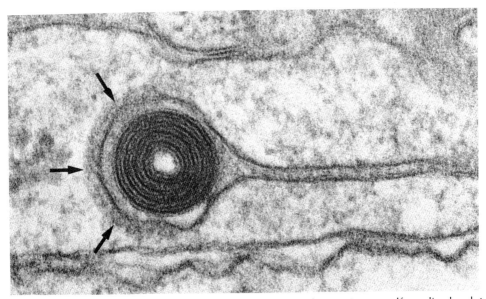

Figure 11.85. Sometimes macrophages engaged in myelin destruction engulf myelin droplets by a process similar to receptor-mediated endocytosis. Here a myelin droplet lies at the end of a crypt within a macrophage where it is closely associated with a coated pit (*arrows*). (Original magnification ×145,000.)

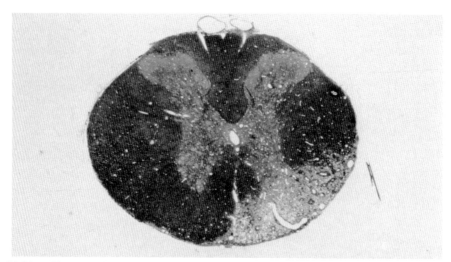

Figure 11.86. Chronic relapsing EAE. A section of thoracic spinal cord from a strain 13 guinea pig with chronic relapsing EAE for 5 months displays a large, chronically demyelinated plaque (*lower right*). Toluidine blue-stained, 1-μm epoxy section. (Original magnification ×22.)

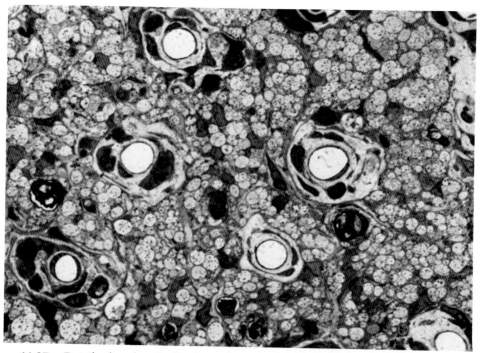

Figure 11.87. Detail of a chronically demyelinated plaque. Note the many naked axons, the fibrotic blood vessels, and the fibrillary gliosis—appearances reminiscent of chronic multiple sclerosis (c.f. Figs. 11.23 and 11.32). (Original magnification ×640.)

cuffing correlates with clinical activity. Plaques tend to be concentrated in the spinal cord, but cerebral lesions are always present. Gliosis, vascular fibrosis, and Schwann cell invasion of chronically de-myelinated areas of the CNS are constant features (115).

Therapeutic trials with myelin-derived compounds have demonstrated that the myelin damage is reversible and accompa-

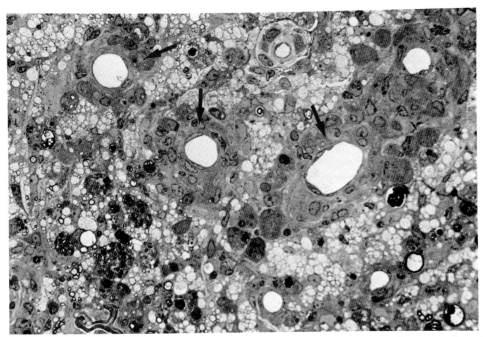

Figure 11.88. An active lesion from a guinea pig with chronic relapsing EAE for 6 months, where the edge of a chronically demyelinated lesion displays recent inflammation (*arrows*). Ongoing myelin breakdown is evident to the lower left. Toluidine blue-stained, 1-μm epoxy section. (Original magnification ×400.)

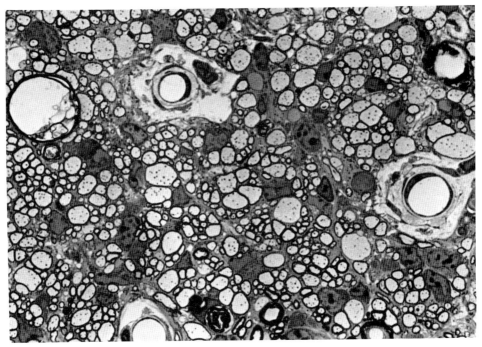

Figure 11.89. A silent lesion from a guinea pig with chronic relapsing EAE shows extensive CNS remyelination and a moderate increase in oligodendroglial and astroglial cells. Blood vessels show fibrotic changes. Toluidine blue-stained, 1-μm epoxy section. (Original magnification ×1,000.)

nied by oligodendroglial proliferation (116, 139). Such studies have led to the rationale that combinations of myelin antigens might have relevance in the causation, and perhaps treatment, of autoimmune demyelination (112).

Immunocytochemical studies on lymphocyte dynamics in acute EAE have demonstrated that prior to the onset of signs, T cells enter the CNS and migrate to the white matter parenchyma. As signs develop, B cells and macrophages appear within the CNS and remain concentrated in perivascular areas. These observations suggest that T and B cells have different mobilities within the CNS (136). Similar studies on T and B cells in chronic relapsing EAE have shown that with each relapse, a fresh influx of T cells into the CNS parenchyma is seen, but with remission most inflammatory cells, except for a few T cells, tend to disappear from the CNS (137). In strain 13 guinea pigs, treatment of chronic relapsing EAE with myelin components results in the almost total absence of T and B cells from the CNS (139).

Experimental Autoimmune Neuritis

First described by Waksman and Adams (149), EAN can be induced in a variety of species by inocula containing either whole peripheral nerve, purified PNS myelin, or the P2 protein of PNS myelin in complete Freund's adjuvant. In most cases, EAN is an acute fatal disease, but some species (e.g., rat) recover from the acute disease. The neuropathology of EAN is strikingly similar to that of idiopathic neuritis, for which it serves as a major experimental analog. With the development of signs (hind limb paralysis) 2–3 weeks postinoculation, small lymphocytes, large mononuclear cells, plasma cells, macrophages, and demyelination appear within the PNS, particularly in radicular regions and ganglia (Figs. 11.90 and 11.91). Myelin stripping by invading macrophages is the predominant change (63) (Figs. 11.92–11.94). Demyelinated axons are rarely damaged and display rapid and total remyelination with clinical recovery. EAN can be therapeutically manipulated with a variety of drugs and myelin preparations.

The pathogenesis of EAN is presumed to be T-cell mediated, and although systemic passive transfer of EAN has not been achieved with lymphocytes, local injection of lymphocytes into the PNS causes demyelination. Injection of serum from animals with EAN into nerve *in situ* also results in demyelination (125).

Canine Distemper Encephalomyelitis

Canine distemper is a naturally occurring, virus-induced demyelinating disease of the CNS of dogs which have not been vaccinated or have lost their immunity to the virus. Distemper encephalomyelitis also occurs in ferrets. The virus is species-specific. Reports exist in the literature which have linked canine distemper encephalomyelitis to multiple sclerosis. The virus causing this canine disease is a paramyxovirus (8), a close relative of measles virus, which produces a systemic infection which precedes the neurologic signs by 1–2 weeks. The disease affects both young and old dogs and can be acute and fatal, or chronic and relapsing. CNS lesions may be visible grossly as large grey areas, sometimes at the floor of the fourth ventricle. Most plaques are inflammatory and demyelinative, although some show severe degeneration and axonal loss. Ultrastructurally, the demyelination is associated with macrophages (Figs. 11.95 and 11.96). Viral nucleocapsids are present within lesions (157) (Fig. 11.97). It has been proposed that the myelin loss may be antibody-mediated, and it has been shown that the virus displays no tropism for any particular cell type within the nervous system, being observed within neurons, astrocytes, and oligodendrocytes (103).

Lesion pathogenesis remains speculative. It is generally believed that the CNS infection induces a local immune response within the CNS and that the observed myelin degeneration is the result of nonspecific myelinotoxic side effects of the products of activated lymphocytes (lymphokines). Selective infection of oligodendroglia or myelin has not been demonstrated. The viral infection has also been associated with an acute lymphopenia and antibodies which have demyelinating properties *in vitro*.

Visna

A naturally occurring disease among Icelandic sheep until eradicated by an inten-

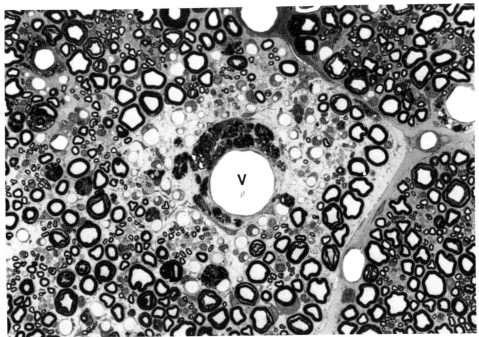

Figure 11.90. Experimental autoimmune neuritis (EAN). A dorsal spinal nerve root from a rabbit with acute EAN displays a ring of demyelinated PNS fibers around a vessel (V) rimmed by macrophages. Toluidine blue-stained, 1-μm epoxy section. (Original magnification ×400.)

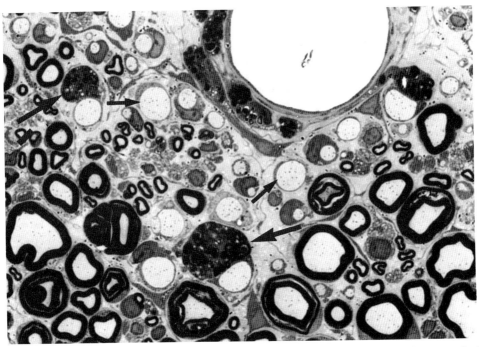

Figure 11.91. Detail from Figure 11.90. Note the naked PNS axons (*small arrows*), some of which are still associated with macrophages containing myelin debris (*large arrows*). (Original magnification ×1,000.)

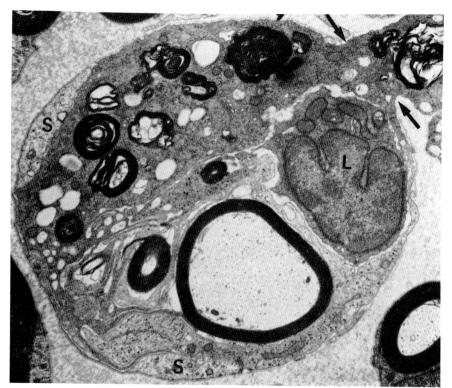

Figure 11.92. Macrophages and a lymphocyte (*L*) have entered the basal lamina of a PNS fiber, pushing the Schwann cell cytoplasm (*S*) to the periphery. One macrophage contains myelin debris and extends a process through a gap in the basal lamina (*arrows*). (Original magnification ×8,400.) (From C. S. Raine (106).)

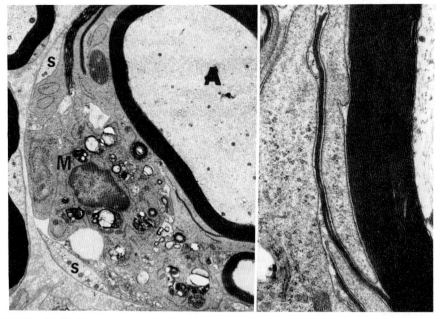

Figure 11.93. (*Left*) Acute EAN—rabbit sciatic nerve. A macrophage has entered this PNS fiber, pushed the Schwann cell cytoplasm (*S*) aside, and extended processes between several layers of myelin around the axon (*A*). (Original magnification ×4,700.) (From C. S. Raine (106).)

Figure 11.94. (*Right*) Detail from Figure 11.93. Note how the process from the macrophage has separated several layers of myelin from the rest of the myelin sheath. (From C. S. Raine (106).)

540

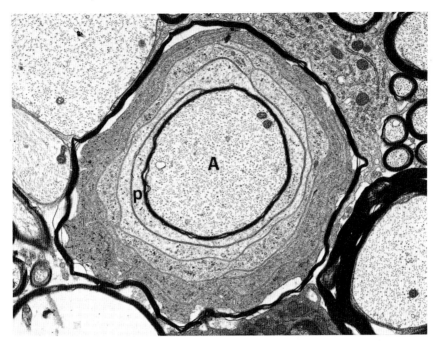

Figure 11.95. Chronic canine distemper encephalomyelitis (CDE). A CNS fiber (axon at *A*) from the spinal cord of a dog with natural CDE for 3 months has its myelin sheath invaded by processes from macrophages, one of which (*p*) is stripping a single layer of myelin from the rest of the sheath. Naked axons lie to the upper left. (Original magnification ×10,200.) (From C. S. Raine (106).)

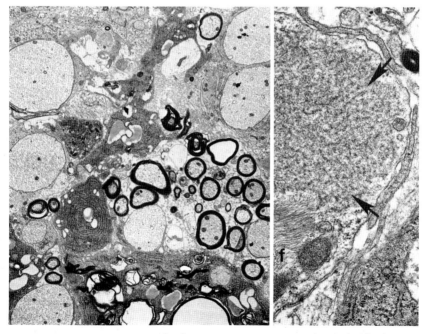

Figure 11.96. (*Left*) Chronic CDE, similar history to Figure 11.95. Several naked axons are seen between normal fibers and myelin-laden macrophages. (Original magnification ×4,800.) (From C. S. Raine (106).)

Figure 11.97. (*Right*) Chronic CDE. Viral nucleocapsid is commonly located in CDE lesions, usually within astrocytes. Here, a group of intracytoplasmic distemper nucleocapsids is seen (*arrows*) within a process from a fibrous astrocyte containing glial filaments (*f*). (Original magnification ×22,000.) (From C. S. Raine (106).)

sive extermination program, visna exists today only as a laboratory model. The disease presents as a paralytic encephalomyelitis, with lesions of the CNS being manifested neuropathologically sometimes as necrotic, degenerative areas. However, some inflammatory demyelinating lesions are seen. There is a predilection for subependymal and subpial involvement. The disease apparently progresses in the presence of an increase in spinal fluid protein and serum antibody, and since the virus (a retrovirus) buds from cell membranes, it has been suggested that antigen-antibody reactions might occur on glial cell membranes, leading to cellular destruction and myelin loss (61). More recent studies on visna have reconfirmed the propensity for demyelination to occur (45), but large scale demyelinated plaques are not a feature.

Coonhound Paralysis

In this condition, there is inflammatory involvement of the PNS leading to demyelination. The disease occurs in dogs (particularly the coonhound breed), which are bitten by a raccoon (28). The cause is probably viral. PNS lesions bear striking resemblances to EAN and the Guillain-Barré syndrome. After an onset of limb weakness, the nerve roots and distal peripheral nerves display inflammation and segmental demyelination. The present consensus is that the disease results from a combination of viral and autoimmune-related phenomena. Virus has not been observed within the PNS.

Marek's Disease

Marek's disease poses a severe economic problem to poultry breeders in North America since it is a major cause of death among chickens. Marek's disease is ostensibly a malignant lymphomatous condition, etiologically related to infection by a herpes virus, but as a secondary complication, a peripheral neuropathy might develop. This neurological condition is typified neuropathologically by the invasion of the PNS by inflammatory cells which seek out and destroy myelin in a manner similar to that reported in EAN and the Guillain-Barré syndrome (100). These appearances might imply a role for autoimmunity, but whether cross-reactivity between viral and myelin antigen occurs, or whether the myelin damage occurs as a nonspecific, bystander event, remains to be proven. Virus has not been observed within the PNS.

Mouse Hepatitis Virus Encephalomyelitis

This disease occurs in mice and shares several neuropathologic features with acute disseminated encephalomyelitis and progressive multifocal leukoencephalopathy. The causative agent, a neurotropic coronavirus (JHM strain of mouse hepatitis virus), was isolated originally from mouse brain tissue (24). This agent is a major problem among mouse colonies and, like Sendai virus (paramyxovirus), is a major bain to the immunologist and geneticist. Selective damage of CNS myelin in this condition was first noted by Waksman and Adams (150), and later defined ultrastructurally by Lampert et al. (66) and Fleury et al. (43). Within lesions, virions are easily identified by several techniques, and there appears to be selective involvement of oligodendrocytes. While mononuclear cells are the effectors of demyelination, an inflammatory response is not always prominent. The observed demyelination has been reported to occur even in immunosuppressed animals (61), thereby ruling out a central role for cell-mediated immunity in lesion development. A delayed onset form of the disease has also been described (80).

Theiler's Virus Encephalomyelitis

Belonging to the enteroviruses, Theiler's virus causes an enteric disease of mice, which sometimes leads to a spontaneous flaccid paralysis as a result of CNS involvement (29, 30, 85). The CNS displays demyelination and inflammation and a pathology similar to canine distemper, albeit to a lesser degree. The virus persists in the CNS. Immunosuppression studies have shown that lesion growth depends upon the presence of an inflammatory response (71).

Diphtheritic Neuropathy

Included only for the sake of completeness, experimental diphtheritic neuropathy is a model of limited relevance to the multiple sclerosis field (being more a model of toxin-induced demyelination) and has proven more useful in physiologic investigations on nerve condition. It can be induced in a number of species by injection of either crude toxoid or incompletely neutralized toxin from *C. diphtheriae*. About 1 week after systemic injection, animals show limb weakness and may die due to respiratory involvement. PNS tissue displays marked demyelinative changes (151, 154). Schwann cells are the major myelin phagocytes, and inflammation is not a feature. The CNS is usually not involved, but demyelinated lesions can be induced in the CNS by infusion of toxin (156). This procedure also leads to CNS and PNS remyelination.

CONCLUSIONS

Thus, the demyelinating diseases of man are an heterogeneous group with, as a common denominator, an acquired etiology of suspected or proven viral association and are epitomized by multiple sclerosis. In most cases, circumstantial evidence for a role for both virus and an autoimmune process against myelin components is implicated, but the specificity of the evidence is frequently equivocal, since similar immunologic phenomena occur ubiquitously in other conditions where white matter destruction is a feature (stroke, systemic degenerative disorders). The availability of sophisticated immunologic markers (monoclonal antibodies), virus isolation techniques, assays for antibody activity, methods to identify different T cell subsets, neuropathologic technology, and a growing battery of good laboratory models, have made significant inroads into problems which, until about 20 yr ago, had witnessed only minor advances since their original delineation more than a century earlier.

ACKNOWLEDGMENTS

I thank my many colleagues at the Albert Einstein College of Medicine, Bronx, New York, for their collaboration, particularly Drs. Robert D. Terry, Asao Hirano, Harry M. Zimmerman, John W. Prineas, Wayne Moore, Dikran S. Horoupian, and Herbert H. Schaumburg, Murray B. Bornstein, and Labe C. Scheinberg. I am especially grateful to Dr. Ute Traugott for her collaboration in the area of neuroimmunology. My technical team of Everett Swanson, Miriam Pakingan, and Howard Finch have proven fundamental to my work, as has the assistance of my faithful secretary, Mary Palumbo. Agnes Geoghan provided invaluable assistance in the preparation of the manuscript.

This work was supported in part by USPHS grants NS08952, NS11920, and NS07098, and by grant RG 1001-D-4 from the National Multiple Sclerosis Society.

The following investigators are thanked for their permission to reproduce illustrations. Where appropriate, the original source is acknowledged, with permission, in the legend. Dr. Stanley Aronson (Brown University), Figure 11.3; Dr. William Schoene (Harvard University), Figure 11.4*A* and *B*; Dr. James Powers (Medical University of South Carolina), Figure 11.7; Elsevier Publishing Company, Amsterdam, Figures 11.8, 11.9, 11.12, 11.18, and 11.34; Dr. Robert D. Terry (Albert Einstein College of Medicine), Figures 11.13, 11.47, and 11.65; Dr. Yoshio Takei (Emory University), Figures 11.53 and 11.54; Dr. Harry M. Zimmerman (Albert Einstein College of Medicine), Figures 11.55–11.57; Dr. Peter W. Lampert (University of California, San Diego), Figure 11.58; Dr. Asao Hirano (Albert Einstein College of Medicine), Figure 11.60; Dr. Nancy Peress (Northport Veterans Administration Hospital, and State University of New York, Stony Brook), Figures 11.61–11.64; Dr. Julio Garcia (University of Alabama), Figure 11.66; Dr. G. R. Wayne Moore (Albert Einstein College of Medicine) and Dr. Sash Chittal (Memorial University of Newfoundland, Canada), Figure 11.69; Dr. Dikran S. Horoupian (Albert Einstein College of Medicine), Figures 11.71 and 11.74; Dr. Herbert H. Schaumburg (Albert Einstein College of Medicine), Figures 11.72 and 11.75; Dr. Gabrielle Zu Rhein (University of Wisconsin), Figures 11.73, 11.76, and 11.77; Dr. Arthur K. Asbury (University of Pennsylvania), Figure 11.78; and Dr. John W. Prineas (New Jersey College of Medicine & Dentistry), Figures 11.80 and 11.81.

References

1. Adams CWM: The general pathology of multiple sclerosis: morphological and chemical aspects of the lesions. In Hallpike JF, Adams CWM, Tourtellotte WW (eds): *Multiple Sclerosis: Pathology, Diagnosis, and Management.* London, Chapman & Hall, 1983.
2. Adams JM, et al: Inclusion bodies in measles encephali-

tis. *J Am Med Assoc* 195:290, 1966.

3. Adams RD: A comparison of the morphology of the human demyelinative disease and experimental "allergic" and encephalomyelitis. In Kies MW, Alvord EC (eds): *"Allergic" Encephalomyelitis*. Springfield, IL, Charles C Thomas, 1959.

4. Adams RD, Kubik CS: The morbid anatomy of the demyelinative diseases. *Am J Med* 12:510, 1952.

5. Adams RD, Sidman RL: Demyelinative diseases. In Adams RD, Sidman RL (eds): *Introduction to Neuropathology*. New York, McGraw-Hill, 1968.

6. Adams RD, Victor M: Multiple sclerosis and allied demyelinative diseases. In Adams RD, Victor M (eds): *Principles of Neurology*. New York, McGraw-Hill, 1977.

7. Albutt TC: On the ophthalmoscopic signs of spinal disease. *Lancet* 1:76, 1870.

8. Appel MJG, Gillespie JH: Canine distemper virus. *Virol Monogr* 11:1, 1972.

9. Arnason BGW: Inflammatory polyradiculoneuropathies. In Dyck PJ, Thomas PK, Lambert EH (eds): *Peripheral Neuropathy*. Philadelphia, WB Saunders, 1975, vol 2.

10. Arnason BGW, et al: Histocompatibility types and measles antibodies in multiple sclerosis and optic neuritis. *J Neurol Sci* 22:419, 1974.

11. Asbury AK, et al: The inflammatory lesion in idiopathic polyneuritis. Its role in pathogenesis. *Medicine* 48:173, 1969.

12. Aström KE, et al: Progressive multifocal leukoencephalopathy. *Brain* 81:93, 1958.

13. Balo J: Encephalitis periaxialis concentrica. *Arch Neurol Psychiatry (Chicago)* 19:242, 1928.

14. Behring E, Kitasato S: Ueber das Zustandekommen der Diphtherie-Immunität und der Tetanus-Immunität bei Thieren. *Deutsch Med Wochenschr* 16:1113, 1890.

15. Berard-Badier M, et al: Comparative clinicopathological study of one early and two late cases of measles encephalitis (with an electroencephalographic study of one case). In Van Bogaert L, Rademeker J, Hozay J, Lowenthal A (eds): *Encephalitides*. Amsterdam, Elsevier, 1961.

16. Bourneville D, Guerard L: *De la Sclérose en Plaques Disseminées*. Paris, A. Delaye, 1869.

17. Brain WR: Critical review: Disseminated sclerosis. *Q J Med* 22:343, 1930.

18. Brieger L, Fraenkel C: Untersuchungen über Bacteriengifte. *Berl Klin Wochenschr* 24:241, 1890.

19. Brosnan CF, et al: Proteinase inhibitors suppress experimental allergic encephalomyelitis. *Nature* 285:235, 1980.

20. Carswell R: *Pathological Anatomy: Illustrations on the Elementary Forms of Disease*. London, Longman, Orme, Brown, Greene, and Longman, 1838.

21. Cavanagh JB, et al: Cerebral demyelination associated with disorders of the reticuloendothelial system. *Lancet* 2:525, 1959.

22. Charcot J-M: Seance du 14 mars. *C R Soc Biol (Paris)* 20:13, 1868.

23. Charcot J-M: Histologie de la sclérose en plaques. *Gaz Hop (Paris)* 41:554, 1868.

24. Cheever FS, et al: A murine virus (JHM) causing disseminated encephalomyelitis with extensive destruction of myelin. I. Isolation and biological properties of the virus. *J Exp Med* 90:181, 1949.

25. Cloys De, Netsky MG: Neuromyelitis optica. In Vinken PJ, Bruyn GW (eds): *Handbook of Clinical Neurology*. Amsterdam, North-Holland, 1970, vol 9.

26. Courville CB: Concentric sclerosis. In Vinken PJ, Bruyn GW (eds): *Handbook of Clinical Neurology*. Amsterdam, North-Holland, 1970, vol 9.

27. Cruveilhier J: *Anatomie Pathologique du Corps Humain*. Paris, JB Bailliere, 1829–1842, vol 2.

28. Cummings JF, Haas DC: Coonhound paralysis: an acute idiopathic polyradiculoneuritis in dogs resembling the Landry-Guillain-Barré syndrome. *J Neurol Sci* 4:51, 1967.

29. Dal Canto MC, Lipton H: Primary demyelination in Theiler's virus infection: an ultrastructural study. *Lab Invest* 33:626, 1975.

30. Dal Canto MC, Lipton HL: Recurrent demyelination in chronic cerebral nervous system infection produced by Theiler's murine encephalomyelitis virus. *J Neurol Sci* 42:391, 1979.

31. Dawson JW: The histology of disseminated sclerosis. *Trans R Soc Edinb* 50:517, 1916.

32. Dejong RN: Multiple sclerosis: History, definition and general considerations. In Vinken PJ, Bruyn (eds): *Handbook of Clinical Neurology*. Amsterdam, North-Holland, 1970, vol 9.

33. Devic E: Myelite subaigue compliquée de nevrite optique (abstr). *Bull Med (Paris)* 8:1033, 1894.

34. Duménil L: Paralysie periphérique du mouvement et du sentiment portant sur les quatres membres. Atrophie des remeaux nerveaux des parties paralysées. *Gaz Hebdom Med Chir* 1:203, 1864.

35. Dyck PJ, et al: Chronic inflammatory polyradiculoneuropathy. *Mayo Clin Proc* 50:621, 1975.

36. Epstein LG, et al: Attachment of myelin to coated pits on macrophages in experimental allergic encephalomyelitis. *J Neurol Sci* 6:341, 1983.

37. Esiri MM, et al: Application of an immunoperoxidase method to a study of the central nervous system: preliminary findings in a study of human formalin-fixed material. *Neuropathol Appl Neurobiol* 2:233, 1976.

38. Eylar EH: Experimental allergic encephalomyelitis and multiple sclerosis. In Wolfram F, Ellison GW, Stevens JG, Andrews JM (eds): *Multiple Sclerosis: Immunology, Virology and Ultrastructure*. New York, Academic Press, 1972.

39. Feasby TE, et al: Passive transfer of demyelinating activity in Guillain-Barré polyneuropathy. *Neurology* 30:363, 1980.

40. Ferraro A: Allergic brain changes in post-scarlatinal encephalitis. *J Neuropathol Exp Neurol* 3:239, 1944.

41. Ferraro A, Jervis G: Experimental disseminated encephalopathy in the monkey. *Arch Neurol Psychiatry (Chicago)* 43:195, 1940.

42. Fisher CM, Adams RD: Diphtheritic polyneuritis - a pathological study. *J Neuropathol Exp Neurol* 15:243, 1956.

43. Fleury HJ, et al: Further ultrastructural observations of virus morphogenesis and myelin pathology in JHM virus encephalomyelitis. *Neuropathol Appl Neurobiol* 6:165, 1980.

44. Frerichs F: Über Hirnsklerose. *Haeser's Arch* 10:334, 1849.

45. Georgsson G, et al: Primary demyelination in Visna. *Acta Neuropathol* 57:171, 1982.

46. Ghatak N, et al: Remyelination in multiple sclerosis with peripheral type myelin. *Arch Neurol* 29:262, 1973.

47. Glanzmann E: Die nervösen Komplikationen der Varizellen, Variola und Vakzine. *Schweiz Med Wochenschr* 57:145, 1927.

48. Greenfield JG, King LS: Observations on the histopathology of the cerebral lesions in disseminated sclerosis. *Brain* 59:445, 1936.

49. Greenfield JG, Norman RM: Demyelinating diseases. In Blackwood W, McMenemey WH, Meyer M, Norman RM, Russell DS (eds): *Greenfield's Neuropathology*. ed 2. London, Arnold, 1971.

50. Grundke-Iqbal I, Bornstein MB: Multiple sclerosis: serum gamma globulin and demyelination in organ cultures. *Neurology* 30:749, 1980.

51. Guillain G, et al: Sur un syndrome de radiculo-nevrite avec hyperalbuminose du liquide cephalo-rachidien sans reaction cellulaire. Remarques sur les caracteres cliniques et graphiques de reflexes tendineux. *Bull Soc Med Hop Paris* 40:1462, 1916.

52. Hallervorden J, Spatz H: Über die konzentrische Sklerose und die physikalisch-chemischen Faktoren bei der Ausbreitung von Entmarkungsprozessen. *Arch Psychiatr*

Nervenkr 98:641, 1933.

53. Hallpike JF, Adams CMW, Tourtellotte WW (eds): *Multiple Sclerosis: Pathology, Diagnosis, and Management.* London, Chapman & Hall, 1983.

54. Haymaker W, Kernohan JW: The Landry-Guillain-Barré syndrome. A clinico-pathologic report of fifty fatal cases and a critique of the literature. *Medicine* 28:59, 1949.

55. Hurst EW: The effects of the injection of normal brain emulsion into rabbits, with special reference to the aetiology of the paralytic accidents of antirabic treatment. *J Hyg (Camb)* 32:33, 1932.

56. Hurst EW: Acute hemorrhagic leucoencephalitis: a previously undefined entity. *Med J Aust* 2:1, 1941.

57. Ibrahim MZM, Adams CWM: The relationship between enzyme activity and neuroglia in plaques of multiple sclerosis. *J Neurol Neurosurg Psychiatry* 26:101, 1963.

58. Ibrahim MZM, Adams CWM: The relationship between enzyme activity and neuroglia in early plaques of multiple sclerosis. *J Pathol Bacteriol* 90:239, 1965.

59. Itoyama Y, et al: Immunocytochemical observations on the distribution of myelin-associated glycoprotein and myelin basic protein in multiple sclerosis lesions. *Ann Neurol* 7:167, 1980.

60. Johnson RT: The possible viral etiology of multiple sclerosis. In Friedlander WS (ed): *Current Reviews. Advances in Neurology.* New York, Raven Press, 1975, vol 13.

61. Johnson RT, Weiner LP: The role of viral infections in demyelinating diseases. In Wolfgram F, Ellison GW, Stevens JG, and Andrews JM (eds): *Multiple Sclerosis: Immunology, Virology and Ultrastructure.* New York, Academic Press, 1972.

62. Krücke W: Die primär-entzündliche Polyneuritis unbekannter Ursache. In Lubarsch O, Henke F, Rössle G (eds): *Erkrankungen der peripheren Nerven. Handbuch der speziellen pathologischen Anatomie und Histologie.* Berlin, Springer Verlag, 1955, part 5, vol 13.

63. Lampert PW: Mechanism of demyelination in experimental allergic neuritis. Electron microscopic studies. *Lab Invest* 20:127, 1969.

64. Lampert PW: Autoimmune and virus-induced demyelinating diseases. *Am J Pathol* 91:176, 1978.

65. Lampert PW: Fine structure of the demyelinating process. In Hallpike JF, Adams CWM, Tourtellotte WW (eds): *Multiple Sclerosis: Pathology, Diagnosis, and Management.* London, Chapman & Hall, 1983.

66. Lampert PW, et al: Mechanism of demyelination in JHM virus encephalomyelitis. *Acta Neuropathol* 24:76, 1973.

67. Landry O: Note sur la paralysie ascendante aigue. *Gaz Hebdom Med Chir* 6:472, 1859.

68. Levine S, Wenk EJ: A hyperacute form of allergic encephalomyelitis. *Am J Pathol* 47:61, 1965.

69. Leyden E: Ueber Poliomyelitis und Neuritis. *Z Klin Med* 1:387, 1880.

70. Link H, et al: Pleocytosis and immunoglobulin changes in cerebrospinal fluid and herpes virus serology in patients with Guillain-Barré syndrome. *J Clin Microbiol* 9:305, 1979.

71. Lipton HL, Dal Canto MC: Theiler's virus-induced demyelination: prevention by immunosuppression. *Science* 192:62, 1976.

72. Lumsden CE: The clinical pathology of multiple sclerosis. In McAlpine D, Compston ND, Lumsden CE (eds): *Multiple Sclerosis.* Edinburgh, Livingstone, 1955.

73. Lumsden CE: The neuropathology of multiple sclerosis. In Vinken PJ, Bruyn GW (eds): *Handbook of Clinical Neurology.* Amsterdam, North-Holland, 1970, vol 9.

74. Marie P: Sclérose en plaques et maladies infectieuses. *Prog Med (Paris)* 12:287, 1884.

75. Martins A, et al: Acute hemorrhagic leukoencephalitis (Hurst) with concurrent primary herpes simplex infection. *J Neurol Neurosurg Psychiatry* 27:493, 1964.

76. McAlpine D, et al: *Multiple Sclerosis. A Reappraisal.* Edinburgh, Churchill Livingstone, 1972.

77. McDonald WI, Kocen RS: Diphtheritic neuropathy. In Dyck PJ, Thomas PK, Lambert EH (eds): *Peripheral Neuropathy.* Philadelphia, WB Saunders, 1975, vol 2.

78. McFarlin DE, McFarland HF: Multiple sclerosis. *N Engl J Med* 307:1183, 307:1246, 1982.

79. Medaer R: Does the history of multiple sclerosis go back as far as the 14th century? *Acta Neurol Scand* 60:189, 1979.

80. ter Meulen V, Stephenson JR: The possible role of viral infections in multiple sclerosis and other related demyelinating diseases. In Hallpike JF, Adams CWM, Tourtellotte WW (eds): *Multiple Sclerosis: Pathology, Diagnosis, and Management.* London, Chapman & Hall, 1983.

81. ter Meulen V, et al: Isolation of infectious measles virus in measles encephalitis. *Lancet* 2:1172, 1972.

82. Miller HG, Evans MJ: Prognosis in acute disseminated encephalomyelitis; with a note on neuromyelitis optica. *Q J Med* 22:347, 1953.

83. Miller HG, et al: Para-infectious encephalomyelitis and related syndromes. A critical review of the neurological complications of certain specific fevers. *Q J Med* 25:427, 1956.

84. Moxon D: Case of insular sclerosis of brain and spinal cord. *Lancet* 1:236, 1873.

85. Olitsky PK: Viral effect produced by intestinal contents of normal mice and of those having spontaneous encephalomyelitis. *Proc Soc Exp Biol Med* 72:434, 1939.

86. Paterson PY: Autoimmune neurological diseases: experimental animal systems and implications for multiple sclerosis. In Talal N (ed): *Autoimmunity: Genetic, Immunologic, Virologic, and Clinical Aspects.* New York, Academic Press, 1977.

87. Perdrau JR: The histology of post-vaccinal encephalitis. *J Pathol Bacteriol* 31:17, 1928.

88. Peters A, et al (eds): *The Fine Structure of the Nervous System: The Cells and Their Processes.* Philadelphia, WB Saunders, 1976.

89. Poser C: Diffuse-disseminated sclerosis in the adult. *J Neuropathol Exp Neurol* 16:61, 1957.

90. Poser CM: Diseases of the myelin sheath. In Baker AB, Baker CH (eds): *Clinical Neurology.* New York, Harper & Row, 1979, vol 2.

91. Prineas JW: Polyneuropathies of undetermined cause. *Acta Neurol Scand* 46:7, 1970.

92. Prineas JW: Acute idiopathic polyneuritis. An electron microscope study. *Lab Invest* 26:134, 1972.

93. Prineas JW: Paramyxovirus-like particles in acute lesions in multiple sclerosis. In Shiraki H, Yonezawa T, Kuroiwa Y (eds): *The Aetiology and Pathogenesis of the Demyelinating Diseases.* Tokyo, Japan Science Press, 1975.

94. Prineas JW: Pathology of the early lesion in multiple sclerosis. *Hum Pathol* 6:531, 1975.

95. Prineas JW: Pathology of the Guillain-Barré syndrome. *Ann Neurol* 9(Suppl):6, 1981.

96. Prineas JW, Connell F: Remyelination in multiple sclerosis. *Ann Neurol* 5:22, 1979.

97. Prineas JW, Graham JS: Multiple sclerosis: capping of surface immunoglobulin G on macrophages engaged in myelin breakdown. *Ann Neurol* 10:149, 1981.

98. Prineas JW, McLeod JG: Chronic relapsing polyneuritis. *J Neurol Sci* 27:427, 1976.

99. Prineas JW, Raine CS: Electron microscopy and immunoperoxidase studies of early multiple sclerosis lesions. *Neurology* 26(Suppl):29, 1976.

100. Prineas JW, Wright RG: The fine structure of peripheral nerve lesions in a virus-induced demyelinating disease in fowl (Marek's disease). *Lab Invest* 26:548, 1972.

101. Prineas JW, Wright RG: Macrophages, lymphocytes, and plasma cells in the perivascular compartment in chronic multiple sclerosis. *Lab Invest* 38:409, 1978.

102. Raine CS: Experimental allergic encephalomyelitis and related conditions. In Zimmerman HM (ed): *Progress in Neuropathology.* New York, Grune & Stratton, 1976, vol 3.

103. Raine CS: On the development of lesions in natural canine distemper. *J Neurol Sci* 30:13, 1976.

104. Raine CS: The etiology and pathogenesis of multiple sclerosis: recent developments. *Pathobiol Annu* 7:347, 1977.

105. Raine CS: Membrane specialisations between demyelinated axons and astroglia in chronic EAE lesions and multiple sclerosis plaques. *Nature* 275:326, 1978.

106. Raine CS: Pathology of demyelination. In Waxman SG (ed): *Physiology and Pathobiology of Axons.* New York, Raven Press, 1978.

107. Raine CS: Multiple sclerosis and chronic relapsing EAE: comparative ultrastructural neuropathology. In Hallpike JF, Adams CWM, Tourtellotte WW (eds): *Multiple Sclerosis: Pathology, Diagnosis, and Management.* London, Chapman & Hall, 1983.

108. Raine CS: The morphology of myelin and myelination. In Morell P (ed): *Myelin,* ed 2. New York, Plenum Press, 1984.

109. Raine CS, Bornstein MB: Experimental allergic encephalomyelitis: an ultrastructural study of experimental demyelination *in vitro. J Neuropathol Exp Neurol* 29:177, 1970.

110. Raine CS, Schaumburg HH: The neuropathology of the diseases of myelin. In Morell P (ed): *Myelin.* New York, Plenum Press, 1977.

111. Raine CS, Stone SH: Animal model for multiple sclerosis. Chronic experimental allergic encephalomyelitis in inbred guinea pigs. *NY State J Med* 77:1639, 1977.

112. Raine CS, Traugott U: The pathogenesis and therapy of multiple sclerosis is based upon the requirement of a combination of myelin antigens for autoimmune demyelination. *J Neuroimmunol* 2:83, 1982.

113. Raine CS, et al: Intranuclear "paramyxovirus-like" material in multiple sclerosis, adreno-leukodystrophy and Kuff's disease. *J Neurol Sci* 25:29, 1975.

114. Raine CS, et al: Immunocytochemical studies for the localisation of measles antigens in multiple sclerosis plaques and measles virus-infected CNS tissue. *J Neurol Sci* 33:13, 1977.

115. Raine CS, et al: Glial bridges and Schwann cell invasion of the CNS during chronic demyelination. *J Neurocytol* 7:541, 1978.

116. Raine CS, et al: Suppression of chronic allergic encephalomyelitis: relevance to multiple sclerosis. *Science* 201:445, 1978.

117. Raine CS, et al: Multiple sclerosis: oligodendrocyte survival and proliferation in an active, established lesion. *Lab Invest* 45:534, 1981.

118. Remlinger P: Les paralysies du trâitement antirabique. *Ann Inst Pasteur (Paris)* 41(Suppl):71, 1927.

119. Richardson EP Jr: Progressive multifocal leukoencephalopathy. *N Engl J Med* 265:815, 1961.

120. Rivers TM, et al: Observations on attempts to produce acute disseminated encephalomyelitis in monkeys. *J Exp Med* 58:39, 1933.

121. Roizin L, et al: Disease states involving the white matter of the central nervous system. In Haymaker W, Adams RD (eds): *Histology and Histopathology of the Nervous System.* Springfield, IL, Charles C Thomas, 1982.

122. Rose AS: Multiple sclerosis: a clinical interpretation. In Wolfgram F, Ellison GW, Stevens JG, Andrews JM (eds): *Multiple Sclerosis: Immunology, Virology and Ultrastructure.* New York, Academic Press, 1972.

123. Ruddle NH, Waksman BH: Cytotoxicity mediated by soluble antigen and lymphocytes in delayed hypersensitivity, Part 1 (Characterization of the phenomenon). *J Exp Med* 128:1237, 1968.

124. Russell D: Nosological unity of acute haemorrhagic leukoencephalitis and acute disseminated encephalomyelitis. *Brain* 78:369, 1955.

125. Saida T, et al: Peripheral nerve demyelination induced by intraneural injection of experimental allergic encephalomyelitis serum. *J Neuropathol Exp Neurol* 38:498, 1979.

126. Saida T, et al: In vivo demyelinating activity of sera from patients with Guillain-Barré syndrome. *Ann Neurol* 11:69, 1982.

127. Schüle H: Beitrag Zur multiplen Sclerosis des Gehirns und Rückenmarks. *Dtsch Arch Klin Med* 7:259, 1870.

128. Schüle H: Weiterer Beitrag Zur Hirn-Rückenmarks-Sclerose. *Dtsch Arch Klin Med* 8:223, 1871.

129. Seguin EC, et al: A contribution to the pathological anatomy of disseminated cerebro-spinal sclerosis. *J Nerv Ment Dis* 5:281, 1878.

130. Seitelberger F, et al: Zur Genese der akuten Entmarkungsencephalitis. *Wien Klin Wochenschr* 70:453, 1978.

131. Shein HM: Oncogenesis, latency, and pathogenetic immune response in chronic virus infections of brain tissues. In Schmitt FO, Worden FG (eds): *The Neurosciences Third Study Program.* Cambridge, MA, MIT Press, 1973.

132. Shiraki H: The comparative study of rabies, post-vaccinal encephalomyelitis and demyelinating encephalomyelitis of unknown origin, with special reference to the Japanese cases. In Bailey OT, Smith DE (eds): *The Central Nervous System.* International Academy of Pathology, Monographs in Pathology, No. 9. Baltimore, Williams & Wilkins, 1968.

133. Steiner G (ed): *Krankheitserreger und Gewebsbefund bei Multiple Sklerose.* Berlin, Springer-Verlag, 1931.

134. Suzuki K, et al: Ultrastructural studies of multiple sclerosis. *Lab Invest.* 20:444, 1969.

135. Traugott U, Raine CS: The neurology of myelin diseases. In Morell P (ed): *Myelin,* ed 2. New York, Plenum Press, 1984.

136. Traugott U, et al: Autoimmune encephalomyelitis: simultaneous identification of T and B cells in the target organ. *Science* 214:1251, 1981.

137. Traugott U, et al: Chronic relapsing experimental allergic encephalomyelitis: identification and dynamics of T and B cells within the central nervous system. *Cell Immunol* 68:261, 1982.

138. Traugott U, et al: Monoclonal anti-T cell antibodies are applicable to the study of inflammatory infiltrates in the central nervous system. *J Neuroimmunol* 3:365, 1982.

139. Traugott U, et al: Chronic relapsing experimental autoimmune encephalomyelitis: treatment with combinations of myelin components promotes clinical and structural recovery. *J Neurol Sci* 56:65, 1982.

140. Traugott U, et al: Multiple sclerosis: distribution of T cell subsets within active chronic lesions. *Science* 219:308, 1983.

141. Traugott U, et al: Multiple sclerosis: distribution of T cells, T cell subsets and Ia-positive macrophages in lesions of different ages. *J Neuroimmunol* 4:201, 1983.

142. Turnbull HM, McIntosh J: Encephalomyelitis following vaccination. *Br J Exp Pathol* 7:181, 1926.

143. Uchimura I, Shiraki H: A contribution to the classification and the pathogenesis of demyelinating encephalomyelitis with special reference to the central nervous system lesions caused by preventive inoculation against rabies. *J Neuropathol Exp Neurol* 16:139, 1957.

144. Uhthoff W: Untersuchungen über die bei der multiplen Herdsklerose vorkommenden Augenstorungen. *Arch Psychiatr Nervenkr* 21:55, 1889.

145. Van Bogaert L: Les manifestations nerveuses au coins des maladies eruptives (varicelle, rougeole, scarlatine). *Rev Neurol (Paris)* 1:150, 1933.

146. Vinken PJ, Bruyn GW (eds): *Handbook of Clinical Neurology.* Amsterdam, North-Holland, 1970, vol 9.

147. Virchow R: Uber das ausgebreitete Vorkommen einer dem Nervenmark analogen Substanz in den tierischen Geweben. *Virchows Arch Pathol Anat* 6:562, 1854.

148. Waksman BH: Experimental study of diphtheritic polyneuritis in the rabbit and guinea pig. III. The blood-nerve barrier in the rabbit. *J Neuropathol Exp Neurol* 20:35, 1961.

149. Waksman BH, Adams RD: Allergic neuritis: experimental disease of rabbits induced by the injection of periph-

eral nervous tissue and adjuvants. *J Exp Med* 102:213, 1955.

150. Waksman BH, Adams RD: Infectious leukoencephalitis. A critical comparison of certain experimental and naturally-occurring viral leukoencephalitides with experimental allergic encephalomyelitis. *J Neuropathol Exp Neurol* 21:491, 1962.

151. Webster HdeF, et al: Phase and electron microscopic studies of experimental demyelination. II. Schwann cell changes in guinea pig sciatic nerves during experimental diphtheritic neuritis. *J Neuropathol Exp Neurol* 20:5, 1961.

152. Weigle O: Analysis of autoimmunity through experimental models of thyroiditis and allergic encephalomyelitis. In Dixon FJ, Kunkel HG (eds): *Advances in Immunology.* New York, Academic Press, 1980, vol 30.

153. Weiner LP, Narayan O: Progressive multifocal leukoencephalopathy. In Thompson RA, Green JR (eds): *Infectious Diseases of the Central Nervous System. Advances in Neurology.* New York, Raven Press, 1974, vol 6.

154. Weller RO: Diphtheritic neuropathy in the chicken: an electron microscopic study. *J Pathol Bacteriol* 89:591, 1965.

155. Westphal C: Beobachtungen and Untersuchungen über die Krankheiten des centralen Nervensystems. *Arch Psychiatrie* 4:335, 1874.

156. Wisniewski H, Raine CS: An ultrastructural study of experimental demyelination and remyelination. V. Central and peripheral nervous system lesions caused by diphtheria toxin. *Lab Invest* 25:73, 1971.

157. Wisniewski H, et al: Observations on viral demyelinating encephalomyelitis—canine distemper. *Lab Invest* 26:589, 1972.

158. Zimmerman HM, Netsky MG: The pathology of multiple sclerosis. Multiple sclerosis and the demyelinating diseases. *Proc Assoc Res Nerv Mental Dis* 28:271, 1950.

159. Zito G, et al: Immunological diseases of the human peripheral nervous system. In Waksman BH (ed): *Clinics in Immunology and Allergy.* Philadelphia, WB Saunders, 1982, vol 2.

160. Zu Rhein GM: Virions in progressive multifocal leukoencephalopathy. In Minckler J (ed): *Pathology of the Nervous System.* New York, McGraw-Hill, 1972, vol 3.

161. Zu Rhein GM, Chou SM: Papovavirus in progressive multifocal leukoencephalopathy. Infectious diseases of the nervous system. *Proc Assoc Res Nerv Ment Dis* 44:307, 1968.

Circulatory Disorders and Their Effects on the Brain

JULIO H. GARCIA, M.D.

INTRODUCTION AND DEFINITIONS

This chapter contains a compendium of information on the effects that various circulatory disturbances, i.e., ischemia, hemorrhage, and edema, exert on the gross appearance and the histologic features of the brain. After a brief introduction that touches on basic mechanisms regulating the circulation of the nervous system, the material is presented in five separate sections: angiopathies affecting the nervous system; ischemic lesions (occlusive and hypotensive); brain (parenchymal) hemorrhages; subarachnoid hemorrhage; and brain edema secondary to the above disturbances. The traditional designation of cerebrovascular disorders adopted in many textbooks has been broadened to emphasize that it is the disturbance in *circulation* that injures the brain. Some vascular diseases, e.g., atherosclerosis, frequently exist in brains whose function and structure are either normal or only slightly abnormal.

The circulation to the central nervous system (CNS) is under the influence of an autoregulatory control that maintains constant an average blood flow of about 55–60 ml/min/100 g in the face of changing values in systemic pressure. The system remains operative as long as the mean arterial pressure is maintained between 45 to 170 mm Hg; these values move upward in patients with longstanding systemic hypertension. This circulatory equilibrium may be altered by systemic or local factors which decrease

the cerebral blood flow (CBF) and make it insufficient to maintain function; such a situation is referred to as one of *ischemia.*

A second type of circulatory disorder results from alterations in the brain blood vessels that lead to extravasation of red blood cells (i.e., *hemorrhage*). This extravasation may accumulate primarily in the subarachnoid space, when the bleeding originates in large arteries, or in the brain parenchyma if the bleeding vessels are small arteries or arterioles. Finally, circulatory alterations may result in marked retention of fluid (water, serum) in the brain parenchyma; this condition is called brain *edema.*

The causes of the above circulatory disorders, which sometimes coexist in the same patient, are myriad; however, they can be classified into four main categories as follows.

(1) Defects in the blood vessel walls, i.e., *angiopathies* may cause either brain *hemorrhage* or brain *infarction*, for example, following the rupture of a saccular aneurysm or after the occlusion of an atherosclerotic artery.

(2) Persons having normal cardiovascular function and intact vasculature may occlude cerebral vessels as a consequence of intravascular thrombosis; alternatively, patients free of angiopathies may bleed either in the brain or the meninges on the basis of *systemic coagulopathies* or blood dyscrasia.

(3) *Systemic hemodynamic failures:*

brain ischemia develops as a result of mean arterial blood pressure drops below 45 mm Hg, as a consequence of abrupt, severe deficits in cardiac output (e.g., after a massive myocardial infarction); as a result of cardiac valvulopathies (e.g., mitral prolapse, aortic stenosis); following disturbances in cardiac rhythm; and secondary to peripheral collapse, i.e., shock.

(4) In addition to the above circumstances, which may apply to any organ, the brain's circulation can be adversely influenced by *increases* in *intracranial pressure.* The effective brain perfusion pressure is approximately equal to the difference between arterial and intracranial pressures. Thus, abrupt increases in intracranial pressure (ICP) which frequently develop after closed head injury, for example, are promptly reflected in decreased brain perfusion pressure. Closed head injury is frequently associated with marked increases in ICP, in part because of the post-traumatic loss of autoregulation and the development of post-traumatic brain edema. This decreased brain perfusion pressure, caused by a rise in ICP, is aggravated by the nonexpansile nature of the adult skull and the minimal difference (less than 5% in the adult) that exists between intracranial volume and cerebral volume.

Disorders of circulation, of which the *ischemic ones* are the most numerous, are the main cause of death and disability in the United States. In recent years systemic hypertension, cardiovascular disease, and stroke have affected at any given time as many as 20 million adult Americans. These same conditions caused approximately 1 million deaths in 1975, a figure representing over one-half of the annual deaths in the U.S. (127). Strokes (ischemic and hemorrhagic) are the most common type of focal organic neurologic disease among adults. Collectively, strokes are responsible for about 10% of the annual deaths in the United States (208).

Stroke and syncope are useful descriptive terms commonly used in epidemiology to designate neurologic deficits of circulatory origin that become manifest in an abrupt, unexpected manner.

Stroke designates a localized neurologic symptom that, usually, appears suddenly, without warning; in most patients the neurologic deficit tends to improve spontaneously within hours or days of the ictus. The nature and type of the neurologic deficit varies enormously, depending on the territory involved, and may include: unilateral blindness, dysarthria, monomelic motor weakness, hemifacial sensory deficit, and numerous other expressions. Regardless of its symptoms, the implied meaning of stroke is that of a *focal* neurologic deficit that can be traced, in most instances, to a local or regional *disturbance* of the brain's circulation.

Epidemiologic analyses and postmortem examinations have shown the distribution of the anatomic lesions among most stroke victims (Table 12.1).

In contrast to the focal nature of stroke, *syncope* implies a generalized but transient loss of several brain functions, especially consciousness. The main causes of such an abrupt loss of brain functions are also circulatory; the generalized functional loss is explained by a circulatory deficit simultaneously affecting the *entire* brain, e.g., during episodic cardiac dysrhythmias.

Traditionally, the brain damage resulting from the above situations has been attributed to *hypoxia* or *anoxia.* Oxygen deficiency only a few minutes in duration is believed to be most damaging to the brain, presumably because this organ cannot metabolize glucose under anaerobic conditions. However, appropriate experiments show that brain energy metabolism is maintained even at pronounced degrees of hypoxic hypoxia (110). This is because during transient interruptions of oxygen intake CBF increases several hundred percent, as demonstrated in human volunteers in whom PaO_2 values had been lowered to 50 mm Hg while the brain functions re-

Table 12.1
Confirmed Cases of Stroke[a,b]

Brain infarction (embolic and thrombotic)	73.3%
Brain (parenchymal) hemorrhage	19.3%
Subarachnoid hemorrhage	7.4%
	100

[a] Adapted from H. R. Müller and E. W. Radu (156).
[b] Diagnosis confirmed either by CT scan or at autopsy.

mained intact (126). In rats, PaO$_2$ values of 22 mm Hg result in a four- to six-fold increase in CBF; the changes in blood flow are unrelated to alterations in either systemic blood pressure or PaCO$_2$ (110).

If the tissue consequences of insufficient CBF (ischemia) were directly related to oxygen deficiency (hypoxia), cerebral oxygen deficit, sufficiently severe as to be symptomatic, might be induced either by decreasing arterial oxygen tension (hypoxemia) or by reducing CBF (ischemia). However, clinical observations and laboratory experiments do not support the assumption that *ischemia* and *hypoxia* exert comparable effects on the brain.

Brain tissues supplied by hypoxic blood for several minutes and evaluated by electron microscopy show no significant alterations (14). Atmospheric hypoxia affecting primarily or exclusively the brain is nearly impossible to create. Experimentally induced CO hypoxia and hypoxemic hypoxia result, within seconds, in severe myocardial and circulatory disturbances (i.e., ischemia) at a time when the electroencephalogram remains unchanged (9, 199). Moreover, chronic CO poisoning induces brain lesions of a magnitude directly proportional to the degree of hypotension brought about by the CO (81, 82). Severe oxygen deficiency (less than 15 mm Hg) of 4–5 min in duration is accompanied by circulatory failure (e.g., cardiac arrhythmias), therefore hypoxemia per se cannot give rise to brain damage (24).

Withholding intake of atmospheric oxygen for several seconds should result in severe functional or structural brain damage. Yet, with appropriate training, professional deep-sea divers make, during consecutive hours, repetitive breath-holding dives, each lasting as long as 150 s. The transient neurologic deficits developing in a minority of these persons are attributed to nitrogen retention and not to hypoxemia (104).

In contrast to the relative tolerance that the adult brain can develop to oxygen deficiency, Rossen et al. (180) showed in healthy human volunteers fixation of eye movements, blurring of vision, unconsciousness, and paresthesias appearing within *6 s* after inducing brain ischemia via an inflatable cuff placed around the neck.

In these individuals, seizures lasting 6–8 s invariably followed momentary loss of consciousness and always occurred during the reperfusion period. Severe brain injury has been documented in normothermic cat brains made globally ischemic through simultaneous carotid arterial occlusion and induction of systemic hypotension of a few minutes' duration (84).

When the metabolic effects of hypoxia and ischemia are separately evaluated at the cellular level, ischemia is characterized by energy metabolite failure, presumably as a result of mitochondrial injury. In contrast, mitochondria quickly adapt to hypoxemic conditions, which prevents or delays energy failure; instead, hypoxia induces neurotransmitter failure (175). Neither hypoxia nor hypercapnia correlate with the extent of brain damage in experiments designed to measure the contribution that each of these conditions make to the injury of ischemia (186). Moreover, the severity and extent of neuronal-glial damage correlates extremely well with the percent drop in local CBF and the *duration* of the same (45, 72).

One final consideration is of importance in establishing a distinction between hypoxic and ischemic injuries. In many experimental situations, the topographically heterogeneous effects of ischemia become apparent during the *reperfusion* period. Brains deprived of circulation for up to 60 min show chemical-metabolic changes that are relatively *minimal* and *homogeneous* throughout the entire brain (41, 116). Pronounced and inhomogeneous structural-metabolic abnormalities have been demonstrated in brains that were injured by ischemia during a period of 5–15 min, followed by *reperfusion* for up to 60 min (109, 211).

ANGIOPATHIES

Structural abnormalities involving the vessels that supply or drain the brain include: variations of the gross anatomical features or congenital defects, as well as acquired angiopathies. Congenital defects of the cervicocranial vessels can be incidental findings unrelated to clinical signs and symptoms; alternately, these anatomical variations may constitute the basis that explains the involvement of specific brain sites after a vascular occlusion (e.g., infarction of both frontal hemispheres after unilateral carotid artery occlusion in persons in whom both pericallosal arteries originate from the same side) (Table 12.2).

Anatomic Variations

The typical aortic anatomic pattern in which the brachiocephalic trunk, the left common carotid artery, and the left subcla-

Table 12.2
Nervous System Angiopathies

A. Anatomical variations
B. Angiomatous malformations
C. Saccular (Berry) and other aneurysms
D. Atherosclerosis
E. Arteriolosclerosis
F. Angiitis (noninfectious)
G. Miscellaneous

vian artery originate separately from the aortic arch exists in about 55–70% of the population. In the remainder, variations of the type shown in Figure 12.1 can be found according to the indicated percentages (203). These anatomic variations may determine blood flow patterns that influence the topographic distribution of ischemic lesions.

The extradural intracranial portion of the internal carotid artery (ICA) normally shows a well-developed external elastic layer and abundant calcium deposits in all three tunicae, unrelated to atherosclerosis or to any systemic disease (172). Compared to extracranial arteries of the same caliber, intracranial arteries (examined by conventional histologic methods) show no external elastic, and both the tunica media and the tunica adventitia have fewer layers of cells and fibers (150).

The following abnormalities of the extracranial internal carotid artery (ICA) are

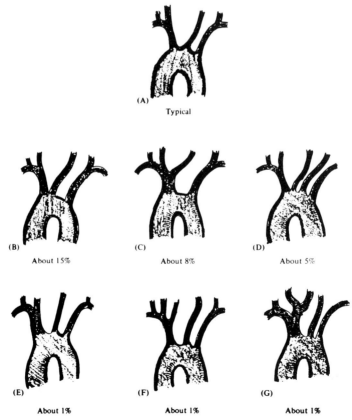

Figure 12.1. Anatomic variations of the aortic arch and its branches. (From J. F. Toole and A. N. Patel (203).)

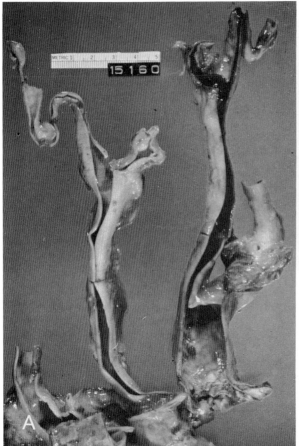

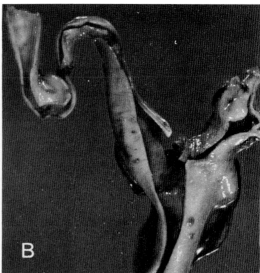

Figure 12.2. (*A*) Bilateral kinking of the distal internal carotid arteries in an elderly woman who apparently suffered no ill effects from this structural abnormality. (*B*) Closeup of left internal carotid artery.

rather frequently demonstrated in angiographic studies: (*a*) coiling; (*b*) kinking of the upper cervical portion (Fig. 12.2); and (*c*) stenosis or hypoplasia, with up to 50% reduction of the lumen. Some authors suggest that these abnormalities may predispose to the development of intracranial saccular aneurysms (190). The cause of kinking of the ICA is unknown; in most cases it seems to be an acquired condition related to advanced age and systemic hypertension. A somewhat comparable deformity of the basilar artery, called *dolichoectasia* (i.e., elongation and distention), may become symptomatic because the artery either compresses cranial nerves or obstructs the CSF circulation, e.g., at one of the lateral recesses (52).

Patients with *hypoplasia* of the cervical portion of the internal carotid artery may suffer from the consequences of episodic cerebral ischemia or cerebral hemorrhage.

The condition may be sporadic or familial (11).

Additional variations in the vascular anatomy of the brain include changes in the symmetry of the circle of Willis; in most instances these variations represent a persistence of embryonal artery-to-artery connections (Table 12.3).

VARIATIONS OF THE CIRCLE OF WILLIS

Slightly less than 50% of the population has a perfectly symmetrical arterial circle at the base of the brain, where pairs of vertebral, posterior communicating, middle cerebral, and anterior cerebral arteries have nearly identical caliber. Significant asymmetries can be found in about 40% of the adult autopsied population (7). In addition to these asymmetries, the arteries of the circle of Willis may show the following variations:

Table 12.3
Persistent Anastomotic Channels in the Arteries at the Base of the Brain[a]

1. Primitive *trigeminal* artery; connects internal carotid to basilar artery (just proximal to PCA takeoff)
2. Primitive *otic* artery; connects internal carotid to basilar artery (midportion)
3. Primitive *hypoglossal* artery; connects internal carotid to basilar artery (just distal to the vertebral arteries)
4. Primitive *stapedal* artery; connects internal carotid to middle meningeal artery
5. Primitive *ophthalmic* artery; connects lacrimal branch of ophthalmic artery to middle meningeal artery
6. Anastomic channels connecting the vertebral arteries with one another
7. Anastomic channels connecting the ophthalmic and the meningeal arteries

[a] Adapted from J. F. Toole and A. N. Patel (203).

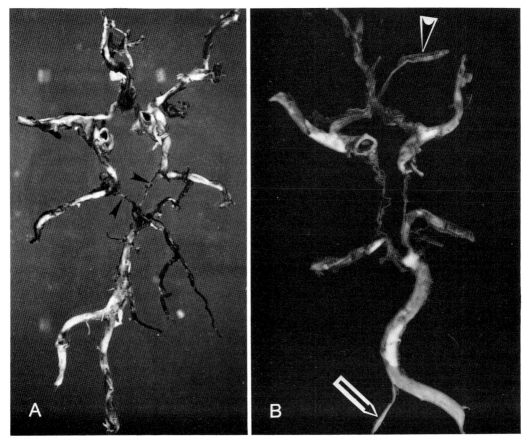

Figure 12.3. Anatomic variations in the circle of Willis. (*A*) The posterior cerebral arteries originate from the internal carotid vessels; thin posterior communicating arteries (*arrowheads*) connect the PCA with the dome of the basilar artery. (*B*) Asymmetry of vertebral arteries (*arrow*) and pericallosal arteries (*arrowhead*). Small atheromatous plaques are seen on the basilar and middle cerebral arteries.

(a) Posterior cerebral artery originates from the internal carotid (Fig. 12.3).
(b) Marked asymmetry exists in the caliber of the posterior communicating arteries. Usually, variations (a) and (b) coexist in the same patient.

(c) Both pericallosal arteries originate from the same anterior cerebral artery.

(d) Posterior communicating artery may be unilaterally absent (203).

Angiomatous Malformations

These include a number of anatomical abnormalities, which in many instances are attributed to persistence of the vascular patterns normally found in the fetal brain, i.e., direct communication between arteries and veins without intervening capillary beds (119); the angiomatous malformations are traditionally divided into:

1. Capillary telangiectasis
2. Cavernous angioma
3. Venous angioma
4. Arteriovenous malformation
5. Varix of the vein of Galen

CAPILLARY TELANGIECTASES

This condition often occurs in the pontine base but also can be found in the white matter of the cerebral hemispheres. These lesions are not identifiable at angiography and frequently are curiosities discovered at necropsy. The average telangiectasis occupies an area measuring approximately 3.0 cm in diameter and may be seen as a pink or pink-gray circular lesion that is sometimes mistaken for a cluster of petechiae. Microscopically, the vessels measure up to 30 μm in diameter; are lined but by one endothelial cell layer; and are separated from one another by normal brain parenchyma (141). Exceptionally, capillary telangiectasis in the lower brain stem may cause slowly progressive neurologic deficit (56). Among young children, acute episodic neurologic "illnesses" have been associated with bleeding angiomatous malformations of the brainstem which sometimes simulate pontine gliomas (221). Capillary telangiectases and similar vascular deformities have been observed in the cerebrum, cerebellum, and brain stem of patients with hereditary hemorrhagic telangiectasia or Osler-Weber-Rendu disease (93, 173).

CAVERNOUS HEMANGIOMAS

The main clinical significance of cavernous hemangiomas stems from their tendency to induce either brain hemorrhages or seizures. Approximately 16% of patients afflicted with cavernous hemangiomas have multiple ones. The lesions are usually dark red or black, well circumscribed, and may show calcification and ossification. Under the microscope, they appear as a collection of large, closely clustered vessels with or without intervening normal brain tissue. Hemosiderin containing macrophages and gliosis may be abundant. The distinction between telangiectasis and cavernous hemangioma may not always be clear, although the age at which the two types of lesions become symptomatic is slightly different. Cavernous hemangiomas usually become manifest in early adolescence, and are characterized by large vessels with thick fibrous walls, as opposed to the one-layer, capillary-like appearance of the telangiectases. Cavernous hemangiomas are rarely associated with similar cutaneous and/or visceral lesions. Intracranial cavernous angiomas may be confined to the dura and/or the skull (129, 142).

VENOUS ANGIOMAS

These lesions are more common in the spinal cord and its meninges than intracranially. When they occur in the cerebrum, venous angiomas appear in angiograms as triangularly shaped structures with the base directed toward the ventricular wall; the vascular components of these angiomas fill during the late arterial or early venous phase of the angiogram. Microscopically, the absence of arteries in the malformation is necessary for the diagnosis. Dilated hypertrophic veins with walls made of a single layer of fibromuscular tissue lined by endothelium with intervening normal brain parenchyma are characteristic (30). Differentiating these lesions from cavernous angiomas and telangiectases may require an integrated study of the anatomic lesion together with the angiographic and scintigraphic patterns.

ARTERIOVENOUS MALFORMATIONS (AVM)

These are the most common of all the congenital vascular anomalies. Hemorrhagic stroke or convulsions usually beginning about the second decade of life are the most frequent clinical manifestations of AVMs. Ninety-three percent of these ab-

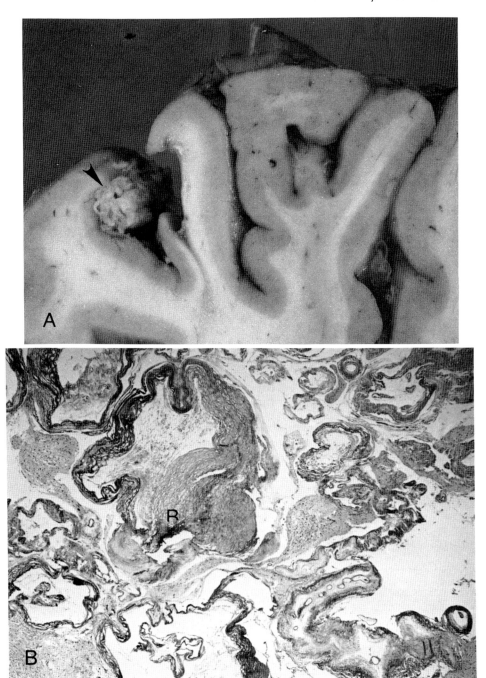

Figure 12.4. A 75-yr-old man had been operated on 26 yr before for an arteriovenous malformation in the right frontoparietal region. (*A*) Large surgically repaired angiomatous malformation of the right cerebral hemisphere (*arrowhead*). (*B*) Histologic view of the same specimen shown in *A*. Verhoeff-Van Gieson. (Original magnification ×100.)

normalities are located supratentorially. Most are placed away from the midline, are supplied by branches of the MCA, and are more common in the frontotemporal lobes than in the rest of the cerebrum. Their gross appearance at autopsy is less impressive than during surgery because of the postmortem collapse of the vessels (Fig. 12.4). AVMs usually have a triangular shape with the base directed towards the meninges. Some are clearly traumatic in origin. Arterial venous malformations in the midbrain (Fig. 12.5) may be associated with lesions in the retina and with cutaneous nevi. Some of the arteriovenous malformations demonstrable by histopathologic means are not visible on angiography (19).

Microscopically, AVMs show many enlarged, engorged vessels of many diameters, walls of irregular thickness, mostly composed of fibrous tissue with occasional smooth muscle fibers, but no elastic layer. Thrombosis, recanalization, calcium deposits, and occasional mural amyloid deposits may be found. Intracranial hemorrhages accompanying AVMs can occur in any compartment, but most are either subarachnoid or intracerebral (143). In general AVMs do not become symptomatic until the early 20s; therefore, it is believed that these congenital lesions progressively enlarge. Spontaneous occlusion of the AVM may lead to either remission of symptoms or to sudden death. Some AVMs may be difficult to differentiate from true vascular neoplasms. Patients who develop symptoms secondary to an intracranial AVM before the first year of life usually have signs of congestive heart failure or, in the case of strategically placed lesions, obstructive hydrocephalus. Children who become symptomatic after the first year of life have symptoms, which resemble those of the adult population, i.e., hemorrhage and seizures (125). AVMs commonly occur near the surface of the cerebral hemispheres (Fig. 12.6); only 6% are located in the posterior fossa, and only 18% are situated deep, near the basal ganglia and internal capsule. Intracranial saccular aneurysms are associated with AVMs in approximately 10% of these patients (193, 194).

The occurrence of a hemorrhagic stroke, particularly a lethal one, among children under the age of 16 should always raise the possibility of a congenital vascular defect as the source for the bleeding into the subarachnoid space, the brain parenchyma, or the cerebral ventricles (Fig. 12.7).

The frequency of spinal AVMs ranges between 3.3 and 11% of all of spinal cord tumors. The incidence might be higher than indicated above because the disorder does not lend itself to easy diagnosis. Spinal AVMs have frequently been found at autopsy among patients who die with a diagnosis of idiopathic diffuse or transverse myelitis (20, 36). Slowly progressive spastic paraplegia, paresthesias, pain, and micturition disturbances are common complaints in these patients (78, 202). The ratio of male:female is almost 2:1; the vast majority of the spinal AVMs occur in the lower thoracic-lumbar segment. AVMs of the cord tend to become symptomatic between the third and sixth decades of life (202). Cutaneous angiomas frequently exist at the same segment where spinal angiomas are subsequently demonstrated at angiographs (48).

Subacute necrotic myelopathy (Foix and Alajouanine) is a progressive thrombotic disorder, involving spinal cord vessels and ultimately leading to fatal complications. In most cases there is an association between the myelopathy and an arteriovenous malformation of the cord. Thrombosis of previously demonstrated spinal cord AVMs has been shown both by angiography and at surgical exploration (214).

VARIX OF THE VEIN OF GALEN

This vascular abnormality is a variant of arteriovenous malformations; in the overwhelming number of reported cases, direct connections can be demonstrated between the dilated vein of Galen and branches of either the posterior cerebral arteries or other arteries of the circle of Willis. The symptomatology varies according to the age of the patient. Thus, signs of congestive heart failure are the usual presentation among newborns while hydrocephalus, convulsions, subarachnoid hemorrhage, and visible distention of the scalp veins are usual in all children up to the age of 10 months. Headaches, vertigo, fatigue, hemiparesis, and subarachnoid hemorrhage are the norm in older children (8, 85, 99).

The *Sturge-Weber syndrome* consists of angiomatosis of the third portion of the trigeminal nerve on the skin of the face and the cerebral leptomeninges with progressive calcification of the underlying cerebral cortex. These abnormalities are usually unilateral. Atrophy of the involved cerebral hemisphere may be present, along with contralateral hemiparesis, focal seizures, and mental retardation (213).

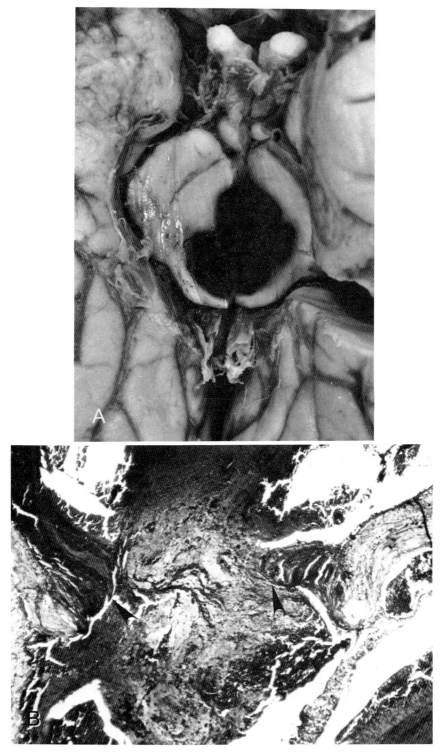

Figure 12.5. (*A*) Large angiomatous malformation in the midbrain of a 62-yr-old man. A stroke occurred about 4 d before death. (*B*) The site of rupture of the AVM shown in *A* is indicated by *arrowheads*. H&E. (Original magnification ×100.)

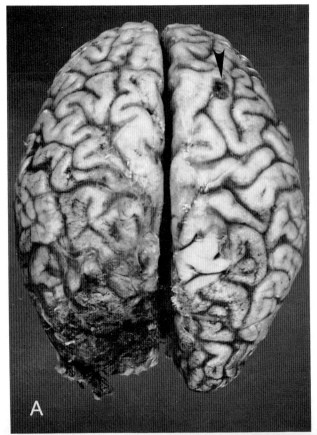

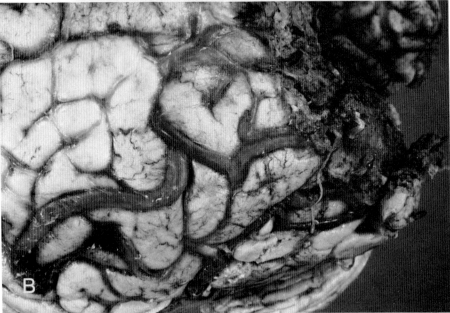

Figure 12.6. (*A*) Operative site of an AVM of the left occipital lobe excised 6 d before death. The patient died of pulmonary thromboembolism. An *arrowhead* points at the site where an intraventricular catheter had been placed. (*B*) Closeup of the same specimen in *A*, showing marked dilatation and early thrombosis of some of the vessels feeding the AVM.

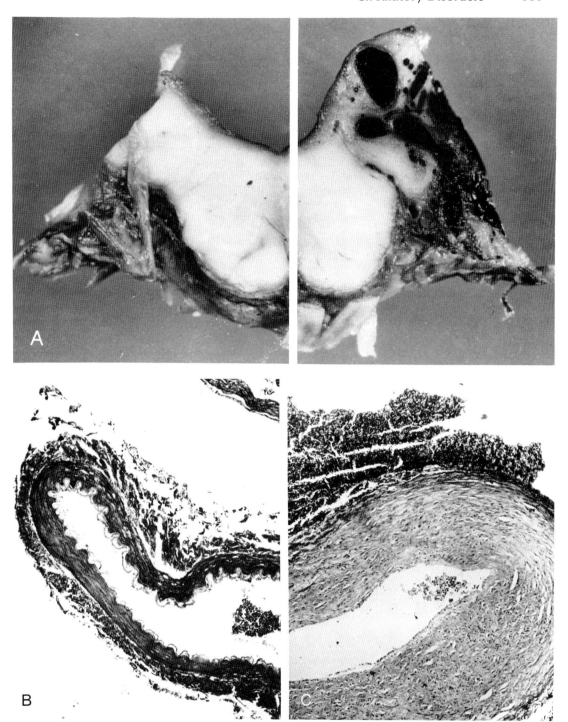

Figure 12.7. A 3-yr-old girl had a stroke 3–4 d before death; she remained in coma. There was massive subarachnoid hemorrhage, especially prominent around the brain stem and cerebellum (see Fig. 12.45). (*A*) Cross-section of medulla; large, anomalous vessels are partly embedded in this portion of the brain stem. (*B*) Normal right vertebral artery with three clearly visible tunicae. (*C*) Detail of the architecture of anomalous vessel: no elastic lamina or smooth muscle fibers are visible. Both light micrographs, H&E. (Original magnification ×40.)

Saccular (Berry) Aneurysms

Localized ectasias of the intracranial arterial walls with the approximate shape of a sac are also called "berry" aneurysms, presumably because of the similarity they offer, when filled with blood, to the fruit of a berry-bearing bush.

Intracranial saccular aneurysms are not found in childhood. Unruptured, asymptomatic aneurysms exist in about 25% of autopsies in persons over the age of 55 (140, 178).

Saccular aneurysms become symptomatic primarily on account of their rupture and subsequent bleeding into either the subarachnoid space or the brain parenchyma. Exceptionally, they may bleed into the subdural space. Large and unruptured saccular aneurysms may become symptomatic by compressing nearby structures (e.g., the cranial nerves or the brain stem) or by interfering with the spinal fluid flow (Fig. 12.8).

The portion of the circle of Willis located rostral to (and including) the posterior communicating arteries harbors many more aneurysms than the posterior fossa arteries, by a ratio of about 5:1. Sites where saccular aneurysms occur most frequently are, in approximate order: (*a*) the internal carotid-posterior communicating-proximal MCA complex; (*b*) the anterior communicating artery; and (*c*) the bifurcation or trifurcation of the MCA (Fig. 12.8). In the vertebral-basilar systems, saccular aneurysms are more common at the apex of the basilar artery and at the site of origin of the posterior-inferior cerebellar artery (Fig. 12.8) (50). Regardless of location, intracranial aneurysms are far more common at arterial branching points. The diameter of *ruptured* saccular aneurysms tends to be larger (greater than 7 mm) than that of the unruptured ones. In autopsy evaluations, increasing age correlates with increasing numbers of saccular aneurysms; up to 22% of patients with saccular aneurysms have multiple ones. Aneurysms predominate in females by a ratio of about 3:2. In one cooperative study, the peak incidence of symptomatic (ruptured) aneurysms occurred at about 54 years of age (140).

Early aneurysmal changes (funnel-shaped dilatations, areas of thinning, and small evaginations) are frequent among persons with a mean age of 57 years. These are associated with severe alterations in the internal elastic lamina, a structure which is usually deficient in the area of thinning (192). Saccular aneurysms arise at the site of substantial breaches in the muscular and elastic layers which normally occur at branching points. The gap in the muscular layer is usually a focus of medial aplasia, which may be substantially enlarged by presumptive degenerative changes (34). Traumatic intracranial aneurysms are rare; only 18 cases have been reported in the literature (1). Solitary aneurysms of the extramedullary arteries of the spinal cord are rare; less than 10 cases have been reported in the recent literature (68).

ANEURYSMS OF THE EXTRACRANIAL PORTION OF THE INTERNAL CAROTID

These are rare lesions. About 30 *fusiform aneurysms* of the extracranial portion of the ICA were encountered among 25 patients whose most frequent complaints were those of brain ischemic symptoms (e.g., transient ischemic attacks, or TIAs). Atherosclerosis, severe hypertension, temporally remote blunt injury to the neck, and previous surgical interventions of the carotid vessels are the most common factors associated with these aneurysms. Large ICA aneurysms in the neck may or may not be pulsatile (155, 176).

Intramural arterial bleeding, or *dissecting aneurysms*, have been documented both in the extra- and intracranial portions of the carotid-vertebral circulations (Fig. 12.9). Hypertensive disease, degenerative changes in the tunica media, blunt trauma (direct or indirect), needle puncture, and pregnancy are some of the factors associated with this condition (89). Dissecting aneurysms of the basilar artery have been described in two patients; in one of these, dissection was associated with extensive atherosclerosis and subarachnoid hemorrhage. The second dissecting aneurysm developed in a young man who had had a 15-year history of migrainous headaches; in this patient, intramural hemorrhage of the basilar artery was accompanied by thrombosis of the lumen and infarctions of the

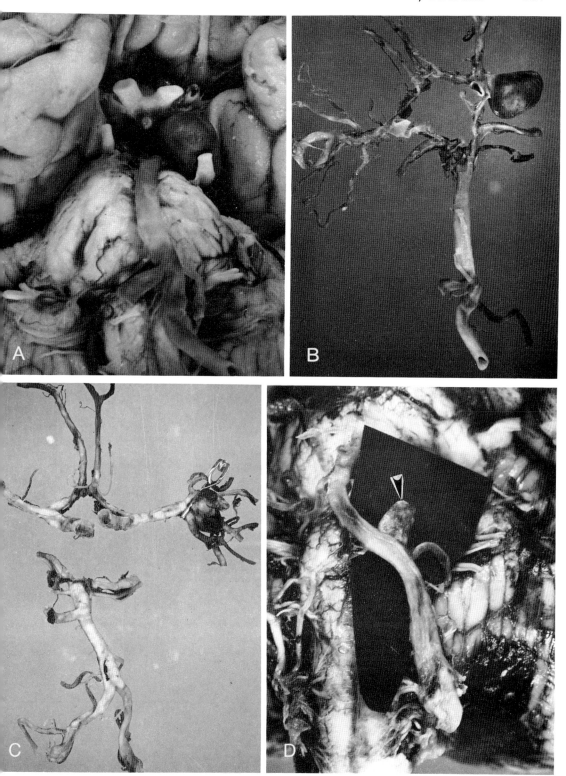

Figure 12.8. (*A* and *B*) Large, unruptured saccular aneurysm at the distal end of the left ICA; there exists a close topographic relationship between the aneurysm, the III and IV cranial nerves, and other neighboring structures. (*C*) Surgically clipped aneurysm at the trifurcation of the left MCA. (*D*) The *arrowhead* points at a ruptured aneurysm of the left vertebral artery.

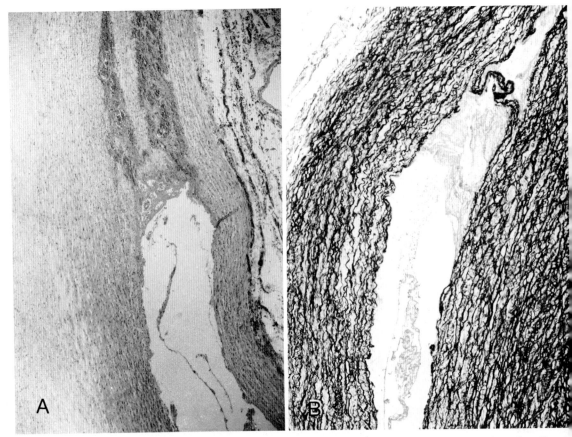

Figure 12.9. Dissecting aneurysms of the extracranial portion of the ICA. (*A*) H&E. (*B*) Verhoeff-Van Gieson. (Original magnification ×100.) (Courtesy of Dr. U. Sandbank, Tel Aviv, Israel.)

rostral pons, midbrain, and nearby brain structures (16). No associated factors are apparent in many patients with dissecting aneurysms of the head and neck vessels.

Atherosclerosis

Atherogenesis is a process characterized by intimal thickening with focal deposition of plasma-derived lipids, smooth muscle proliferation, and influx of blood monocytes and connective tissue formation. In human samples, one of the cells showing earliest lipid deposits is the subintimal smooth muscle fiber (79). Among the brain vessels atherosclerosis tends to be more severe and to become symptomatic at these *sites*: the origin of the internal carotid artery, the intracranial segment of the vertebral arteries, the midportion of the basilar artery (Fig. 12.10), and the initial segment of the MCA (13, 150). The morpho-

logic features of atherosclerosis in the extracranial cerebral arteries more closely resemble those of other systemic arteries (150) (Fig. 12.11).

Three factors influence the progression of atherosclerosis of the cervicocranial vessels: aging, hypertensive disease, and diabetes mellitus (102). Traditionally, the disease is said to evolve through three stages, i.e., fatty streak, fibrous plaque, and complicated (ulcerated) plaque. The first two stages of this lesion are asymptomatic. The ulcerated plaque may become symptomatic in two ways.

Obstruction of Blood Flow. This occlusion of the lumen may come about either through the local formation of a thrombus (Fig. 12.12) or by development of a mural hemorrhage from one of the plaque's newly formed capillaries. In a comprehensive analysis, conducted by a single observer, of over 200 brains with infarctions and the

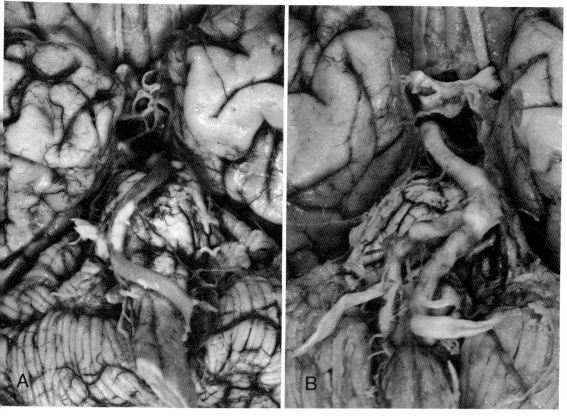

Figure 12.10. (*A* and *B*) Atheromatous plaques and elongation-ectasia of the basilar artery. The latter is more commonly seen in elderly, hypertensive persons.

respective arterial tree, more sites of occlusion were found intracranially than in the cervical portion of the carotid vertebral arteries (151, 152).

Becoming a Source of Embolism. Fibrin and platelet thrombi, as well as fragments of the plaque itself (e.g., cholesterol crystals), may enter the circulation and occlude more distally located arteries.

Arteriolar Disease (Small Blood Vessel Disease)

Increased blood pressure alters brain function by accelerating cerebral atherosclerosis and by initiating a series of changes in the small parenchymal small arteries and arterioles, i.e., arteriolosclerosis. Similar but less pronounced alterations may be induced in arterioles by long-standing diabetes mellitus and aging. The result of these vascular derangements are: small brain infarctions (or lacunes) and

brain (parenchymal) hemorrhages; these lesions are more common and abundant among hypertensive brains. Therefore, treatment of asymptomatic systemic hypertension is associated with reduced neurologic morbidity and decreased incidence of strokes (181).

In addition to localized or focal lesions, high blood-pressure crises may induce generalized brain disturbances. The dominant CNS symptoms in *hypertensive encephalopathy* are altered state of consciousness and severe headache. Nausea, vomiting, visual disturbances, seizures, and focal signs are much less common. The encephalopathy is invariably accompanied by characteristic ophthalmoscopic expressions of malignant hypertension and by uremia. The brains in these patients show severe vascular alterations (fibrinoid necrosis, thrombosis of arterioles, and capillaries) and parenchymal lesions (cortical or subcortical microinfarctions, petechiae, and

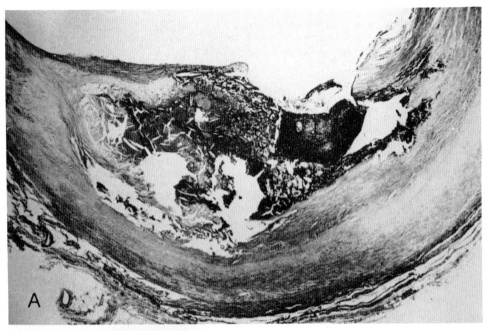

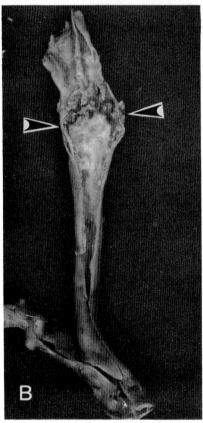

Figure 12.11. (*A*) Cross-section of same lesion shown in *B*; the crater of the ulcerated plaque contains fibrin, platelets, calcium, cholesterol crystals, and cellular debris. Any of these materials may embolize into distal intracranial branches. H&E. (Original magnification ×40.) (*B*) Large, calcific ulcerated atheromatous plaque at the site of origin of the internal carotid artery (*arrowheads*).

basal ganglia cavities (lacunes)). Vascular changes affect, in addition to the brain, the eyes, the kidneys, and other organs. In the CNS, the cerebrum is most severely affected by hypertension (37).

Four different types of structural abnor-

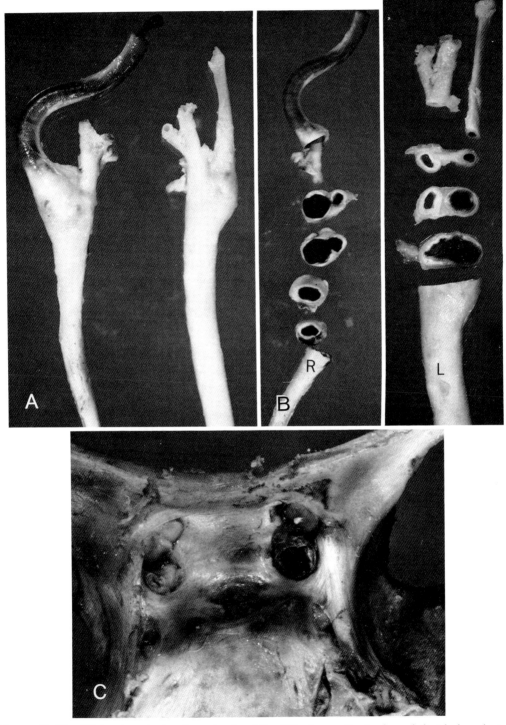

Figure 12.12. Bilateral occlusive thrombosis of the ICAs in a patient whose left-sided occlusion (and stroke) occurred about 9 months before; the right-sided occlusion developed 3 d before death. (*A*) External view of both arteries. (*B*) Cross-sections of ICAs showing old (*R*) and recent (*L*) thrombosis. (*C*) View of the ICAs as they emerge from the cavernous sinuses.

malities are described in the parenchymal brain arterioles (or small arteries) of hypertensive individuals: (*a*) *miliary saccular aneurysms* (300–1100 μm) involve arterial branches measuring 40–160 μm. (*b*) Miliary aneurysms and "lipohyalinosis," also called *"fibrinoid necrosis,"* involve vessels ranging in diameter from 80 up ot 300 μm with the sites of predilection being the putamen, thalamus, pons, cerebellum, and cerebral cortex. These are the same regions where the incidence of hypertensive hemorrhage and lacunar infarctions is highest. This type of angiopathy (i.e., "lipohyalinosis") is almost exclusively limited to cerebral arteries. (*c*) Asymmetric *fusiform miliary aneurysms* are found in penetrating arteries of approximately 150 μm in diameter. (*d*) *Bleeding globes*, fibrin globes, or pseudoaneurysms consist of masses of red blood cells enclosed or enveloped in concentric rings of fibrin emanating from breaks in the arteriolar wall (63).

Brains from 100 hypertensives and 100 age- and sex-matched normotensives were examined for intracerebral microaneurysms. Forty-six hypertensive and 7 normotensive had microaneurysms measuring up to 2 mm in diameter. The majority occur in vessels below 200 μm in diameter and the minority on arterial vessels of up to 400 μm in diameter. These aneurysms occur at a rate of 71% in hypertensives over the age of 60 while only 2 of 21 hypertensives under 50 years of age showed aneurysms. All microaneurysms in normotensives were found among people over the age of 65. Cerebral hemispheres were involved in all 53 affected cases; the main site where microaneurysms were found was the basal ganglia, but the subcortical white matter, pons, and cerebellum were also involved. Massive brain hemorrhage occurred in 20 hypertensives, 18 of whom had aneurysms. Massive hemorrhage also occurred in one normotensive without microaneurysms (39).

Fibrinoid changes may develop in the parenchymal arterial vessels of hypertensive patients with and without concomitant hemorrhage. These arteriolar changes are not necessarily present in other organs (58). The deep cerebral white matter of hypertensives contains significantly more water than appropriate control samples and shows histologic changes suggestive of actual or antecedent cerebral edema. In contrast the cortex, arcuate fibers of the white matter, and corpus callosum are essentially similar in the normotensive and hypertensive brains (2). Moderate intermittent hypertension and rapidly progressive and profound dementia without localizing neurologic signs may be the clinical expression of vascular alterations and diffuse white matter changes which characterize *subcortical arteriosclerotic encephalopathy* (Binswanger's disease) (27). The clinical picture of subcortical arteriosclerotic encephalopathy includes: persistent hypertension and systemic vascular disease, history of acute strokes, subacute accumulation of multifocal neurologic symptoms, long latent periods, lengthy clinical course, dementia, prominent signs of pseudobulbar palsy, and ventricular dilatation (32) (Fig. 12.13).

Angiitis (Noninfectious)

Polyarteritis nodosa (and its variants) (PAN)
Hypersensitivity angiitis (HSA)
Wegener's granulomatosis (WG)
Lymphomatoid granulomatosis (LYG)
Giant-cell arteritis (GCA)
Takayasu arteritis
Thromboangiitis obliterans (TAO)
Angiitis of systemic disease, e.g., lupus erythematosus (SLE)

Segmental inflammation and necrosis of the vessels are the common denominator of these conditions. A substantial proportion of these angiitis is closely associated with immunopathogenetic mechanisms and possibly with hypersensitivity. Deposits of immune complexes in the blood vessel walls and increased vascular permeability are important antecedents in the development of the vascular abnormality. Among the noninfectious angiitis, the only two that may involve the brain parenchymal vessels are SLE and LYG. Others (PAN, WG, and GCA) involve vessels in the subarachnoid space, the peripheral nervous system, or the extracranial vessels. Vascular histologic abnormalities in patients afflicted with angiitis are better interpreted after establishing the clinical features, i.e., is there systemic connective tissue disease? Hepatitis B infection? The histologic findings must be analyzed also in conjunction with the

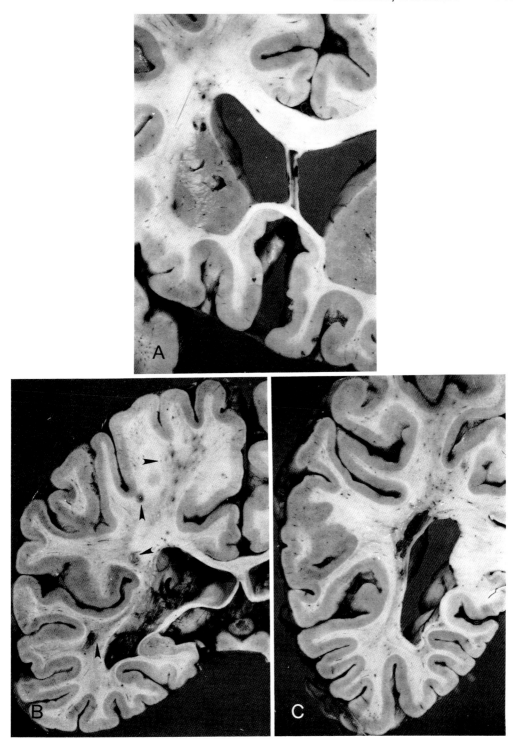

Figure 12.13. The effects of long-standing systemic hypertension are visible at various sites in this brain. (A) Multiple "lacunae" in the head of the caudate nucleus. (B) Multiple sites of cavitation/softening (*arrowheads*) in the parietal white matter. (C) confluent cavities in a periventricular location.

laboratory and immunofluorescence findings.

The experimental induction of immune-complex-mediated angiitis requires: (*a*) circulation of soluble immune complexes with a size greater than 19S; (*b*) Increased vascular permeability leading to filtration of immune complex by the elastic lamina or the venous basement membrane; (*c*) activation of complement and attraction of leukocytes (especially neutrophils); and (*d*) release of proteases by neutrophils with consequent damage to the vessel wall (149).

Classic polyarteritis nodosa (PAN) is a disease of medium-sized muscular arteries. The nervous system is usually involved in the form of *mononeuritis multiplex.* Aneurysms of up to 1.0 cm in diameter are common in the renal, hepatic, and visceral arteries. The inflammatory process in the vascular wall is not granulomatous, and glomerulonephritis is common (Fig. 12.14) PAN may be associated with hepatitis B antigen, rheumatoid arthritis, or SLE. Occasionally, PAN may be the cause of subarachnoid hemorrhage.

Neurologic dysfunction occurs in 80% of patients with PAN and fewer than 10% of patients with *hypersensitivity vasculitis* (HSA). The mechanism of neurologic dysfunction in both conditions is tissue ischemia. Mononeuritis multiplex, polyneuropathy, and stroke are frequent complications, but encephalopathies, cranial neuropathies, and brachial plexopathies are also seen (149). *Wegener's granulomatosis* (WG) in the nervous system usually becomes manifest in the form of mononeuritis multiplex involving spinal or cranial nerves. Necrotizing granulomatous vasculitis is common; the condition is exquisitely sensitive to cyclophosphamide therapy. Extravascular granuloma are very common, but typical tubercles are rare. In some biopsies only extravascular granulomata are visible, in which case rebiopsy may be indicated. The diagnosis of this condition is based entirely on histologic criteria, of which the most reliable one is the type of inflammatory lesion of vessels: phlebitis, and necrotizing arteritis (Fig. 12.15) (57).

Lymphomatoid granulomatosis (LYG) usually presents as a multinodular pulmonary infiltrate which microscopically is characterized by an angiodestructive and infiltrative process composed of small lymphocytes, plasma cells, histiocytes, and atypical lymphoreticular cells. Involvement of the CNS occurs in about 20% of the cases, and it results in a variety of syndromes such as: stroke, brain tumor, and encephalopathy (105).

Giant cell (cranial) arteritis (GCA) may be a component of polymyalgia rheumatica and usually involves the temporal artery in people over the age of 55. Absence of inflammation in one horizontal segment of the artery does not rule out the diagnosis. Blindness, secondary to involvement of the ophthalmic artery, is a definite risk (Fig. 12.16). Involvement of intracranial vessels by GCA is uncommon (57).

Takayasu arteritis is more common in young females. Although usually it can be a panarteritis, the inflammatory response rarely includes giant cells. Progressive intimal proliferation with luminal occlusion and stroke involving the aortic arch and its branches are the most characteristic presentations (Fig. 12.17). Takayasu's disease and thromboangiitis obliterans may involve the brain through the induction of ischemic changes (139).

Thromboangiitis obliterans (TAO) affects males between 20 and 40 years of age. It is a true angiitis of intermediate- and small-sized arteries. Inflammation and thrombosis almost always coexist (Fig. 12.18) The thrombus may contain microabscesses which lead to chronic inflammation which leads to occlusion and recanalization. No immune phenomena have been demonstrated in patients with TAO an entity that is almost exclusively confined to heavy smokers (57).

In most large series, two of three patients with *systemic lupus erythematosus* (SLE) develop neurologic symptoms (especially seizures, hemiparesis, and cranial neuropathies). These symptoms can be attributed, in most instances, to one or more of these lesions: brain infarctions (large and small); hemorrhages (parenchymal, subarachnoid, or subdural); and various CNS infections. The underlying structural alterations present in the brain blood vessels of these patients include: hyalinization, perivascular inflammation, endothelial hyperplasia, thromboembolism, and noninfectious angiitis (52a). Deposition of soluble

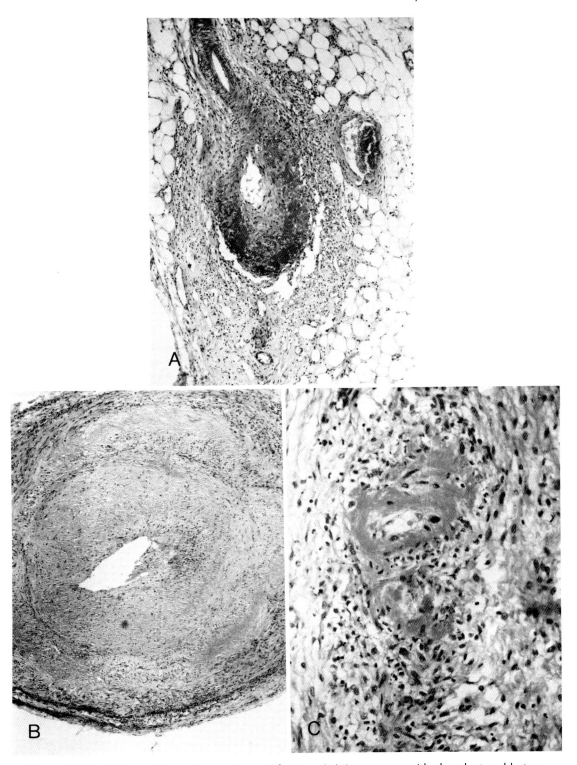

Figure 12.14.   Polyarteritis nodosa: extracranial artery. (*A*) Acute stage with abundant and heterogeneous leukocytic infiltrates. (*B*) Healed stage showing extensive fibrosis. (*C*) Fibrinoid necrosis and leukocytic inflammation of acute stage. (Courtesy of Dr. U. Sandbank, Tel Aviv, Israel.)

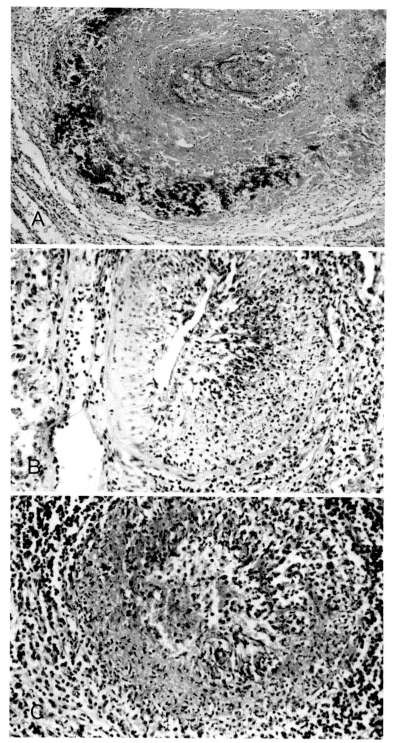

Figure 12.15. Wegener's granulomatosis: peripheral nerve artery. The leukocytic inflammatory picture and the fibrinoid necrosis in this condition are very similar to those of polyarteritis nodosa. Granulomas sometimes may be seen close to the involved vessels. (Courtesy of Dr. U. Sandbank, Tel Aviv, Israel.)

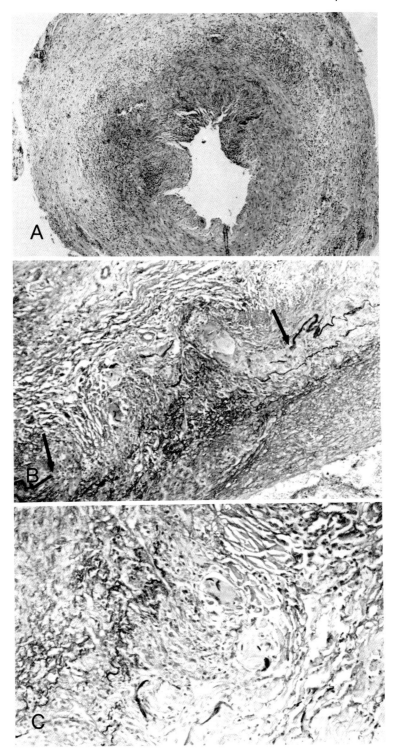

Figure 12.16. Giant-cell arteritis: temporal artery. The circumferential involvement of the vessel with most inflammatory cells being close to the intima is shown in *A*. (*B*) Interrupted internal elastic layer (*arrows*) with (*C*) granulomas containing multinucleated giant cells. (Courtesy of Dr. U. Sandbank, Tel Aviv, Israel.)

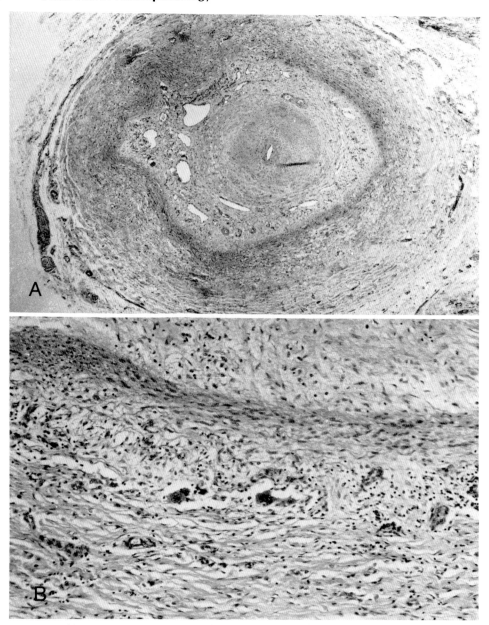

Figure 12.17. Takayasu arteritis in an extracranial vessel. (*A* and *B*) Recanalized thrombus and preferential involvement of the adventitia and outer tunica muscularis contrast with the granulomatous inflammation and involvement of the inner arterial layers which is characteristic of GCA. In advanced, chronic cases, considerable overlap may exist between the structural features of these two entities. (Courtesy of Dr. U. Sandbank, Tel Aviv, Israel.)

antigen-antibody complexes in the choroid plexus may reflect another abnormality by which brain functions become altered in patients with SLE.

Miscellaneous

Spontaneous occlusion of the branches of the circle of Willis and the development of abnormal vascular networks, both at the base and on the convexity of the brain, were first described in 1956 (131). The hazy angiographic appearance of these abnormal vascular networks, resembling a puff of smoke, has given rise to the Japanese designation of moyamoya. In 19 fatal cases of *moyamoya* angiopathy among adults, fresh

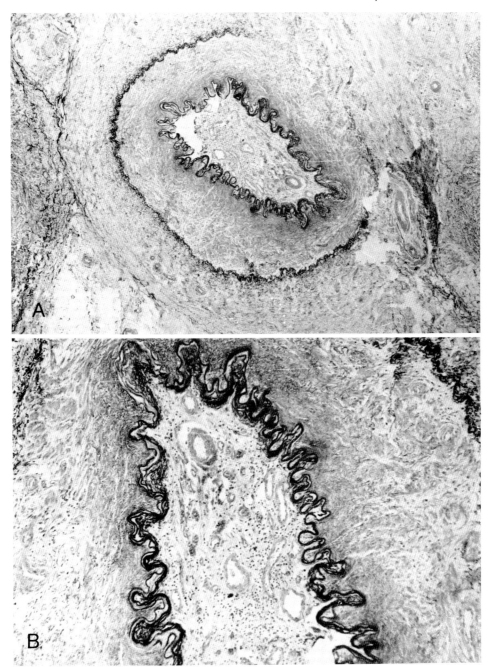

Figure 12.18. Thromboangiitis obliterans. Extracranial artery. Fibrosing granulomas and recanalized thrombus in an artery showing the healed stage of TAO. (Courtesy of Dr. U. Sandbank, Tel Aviv, Israel.)

and massive brain hemorrhage was found in the basal ganglia, thalamus, and hypothalamus of 9, and in the thalamus, peduncle, and midbrain of 5. Cerebral infarcts were found in four children. Saccular aneurysm of cerebral arteries in the subarach-

noid space was present in 2 of 19 patients (165). The structural alterations in this disease are confined to the vascular system, particularly to the arteries of the brain and heart. Concentric intimal thickening with severe narrowing or obstruction of the lumen, infolding of the internal elastic lamina, and decreased caliber of the vessel is common in all cases examined postmortem or by biopsy of the external carotid artery branches. Lipid or calcium deposits are exceptional. Presence of immunoglobulins or complement components cannot be demonstrated. The increased and abnormal networks of thin-walled vessels are interpreted as secondary collaterals that develop as a result of progressive multiple vascular narrowings or occlusions (91).

Fibromuscular dysplasia of the cervical portion of the carotid, vertebral arteries and, sometimes, the intracranial arteries, is a condition having a characteristic angiographic pattern (i.e., multiple segmental narrowings of the involved vessel) that is explained by the distortion of the mural architecture. Numerous irregular patches of fibrous tissue are visible in the subintimal space or in the tunica media; these form ridges that protrude into the vascular lumen and cause segmental stenoses (182).

Among persons over the age of 60, *amyloid angiopathy* may be an important, although rare, cause of repeated intraparenchymal or subarachnoid hemorrhage and multiple cortical infarctions. Large- and medium-sized meningeal and cortical arteries can be the site of focal or diffuse amyloid infiltration with secondary lumen stenosis. Fibrinoid change and microaneurysm formation may also be present in some of the involved vessels (166).

Mineralization of the blood vessels is a common autopsy finding in human brains, especially frequent in persons dying after the age of 65. These irregularly shaped, granular deposits may exist both in the blood vessel walls (arteries, veins, and capillaries) and in the brain parenchyma. The most common sites where these mineral deposits can be found are: the hippocampal gyrus; the putamen-globus pallidus; and the cerebellar white matter near the dentate nucleus. Mineral salts present at these deposits are primarily made of iron. The existence of these mineral deposits is not associated with any known neurologic syndrome, and the mechanism by which they deposit in many brains is unknown.

Deposits of calcium-rich salts, having an appearance similar to that described before but usually present throughout the cerebral hemispheres, are frequently associated with parathyroid gland disorders. A third category of conditions, characterized by progressive neurologic deficits and widespread mineralization of blood vessels and brain parenchyma, is known under the eponymic designation of *Fahr's disease.*

Mineral deposits of a similar nature (in terms of the microscopic appearance) but confined to the cerebral cortex and coexisting with a facial cutaneous hemangioma are part of the *Sturge-Weber syndrome.*

ISCHEMIA

Ischemia is a condition in which the blood low (BF) is sufficiently decreased as to result in either temporary or permanent loss of organ function. Normally, and within a well-defined range of blood pressure changes (45–170 mm Hg mean arterial blood pressure), the flow of blood to the brain is maintained constant (average value: about 55 ml/100 g/min) through a system of autoregulation that presumably is dependent on arteriolar myogenic responses to changes in $PaCO_2$ and luminal pressure.

Among patients subjected to carotid occlusion (in the course of therapeutic endarterectomy), the critical blood flow required to maintain a normal electroencephalographic tracing is about 30% of normal. After the functional injury appears in the form of an isoelectric EEG tracing, this type of ischemia must persist for an as yet undetermined period (about 30–60 min) before the loss of function becomes irreversible (198). Neuronal function is maintained when cerebral BF is at 15–20 ml/100 g/min; flows below 15 ml/100 g/min result in rapid changes in function (197). Experimentally the flow at which individual neurons cease spontaneous activity is 0.18 ml/100 g/min, but a high interneuronal variability exists. The upper level of flow is called neuronal function threshold, the lower one membrane failure threshold (95). In addition to the absolute figures of blood flow, duration of the ischemic episode is very important. Thus, a close mathematical correlation has been demonstrated between percent of necrotic neurons at a given site and *degree* or *severity* of ischemia, i.e., local BF × time (75).

Ischemic injuries to the human brain can be of many types and include those secondary to absolute ischemia (i.e., postmortem effects); progressive ischemia secondary to the circulatory failure characteristic of prolonged agony, which is common to many persons who die in a hospital; abrupt and global (but transient) ischemia of patients who suffer *syncopal* episodes; and regional (or focal) ischemia secondary to vascular occlusion (arterial, arteriolar, venous) (76). Most brain ischemic lesions are characteristically *incomplete*, either because they are transient or because after a vascular occlusion, residual flow is maintained through the numerous end-to-end anastomoses that connect various vascular systems in the human brain. Depending on the causative mechanism and the percent decrease in blood flow, at least five varieties of ischemic injuries are recognized (Table 12.4).

Complete (Irreversible) Ischemia

The interpretation of cellular abnormalities induced by ischemia (particularly those of a recent type) may be blurred by *artifacts,* i.e., postmortem alterations of the structural features. These artificial changes may be a result of one or more of the following: (*a*) handling an unfixed organ; (*b*) long delays in tissue fixation (i.e., postmortem ischemia); (*c*) use of fixatives with the wrong composition; and (*d*) faulty tissue processing.

The cellular conditions created by the complete absence of circulation are sometimes called autolysis, i.e., the process of cellular self-destruction attributed to the activation of lysosomes; however, that such

a process is not activated until several hours after the circulation stops (55) is suggested by the ability to transplant cadaver organs as late as 2 h after death; therefore, the cellular changes occurring in the immediate postmortem period might be described more accurately as those of *postmortem ischemia.*

It is uncommon (except in forensic pathology) for pathologists to evaluate the brain of persons in whom the transition from life (normal circulation) to death (absence of circulation) occurs in a matter of seconds or minutes. Instead, the process of dying in most hospitals evolves over a matter of hours or days, during which time the CBF probably fluctuates widely. Evaluating the effects of these circulatory changes in most human brains is usually modified by an additional period of total ischemia, i.e., the death-fixation interval (average, 8 h). The effects of this period of ischemia at a temperature of 4°C are relatively minimal (115). Total brain ischemia (room temperature) of up to 2 h duration induces minor structural and biochemical alterations (41). The use of buffered formalin solutions (4%) to fix human brains for periods of 7–10 days (before attempting dissection) is as widespread as is the standardization of methods for embedding, cutting, and staining. Therefore, unless the tissue processing conditions are extraordinary, the introduction of artifacts in histologic preparations of human brains should be the exception rather than the rule.

Cellular responses to the complete absence of circulation include changes in the distribution of nuclear chromatin, disintegration of polyribosomes (with consequent

Table 12.4
Types of Ischemic Injury and Their Anatomic Counterpart

A. Complete irreversible ischemia	1. Somatic death: ischemic cellular changes precede autolysis by several hours.
B. Global ischemia with various degrees of either reperfusion or incomplete ischemia	2. Brain death; cardiac arrest, severe hypotension; strangling closed head injury; cardiac valvulopathies
C. Regional (arterial) ischemia: thrombotic, embolic	3. Brain infarctions: ischemic or hemorrhagic.
D. Regional (venous) ischemia	4. Brain infarction: hemorrhagic
E. Regional (arteriolar) ischemia	5. Brain infarction: lacunae and other microinfarctions.

loss in the stainability of nucleic acids), and deposition of mineral salts, usually calcium carbonate, in the mitochondrial matrix (90, 204). One of the earliest signs of cell death is reflected in the influx of calcium salts into the mitochondria; however, the death of numerous cells may be compatible with recovery of organ function. Thus, in organs containing abundant epithelial cells (i.e., the intestinal mucosa), functions may be reestablished by means of cell division and replacement of the lost cells.

Cellular changes similar to those described in liver and other organs have been induced by keeping normal animal brains absolutely ischemic for up to 2–3 h (19°C) (41, 116). As long as the circulation is promptly terminated and the tissues are fixed by cardiovascular perfusion, the effects of complete ischemia are the same on all the cells, i.e., neurons, glia, and vascular elements all display, at a given moment, comparable structural changes, including peripheral clumping of chromatin granules, dispersion of ribosomes, and dilatation of endoplasmic reticulum cisternae. Probably some of these cellular alterations can be reversed by reperfusion (41, 116). Interestingly, reperfusing a brain for 60 min after keeping it completely ischemic for 15 min induces heterogeneous abnormalities that can be demonstrated by structural and biochemical methods (109, 211). A somewhat comparable observation had been made earlier: normal brains fixed by cardiovascular perfusion contain homogeneously staining neurons, whereas normal animal brains fixed by immersion (after being kept ischemic for a period of minutes) contain foci where "dark" neuronal profiles are visible (31). The author attributed this phenomenon to the effects of manipulating an incompletely fixed brain. These observations have been extended to demonstrate that in poorly stabilized (fixed) samples of normal brain, individual neurons adopt a "dark" appearance when they are exposed to hyperosmolar solutions (168).

Global (Incomplete) Ischemia

DEFINITION

Disorders of systemic circulation may either *reduce* the entire cerebral blood flow,

below the levels of autoregulatory mechanisms, or may *interrupt* completely but transiently the CBF. This condition is clinically expressed in the form of a syncope or a sudden and transient loss of consciousness. Cardiac dysrhythmias, shock, hypotension, and conditions that increase the intracranial pressure (e.g., closed head injury) can all result in severe reduction of CBF. Cardiac standstill induces a form of ischemia that is *incomplete* because the circulatory interruption is transient. Since all these mechanisms of ischemia simultaneously affect all brain components, the condition is described as one of *global* ischemia (70).

In addition to those afflicted by cardiac arrest, hypotension, and cardiac dysrhythmias, at least four other groups of patients can be victims of transient global ischemia, i.e., patients undergoing open cardiac surgery, persons with massive increases in intracranial pressure (usually after blunt head injury), victims of large subarachnoid hemorrhage, and survivors of either hanging (strangulation) or near drowning.

Symptoms. The neurologic consequences of episodic cardiac arrest vary enormously, depending on factors such as the duration of the circulatory crisis, age of the patient (children and young persons withstand this injury better than adults), body temperature (hypothermia lengthens the tolerable period of total ischemia), and the anatomic condition of the vasculature. Adults who coincidentally become hypothermic [or who purposely are made hypothermic (18°)] at the time of a prolonged (up to 25 min) cardiac standstill may recover entirely their brain functions (185).

Behavioral and neurologic abnormalities (e.g., transient visual agnosia) are common among patients subjected to open heart surgery in the immediate postoperative period. The degree of cerebral injury correlates with the patients' advanced age and the low levels of blood pressure; moreover, the symmetrical brain lesions that develop under the above conditions are identical to those induced by hypotension (205). Some of the brain lesions found among open heart surgery patients may be of embolic origin (25, 80). In patients undergoing cardiac operations with pulmonary bypass, a linear correlation can be established among the degree and duration of intraoperative hypotension, the time when certain types of EEG abnormalities become detectable, and the extent of ischemic lesions in the brain arterial border zones (195).

Patients recovering from episodic cardiac arrest may suffer from transient or persistent amnestic syndromes, miscellaneous motor deficits, cortical blindness, ataxia, and other neurologic symptoms that reflect the involvement by ischemia of multiple nervous system sites (Table 12.5). In all of the above circumstances the brain injured by ischemia is reperfused either spontaneously or as a result of vigorous therapeutic efforts. Thus, the average type of injury evaluated in most human brains consists of ischemia and reperfusion. Many of the anatomic patterns of ischemic injury become grossly visible only after a significant period of reperfusion. Multiple sites of focal hemorrhagic softening are more readily demonstrated in a patient who survives cardiorespiratory arrest for 3 days, for example (Fig. 12.19), than in one who dies within the first 30 min after the ictus. The inhomogeneous and unpredictable patterns of multifocal brain softening are attributable, in part, to the variable anatomical patterns of the brain vessels and to intrinsic factors known as *selective vulnerability*.

After episodic global ischemia, the extent of brain injury among some of the survivors may be such as to necessitate mechanical takeover of their breathing function. In these cases, the usual sequence of events includes cardiorespiratory arrest (i.e., global brain ischemia) leading to brain edema and massive increases in intracranial pressure. The latter may equal or exceed the systolic pressure, thus effectively cutting off the brain circulation, as demonstrated by angiographic and scintigraphic methods (94, 128), and injuring the respiratory center, among others. Brain tissue pressure remains markedly increased, as evidenced by the mushrooming of brain tissues when craniotomy is attempted in these patients. Maintenance of the ventilatory thoracic functions by mechanical means leads to a situation in which the extracranial circulation is maintained while the intracranial contents (including the pituitary gland) remain devoid of effective blood flow and at a temperature of 37°C; within a few days, these conditions lead to profound structural abnormalities (i.e., extensive cell membrane disintegration) commonly but incorrectly designated "*respirator brain*" (207).

The clinical counterpart of this circulatory disturbance constitutes one of the most frequently encountered types of "*brain death*" (Table 12.5), or a situation in which brain tissues disintegrate in a patient whose other tissues are relatively intact. That the disintegration of the brain in such cases precedes death can be demonstrated by finding macerated brain tissues when the autopsy is completed within a few minutes of death (115). The pattern of coagulation necrosis involving the adenohypophysis, in cases of global intracranial ischemia, is similar to that found after transection of the pituitary stalk (45).

Table 12.5
Postcardiac Arrest: Prototypical Neurological Syndromes[a]

A. Minimal or no structural damage (coma less than 12 h)
    Complete recovery; transient amnesia
B. *Multifocal* structural damage (coma longer than 12 h)
    Cerebral cortex:
        Amnesia; dementia
        Bibrachial paresis; quadriparesis
        Cortical blindness; visual agnosia
    Spinal cord: paraparesis
    Other: ataxia, seizures, myoclonus, extrapyramidal signs
C. Extensive global damage (no recovery of consciousness)
    Cortex: vegetative state; neocortical death (apallic state)
    Cortex + brain stem ± spinal cord: brain death

---

[a] Adapted from J. J. Caronna and S. Finkelstein (35).

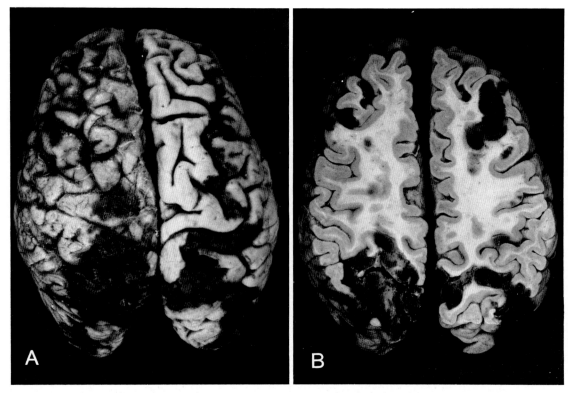

Figure 12.19. The anatomical distribution of the arterial border zones between MCA and ACA is visible in this specimen from a patient who suffered cardiac arrest 7 d before; normal BP was reestablished after several minutes, and this explains the marked hemorrhagic nature of the lesions; however, the patient did not regain consciousness.

STRUCTURAL FEATURES

Global (incomplete) brain ischemia induces a wide variety of structural changes; however, during the acute state (i.e., the first hour of reperfusion) these changes may not be readily apparent to the naked eye. One of the best known effects of ischemia is the induction of *energy failure*; as a consequence of this, there is an almost immediate escape of intracellular K^+ with concomitant intracellular entry of Na^+ and water; alterations in the compartmental distribution of Ca^{2+} also develop quickly and may accelerate the demise of ischemic cells (95). As a result of these ionic exchange abnormalities, brain ischemia induces brain edema that is translated into narrowing of the ventricular cavities and sulci of the subarachnoid space; in addition, capillary dilatation and congestion impart a dusky discoloration to isolated foci of the cerebral and cerebellar cortices (Fig. 12.20). The ischemic edematous brain which initially is tense and firm becomes flabby and mushy, once the distintegration of the cell membranes becomes widespread. Abnormalities consistently observed in specimens obtained from patients dying after global brain ischemia with survival of several days include: increased brain weight; diffuse softening; congestion; dusky discoloration in isolated foci of the cortex and white matter (usually more apparent at the bottom of cortical gyri); and brain herniations (uncinate and cerebellar) (207). The latter sometimes are sufficiently pronounced as to result in sloughing of cerebellar cortex fragments into the spinal subarachnoid space (98).

The topographic distribution of the lesions of global ischemia is extremely variable; the multifocal circumscribed lesions usually found in these cases may involve various portions of the cerebral cortex (especially Sommer's sector of the hippocampus), cerebral white matter, basal ganglia, thalamus, cerebellum, brain stem, and

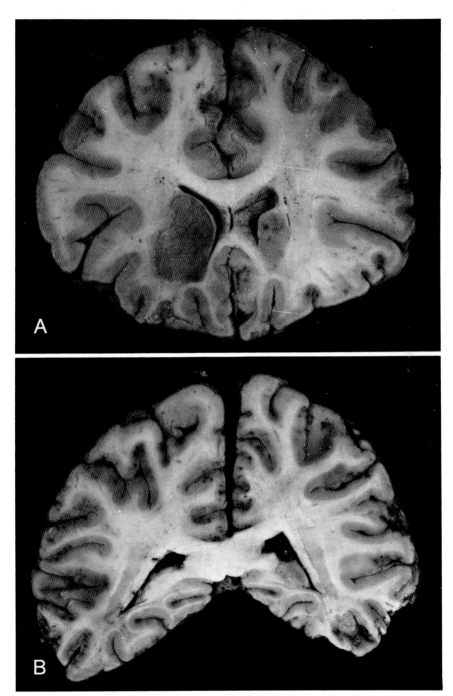

Figure 12.20. Six-day survival of cardiac arrest. An 80-yr-old woman underwent cardiorespiratory arrest and irreversible coma 4 d before death. Microscopically, the brain showed typical pseudo-laminar necrosis and the adenohypophysis was completely necrotic. (A) Coronal section of cerebrum at the level of the head of the caudate nuclei and (B) at the level of the splenium to illustrate multifocal sites of abnormal color and texture in the cerebral cortex; a few petechiae are also visible in the cortex.

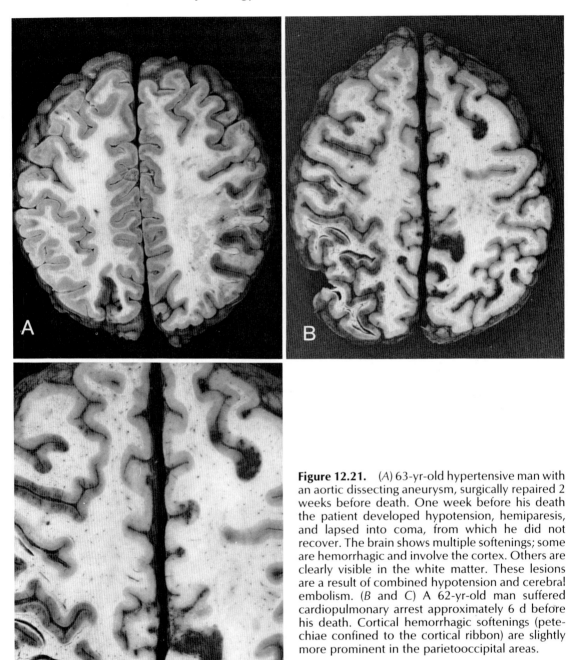

Figure 12.21. (*A*) 63-yr-old hypertensive man with an aortic dissecting aneurysm, surgically repaired 2 weeks before death. One week before his death the patient developed hypotension, hemiparesis, and lapsed into coma, from which he did not recover. The brain shows multiple softenings; some are hemorrhagic and involve the cortex. Others are clearly visible in the white matter. These lesions are a result of combined hypotension and cerebral embolism. (*B* and *C*) A 62-yr-old man suffered cardiopulmonary arrest approximately 6 d before his death. Cortical hemorrhagic softenings (petechiae confined to the cortical ribbon) are slightly more prominent in the parietooccipital areas.

spinal cord (Fig. 12.21). When the period of survival, after global ischemia, extends over several weeks, i.e., when the injury is chronic, the sites of brain softening may be visible in the cerebral cortex in the form of either linear or irregular areas of tissue destruction, i.e., *laminar* and *pseudolaminar* necrosis (Fig. 12.22). The arterial border zones, the hippocampus, the cerebellar cortex, and the pontine base are among the sites most constantly involved by global ischemic injury. Grossly visible changes in the brains of cardiac arrest survivors (lasting 2–15 min) may affect the striatum, basal ganglia, parietal occipital cortex and, particularly, the precentral and calcarine cortex (191).

Postmortem brain analyses among patients who, in the course of surgical interventions, suffer cardiac arrest and survive at least 6½ hours disclose edema, multifocal areas of cortical pallor, neuronal necrosis, and astrocytic proliferation that are more pronounced at, or near, the parietooccipital notch. This location corresponds to the "terminal field" of all three hemispheric arteries, and for this reason the tissues at the parietooccipital notch may be more vulnerable to hypotension. Focal necrosis of this type can also be seen in the basal ganglia, thalamic nuclei, cerebellar cortex, brain stem (especially pontine neurons), and, less commonly, in the cerebral white matter (Fig. 12.23) (25, 133, 191).

Among surviving victims of strangling (i.e., global ischemia with arterial and venous involvement), two features have been emphasized: an initial asymptomatic period, sometimes lasting several days, and bilateral symmetrical softening of basal ganglia structures (47).

Multifocal softening of cerebral and cerebellar *white matter* (some times hemorrhagic) has been observed in survivors of hanging, strangulation, and hypotensive crises (191). Some authors (28) attribute these white matter lesions to the effects of edema and vasospasm. Others emphasize the rarity of predominant white matter involvement in cases of "pure" ischemia and suggest that perhaps three factors must operate sequentially before this *leukoencephalopathy* develops: preexisting hypoxemia (as observed after respiratory depression); global ischemia; and reperfusion (i.e., several days survival) (83). Experimentally, subcortical leukoencephalopathy or white matter "infarction" has been induced after occluding an artery (for about 6 h) and reperfusing for a minimum of 24 h (118). Predominant involvement of white matter,

as a consequence of circulatory derangements, has been traditionally known as "edema necrosis." Among newborns, lesions having similar features are designated: periventricular leukomalacia.

Regardless of the sites of involvement, ischemic lesions (i.e., infarctions) that are of a similar age and are symmetrically distributed in the left and right sides of a brain in which there are no demonstrable vascular occlusions should be interpreted as being the consequence of global incomplete ischemia (Fig. 12.24). Relatively symmetrical brain softenings involving the arterial border zones are associated either with simultaneous bilateral occlusion of large cervical arteries or with decreased cardiac output and systemic hypotension (3, 25, 138, 159, 170, 179).

Wide variability in the distribution of the brain lesions has been observed in experimental models of transient global ischemia. Some authors emphasize involvement of the arterial border zones; others stress the involvement of the occipital lobes and certain brain stem nuclei (162). Considerable interest has been elicited by the observations that, in experimental animals, the extent of brain damage attributable to global ischemia can be reduced by any one of these three: barbiturate administration, induction of hypothermia, and lowering the serum glucose levels (158).

SELECTIVE VULNERABILITY

Various brain components react in different or selective ways to the same ischemic injury. This traditional concept of *selective vulnerability* may be applied to three different situations.

(1) There are certain *sites* in the brain where the lesions of hypotension or cardiac arrest are more likely to develop. These areas are unpredictable in a given individual, but as a general rule the most distal arterial territories (i.e., "arterial border zones," boundary zones, or "watershed areas"), the hippocampus, and the cerebellum, are more susceptible to the same degree of ischemia than the rest of the brain. Likewise, cerebral cortical layers III, IV, and V are said to be more susceptible to the same ischemic insult than layers I, II, and VI (191).

(2) *Neurons,* as a group, are more suscep-

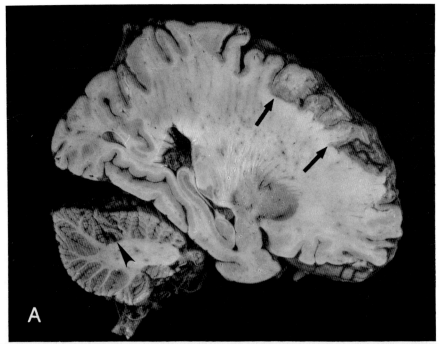

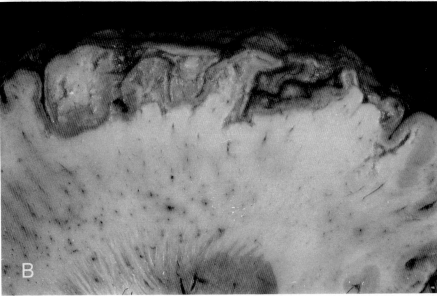

Figure 12.22.   Three different views of a specimen from a patient who died several weeks after a prolonged episode of cardiac arrest. (*A*) Selective destruction of the cortical ribbon in the arterial border zones of cerebrum (*arrows*) and cerebellum (*arrowhead*). There is no overt necrosis of hippocampus. (*B*) Closeup of same area shown in *A* to illustrate laminar or pseudolaminar necrosis. (*C*) The same specimen was reconstructed to show, in the CT scan plane of section, the haphazard distribution of ischemic cortical lesions (*arrowheads*).

tible to ischemia than oligodendrocytes, and these are more vulnerable than astrocytes.

(3) Within a single homogeneous neu-

ronal population, e.g., pyramidal cell layer of the hippocampus, *certain neurons* either are more susceptible to the same ischemic conditions or react with a different struc-

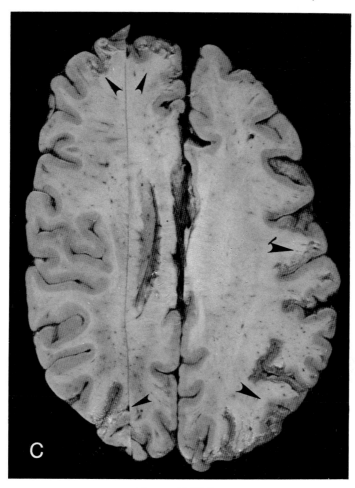

Figure 12.22C

tural expression to the same degree of injury. Thus, neurons in Sommer's sector of the hippocampus are more susceptible to changes in blood flow than the remaining pyramidal cells of this structure. Neither regional differences in blood flow nor in oxidative enzyme activities adequately explain these different neuronal responses (51). In experimental global ischemia, this selective neuronal response becomes apparent only in areas where either some residual circulation persists or when brains made ischemic for 15 min are reperfused for about 1 h (109).

Microscopically, pallor of red blood cells, lack of nuclear stainability, pale eosin stainability of myelin sheaths, and near absence of cellular inflammatory response are characteristic of severe, global brain ischemia (i.e., brain death). Some sites,

such as the internal granule-cell layer of the cerebellum and the neurons of the pontine base, are more extensively injured than other brain stem nuclei. Some of the large neurons in periventricular nuclei, brain stem, and spinal cord tend to retain their normal stainability after severe ischemic injury to the entire brain. This has been interpreted as indicative of their relative resistance to the effects of ischemia.

Several of the *microscopic* features of transient global brain ischemia (especially during the acute period) are indistinguishable from those observed after an arterial occlusion. For this reason, these cellular alterations are described together below.

Regional Ischemia

Brain infarction is a localized area of tissue necrosis that results from the prolonged

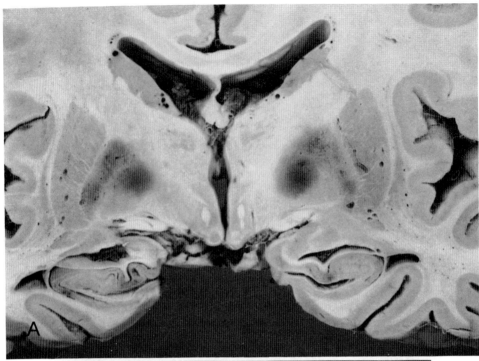

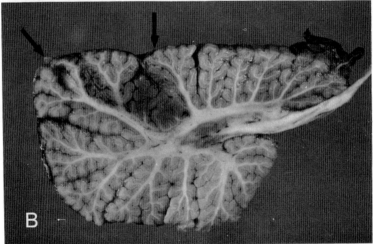

Figure 12.23. Effects of global ischemia on the basal ganglia, hippocampus, and cerebellum. (A) Coronal view of cerebral hemispheres showing bilateral, symmetrical, and partly hemorrhagic softening of globus pallidus and hippocampus. The patient suffered a severe hypotensive crisis about 7 d before death when he bled massively from esophageal varices. Death supervened as a result of a second bleeding episode. (B) Detail of softening in cerebellar arterial border zone (*arrows*) in a survivor of a hypotensive crisis.

occlusion of a vessel, either arterial or venous. This traditional definition may be extended to include focal brain lesions of ischemic origin, associated with vascular narrowing, hypotension, and vasospasm.

Occluding the *terminal* portion (i.e., dis-

tal to the collateral connections with other brain arteries) of a cerebral hemispheric artery induces local circulatory deficits and contralateral focal neurologic symptoms that disappear promptly when the regional ischemia is compensated for by collateral

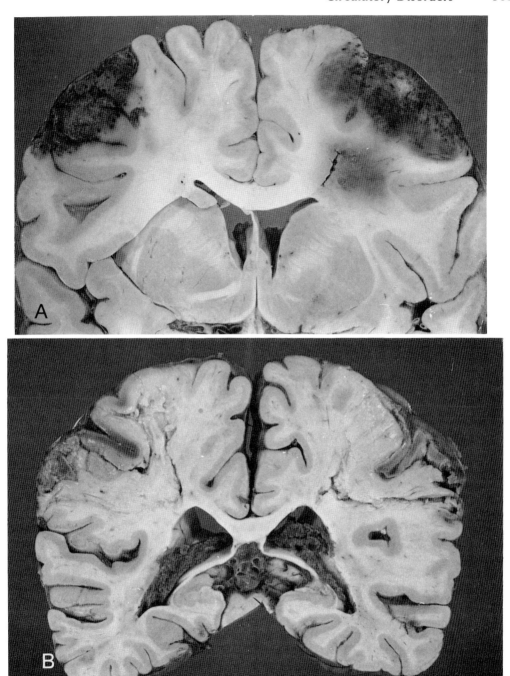

Figure 12.24. Examples of "watershed" infarcts. (A) Embolic, hemorrhagic infarctions in a patient with aplastic anemia and disseminated aspergillosis. (B) Bilateral, symmetrical, subacute infarctions in a patient who had a severe hypotensive crisis 12–14 d before death. The areas involved are variously called: boundary zones, watershed zones, and arterial border zones.

flow or by terminating the arterial occlusion before 1–2 h. This suggests that the initial neurologic deficit reflects a sublethal injury to the brain regions normally supplied by the occluded artery. The neurologic deficit, and therefore the neuronal injury, become irreversible only after a relatively prolonged time (154). The designation of *infarction* is commonly applied to lesions of ischemic origin that have reached irreversibility and are grossly apparent as sites of marked softening.

RISK FACTORS

Conditions associated with brain infarction include cardiac disease, hypertension, diabetes mellitus, and hypotensive episodes (188). Both high blood pressure and diabetes mellitus accelerate the rate of atherosclerosis and thus increase the risk of brain infarction. Anomalies of the circle of Willis are more common among persons with brain infarctions than among appropriate controls (18).

CAUSES

In adult autopsy studies, between 55 and 90% of the lesions having the gross appearance of large brain infarcts are caused by *thromboembolic occlusion* of the respective vessels. Atherosclerotic narrowings accompanied by transient systemic circulatory failure (dysrhythmia, hypotension) are responsible for a minority of the brain infarcts (112). Nearly one-third of the thromboembolic occlusions demonstrated at necropsy are located in the extracranial portion of the carotid or vertebral arteries (112). This is in agreement with the findings by Moossy (151), who reported more occlusions in the intracranial than in the extracranial vasculature of 204 brains with recent infarctions. Occlusions of the internal carotid, below the clinoid processes, occur more frequently in patients over the age of 40. Arterial occlusions in the carotid system, above the clinoid, and occlusions of the MCA are more common among patients below the age of 40 (189). Brain infarcts associated with embolism are preferentially located in the territory of the MCA. Platelet aggregates are more prevalent in cases of embolism, and embolism is commonly reflected in an infarct that has hemorrhagic features (113).

SPONTANEOUS FORMATION OF INTRAVASCULAR THROMBI: (Table 12.6)

Atherosclerosis, associated with thrombus formation and brain infarction is most common at the origin of the internal carotid artery (Fig. 12.11). Spontaneous thrombosis in the absence of significant angiopathy occurs in persons with "hypercoagulable states," which may be variously associated with neoplasia (e.g., thrombosis associated with carcinoma of the pancreas), bacterial infection (septicemia), and other less well-defined conditions. The association between septicemia, shock, and disseminated intravascular coagulation (DIC) has been attributed to hypofibrinogenemia, which is usually accompanied by platelet depletion. Thus, in addition to small fibrin thrombi, petechiae are common among patients with DIC and brain involvement. Most of these patients are victims of leukemia, lymphoma, and other neoplastic processes. The main lesions found in these brains are multiple brain infarctions, all of which have comparable age, and usually measure less than 1.0 cm in diameter. Thrombi may be found also in arteries, veins, and sinuses (40).

SOURCES OF BRAIN EMBOLISM (Table 12.7)

The identification of brain lesions whose gross features suggest an embolic origin should be accompanied by careful evaluation of the aortic-mitral valves in search of vegetations; in addition to those of bacterial endocarditis, small and friable, easily detached vegetations can be found in cases of nonbacterial endocardiopathy, i.e., "mar-

Table 12.6
Conditions Associated with Thrombotic Occlusion of Craniocervical Arteries

Atherosclerosis:
Endothelial injury, especially if accompanied by distal slowing of blood flow
Trauma (blunt, needle puncture)
Dissecting aneurysms
Miscellaneous angiopathies, e.g., Moyamoya syndrome
Hypercoagulability (DIC)

Table 12.7
Source of Embolism to the Craniocervical Arteries

Atrial fibrillation[a]
Mitral and aortic valves vegetations
Mural thrombi at the site of transmural myocardial infarction
Ulcerated atheromatous plaques in the aortic arch and at the origin of the internal carotid
Pulmonary veins' thrombi
Circulating adipose tissue
Foreign substances such as air introduced in the circulation after invasive intravascular procedures

[a] From P. A. Wolf et al. (216).

antic" endocardiopathy. Ulcerated atheroma involving the ascending aorta and the origin of the internal carotid is another source of embolism into the arteries of cerebral hemispheres. Procedures involving cannulation of large arteries or surgical opening of the heart increase the frequency of artery-artery embolism (22). Fractures involving the shaft of long bones have been associated with the condition of cerebral fat embolism (117).

Yates and Hutchinson (220) concluded that cerebral infarction rarely has a single cause; usually, it is the result of a combination of systemic disease and stenosis of extracranial and intracranial cerebral arteries. In this analysis of 100 brains, large cerebral infarctions were most frequently associated with atherosclerosis of the extracranial arteries than with disease of intracranial arteries (220).

Unusual causes of ischemic stroke among young people include migraine, vasculitis, hematologic disorders, and congenital vascular defects (134). Trauma to the neck, puerperium, granulomatous arteritis, and systemic lupus erythematosus are additional uncommon causes of brain infarction (4). Occlusion of the initial segment of a MCA has been documented in persons who suffered head trauma up to 5 days before the onset of unilateral neurologic deficits (103). Transient ischemia involving brain stem and cerebellum may be caused by extracranial vertebral artery stenosis (occlusion) frequently attributed to atlantoaxial instability, which in turn can be induced by rheumatoid arthritis (65). Cervical manipulation (e.g., chiropractic maneuvers) can be one of the major factors determining the development of ischemic stroke among these patients (130).

Mitral valve prolapse (demonstrated by echo cardiography) is a probable cause of transient cerebral ischemia among patients under the age of 40 (16). Intracranial venous and sinus thrombosis (associated with brain infarction) seem to be more common among women of childbearing age; however, the mechanism(s) responsible for thrombosis in these patients is unknown (12, 54). The causes of ischemic strokes among pregnant or puerpural women are similar to those prevailing among nonpregnant women of the same age. Over 70% of ischemic strokes in pregnancy are associated with occlusive arterial disease or other mechanisms unrelated to thrombosis of the venous system (44).

Finally, local brain ischemic lesions have been associated with angiographically evident *arterial spasm* in two types of conditions: following subarachnoid hemorrhage (from a ruptured aneurysm) (184) and after blunt head injury (147).

CLINICAL FEATURES

Brain infarctions become manifest in the form of localized neurologic deficits that are usually designated *ischemic stroke*. Deficits of this type that disappear before 24 h, usually within 30 min, are called transient ischemic attack (TIA) (Table 12.8). A completed stroke signifies a focal neurologic deficit (usually of ischemic origin) that has ceased to improve. Temporary localized motor-sensory deficits, monocular blindness, and dysphasia are common among patients with infarctions in the carotid distribution. Transient dizziness, ataxia, diplopia, binocular blindness, and dysarthria (with or without motor-sensory deficits) are common complaints among patients with vertebrobasilar artery insufficiency (74).

Transient ischemic attacks (TIA) can be

Table 12.8
Conditions Associated with Transient Cerebral Ischemic Attacks[a]

1. Abnormalities of cervical *blood vessels* that promote thrombosis (atherosclerosis, fibromuscular dysplasia, arteritis, dissection, and Moyamoya syndrome)
2. *Cardiac* abnormalities (ischemic heart disease, rheumatic heart disease, endocarditis, myxoma, mitral prolapse)
3. *Hematologic* abnormalities, e.g., thrombotic thrombocytopenic purpura
4. Altered *circulation* (hypotension; cervical spondilosis with vertebral compression)
5. *Miscellaneous* conditions (migrainous hemiplegia, contraceptives, hemorrhagic telangiectasis, and complications of angiography)

[a] Adapted from J. W. Schmidley and J. J. Coronna (183).

considered incomplete or embryonal infarctions; they are powerful predictors of stroke; within 5 years of the initial TIA, about 30% of these individuals will have a lethal or incapacitating stroke; 30% will have more TIAs but no stroke; 30% will have no more trouble; and 10% will either have a myocardial infarction or some other significant cardiovascular illness (146). The average annual incidence rate for first episodes of TIA is about 31/100,000 population. There is a marked increase in the number of brain infarctions among persons with TIA, as compared to persons of the same age (212). TIAs are rare in patients who have episodes of cardiac dysrhythmia of the type associated with reduction of cardiac output. Among patients who receive pacemakers for disturbances of rhythm or conduction, *focal* neurologic symptoms or signs are rare. The vast majority of such patients have symptoms of generalized brain ischemia, i.e., *syncope* (174).

GROSS FEATURES

Brain infarctions of arterial origin may be *pale (ischemic)* or *red (hemorrhagic)*. Brain infarctions of the former variety are difficult to visualize in their fresh state (Fig. 12.25). The differences that exist between infarcts and the surrounding nonischemic tissue include the blurring of the cortical-medullary boundaries and the decreased consistency of the ischemic tissues commonly designated *encephalomalacia*. Large fresh infarctions in the cerebrum are accompanied by displacement of midline structures, deformity of the ventricles, and herniations of the uncinate and cingulate gyri (Fig. 12.26). All of these abnormalities can be readily explained by the retention of water (commonly attributed to metabolic energy failure) in the ischemic tissues. Swelling of the infarcted hemisphere, manifested by shift of the midline structures, continues to develop during the first 3–5 days, when it reaches a maximum. Hemispheric swelling disappears after about 2 weeks (187). The rapidly fatal outcome of large hemispheric infarcts is related to the acute hemispheric swelling, and the resulting transtentorial herniation with consequent brain stem infarction or hemorrhage (163).

Red (hemorrhagic) infarctions of arterial origin differ from pale ones only by the numerous petechiae (usually confined to the gray matter, especially the cortex) that allow their ready identification (Fig. 12.26). There is no explanation for the selective localization of the petechiae to the gray matter. Hemorrhagic infarctions on the mesial surface of the occipital lobes are frequent in brains showing evidence of massive swelling and uncinate herniation. In such cases, the infarction is attributed to the extrinsic compression of the posterior cerebral artery by the herniated uncus against the edge of the tentorial incisura. The hemorrhagic component is explained by the fact that extrinsic arterial pinching probably results in incomplete occlusion of the lumen; in this situation, the residual flow is inadequate to prevent tissue necrosis but sufficient to allow bleeding into the ischemic territory. A comparable situation can be observed in patients with dissecting aneurysms of the cervical arteries (Fig. 12.27).

A second variety of hemorrhagic infarction develops in areas where arteries are occluded by emboli. Regional CBF studies strongly support the view that cerebral arterial occlusions frequently are transient

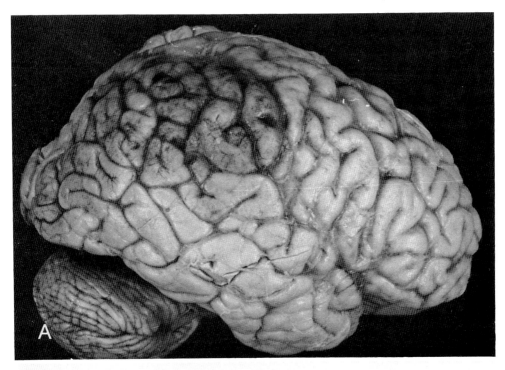

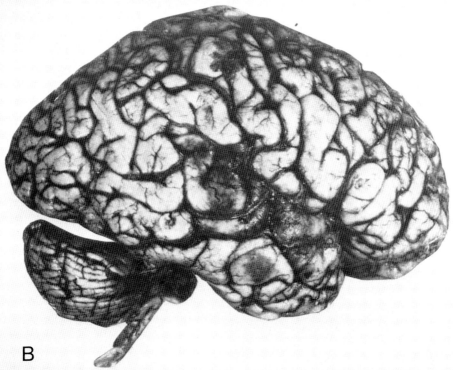

Figure 12.25. Cerebral fresh infarctions. Recent (i.e., about 1 week) embolic infarctions in the cerebral cortex. (A) Involvement of parietal lobule secondary to embolism originating from the ascending aorta, following attempted surgical repair of aortic dissecting aneurysm. (B) Hemorrhagic infarction in the right temporal lobe; embolism originated from aortic valve in a patient with nonbacterial, marantic endocardiopathy.

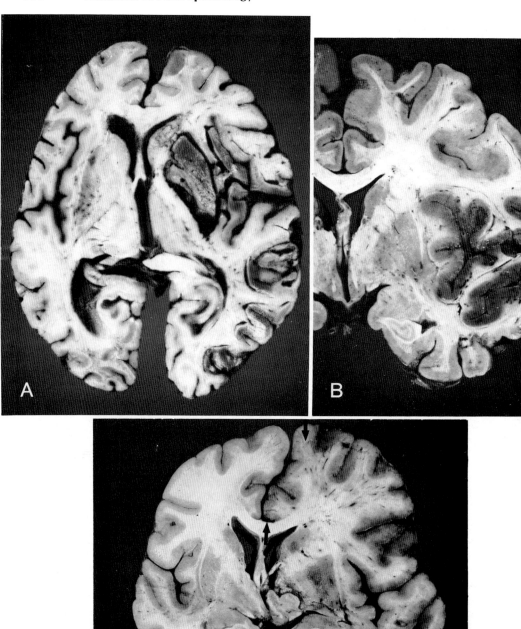

Figure 12.26.   Acute large infarctions with massive swelling. (*A*) Large, pale, recent (about 5 d old) infarction in the territory of the right MCA; extreme fragility of the white matter results in easy fragmentation. Swelling of the infarcted hemisphere has peaked. (*B*) Hemorrhagic infarction (same as in Fig. 12.25*B*). The picture demonstrates the confinement of petechiae to the cortical ribbon. (*C*) Massive swelling of right hemisphere, secondary to recent arterial occlusion and infarction, resulted in marked shift of midline structures, including subfalcial herniation of the cingulum (*arrows*) and asymmetry of lateral ventricles.

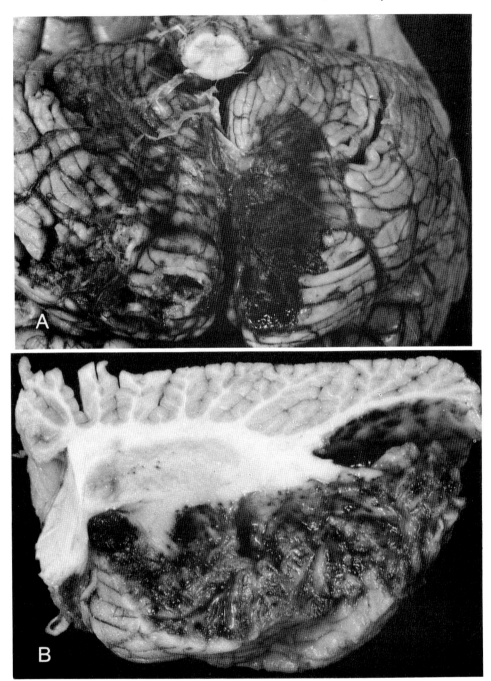

Figure 12.27. Hemorrhagic infarctions of the cerebellum in 64-yr-old person with bilateral dissecting aneurysms of veretebral arteries.

and secondary to emboli that fragment and move distally (169). Postmortem and angiographic observations also suggest that arterial occlusions secondary to embolism are frequently transient; angiography in 86 patients with acute stroke showed that of 31 patients with demonstrable arterial occlusion, 10 had lysed or mobilized the clot at the time of a reexamination, i.e., second angiography or autopsy (59). Therefore, the hemorrhagic component of an arterial brain infarction of embolic origin is ascribed to the effects of reperfusion, a concept that has been corroborated in experimental studies during which the artery is reopened after 6 h, and reperfusion of the ischemic tissues is allowed for at least 24 h (118). In certain instances of surgical reopening of the internal carotid artery, preexisting brain infarctions convert into a large parenchymal hemorrhage. The latter may represent a confluency of numerous hemorrhages in an infarction. Brain infarctions associated with embolism are preferentially distributed through the territory of the MCA and are almost always hemorrhagic (113). Brain infarctions caused by septic embolism (bacterial or fungal) tend to be hemorrhagic, in part because of the necrotizing effect that many of these microorganisms have on blood vessel walls.

HEMORRHAGIC INFARCTIONS SECONDARY TO VENOUS/SINUS OCCLUSIONS

The topography of brain softenings secondary to venous (sinus) occlusion corresponds (roughly) to that of one of the major venous territories. In the cerebral hemispheres, the lesions have two distributions: those deep-seated, bilateral, and close to the midline softenings are secondary to occlusions involving the internal cerebral veins and the vein of Galen or their tributaries. Softenings associated with occlusion of the superficial cortical veins are usually unilateral and involve mainly the cortical and subcortical structures (Fig. 12.28). Occlusion of the superior sagittal sinus is usually fatal within a short period; this lesion may be accompanied by extensive bilateral and subcortical hemorrhagic softenings of

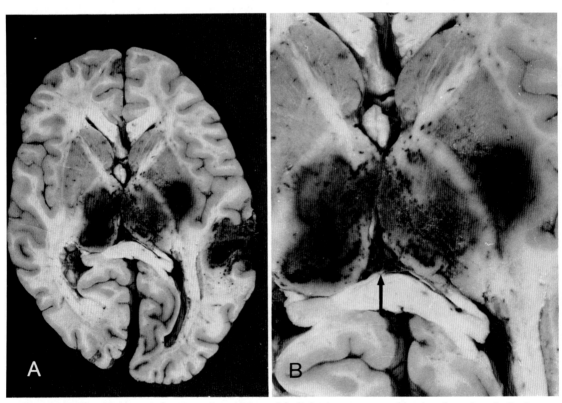

Figure 12.28. Venous infarctions in a 26-yr-old diabetic woman who developed polydipsia, polyuria, increased headaches and, eventually, coma; she died on the 7th hospital day. (*A*) CT scan plane of section shows hemorrhagic softening of the thalamic nuclei and right basal ganglia; an additional lesion is seen in the right temporal lobe where a large cortical vein was thrombosed. (*B*) Closeup of *A* to show thrombosed internal cerebral veins; the veins of Rosenthal, the vein of Galen, and several posterior fossa sinuses were also occluded by organizing thrombi.

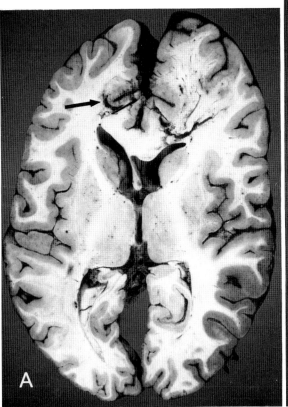

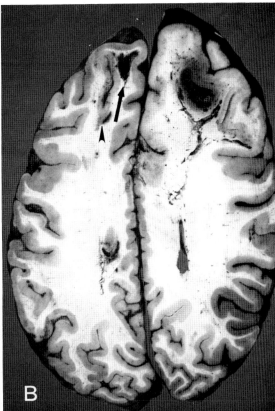

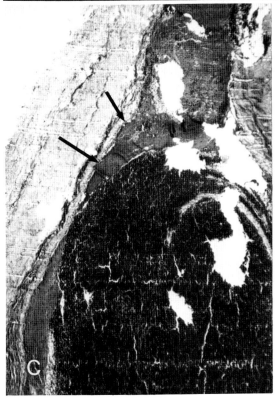

Figure 12.29. The effects of occluding the rost
three-fourths of the superior sagittal sinus in a 7-ɣ
old afflicted with sickle cell disease can be appreciat
in these views of the cerebral hemispheres. Surviv
after the stroke, was about 5 d. Subarachnoid her
orrhage, subcortical brain hemorrhages (*arrows*), a
marked softening of right frontal white matter a
visible in *A* and *B*. (C) Cross-section of superior sagit
sinus showing incomplete occlusion by organizi
thrombus (*arrows*). H&E. (Original magnificati
×250.)

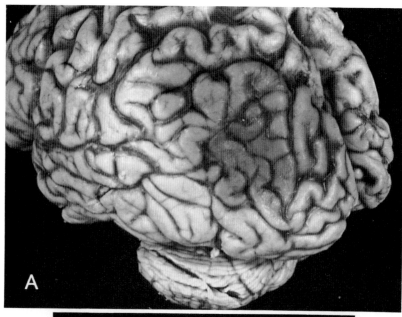

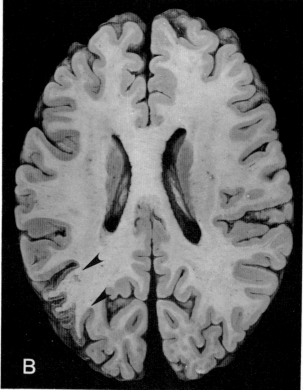

Figure 12.30.   Healing (or subacute) infarction in the left hemisphere, as seen on the brain surface (A) and on the CT plane of section (*arowheads*) (B). (C) Multiple cortical infarctions, either healed or healing. Acute ischemic injury is also apparent in the MCA-ACA border zones.

the frontal-parietal lobes in particular. Among young children and infants, the typical perivenous ring hemorrhages may not be readily apparent; instead, there may be confluent myelin breakdown and even liquefaction of white matter with sparing of

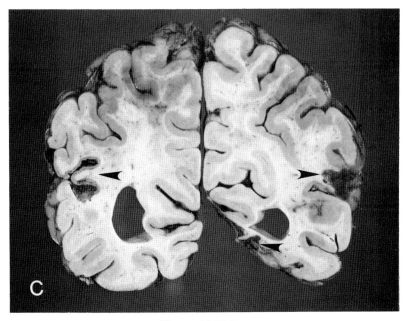

Figure 12.30C

cortex and basal ganglia (114) (Fig. 12.29). Numerous predisposing factors for intracranial venous thrombosis have been reported, among which infections and dehydration are preeminent (15, 107). Few of these reports have shown a causative association between the thrombosis and the presumptive risk factor. A syndrome of raised intracranial pressure, without detectable changes in brain parenchyma, has been associated with thrombosis of the lateral and posterior sagittal sinus (114). In addition to their typical topographic distribution, venous infarctions differ from those of arterial origin in that they are accompanied by early severe edema and by hemorrhages that are larger and more extensive (they extend into the white matter) than those of arterial infarctions. Leukocytic infiltrates are very abundant in infarctions of venous origin, probably because their entry into the area of necrosis is facilitated by the patency of the arterial vessels.

The *anatomic features* of brain infarctions are influenced by two factors: the caliber-location of the occluded vessel and the time evolved between the stroke and death. The topography of brain infarction is determined by the *site of the vascular occlusion;* infarctions resulting from occlusions of either the anterior cerebral artery or one of the pericallosal arteries primarily

cause softening in the rostral cingulum and a portion of the head of the caudate nucleus. Occluding the initial segment of the MCA results in softening of numerous structures, including the lateral portion of the head of caudate nucleus, anterior limb of the internal capsule, globus pallidus, putamen, insula, middle and inferior frontal gyri, most of the pre- and postcentral gyri, superior temporal gyrus, and a portion of the parietal lobe (Fig. 12.26). Internal carotid occlusions (at the intracranial segment) usually result in infarction of both ACA and MCA territories.

The main structures supplied by the posterior cerebral artery (PCA), which would become ischemic during occlusion of this vessel, are: middle and inferior temporal gyri; hippocampal gyrus; thalamus; and occipital pole, including the calcarine fissure. Occlusion of a single ICA can result in infarction of all three territories (ACA, MCA, and PCA) in persons in whom the PCA originates from the ICA. Also, bilateral frontal pole infarction can develop after unilateral ICA occlusion in patients in whom both ACA fill from the same side.

Acute infarction with involvement of one cerebellar hemisphere only can be the result of PICA occlusion. Massive cerebellar infarction that predominantly involves the posterior-inferior half of one hemisphere can be fatal within a period of 5–6 d. The infarction is of the hemorrhagic type in about one-fourth of the cases (200).

Occlusions of the vertebral artery or the posterior-inferior cerebellar artery (PICA) are associated with specific syndromes, e.g., Wallenberg syndrome, a clinical situation reflecting the involvement of lateral medullary structures located dorsal to the inferior olivary nucleus (60).

CAUSES OF DEATH

The overall number of deaths among patients with large infarctions in the distribution of the carotid-middle cerebral arteries during the acute stage (i.e., first week) is about 11%. However, a higher mortality (41%) prevails among patients who become unconscious and hemiplegic shortly after the stroke (111).

Cardiovascular failure (usually reflecting the involvement of the heart and large vessels by hypertension and atherosclerosis), renal failure, pulmonary thromboembolism, and pneumonitis are some of the leading extracranial causes of death among patients with brain infarction. Intrinsic or intracranial factors that may cause the death of brain infarction patients during the acute stage include brain edema and neurogenic failure. The latter is particularly significant in cases in which brain stem and diencephalon are directly involved by the infarction. Cerebral hemispheric edema or swelling can induce unconsciousness and death by creating conditions that interfere with the blood supply to the tegmentum of midbrain and pons (see below under Brain Edema). Large cerebellar infarction may be fatal during the acute stage, seemingly because of the compression that the swollen cerebellar hemisphere exerts on the medulla oblongata.

SUBACUTE BRAIN INFARCTION

Once the swelling of incomplete ischemia subsides (about the 6th to the 10th day), brain infarctions become sharply separated from the surrounding brain tissues; the white matter fragments easily; and the gray matter takes on a granular, slightly orange appearance. By this time, infarcted brain tissues begin to look smaller than tissues located in homotopic sites (Fig. 12.30). Almost all subacute brain infarctions are de-

monstrable by means of computerized axial tomography. Ischemic lesions of the cerebral hemispheres are more easily seen by CT scan than those involving the posterior fossa tissues, regardless of age and location.

HEALED BRAIN INFARCTION

The time elapsed between the stroke and the final stage of healing of the infarction is directly proportional to the volume of tissue destroyed by the regional ischemia. Completely healed brain infarctions (especially those located in the cerebral hemispheres), unlike those in other organs, are converted into a fluid-filled cavity that has sharply circumscribed edges. In the cerebellum, cavity formation is rare, possibly because most chronic infarctions here and in the brain stem are of a small size (Figs. 12.31 and 12.32).

Lacunes are destructive brain lesions, usually of ischemic origin (i.e., infarctions) that occur almost exclusively in one or more of these locations: basal ganglia, internal capsule, thalamic nuclei, base of the pons, and convolutional white matter. In addition to the location, lacunes are defined by their size: 0.2–15 cu mm. Because of their size, recent lacunes are probably easily overlooked at autopsy. Once the process of healing is completed, lacunes become visible in the form of a cavity having a sharply circumscribed edge and a roughly spherical shape (Fig. 12.33). Lacunes are associated with occluded penetrating small arteries or arterioles which branch out at right angles from relatively large caliber vessels (MCA or basilar arteries); these penetrating vessels have a mean diameter of 100–200 μm (upper limit: 500 μm) and represent end arteries, i.e., they are non-anastomosing. The size of lacunes is determined by the caliber of the involved vessel and the distance from the ostium at which the occlusion occurs. Numerous clinical syndromes have been described in patients with lacunes. Particularly frequent are: pure motor stroke, pure sensory stroke, and hemichorea-hemiballismus (64, 148). Atheromatous disease of the MCA and basilar arteries, with narrowing of the ostia of the perforating vessels and arteriolosclerosis of intraparenchymal arteries are the most common causes of small infarctions (lacunae) in the basal ganglia and pontine base (61).

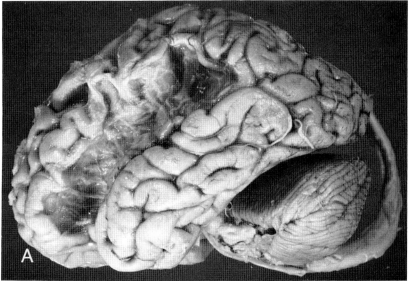

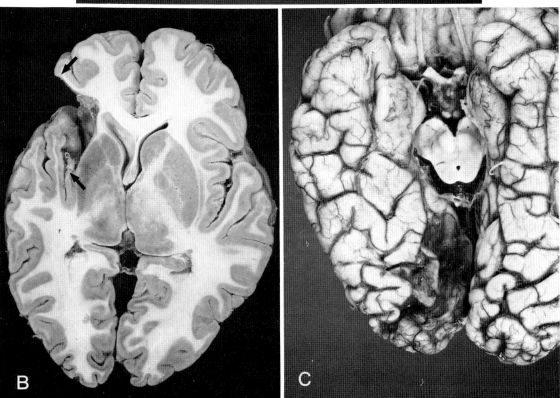

Figure 12.31. (*A*) Several years before death, this 54-yr-old woman with aortic stenosis suffered a stroke which resulted in expressive aphasia and seizures. The photograph shows the typical appearance of a healed infarction in the distribution of an MCA branch. (*B*) CT plane of section of same specimen shown in *A*. The *arrows* point to the sites of tissue destruction. (*C*) Healed infarction, the result of occluding a PCA branch.

Spinal Cord Infarction

The causes of this lesion are varied and abundant; they range from occlusion of seg- mental, medullary, and spinal arteries (sometimes by fibrocartilaginous tissue) to aortic dissecting aneurysms, cardiac arrest, and the effects of angiography (153). The

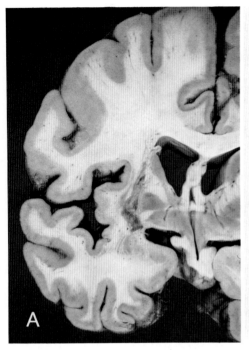
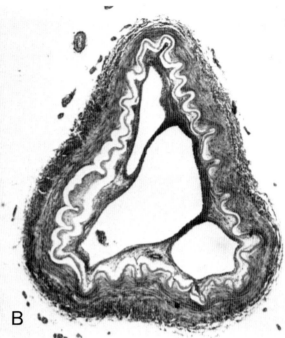

Figure 12.32. Healed infarctions, small. (*A*) Coronal section of hemisphere from a 27-yr-old woman with a history of stroke 1 yr before death; residual deficits included: expressive dysphasia, seizures, and right hemiparesis. The infarction involves the left striatum and internal capsule fibers. (*B*) Cross-section of the left MCA in same patient to show recanalization of the lumen; the embolus originated from mural thrombi in the left cardiac ventricle. Masson trichrome. (Original magnification ×10.)

sequence of cellular events in spinal cord infarction duplicates that seen in cerebral infarctions (153). In rare instances, the embolic occlusion of the anterior spinal artery may result in medial medullary infarction (122).

MICROSCOPIC FEATURES OF BRAIN INFARCTION

A description of these is preceded by a summary of observations made in experimental animals in which a prospective analysis of the local changes in cerebral blood flow has been associated with the structural abnormalities.

Experimental occlusion of an intracranial artery (e.g., MCA) induces multifocal, patchy areas of ischemia-hyperemia that over a period of 2–3 h coalesce into a large pale area of brain "infarction" (196). The changes in blood flow, induced by an arterial occlusion, are progressive rather than abrupt and uniform. Two to three hours after the arterial occlusion, an increasing number of neurons succumbs to the local ischemic conditions. Thus, multifocal heterogeneity is the rule in an area of evolving infarction. The heterogeneous nature of the changes of cerebral BF (amply demonstrated in experimental occlusion of a single brain artery) (77) has been assumed to be responsible for the development of three roughly concentric zones, each having characteristic microscopic features. These zones (*central reactive* and *marginal*) become clearly apparent approximately 3 h after the arterial occlusion (69).

In patients with documented occlusion of the MCA, focal disturbances of regional cerebral BF appear mostly in the form of ischemic foci, but some patients also show hyperemic areas (169). These local hyperemic values within areas of ischemia correlate with the angiographic finding of early filling veins and focal loss of autoregulation, a condition sometimes described under the designation of "luxury perfusion syndrome" (101).

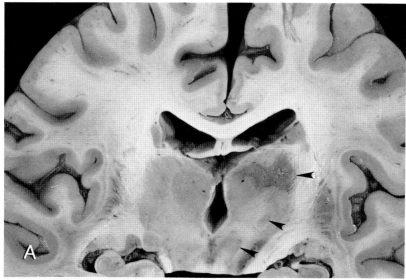

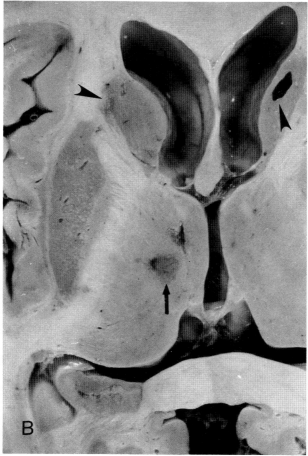

Figure 12.33. (*A*) Three small areas of recent infarction (*arrowheads*) are shown in the brain of a victim of polycythemia rubra vera. The vessels occluded by immature circulating white blood cells were all either small arteries or arterioles. (*B*) Two typical lacunes are seen in the caudate nuclei (*arrowheads*); two additional ones are seen in the left thalamus (*arrow*). The patient with lacunes had long-standing hypertensive disease.

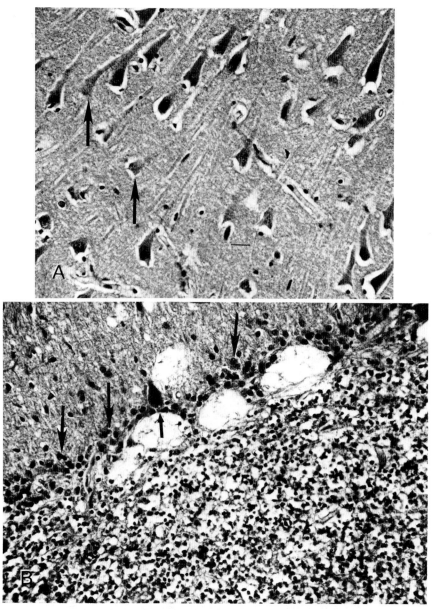

Figure 12.34. Acute neuronal injury. (*A*) Effects of *global ischemia* in cerebral cortex. Some neuronal perikarya are barely stainable (*arrows*); others are markedly dark. (*B*) In the same patient, changes in the cerebellar cortex include: necrosis of neurons in granule cell layer, marked shrinkage of Purkinje cell (*short arrow*), and proliferation of Bergmann glia (*long arrows*). Both preparations H&E. (Original magnification ×63.) (*C*) Normal cerebral cortex from subhuman primate to compare with (*D*) cerebral cortex from subhuman primate injured by irreversible ischemia of 60 min duration at 37°C. There are homogeneous changes in stainability of neuronal perikarya, astroglia, and neuropil. Both preparations, H&E. (Original magnification ×63.) (*E*) Effects of *regional ischemia* (subhuman primate) heterogeneous responses in neurons of basal ganglia, 90 min after MCA occlusion; profile of large, unstained neuron (*arrow*). H&E. (Original magnification ×63.) (*F*) Basal ganglia, from same animal as in *E* showing neuropil sponginess and contrasting responses in neuronal and astrocytic nuclei. Toluidine blue. (Original magnification ×100.) (*G* and *H*) Effect of *regional ischemia*: Basal ganglia of subhuman primates (MCA occlusion 2 h followed by 24-h reperfusion). Neuronal scalloping is clearly visible. Both preparations H&E. (Original magnification, ×100.)

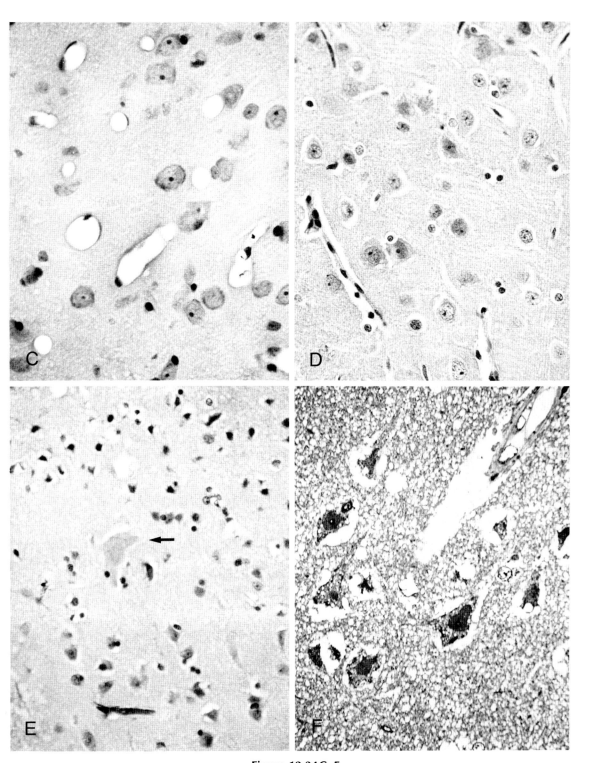

Figure 12.34*C–F*

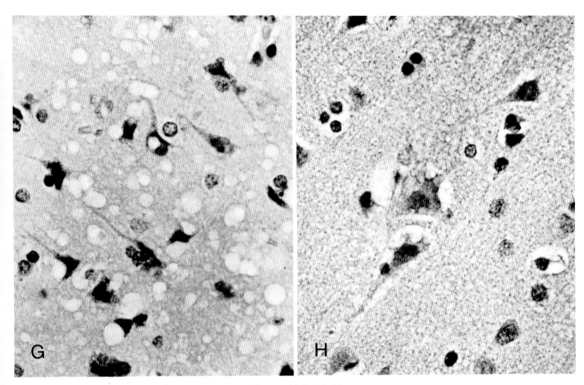

Figure 12.34*G–H*

Neurons

The number of structural alterations that ischemic neurons display is extremely varied; neuronal alterations in brains made ischemic by either arterial ligation or hypotension include: pallor of nuclear and cytoplasmic nucleic acids (ghost neurons); shrinkage and condensation of the perikaryon (dark neurons); nuclear pyknosis with cytoplasmic eosinophilia (red neurons); precipitation of formaldehyde pigment on the neuronal perikaryon (incrustation); neuronal scalloping; neuronal vacuolation; development of a perineuronal halo; and many others that probably are determined by the severity-duration of the ischemia and the reperfusibility of the ischemic territory (Figs. 12.34 and 12.35) (72, 76). Because these changes are highly heterogeneous (both chronologically and spatially) and because it is unlikely that they are specific for ischemia, the designation of ischemic cell injury, originally suggested by Coimbra (38) may be substituted for *acute neuronal injury*. This signifies that the time elapsed between the neuronal insult and the patient's death was but a few hours or days. Some ischemically injured neurons are surrounded by inflammatory cells (i.e., satellitosis) while others simply disintegrate locally or are phagocytized (Fig. 12.36). Studies conducted in an experimental stroke model show that neurons located within brain territories made partially ischemic for periods of up to 2 h and reperfused for 24 h display structural alterations (i.e., scalloping) that seemingly represent the first stage of what eventually is irreversible cell damage. These neuronal changes develop concomitantly with progressive local edema (75).

The typical large cerebral hemispheric infarction secondary to the occlusion of a large artery shows, during the *subacute stage* (ca. 7th–10th d), three easily visualized zones. First there is a central one, where the BF is presumably lowest and *coagulation necrosis* of all tissue components is visible. Peripheral to this zone, and after a period of a few hours, there appear regenerated capillaries (recognizable by their thickened endothelial lining with prominent nuclei); abundant inflammatory cells (mostly mononuclear), including

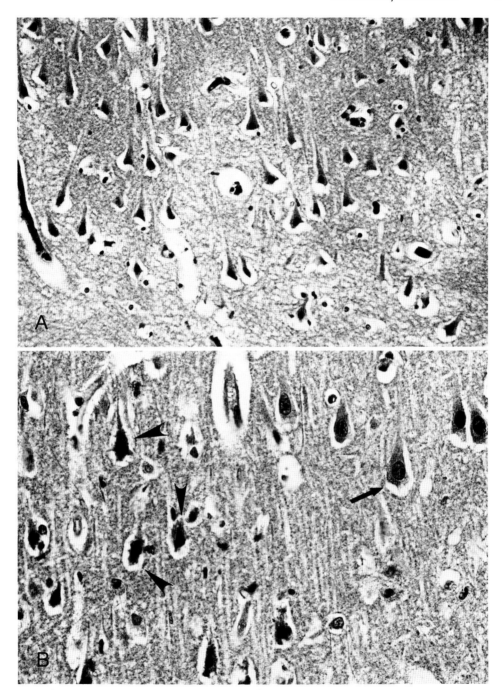

Figure 12.35. (A) Typical appearance of acute (about 24 h) ischemic injury to the cerebral cortex, after episodic cardiac arrest. All neuronal perikarya are markedly shrunken and surrounded by a halo. Intervening neuropil is severely vacuolated. (B) Closeup of a cerebral cortex segment showing "selective vulnerability," i.e., different responses in neurons at right (arrow) compared to those at the extreme left of field (arrowhead).

phagocytic histiocytes; and reactive astrocytes (Fig. 12.37). Peripheral to the reactive zone, there are: round, seemingly empty vacuoles (about 25 μm in average diameter) that probably represent sites of water accumulation; pale pink fragments of swollen

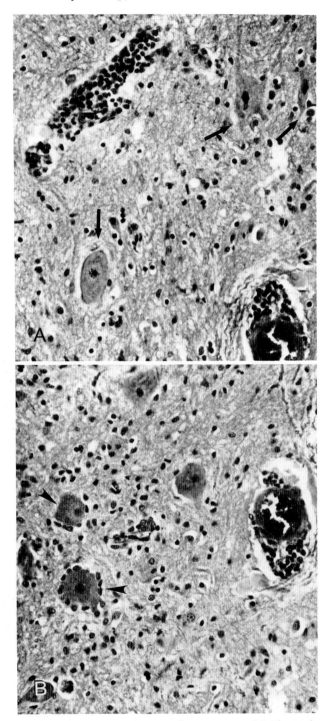

Figure 12.36. Cellular inflammatory response to ischemic injury. (*A*) Three-day survival following transient cardiorespiratory arrest induced extensive neuronal necrosis in the spinal cord as indicated by the homogenizing appearance of the cytoplasm, the nuclear pyknosis, and the shrinkage of the neuronal perikarya (*arrows*). A few mononuclear cells are visible in a perivascular location at the *left upper corner*. (*B*) Another field of the same specimen showing satellitosis/neuronophagia, i.e., lethally injured neuronal perikarya surrounded by mononuclear cells (*arrowheads*). H&E. (Original magnification ×40.)

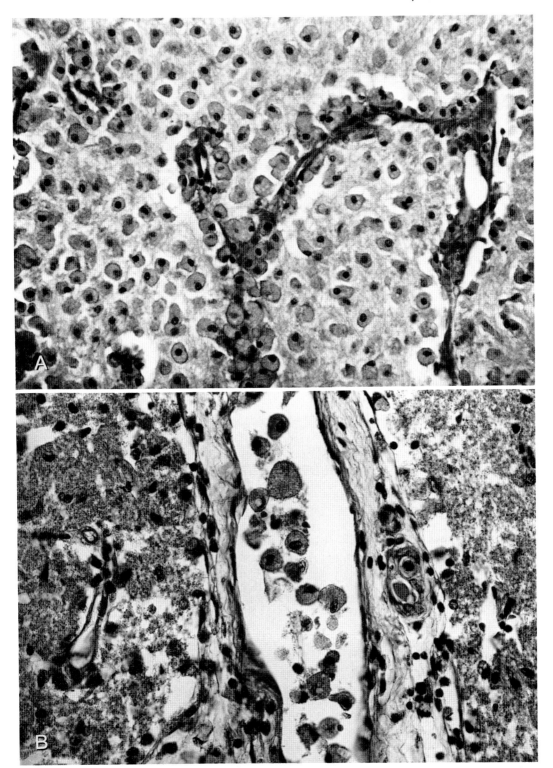

Figure 12.37.   Abundant lipid-laden macrophages are shown in a healing brain infarction (about 6 weeks old); their distribution around venules (*A*) and in the lumen of venules (*B*) suggests that these cells return to the circulation after completing their phagocytic function.

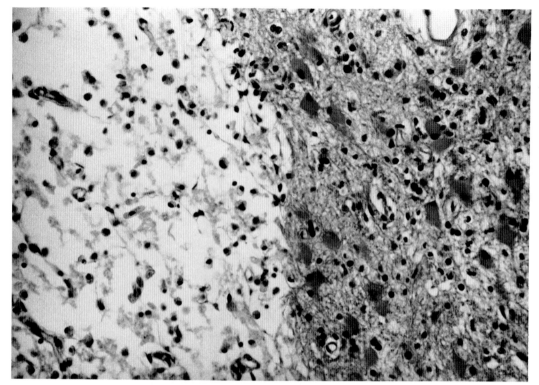

Figure 12.38.   Sharp edge of several months old brain infarction, where astrocytes remain "activated" indefinitely. H&E. (Original magnification ×63.)

axons ("spheroids") measuring about 15 μm in average diameter; and selected neurons showing signs of acute injury. The considerable heterogeneity of tissue changes frequently seen in an infarction may reflect either vastly inhomogeneous changes in local BF, or occlusion of several small arterial branches at different time intervals. Multifocal heterogeneity is frequently demonstrable in large infarctions of the cerebral hemispheres. For this reason, determining the age of an infarction by the study of the histologic features requires adequate sampling from multiple areas.

Astrocytes

In contrast to the degenerative changes that neurons undergo in areas of ischemia, astrocytes show early signs of activation (4–6 h after the ischemic injury), which some authors believe may be triggered by the increased content of K$^+$ in the extracellular space. Under conditions of partial ischemia, astrocytes increase in number and in volume (Figs. 12.38 and 12.39); their cytoplasm becomes hyperplastic and easily

stained with eosin, partly as a result of plasma proteins adsorption. Astrocytic division is suggested by the presence of numerous side-to-side astrocytic nuclei. The reactive plump astrocyte and the large spherical vacuole, filled with protein-free fluid, are two of the most durable indicators of incomplete ischemic brain injury. Both abnormalities can be detected, at the periphery of a brain infarction, several months after the original stroke (Fig. 12.39).

Oligodendrocytes

Next to the neurons, these cells are among the most vulnerable to the effects of ischemia. However, in an area of evolving infarction, a lapse of several hours exists between the time when the first group of neurons display lethal injury and the oligodendrocytes begin to disintegrate.

Myelin

Approximately 8–12 h after occluding an artery, the myelin sheaths of the corresponding area begin to show changes in

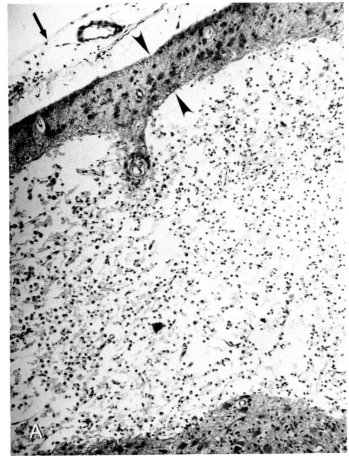

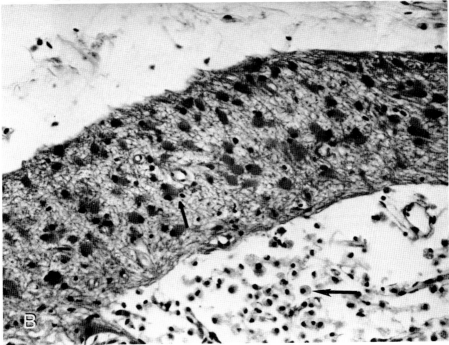

Figure 12.39. (*A*) In most healed, old infarctions, the molecular cortical layer (*arrowheads*) beneath the arachnoid (*arrow*) remains intact while the rest of the cortex is reabsorbed and replaced by a fluid-filled cavity. (*B*) Closeup of reactive astrocytes and lipid-laden macrophage or "gitter" cell (*arrows*).

stainability (pallor) which initially are due to primarily to the separation of myelinated tissues by interstitial edema. Disintegration of myelin sheaths can be visualized after two to three days.

Capillaries

Functional derangement, i.e., abnormalities in water transport, are demonstrable soon after the induction of ischemia; necrosis and regeneration of endothelial cells can be demonstrated abundantly after day 2 of the beginning of ischemia.

Cellular Inflammation

Neutrophils may be seen in the vascular lumen of capillaries and venules within 18 h of a stroke; in the ischemic tissues neutrophils usually disintegrate within 24–36 h. At this time, mononuclear cells (monocytes) arrive in abundance and are promptly (about 5–7 days) transformed into macrophages (gitterzelles) that ingest fragments of necrotic brain cells and erythrocytes (Fig. 12.37). The presence of macrophages in large numbers can be demonstrated with ease, beginning on day 7 after the ischemic stroke (69). The progressive disappearance of these phagocytes coincides with the formation of a fluid-filled cavity. Phagocytes have a relatively short half-life; finding them in large numbers at sites of old (several years) tissue destruction is suggestive of their continuous arrival at the infarction site (Fig. 12.39) (Table 12.9).

BRAIN (PARENCHYMAL) HEMORRHAGE

Definition

Bleeding into the brain parenchyma must be distinguished from hemorrhages that originate outside the dura (i.e., epidural hemorrhages), in the subdural compartment, in the subarachnoid space, or in the cerebral ventricles. Although parenchymal hemorrhages occur in isolated sites of the cerebrum, cerebellum, and brain stem, it is common to designate them *intracerebral* hemorrhages; this may be incorrectly interpreted as applying only to bleeding in the parenchyma of the cerebrum. Therefore, the designation *brain (parenchymal) hemorrhage* is adopted in an effort to avoid ambiguity.

Nontraumatic or spontaneous brain hemorrhages among adults may be of two types: large or massive (usually single) and small (frequently multiple). The latter tend to occur simultaneously at various sites in the brain parenchyma; the gross appearance of brains with multiple petechiae diffusely scattered throughout the white matter is designated *brain purpura*. The presence of multiple simultaneously occurring hemorrhages in the brain parenchyma can be associated with: (*a*) blood dyscrasias (e.g., leukemia); (*b*) immunologic disorders associated with demyelinating conditions (e.g., acute hemorrhagic encephalomyelitis); (*c*) fat embolism; (*d*) infections involving either the endothelial cells (e.g., rickettsiae) or the erythrocytes (e.g., malaria);

Table 12.9
Cerebral Infarction: Histological Features of Brain after Unilateral MCA Occlusion[a,b]

Duration of MCA clipping	Degree of nerve cell damage			Hemispheric swelling	Axonal swelling	PMN	Macrophages	Newly formed capillaries	Astrogliosis	Contralateral
	M	R	C							
2½ h	(See text)			−	−	−	−	−	−	−
12 h	±	±	+	+	−	−	−	−	−	+
18 h	+	+	+	+++	±	−	−	−	−	+
24 h	+	+	+	++++	+	±	−	−	−	++
2 d	+	+	+	+++	++	+	−	−	−	+
3 d	+	+	+	+++	+++	++	±	−	−	+
7 d	+	+	+	++	++++	+	++	+	±	+
16 d	±	+	+	−	++++	−	++	++	++	?

[a] From J. H. Garcia and Y. Kamijyo (69).
[b] All observations are based on paraffin-embedded material stained with hematoxylin and eosin.

and (e) the effects of substances either accidentally ingested (e.g., arsenic) or therapeutically administered (e.g., anticoagulants).

Brain purpura is said to be associated with a number of other miscellaneous conditions, e.g., head trauma and heat stroke. The multiple brain hemorrhages found in such cases probably are in fact a reflection of transient systemic circulatory disorders (i.e., global ischemia). The hemorrhages probably occur, during the reperfusion stage, at sites where capillaries may have undergone earlier ischemic injury. Multiple small brain hemorrhages can be a prominent feature of some brain infarctions caused by arterial or venous occlusions.

The condition of multiple, primary, small brain hemorrhages, i.e., brain purpura, becomes clinically expressed in the form of a progressive loss of brain functions, especially consciousness (i.e., first stupor, then coma). These hemorrhages may escape clinical notice in patients in whom there is multiple organ involvement by a systemic disease, e.g., leukemics with systemic fungal or bacterial infections.

Large or *massive* brain hemorrhage is defined as a parenchymal collection of blood where the largest diameter measures a minimum of 3.0 cm in the cerebral hemispheres, 2.0 cm in the cerebellum, and 1.0 cm in the brain stem. This type of hemorrhage, which is usually single, tends to express itself in the form of an abruptly developing localized neurologic deficit, i.e., a stroke.

The majority (about 52%) of these *large* brain hemorrhages are associated with systemic hypertension and the angiopathic changes that this condition induces in the arterial vessels of the brain, i.e., arteriolosclerosis. Many other local and systemic conditions can be associated with the development of large and small brain hemorrhages; in a significant percent of cases, the cause of the hemorrhage is not demonstrable, even at autopsy, probably because the bleeding obscures its underlying cause (Table 2.10) (144). On the basis of meticulous postmortem studies, some authors have suggested that the causative role of hypertension in large brain hemorrhages may be exaggerated (145).

Arterial and venous occlusions cause brain infarctions that can be accompanied by multiple brain hemorrhages (usually of petechial size). In the case of hemorrhagic infarctions involving the cerebrum, the petechiae are almost exclusively confined to gray matter structures (especially cortex) in instances in which the infarction is produced by a *transient* arterial occlusion, as is frequently the case in embolism (169).

The brain hemorrhages of venous infarctions tend to be larger than those of arterial infarctions; these hemorrhages have a different topographic distribution, i.e., they are not confined to any arterial territory and may involve equally white and gray substances (Fig. 12.40).

The evidence for the association between *systemic hypertension* and brain hemorrhage is derived from analysis of postmor-

Table 12.10
Brain (Parenchymal) Hemorrhage-Associated Conditions[a]

1. Arterial and venous occlusion
2. Arteriolosclerosis, especially if associated with systemic hypertension
3. Blood dyscrasias, e.g., anemia (sickle-cell), leukemias
4. Demyelinating conditions
5. Drugs (miscellaneous ones)
6. Extrinsic compression of arteries and veins
7. Inflammatory angiitis
8. Intraparenchymal neoplasms
9. Open-heart surgery, carotid endarterectomy
10. Ruptured intracranial aneurysms and angiomatous malformations
11. Blunt trauma, especially when directed to the head
12. Miscellaneous angiopathies
13. Hypoxia-ischemia in the newborn

[a] Adapted from J. H. Garcia and H. Mena (71).

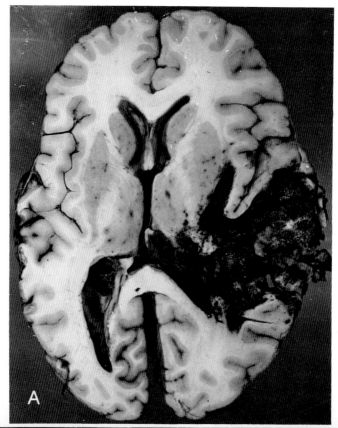

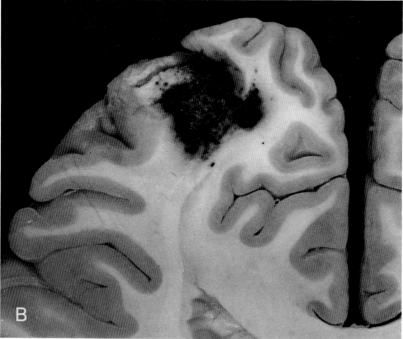

Figure 12.40. (A) This atypical brain hemorrhage (white matter of right parietal lobe) was associated with cortical vein thrombosis and hemorrhagic softening of the underlying cortex. (B) Superficial hemorrhagic softening in a patient with aspergillosis.

tem heart weight (23), the necropsy demonstration of nephroarteriolosclerosis, the decline of brain hemorrhages as a result of antihypertensive therapy (10), and the greater frequency with which hypertensive angiopathic changes (cerebral arteriolosclerosis) are found among brains with hemorrhages when compared with age- and sex-matched brains without hemorrhages (Fig. 12.41) (39). Hypertensive crises associated with pregnancy, i.e., eclampsia and preeclampsia, are a well-known cause of brain hemorrhage in young women (Fig. 12.42).

Multiple parenchymal hemorrhages with a propensity for the white matter of the cerebral hemispheres have been reported in as many as 49% of *leukemics* examined at autopsy. Acute lymphocytic leukemia (86) and acute myelogenous leukemia were associated with brain hemorrhages in two separate autopsy studies. In these studies brain hemorrhage predominated among patients dying with high terminal white blood cell count. In contrast, subarachnoid and subdural hemorrhages correlated with marked thrombocytopenia (171). Sickle cell disease may induce bleeding in the brain parenchyma and subarachnoid space; sickle cell disease may also lead to occlusion of major arteries or veins with secondary brain infarction.

The immunologic disorder confined to the white matter of the brain and myelin called *acute hemorrhagic leukoencephalopathy* may be accompanied by numerous white matter petechiae, which on occasion may be confined to a single cerebral lobe (see Chapter 11).

Patients undergoing therapy with anticoagulants (e.g., urokinase) for acute ischemic stroke may develop intracerebral hemorrhage at the ischemic site (92). Massive intracerebral hemorrhage in drug addicts has been associated, among others, with amphetamines and phencyclidine (21).

Multiple hemorrhages (and infarctions) in the brain stem, especially those located near the midline of midbrain and pontine tegmentum, can be traced to the extrinsic compression of mesencephalic vessels (arteries and veins) secondary to the transtentorial herniation of the uncinate and parahippocampal gyri. These are sometimes called Duret hemorrhages.

Spontaneous brain hemorrhages (especially those peripherally located in the cerebral hemispheres) have been described among normotensive patients afflicted with bacterial endocarditis. In such cases, the bleeding probably originates at the site of a "mycotic" aneurysm formed by bacterial colonization usually involving a branch of the MCA (217). Among the noninfectious systemic angiitis, two conditions may become clinically manifest by bleeding inside the brain: systemic lupus erythematosus (usually in the form of petechiae in gray matter structures) and lymphomatoid granulomatosis (105, 149).

Brain hemorrhage (both supra- and infratentorial) can occur at the site of brain neoplasms. Oligodendroglioma and glioblastoma multiforme are prominent among the primary tumors that bleed and manifest themselves as a hemorrhagic stroke. Bronchogenic carcinoma, melanoma, and choriocarcinoma are common among the metastatic tumors that bleed in the brain. The frequency of brain hemorrhage at the site of a tumor may have been underestimated in the era anteceding the CT scan (136).

Massive intracerebral hemorrhage in normotensive patients is a rare complication of open heart surgery. Drug-induced hypertension, systemic heparinization, and preexisting brain infarctions may be factors associated with the induction of this lesion. Intracranial hemorrhage has been recorded in children following cardiac surgery. The lesions encountered include: subdural hematomas; massive extradural hemorrhages; and intracerebral bleeding (108). Endarterectomy to relieve stenosis or occlusion of the internal carotid artery stenosis is complicated in about 0.3% of the cases by postoperative intracerebral hemorrhage (26). Four to five weeks after repair of tight internal carotid artery stenosis, patients may develop intracerebral hemorrhage. Systemic hypertension is a significant complication of cartoid endarterectomy and may be a prominent factor in the development of intracerebral hemorrhage after carotid endarterectomy (33).

Brain hemorrhages not attributable to hypertensive angiopathy, i.e., cerebral arteriolosclerosis, may be associated with *saccular aneurysms* of the circle of Willis vessels and with *angiomatous malformations* of the intraparenchymal vessels. This is particularly true of frontal-temporal lobar hemorrhages. Although saccular aneurysms and many vascular malformations usually bleed into the subarachnoid space, some aneurysmal sacs (for example, those originating at the MCA bifurcation or those that form at the anterior communicating-pericallosal arteries) may have their apical portion embedded into the brain parenchyma. Thus, when these aneurysms rupture, the bulk of the hemorrhage accumulates in the brain parenchyma, rather than in the subarachnoid space (145). Developmental defects in the large subarachnoid blood vessels can frequently be demonstrated at the site of either brain parenchymal or subarachnoid hemorrahges occurring among young persons, i.e., under the age of 25 (164).

Brain hemorrhages associated with *blunt head injuries* are frequently multiple and associated with hemorrhages in the meninges or at multiple sites in the brain (see Chapter 17).

The vascular changes characteristic of moyamoya syndrome are accompanied in children by ischemic brain changes. Brain hemorrhages are a more common manifestation of moyamoya angiopathy among adults (91).

Anatomic Features

Brain hemorrhages of hypertensive origin are traditionally labeled according to the site where bleeding presumably starts. These sites are: basal ganglia; thalamus; cerebral white matter; cerebellum; and pons. In some instances the site of origin may be impossible to determine because more than one of the above sites is involved by the hemorrhage (Fig. 12.41).

Among 131 instances of spontaneous *large* intracerebral hemorrhages studied postmortem by Mutlu et al. (157), bleeding was more common in the cerebrum-cerebellum (94%) than in the brain stem, which was selectively involved in only 6% of the cases. Ventricular extension occurs in about 75% of the fatal cases. In supratentorial hemorrhages the basal ganglia (mainly the putamen) is involved in 74% of cases. Extension to the subarachnoid space by destruction of the cortex is rare (about 3% of the cases). Thirty-four percent of the basal ganglia hemorrhages are laterally

placed, i.e., they involve the claustrum, extreme capsule, and a portion of the putamen. The mesial portion of the thalamus and adjacent structures are involved in 12% of the basal ganglia hemorrhages.

Arterial groups implicated in spontaneous large brain hemorrhages include striate branches of the MCA, thalamic branches of the posterior cerebral artery, mesencephalic branches of the basilar-posterior cerebral arteries, and branches of the cerebellar arteries supplying cerebellar white matter and dentate nucleus. Large brain hemorrhages (of hypertensive origin) that prove lethal within 3–4 d of the stroke involve the following sites: striate body and adjacent structures (42%); pons (16%); thalamus (15%); cerebellum (12%); cerebral white matter (10%); and other sites (5%). Three percent of the above brains showed multiple and simultaneous bleeding sites. Death supervenes more promptly (24 h) among patients with pontine hemorrhage than among those with supratentorial hemorrhages. Those in the latter group typically die on the 3rd–4th hospital day (66).

Excellent correlation exists between CT scans and the location and extent of intraparenchymal hemorrhages. CT scan is superior to angiography and radionuclide brain scanning in diagnosing intracerebral bleeding and in determining the extent of hemorrhage and the associated ventricular size (29). CT scans permit the accurate determination of the site, size, and extension of *thalamic hemorrhages*. All hemorrhages in this location larger than 3.0 cm in diameter are acutely fatal. The clinical manifestations of thalamic hemorrhage include sensory motor hemiplegia, limitation of vertical gaze, downward deviation of the eyes, and small unreactive or sluggish pupils (17, 209). Factors related to a fatal outcome in *thalamic hemorrhage* include: (*a*) decreased level of consciousness; (*b*) bilateral Babinski sign; (*c*) hematoma confined to the thalamic nuclei: (*d*) hematoma volume larger than 10 ml; (*e*) largest dimension of hematoma exceeding 30–35 mm; and (*f*) dilatation of the ventricles (132).

Seventy-four patients with hypertensive *putaminal hemorrhage* were followed at least 6 months after treatment. Analysis of

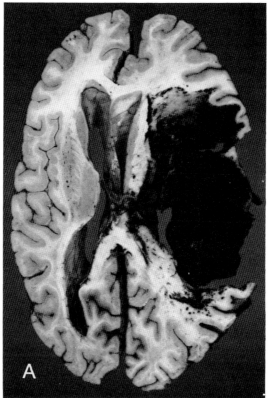

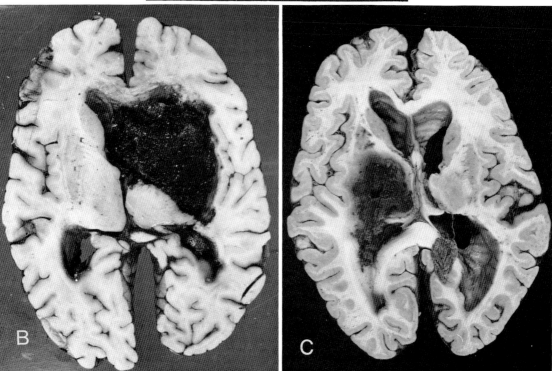

Figure 12.41. (A) Atypical brain hemorrhage (because of extensive cortical involvement) in a patient with carcinomatosis and multiple intracranial vein and sinus thromboses. (B) Typical, acute brain hemorrhage in a hypertensive patient with extensive destruction of striatum, globus pallidus, and a portion of the thalamus. Death occurred 3 d after the stroke. (C) Thalamic brain hemorrhage in a 80-yr-old person who suffered a stroke and underwent surgical drainage of the hemorrhage, 25 d before death.

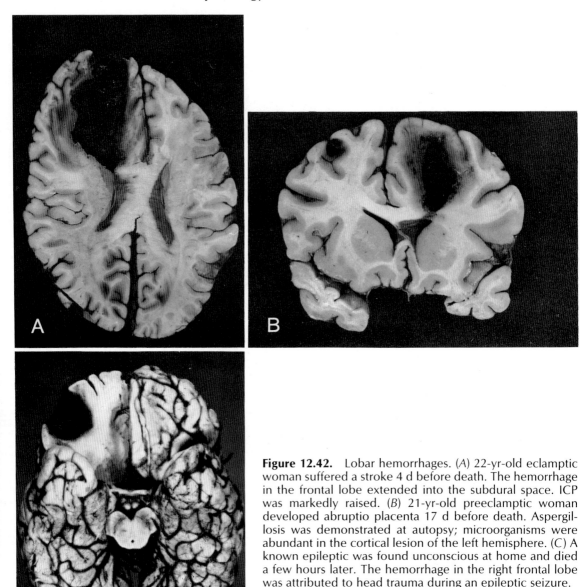

Figure 12.42. Lobar hemorrhages. (*A*) 22-yr-old eclamptic woman suffered a stroke 4 d before death. The hemorrhage in the frontal lobe extended into the subdural space. ICP was markedly raised. (*B*) 21-yr-old preeclamptic woman developed abruptio placenta 17 d before death. Aspergillosis was demonstrated at autopsy; microorganisms were abundant in the cortical lesion of the left hemisphere. (*C*) A known epileptic was found unconscious at home and died a few hours later. The hemorrhage in the right frontal lobe was attributed to head trauma during an epileptic seizure.

the results does not support the view that surgical treatment of hypertensive putaminal hemorrhages is superior to the conservative one (206).

Lobar hemorrhages constitute 26% of all massive brain hemorrhages; they occur independently in the *white matter* of frontal,

parietal, occipital, or temporal lobes. Their frequency is exceeded only by that of hemorrhages in the putamen. The parietooccipital area or the caudal half of the hemisphere is involved in about 80% of the cases. Systemic hypertension is the leading associated factor. As in other parenchymal

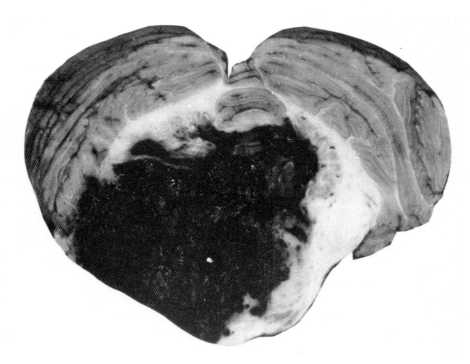

Figure 12.43   Pontine-cerebellar hemorrhage in a 54-yr-old patient with lymphomatoid granulomatosis.

hemorrhages the outcome is linked to the volume of the hemorrhage (Fig. 12.42) (121).

Among patients with *cerebellar hemorrhage* the mean age is 64 years. Hypertension, usually of several years' duration, is the associated condition in almost 90% of the adults evaluated at necropsy. The white matter, near the dentate nucleus, is a frequent site of origin for the hemorrhage; a minority of these hemorrhages may be confined to the vermis. The vessel commonly implicated as the source of parenchymal blood is a branch of the superior cerebellar artery. Most cerebellar hemorrhages extend into either the fourth ventricle or the subarachnoid space (46). They frequently are accompanied by herniation of cerebellar tissue through the foramen magnum. The diagnosis of primary cerebellar hemorrhage is extremely difficult without CT scan. Children may develop spontaneous cerebellar hemorrhage at the site of neoplastic growths such as ependymoma and astrocytoma (124).

Primary *pontine hemorrhages* are the least common of all hypertensive brain hemorrhages (Fig. 12.43). The majority originate at midpontine level, near the midline of the basis pontis, and may extend rostrally to the anterior hypothalamus. Caudal extension into the medulla is rare, while rupture into the fourth ventricle is common (46). Typical signs of pontine hemorrhage (coma, pinpoint pupils, and hyperthermia) may be absent in those instances in which only one-half of the pons is involved (120). Primary pontine hemorrhages are acutely fatal in about 72% of these patients (160). The primary rupture (in the absence of aneurysm formation) of an artery 200 μm in diameter may cause a fatal pontine hemorrhage (62).

Studies based on the use of erythrocytes labeled with a radionuclide (injected shortly after the stroke) suggest that brain bleeding in hypertensives occurs over a short period of time and that there is no rebleeding. Brain stem hemorrhages (secondary to uncinate herniation) seem to develop as an almost immediate consequence of the primary hemispheric hemorrhage. This is in contrast to brain hemorrhages secondary to either a ruptured aneurysm or an arteriovenous malformation, which appear to accumulate over an extended period of time (96).

Healing of brain hemorrhages was evaluated in 70 brains from patients who survived a minimum of 2 d. After 2–4 d there was extensive leukocytic infiltration, especially in tissues bordering directly the hemorrhage. Monocytes are numerous, and perineuronal satellitosis is common. After 5–20 d, occasional fibroblasts (presumably derived from monocytes) appear in the margins of the hemorrhage. Outside the layer of macrophages, plump astrocytes are numerous, and the vascular network becomes more apparent. When survival exceeds 21 d, abundant macrophages in contact with extravasated erythrocytes are laden with orange and brownish-green pigment (i.e., hemosiderin). In addition, large amounts of golden-yellow pigment (hematoidin) are seen extracellularly, while strands of fibroblasts with blood vessels are visible also at the periphery (215). The process by which brain hemorrhages heal appears to be very similar to that operating in an infarction. Evidence of either old infarction or hemorrhage, i.e., a golden yellow stained cavity wall, is found in about 24% of the brains evaluated at autopsy for acute brain hemorrhage (157).

Secondary Effects

The natural history of spontaneous intracerebral (and subarachnoid) hemorrhage is devastating. Of 138 patients with *hemorrhagic* stroke admitted to a single hospital, 64% had intraparenchymal hemorrhage; the remainder had subarachnoid hemorrhage. Hypertension is associated with 43% of the parenchymal hemorrhages, while aneurysms are demonstrated in 74% of the subarachnoid hemorrhage patients. Survival is only 14% for patients requiring emergency surgery. The overall mortality for intracerebral hemorrhage is 58%, and for subarachnoid hemorrhage it is 74% (218, 219). During the acute postictal stage death may supervene in patients with brain hemorrhage because of internal cerebral or cerebellar herniations (see below under Brain Edema), hemorrhagic destruction or inhibition of vital centers in the brainstem and *massive* blood flooding of the ventricular system. Although CT scan has shown

that small amounts of blood in the ventricular system are compatible with life, sudden entry of large hemorrhages into the ventricles apparently is lethal. Other undesirable effects of large brain hemorrhages include rapid and marked increases in ICP which usually lead to marked decrease (sometimes global) in perfusion pressure and, therefore, in global ischemia.

The disturbances of cerebral circulation secondary to intraparenchymal bleeding correlate particularly well with altered levels of consciousness. Mean cerebral BF values are lowest among patients whose consciousness is most impaired. Patients in whom the CT shows large hemorrhages have mean CBF values significantly lower than the group with smaller hemorrhages (123).

Secondary brain stem hemorrhages and infarctions are demonstrable in about 54% of brains having acute lethal supratentorial hemorrhages. Preexisting lesions of presumed vascular origin (infarctions or hemorrhages) are demonstrable in a small minority (25%) of brains harboring massive lethal hemorrhages (66).

PRIMARY SUBARACHNOID HEMORRHAGE

Bleeding into the subarachnoid space can occur in association with a variety of conditions (Table 12.11).

Trauma to the head (including the trauma associated with vaginal delivery) is a prominent cause of subarachnoid hemorrhage. However, in the vast majority of cases, subarachnoid bleeding of traumatic origin is accompanied by hemorrhages in other compartments (e.g., subdural, intraparenchymal) or by additional traumatic injuries to the head, e.g., skull fractures and brain contusions. Only under extraordinary circumstances is subarachnoid hemorrhage *the only* manifestation of trauma to the head (201).

This portion of the chapter deals primarily with subarachnoid hemorrhage (SAH) that develops spontaneously, i.e., in the absence of traumatic injury. This type of bleeding is sometimes designated *primary* SAH to signify its occurrence in the absence of trauma to either the head or the trunk.

Table 12.11
Subarachnoid Hemorrhage: Associated Conditions[a]

1. Angiitis, noninfectious, e.g., polyarteritis nodosa
2. Blood dyscrasias, e.g., anticoagulant therapy, leukemia
3. Drugs, e.g., insulin
4. Infections, leptomeningeal
5. Neoplasms, e.g., pituitary adenoma
6. Occlusive cerebrovascular disease, especially venous
7. Ruptured aneurysms and arteriovenous malformations
8. Trauma especially to the head
9. Unknown

[a] Adapted from J. H. Garcia and H. Mena (71).

The annual incidence of SAH varies somewhat, depending on the accuracy of the diagnosis. The latter tends to improve in large urban centers where SAH occurs at a rate of about 17/100,000/yr (88, 97, 167). Ruptured saccular aneurysms are responsible for about 65% of the SAH, while arteriovenous malformations (AVM) are demonstrated in about 10% of the patients. Small superficially placed parenchymal bleeds that break through the pia can be the source of some SAH, but in a significant number of patients (ca. 20%) who are evaluated clinically, the final diagnosis may read "SAH of undetermined origin." In contrast to the conditions prevailing in patients with ruptured aneurysms, SAH secondary to ruptured AVM has its highest incidence during the first decades of life (167).

The peak incidence of SAH (secondary to ruptured saccular aneurysm) occurs between ages 50 and 54; women are more prone to suffer from SAH then men by a ratio of 3:2. Approximately one-third of the SAH are said to be initiated during strenuous activities, such as bending, straining, or lifting heavy objects, but another significant percent seemingly develops during sleep (135). The initial symptoms of SAH include severe headache, nausea, vomiting, brief unconsciousness or confusion, meningismus (i.e., reflex spastic contractions of cervical muscles, also called nuchal rigidity), and isolated cranial nerve palsies or other focal neurologic deficits directly attributable to local pressure caused by the aneurysm itself, e.g., unilateral third cranial nerve palsy caused by pressure from a saccular aneurysm of ICA-posterior communicating artery complex.

The clinical recognition of SAH is not easy. As many as 22% of the patients admitted to a major medical center because of headache, confusion, and vomiting were initially assigned to an incorrect diagnostic category, such as infectious meningoencephalitis (5). Almost 40% of catastrophic SAH are preceded 2–4 weeks earlier by a "warning leak", i.e., mild meningismus attributed to a small hemorrhage in the subarachnoid space. The *risk factors* for SAH, associated with ruptured saccular aneurysm, are unknown in the vast majority of patients. Heros and Kistler (97) have suggested that the following may apply to a small percent of cases: history of ruptured aneurysm in a member of the family; evidence of fibromuscular dysplasia; polycystic kidney; coarctation or hypoplasia of the aorta; Ehlers-Danlos syndrome; Marfan syndrome; and pseudoxanthoma elasticum.

About 20% of those who suffer SAH associated with ruptured aneursym die before reaching the hospital. Of those who are admitted to the hospital, 30% die in the ensuing days to months as a result of the SAH or its complications. Even at the end of 6 months, patients who spontaneously recover from an initial SAH continue to have 3%/year chance of a second (usually lethal) hemorrhage (97).

Mechanisms of Brain Injury in SAH

The presence of blood in the subarachnoid space can be extremely hazardous, as well as uncomfortable. The severe headache in these patients is attributed to the stimulation of abundant pain fibers that exist in the adventitia of the large intracranial blood vessels, especially arteries. The irritation caused by blood is sufficient to mimic a meningeal bacterial infection, even in the way the process heals. The presence of leukocytes in the subarachnoid space and the development of fibrous adhesions between the arachnoid and the pia may be sufficiently extensive as to interfere with the normal flow of spinal fluid. Thus, ventricular dilatation (or hydrocephalus) and increased levels of ICP, which result from the former, are common features of SAH. This situation may be sufficiently severe to reduce cerebral perfusion pressure, thereby causing global cerebral ischemia.

A second undesirable effect of SAH is the constricting decrease in arterial lumen (i.e., *vasospasm*), a condition currently attributed to the effect of a variety of blood products, including serotonin, angiotensin, prostaglandins, and thromboxanes (222). Symptomatic vasospasm characteristically develops in a delayed fashion (4–12 d after the hemorrhage) and may involve only the region of the ruptured aneurysm, or it may affect the entire cerebral arterial tree. The main consequence of vasospasm is the induction of a severe drop of cerebral blood flow.

The development of brain infarctions among patients with ruptured aneurysm correlates with: degree of atheroma of the cerebral arteries; narrowed posterior communicating arteries; hemorrhage in the perivascular sheaths of the perforating ganglionic arteries; large subarachnoid hemorrhage; systemic hypotension; angiographically visible arterial spasm; and direct surgical attack on the aneurysm (43).

Arterial spasm in primary SAH is demonstrable in 62% of patients with brain infarctions, but spasm also exists in 57% patients without such lesions. However, there may be more than one type of spasm; narrowing of the vascular lumen by more than 60%, and diffuseness of the spasm have greater significance in terms of being more likely to decrease the CBF. Middle cerebral and anterior cerebral artery aneurysms are commonly associated with the second type of spasm, and cerebral infarctions almost always occur in territories supplied by the spastic vessels. Spasm is more common under the age of 50 than above this age (184). In several of these patients, there is a 58% increase in cerebral blood volume, which seems to reflect a massive transfer (and stagnation) of blood from subarachnoid vessels into the intraparenchymal vascular compartment (87).

A third undesirable effect of SAH is the widespread hypothalamic dysfunction that is usually reflected in cardiac arrhythmias and serum electrolyte imbalances. Of the latter, the most frequent one is hyponatremia, low serum osmolality with increased urinary sodium and osmolality (97). Thus, the combination of increased intracranial pressure (with concomitant decreased perfusion pressure), vasospasm, and cardiac dysrhythmias is usually reflected in a complex clinical picture associated with several interrelated anatomic abnormalities such as brain edema (and its consequences), dilated ventricles, intraparenchymal hemorrhage and neuronal injury secondary to either global brain ischemia or regional brain ischemia, or both (197).

SAH may be massive and primarily confined to the base of the brain (where the large arteries of the circle are located), or it may be loculated and mostly circumscribed to the area where the ruptured aneurysm is located, e.g., the Sylvian cistern in cases of ruptured aneurysm at the trifurcation of the MCA (Fig. 12.44).

Cardiac dysrhythmias, with evidence of hypothalamic dysfunction, may be the cause of death in some patients with SAH (53). Localized areas of myocardial ischemic necrosis and/or petechiae have been demonstrated in the majority of SAH patients who had evidence of hypothalamic dysfunction. These myocardial lesions were not found among appropriately matched controls (49). Similar myocardial lesions have been induced in animals by intravenous infusion of either norepinephrine or acetylcholine, and by electrical stimulation of the stellate ganglion, vagus nerve, or mesencephalic reticular formation. The above myocardial damage could be prevented by blocking the autonomic system (Fig. 12.45 and 12.46) (210).

BRAIN EDEMA

Definition

Brain edema consists of marked increase in brain volume (localized or generalized) secondary to the retention of either water

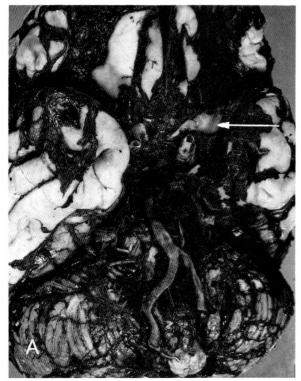 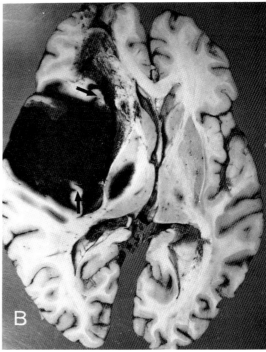

Figure 12.44. (A) Recent subarachnoid hemorrhage secondary to the rupture of a large aneurysm (arrow). (B) Ruptured aneurysms at the site of the MCA bifurcation may result in the formation of a localized hematoma at the insular cistern; the cortical ribbon has been broken by the expanding hematoma (arrows).

or protein-rich fluid. Brain weight alone cannot be used as an indicator of edema because there exists a wide range of normal values that must be adjusted for the age, sex, and race of the individual (100). A discussion of the various types of brain edema is included elsewhere in this textbook. In this section of this chapter, the features of only one type of brain edema are illustrated, i.e., ischemic or postischemic brain edema (73).

Experimentally induced brain ischemia is characterized by prompt failure of cellular functions that are dependent on high-energy compounds. This is reflected in vasoparalysis and retention of fluid in the cellular compartment, especially in the astrocytes. This mechanism of edema has been associated with initial intracellular retention of Na$^+$ (106).

Localized brain edema in cases of circulatory disorders is characteristic of those conditions in which there is either regional brain ischemic injury or large parenchymal hemorrahge. This type of edema is accompanied by herniation (or displacement) of portions of the brain that are topographically related to the site of injury, e.g., the rostral part of the right cingulum herniates in cases in which there is an infarction (or hemorrhage) localized to the right frontal lobe.

Generalized ischemic brain edema is found under conditions of diffuse circulatory injury to the brain, e.g., after transient global ischemia and primary subarachnoid hemorrhage. Under these circumstances there is usually no midline displacement of brain tissues. Instead, the main type of herniation develops at the foramen magnum, where portions of cerebellar cortex may be impacted in such a manner as to interfere with the blood supply to the medulla (Fig. 12.47).

Anatomic Features

Depending on the duration of the injury, postischemic edema may be reflected into

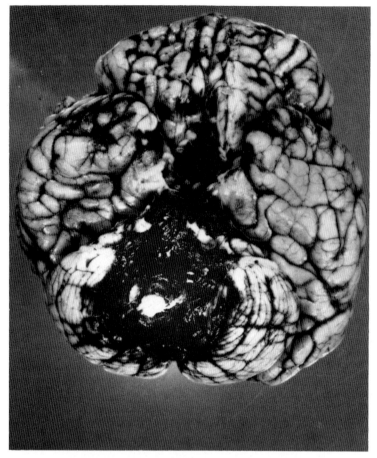

Figure 12.45. (A) Recent subarachnoid hemorrhage in a 3-yr-old child, who had a ruptured anomalous vessel close to the vertebral artery (see Fig. 12.7).

either *increased* brain consistency (when the process is relatively acute) or *decreased* brain consistency, which is typical of instances in which ischemic injury has progressed to a state of widespread cell membrane distintegration. The latter condition, often seen in persons in whom the cardiorespiratory functions need to be mechanically supported, has been erroneously designated "respirator brain" (207).

In very edematous brains, the subarachnoid space (between gyri) and the ventricular cavities are narrowed because of the increased volume of the surrounding tissues (Fig. 12.47). Swollen brain parenchyma and brains covered by abundant subarachnoid blood take a longer time to fix. It is assumed that under the above circumstances the penetration of the fixative is significantly delayed. Therefore, the fresh cut surfaces of these swollen brains frequently have

large pink-colored areas of incompletely fixed tissue that are located approximately in the center of each cerebral hemisphere.

The adult human brain is normally contained in a nonexpansile skull, the volume of which is only slightly larger than that of the brain. Because of this, marked increases in brain volume promptly induce displacement of brain tissues either outside of the skull (e.g., through the foramen magnum) in what is called an *external herniation* or within the intracranial compartments (e.g., across the midline) in an *internal herniation*.

The type of herniation developing in a given case is determined by the topography of the local brain swelling (or edema); thus, the presence of a large brain hemorrhage in the right insula and adjacent temporal lobe will result in swelling, primarily confined to that area, with consequent hernia-

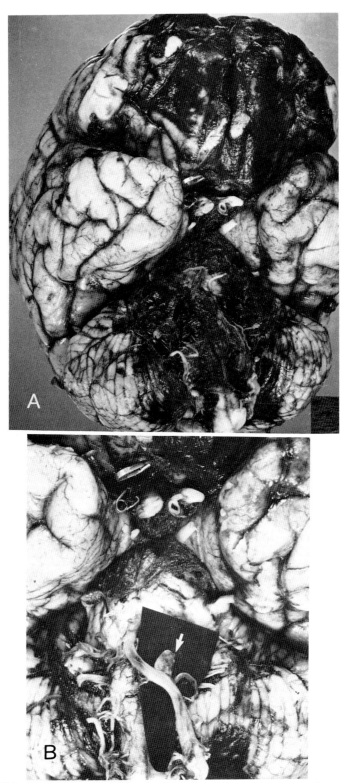

Figure 12.46. (*A*) Recent subarachnoid hemorrhage in a 55-yr-old woman who underwent surgical clipping of three aneurysms of the MCA and ACA about 10 d before death. (*B*) A fourth vertebral artery aneurysm bled profusely on the eve of her death (*arrow*).

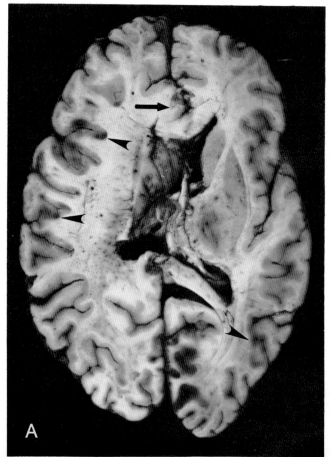

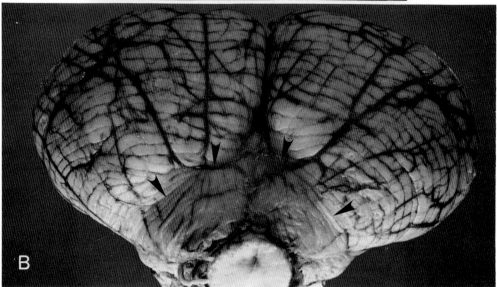

Figure 12.47. (*A*) A large left-sided subdural hemorrhage had been evacuated 40 h before death. Extensive ischemic injury and edema are apparent in the underlying cortex (*arrowheads*). Ipsilateral cingulate herniation is also visible (*arrow*). (*B*) Recent cerebellar herniation; *arrowheads* show the line of indentation caused by the pressure against the edge of the foramen magnum.

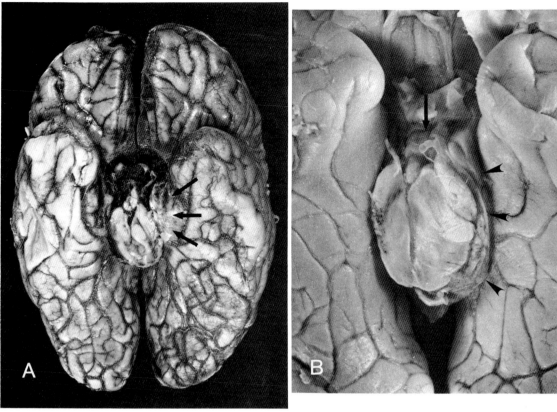

Figure 12.48. (*A*) Acute herniation of the left uncus (*arrows*) in a person with brain hemorrhage (after a gunshot wound to the head 12 h before death). (*B*) Chronic herniation of the uncus (*arrowheads*) has caused marked displacement of the midline structures (*arrow*). The surface of the midbrain contralateral to the site of herniation shows softening and petechiae caused by the pressure of the edge of the tentorial notch. This lesion is sometimes called Kernohan's notch.

tion of the ipsilateral uncus, i.e, *uncinate herniation* (Fig. 12.48).

A second variety of internal herniation involves the displacement, across the midline, of the rostral portion of the cingulum. Swelling affecting the dorsoventral part of the frontal lobe frequently results in herniation of the cingulate gyrus under the rostral most part of the dural falx. *Cingulate herniation* (also called subfalcial) is reflected in a marked shift of the midline structures, which angiographically can be easily appreciated by the characteristic displacement of the pericallosal arteries (Fig. 12.49).

Herniation of the uncus may be accompanied by downward displacement (through the tentorial notch) of a portion of the temporal cortex, commonly known as "parahippocampal gyrus." This is com-

mon in cases in which the cerebral hemispheric swelling is especially severe in the parietooccipital area. Because of the close proximity that exists among the uncus, the cerebral peduncle, the origin of the posterior cerebral artery, the third cranial nerve, and the posterior communicating artery, uncinate herniation frequently leads to mechanical compression of the third nerve (especially the superficially placed parasympathetic fibers) and the posterior cerebral artery. This vessel is usually pinched between the herniated uncus and the sharp edge of the tentorial notch (or incisura) at a point located a few centimeters distal to the site of origin of posterior cerebral artery (Fig. 12.48*B*). The consequence of this arterial extrinsic pressure is the development of an infarction in the corresponding arterial territory. The infarction, very fre-

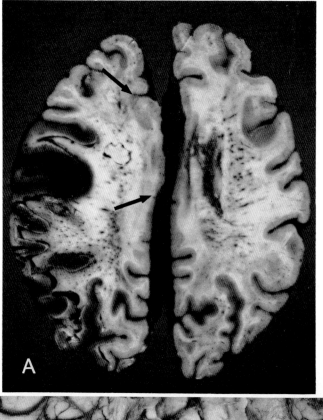

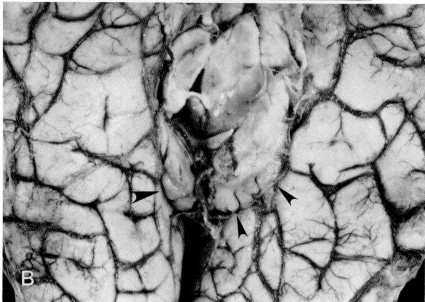

Figure 12.49. (A) Unilateral herniation of cingulate gyrus (*arrows*). (B) Bilateral herniation of parahippocampal gyri (*arrowheads*). (C) Secondary effects of uncinate herniation: bilateral hemorrhagic infarctions of occipital cortex and pulvinar (*arrowheads*).

quently, is of a hemorrhagic nature, i.e., it contains abundant petechiae that, by and large, are confined to the occipital cortex.

The hemorrhagic nature of this type of infarction is generally attributed to the fact that although the extrinsic pressure is suf-

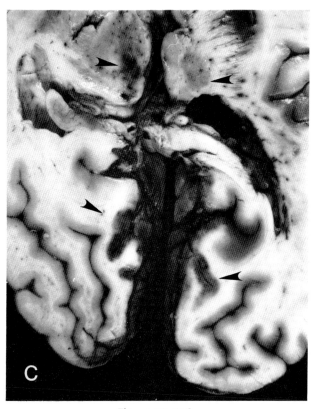

Figure 12.49C

ficiently severe to cause ischemic necrosis, it is also compatible with residual blood flow that gives the hemorrhagic character to the area of softening.

Another circulatory abnormality caused by uncinate gyrus herniation is the necrotizing compression of mesencephalic arterial branches originating from the initial segment of the PCA or the terminal portion of the basilar artery. These mesencephalic vessels supply the bulk of the midline structures located in the tegmentum of the midbrain and pons. Their necrotizing compression (brought about by the displaced swollen brain tissues) results in tegmental infarctions and hemorrhages. The latter are sometimes designated Duret's hemorrhages, after the author of one of the original descriptions of these lesions secondary to uncinate herniation (Fig. 12.50).

Kernohan's name is associated with lesions appearing on the surface of the cerebral peduncle opposite to the side of the uncinate herniation (Fig. 12.48B). This lesion was ascribed by Kernohan to the effects of displacing the midbrain across the midline in such a manner that the brain stem surface is driven against the sharp edge of the tentorial notch (Figs. 12.48–12.50). Such an effect cannot occur on the side of the uncinate herniation, among other reasons, because on the ipsilateral side, the herniated uncus is interposed between the brain stem and the cerebellar tentorium. In summary, *uncinate herniation* can induce any or all of the following: (*a*) functional injury to the ciliary parasympathetic fibers of the ipsilateral third cranial nerve; (*b*) ipsilateral hemorrhagic infarction in the territory of the posterior cerebral artery (a lesion that can aggravate the uncinate herniation); (*c*) infarctions and hemorrhages in the upper brain stem tegmentum; and (*d*) rarely, hemorrhagic softening on the cerebral peduncle contralateral to the side of the herniation.

Among 435 autopsies in patients dying of stroke, secondary brain stem hemorrhages are found in 45% of cerebral hemorrhages, 15% of large cerebral infarctions, and 36% of ruptured aneurysms. In the

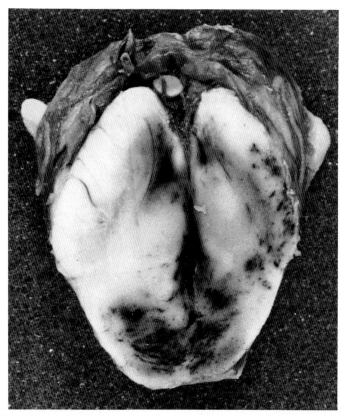

Figure 12.50.   The effects of unilateral uncinate herniation can be appreciated in this cross-section of midbrain. There is narrowing of interpeduncular fossa, softening of petechiae on the lateral surface of the brain stem, as well as multiple bleeding sites in the tegmentum and tectum.

majority of cases the secondary brain stem hemorrhages occur a few days after the onset of strokes, about 2 days in cases of brain hemorrhage and 4 days after ruptured aneurysm or cerebral infarction. Secondary brain stem hemorrhages are significantly less frequent in patients younger than 20 years of age. Secondary occipital lobe infarction was present in 3.5% of the patients (161).

Sphenoid herniation consists of a displacement (usually unilateral) of a portion of the ventral part of the frontal lobe into the medial cranial fossa and over the anterior edge of the greater wing of the sphenoid bone.

Brains of patients who develop edema that simultaneously affects all brain components (e.g., patients dying of Reye's syndrome) show a pronounced downward displacement of the mamillary bodies and other hypothalamic structures. The clinical manifestations of this anatomical deform-

ity are designated, by some authors, *central herniation*.

Cerebellar hemorrhage, cerebellar infarction, and generalized swelling of cerebellar tissue can all result in displacement of cerebellar tissues in either (or both) of two directions: (*a*) upward displacement of the dorsal vermis and the cerebellar tentorium that places the vermis in a mesial position with respect to the two occipital lobes of the cerebral hemispheres. A downward displacement of cerebellar tissues through the foramen magnum may occur under two separate circumstances: (*a*) as a result of congenital deformities, there may exist "chronic" *cerebellar herniations* with or without medullary deformity (67). (*b*) Acute cerebellar tissue herniation can be the consequence of either generalized increase in brain volume, or it may be the result of processes that selectively increase the volume of the posterior fossa contents, i.e., subdural hemorrhage, tumors, abscesses, cerebellar hemorrhage, and cerebellar infarctions. The anatomic consequences of acute *cerebellar herniation* include the formation of a groove on the surface of the herniated cortex, the eventual necrosis (and sloughing) of cerebellar tissues, and the pressure-deformity of the lower medulla, upper cervical cord (Fig. 12.47).

ACKNOWLEDGMENTS

Financial support for the production of this chapter was derived from funds made available through USPHS Grant NS-08802 and a grant from the Department of Pathology, University of Alabama in Birmingham.

I am very pleased to acknowledge the help I received from various friends and colleagues; in particular, I wish to thank the following persons: Dr. Jack C. Geer (Birmingham, AL) for a critical review of the initial draft; Dr. Uriel Sandbank (Tel Aviv, Israel) for contributing several illustrations of angiopathies; and Drs. John Moossy (Pittsburgh, PA) and José Bonnin (Birmingham, AL) for their encouraging comments.

Mrs. Sharon Mardis provided invaluable secretarial support, and Mr. Ralph Roseman was responsible for the production of the illustrations. My special thanks to them.

References

1. Acosta C, et al: Traumatic aneurysms of the cerebral vessels. *J Neurosurg* 36:531, 1972.
2. Adachi M, et al: Hypertensive disease and cerebral oedema. *J Neurol Neurosurg Psychiatry* 29:451–455, 1966.
3. Adams JH, et al: The effects of systemic hypotension upon the human brain. Clinical and neuropathological observations in 11 cases. *Brain* 89:235–268, 1966.
4. Adams HJ, Graham DI: Twelve cases of fatal cerebral infarction due to arterial occlusion in the absence of atheromatous stenosis or embolism. *J Neurol Neurosurg Psychiatry* 30:479, 1967.
5. Adams HP, et al: Pitfalls in the recognition of subarachnoid hemorrhage. *JAMA* 244:794, 1980.
6. Alexander CB, et al: Dissecting aneurysms of the basilar artery in two patients. *Stroke* 10:294, 1979.
7. Alpers BJ, et al: Circle of Willis in cerebral vascular disorders. The anatomical structure. *Arch Neurol* 8:398, 1963
8. Amacher AL, Shillito J: The syndromes and surgical treatment of aneurysms of the great vein of Galen. *J Neurosurg* 39:89, 1973.
9. Aronow WS, et al: Carbon monoxide and ventricular fibrillation threshold in dogs with acute myocardial injury. *Am Heart J* 95:754, 1978.
10. Aurell M, Hood B: Cerebral hemorrhage in a population after a decade of active antihypertensive treatment. *Acta Med Scand* 176:377, 1964.
11. Austin JH, Stears JC: Familial hypoplasia of both internal carotid arteries. *Arch Neurol* 24:1, 1971.
12. Averback P: Primary cerebral venous thrombosis in young adults. The diverse manifestations of an under recognized disease. *Arch Neurol* 37:126, 1980.
13. Baker AB, et al: Cerebrovascular disease. Etiologic factors in cerebral infarction. *Neurology* 13:445, 1963.
14. Bakay L, Lee JC: The effect of acute hypoxia and hypercapnia on the ultrastructure of the central nervous system. *Brain* 91:697, 1968.
15. Barnett HJM, Hyland HH: Non-infective intracranial venous thrombosis. *Brain* 76:36, 1953.
16. Barnett HJM, Hyland HH: Further evidence relating mitral-valve prolapse to cerebral ischemic events. *N Engl J Med* 302:139, 1980.
17. Barraquer-Bordas L, et al: Thalamic hemorrhage: a study of 23 patients with diagnosis by computed tomography. *Stroke* 12:524–527, 1981.
18. Battacharji SK, et al: The circle of Willis—the incidence of developmental abnormalities in normal and infarcted brains. *Brain* 90:747, 1967.
19. Becker DH, et al: Occult cerebrovascular malformations. A series of 18 histologically verified cases with negative angiography. *Brain* 102:249, 1979.
20. Bergstrand A, et al: Vascular malformations of the spinal cord. *Acta Neurol Scand* 40:169, 1964.
21. Bessen HA: Intracranial hemorrhage associated with phencyclidine abuse. *JAMA* 248:585, 1982.
22. Bounds JV, et al: Fatal cerebral embolism following aorto-coronary bypass graft surgery. *Stroke* 7:611, 1976.
23. Brewer DB, et al: A necropsy study of non-traumatic cerebral hemorrhages and softenings, with particular reference to heart weight. *J Pathol Bacteriol* 96:311, 1968.
24. Brierley JB: Cerebral hypoxia. In Blackwood W, Corsellis JAN (eds): *Greenfield's Neuropathology*, ed 3. London, E. Arnold, 1976, pp 43–85.
25. Brierley JB: Neuropathological findings in patients dying after open-heart surgery. *Thorax* 18:291, 1963.
26. Bruetman ME, et al: Cerebral hemorrhage in carotid artery surgery. *Arch Neurol* 9:458, 1963.
27. Burger PC, et al: Subcortical arteriosclerotic encephalopathy (Binswanger's disease): a vascular etiology of dementia. *Stroke* 7:626–631, 1976.
28. Burger PC, Vogel FS: Hemorrhagic white matter infarction in three critically ill patients. *Hum Pathol* 8:121, 1977.
29. Butzer JF, et al: Computerized axial tomography of intracerebral hematoma. A clinical and neuropathological study. *Arch Neurol* 33:206, 1976.
30. Cabanes J, et al: Cerebral venous angiomas. *Surg Neurol* 11:385, 1979.
31. Cammermeyer J: Is the solitary dark neuron a manifestation of postmortem trauma to the brain inadequately fixed by perfusion? *Histochemistry* 56:97, 1978.
32. Caplan LR, Schoene WC: Clinical features of subcortical arteriosclerotic encephalopathy (Binswanger disease). *Neurology* 28:1205, 1978a.
33. Caplan LR, et al: Intracerebral hemorrhage following carotid endarterectomy: a hypertensive complication? *Stroke* 9:457, 1978b.
34. Carmichael R: The pathogenesis of non-inflammatory cerebral aneurysms. *J Pathol Bacteriol* 62:1, 1950.
35. Caronna JJ, Finklestein S: Neurological syndromes after cardiac arrest. *Curr Concepts Cerebrovas Dis Stroke* 13:9, 1978.
36. Caroscio JR, et al: Subarachnoid hemorrhage secondary to spinal arteriovenous malformation and aneurysm. *Arch Neurol* 37:101, 1980.
37. Chester EM, et al: Hypertensive encephalopathy: a clinicopathologic study of 20 cases. *Neurology* 28:928–939, 1978.
38. Coimbra A: Nerve cell changes in the experimental occlusion of the middle-cerebral-artery. Histological and histochemical study. *Acta Neuropathol* 3:547–557, 1964.
39. Cole FM, Yates PO: The occurrence and significance of intracerebral microaneurysm. *J Pathol Bacteriol* 93:393, 1967.

40. Collins RC, et al: Neurologic manifestations of intravascular coagulation in patients with cancer: a clinicopathologic analysis of 12 cases. *Neurology* 25:795, 1975.

41. Conger KA, et al: The effect of aldehyde fixation on selected substrates for energy metabolism and amino acids in mouse brain. *J Histochem Cytochem* 26:423, 1978.

42. Conger KA, et al: Persistent dendritic swelling following transient brain ischemia in the rat. *Int J Neurol*, in press, 1984.

43. Crompton MR: The pathogenesis of cerebral infarction following the rupture of cerebral berry aneurysms. *Brain* 87:491, 1964.

44. Cross JN, et al: Cerebral strokes associated with pregnancy and the puerperium. *Br Med J* 3:214, 1968.

45. Daniel PM, et al: Pituitary necrosis in patients maintained on mechanical respirators. *J Pathol* 111:135, 1973.

46. Dinsdale HB: Spontaneous hemorrhage in the posterior fossa. *Arch Neurol* 10:200, 1964.

47. Dooling EC, Richardson EP: Delayed encephalopathy after strangling. *Arch Neurol* 33:196–199, 1976.

48. Doppman JL, et al: Value of cutaneous angiomas in the arteriographic localization of spinal-cord arteriovenous malformations. *NEJM* 281:1440, 1969.

49. Doshi R, Neil-Dwyer G: A clinicopathological study of patients following a subarachnoid hemorrhage. *J Neurosurg* 52:295, 1980.

50. Duvoisin RC, Yahr MD: Posterior fossa aneurysms. *Neurology* 15:231, 1965.

51. Eadie MJ, et al: Selective vulnerability in ischaemia: studies in quantitative enzyme cytochemistry of single neurons and neuropil. *Brain* 94:647, 1971.

52. Ekbom K, et al: Hydrocephalus due to ectasia of the basilar artery. *J Neurol Sci* 8:465, 1969

52a.Ellis SG, Verity MA: Central nervous system involvement in systemic lupus erythematosus: A review of neuropathologic findings in 57 cases, 1955–1977. *Semin Arthritis Rheum* 8:212–221, 1979.

53. Estanol BV, Marin OSM: Cardiac arrhythmias and sudden death in subarachnoid hemorrhage. *Stroke* 6:382, 1975.

54. Estanol B, Rodriguez A, Conte G, et al: Intracranial venous thrombosis in young women. *Stroke* 10:680–684, 1979.

55. Farber JL, et al: The pathogenesis of irreversible cell injury in ischemia. *Am J Pathol* 102:271, 1981.

56. Farrell DF, Forno LS: Symptomatic capillary telangiectasis of the brainstem without hemorrhage. *Neurology* 20:341, 1970.

57. Fauci AS, et al: The spectrum of vasculitis. Clinical, pathologic, immunologic, and therapeutic considerations. *Ann Intern Med* 89(Part I):660, 1978.

58. Feigin I. Prose P: Hypertensive fibrinoid arteritis of the brain and gross cerebral hemorrhage. *Arch Neurol* 1:98–110, 1959.

59. Fieschi C, Bozzao L: Transient embolic occlusion of the middle cerebral and internal carotid arteries in cerebral apoplexy. *J Neurol Neurosurg Psychiatry* 32:236, 1969.

60. Fisher CM, et al: Lateral medullary infarction–the pattern of vascular occlusions. *J Neuropathol Exp Neurol* 20:323, 1961.

61. Fisher CM: Capsular infarcts. The underlying vascular lesions. *Arch Neurol* 36:65, 1979.

62. Fisher CM: Pathological observations in hypertensive cerebral hemorrhage. *J Neuropathol Exp Neurol* 24:536–550, 1971.

63. Fisher, CM: Cerebral miliary aneurysms in hypertension. *Am J Pathol* 66:313–324, 1972.

64. Fisher CM: Lacunar strokes and infarcts: a review. *Neurology* 32:871, 1982.

65. Fraser RAR, Zimbler SM: Hindbrain stroke in children caused by extracranial vertebral artery trauma. *Stroke* 6:153, 1975.

66. Freytag E: Fatal hypertensive intracerebral haematomas: a survey of the pathological anatomy of 393 cases. *J Neurol Neurosurg Psychiatry* 31:616, 1968.

67. Friede RL, Roessmann U: Chronic tonsillar herniation. An attempt at classifying chronic herniations at the foramen magnum. *Acta Neuropathol* (Berlin) 34:219, 1976.

68. Garcia CA, et al: Ruptured aneurysm of the spinal artery of Adamkiewicz during pregnancy. *Neurology* 29:394, 1979.

69. Garcia JH, Kamijyo Y: Cerebral infarction. Evolution of histopathological changes after occlusion of a middle cerebral artery in primates. *J Neuropathol Exp Neurol* 33:409, 1974.

70. Garcia JH, et al: Cerebral ischemia. The early structural changes and correlations of these with known metabolic and dynamic abnormalities. In Whisnant JP, Sandok B (eds): *Cerebral Vascular Diseases. Ninth Conference.* New York, Grune & Stratton, 1975, pp 313–323.

71. Garcia JH, Mena H: Circulatory disorders of the central nervous system. (a tabulation). In Altman PL, Katz DD (eds): *Human Health and Disease.* Bethesda, MD, FASEB, 1977, pp 282–288.

72. Garcia JH, et al: Neuronal ischemic injury: light microscopy, ultrastructure and biochemistry. *Acta Neuropathol (Berl)* 43:85, 1978.

73. Garcia JH, et al: Post-ischemic brain edema: quantitation and evolution. In: Cervos-Navarro J, Ferszt R: *Advances in Neurology.* New York, Raven Press, 1980, vol 28, pp 147–69.

74. Garcia JH: A concept of stroke. In: *Current Concepts.* Kalamazoo, MI, Upjohn Company, 1983.

75. Garcia JH, et al: Transient focal ischemia in subhuman primates: neuronal injury as a function of local cerebral blood flow. *J Neuropathol Exp Neurol* 42:44, 1983.

76. Garcia, JH: Ischemic injuries of the brain: morphologic evolution. *Arch Pathol Lab Med* 107:157–161, 1983.

77. Garcia JH: Experimental ischemic stroke: a review. *Stroke* 15:5–14, 1984.

78. Garcin R, Lapresle J: Sur une observation d'angiome de la moelle dorsale s'etant manifeste cliniquement pendant 24 ans sous les traits d'une paraplegie spamodique d'etiologie indeterminee. *Ceskoslovenska Neurol* 28:95, 1965.

79. Geer JC, Garcia JH: Atherosclerosis. In Wilkins R, Rengachary SS (eds): *Neurosurgery.* New York, McGraw-Hill, in press, 1984.

80. Gilman S: Cerebral disorders after open-heart operations. *N Engl J Med* 272:489, 1965.

81. Ginsberg MD, Myers RE: Experimental carbon monoxide encephalopathy in the primate. Part I. *Arch Neurol* 30:202–208, 1974.

82. Ginsberg MD, Myers RE: Experimental carbon monoxide encephalopathy in the primate. Part II. *Arch Neurol* 30:209–216, 1974.

83. Ginsberg MD, et al: Hypoxic-ischemic leukoencephalopathy in man. *Arch Neurol* 33:5–14, 1976.

84. Ginsberg MD, et al: Diffuse cerebral ischemia in the cat. III. Neuropathological sequelae of severe ischemia. *Ann Neurol* 5:350, 1979.

85. Gold AP: Vein of Galen malformation. *Acta Neurol Scand* 40(Suppl 2):1–31, 1964.

86. Groch SN, et al: Cerebral hemorrhage in leukemia. *Arch Neurol* 2:439, 1960.

87. Grubb RL, et al: Effects of subarachnoid hemorrhage on cerebral blood volume, blood flow, and oxygen utilization in humans. *J Neurosurg* 46:446, 1977.

88. Gudmundsson G: Primary subarachnoid hemorrhage in Iceland. *Stroke* 4:764, 1973.

89. Guthrie W, Maclean H: Dissecting aneurysms of arteries other than the aorta. *J Pathol* 108:219–235, 1972.

90. Hagler HK, et al: Effects of different methods of tissue preparation on mitochondrial inclusions of ischemic and infarcted canine myocardium: transmission and analytic electron microscopic study. *Lab Invest* 40:528, 1979.

91. Haltia M, et al: Spontaneous occlusion of the circle of Willis (moyamoya syndrome). *Clin Neuropathol* 1:11, 1982.

92. Hanaway J, et al: Intracranial bleeding associated with

urokinase therapy for acute ischemic hemispheral stroke. *Stroke* 7:143, 1976.

93. Heffner RR, Solitaire GB: Hereditary haemorrhagic telangiectasis: neuropathological observation. *J Neurol Neurosurg Psychiatry* 32:604, 1969.

94. Heiskanen O: Cerebral circulatory arrest caused by acute increase of intracranial pressure. A clinical and roentgenological study of 25 cases. *Acta Neurol Scand Suppl (7)* 40:1–89, 1964.

95. Heiss WD: Flow thresholds of functional and morphological damage of brain tissue. *Stroke* 14:329, 1983.

96. Herbstein DJ, Schaumburg HH: Hypertensive intracerebral hematoma. An investigation of the initial hemorrhage and rebleeding using chromium Cr 51-labeled erythrocytes. *Arch Neurol* 30:410, 1974.

97. Heros RC, Kistler JP: Intracranial arterial aneurysm—an update. *Stroke* 14:628, 1983.

98. Herrick MK, Agamanolis DP: Displacement of cerebellar tissue into spinal cord. A component of the respirator brain syndrome. *Arch Pathol* 99:565, 1975.

99. Hirano A, Solomon S: Arteriovenous aneurysms of the vein of Galen. *Arch Neurol* 3:589, 1960.

100. Ho K-C, et al: Analysis of brain weight. *Arch Pathol Lab Med* 104:640, 1980.

101. Høedt-Rasmussen K, et al: Regional cerebral blood flow in acute apoplexy. *Arch Neurol* 17:271, 1967.

102. Hollander W, et al: Aggravation of cerebral atherosclerosis by hypertension. *Circulation* 68:III-190, 1983.

103. Hollin SA, et al: Post-traumatic middle cerebral artery occlusion. *J Neurosurg* 25:526, 1966.

104. Hong SK: The physiology of breath-hold diving. In Straus RH (ed): *Diving Medicine.* New York, Grune & Stratton, 1976, pp 269–286.

105. Hood J, et al: Lymphomatoid granulomatosis manifested as a mass in the cerebellopontine angle. *Arch Neurol* 39:319, 1982.

106. Hossmann KA, Sato K: Recovery of neuronal function after prolonged cerebral ischemia. *Science* 168:375, 1970.

107. Humphrey PRD, et al: Cerebral venous thrombosis. In Harrison MJG, Dyken ML (eds): *Cerebral Vascular Disease. Butterworths International Medical Reviews. Neurology 3.* Boston, Butterworth, 1983, pp 309–319.

108. Humphreys RP, et al: Cerebral hemorrhage following heart surgery. *J Neurosurg* 43:671, 1975.

109. Jenkins LW, et al: The role of postischemic recirculation in the development of ischemic neuronal injury following complete cerebral ischemia. *Acta Neuropathol (Berl)* 55:205, 1981.

110. Johansson H, Siesjo BK: Cerebral blood flow and oxygen consumption in the rat in hypoxic hypoxia. *Acta Physiol Scand* 93:269, 1975.

111. Jones HR, Millikan CH: Temporal profile (clinical course) of acute carotid system cerebral infarction. *Stroke* 7:64, 1976.

112. Jörgensen L, Torvik A: Ischaemic cerebrovascular diseases in an autopsy series. Part 1. Prevalence, location and predisposing factors in verified thrombo-embolic occlusions, and their significance in the pathogenesis of cerebral infarction. *J Neurol Sci* 3:490, 1966.

113. Jörgensen L, Torvik A: Ischaemic cerebrovascular diseases in an autopsy series. Part 2. Prevalence, location, pathogenesis, and clinical course of cerebral infarcts. *J Neurol Sci* 9:285, 1969.

114. Kalbag RM, Woolf AL: *Cerebral Venous Thrombosis.* London, Oxford University Press, 1967.

115. Kalimo H, et al: Cellular and subcellular alterations of human CNS: studies utilizing *in situ* perfusion-fixation in immediate autopsies. *Arch Pathol* 97:352, 1974.

116. Kalimo H, et al: The ultrastructure of "brain death". II. Electron microscopy of feline cortex after complete ischemia. *Virchows Arch B Cell Pathol* 25:207, 1977.

117. Kamenar E, Burger PC: Cerebral fat embolism: a neuropathological study of a microembolic state. *Stroke* 11:477, 1980.

118. Kamijyo, et al: Temporary MCA occlusion: a model of hemorrhagic and subcortical infarction. *J Neuropathol*

Exp Neurol 36:338, 1977.

119. Kaplan HA, et al: Vascular malformations of the brain. An anatomical study. *J Neurosurg* 27:630, 1961.

120. Kase CS, et al: Partial pontine hematomas. *Neurology* 30:652, 1980.

121. Kase CS, et al: Lobar intracerebral hematomas: clinical and CT analysis of 22 cases. *Neurology* 32:1146, 1982.

122. Kase CS, et al: Medial medullary infarction from fibrocartilaginous embolism to the anterior spinal artery. *Stroke* 14:413, 1983.

123. Kawakami H, et al: Regional cerebral blood flow in patients with hypertensive intracerebral hemorrhage. *Stroke* 5:207, 1974.

124. Kazimiroff PB, et al: Acute cerebellar hemorrhage in childhood: etiology, diagnosis, and treatment. *Neurosurgery* 6:524, 1980.

125. Kelly JJ, et al: Intracranial arteriovenous malformations in childhood. *Ann Neurol* 3:338, 1978.

126. Kety SS, Schmidt CF: The determination of cerebral blood flow in man by the use of nitrous oxide in low concentrations. *Am J Physiol* 143:53, 1945.

127. Kolata GB, Marx JL: Epidemiology of heart disease: searches for causes. *Science* 194:509, 1976.

128. Korein J, et al: Radioisotope bolus technique as a test to detect circulatory deficit associated with cerebral death. *Circulation* 51:924, 1975.

129. Kosnik EF, et al: Dural arteriovenous malformations. *J Neurosurg* 40:322, 1974.

130. Krueger BR, Okazaki H: Vertebral-basilar distribution infarction following chiropractic cervical manipulation. *Mayo Clin Proc* 55:322, 1980.

131. Kudo T: Spontaneous occlusion of the circle of Willis. A disease apparently confined to Japanese. *Neurology* 18:485, 1968.

132. Kwak R, et al: Secondary brainstem hemorrhage in stroke. *Stroke* 14:493, 1983.

133. Laprèsle PJ, Milhaud M: Lesions du systeme nerveux central après arret circulatoire. Etude de 10 cas. *La Presse Medicale* 70:429, 1962.

134. Levine J, Swanson P: Diagnosis and treatment. Nonatherosclerotic causes of stroke. *Ann Intern Med* 70:807, 1969.

135. Locksley HB: Report on the cooperative study of intracranial aneurysms and subarachnoid hemorrhage. *J Neurosurg* 25:219–240 and 321–368, 1966.

136. Little JR, et al: Brain hemorrhage from intracranial tumor. *Stroke* 10:283, 1979.

137. MacPherson P, Graham DI: Arterial spasm and slowing of the cerebral circulation in the ischaemia of head injury. *J Neurol Neurosurg Psychiatry* 36:1069, 1973.

138. Mandel MM, Berry RG: Human brain changes in cardiac arrest. *Surg Gynecol Obstet* 108:692, 1959.

139. McCluskey RT, Fienberg R: Vasculitis in primary vasculitides, granulomatoses, and connective tissue diseases. *Hum Pathol* 14:305–315, 1983.

140. McCormick WF, Nofzinger JD: Saccular intracranial aneurysms. An autopsy study. *J Neurosurg* 22:155, 1965.

141. McCormick WF, Nofzinger JD: "Cryptic" vascular malformations of the central nervous system. *J Neurosurg* 24:865, 1966a.

142. McCormick WF, Boulter TR: Vascular malformations ("angiomas") of the dura mater. Report of two cases. *J Neurosurg* 25:309, 1966b.

143. McCormick WF: The pathology of vascular "arteriovenous" malformations. *J Neurosurg* 24:807, 1966c.

144. McCormick WF, Rosenfield DB: Massive brain hemorrhage: a review of 144 cases and an examination of their causes. *Stroke* 4:946, 1973.

145. McCormick WF, Schochet SS, Jr: *Atlas of Cerebrovascular Disease.* Philadelphia, WB Saunders, 1976.

146. McDowell FH: Transient cerebral ischemia: diagnostic considerations. *Prog Cardiovasc Dis* 22:309, 1980.

147. MacPherson P, Graham DI: Arterial spasm and slowing of the cerebral circulation in the ischemia of head injury. *J Neurol Neurosurg Psychiatry* 36:1069–1072, 1973.

148. Mohr JP: Progress in cerebrovascular disease. Lacunes.

Stroke 13:3, 1982.

149. Moore PM, Cupps TR: Neurological complications of vasculitis. *Ann Neurol* 14:155, 1983.

150. Moossy J: Morphology, sites and epidemiology of cerebral atherosclerosis. *Assoc Res Nerv Ment Dis* 41:1–22, 1966a.

151. Moossy J: Cerebral infarction and intracranial arterial thrombus. *Arch Neurol Psychiatry* 14:119, 1966b.

152. Moossy J: Cerebral infarcts and the lesions of intracranial and extracranial atherosclerosis. *Arch Neurol Psychiatry* 14:124, 1966c.

153. Moossy J: Vascular diseases of the spinal cord. In Baker AB (ed): *Clinical Neurology*. Hagerstown, MD, Harper & Row, 1976, ch 34, pp 1–17.

154. Morawetz RB, et al: Cerebral blood flow determined by hydrogen clearance during middle cerebral artery occlusion in unanesthetized monkeys. *Stroke* 9:143, 1978.

155. Mokri B, et al: Extracranial internal carotid artery aneurysms. *Mayo Clin Proc* 57:310, 1982.

156. Müller HR, Radu EW: Intracerebral hematoma. In Harrison MJG, Dyken ML (eds): *Cerebral Vascular Disease. Butterworth's International Reviews. Neurology 3*. Boston, Butterworth, 1938, pp 320–350.

157. Mutlu N, et al: Massive cerebral hemorrhage: clinical and pathological correlations. *Arch Neurol* 8:644, 1963.

158. Myers RE: A unitary theory of causation of anoxic and hypoxic brain pathology. *Adv Neurol* 26:195, 1979.

159. Neubuerger KT: Lesions of the human brain following circulatory arrest. *J Neuropathol Exp Neurol* 13:144, 1954.

160. Nakajima K: Clinicopathological study of pontine hemorrhage. *Stroke* 14:485, 1983.

161. Nedergaard M, et al: Secondary brainstem hemorrhage in stroke. *Stroke* 14:501, 1983.

162. Nemoto EM, et al: Global brain ischemia: a reproducible monkey model. *Stroke* 8:558, 1977.

163. Ng LKY, Nimmannitya J: Massive cerebral infarction with severe brain swellings: a clinicopathological study. *Stroke* 1:158, 1970.

164. Ojemann RG, Heros RG: Spontaneous brain hemorrhage. *Stroke* 14:458, 1983.

165. Oka K, et al: Cerebral haemorrhage in moyamoya disease at autopsy. *Virchows Arch [Pathol Anat]* 392:247, 1981.

166. Okazaki H, et al: Clinicopathologic studies of primary cerebral amyloid angiopathy. *Mayo Clin Proc* 54:22, 1979.

167. Pakarinen S: Incidence, aetiology, and prognosis of primary subarachnoid haemorrhage. A study based on 589 cases diagnosed in a defined urban population during a defined period. *Acta Neurol Scand* Suppl (29) 43:113, 1967.

168. Paljärvi L, et al: The efficiency of aldehyde fixation for electron microscopy: stabilization of rat brain tissue to withstand osmotic stress. *Histochem J* 11:267, 1979.

169. Paulson OB: Regional cerebral blood flow in apoplexy due to occlusion of the middle cerebral artery in ten patients. *Neurology* 20:63, 1970.

170. Petrov V, et al: Post-traumatic thrombosis of the carotid artery. *Acta Neurol Belg* 73:110, 1973.

171. Phair JP, et al: The central nervous system in leukemia. *Ann Intern Med* 61:863, 1964.

172. Ratinov, G: Extradural intracranial portion of carotid artery. A clinicopathologic study. *Arch Neurol* 10:66–73, 1964.

173. Reagan TJ, Bloom WH: The brain in hereditary hemorrhagic telangiectasia. *Stroke* 2:361, 1971.

174. Reed RL, et al: Rarity of transient focal cerebral ischemia in cardiac dysrhythmia. *JAMA* 23:893, 1973.

175. Rehncrona S, Siesjö BK: Metabolic and physiologic changes in acute brain failure. In Grenvik A, Safar P (eds): *Brain Failure and Resuscitation*. New York, Churchill-Livingstone, 1981, pp 35–54.

176. Rhodes EL, et al: Aneurysms of extracranial carotid arteries. *Arch Surg* 111:339, 1976.

177. Robins M, Baum HM: The National Survey of Stroke Incidence. *Stroke* 12:I–45, 1981.

178. Rodda R: The necropsy demonstration of cerebral aneurysms by intra-arterial injection. *Proc Aust Assoc Neurol* 7:115, 1967.

179. Romanul FC, Abramowicz A: Changes in brain and pial vessels in arterial border zones. *Arch Neurol* 11:40, 1964.

180. Rossen R, et al: Acute arrest of cerebral circulation in man. *Arch Neurol Psychiatry* 50:510, 1943.

181. Sandok, BA, Whisnant, JP: Hypertension and the brain. *Arch Intern Med* 133:947–954, 1974.

182. Sato S, Hata J: Fibromuscular dysplasia. Its occurrence with a dissecting aneurysm of the internal carotid artery. *Arch Pathol Lab Med* 106:332–335, 1982.

183. Schmidley JW, Caronna JJ: Transient cerebral ischemia: pathophysiology. *Prog Cardiovasc Dis* 22:325, 1980.

184. Schneck SA, Kricheff II: Intracranial aneurysm, rupture, vasospasm and infarction. *Arch Neurol* 11:668, 1964.

185. Sekar TS, et al: Survival after prolonged submersion in cold water without neurologic sequelae. Report of two cases. *Arch Intern Med* 140:775, 1980.

186. Selkoe DJ, Myers RE: Neurologic and cardiovascular effects of hypotension in the monkey. *Stroke* 10:147, 1979.

187. Shaw C-M, et al: Swelling of the brain following ischemic infarction with arterial occlusion. *Arch Neurol* 1:161, 1959.

188. Silverstein A, Doniger DE: Systemic and local conditions predisposing to ischemic and occlusive cerebrovascular disease. *J Mount Sinai Hosp* 30:435, 1963.

189. Sindermann F, et al: Occlusions of the internal carotid artery compared with those of the middle cerebral artery. *Brain* 93:199, 1970.

190. Spallone, A, Cantore, G: Extracranial carotid abnormalities and intracranial aneurysms. *J Neurosurg* 55:693–700, 1981.

191. Steegmann AT: The neuropathology of cardiac arrest. In Minckler J (ed): *Pathology of the Nervous System*. New York, McGraw-Hill, 1968, vol 1.

192. Stehbens WE: Histopathology of cerebral aneurysms. *Arch Neurol* 8:272, 1963.

193. Stein BM, Wolpert SM: Arteriovenous malformations of the brain. I. Current concepts and treatment. *Arch Neurol* 37:1, 1980.

194. Stein BM, Wolpert SM: Arteriovenous malformations of the brain. II. Current concepts and treatment. *Arch Neurol* 37:69, 1980.

195. Stockard JJ, et al: Hypotension-induced changes in cerebral function during cardiac surgery. *Stroke* 5:730, 1974.

196. Sundt TM, et al: Restoration of middle-cerebral-artery flow in experimental cerebral infarction. *J Neurosurg* 31:311–322, 1969

197. Sundt TM, et al: Results and complications of surgical management of 809 intracranial aneurysms in 722 cases. Related and unrelated to grade of patient, type of aneurysm, and timing of surgery. *J Neurosurg* 56:753, 1982.

198. Sundt, TM, et al: Correlation of cerebral blood flow and carotid endarterectomy with results of surgery and hemodynamics of cerebral ischemia. *Mayo Clin Proc* 56:533–543, 1981.

199. Sylvester JT, et al: Hypoxic and CO-hypoxia in dogs: hemodynamics, cartoid reflexes, and catecholamines. *Am J Physiol* 218:H22, 1979.

200. Sypert GW, Alvord EC, Jr: Cerebellar infarction. A clinicopathological study. *Arch Neurol* 32:357, 1975.

201. Tatsuno Y, Lindenberg R: Basal subarachnoid hematomas as sole intracranial traumatic lesions. *Arch Pathol* 97:211, 1974.

202. Tobin WD, Layton DD: The diagnosis and natural history of spinal cord arteriovenus malformations. *Mayo Clin Proc* 51:637, 1970.

203. Toole JF, Patel AN: *Cerebrovascular Disorders*, ed 2. New York, McGraw-Hill, 1973.

204. Trump BF, Arstila A: Cellular reaction to injury. In LaVia MF, Hill RB (eds): *Principles of Pathobiology*, ed 2. New York, Oxford University Press, 1975, pp 9–96.

205. Tufo H, et al: Central nervous system dysfunction fol-

lowing open-heart surgery. JAMA 212:1333, 1970.

206. Waga S, Yamamoto Y: Putaminal hemorrhage: treatment and results. Is surgical treatment superior to conservative one? *Stroke* 14:480, 1983.

207. Walker AE: Pathology of brain death. *Ann NY Acad Sci* 315:272–279, 1978.

208. Walker GB, Marx JL: The National Survey of Stroke: clinical findings. *Stroke* 12(1):I-13–I-31, 1981.

209. Walshe TM, et al: Thalamic hemorrhage: a computed tomographic-clinical correlation. *Neurology* 27:217, 1977.

210. Weidler DJ: Myocardial damage and cardiac arrhythmias after intracranial hemorrhage. A critical review. *Stroke* 5:759–764, 1974.

211. Welsh FA, et al: Diffuse cerebral ischemia in the cat. II. Regional metabolites during severe ischemia and recirculation. *Ann Neurol* 3:493, 1978.

212. Whisnant JP, et al: Transient cerebral ischemic attacks in a community. Rochester, Minnesota, 1955 through 1969. *Mayo Clin Proc* 48:194, 1973.

213. Wilkins RH, Brody IA: Sturge-Weber syndrome. *Arch Neurol* 21:554, 1969.

214. Wirth FP, et al: Foix-Alajouanine disease. *Neurology* 20:1114, 1970.

215. Wisniewski H: The pathogenesis of some cases of cerebral hemorrhage (a morphological study of the margins of hemorrhagic foci and areas of the brain distant from the hemorrhage). *Acta Med Polona* 2:379, 1961.

216. Wolf PA, et al: Epidemiologic assessment of chronic atrial fibrillation and risk of stroke: The Framingham Study. *Neurology* 28:973, 1978.

217. Yarnell PR, Stears J: Intracerebral hemorrhage and occult sepsis. *Neurology* 24:870, 1974.

218. Yarnell PR: Neurological outcome of prolonged coma survivors of out-of-hospital cardiac arrest. *Stroke* 7:279, 1976.

219. Yarnell P, Earnest MP: Primary non-traumatic intracranial hemorrhage. A municipal emergency hospital viewpoint. *Stroke* 7:608, 1976.

220. Yates PO, Hutchinson EC: Cerebral infarction: the role of stenosis of extracranial cerebral arteries. London, Privy Council, Medical Research Council Special Report Series, No. 300, Her Majesty's Stationary Office, 1961.

221. Zeller RS, Chutorian AM: Vascular malformations of the pons in children. *Neurology* 25:776, 1975.

222. Zervas NT, et al: Reduced incidence of cerebral ischemia following rupture of intracranial aneurysms. *Surg Neurol* 11:339–344, 1979.

CHAPTER 13

Neurologic Infections due to Bacteria, Fungi, and Parasites

JOSEPH C. PARKER, Jr., M.D.
MICHAEL L. DYER, M.D.

OVERVIEW*

Histologic evaluation of any infectious process requires assessment of the inflammatory cellular reaction, the character of any necrosis, and recognition of the infectious agent. These features vary with time, the ability of the host to react, and the nature of the infectious agent itself. This relationship is expressed in the following equation:

$$\int_{t_1}^{t_2} f(a, b) = c$$

where the tissue response (c) depends on the integral of time (t), the ability of the host to respond (a), and the inciting agent (b).

Terminology for inflammatory infections in the central nervous system is confusing. Meningitis refers to leptomeningitis which is confined by the pial and arachnoidal membranes and can be acute or chronic. The former is characterized by neutrophils in the subarachnoid space, and the latter by mononuclear inflammatory cells, particularly lymphohistiocytes. Arteries coursing through this inflammatory exudate may be

involved with the process possessing microbes or sterile vascular inflammation, or demonstrating reactive intimal changes known as endarteritis obliterans. This latter vasculopathy can be seen in tuberculous meningitis and meningovascular neurosyphilis (Fig. 13.1). Focal inflammation scattered through the neuraxis or localized to a particular portion of the cerebrum, brain stem, or both is called cerebritis. Cerebritis and myelitis are comparable terms for inflammation in the cerebrum and spinal cord, respectively. This process seen around an evolving abscess may be infected or sterile. Encephalitis is distinct from cerebritis and is associated with viral or rickettsial infections unless otherwise qualified. Encephalitis is characterized by diffuse inflammation throughout the cerebral hemispheres with or without involvement of the cerebellum and brain stem. An intracranial abscess is a clinicomorphologic entity manifested by an inflammatory process with liquefactive necrosis and predominant neutrophils encased by granulation tissue. The thickness and integrity of the granulation tissue varies with the severity of the inciting agent, the ability of the host to respond, and the length of time the process has been present. In many patients with leptomeningitis, their pial barriers are invaded by the inflammatory infectious process, creating an adjacent neuroparenchymal infection referred to as meningocerebritis or meningoencephalitis.

---

* References pertaining to Overview section are 2, 3, 10, 18, 19, 25, 28, 29, 33, 40, 41, 43, 48, 60–62, 65, 67, 68, 74, 76, 87, 91, 99, 1901, 111, 134, 141, 142, 167, 179, 184, 193, 195, 200, 217, 221, 227, 247, 249, 253, 254, 273, 276, 281, 282, 283, 301, 311, 317, 318, 325, 332, 342, 343, 360.

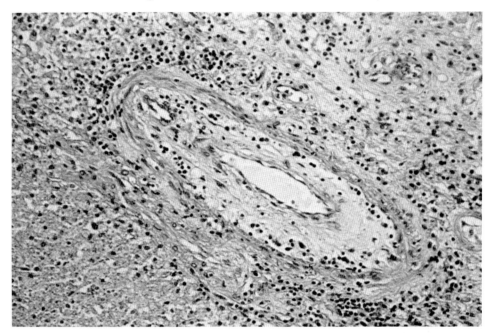

Figure 13.1. Severe endarteritis obliterans is produced in the brain of a patient with neurotuberculosis. H&E. (Original magnification ×200.)

Host Factors

The ability of the individual to respond to an infection is related to the host's nutritional status and general health (2, 3, 10, 19, 25, 28, 33, 40, 41, 43, 48, 60–62, 65, 74, 76, 87, 91, 101, 134, 142, 167, 179, 184, 193, 195, 200, 217, 221, 227, 254, 281–283, 301, 311, 325, 332, 342, 343, 360). Age is a significant factor in determining this response. In utero, the embryo and early fetus cannot produce an inflammatory response until the second trimester. It increases in its intensity with fetal maturation. In the elderly, the inflammatory reaction is reduced as a consequence of intrinsic vessel disease, changing cellular characteristics of the bone marrow, and other age-related factors. The most common deficiency in this host response to an infectious agent is produced by iatrogenic manipulations, such as drug therapy and surgery (10, 19, 28, 48, 61, 74, 91, 142, 167, 184, 193, 195, 332). Antibiotics change the intrinsic bacterial flora, allowing resistant bacteria and fungi to express themselves as opportunistic infections not known prior to widespread use of antimicrobial agents (1, 19, 28, 29, 142, 221, 249, 254, 273). Similarly, toxic chemicals used to treat malignancies compromise

the host's ability to respond to infectious agents, making him susceptible to unusual microorganisms (3, 19, 29, 40, 41, 48, 60, 111, 134, 142, 221, 249, 273, 301, 332).

Tissue changes in the host can be used to determine the inciting agent and the integrity of the host's innate resistance (2, 68, 99, 111, 141, 179, 249, 282, 283, 318, 342, 343, 360). Necrosis, recognized as soft, yellow-tan tissue, is characterized microscopically as (1) *coagulative necrosis* when produced by altered vascular supply to the affected tissue, as seen in an infarct; (2) *liquefactive necrosis* when lysosomal digestion of tissue occurs by inflammatory and noninflammatory cells, as seen in an abscess; (3) *caseous or gummatous necrosis*, which is seen in granulomas induced by fungi, mycobacteria, and *Treponema pallidum*; and (4) *enzymatic necrosis*, as seen in trauma to soft tissues or the pancreas. Recognition of these forms of necrosis provide insight into their pathogenesis.

The inflammatory response, which varies with time and the intrinsic ability of the host to react to the inciting agent, offers insight into the likely causative microbes. For example, in an intact host with multiple intracranial abscesses, inciting agents include such pyogenic bacteria as staphylococci, streptococci, and meningococci. On the other hand, these same agents in a host compromised by chemotherapy for a malignancy may not have enough neutrophils to produce abscesses. Problems within the host, like granulomatous disease of childhood, produce granulomatous inflammatory response to most infectious agents, including pyogenic bacteria (2, 29, 33, 43, 65, 76, 179, 253, 282, 283, 311, 317, 318, 360).

The Infectious Agent

Any infectious agent accessible to the nervous system can infect it. Typically, these microbes are considered pathogenic when a normal individual is infected by an adequate inoculum, and opportunistic when the host is compromised before the less virulent infectious agent creates any injury. Experimentally, opportunistic microbes can infect a normal host when the inoculum is massive (18, 29, 48, 179, 247, 253). Most infectious agents reach the central nervous system through the blood stream, which includes arteries and veins. Any bacteremia may infect the CNS through the four major arteries. The extensive, valveless venous plexus around the spinal column (Batson's venous plexus) provides another hematogenous route to the brain for infectious agents involving the retroperitoneum and retromediastinum. These inflammatory processes can present as paradural empyemas anywhere along the neuraxis with subsequent spread to the leptomeninges. Other infectious routes for microbes into the nervous system include direct inoculation by surgical or nonsurgical trauma or direct invasion from contiguous infected foci, such as sinuses in the base of the skull. In some viral infections, spread through the axoplasm in the peripheral nerves can lead to infection in the CNS (29, 179, 253).

Since the nature of infectious inflammation depends on the host's ability to react to the inciting agent and how long the process has been evolving, i.e., $\int_{t_1}^{t_2} f(a, b) = c$, an approach recognizing the typical infection can be developed (Table 13.1). Small infectious organisms (less than 10 μm) produce host tissue alterations that differ from intermediate, irregular agents (over 10 μm) like pseudohyphae or bacteria within small thrombi, and the larger metozoan parasites and hyphal fungi. These three types of infectious particles produce predictable inflammatory lesions in the nervous system. *Small infectious particles*, like bacteria and yeasts, have easy access to the microcirculation in the neuraxis and can infect the subarachnoid space from this site (Fig. 13.2). Individuals with these infections develop meningeal irritation due to leptomeningitis. The latter may be characterized by neutrophils, mononuclear cells, or mixtures of both. The cellular response depends on how long the infection has been present, as well as the type of infectious agent. *Intermediate size infectious particles*, characterized by candidal pseudohyphae and small thromboemboli with bacteria, produce focal necrosis in the area around the microcirculation with subsequent spread through the damaged vessel

Table 13.1
Infectious Agents

Size	Type	Usual location	Histopathological features
Small (10 μm or less)	Bacteria Yeasts Protozoans	Leptomeninges	Meningitis
Intermediate (10–20 μm)	Infected thromboemboli Pseudohyphae	Neuroparenchyma	Microabscesses Cerebritis
Large (over 20 μm)	Infected thromboemboli Fungal hyphae Metazoans	Neuroparenchyma	Abscesses Septic infarcts

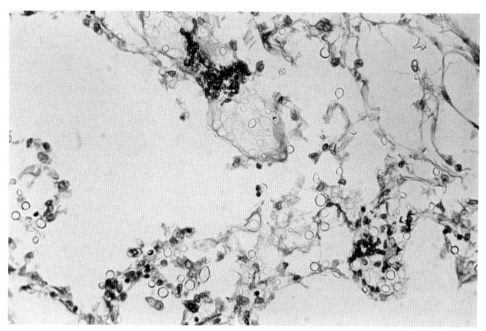

Figure 13.2. Minimal reaction in the subarachnoid space is associated with yeasts (clear oval bodies) of *Cryptococcus neoformans*. Like other small infectious particles, these microbes have easy access to the microcirculation in the CNS and, therefore, infect the leptomeninges. H&E. (Original magnification ×200.)

wall into the necrotic adjacent neuroparenchyma (Fig. 13.3). Microabscesses produced by intermediate infectious particles usually do not create any neuropsychiatric deficits. Nevertheless, these individuals may manifest encephalopathic clinical features. Meningitis is not evident. *Larger infectious particles*, typified by fungal hyphae, infected thromboemboli over 20 μm, and large parasites, occlude larger arteries, producing coagulative necrosis that may develop into an infectious, liquefactive necrosis or septic infarct (Fig. 13.4). These tissue responses are associated with adjacent leptomeningitis, which may be apparent on cerebrospinal fluid examination, but often do not cause recognizable CSF changes (3, 18, 29, 111, 141, 247, 249).

Diagnosis

The final diagnosis of any infectious process resides in the microbiology laboratory. Even though CSF is the most common source for recovering and identifying infectious agents in the CNS, some infectious processes can be recognized accurately in tissue sections (3, 18, 29, 60, 11, 249). The genera of many fungi can be identified by their characteristic morphology (Table 13.2). On the other hand, fungal infections characterized by septate hyphae in tissue cannot be evaluated without culturally recovering the organism or specific immunologic tissue identification. Viruses and other parasites can be determined by their morphology and immunologic techniques as well. Since speciation of any infectious agent requires microbiologic techniques, suspected or known infectious processes must have material adequately collected and handled.

Because CSF is so accessible for culture of potential infections in the neuraxis, suspected individuals with potentially increased intracranial pressure must have this fluid obtained to characterize their inciting microbes, which may be lethal unless treated promptly and vigorously. Changes within the subarachnoid space in the young and elderly can hamper accurate recognition of the infection (29, 101, 247, 249, 253).

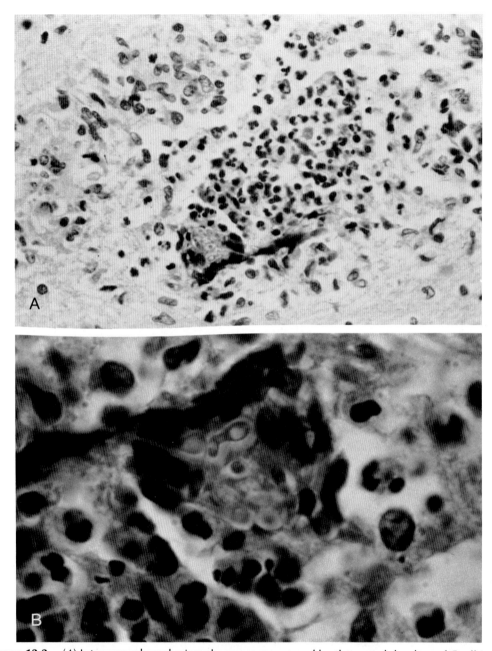

Figure 13.3. (*A*) Intraparenchymal microabscesses are caused by the pseudohyphae of *C. albicans* seen in a multinucleated giant cell (midlower field) H&E. (Original magnification ×250.) (*B*) Phagocytosed pseudohyphae of *C. albicans* are seen in a multinucleated giant cell. H&E. (Original magnification × 900.)

Nonspecific leptomeningeal fibrosis found in the subarachnoid space increases with age and may create loculated areas, preventing accurate reflection of the infectious process by a lumbar puncture. Likewise, previous bleeding anywhere in the neuraxis may contaminate the CSF and, subsequently, produce reactive fibrosis with hemosiderin deposits interfering with CSF flow around the brain and spinal cord.

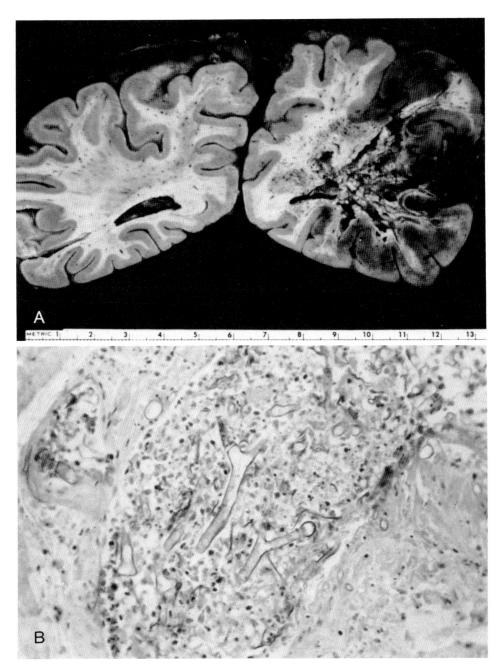

Figure 13.4.   Coronal section of the posterior cerebrum demonstrates a hemorrhagic septic infarct (A) in the right parietooccipital lobe caused by intravascular obstructing phycomycotic hyphae (B). H&E. (Original magnification ×200.)

Table 13.2
Fungal Morphology in Neural Tissue

Form	Fungal genera
Yeasts	*Blastomyces*
	Candida
	Coccidioides
	Cryptococcus
	Histoplasma
	Paracoccidioides
	Sporotrichum
	Torulopsis
Septate hyphae	*Aspergillus*
	Cephalosporium
	Cladosporium
	Diplorhinotrichum
	Hormodendrum
	Paecilomyces
	Penicillium
Nonseptate hyphae	*Absidia*
	Basidiobolus
	Cunninghamella
	Mortierella
	Mucor
	Rhizopus

BACTERIAL INFECTIONS†

Under appropriate circumstances, any bacteria which include prokaryotic ("before the nucleus"), arachaebacteria, and eubacteria when introduced into the central nervous system can infect it. As with other infectious organisms, smaller inocula of some bacteria like *Neisseria meningitidis* in uncompromised hosts can establish an infection. Bacterial infections in the central nervous system are found typically in individuals compromised by endogenous or exogenous mechanisms. These microorganisms usually arrive by a hematogenous route that includes arterial spread through the four great neck vessels from the arch of the aorta, venous spread through Batson's extensive valveless venous plexus around the spinal cord, or both. Direct inoculation of bacteria through contaminated surgical wounds or compound skull fractures is also a well-recognized route for bacterial invasion into the central nervous system.

---

† References pertaining to Bacterial Infections are, 11, 14, 17, 41, 46, 49, 60, 69, 78, 89, 106, 108, 110, 116, 132, 133, 135, 136, 139, 159, 160, 166, 167, 178, 181, 182, 197, 204, 205, 218, 228, 229, 233, 236, 244, 245, 252, 254, 266, 287, 296, 300, 302, 303, 304, 322, 337, 351, 355, 359.

Lesions produced by bacteria in the central nervous system depend upon such factors as the ability of the host to respond to the inciting organism, the nature of the infectious agent itself, its portal of entry into the central nervous system, and the level at which the host's circulation is invaded by the bacteria. Microbes that are accessible to the microcirculation rapidly involve the leptomeninges, whereas those that enter the central nervous system through larger septic thromboemboli produce intraparenchymal abscesses without extensive purulent leptomeningitis (Table 13.1). Organisms invading directly into the central nervous system from adjacent sinuses and paradural foci can produce epidural empyemas, subdural empyemas, or both. Reactive acute sterile leptomeningitis may occur as a response to the adjacent paradural infection. In addition, bacteria may compromise the host by creating a disseminated intravascular coagulopathy, septic shock, or toxins that directly affect the central nervous system without producing a septic inflammatory process.

Leptomeningitis (14, 17, 89, 108, 133, 136, 159, 166, 181, 182, 197, 233, 245, 254, 300, 303, 304, 359)

This inflammatory process involves the meningeal coverings of the brain and spinal cord and indicates inflammation of the pia-arachnoid membranes or leptomeninges. In contrast, pachymeningitis implies dural inflammation. Leptomeningitis maybe acute, subacute, or chronic, depending upon its causation, duration of infection, and previous treatment. In addition, the process may be suppurative or nonsuppurative, depending upon the character of the infectious microbes.

Acute leptomeningitis implies an infection present for hours to days and is characterized morphologically by an outpouring of polymorphonuclear neutrophils. Bacteria producing this form of infection are pyogenic organisms and include *Haemophilus influenzae*, *N. meningitidis*, *Staphylococcus aureus*, *Streptococcus pneumoniae*, and other *streptococci*. The initial inflammatory reaction for most invasive microbes in the central nervous system, including viruses, is a transient outpouring of polymorphonuclear neutrophils. Subacute leptomeningitis is a poorly defined and rarely used term that implies an inflammatory process of days to weeks duration manifested by a mixed inflammatory exudate of neutrophils, lymphocytes, plasma cells, and mononuclear phagocytes. Chronic leptomeningitis implies an inflammatory reaction of weeks to months duration, characterized by mononuclear phagocytes and lymphoid cells with proliferative changes, including granulation tissue and fibrosis. These reactions in the leptomeninges are caused not only by microorganisms but also their toxins, nonseptic irritants, trauma, and foreign substances introduced into the subarachnoid space.

In uncompromised hosts, any microorganism may produce a leptomeningitis, but, when dealing with the compromised host, specific pathogenic bacteria may create acute leptomeningitis under different clinical circumstances. Antibiotic and antineoplastic therapy have increased the varieties of leptomeningitis. Previous nonpathogenic organisms are now recognized as opportunistic bacteria that can produce leptomeningitis. Different inciting organisms create varying appearances in the consistency and color of the exudate which is distributed irregularly in the subarachnoid space. Initially, the pia-arachnoid is congested and hyperemic, and the subarachnoid space is distended with an exudate. Some bacteria, such as *H. influenzae*, produce a heavy exudate located in the basal cistern, Sylvian fissure, and adjacent sulci. On the other hand, *S. pneumoniae* may extend directly from an adjacent paraneural focus, infecting the underlying brain and its coverings. Before antibiotic therapy, microorganisms are seen in the intercellular spaces and in clusters within neutrophils. After about 2 h of infection, mononuclear phagocytes are evident and apparently are derived from pial cells, adventitial cells, microglia, and circulating monocytes. After 48 h, mononuclear phagocytes with bacteria and cellular debris are seen. During the early period of suppurative leptomeningitis, no reaction in the adjacent neuroparenchyma is noted. However, after 2 to 3 d, subpial astrogliosis becomes apparent. Blood vessels engulfed in this purulent process become altered after several days, probably as a result of associated immune complexes

and chemical stimulation of the intimal and subintimal cells to isolate the inflammatory process. This endarteritis obliterans is striking in subacute or chronic inflammatory processes due to tubercle bacilli and spirochetes (Fig. 13.5).

As the inflammatory process develops, the cellular exudate changes from neutrophils to a predominant mononuclear cellular response of lymphocytes, monocytes, plasma cells, histiocytes, and fibroblasts. Fibrin, which aids phagocytes in their activities, also contributes to the organization and repair processes. Final repair, weeks later, may result in a dense fibrous scar. The subarachnoid space, ventricular lining, and choroid plexi may be affected. Without successful treatment, the inflammatory process can become densely organized and, within the subarachnoid space, may extend into the Virchow-Robin spaces, penetrating the pia and producing adjacent cerebritis (Fig. 13.6). Individuals with acute purulent leptomeningitis develop massive cerebral edema during the first few days and may die as a consequence of this mass effect with brain stem ischemia and cardiorespiratory arrest. Appropriate antibiotic therapy, which usually avoids this complication, is the major indication for an aggressive, early evaluation of spinal fluid from a diagnostic lumbar puncture done carefully, even in the presence of cerebral edema.

A massive inoculum of nonpathogenic bacteria into the central nervous system can infect it. A smaller inoculum of pathogenic bacteria in the same host may create an overwhelming infectious process. Specific bacteria tend to cause leptomeningitis in different hosts under different circumstances. The uncomprised neonate with placentally transferred IgG from his mother is thereby provided protection from many bacteria. Since *Escherichia coli* and other gram-negative organisms require IgM for their neutralization and, since this immunoglobulin is not made by the neonate or transferred to him from his mother, acute leptomeningitis in the neonate is most often caused by gram-negative bacteria like *E. coli*, normally found in the perineal region. In infants born vaginally, organisms found in large quantities in the birth canal may infect the neonate. Group B-streptococci have become important

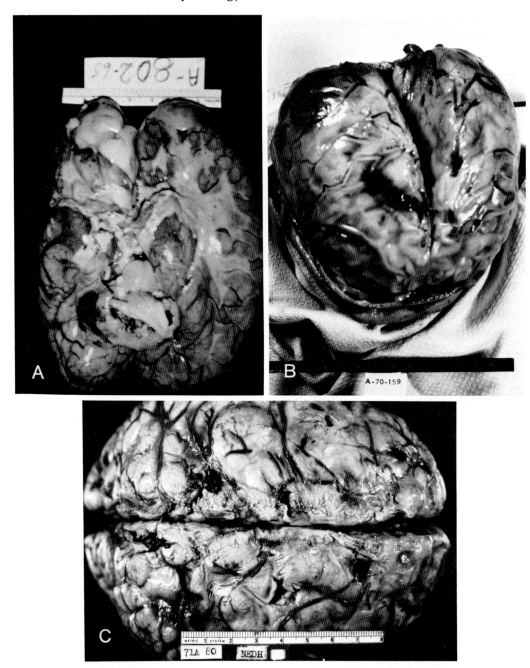

Figure 13.5. (A) Purulent leptomeningitis, which occurs in all age groups, is often caused by specific microorganisms in different age groups. (B) This neonate has acute hemorrhagic and purulent leptomeningitis due to *E. coli*. (C) Older individuals compromised by chronic alcoholism are susceptible to pneumococcal leptomeningitis which can produce an acute purulent exudate in the subarachnoid space with associated vasculitis.

causes of neonatal meningitis by colonizing the birth canals of some mothers. Similarly, candidal and herpes simplex infections are transferred from the mother to her baby when passed through an infected birth canal. During infancy and childhood, even though humoral and cellular immunity are adequate, exposure to a ubiquitous, infec-

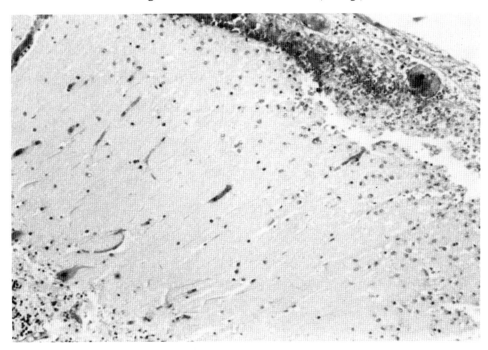

Figure 13.6. Acute purulent leptomeningitis may disrupt the underlying pia causing acute cerebritis. This inflammatory process can produce focal neurological deficits. H&E. (Original magnification × 150.)

tious, pathogenic antigen like *H. influenzae* for the first time, particularly in large doses, allows this agent to cause more acute leptomeningitis in this age group than any other bacteria.

Older healthy children and young adults during their teens and twenties are more susceptible to *N. meningitidis* (meningococcus) due to exposure to this organism in large quantities without adequate immunologic protection. The older adult is immune to most bacterial pathogens; however, *S. pneumoniae* becomes an important cause of meningitis in this group of individuals because of their susceptibility to aspiration bronchopneumonia, lobar pneumonia, and infections in the upper air passages. Subsequent pneumococcal bacteremia can lead to purulent leptomeningitis. Whenever the host is compromised by disease, iatrogenic measures, or both, infections are produced by those microbes in the environment that, at the time, are most pathogenic and most accessible to the host. So-called nonpathogenic bacteria, like most gram-negative organisms in the human gastrointestinal tract, may behave in a malignant fashion in the compromised host, as

illustrated by those patients with the acquired immunodeficiency syndrome. Different varieties of bacterial leptomeningitis, classified according to their etiologic agents, may produce similar complications and clinical manifestations.

HEMOPHILUS INFLUENZAE (14, 108, 229, 252)

This minute gram-negative aerobic rod is a leading cause of purulent meningitis in children between 4 months and 3 yr of age. The hemolytic character of *H. influenzae* is due to its requirement for factors V and X in whole blood for growth. *Haemophilus parainfluenzae* and *H. influenzae* include a, b, c, d, e, and f. Type b is responsible for most cases of meningitis caused by the organism. *H. influenzae* meningitis is rare after age 4 yr. Transferred maternal IgG antibodies protect infants for the first two months after birth, but this protection is lost by 4 months of age. From 2 months to 3 yr of age, little host cellular activity against *H. influenzae* is present. Once protective cellular activity is acquired, permanent resistance persists.

After 5 yr of age, *H. influenzae* becomes

less frequent and is extremely unusual after 10 yr of age but does occur in adults with predisposing factors, including diabetes mellitus, nephrosis, chronic alcoholism, agammaglobulinemia, or cerebrospinal fluid fistulae. A lack of bacterial cellular antibodies against this organism is a major factor in predisposing adults and children to influenzal meningitis.

N. MENINGITIDIS (160, 166, 167, 205, 197, 229, 322, 355)

This gram-negative micrococcus, which usually appears in pairs, includes different strains that can be isolated from the oral cavity in healthy carriers and may produce fulminating meningococcemia with meningitis. Meningococcal meningitis occurs throughout the world, but most commonly in large cities in the northern latitudes. This leptomeningitis appears year after year in crowded communities and may become epidemic after 10- to 12-yr intervals. About 10% of people in contact with the disease become healthy carriers, the organism residing in the nasopharynx. During epidemics, carrier rates rise to over 80%. The incubation period is 1 to 7 d with an average of 3. Any age level can be affected, but over 40% of all cases are seen in children under age 5 yr.

Meningococcal meningitis is similar to other purulent meningitides, being extremely severe and potentially lethal. The initial subarachnoid exudate may be minimal and associated with hyperemic and congested leptomeninges. A yellow, white to green, creamy material accumulates in the subarachnoid space and ventricles. The subarachnoid exudate may cover both cerebral hemispheres and be particularly excessive around the base of the brain and in the Sylvian fissures. Massive cerebral edema which develops over the first several days may kill the patient. Petechial hemorrhages are common. Thromboses of pial veins and dural sinuses occur. Cranial and spinal nerves commonly become engulfed in the exudate. After several days, the inflammatory exudate converts from predominant neutrophils to monocytic phagocytes, lymphocytes, plasma cells, and histiocytes. Meningococci are present in the exudate and within macrophages, unless previously treated. The ependymal lining may be denuded, and the choroid plexi swollen and encased in fibrinopurulent exudate. Cerebrospinal fluid, which reflects these changes, enables early recognition of the infecting agent by a carefully performed lumbar spinal puncture.

After circulatory collapse, death generally intervenes promptly. At autopsy, intravascular coagulopathy may be manifested by hemorrhage in the adrenals (Waterhouse-Friederichsen syndrome) and petechiae in other organs, including the central nervous system (Fig. 13.7). Most patients are infants and young children infected with the disease during an epidemic. Subacute and chronic meningococcal meningitides develop over periods of weeks to months. The organism in these patients appears less virulent with increased host resistance, and features may mimic a tuberculous meningitis. Hydrocephalus and spinal and cranial nerve defects may be apparent. Multiple attacks by the organism occur in some individuals in whom an infected focus in the central nervous system may be reactivated. Neurological sequelae from meningococcal meningitis are significant and frequent and can affect any area of the central nervous system. Early diagnosis and treatment prevent most complications.

S. PNEUMONIAE (17, 133, 167, 181, 254)

Any of the 70 or more varieties of pneumococci can produce meningitis. S. pneumoniae is a gram-positive, encapsulated coccus, usually arranged in pairs. More than 75 types of pneumococcus are recognized by their immunologically distinct capsular polysaccharides. At any age beyond infancy, pneumococcal meningitis is the most common form of purulent meningitis and produces an inflammatory response in the central nervous system similar to any other purulent leptomeningitis. The distribution and character of the inflammatory exudate may be yellow-green and located over the cerebral convexities, but this is not specific and can be found in any infectious leptomeningitis. Etiologic recognition requires cultural identification. Pneumococcal meningitis is rare in the newborn, but from 4 months until 3 yr of

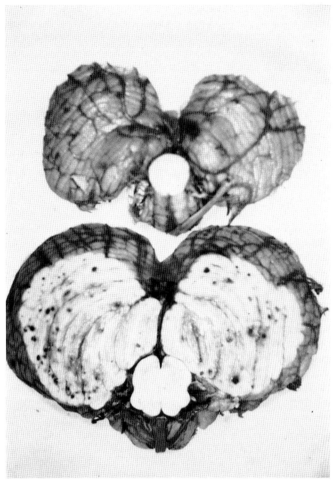

Figure 13.7. Meningococcemia produces disseminated intravascular coagulation which can involve the entire body, including the central nervous system. Sections of the cerebellum demonstrate discrete petechial hemorrhages associated with meningococcal meningoencephalitis.

age is second only to influenzal meningitis. It shows a predisposition for the 1st and 2nd years of life, as well as for older adults and is characterized by a purulent exudate similar to meningococcal meningitis. It is life-threatening, particularly in individuals over 40 yr. New therapeutic measures, however, have reduced this mortality rate.

Usually, this meningitis is associated with a suppurative focus and an underlying systemic disorder or some structural defect permitting communication of the subarachnoid space with the exterior. Lobar pneumococcal pneumonia has been a common primary focus for this meningitis, but otitis media has become a more commonly identified primary focus in children. Splenec-

tomy appears to predispose individuals to pneumococcal infections as do systemic disorders with immunological defects, such as histiocytosis, Wiskott-Aldrich syndrome, thalassemia major, nephrosis, and sickle cell disease. Any individual with previous head trauma and skull fracture may develop pneumococcal meningitis. Congenital defects and disturbances in the cribriform plate, middle ear, and nasopharynx can create communications between the subarachnoid space and the exterior, providing a portal of entry for pneumococci. Searching for these abnormalities is important in individuals with recurrent pneumococcal meningitis or other inflammatory meningitides.

MYCOBACTERIUM TUBERCULOSIS (78, 266, 302, 337)

These slow-growing, gram-positive rods measuring 1 to 3 μm are resistant to acid discoloration when stained with aniline dyes. Their lipid wall contributes to this acid-fast quality, whereas their tuberculoproteins are associated with tissue hypersensitivity. Tuberculous meningitis has accounted for less than 10% of all forms of bacterial meningitis in all age groups. The influx of refugees from third world countries has increased the frequency of tuberculous meningitis. The tubercle bacilli enter the host through the respiratory system by inhalation. After the initial pulmonary infections, phagocytes carry these microbes to regional lymph nodes, which enlarge due to chronic inflammation. This primary complex, consisting of the parenchymal lung lesion and involved regional lymph nodes, represents primary pulmonary tuberculosis. Spontaneous recovery from the initial primary pulmonary tuberculosis often occurs, but in some altered hosts it may be disseminated throughout the body, including the central nervous system. Generalized dissemination of tubercle bacilli with diffuse pulmonary infiltrations and widespread organ infections is referred to as miliary or disseminated tuberculosis, which is fatal unless treated early.

Tuberculous leptomeningitis results from the hematogenous spread of tubercle bacilli to foci in the central nervous system which then infect the circulating cerebrospinal fluid. Rich and McCordock (266) emphasized the virulent, allergic reaction in the acute phase of tuberculous meningitis but felt that massive numbers of mycobacteria invading the subarachnoid space by hematogenous dissemination could not produce such a response. Sensitized animals injected intravenously with heavy doses of tubercle bacilli did not develop an acute exudative meningitis. Nevertheless, Rich and McCordock found caseous tuberculous foci adjacent to the subarachnoid space in 77 of 82 patients with tuberculous meningitis at autopsy and attributed diffuse tuberculous meningitis to discharge of the organisms from these sites. Tubercles were 3–5 mm in diameter and found either in the meninges or neuroparenchyma itself adjacent to the subarachnoid space. These tuberculous foci, resulting from previous hematogenous spread of mycobacteria to the central nervous system, remained silent for varying periods before depositing organisms into the cerebrospinal fluid. This mechanism explains the occurrence of tuberculous meningitis months or years following previous pulmonary tuberculosis. Tubercle bacilli in the spinal fluid of rabbits produce an immediate inflammatory meningeal response only in those animals previously sensitized to tuberculoprotein.

Morphologically, tuberculous leptomeningitis is associated with cerebral edema, astrocytic proliferation, and diffuse grey opacity of the leptomeninges. This opacity is due to a thick, gelatinous, and fibrotic infiltrate around the base of the brain extending into the basilar cisterns. Lymphocytes, plasma cells, and multinucleated giant cells are scattered among areas of caseous necrosis (Fig. 13.8). Tubercle bacilli may be seen in large numbers or may be difficult to recognize. Meningeal vessels may be intact or altered directly by the infectious inflammatory exudate, indirectly by reactive endarteritis obliterans, or by both processes (Fig. 13.9). Vessels traversing the basilar tuerculous exudate are involved most profoundly. Complications include subdural effusion, communicating hydrocephalus, neuroparenchymal destruction, and intracranial calcifications.

Tuberculous spondylitis may involve any portion of the spine, but the lower thoracic region is most commonly affected. Several adjacent vertebral bodies may be affected, or multiple areas in one vertebra may show damage from the disease. The initial location of the process is the vertebral body itself; less frequently, the laminar arches of the spine are involved. Spread from one vertebral body to another may occur under the anterior spinal ligament or through the intervertebral disc, resulting in reduction of the disc space. A paravertebral soft tissue abscess may develop. Resulting complications of the spinal cord include direct compression, ischemic changes, or both. Spinal cord compression occurs only in patients who had spondylitic disease caused by the tubercle bacillus. Pott's disease, which is paraparesis or paraplegia secondary to vertebral tuberculous involvement, occurs in

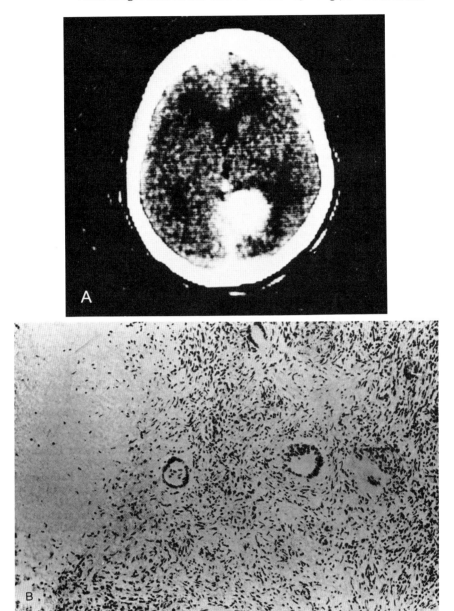

Figure 13.8. Tuberculosis can produce acute leptomeningitis and tuberculomas. (*A*) This computerized tomogram demonstrates a discrete mass in the right posterior brain above and below the tentorium. (*B*) The histomorphologic evaluation shows discrete caseating granulomas without demonstrable organisms. H&E. (Original magnification ×450.) (From DeAngelis LM: *Neurology* 31:1135, 1981.)

about 15% of these patients. Pain and localized spinal tenderness are prominent symptoms in this illness and may eventually result in vertebral destruction with gibbous formation, complete paraplegia, and sphincter paralysis. Radicular pain may also develop.

The cerebrospinal fluid may be opaque and under increased pressure with varying numbers of inflammatory cells. Early, the cerebrospinal fluid contains many neutrophils, but later lymphocytic pleocytosis develops. Rarely does the cell count exceed 500 cells/cu mm. The cerebrospinal fluid

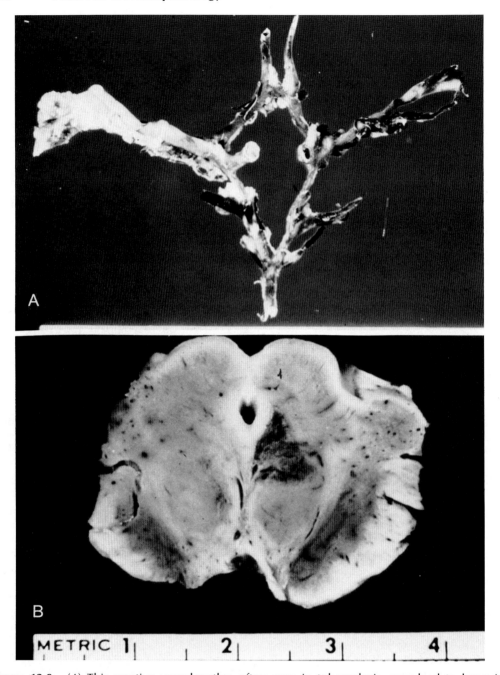

Figure 13.9. (*A*) This reactive vasculopathy, often seen in tuberculosis, may lead to hypoxic-ischemic changes in the adjacent neuroparenchyma. (*B*) This lesion is an evolving infarct in the tegmentum of the midbrain caused by tuberculous vasculopathy.

sugar may be between 15 and 35 mg/dl, and spinal fluid protein may be normal or slightly increased in early stages, but later elevated to 100–400 g/dl. Acid-fast bacilli may be found on stained smears of the fluid and should be looked for in the pedicle

formed after the fluid stands for awhile (Fig. 13.10). Gram stains should be done on all specimens, for occasionally mixed infections of tubercle bacilli with other bacteria occur. Recovery of tubercle bacilli, which confirms the diagnosis of tuberculosis, can

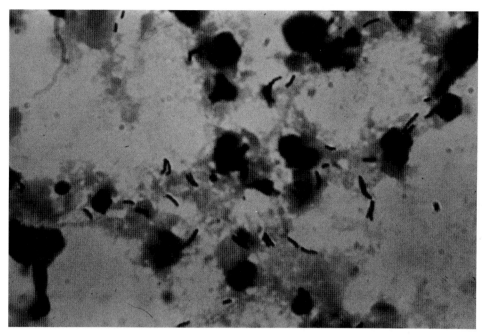

Figure 13.10. Aggressive evaluation of the cerebrospinal fluid is indicated in any potential infectious process in the central nervous system. This cerebrospinal fluid smear demonstrates acid-fast bacilli in a patient with tuberculous leptomeningitis.

be achieved by cultural techniques as well as by guinea pig inoculations of spinal fluid specimens. Isolation of the tubercle bacilli from the cerebrospinal fluid is accomplished in about half of the patients.

MISCELLANEOUS BACTERIA (136, 139, 159, 178, 197, 233, 245)

Any bacteria with access to the subarachnoid space or the neuroparenchyma may infect it. Increasing number of compromised hosts created by modern therapies have developed patients with leptomeningitis produced by bacteria previously considered nonpathogenic, such as *Serratia marcescens* and the endogenous aerobic and anaerobic eubacteria in the gastrointestinal tract. Recognition of any bacterial leptomeningitis requires accurate identification of the organism in the microbiological laboratory. Under appropriate circumstances, aerobic and anaerobic eubacteria, including bacilli, cocci, mycoplasma, protoplasts ("L" forms), and spirochetes may be recovered from the cerebrospinal fluid. Any organism that can produce a bacteremia can infect the leptomeninges. Gonococcal meningitis

caused by the gram-negative diplococcus, *Neisseria gonorrheae*, illustrates this point.

Brucella species are recognized rarely as a cause for leptomeningitis in the United States. These small, gram-negative coccobacilli have been recovered from the cerebrospinal fluid and neural tissue. Some individuals with *Brucella* meningitis have been recognized by specific agglutination techniques in the spinal fluid. Meningoencephalitis with abnormal cerebrospinal fluid has been recognized in patients with undulant fever caused by *Brucella abortus*, as well as *Brucella canis*, *Brucella melitensis*, *Brucella neotomae*, and *Brucella suis*. These microbes can produce abscesses and granulomas throughout the body. Leptomeningitis produced by *Bacillus anthracis*, a large, gram-positive spore-forming rod, has been described in neonates and the elderly. Males predominate in this fulminating disorder, which usually has a short duration and terminates fatally within 1–4 d. Pathologically, diffuse hemorrhages are associated with an acute inflammatory response scattered through the subarachnoid space. The incriminating organism can be found in the subarachnoid space, which is filled not only with erythrocytes but also with neutrophils. Cerebrospinal fluid protein is markedly increased, and spinal glucose and chloride levels are reduced. Large, gram-positive rods can be found in smears of the cerebrospinal fluid.

Leptomeningitis can be created by *Listeria monocytogenes*, which can attack any individual of any age. This gram-positive diptheroid bacillus can be recovered in smears or culture as a motile, nonacid-fast, microaerophilic and nonsporulating bacillus. Typically, extensive meningoencephalitis with associated ependymitis occurs in infants, children, and adults that are compromised. The meningeal changes are seen at the base of the brain and are associated with mononuclear phagocytes and scattered neutrophils. Lymphocytes and plasma cells may be noted. Cystic destruction may occur in infantile brains, but leptomeningitis is the dominant form of listeriosis in man. The organism may be transferred directly from mother to her fetus. The most common residual complication in infants is hydrocephalus. *Staphylococcus aureus* or *Staphylococcus epidermidis* can be introduced directly into the central nervous system through operative intervention, monitoring equipment, or other iatrogenic procedures. Suspicion of infectious leptomeningitis should be maintained in order to avoid missing a potentially treatable and reversible condition that, unless appreciated, can kill the patient.

Gram-Negative Bacteria (89, 108, 132, 135, 160, 166, 197, 204, 245, 296, 300)

Many different gram-negative organisms are known to cause purulent leptomeningitis. *Citrobacter* has caused necrotizing meningoencephalitis with subsequent cystic gliotic changes in neonates and infants (Fig. 13.11). In the newborn, *E. coli* (the colon bacillus) is the most frequent cause of purulent meningitis, yet it is rarely observed in older children and adults. This small, nonspore-forming, gram-negative rod measures 1–3 μm and can be cultured easily on appropriate media. *Klebsiella pneumoniae* can cause middle ear infections, mastoiditis, nasal sinusitis, or even pneumonia with subsequent hematogenous spread to the meninges. This pyogenic meningitis, which may be similar to other pyogenic bacterial meningitides, produces a mucoid appearance to the cerebrospinal fluid from the bacterial capsular material. *Mima polymorpha* may be mistaken for *N. meningitidis*, *N. gonorrhoeae*, and *H. influenzae*. This meningitis originates from wounds and intravenous catheters contaminated by *M. polymorpha* and usually occurs as sepsis in the very young or very old. The organism causes abscesses, cellulitis, conjunctivitis, endocarditis, pneumonitis, pyelonephritis, urethritis, and vaginitis, as well as meningitis. Thirty per cent of these patients with meningitis have a petechial rash that can be confused with meningococcal meningitis. Although most patients with *M. polymorpha* meningitis have a relatively benign course, a fulminating course, terminating in Waterhouse-Friderichsen syndrome, has been identified. Meningitis due to *Proteus vulgaris* can occur at any time during life and generally enters the body from a specific focus, often in the abdomen, then spreads by the bloodstream to the central nervous system. *Pseudomonas aeruginosa* has been seen frequently in patients with gram-negative sepsis and can infect their leptomeninges. At autopsy, neutrophils are not uncommonly scattered through the subarachnoid space and associated with congested vessels and scanty gram-negative organisms culturally recognized as a variety of different gram-negative bacilli, including *Pseudomonas aeruginosa* and *Proteus* species. These organisms may contaminate the subarachnoid space through a spinal puncture or shunt. They may produce a gram-negative vasculopathy, with many bacilli replacing the vascular media without any inflammation (Fig. 13.12). Clinically, *P. aeruginosa* meningitis may be acute, subacute, or chronic, but typically is purulent and may continue for days or weeks. The infection is resistant to therapy and has a high mortality. A bluish-green to yellow exudate reflects the pigment produced by this gram-negative organism. Despite the ubiquitous nature of *Salmonella* organisms, meningitis due to the microbe is uncommon. Its incidence is highest in children. Mortality rate among newborns is over 90% with decreasing mortality (over 75%) at and beyond age 15 yr. Meningitis may complicate typhoid fever during any part of its course and is associ-

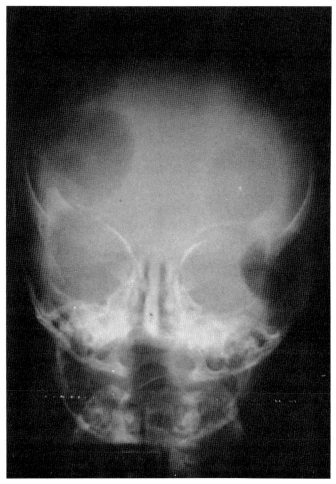

Figure 13.11.   Cystic gliotic intracerebral lesions can be produced in infants by *Citrobacter* species and here caused large intracerebral cavities above each orbit.

ated with a high mortality rate. Cerebrospinal fluid demonstrates increased pressure, turbid fluid, and predominant neutrophils with over 1,000 cells/cu mm. In addition, prominent protein, reduced sugar, and normal chlorides are associated with gram-negative rods on smears. Some other gram-negative organisms have been incriminated with purulent leptomeningitis and include *Acinetobacter* species (*Achromobacter, Moraxella, Herellea* and *Mima*), *Actinobacillus, Aeromonas, Alcaligenes, Arizona, Bacteroides, Borrelia, Branhamella, Campylobacter, Cardiobacterium, Chromobacterium, Comamonas, Edwardsiella, Eikenella, Enterobacter, Erwinia, Flavobacterium, Fusobacterium, Moraxella, Pasteurella, Providencia, Rickettsia, Serratia, Treponema* and *Yersinia.*

Gram-Positive Bacteria (17, 133, 181)

Many other gram-positive bacteria have also been recovered from the central nervous system, including genera of *Actinomyces, Clostridium, Corynebacterium, Eubacterium, Gaffkya, Leptospira, Nocardia, Peptococcus, Peptostreptococcus, Propionibacterium, Streptococcus,* and *Streptomyces.*

Paradural Empyemas (69, 106, 116, 304)

The central nervous system is protected from infections by membranous coverings, including the pachymeninx (dura) and leptomeninges (pia-arachnoid). The dura has dense fibrocollagenous tissue with few blood vessels and peripheral nerves and is

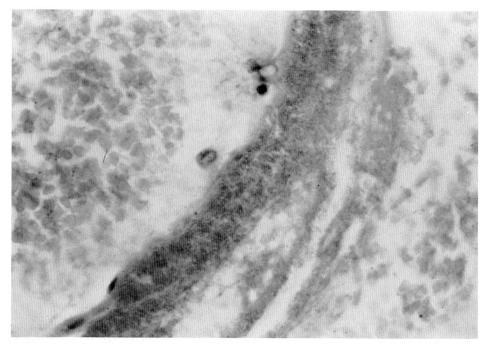

Figure 13.12.   Gram-negative sepsis can cause vasculitis with many gram-negative organisms replacing the media without inflammation. This blood vessel possesses *Pseudomonas* organisms replacing almost the entire media.

adherent to the periosteum in the newborn and elderly. It develops a potential space easily demonstrated at autopsy in older children and young adults. In addition to the bony skull, the dura provides an effective barrier, although emissary veins may carry infection through it to the brain. This barrier function of the dura is particularly evident around the spinal cord where bony attachments are not present, and a large epidural space in the spinal canal separates the vertebrae from the spinal cord. The external mesothelioid cell layer of the arachnoid provides another protective covering that prevents infectious agents from invading either into or out of the subarachnoid space. Infections near the dura occur either outside the dura (epidural infections) or inside the dura (subdural infections) and can be referred to collectively as paradural infections or empyemas. A sterile acute or chronic leptomeningitis may be evident in some people as a "sympathetic" or indirect, reactive, noninfectious inflammatory response to any paradural extraarachnoidal infectious inflammation.

Infections in the intracranial epidural space may produce small abscesses flat-

tened between the bone and dura. Epidural infections are caused usually by previous infections in air sinuses, adjacent bones (osteomyelitis), or both. Frontal and mastoid sinusitis produces epidural abscesses in the anterior and posterior fossae, whereas infections in other air sinuses may burst through the dura into the adjacent subdural or subarachnoid space. This is related to the firm dural attachment to adjacent bones in these regions at the base of the skull. If the dura is adherent to the adjacent bone, the dura can be breached, creating subdural infections.

Epidural infections in the spine are usually secondary to osteomyelitis involving adjacent vertebrae and are most often caused by *S. aureus*. Initially, the abscess develops with many neutrophils, eventually replaced by granulation tissue with fibrosis, isolating the abscess into an inflammatory, fibrotic mass. As a rule, these abscesses are seen in the thoracic area, extending over several segments of the spinal cord. The pus may spread throughout the epidural space, creating purulent collections in the lumbar region. The initiating focus of osteomyelitis may not be evident but includes any source for intravascular bacteremia, including intravenous drug abuse. The initiating focus of osteomyelitis may not be evident. *Salmonella typhi,* as well as other infectious agents, can produce epidural abscesses after infecting vertebral bodies or adjacent soft tissue, extending into the epidural space. Infections of the retromediastinal or retroperitoneal areas can extend through adjacent intervertebral foramina into the spinal epidural space, producing epidural inflammatory lesions. Infections do not tend to spread in the reverse directions from the epidural space to the retroperitoneal or retromediastinal areas.

Subdural empyemas are usually widespread throughout the subdural space and complicate infections in the paranasal air sinuses. Venous spread through adjacent bones may give rise to subdural empyemas which can be associated with adjacent venous thromboses. Sphenoid sinusitis and osteomyelitis of cranial bones can lead to subdural infections which tend to spread diffusely and cause phlebitis of adjacent and distant veins. Pus usually collects most intensely near the initial infecting focus, which can indicate the portal of entry. Occasionally, the pus accumulates in areas difficult to drain, especially along the falx cerebri or upper tentorium. Since the dura is poorly vascularized, antibiotic therapy has little access to the region.

Neuroparenchymal Infections (46, 49, 89, 110, 116, 296)

Infectious inflammatory infiltrates involving the entire neuroparenchyma to some degree, including the cerebrum, deep basal nuclei, brain stem, and cerebellum, have been called encephalitis. Unqualified, this term implies a viral infection, but pathologically, indicates inflammation of the cerebrum or encephalon. Focal inflammatory infiltrates in the neuroparenchyma, on the other hand, are known as cerebritis, which can be seen around septic thromboemboli, cerebral abscesses, infarcts, and traumatic lesions. Inflammation in the spinal cord, called "myelitis," may be local or diffuse. Bacterial infections in the neuroparenchyma include: (1) focal pyogenic encephalitis (cerebritis); (2) widespread or diffuse embolic suppurative encephalitis, or

(3) localized cerebral abscess. The latter can be associated with open skull fractures, septic thromboemboli, contaminated surgical fields, or direct spread from infected foci around the neuraxis. Secondarily infected metastatic carcinoma, particularly from the gastrointestinal tract, may also present as a cerebral abscess. The infective organisms are usually gram-negative rods that enter the brain from outside sources through the bloodstream, even though the primary lesion may not be evident. Sepsis within the central nervous system can complicate any bacteremia. Local venous spread is a rarer vascular infectious route into the central nervous system. Adjacent, destructive, purulent foci in bones around the brain and spinal cord may bridge the bony and meningeal barriers, providing entry for pyogenic microbes. Trauma is an obvious mechanism for infecting the brain and spinal cord with contaminated foreign material, osseous fragments, and necrotic debris, providing for spread of bacteria. Antibiotics have not only altered the frequency and character of abscesses in the brain but also reduced their mortality rates.

Embolic suppurative encephalitis is characterized by many microabscesses and rare macroabscesses. At autopsy, most individuals with suppurative bacterial encephalitis are over 50 yr of age and are older than those with discrete isolated cerebral abscesses. Prior to the antibiotic era, abscesses in the brain at autopsy were seen more commonly. The heart continues to be the most common source for infected thromboemboli, followed by septicemia and lung infections. Leptomeningitis may complicate these infections. *Streptococcus viridans,* which can be found in the mouth and upper respiratory tract, is a common organism in cerebral abscesses in people with bacterial endocarditis. Enterococci are gram-positive cocci that can invade the bloodstream after genitourinary tract manipulations. Transient bacteremia may result from any focal infection in any part of the body and subsequently infect the neuraxis.

Metastatic or embolic bacterial encephalitis is characterized by diffuse congestion and hyperemia of the leptomeninges and neuroparenchyma occurring agonally in patients with bacteremia. Focal subarachnoid hemorrhage may be associated with some degree of cerebral edema. Extensive subarachnoid hemorrhage can result from a ruptured mycotic aneurysm, usually located in the distribution of the middle cerebral arteries and potentially a complication of almost any infectious agent. Grossly, the brain shows punctate congestion and red-grey-tan lesions scattered through the neuroparenchyma, primarily in the grey matter, grey-white cerebral junctions, and brain stem. These lesions may be difficult to separate from petechial hemorrhages or congestion. Multiple microabscesses may be evident. Healed foci appear as minute scars in the cortex and underlying white matter. Microscopically, focal acute leptomeningitis may be seen over areas of suppurative encephalitis. Most leptomeningeal infiltrates are localized to the Virchow-Robin spaces in the brain. Gram-negative bacterial vasculopathy in some patients is typified by gram-negative rods replacing the media without any inflammation (Fig. 13.12). Early lesions vary from small collections of neutrophilic leukocytes with microglia and bacteria to miliary discrete abscesses with scattered erythrocytes and a predilection for the grey-white cerebral junctions. The smaller lesions may be a few micrometers in maximum diameter and contain scattered neutrophils and a few bacteria. A small blood vessel may be seen in the center or adjacent to the lesions and can be occluded by a thromboembolus. Multiple microabscesses coalesce in some individuals, producing a discrete macroabscess with adjacent granulation tissue, astrogliosis, and cerebral edema. The resulting mass effect can be lethal. After several days, the predominant mononuclear cell response is associated with astrocytosis. All lesions appear to be the same age. Since some yeast fungi like *Candida albicans* can mimic these acute bacterial lesions, multiple stains including periodic acid-Schiff and methenamine silver can exclude these organisms.

BRAIN ABSCESS (46, 49, 89, 110, 218, 296)

Prior to antibiotic therapy, cerebral abscesses were found in about 1% of all autopsies, but subsequently, even though they were recognized more frequently clinically, their incidence at autopsy has decreased. Predisposing factors include congenital cyanotic heart disease complicated by cerebral abscesses in about 10% of these patients, pulmonary infections, and sinusitis. Cerebral abscesses occur in all age groups, with patients ranging from newborn into the ninth decade. Their source correlates with the age of the patient. The peak frequency appears in young and older adults due to increased pulmonary disorders and infective endocarditis, particularly related to intravenous drug abuse. During infancy, most cerebral abscesses are caused by septic thromboemboli, and after 2 yr of age, are related to cyanotic congenital heart disease.

Brain abscesses can be produced by direct penetrating injuries to the central nervous system and can appear from 2 weeks to 6 months after the trauma. Some nontraumatic cerebral abscesses appear within 2 months after the primary infection. With more aggressive and reliable microbiological culture techniques, the bacteria recovered from cerebral abscesses include multiple aerobic and anaerobic rods and cocci. Since antibiotic usages can yield sterile cultures, it should be avoided before determining the infectious agents unless life-threatening events occur. Previously, the most common organism in cerebral abscesses was *Staphylococcus*, which is still common in children. Other bacteria recovered from cerebral abscesses include the pneumococcus and *Streptococcus viridans*. In the preantibiotic era, the most frequent organisms recovered from brain abscesses were β-hemolytic streptococci and *H. influenza*, associated with congenital heart disease. In traumatic cerebral abscesses, staphylococci continue to predominate, but in hospitalized patients with hematogenously disseminated cerebral abscesses, mixed aerobic and anaerobic bacterial flora, particularly gram-negative organisms, have become important.

Four types of brain abscesses include: (1) embolic cerebral abscesses from infected foci elsewhere in the body; (2) direct-extension cerebral abscesses from adjacent infectious foci, such as the ear, mastoid, or paranasal sinuses; (3) trauma-related cerebral abscesses; and (4) idiopathic cerebral abscesses where no originating infectious focus is evident. *Embolic cryptogenic ab-*

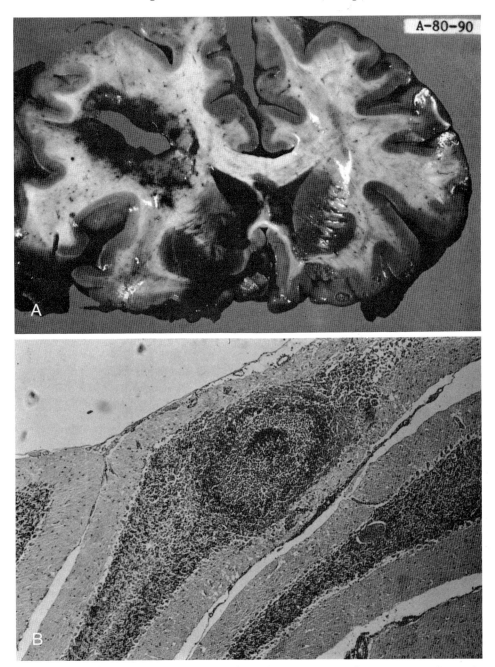

Figure 13.13.   (A) This necrotic and congested cavity representing a hematogenous brain abscess is located in the left centrum semiovale. (B) A microabscess produced by *C. albicans* is located in the cerebellar folium. H&E. (Original magnification ×150.)

scesses, which may be multiple or solitary, account for about 40% of all brain abscesses. More than half of the metastatic and cryptogenic cerebral abscesses are solitary. These abscesses are primarily located in the anterior and middle cerebral arterial distributions involving both cerebral hemispheres (Fig. 13.13). The frontal lobes are involved most often by metastatic cerebral abscesses which at autopsy appear at the grey-white junction invading the underlying white matter and extending towards the ventricles. Other lobes of the brain are infected less frequently. The temporal lobes are affected more often than either the parietal or occipital lobes due to direct extension from adjacent infected bones, sinuses, and soft tissues. The cerebellum, basal ganglia, brain stem, and thalamus rarely have abscesses. Most metastatic brain abscesses originate from the lungs or heart; however, bacteremia from any cause can produce a brain abscess. Bronchiectasis, pulmonary abscess, and empyemas are associated with intracranial abscesses. Most cryptogenic abscesses in the cerebral arterial distribution are associated with transient bacteremias. Iatrogenic manipulations in any site can led to a transient bacteremia. Infected small thromboemboli may enter the brain through the internal carotid arterial system, lodging in the cerebral hemispheres or enter through the paravertebral venous plexus of Batson. Arterial thromboembolism is the most likely source for most metastatic cryptogenic cerebral abscesses.

Direct extension cerebral abscesses arise by continuous spread from adjacent infected foci around the mastoid air cells and cranial sinuses. Aggressive antibiotic therapy has created a marked reduction in these abscesses by early successful treatment of infections in the ears, sinuses, and mastoid. Most direct extension abscesses are located in the temporal lobe and less often in the cerebellum and cerebellopontine angle. Microbes in infected bones can invade the adjacent meninges, producing epidural and subdural abscesses. Once the arachnoid is breached by the bacteria, the neural parenchymal can be infected through extension into the Virchow-Robin perivascular spaces and, finally, pial invasion. A retrograde infected thrombophlebitis may also provide an infectious route. With development of the cranial air sinuses by about 8 yr of age, infective sinusitis can lead to adjacent cerebral abscesses.

Traumatic brain abscesses account for about 30% of intracerebral abscesses and are a particular problem after head injuries from any cause. Latency from the time of injury to subsequent infection may be associated with retained fragments of necrotic tissue, bone, and foreign material, providing a nidus for development of an intracranial abscess that may be indolent, requiring operative intervention.

A brain abscess may be a huge macroscopic lesion or so small as to be appreciated only by careful microscopy. Necrotic neuroparenchyma created by an infected thromboembolus provides a medium for supporting the multiplication of contaminating microbes, which reach the brain through hematogenous routes, direct invasion, or traumatic inoculation. With reduced oxygen tension and altered local and primary defense mechanisms in the host, the organisms replicate with the necrotic, poorly demarcated focus of septic, acute cerebritis, creating softening, hyperemia, and neutrophilic infiltrates. Necrotic changes occur centrally and are followed by liquefaction and purulent exudate (Fig. 13.13). During this phase, the excessive neutrophils can be seen grossly as yellow purulent abscesses, typically located at the grey-white junction and invading the adjacent white matter. If the septic thromboembolus is small, the early abscess is also small. A larger septic thromboembolus produces a larger abscess. After 2 d, the inflammation includes some mononuclear phagocytes, lymphocytes, and plasma cells mixed with many neutrophils. By 5 to 7 d, capillaries proliferate at the margin of the liquefactive necrosis and are associated with fibroblasts, slight collagen, and some reactive astrocytes in the adjacent neuroparenchyma. At this time, the abscess can be visualized by enhancing radiographic techniques in the computerized axial tomogram. As its granulation tissue increases over the next 2–3 weeks, a mass effect may become apparent clinically and radiographically. Granulation tissue and fibroblastic activity around the abscess results in encapsulation, and, with continued expansion, profound edema can occur around the abscess extending several centimeters from its periphery. Multiple microabscesses may coalesce to produce a single lobulated macroabscess. Metastatic (thromboembolic) cerebral abscesses dissect towards the ventricles rather than the overlying, more resistant vascular cerebral cortex. When these abscesses rupture, they tend to spread through the ventricular system rather than the subarachnoid space due to the unique difference in vascularity between the cerebral cortex and its less vascular underlying white matter. Cultures identify the inciting bacteria in most abscesses. Frequently recovered organisms include streptococci, staphylococci, and pneumococci. Gram-negative organisms, such as *E. coli, H. influenzae, Proteus,* and *Pseudomonas,* are recognized less frequently. Since anaerobic bacteria have been identified in brain abscesses, techniques for both aerobic and anaerobic cultures should be performed in any cultural attempt. Many nonbacterial infectious agents have also produced intracranial abscesses. Fungi, actinomycetes, and amebae can create brain abscesses, especially in patients debilitated by chronic disease or immunosuppressive therapy.

Clinical manifestations of a brain abscess depend on the age of the host, mass location, size, multifocality, growth rate, and associated cerebral edema. The most serious manifestations are related to mass effect rather than to the infection itself. Abscesses in the brain stem occur infrequently, but develop either from hematogenous spread or invasion from an otogenic source. Sudden deterioration suggests internal herniations or spontaneous rupture of the abscess into the ventricles. Although not invariably fatal, these complications worsen the prognosis and indicate the desirability of prompt diagnosis and treatment before such a catastrophe occurs. Another fatal event in a cerebral abscess is massive hemorrhage. Cerebrospinal fluid is usually clear and colorless without any organisms, unless rupture of the lesion has produced leptomeningitis. Elevation of the cerebrospinal fluid pressure is usually present. The protein content is often modestly elevated. Leukocytic counts may be normal, although 10–100 lymphocytes and neutrophils per cubic millimeter may be noted. With more chronic encapsulated cerebral abscesses, a lymphocytic pleocytosis may be evident. When an abscess is suspected and meningitis can be excluded with reasonable certainty, a lumbar spinal tap should be avoided to prevent the potential hazard of tonsillar herniation. With the advent of cerebral computerized axial tomography, evaluation of intracranial masses can be done before a spinal tap is required.

SPECIFIC INFECTIONS

Actinomycosis (94, 171, 183, 196, 207, 315)

Actinomycosis primarily causes abscesses in the mandible and other bones with draining sinuses and fistulae possessing yellow granules or "sulfa (sulfur) granules." It is a chronic suppurative disorder, characterized by extensive purulent exudate with yellow granules of thin (less than 1 μm), branching gram-positive actinomycetic filaments in matted tangles. This infection involves not only the jaw but also the gastrointestinal tract, liver, lung, and occasionally the central nervous system. These thin branching filaments are higher forms of microaerophilic, gram-positive bacteria. A granule from the purulent exudate can be examined in unstained and gram-stained preparations to demonstrate the branching organisms. Most human infections are produced by *Actinomyces israelli* and *Actinomyces bovis* which can be seen in hematoxylin and eosin- and silver methenamine-stained sections (Fig. 13.14).

Actinomycosis in the central nervous system is acquired from microbes originating from the oral cavity or gastrointestinal tract invading underlying tissues through breaks in the mucosa. The cervicofacial variety of actinomycosis may develop several weeks following a dental extraction. The gastrointestinal variety may be associated with abdominal abscesses following perforation of the appendix. Hematogenous spread of the actinomycetes to the central nervous sytem can be associated with direct extension from adjacent infected structures at the base of the skull or around the spine. In cervicofacial actinomycosis, the meninges may be invaded through associated fascial planes from the cervical region, creating epidural and subdural empyemas. Actinomycetic abscesses possess central liquefactive necrosis and many neutrophils surrounded by mononuclear cells, granulation tissue, and dense fibrosis with branching gram-positive filaments (Fig. 13.14). Although lymphoplasmacytes and monocytes are found in the abscesses with multinucleated giant cells, granulomas are unusual. Paradural inflammations with adjacent cerebral abscesses may appear.

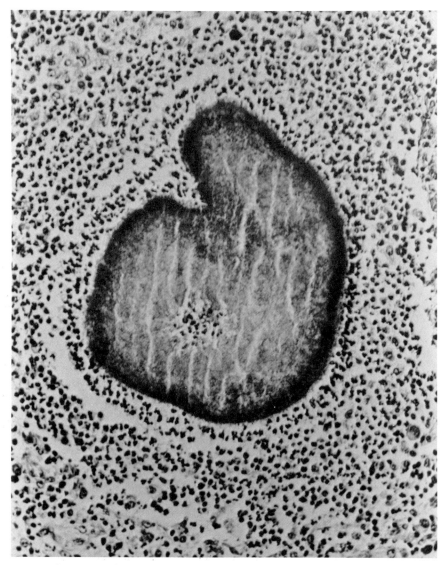

Figure 13.14. Actinomycetes are gram-positive and silver-positive, thin branching bacteria which produce discrete granules. GMS. (Original magnification ×500.)

Mycobacterosis (77, 78, 185, 266, 302, 331, 337, 348)

Intraparenchymal tuberculous lesions occur in all patients with tuberculous meningitis but may be difficult to discern if small. Associated bacterial encephalitis due to *Mycobacterium tuberculosis* is well established, yet other mycobacteria rarely, if ever, infect the central nervous system. *Mycobacterium leprae* commonly involves the peripheral nervous system. Sarcoidosis, which is well known to affect the neuraxis and its coverings, has been related to typical and atypical mycobacteriosis but is a diagnosis of exclusion. Its etiology is still not known.

Vascular proliferations and vasculitis in the central nervous system can be produced by *M. tuberculosis*. The induced acute and chronic inflammation causes associated vascular changes that, in turn, lead to ischemic necrosis and tuberculous abscesses. Endarteritis obliterans may produce severe ischemia and is a consequence of direct tuberculous vasculopathy with necrotizing vasculitis as well as reactive vascular changes in resolving meningitis (Fig. 13.9). The parenchymal tubercle derived from hematogenous spread from the lungs of *M. tuberculosis* is the primary lesion for neutrotuberculosis and can lead to diffuse tuberculous leptomeningitis. A discrete mass effect can be produced with coalescence and expansion of intraparenchymal tubercles, producing a tuberculoma. This is usually an irregular, round, firm mass with a yellow-tan-white discoloration and a soft, caseous center (Fig. 13.8). The latter is surrounded by epithelioid and spindle-shaped nucleated cells with multinucleated giant cells and adjacent inflammatory cells, including mononuclear phagocytes, lymphocytes and plasma cells. Fibrocollagenous tissue may be seen around the periphery of the granuloma. Chronic tuberculomas can possess markedly reduced inflammatory response, scattered calcification, and even ossification. Rarely, cystic changes appear in the center of the tuberculomas. Within the United States, tuberculomas are uncommon in the central nervous system; however, in less well-developed and third-world countries, tuberculosis is a prominent public health problem, and infections in the central nervous system are not uncommon. In India, tuberculomas constitute the most common intracranial mass in children.

Neurosyphilis (27, 50, 86, 114, 128, 146, 149, 161, 211, 212, 237, 239, 269, 277, 310, 329)

Syphilis is caused by the *Treponema pallidum*, a thin spiral organism, varying between 5 and 15 μm in length. *T. pallidum* can pass through intact mucosal membranes and the compromised skin and is transmitted in humans by venereal contact in most cases.

Congenital syphilis is caused by spirochetes transferred transplacentally from the mother to her infant. It can result in abortions, stillbirths, or active infections in live neonates. The fetus is protected against infection in the first 4 months of pregnancy because of the Langhans' cell layer in the early placenta, which provides a barrier against transplacental passage of treponemes. At about 16–18 weeks gestation, this barrier is dissolved, and the fetus becomes susceptible to syphilis and remains so for the remainder of the pregnancy. Penicillin therapy in early pregnancy will prevent fetal infection and treatment of the mother late in pregnancy can bring about cure of the infected fetus. The later in pregnancy therapy is started, the greater are the chances that the infant will subsequently demonstrate stigmata of intrauterine acquired syphilis, even though the active infection is cured. Congential syphilis may create neuroparenchymal lesions similar to the acquired form. Basal meningitis can lead to infantile hydrocephalus, and general paresis may occur at the end of the first or second decade of life. Tabes dorsalis is rare. Pathological changes which are seen throughout the neuraxis in congential syphilis include degenerative changes in the cerebral cortex, Purkinje cell loss, and internal granular cell loss with shrunken atrophic cerebellar gyri and dense neuroglial overgrowths throughout the cortex.

In many individuals with syphilis, the illness is self-limited after the initial stage, which may go undetected. In others, the disorder progresses over many years to lead to devastating consequences known as late or tertiary syphilis, which is usually preventable by treating primary or secondary syphilis. In congenital and acquired syphilis, the cutaneous lesions represent the secondary stage of the disease. In addition, hypersensitivity conditions, like interstitial keratitis and joint changes, may occur in spite of therapy in the neonatal period. Usually, when therapy is begun later, response is less effective. Patients infected for 2 to 3 yr before receiving treatment may remain seropositive for life. Syphilis can infect the nervous system as acute leptomeningitis in secondary syphilis, meningovascular tertiary neurosyphilis, parenchymatous tertiary neurosyphilis, syphilitic vascular disease, tabes dorsalis, and gumma. With effective antisyphilitic medications, neurosyphilis has been reduced drastically. After infection with *T. pallidum*, many patients have their meningeal spaces invaded by the organism. Approximately 50% of all infected individuals show changes in their cerebrospinal fluid, which vary with the adequacy of early treatment and infective stage when therapy is started. Increased leukocytes in the cerebrospinal fluid may be associated with increased protein. These changes disappear during treatment and do not reappear after therapy is completed. Tertiary neurosyphilis is a rare phenomenon in such treated patients.

Meningeal invasion by *T. pallidum* in secondary or latent syphilis is typically asymptomatic. In these individuals, the cerebrospinal fluid shows inflammatory features with several hundred leukocytes per cubic millimeter, increased globulins, and a positive VDRL test. Even with treatment, tertiary neurosyphilis can occur. Neurosyphilis involves primarily the meninges, blood vessels, neuroparenchyma, or some combination of these structures. Characteristic features include thickened meninges, lymphocytic meningeal infiltrates, and lymphocytic perivascular infiltrates around small blood vessels. Meningovascular syphilis, which is distinct from parenchymatous neurosyphilis (tabes dorsalis and paretic dementia), demonstrates similar vascular changes observed in the rest of the body of patients with tertiary syphilis. Diffuse, proliferative inflammatory changes in the cerebral cortex with many spirochetes are found typically in general paralysis, affecting the prefrontal cortex and corpus striatum most severely and rarely associated with either miliary (small) or larger gummata. Tabes dorsalis is a variety of parenchymatous neurosyphilis with lesions in dorsal root ganglia and posterior spinal columns. Primary optic atrophy is associated commonly with tabes dorsalis and meningovascular syphilis but rarely with general paralysis.

Neurosyphilis is seen in patients with secondary syphilis, which occurs from several weeks to several months after the primary chancre and is a variety of lymphoplasmacytic leptomeningitis. Secondary syphilis includes cutaneous and mucous membrane lesions and macular and papulosquamous eruptions and vesicular and bullous lesions. Cutaneous lesions on the palms and soles may occur with focal alopecia and hair loss from the eyebrows. The meninges may be involved and appear cloudy during this phase, but often go undetected clinically. Latent syphilis is associated with reactive serologic tests but no clinical manifestations or cerebrospinal fluid abnormalities. Late or tertiary neurosyphilis occurs in about 8% of patients

with untreated syphilis. Some patients have both tabes dorsalis and general paresis, and all types of neurosyphilis are preceded by asymptomatic neurosyphilis which is usually prolonged. During this period, the cerebrospinal fluid possesses increased mononuclear cells, increased protein, and reactive serologic tests. Meningovascular syphilis is characterized by headache and increased intracranial pressure, but in infants with congenital syphilis, meningeal proliferative changes result in progressive head enlargement. Chronic syphilitic meningeal inflammation with syphilitic vasculitis characterized by endarteritis obliterans occurs in middle age and elderly adults producing multiple clinical features, depending on the location and extent of the infarcted lesions. Progressive arachnoiditis may produce multiple cranial nerve palsies, a spinal cord syndrome, or occlusive vascular disease involving any portion of the brain, brain stem, or cerebellum in either an acute or chronic progressive fashion.

General paresis is a late form of neurosyphilis that occurs 15–20 yr after the initial infection and is more common in men. This disorder is usually progressive and ends in death after 2–10 yr, unless the course is interrupted by penicillin therapy. It is a chronic syphilitic meningoencephalitis associated with spirochetes in the cortical grey matter. Morphologically, these brains possess opacified leptomeninges, cortical atrophy, and a granular ependymitis. Cortical perivascular infiltrates with lymphocytes and plasma cells occur with degenerative neuronal changes, gliosis, and scattered microglia (rod) cells which are large and elongated (Fig. 13.15). Iron deposit in the brain has been observed, particularly in the frontal regions. A syndrome associated with convulsions, focal neurological signs, and progressive dementia is known as Lissauer's general paralysis. Untreated neuroparenchymal tertiary neurosyphilis is slowly progressive, with declining neurological and mental functions, diffuse spasticity, and profound retardation. Treatment with penicillin during the early stages may reverse the process, although most patients continue to worsen despite adequate therapy. In congenital syphilis, a juvenile syphilitic encephalitis is a late

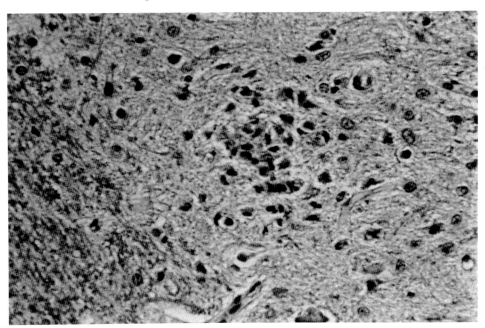

Figure 13.15. Infections in the central nervous system produced by viruses, rickettsia, and spirochetes are associated with discrete microglial nodules with rod cells. In children, hypoxic-ischemic alterations can cause the same lesions. H&E. (Original magnification ×500.)

complication in rare instances, and general paresis can develop during the first and second decades progressing to dementia. Cerebrospinal fluid reveals increased mononuclear cells, increased protein, and altered γ-globulin concentrations reflected by a first zone rise in the colloidal gold curve. Nontreponemal serologic tests in the cerebrospinal fluid are usually positive, but not always. The fluorescent treponemal antibody absorption (FTA-ABS) is virtually always positive. Spirochetes can be demonstrated by dark field examination from the surface of early syphilitic lesions or from material obtained from an infected lesion. *T. pallidum* is recognized by its peculiar structure and characteristic rotary motility along its long axis with undulations from side to side.

Tabes dorsalis is a tertiary form of neurosyphilis associated with atrophic, degenerated, and demyelinated dorsal roots and posterior spinal columns. This myelopathy follows primary syphilitic infection from several years to more than 20 yr. The primary insult is an inflammatory process in dorsal roots and ganglia. The dorsal spinal column involvement is a secondary degeneration of ascending neurites from the dam-aged dorsal roots. Ataxia is a common manifestation caused by position-sense loss and is most profound in the lower extremities. Severe sensory denervation may lead to damaged weight-bearing joints that sustain repeated unrecognized trauma, producing the neuropathic arthropathy known as Charcot joints. Knees and ankles are most severely affected, but the spine and larger joints in the upper extremities may be affected. The morphologic lesion for the Argyll-Robertson pupil may be in the tectal or pretectal area of the brain stem, the upper brain stem, or the ciliary reflex fibers of the iris itself. It is most often associated with tabes dorsalis but can be seen in other forms of neurosyphilis. Similar pupillary abnormalities have been recorded with tectal neoplasms, following encephalitis, and in chronic alcoholics. Tabes dorsalis may be associated with congenital neurosyphilis but is extremely uncommon.

The cerebral gumma is a most uncommon lesion and was uncommon when neurosyphilis was more frequently identified. These unusual masses can be scattered through the neuraxis, but are often identified over the surface of the brain or spinal cord. The cerebral cortex is the most commonly involved site, but other locations include the cerebral peduncles, hypothalamus, and spinal cord. Gummata tend to locate near the surface since they originate from meningeal connective tissue and blood vessels. They vary from 1 mm to 4 cm, creating a mass effect, and are usually round, discrete, red-tan-grey lesions that are focally hard with a central area of softening. Histologically, cerebral gummas are similar to gummas in the rest of the body. There is central caseous or gummatous necrosis surrounded by multiple dense cellular epithelioid cells and spindle fibroblasts intermingled with scattered multinucleated giant cells. Focal fibrosis surrounds the cellular wall which has lymphocytes, plasma cells, and multinucleated giant cells. The adjacent vascularity may be marked, and the overlying leptomeninges may be focally thickened and fibrotic. Spirochetes are rarely demonstrated in gummas.

Nocardiosis (20, 262, 297, 320, 356)

This uncommon disorder is associated with acute or chronic pulmonary infection, a chronic granulomatous suppurative disease of the skin or bone, a disease with predominant central nervous system signs, and a widely disseminated illness with multiple organ-system involvement. The organism is a thin, less than 1 μm thick, gram-positive branching filament which produces cerebral abscesses and primarily involves the lungs, subcutaneous tissue, and brain. *Nocardia asteroides* is the infectious agent most likely incriminated in the central nervous system and is aerobic, gram-positive, and focally acid-fast. These organisms cannot be appreciated with routine hematoxylin and eosin sections, but are easily noted in sections stained with gram and methenamine silver stains. *Nocardia*, which is commonly found in the soil all over the world, is easily cultured on Sabouraud's or beef infusion glucose agar. One to four weeks are needed for cultural identification. Although *N. asteroides* causes most human infections, *Nocardia brasiliensis* is also a pathogen, particularly in Central and South America.

From the initial pulmonary lesions, the bacteria spread through the bloodstream to the brain, producing multiloculated, solitary, or multiple abscesses. These are poorly or partially encapsulated and possess thick yellow-green, purulent exudate. Microabscesses in the central nervous system are surrounded by dark red margins and contain neutrophils, scattered mononuclear cells, liquefactive necrosis, and gitter cells with reactive astrocytosis and fibrosis. Chronic granulomatous change adjacent to the abscesses may have occasional giant cells. Meningitis infrequently coexists with parenchymal abscesses. These patients have a rapidly progressive clinical course with focal neurological deficits, depending upon the location of the lesion. Increased intracranial pressure may appear. Cerebrospinal fluid shows few abnormalities unless meningitis coexists with the abscesses. Surgical drainage is often necessary.

Whipple's Disease (63, 112, 131, 157, 169, 226, 288, 346, 354)

This disorder is associated with steatorrhea, malabsorption, and joint abnormalities complicated by cerebral involvement with psychiatric manifestations resembling Wernicke's encephalopathy. Whipple's disease has been associated with phagocytized bacteria similar to *Corynebacteria* in the lamina propria of the small bowel and other parts of the body, including the brain. Its pathogenesis is not known. Demonstration of macrophages with intracytoplasmic diastase-resistant, periodic acid-Schiff-positive inclusions in the lamina propria of the small intestine provides the diagnosis. Ultrastructural studies within and outside the brain reveal these inclusions to be degenerating 1.5 × 0.2 μm bacilli and fine fibrillar material within phagolysosomes, considered to be bacterial material. Cultivation with transmission of Whipple's bacilli to laboratory animals has been done. Humoral and cellular immunological deficiencies have been observed as well.

Similar organisms stained with the periodic acid-Schiff can be found within macrophages around blood vessels throughout the central nervous system (Fig. 13.16). These phagocytes tend to aggregate within the neuraxis into granular foci containing gram-positive particles in their cytoplasm. Whipple's disease, which may present rarely as a primary neurological disorder,

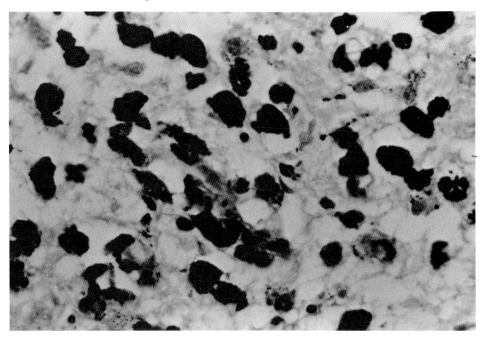

Figure 13.16. Whipple's disease is associated with *Corynebacterium species* that disseminate throughout the body. These phagocytized organisms in the central nervous system can be stained by periodic acid-Schiff stain. PAS. (Original magnification ×100.)

often involves the central nervous system secondarily. Clinical manifestations include progressive dementia, myoclonus, visual impairment, ophthalmoplegia, coma, seizures, and various brain stem syndromes. Untreated cerebral Whipple's disease may progress to death within 6–12 months and requires early establishment of its diagnosis for antibiotic treatment to reverse the process, although occasional resistance occurs.

Indirect Effects (120, 257)

Bacteria can involve the central nervous system by direct invasion, their indirect effects, or both. Toxic bacterial substances affect the central nervous system, causing neuropsychiatric deficits and even death. Neurotoxins produced by *Clostridium tetani* cause tremendous neurological deficits with effects on the spinal cord and brain stem, producing muscle rigidity and spasms. Morphologic changes in the central nervous system may not be apparent. Likewise, *Clostridium botulinum* can cause a life-threatening disorder due to its toxin, botulin, known to occur in some contaminated canned foods. Botulism is caused by

consumption of inadequately cooked food contaminated by *C. botulinum* and its exotoxin. This disease can be contracted from contaminated wounds. The toxin is absorbed from the gastrointestinal tract and carried in the bloodstream to its site of action at neuromuscular junctions. Outbreaks in the United States often result from home canned foods that stand for long periods of time and are eaten without further cooking. The toxic effects on peripheral neuromuscular junctions interfere with conduction at terminal motor nerves, proximal to the site of acetylcholine release, causing weakness, bowel disturbances, headache, sweating, malaise, visual disturbances, difficulty in swallowing, and an inability to speak properly. Generalized weakness is apparent in all extremities, particularly in the neck muscles, and respiratory difficulties become apparent. Body temperatures are usually normal, although subnormal temperatures may occur in some individuals. The morphologic changes are not characteristic and represent secondary complications due to the chemically induced altered neural transmissions. Any foreign bacterial proteins can have a toxic effect on the central and peripheral nervous systems and may produce septic shock, which can cause hypotensive lesions in the central nervous system. Bacterial proteins may accelerate the intrinsic clotting mechanism causing infarcts throughout the body. Effective antibiotic therapy can avoid these problems.

Complications (1, 107, 120, 257, 293, 313)

Bacterial infections give rise to early and late complications. Early complications result from direct invasion by the microbes into the nervous system, affecting different foci in the brain and producing appropriate neuropsychiatric deficits. Indirect early effects are caused by bacterial toxins, their antigenic proteins, or both, which can accelerate intravascular clotting. Any portion of the nervous system may be involved. Late complications of bacterial infections may be a consequence of direct damage by the organism with cystic gliotic lesions that may cause neuropsychiatric deficits varying with the affected area in the central nervous system. Leptomeningitis may resolve with severe obstructive fibrosis, causing communicating hydrocephalus, further compromising the central nervous system months to years after the infection. Dense fibrosis around cranial and spinal nerves may create nerve palsies. Early recognition of the inciting agent producing the infection can prevent these bacterial complications. Examination of the cerebrospinal fluid may identify most microbes, although recognition by culture allows proper antibiosis. A negative cerebrospinal culture does not exclude an infectious process in the central nervous system. Evaluation of the complete host is required to determine the likelihood of an infectious process involving the central nervous system. In some circumstances, appropriate therapy for the most likely agent, which may not be cultured, can prevent complications.

An altered host response to some infectious antigen may be the cause for sarcoidosis. This typically noncaseating granulomatous disorder can involve any part of the nervous system and may be confused with a neoplasm clinically. Sarcoidosis is a diagnosis of exclusion, following negative cultures and histologic studies for recognizable infectious agents.

Recently, an infectious agent, probably human T-cell leukemia-lymphoma virus, seems to be transmitted by contaminated blood, its products, sexual contact, or some combination of these, producing an acquired immunodeficiency syndrome (AIDS). This disorder occurs in homosexual and bisexual males, hemophiliacs, intravenous drug abusers, and others with intimate contact with these victims. In the central nervous system, primary lymphomas and unusual opportunistic infectious agents, including toxoplasmosis, herpesviruses, PAPOVA viruses, fungi, mycobacteria, and other bacteria, have been recognized in AIDS victims. The mortality approaches 50%.

FUNGAL INFECTIONS

Pathobiologic Features (18, 19, 28, 60, 68, 71, 74, 99, 111, 142, 273, 290, 319, 332, 336, 358)

Within human tissues, fungi are found as one of three major forms: (1) yeasts varying from several to 20 μm in diameter; (2) variable sized, branching hyphae; or (3) pseudohyphae. Mycotic lesions in the central nervous system vary with these tissue fungal elements and include three distinct clinicomorphologic patterns (Figs. 13.17). First, acute and chronic leptomeningitis produced by pure yeasts in the central nervous system is seen in blastomycosis, cryptococcosis, and histoplasmosis. These organisms have access to the cerebral microcirculation from which they infect the subarachnoid spaces (Figs. 13.2, 13.18–13.20). Second, septic infarcts with coagulative necrosis are caused by hyphal fungi that obstruct large and intermediate arteries and can be found in aspergillosis and phycomycosis (Figs. 13.4, 13.21). Third, abscesses produced by pseudohyphae are observed in cerebral candidosis. Pseudohyphae are larger and more irregular than yeasts, yet smaller than true hyphae. They occlude small blood vessels (arterioles) in the microcirculation, producing adjacent tissue necrosis that rapidly converts to microabscesses (Figs. 13.3, 13.22, 13.23). As these distinctive clinicomorphologic syndromes

PATHOBIOLOGY OF CEREBRAL MYCOSES
(39 PATIENTS)

FUNGAL FORMS	PROTOTYPE MYCOSIS	DIFFUSE MENINGITIS	STROKE	DEEP CEREBRITIS	NON-CNS MYCOTIC LESIONS
YEASTS	CRYPTOCOCCOSIS	+	+	+	+
HYPHAE	ZYGOMYCOSIS	O	+	+	+
PSEUDO-HYPHAE	CANDIDOSIS	O	O	+	+

Figure 13.17.   Mycotic lesions in the central nervous system vary with the fungal forms. Smaller yeasts have access to the microcirculation and produce diffuse leptomeningitis. Larger filamentous forms, like *Aspergillus*, embolize through blood vessels, obstructing major arteries and their branches, and producing infected strokes. Pseudohyphae of *Candida* species, on the other hand, cause small abscesses with limited access to the subarachnoid space or ventricular system. These latter individuals manifest encephalopathic features.

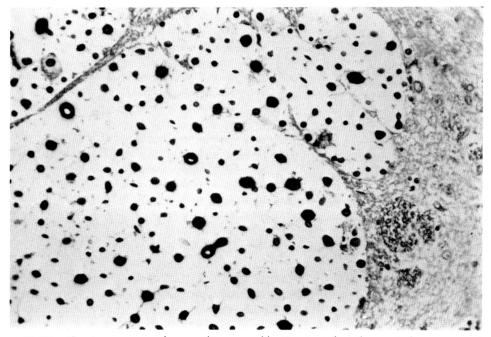

Figure 13.18.   *Cryptococcus neoformans* has a predilection to infect the central nervous system. This yeast involves the leptomeninges extending into and expanding the Virchow-Robin spaces, ultimately invading the pia and adjacent neuroparenchyma. Mucicarmine. (Original magnification ×200.)

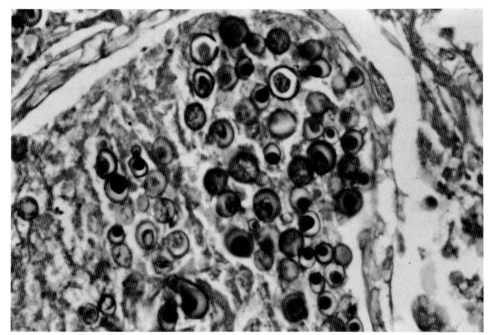

Figure 13.19.   Yeasts with single buds and recognizable cytoplasmic material are *Blastomyces dermatididis*, which can produce leptomeningitis. PAS. (Original magnification ×450.)

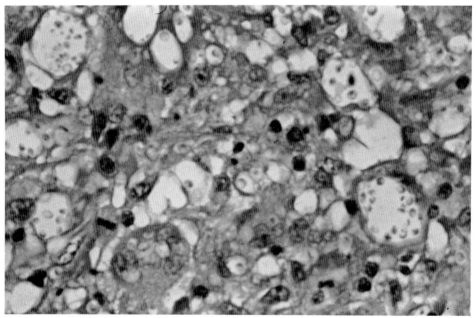

Figure 13.20.   Histoplasmosis in the central nervous system can mimic other intracellular infections, such as leishmaniasis and toxoplasmosis. *H. capsulatum* is PAS-positive and silver-positive and rarely infects the central nervous system. H&E. (Original magnification ×450.)

persist, granulomatous inflammation occurs in adjacent leptomeninges, neural parenchyma, or both. Realizing the relationship in the central nervous system between fungal elements and tissue lesions, insight into the inciting infectious agent can be achieved by evaluating the reaction produced by the infected host.

Fungi are larger and more complicated organisms than bacteria and can adapt to a changing environment. The phyllum *Thallophyta* includes plants without leaves, stems, or roots, such as algae and fungi (mycetes). The former contain chlorophyll and synthesize food from carbon dioxide and water with sunlight. *Protheca,* blue-green algae, have infected man and lower animals and have involved the central nervous system in animals. Fungi do not contain chlorophyll, are saprophytic, and include two large groups. The Pseudomycetes are slime molds and higher bacteria about the same thickness as tubercle bacilli with associated branching. The other group, Eumycetes or true fungi, include organisms with thick hyphae (filaments) and oval structures or spores. They may have non-septate mycelia like the Phycomycetes, or septate mycelia like the Ascomycetes, Basidiomycetes, and Fungi Imperfecti. Human fungal infections or mycoses constitute an increasingly important group of infectious diseases that may be superficial, deep, or both. Superficial mycoses are confined to lining surfaces, like the skin or aerodigestive lining, and do not involve blood vessels or deep parenchymal organs, such as the brain, heart, and kidney. Deep mycoses are caused by many different fungi that can infect the nervous system. The most common cerebral mycoses are aspergillosis, candidosis, cryptococcosis, and phycomycosis.

Common Cerebral Mycoses

ASPERGILLOSIS (6, 23, 60, 151, 155, 164, 208, 223, 231, 294, 357)

In recent years the frequency of aspergillosis has increased in the United States due primarily to large numbers of variously compromised patients. This opportunistic fungal infection is created by an organism that is usually saprophytic, growing in a debilitated host. Predisposing factors include immunosuppression, leukemia, diabetes mellitus, chronic pulmonary disease, the use of steroids, alcoholism, intravenous drug abuse, and general malnutrition. The primary portal of entry for *Aspergillus* is the respiratory tract with subsequent hematogenous spread to the central nervous system. Most human infections occur initially in the lung.

Aspergillosis is caused by a fungus with filaments or hyphae varying from 4 to 12 μm in width. Multiple cross-septa are seen at regular intervals in this organism (Figure 13.21) and are quite distinctive from the larger, thicker, more perpendicularly branching hyphae of the phycomycetes. Hyphal branching in the *Aspergillus* species are acute and occur in the same direction as the main hypha. In an air-filled space, oxygen encourages the fungus to produce fruiting heads as seen in artificial cultures. Organisms normally grow rapidly in culture and produce black-green or yellow mycelia. The usual human pathogens include *Aspergillus fumigatus, Aspergillus niger,* and *Aspergillus flavus.* Since aspergilli are ubiquitous and may be contaminants in the microbiology laboratory, the concentration of their recovery, presence of septate hyphae in tissue, and clinical correlation determine their significance.

Manifestations of cerebral aspergillosis are related to the onset of focal neurological deficits that commonly involve areas of the anterior and middle cerebral arterial distributions. The evolving hemorrhagic infarcts convert into septic infarcts with associated abscesses and cerebritis. Granulomatous inflammation is not usually seen in these lesions. The fungal hyphae are found in large, intermediate, and small blood vessels, with invasion through vascular walls into adjacent tissue. Acute cerebritis may be associated with vasculitis. Organisms are evident in sections stained with hematoxylin and eosin, periodic acid-Schiff, and methenamine silver. They are not usually found in cerebrospinal fluid.

CANDIDOSIS (22, 37, 38, 74, 83, 95, 190, 213, 224, 232, 246, 248, 249, 259, 272, 291, 316)

Candida grow as pseudohyphae with periodic constrictions at septation points (Fig. 13.22). These pseudohyphae represent a succession of individual cells and are distinct from true hyphae or filaments, which do not have these "pinching" points at septa unless altered by chemical damage, degenerative changes, or both. In candidosis, pseudohyphae are associated with 2-

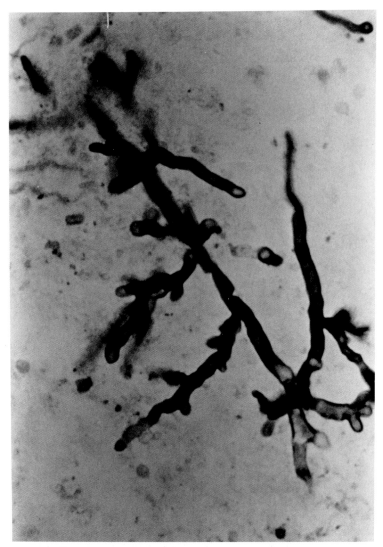

Figure 13.21. *Aspergillus* species possess branching septate hyphae. Grocott's methenamine silver. (Original magnification × 100.) (From B. F. Felter et al. (111).)

to 3-μm oval spores or blastospores. These elements can be seen in deep tissues or on surface linings. The fungus originally infects the human gastrointestinal tract following antibiotic treatment, then invades submucosal blood vessels, and finally disseminates hematogenously throughout the body infecting any organ. At autopsy, gross lesions often are not apparent; microscopically, however, microabscesses in the distribution of the anterior and middle cerebral arteries may be evident (Fig. 13.23). These lesions can involve any part of the central nervous system and are associated initially with yeasts and pseudohyphae.

The abscesses possess mononuclear inflammatory cells approaching a granuloma after 5–7 d. Eventually, the lesions may resolve. Macroabscesses and leptomeningitis are unusual. Pseudohyphae and blastospores can be visualized by methenamine silver and periodic acid-Schiff (PAS) stains. Although clinical meningitis is well documented in candidal infections, at autopsy this is an unusual finding. Most patients with cerebral candidosis are not recognized until postmortem examination. Autopsy studies have demonstrated convincingly that the most common cerebral mycosis is caused by *Candida* species. In man, this

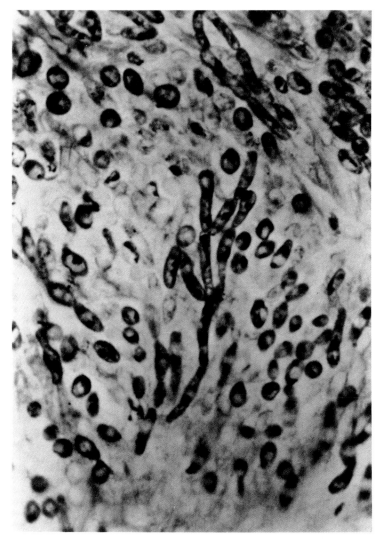

Figure 13.22. *Candida* are characterized by yeasts and pseudohyphae. MacCallum-Goodpasture's bacterial stain. (Original magnification ×1000.) (From B. F. Fetter et al. (111).)

fungus is present normally in the oral cavity and gastrointestinal tract and can invade tissues when overwhelming numbers are present. Deep candidosis affects the kidneys (80%), brain (50%), and heart (40%), but no tissue is exempted.

CRYPTOCOCCOSIS (26, 88, 97, 126, 143, 186, 206, 267, 298, 308, 327)

The most commonly recognized clinical cerebral mycosis is cryptococcosis. This disease primarily infects the host's lung, subsequently spreading hematogenously to the central nervous system. The causative organism is a budding yeast that varies

from 5–20 μm in maximum dimension. Originally referred to as *Torula histolytica*, currently it is known as *Cryptococcus neoformans*. These organisms can be cultured easily, as well as recognized by their characteristic antigen in the cerebrospinal fluid (CSF). These fungi produce an inflammatory response recognized throughout the subarachnoid space. India ink preparations of the spinal fluid can demonstrate the mucoid capsules which are shown well in tissue with mucicarmine (Fig. 13.24). Like other fungi, cryptococci can be seen in tissues with routine hematoxylin and eosin, periodic acid-Schiff, and methenamine sil-

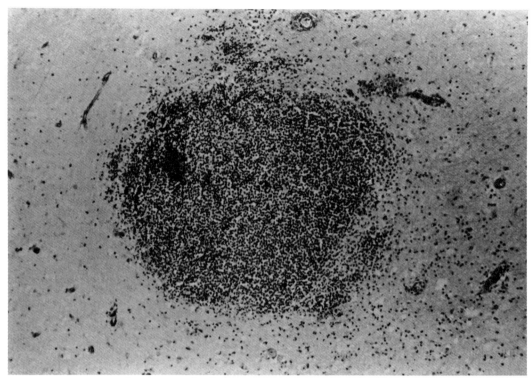

Figure 13.23.   Microabscesses in the brain are seen in cerebral candidosis. (From B. F. Fetter et al. (111).)

ver stains. CSF smears are made by diluting ordinary India ink with water, mixing this solution with spinal fluid or pus, and then examining it directly in a wet preparation under reduced light in the microscope. The same procedure can be applied to the cut surface of the brain, scraping across the surface of the involved brain or meninges with a scalpel and obtaining a drop of the material, subsequently mixing it with India ink to show the thick capsules of the yeasts.

Cryptococcosis is a worldwide infection that can develop spontaneously in individuals considered healthy. In about 30%, predisposing factors include lymphoproliferative diseases, prolonged steroid therapy, and generalized malnutrition. The primary portal of entry is the lung. Pulmonary lesions due to cryptococcosis do not tend to calcify and hence do not leave significant traces of their previous activity, as seen in histoplasmosis and coccidioidomycosis.

These yeasts produce disseminated leptomeningitis, usually associated with minimal inflammatory response. Adjacent neuroparenchymal lesions may be seen with the leptomeningitis. Granulomas are rarer late reactions that can mimic tubercles. Secondary ventricular dilatation is present in individuals with chronic fibrosing leptomeningitis. Multiple cysts related to exuberant capsular material produced by the proliferating cryptococci create honeycomb cystic cerebral changes. Rare cryptococcomas may develop when masses of the fungi aggregate in an inflammatory lesion. Individuals with minimal inflammation to cryptococci may be compromised, while, in others, the fungus produces a chronic infection with an inflammatory response including granulomas. The organisms in these individuals are found within multinucleated giant cells and possess minimal capsules. Mucicarmine and Alcian blue stains provide easy recognition of the capsule of *C. neoformans*.

PHYCOMYCOSIS (4, 42, 57, 79, 85, 137, 138, 152, 188, 203, 210, 214, 260)

Phycomycosis includes mucormycosis and zygomycosis and in the brain is a unique disease widely observed in the

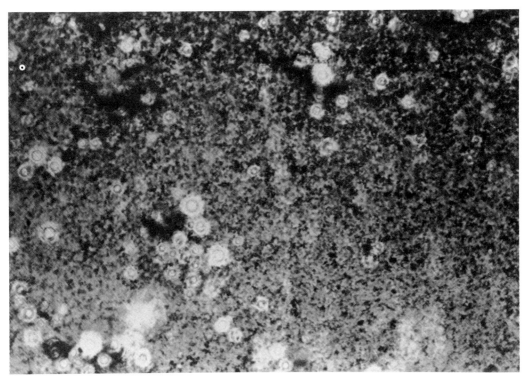

Figure 13.24. India ink preparation demonstrates a pale, thick capsule of *C. neoformans.* (From B. F. Fetter et al. (111).)

United States and often associated with diabetic ketoacidosis. This acute fulminating disorder is caused by direct invasion or hematogenous spread of nonseptate irregular hyphae of several phycomycetes, including *Rhizopus, Mucor,* and *Absidia,* to the central nervous system. Phycomycosis occurs in the rhinosinoorbital region, pulmonary areas, and gastrointestinal system, as well as a focal or a disseminating disease in the skin.

Rhizopus, the genus recovered from cerebral phycomycosis, grows rapidly on Sabouraud's agar, filling a Petri dish in 2 or 3 d with a fluffy white growth. This becomes dark due to production of spores. The fungus consists of filaments or stolons from which root-like structures or rhizoids grow. From these rhizoids, sprouts or sporangiophores bearing sacs (sporangia) develop. These contain brown spores about 7 μm in diameter.

This mycosis is associated with broad, nonseptate tissue hyphae with a mixed inflammatory response (Fig. 13.25). Granulomas are not evident as a rule. The hyphae occlude and penetrate vascular walls, causing thrombosis, associated infarction, and adjacent inflammation. Within the central nervous system, hemorrhagic infarcts are associated with broad, nonseptate hyphae, measuring from 6 to 20 μm in diameter, obstructing blood vessels, and extending into adjacent damaged tissue (Fig. 13.25). Acute and chronic cerebritis are present. Initially, the phycomycetes infect the nasal mucosa, which becomes swollen and dark red-brown. Subsequent invasion of the antrum, periorbital region, adjacent orbital arteries, and internal carotid artery may occur. The frontal lobes are involved by direct hematogenous spread or associated invasion through the orbital plate. Even though the prognosis in this infection is usually poor, improvement can occur after tratment of the diabetic ketoacidosis. Likewise, aggressive surgical extirpation with subsequent antifungal agents have aided these patients. The diagnosis can be recognized by the appropriate clinical syndrome and examining the biopsied nasal material or scrapings from the diseased an-

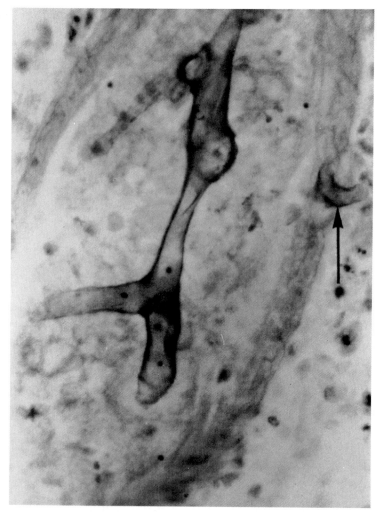

Figure 13.25.   In phycomycosis, large nonseptate and irregular hyphae appear in a thrombosed blood vessel. PAS. (Original magnification ×1000.) (From B. F. Fetter et al. (111).)

trum. The characteristic nonseptate hyphae with right angle branches are diagnostic.

Unusual Cerebral Mycoses

These mycoses include blastomycosis, coccidioidomycosis, histoplasmosis, and paracoccidioidomycosis. Fungal infections such as histoplasmosis and blastomycosis in the southeastern United States and Coccidioidomycosis in the southwestern United States occur with increased frequency in the general population, yet rarely infect the central nervous system. Their lack of neurotrophism, as compared to cryptococcosis, is not understood.

BLASTOMYCOSIS (56, 81, 93, 118, 125, 129, 140, 180, 189, 261, 286, 350)

North American blastomycosis is less common than histoplasmosis and coccidioidomycosis. The portal of entry for blastomycosis has not been well established. The fungus causing this mycosis is maintained in decayed wood and may have a natural reservoir in dogs. *Blastomyces dermatitidis* has been isolated from the soil and produces a fluffy white mycelium with hyphae and conidia on short lateral conidiophores. At 37°C, this fungus makes yeasts on blood agar. In H&E sections, the organism is readily identified by its central protoplast with a surrounding space and well-defined wall. Special stains, like PAS and methenamine silver, easily demonstrate the organism. With reduced light and careful observation, the fungus can be recognized in H&E preparations and unstained wet preparations by its characteristic, single thick-necked buds and distinctive protoplasmic body (Fig. 13.19).

Initial infection in the lung can allow the yeasts to spread through blood vessels to the central nervous system. The skin may also be a portal of entry. Debilitating disorders and other predisposing conditions are not necessary for the establishment of blastomycosis in the central nervous system. Typically, cerebral blastomycosis produces leptomeningitis and adjacent abscesses. Granulomatous responses with caseous or liquefactive necrosis have been seen with granulomatous abscesses. Fibrosis can occur in the subarachnoid space, leading to hydrocephalus. Intraparenchymal abscesses with or without granulomas may appear anywhere within the central nervous system associated with abscesses, epithelioid histiocytes, multinucleated giant cells, caseous necrosis, and large, 10- to 15-μm yeasts without hyphae or pseudohyphae.

Neuropsychiatric manifestations can appear, depending upon the infected area. Individuals susceptible to blastomycosis are usually males who work with the soil. The disease is more common in the southeastern part of the United States, and its diagnosis may be made during examination of the cerebrospinal fluid or by histological evaluation of a granuloma from the intracranial contents. The incidence of this disease is low, even in an endemic population.

COCCIDIOIDOMYCOSIS (59, 80, 82, 153, 154, 156, 170, 238, 265, 305)

This mycosis is endemic in the southwestern United States, Mexico, and South America. Its distribution corresponds to the sonora life belt where certain temperatures and moist conditions exist. Arthrospores are breathed into the lungs with infected dust. Rodents and cattle are commonly infected. The fungus is typified by large round spherules, varying from 40–50 μm in diameter. This structure is seen easily on routine H&E stains (Fig. 13.26). Within the spherules, smaller yeasts with distinctive walls and protoplasts vary from 2–5 μm in diameter. These endospores are released into the tissue after the spherules rupture. The fungus can be recovered as a fluffy mycelium with arthrospores that are extremely infectious to laboratory workers. On the other hand, a suspected pus or spinal fluid from a patient with coccidioidomycosis can be inoculated intraperitoneally into a rodent with subsequent tissue sections of the abdominal wall examined about a week after the animals are sacrificed. Complement fixation tests on serum are helpful in recognizing this mycosis.

Tissue response is neutrophilic with pus production as well as necrotizing granulomas. Multinucleated giant cells are present. Coccidioidomycosis begins in the lung with primary calcified lesions and minimal lymph node response. Progressive disease involves the bones, central nervous system, joints, lungs, pericardium, and skin. About 100 individuals die in the United States yearly from coccidioidomycosis, and the CNS plays a major role in their deaths. Typically, the central nervous system possesses meningeal inflammation with infectious purulent and caseous granulomas. Thickened, cloudy, opacified leptomeninges, particularly around the base of the brain, may lead to fibrosis and subsequent obstructive hydrocephalus. Multiple abscesses, as well as abscesses in granulomas, are observed.

Patients with meningeal coccidioidomycosis may live for weeks to many months. Manifestations are similar to other chronic meningitides and vary with the damaged area of the CNS. Usually, the organism can be recognized in wet preparations of the spinal fluid, which can show endosporulating spherules and scattered endospores.

HISTOPLASMOSIS (70, 72, 73, 96, 100, 122, 124, 162, 163, 235, 289, 306, 340)

Even though about 25% of the population in the United States have positive histoplasmin skin tests, CNS involvement is rare. Dead organisms can be demonstrated in calcified nodules in the lungs and mediastinal lymph nodes in up to 85% of autopsied patients. Five percent of people with histoplasmosis in the United States have active disease. The organism, *Histoplasma capsulatum*, is a budding yeast mea-

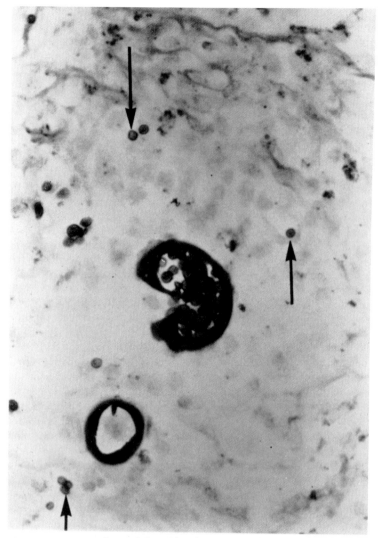

Figure 13.26.   A mature sporangium of *Coccidioides immitis* is surrounded by endospores (*arrows*) dispersed in the brain. GMS. (Original magnification ×1000.) (From B. F. Fetter et al. (111).)

suring 2- to 5-μm in human tissue and in blood agar at 37°C. With active disease, yeasts are found in macrophages, but when cultured on corn meal agar at room temperature, the fungus is a fluffy mycelium with tuberculated chlamydospores.

In adults, histoplasmosis can resemble pulmonary tuberculosis and often is associated with widespread calcifications in the lungs and reticuloendothelial system, particularly the spleen. Disseminated histoplasmosis in infancy or childhood involves macrophages of the reticuloendothelial system. Rarely, mononuclear phagocytes contain these fungi in the leptomeninges. *H.*

capsulatum can be found in macrophages in the liver, spleen, lymph nodes, and bone marrow, and may produce hepatosplenomegaly. Lesions in the neural parenchyma due to histoplasmosis are rare, even though the portal of entry is the lung where infection is ubiquitous in endemic areas. Organisms are inhaled in infected dust contaminated by chicken, bird, or bat excreta. In the United States, histoplasmosis occurs in the central and east-central regions, but a worldwide distribution has been recognized.

Diffuse leptomeningitis or discrete granulomas appear in histoplasmosis. Inflammatory response can occur anywhere in the central nervous system and is typified by mononuclear phagocytes with intracytoplasmic organisms (Fig. 13.20) and rarely histoplasmomas. Microscopically, caseous necrosis in the evolving granulomas is associated with epithelioid macrophages, scattered multinucleated giant cells, and lymphoplasmacytic infiltrates. Adjacent reactive gliosis and fibrosis may be noted. Central nervous system involvement in histoplasmosis is evident in less than 10% of patients with active histoplasmosis and includes perivenous miliary granulomas, parenchymal granulomatosis, meningitis, histoplasmomas, and histiocytic histoplasmosis.

Clinical manifestations depend upon the affected area in the central nervous system. The disorder is a rare mycosis of the central nervous system and in an endemic population was seen in only autopsied individuals compromised by burns, antibiotics, and steroid therapy.

PARACOCCIDIOIDOMYCOSIS (21, 90, 111, 174, 251, 263, 284)

South American blastomycosis or paracoccidioidomycosis is recognized in South and Central America. The causative organism is known as *Blastomyces braziliensis* and has multiple thin-neck buds arising from a single yeast (Fig. 13.27). This organism is dimorphic, with a mycelial phase at room temperature and yeast phase at 37°C. In tissue, yeasts possess round to oval bodies, varying from 10- to 20-μm in diameter with single to multiple, attached thin-neck buds.

Cerebral lesions in this disorder are associated with leptomeningitis, and the inflammatory response becomes a lymphohistiocytic infiltrate with granulomas. Tuberculoid granulomas can be associated with adjacent chronic inflammation and fibrosis in the leptomeninges and neuroparenchyma. Routine H&E sections and special stains, including PAS and methenamine silver, demonstrate these organisms.

Clinical manifestations of this deep mycosis are variable, depending on the involved site in the central nervous system. Leptomeningitis may lead to obstructive hydrocephalus.

Miscellaneous and Rare Cerebral Mycoses (5, 16, 30, 32, 34, 39, 64, 92, 105, 111, 115, 117, 150, 168, 202, 209, 225, 230, 243, 268, 292, 295, 324, 338, 352)

Any fungus accessible to the central nervous system can infect it. Limiting factors include availability of the organism to the central nervous system, pathogenicity of the fungus, amount of infectious inoculum, and ability of the host to react. With medical manipulations, suspicion of unusual infections, like the mycoses, should be maintained for any compromised patient. Some fungi that rarely infect the central nervous system include such opportunistic mycoses as allescheriosis, cephalosporiosis, chromoblastomycosis, dermatophytosis, paecilomycosis, penicilliosis, rhinosporidiosis, sporotrichosis, streptomycosis, torulopsiosis, and ustilagomycosis.

ALLESCHERIOSIS (7, 12, 98, 192)

Allescheriosis or monosporiosis presents as a mycetoma, but has been identified in the central nervous system. This fungus occurs in tissue as septate hyphae and is a rare cerebral mycosis in markedly compromised individuals. Typically, mass lesions result from the fungal elements, producing hemorrhagic infarcts with associated leptomeningitis. These hemorrhagic infarcts may be converted into cerebral abscesses requiring surgical intervention.

CEPHALOSPORIOSIS (44)

Any infectious agent introduced directly into the central nervous system through contaminated procedures, equipment, or injuries can create an infection. When this phenomenon occurs, yeasts and fungal filaments may be scattered throughout the subarachnoid space. Granulomatous leptomeningitis has been caused by *Cephalosporium* species in immunocompromised individuals following a spinal infection.

CHROMOBLASTOMYCOSIS (8, 349)

These dematiaceous fungi cause cutaneous infections in the tropics and may be associated with verrucous, black-brown pigmented lesions. The organisms possess floccose hyphae as indicated by the term

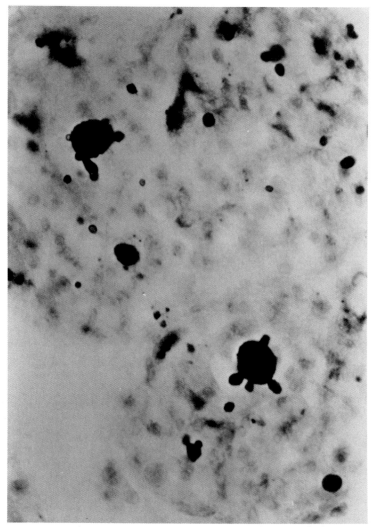

Figure 13.27. Numerous yeasts of *B. brasiliensis* contain multiple budding yeasts. GMS. (Original magnification ×1000.) (From B. F. Fetter et al. (111).)

"dematiaceous." The infectious agents possess brown pigment in cultures and tissue lesions inside and outside the central nervous system. PAS and methenamine silver stains may obscure the color; consequently, tissues should be examined in unstained preparations. Cerebral chromoblastomycosis arises from a nonneural infected site and hematogenously spreads to the brain. It is caused by many different pigmented fungi, including *Cladosporium*, *Hormodendrum*, and *Phialophora*. Hyphae of these fungi vary from 2–3 μm in thickness with slightly pinched-in septations occurring at every 3- to 15-μm interval. Branching may be apparent. Some heavily pigmented chla-

mydospores appear split apart. Their specific identification requires cultural studies. They grow slowly on Sabouraud's glucose agar, so by 3 weeks the fungal colony may have a diameter of only 2 cm. Microscopically, the hyphae and conidiophores are 3- to 4-μm in thickness and incude chains of single cell conidia which are elliptical. The terminal conidia are smaller than the basal ones and represent young, immature cells. Abscesses produced by these fungi are larger than the microabscesses caused by the pseudohyphae of *Candida* species. Tissue reactions are primarily intraparenchymal abscesses associated with acute and chronic inflammation with focal multinucleated giant cells. Hyphal aggregates are seen in most cerebral abscesses that have been converted from earlier septic infarcts. Granulomatous response may be minimal. The most likely portal of entry is the lung, but, in some instances, the site is not apparent. Typically, abscesses in the brain can extend into the subarachnoid space or ventricles, producing leptomeningitis and ventriculitis, respectively. Headache, coma, and localizing neurological signs may be associated with fever and a mass effect.

MISCELLANEOUS MYCOSES

Rare mycoses with hyphae, such as dermatophytes, *Paecilomyces* and *Penicillium*, spread to the brain hematogenously as intermediate size or large, infected thromboemboli to produce hemorrhagic infarcts that later become abscesses. These lesions are distributed in the area supplied by the internal carotid arteries. Individuals who are often compromised can be infected with these unusual rare fungi by having the organism directly inoculated into their central nervous system, circulatory system, or both. Accurate identification of these infectious agents requires cultural studies. Rare and unusual mycotic agents, including *Sporotichum shenckii*, *Streptomyces*, and *Toruloposis glabrata*, produce meningitis, microabscesses, or both. The phytopathogen, *Ustilago*, which has produced chronic leptomeningitis and ependymitis, has similar morphologic features to yeast fungi. All these organisms require host susceptibility and a moderate inoculum to establish infection in the central nervous system.

PARASITIC INFECTIONS

Approach (47, 104) (Table 13.3)

Compared with neurologic infections caused by bacteria, cerebral parasitosis in the United States is uncommon. Its frequency in North America is significantly lower than in other, less developed areas in the world. Easy accessibility by air travel to any part of the world increases the likelihood of these diseases in nonendemic areas. Predisposing factors for parasitic infections include poverty, poor living conditions, and availability of the parasites, their vectors, and intermediate hosts. Any

Table 13.3
Neurologic Infections Due to Parasites

Protozoa (genera)
Acanthamoeba
Entamoeba
Naegleria
Plasmodium
Trypanosoma
Toxoplasma
Metazoa (genera)
Angiostrongylus
Echinococcus
Onchocerca
Paragonimus
Schistosoma
Sparganum
Stronglyoides
Taenia
Toxocara
Trichinella

protozoan or metazoan parasite accessible to the central nervous system can infect it.

The size of parasites infecting the central nervous system help to determine the tissue lesions (Table 13.1). Small protozoans with access to the microcirculation are associated with intraparenchymal microabscesses with adjacent leptomeningitis. Larger parasites or metazoans can obstruct blood vessels, actively migrate into the neuroparenchyma, or both. These organisms include round worms (nematohelminthes) and flat worms (platyhelminthes, including tapeworms and flukes) that are often confined to the neuroparenchyma. In the uncompromised host, circulating blood changes, such as eosinophilia, can suggest parasitism. In chronic or inactive parasitic infections in the nervous system, eosinophils may not be present in large numbers in either the blood or cerebrospinal fluid. The cerebrospinal fluid in some patients may demonstrate the infectious agent, particularly in primary amebic meningoencephalitis. Serologic examinations are also helpful in recognizing some parasitic infestations.

PROTOZOAL INFECTIONS

Although any protozoan can infect the nervous system, the most significant infections include *Acanthamoeba, Entameba, Naegleria, Plasmodium falciparum, P. vi-*

vax, *Toxoplasma gondii, Trypanosoma gambiense*, and *Trypanosoma rhodesiense*. Trichomonads were recovered from the spinal fluid in a patient with an esophageal fistula.

AMEBIASIS (51–54, 58)

Two distinctive varieties of amebiasis affect the central nervous system. Primary amebiasis is usually rapidly progressive and lethal, whereas secondary cerebral amebiasis is manifested by discrete, chronic abscesses distributed in the area of the anterior and middle cerebral arteries. Its course is not rapidly deteriorating.

Primary Amebic Meningoencephalitis

In 1959, free-living, soil, and water amebae were demonstrated experimentally to produce severe acute meningoencephalitis in mice. These amebae belonged to the genera of *Hartmanella* and *Acanthamoeba*. Through intranasal inoculations, they invaded olfactory nerves and created a rapidly fatal purulent leptomeningitis. In 1964, these ubiquitous, free-living amebae were demonstrated to infect humans. The illness is seen in children and young adults who are otherwise healthy. Typically, they have been exposed to fresh water swimming associated with much diving, but the infection has occurred in individuals swimming in treated pool water. This amebiasis progresses rapidly to death within a few days following the passage of the amebae through the cribriform plate via the olfactory nerves.

The infection has been recognized throughout the world, including Australia, Czechoslovakia, England, and North America, particularly the southeastern United States. Three different genera of free-living amebae, including *Acanthamoeba*, *Hartmanella*, and *Naegleria*, have been incriminated in primary cerebral amebiasis. The rapidly progressive, potentially lethal primary amebic meningoencephalitis is caused by *Naegleria* species. In tissues, trophozoites of *Naegleria* measure 10–18 μm, whereas *Acanthamoeba* are larger (Fig. 13.28). Cysts with wrinkled, double walls in tissue are found only with *Acanthamoeba*. A distinctive feature of *Naegleria* is its ability to convert from a trophozoite to a flagellate, which can be induced by dilution of the culture with water. In cerebrospinal fluid, the amebae may be confused with leukocytes, but can be identified in un-

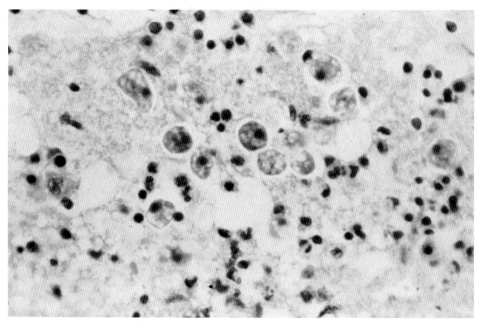

Figure 13.28. Primary amebic meningoencephalitis is caused by protozoans with distinctive karyosomes (nucleoli). These amebae may be confused with macrophages. H&E. (Original magnification ×800.)

stained, warm, wet preparations by its motility and altered shape and configuration. A drop of 1% cresyl violet stain to cerebrospinal fluid aids in visualization of the amebic nucleus by producing a distinct purple nuclear membrane and karyosome.

Primary amebic meningoencephalitis can be an acute, rapidly progressive, fulminating disorder in previously healthy children and young adults, or it may be a chronic granulomatous mass involving the neuroparenchyma in compromised hosts. The aggressive variety of primary amebic meningoencephalitis occurs in young individuals, often after swimming in fresh water 7–14 d before onset of their symptoms. Clinical manifestations, including headache, fever, pharyngitis, nasal stuffiness, and nasal obstruction, can be abrupt and variable. A nasal discharge may develop. Subsequent vomiting occurs with headaches and fever. Within 2–4 d after onset, drowsiness appears with confusion and neck stiffness. Finally, convulsions develop and progressively lead to coma with occasional focal neurological signs. Most patients die 1–2 weeks after the onset of their symptoms. A peripheral leukocytosis is ap-

parent, and the cerebrospinal fluid shows purulent exudates with many neutrophils and absent bacteria. Hemorrhage may be associated with the purulent exudate. Protein content is generally elevated in the cerebrospinal fluid, whereas glucose is usually reduced. A less aggressive variety of primary amebic meningoencephalitis is produced by *Acanthamoeba* and *Hartmanella* in immunocompromised hosts and includes discrete, mass-like lesions with amebic cysts and granulomatoid reactions.

At autopsy, fulminating primary amebic meningoencephalitis produces marked cerebral edema with purulent exudates and hemorrhages scattered over the base of the brain, brain stem, and cerebellum. In rare cases, the amebae can be recovered from the liver, spleen, lungs, and brain. The olfactory bulbs tend to be inflamed, soft, and hemorrhagic and may be destroyed by the exudate. The leptomeninges are filled with inflammatory cells (neutrophils and monocytes) and amebae. An underlying cortical cerebritis is seen when the pia is violated (Fig. 13.6). The benign form of primary amebic meningoencephalitis, caused by *Acanthamoeba* and *Hartmanella*, is associ-

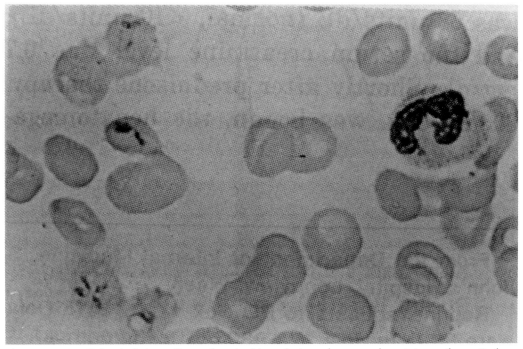

Figure 13.29. Babesiosis is easily confused with malaria and can produce intraerythrocytic forms in a tetrad maltese cross-configuration. Wright stain. (Original magnification ×1000.) (From A. B. Bredt et al. (45).)

ated with multiple, small, hemorrhagic abscesses, particularly in the distribution of anterior and middle cerebral arteries, and is associated with granulomatoid changes in immunocompromised individuals.

Cerebral Amebic Abscess

Amebic abscesses of enteric origin can occur in the central nervous system and are observed in endemic areas, such as Latin America. Among 220 patients with fatal amebiasis, cerebral involvement was evident in 2 (0.9%). High incidences are reported from Mexico, where 8.1% of 210 autopsied confirmed cases of amebiasis were demonstrated in the central nervous system. Trophozoites of *Entamoeba histolytica* invade the central nervous system through hematogenous routes. Initial lesions in this disorder develop in the intestinal tract and, subsequently, infect the liver and lungs. Coexistent amebic abscesses in the liver are found in patients with cerebral amebiasis. As in many other opportunistic infections, cerebral involvement in patients with amebiasis occurs as a late complication.

As expected in a disorder hematogenously spreading to the central nervous system, the most common locations for amebic lesions include grey-white junctions of the cerebral hemispheres and the basal ganglia in the distribution of the anterior and middle cerebral arteries. Abscesses may be single or multiple and are soft, red-tan, discrete masses with scattered petechiae. Necrosis gradually becomes evident, and cavitation appears later. These lesions are associated with tremendous numbers of neutrophils and, eventually, histiocytes, lymphocytes, and plasma cells. The thickness of the abscess wall depends on its age. The amebae are found typically at the edge of the abscess within the necrotic purulent material. The overlying meninges may be secondarily involved with the inflammatory response. Edema can occur adjacent to the lesions. Histomorphologic features for amebic abscesses are similar to bacterial abscesses. Necrosis adjacent to the inner wall of granulation tissue is evident. Early inflammatory reactions include neutrophils, which are later replaced by lymphocytes, histiocytes, and plasma cells. Reacting astrocytes, including gemistocytes and fibrillary astrocytes, are seen adjacent to the granulation tissue. Recognition of the trophozoites of *E. histolytica* in the necrotic area or abscess wall is required for diagnosis. Other gastrointestinal protozoans have been incriminated in abscesses within the central nervous system, but they are uncommon and inadequately documented.

BABESIOSIS (45, 75, 102, 145, 278, 279, 330)

The protozoans of the genus *Babesia* are transmitted by ticks to wild and domesticated animals. Seventy-one species of *Babesia* are scattered throughout the world and can infect birds, cats, cattle, dogs, goats, horses, rodents, and sheep. They infect erythrocytes and can be confused with malarial protozoa. Babesiosis is maintained in rodents by the northern deer tick of *Ixodes* species. Principal hosts for the adult tick are deer, while larvae and nymphs are found in mice and deer. The nymphs can transmit *Babesia* to man by feeding on him. *Babesia microti* may be transmitted transstadially from larva to the nymph, but not transovarially. Infectious nymphs feed from May to September, producing human infections 1–3 weeks after biting susceptible hosts.

Human infection includes two patterns. With an intact spleen, the host may demonstrate an asymptomatic infection or a moderately severe, febrile, hemolytic disease. These individuals recover with only symptomatic care. On the other hand, persons without their spleens develop overwhelming intraerythrocytic infections with high fever, toxic reactions, and renal and liver failure, even leading to death. Less than 40 human cases have been recognized throughout the world. Babesiosis, which mimics malaria, can produce severe illnesses in both spleen-intact and splenectomized individuals. Recent exposure to areas where ticks can transmit the disease suggests the diagnosis in individuals with moderate toxicity, fever, hemolytic anemia, anorexia, prostration, and vague neurological symptoms, including headache and myalgia. Parasites found in the circulating erythrocytes may involve blood vessels throughout the body, including the central nervous system. The intraerythrocytic parasites have a characteristic tetrad form and lack schizonts, gametocytes, and hemazoin pigment (Fig. 13.29). Serologic diagnosis of clinical babesiosis is possible at its onset, and the parasite can be isolated and identified by hamster inoculation. Mild infections can be treated symptomatically, but moderate to severe infections may require transfusions and therapy, including guanine and pyrimethamine. Prevention consists of avoiding contact with the nymphal stage of the vector ticks, *Ixodes dammini.*

MALARIA (66)

The most important parasitic disease of man is malaria. At least 100 million persons throughout the world are infected by this parasite, and about 1 million die from the illness each year. Primary cases of malaria are found in tropical and subtropical regions, but because of extensive international travel, may be found anywhere in the world. The disease is acquired by the bite of an infected *Anopheles mosquito.* This insect inoculates the sporozoite into its human victim where the parasite infects the liver, develops into a cryptozoite and then a merozoite, which ruptures from the liver cells. Invasion of human erythrocytes by these liberated merozoites results in the ring forms or trophozoites, which subsequently produce schizonts. After maturation, the schizont splits into merozoites, liberated with red cell rupture, and then reenters other erythrocytes to repeat the schizogonic cycle.

The most common type of malaria is caused by *Plasmodium falciparum,* which has an incubation period of 1 to 3 weeks. *Plasmodium vivax* infection has an incubation period of several months, and *P. ovale* and *P. malarie* infections are even longer. The most serious complication of malaria is cerebral involvement, which occurs most often in individuals not immune to this parasite. Consequently, children between 6 months and 4 yr of age or adults foreign to the endemic area are most susceptible to cerebral malaria with their first exposure. Sickle cell trait or disease provides some protection against cerebral malaria. One to 2% of all patients with falciparum malaria have cerebral involvement with generalized mild cerebral edema and petechial hemorrhages, especially in the white matter of the cerebrum and cerebel-

lum. Some petechiae may be seen in the grey matter. Microscopically, these lesions appear as ring hemorrhages, with the central vessel engorged with erythrocytes, thromboses, and pericapillary necrosis and edema with adjacent erythrocytes in the neuropil (Fig. 13.30). Mononuclear phagocytes may be present. A glial nodule reacting to a ring hemorrhage has been referred to as a Durck granuloma, which may be associated with severe astrogliosis. Malarial pigments are anisotrophic crystals lining the perivascular spaces in some instances. The entire capillary system of the brain may possess parasitized erythrocytes, which are associated with ring hemorrhages similar to those seen in fat embolism. Venous congestion is associated with endothelial proliferation and occlusion of some small blood vessels by parasitized erythrocytes. Cerebral dysfunction is attributed to the vascular compromise, associated anemia, and hyperthermia.

The initial manifestations of cerebral malaria include listlessness, headache, and subsequent fever. A rapid rise in temperature may be associated with convulsions. Early in the disease, fever may be prolonged so that peaks of temperature elevation emerge in characteristic patterns, distinct for the different forms of malaria. Eventually, recurrent fevers at 1- to 2-d intervals become established with falciparum infections. The acute illness is more severe with falciparum malaria than with either vivax or quartan infections. Death in the acute phase is associated with cerebral involvement in "black water" fever, produced by infection with *Plasmodium falciparum.* The other forms of malaria have an abrupt, dramatic onset, and several days after the acute illness, headache, fever, and disturbances in responsiveness are noted. Prolonged and repeated generalized convulsions may occur. Occasional disorientation, confusion, obtundation, tremulousness, or other movement disorders precede the convulsions. Status epilepticus with hyperthermia may precede death. Appropriate therapy can result in complete recovery.

TOXOPLASMOSIS (109, 123, 280, 299)

This protozoal infection can produce a devastating congenital infection leading to hydrocephalus, cerebral calcifications, and

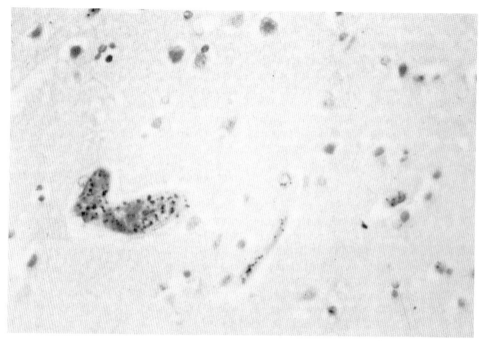

Figure 13.30. Malaria causes diffuse intraerythrocytic parasitemia which can obstruct blood vessels creating hemorrhages, necrosis, and edema in the central nervous system. The dark pigment (*left*) represents degenerated hemoglobin in previously parasitized erythrocytes in a patient with cerebral malaria. H&E. (Original magnification ×800.)

chorioretinitis. Recently, *Toxoplasma* have been known to cause a subclinical infection in the compromised host and are organisms which are obligatory intracellular opportunistic parasites with a propensity for the nervous system. This protozoan exists in birds and mammals and can infect any cell except for nonnucleated erythrocytes. Free trophozoites are concentric or oval in tissue and measure 4–7 μm in length. Wright-Giemsa stains reveal a red to pink nucleus and pale blue cytoplasm. In tissues, including infected human tissue and tissue cultures, *Toxoplasma* can survive for years and occur in clusters with a discrete limiting membrane previously called a "pseudocyst," but now known as a "true cyst" (Figs. 13.31 and 13.32).

Toxoplasmosis in man is either acquired or congenital. Acquired toxoplasmosis is a worldwide infection, with about 25% of all adults in the United States having positive dye-test antibody titers indicating previous infection with *Toxoplasma gondii*. Fifty percent of blood donors in England have been found to have positive dye-test titers. Patients with acquired toxoplasmosis may

be asymptomatic or possess mild manifestations due to widespread distribution of the parasite throughout the body. The parasites encyst and then may persist in tissues for the life of the individual with minimal host cellular reaction. After encystment, antibody titers may decline to lower levels, despite persistence of viable organisms. A benign, transient, acquired toxoplasmosis is manifested by a diffuse maculopapular rash, malaise, and muscle pain. An inflammatory myopathy has been associated with elevated *Toxoplasma* titers and can mimic polymyositis. Lymphadenopathy may be associated with fever and can easily be confused with infectious mononucleosis; however, the latter does not demonstrate a positive serology to *T. gondii* and has a positive heterophile reaction. Other conditions described in patients with acquired toxoplasmosis include myocarditis, acute hepatitis, and meningoencephalitis. The latter is rare but has been recognized in children and adults. The neurological abnormalities may coexist with a rash, generalized adenopathy or both. Ocular disease has been related to acquired toxoplas-

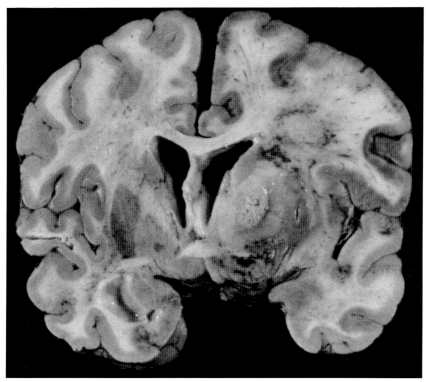

Figure 13.31. Cerebral toxoplasmosis appears in compromised patients producing discrete necrotic and hemorrhagic lesions with free or phagocytized toxoplasmic organisms.

mosis but is more of a problem in the congenital variety. Uveitis can complicate acquired toxoplasmosis in the adult. Acquired toxoplasmosis is one of several diseases, including gram-negative bacterial infections, herpes viral infections, and opportunistic fungi, such as *Candida* and *Aspergillus* species, that have emerged as important pathogens in impaired hosts. *Pneumocystis carinii* is a similar secondary invader but does not cause direct neurological disease.

Toxoplasmosis is a special hazard in patients compromised by hematologic malignancies and immunosuppressive therapy. Susceptibility of the brain to congenital toxoplasmosis is due to the lack of antibodies in this organ and a defect in delayed hypersensitivity. The predilection of acquired toxoplasmosis in the compromised host for the central nervous system indicates the uniqueness of this system, allowing the organism to grow and may be related to the blood-brain barrier. Both diffuse and focal cerebral disease have been associated with cerebral toxoplasmosis

complicated by headaches, drowsiness, and disorientation. Occasionally, increased intracranial pressure may be associated with progressive focal deficits, suggesting a cerebral neoplasm. Cerebrospinal fluid may show elevated pressure and increased protein content in some patients. Glucose in the spinal fluid is normal, and the cell count may be normal or moderately increased with a predominance of mononuclear phagocytes. Necrotizing toxoplasmic encephalomyelitis with minimal leptomeningeal changes may be associated with localized, soft, discrete lesions associated, with abundant *Toxoplasma* organisms evident microscopically as free and cyst forms (Fig. 13.32). This disorder has been recognized in AIDS patients. Multifocal lesions may be distributed in the anterior and middle cerebral arterial zones suggesting metastatic tumors. Inflammatory reactions in these compromised hosts may be absent or minimal. Toxoplasma encephalitis may be life-threatening but responds to appropriate therapy.

Congenital toxoplasmosis is transmitted

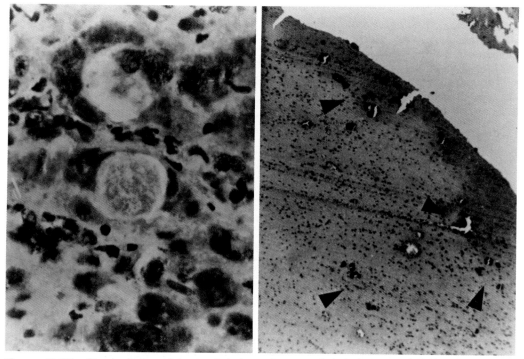

Figure 13.32. *T. gondii* found intracellularly and extracellularly possess darkly stained nuclei. Parasitic cysts are common. H&E. (Original magnification ×1000.) (From F. Tognetti: *J Neurosurg* 56:718, 1982.)

from the mother to her fetus, that may be an aborted stillborn or a newborn infant with severe tissue damage. Most neonates with congenital toxoplasmosis are not recognized at birth. Clinical cases are estimated to be 1 per 4,000 births in the United States and up to 1 per 1000 births in France. Women who acquire toxoplasmosis during pregnancy possess infected placentas in about 25% of cases. Transmission of the parasites to the fetus may occur any time during pregnancy but appears most serious during the latter part of the first trimester and second trimester. Subsequent pregnancies in women who have been infected with toxoplasmosis do not appear at risk, although exceptions have been noted. A child with convulsions and increased head size is a potential host infected with toxoplasmosis. In some, chorioretinitis may be the only manifestation. Congenital toxoplasmosis is associated with chorioretinitis in about 75% of patients, neurological dysfunction in 50%, and abnormal intracranial volume with either hydrocephalus

or micrencephaly in 25%. Over 60% of the patients have jaundice and enlarged liver and spleen. Prematurity is also increased in fetuses with intrauterine toxoplasmosis. Generally, cerebral calcifications are scattered throughout the brain as compared to congenital cytomegaloviral encephalitis which has primary periventricular calcifications. Developmental and mental retardation may be associated with bilateral chorioretinitis and microophthalmia. Disseminated toxoplasmosis in neonates can produce thrombocytopenia, elevated bilirubin, increased serum IgM, and xanthochromic cerebrospinal fluid with an elevated protein level. Inflammatory cells in the spinal fluid vary from several to 300/cu mm. Occasional *Toxoplasma* may be seen. The leptomeningeal exudate includes lymphocytes, plasma cells, and occasional neutrophils. Neuroparenchymal lesions in the cerebrum and basal ganglia show coagulative necrosis with cerebritis (Fig. 13.31) and focal calcifications. Free toxoplasma and parasite-laden cysts are found in the lesions and meningeal exudate. Periependymal and aqueductal granulation tissue may lead to aqueductal occlusion.

Maternal toxoplasmic infection can spread through the bloodstream, subsequently infect the placenta, and then gain entrance to the fetal circulation where potentially any tissue, including the central nervous system, can be infected. Consumption of uncooked or poorly cooked infected meat accounts for acquired human infections with *T. gondii*. Serologic conversions have been demonstrated in individuals ingesting poorly cooked meats. Pregnant women, in particular, should avoid exposure to cats, which have been incriminated as a source for human toxoplasmosis. Leukocyte transfusions may be an additional mode of transmitting human toxoplasmosis. Postnatally acquired toxoplasmosis in the normal or compromised host may be associated with discrete neuroparenchymal lesions as well as diffuse leptomeningeal opacity. Intrauterine acquired toxoplasmosis shows hydrocephalus, intracranial calcifications, and bilateral chorioretinitis in the newborn; yet most cases are acquired postnatally. In older children or adults, persistent unexplained fever or the development of progressive neurological deficits with inflammation suggests toxoplasmosis. In newborns, chorioretinitis with or without intracranial calcifications is consistent with toxoplasmosis. Confirmation requires demonstration of toxoplasma in the tissue or cerebrospinal fluid. Serologic measures can suggest the infection and require two serum specimens obtained at least 2 weeks apart. A rising titer indicates a recently acquired infection, while a stable titer from serial specimens indicates previous infections. Antibodies are detected by this method 2–3 weeks after the onset of symptoms and gradually diminish over ensuing years. The Sabin dye test is sensitive and specific, but technically demanding and hazardous to laboratory workers. A complement fixation test has advantages, since live organisms are not used, but the complement-fixing antibodies develop slower than those of the dye test. A hemagglutination test is the routine screening procedure that uses nonviable antigen and correlates well with the methylene blue dye test. The indirect fluorescent antibody method and the IgM fluorescent antibody technique are helpful in recognizing congenital toxoplasmosis. *T. gondii* can be isolated in tissue culture, and the acquired variety shows characteristic lymph node changes manifested by reactive follicular hyperplasia with irregular epithelioid histiocytes in cortical and paracortical zones.

TRYPANOSOMIASIS (9, 35, 55, 144, 191, 198, 199, 339)

These generalized infections are commonly seen in Africa and South America and often infect the central nervous system during their course. The pathogenic protozoans in this family include *Trypanosoma cruzi*, *Trypanosoma gambiense*, and *Trypanosoma rhodesiense*. Although *T. gambiense* and *T. rhodesiense* produce different clinical diseases and are transmitted by the tsetse (Glossina) fly, they are indistinguishable from one another morphologically. These trypanosomes infect man, horses, camels, dogs, sheep, goats, and pigs, and may have originated from *T. brucei* infecting herbivorous animals. In blood and tissue fluids, *T. gambiense* and *T. rhodesiense* are thin flagellates, measuring 10–30 μm. Unlike *T. cruzi*, there are no tissue leishmanoid forms. Man appears to be the primary reservoir for *T. gambiense*, whereas wild animals appear to be the reservoir for *T. rhodesiense*. *T. cruzi* occurs throughout Central and South America, except for Honduras and the Guianas, and causes American trypanosomiasis. It resembles the African trypanosome measuring 15–20 μm in length, but does not propagate in the blood, only tissue cells. A few flagellated forms of this organism can be found in the peripheral blood. The organisms multiply as leishmania in the viscera, particularly bones and cardiac muscle. Infected host cells possess peripherally displaced and flattened nuclei caused by the intracytoplasmic leishmanial cysts occurring in all tissues. The most striking lesions are encountered in the heart and brain. Vectors of Chagas' disease or American trypanosomiasis are large reduviid bugs (*Trotoma magista*), that may infect wild and domesticated animals, important reservoirs for the infections.

Chagas' disease or American trypanosomiasis may be an acute or chronic disorder infecting the central nervous system early. Fever, swollen eyelids and face, and conjunctivitis may be associated with anasarca, hepatomegaly, splenomegaly, and enlarged lymph nodes. Encephalitis can develop, causing a poor prognosis. Chronic forms occur in older children and adults and are associated with myocarditis. The central nervous system may also be infected, although less frequently than in the acute form. Macroscopically, the brain has congested leptomeninges and small petechial hemorrhages in the centrum semiovale. Acute and chronic inflammatory cells can be found in the subarachnoid space. A widespread encephalomyelitis is apparent during active trypanosomiasis, characterized by microglial nodules that vary in size and include microcytes, mononuclear phagocytes, reactive astrocytes, lymphocytes, and plasma cells (Fig. 13.33). Most microglial nodules are adjacent to capillaries throughout the cortex and white matter of the entire neuraxis. Parasites are difficult to find in microglial nodules but can be observed during active degenerative and necrotic changes. Other histological abnormalities include lymphocytic perivascular infiltrates with occasional neutrophils, focal perivascular hemorrhages, and swelling and proliferation of vascular elements. Extensive tissue necrosis is not common, but may be associated with many parasites. In late infections, the organisms disappear. Calcification around the ventricles may be seen with cysts and diffuse astrogliosis. The parasites observed in the central nervous system are leishmania, which are found intracellularly and extracellularly. Astrocytes may be filled with these organisms in their cytoplasm. Leishmania may also be seen in endothelial cells, microglia, and, rarely, neurons. In American trypanosomiasis, intraparenchymal central nervous system lesions may be related to liberated toxins from infected dead cells and dead parasites. These produce parenchymal necrosis with a cellular response, including microglia, astrocytes, histiocytes, and few leukocytes. The central nervous system is not always infected in Chagas' disease. Commonly involved organs include the

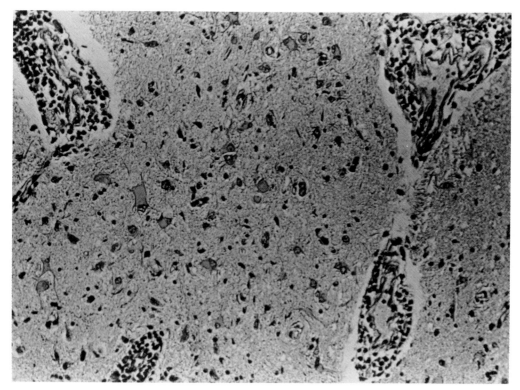

Figure 13.33. In trypanosomiasis, the brain may have plump astrocytes and perivascular chronic inflammation. Armed Forces Institute of Pathology (AFIP).

skin, heart, skeletal muscle, and gastrointestinal tract. Chagomas, which are red cutaneous nodules, constitute either primary lesions, resulting from invasion by the parasites, or lymphatic or hematogenous transport of the organisms into the skin. Morphologically, the cutaneous lesions include mononuclear phagocytes, focal fat necrosis, and scattered leishmania with a characteristic kinetoplast in the protozoan. Romaña's sign, which is edema of the eyelids and unilateral conjunctivitis, occurs early in the infection. Myocarditis is a common complication of Chagas' disease and is associated with mononuclear inflammatory infiltrates and intracellular organisms in the cardiac muscle. The myenteric plexi and visceral organs may be damaged by infection with the leishmania and can lead to an enlarged esophagus, stomach, and large bowel.

African trypanosomiasis is produced either by *T. rhodesiense* or *T. gambiense*. Rhodesian trypanosomiasis is more fulminating and can cause death within 2–3 months. Cardiac complications are seen more often in this variety as well. Grossly, a slight clouding to the leptomeninges is evident, but microscopically, widespread lymphocytic meningitis with focal accumulations in various portions of the central nervous system are evident. Eosinophilic bodies have been noted in the meninges and perivascular mononuclear cell infiltrates in the neuroparenchyma. Patients with Rhodesian trypanosomiasis may show lymphocytic and plasma cell exudates throughout the central nervous system associated with macrophages and morular cells in the leptomeninges, perivascular spaces, and brain parenchyma itself. Microglial nodules and lymphophagocytosis may be striking features in this variety of sleeping sickness. Perivascular demyelination may be associated with inflammatory and reactive responses in the central nervous system. Inflammation within the neuroparenchyma involves both grey and white matter and is prominent in deep cortical layers and at the corticomedullary junctions. Cellular infiltrates are seen around both arteries and veins throughout the neuraxis. The heart often has scattered subacute and chronic inflammatory changes in the myocardium. Malaria-like pigment may be evident. Enecephalopathic changes are less intense in Gambian encephalitis and not as widespread. Gambiense trypanosomiasis has an incubation period of 14 d with a local cutaneous trypanosome chancre. Vascular invasion occurs soon after the infecting bite, and organisms may be present in the blood for 3 weeks. Fever may be accompanied by erythema, edema, and hyperesthesia (Kerandel's signs). Pathologically, the changes in gambiense trypanosomiasis are similar to those in the rhodesiense variety; however, meningitis is milder, and less inflammatory infiltrates are noted. Lymphophagocytosis is unusual in gambiense trypanosomiasis.

The term "sleeping sickness" describes the trypanosomal encephalitides, which are characterized by fever, cutaneous lesions, cardiac arrhythmias, debilitation, anemia, and weakness. Hepatosplenomegaly and lymphadenopathy may be present. In the posterior neck, enlarged lymph nodes have been called Winterbottom's sign in patients with gambiense trypanosomiasis. Sleeping sickness symptoms develop acutely or progressively, showing a chronic course with increasing debility, slow gait, mask-like expressions, and restlessness at night. Speech disturbances and mental and personality changes have been described. Tremors of the hands, chorea, temporary paralysis, and convulsions are also evident. The condition may last for weeks, months, or years. Spontaneous death of the parasites does occur. Death is more rapid in patients with rhodesiense than with gambiense trypanosomiasis. Meningoencephalitis is a characteristic feature in both rhodesiense and gambiense trypanosomiasis and can be easily confused with viral infections of the central nervous system. The organisms are not readily apparent in the central nervous system, but trypanosomes are found in the blood, cerebrospinal fluid, and lymph nodes.

METAZOAL INFECTIONS

ANGIOSTRONGYLIASIS (104, 172, 274, 275, 345)

This metastrongylial lung nematode of rats has been identified in the brain, meninges, and eye. *Angiostrongylius cantonen-*

sis is a nematode that has been recognized throughout the neuraxis, including the cerebrospinal fluid. Humans may acquire the infection from ingestion of uncooked terrestrial snails or slugs that serve as intermediate hosts to the larvae. Clinical manifestations include diffuse meningeal signs with encephalopathic features, including behavioral disturbances. The cerebrospinal fluid possesses increased cells with many eosinophils, increased protein, and low sugar. More than 90% of the cerebrospinal fluid cells can be eosinophils, providing the diagnosis of eosinophilic leptomeningitis or meningoencephalitis. Patients with unexplained eosinophilic meningitis have been considered to have angiostrongyliasis. The inflammatory exudate is particularly prominent around blood vessels near the invading worms and includes mononuclear phagocytes, plasma cells, lymphocytes, and eosinophils, which can be seen around the parasite itself. Occasional granulomas with lymphocytes, eosinophils, neutrophils, plasma cells, and a few multinucleated giant cells are most evident after the nematodes have died. Experimentally, *A. cantonensis* has produced similar lesions in lower primates that also develop severe eosinophilic meningoencephalitis and myelitis.

COENUROSIS (24, 31, 47, 103, 104, 147, 158, 173, 175, 215, 270, 335, 341)

Coenurus cerebralis is the larval stage of the dog tapeworm. The intermediate host for this worm is the human or sheep infected after ingesting food contaminated with the ova of these parasites from canine feces. The adult tapeworm, *Multiceps (Taenia) multiceps,* measures up to 60 cm in length and inhabits the intestinal tract of coyotes, dogs, or foxes. Eggs are intermittently shed in the stools from these animals. The coenurus is a delicate, semitransparent bladder filled with water-clear fluid and as many as 400 scoleces attached to the inside of its wall (Fig. 13.34). Infection with the larval stage follows oral ingestion of the ova. The onchospheres hatch in the intestine of the secondary host, penetrate the intestinal wall, and reach the circulation where they are distributed to the brain, spinal cord, and other tissues. Within the tissue, the larva develops into a coenurus. Unlike the cysticercus, which has a single scolex, the coenurus possesses multiple (several hundreds) scoleces invaginated into its wall. In addition, the coenurus can become extremely large, measuring up to 5 cm in diameter within a year.

The disease has been recognized in the Caribbean and South Africa. In most individuals, one cyst develops, but occasionally multiple cysts occur. The parasitic cyst can be found in the cerebral ventricles, subarachnoid space, or the neuroparenchyma and may enlarge in the cisterna basalis, developing lobulations similar to the racemose cysticercus. Cyst walls of the coenurus and cysticercus may be similar. The initial inflammatory response in the neuraxis includes lymphocytes, neutrophils, and eosinophils. When the onchospheres or larvae disintegrate, inflammation becomes more intense. Mature coenuri are associated with astrocytic proliferation and fibrocollagenous tissue in the adjacent neuroparenchyma. Mild chronic inflammation and occasional giant cells may be evident. The outer layer of the cyst is a thin shell with an inner germinal layer from which scoleces develop. When the coenurus degenerates, collagen tends to replace it and may be associated with seizures.

Coenurosis of the central nervous system is uncommon. The cysts occur in the fourth ventricle or basal cistern and produce increased intracranial pressure due to obstructive hydrocephalus. Cerebellar disturbances may be apparent. The cerebral hemispheres may be rare sites for cyst formation, and intraocular cysts may appear. Cerebrospinal fluid can show increased mononuclear cells and moderately elevated protein. The coenurus in the cerebral hemispheres is unilocular and oval or circular, while in the fourth ventricle, it is irregular and racemose, resembling a cysticercus. Excised tissue can provide a specific diagnosis with identification of multiple scoleces. Surgical intervention is required for the associated obstructive features and seizures.

CYSTICERCOSIS (36, 47, 113, 148, 177, 187, 194, 241, 264, 314, 326, 333, 345a)

This infection is caused by *Cysticercus cellulose*, which is the larval form of the pork tapeworm, *Taenia solium*. Man is the

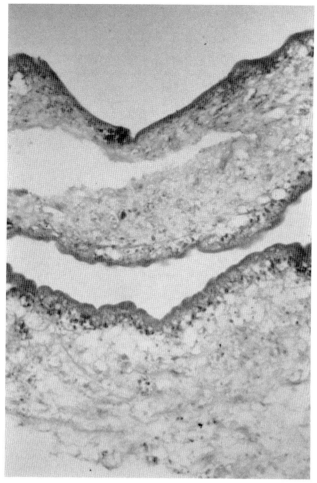

Figure 13.34.   In coenurosis, papillary villi are seen inside the parasitic cyst (coenurus) produced by *T. multiceps*. H&E. (Original magnification ×160.)

definitive host and harbors the adult tapeworm in the upper small intestine. Proglottids ladened with eggs are eliminated intermittently in the feces. If consumed by the intermediate host, the hog, the ova will develop into larvae or onchospheres that penetrate the intestinal wall, then invade the lymphatics and veins, and disseminate into skeletal muscles and other tissues. Man becomes infected when he ingests poorly cooked, infected pork. The consumed cysticercus develops an evaginated scolex that attaches to the jejunal mucosa and develops into an adult worm in the human intestine, completing its life cycle. Acquisition of larval forms producing cysticercosis occurs after ingestion of *T. solium* eggs in food or water contaminated with infected feces. The ova can also be acquired by oral transmission from unclean hands of carriers of the adult tapeworm. Internal autoinfection is possible by regurgitation of eggs from the jejunum into the stomach through reverse peristalsis. Onchospheres, once outside the gastrointestinal tract, invade other tissues and become mature cysticerci, which are oval, translucent cysts, containing a single scolex bearing four suckers. Within 12 weeks, the cysticerci mature and are primarily observed in skeletal muscle. Other infected organs include the brain, eyes, liver, lung, and subcutaneous tissues. In the United States, these infections are rare, since hogs have limited access to human excreta. The infection is common in Mexico, South America, India, and certain European countries and has been reported in border states like Texas and California.

Cysticerci develop in skeletal muscle, which may be tender and mildly painful. Multiple, nontender nodules of varying size can develop within the infected skeletal muscle. Generalized muscle enlargement may be associated with progressive muscle weakness. Subcutaneous and muscular cysts eventually calcify and can be seen roentgenographically. After skeletal muscle infestation, the brain is most often involved with these parasitic cysts (Figs. 13.35 and

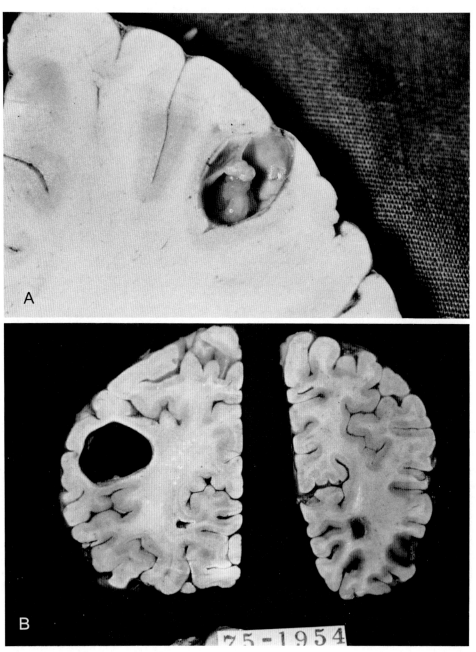

Figure 13.35. Cysticercosis is caused by the larvae of *T. solium*, which infect tissues throughout the body, including the central nervous system. Occasionally, the single bladder-filled cysticercus possesses a larva (*A*), but usually multiple cysts (*B*) are seen.

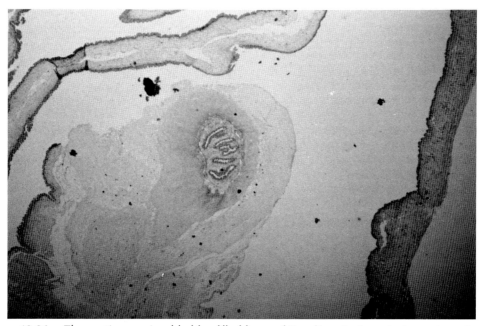

Figure 13.36.   The cysticercus is a bladder-filled larva of *T. solium*. Its intestinal tract is evident in cross-section. H&E. (Original magnification ×250.)

13.36). Clinical manifestations usually do not occur until the parasite evokes an inflammatory response as it dies. Neurological deficits may be delayed for many years after the acquired infection. Altered ocular movement with cysticercosis can result from cyst formation in the extraocular muscles or the orbit. Intracranial infestation is the most serious component of the disease, although cysts can occur in the brain without associated manifestations. Cysts are primarily observed in the cerebral grey matter but have been observed in the brain stem, cerebellum, and meninges. The ventricular system or cerebellopontine angle may be infected, creating obstructive hydrocephalus. Cysticerci within the brain create an inflammatory response with fibroconnective tissue, adjacent granulation tissue, and chronic inflammation including monocytes, lymphocytes, plasma cells, and focal eosinophils. Within the ventricular system, the cysticercus can enlarge and proliferate to a large irregular (racemose) size with numerous projections and loculations and little inflammatory reaction. The racemose cysticercus is large, thin-walled, translucent, and multilocular. Its shape adapts to the side of the ventricles.

Clinical manifestations due to infections in the central nervous system depend upon the site, number, and location of the cysts. Recurrent, focal, and generalized convulsions may be associated with progressive dementia. Other localizing deficits depend on the sites of the lesions. A posterior fossa syndrome may be produced by the racemose cysticercus in the fourth ventricle. Headache, vomiting, papilledema, and ataxia are produced by intermittent obstructive hydrocephalus. Bruns' syndrome is associated with cysticerci in the fourth ventricle with intermittent obstructive hydrocephalus and vertigo caused by abrupt movements of the head. Cerebrospinal fluid may show only slightly elevated protein, normal to slightly reduced glucose, and some eosinophils. When subcutaneous nodules are present, they provide an available source for histological confirmation of the parasite. Multiple calcified, soft tissue lesions can be demonstrated on x-ray, suggesting cysticercosis. Serological tests of the cerebrospinal fluid may help diagnose the condition, but overlapping reactivity with coenurosis and echinococcosis occurs. Surgical intervention can be required for the obstructive hydrocephalus. Attempts must be made not to release the contents of the cysticerci, which can produce an exuberant, acute inflammatory response leading to death.

ECHINOCOCCOSIS (15, 84, 130, 165, 176, 220, 250, 255, 271, 285, 353)

The larval stage of *Taenia echinococcus* occurs in man after ingesting ova-infected food or by accidental contamination of hands with canine feces harboring the adult tapeworm—*Echinococcus granulosus*. Most cases of hydatidosis are seen in children. The usual definitive host is sheep. After ingestion, ova hatch in the gastrointestinal tract, liberating larvae that invade the circulatory system and are distributed throughout the body. The larvae develop into encysted embryos, producing a primary hydatid cyst in the liver (75%) and the lungs (15%). Involvement of the central nervous system has been called encephalic hydatidosis. Bone involvement in hydatidosis has been seen in the skull and vertebrae. About 2–5% of all patients with echinococcosis develop hydatid cysts in the brain. Cerebral hydatid cysts are more frequent in children than in adults, yet skull lesions are seen equally in adults and chil-

dren. Vertebral hydatidosis is typically found in adults.

Hydatid cysts are characterized by an amorphous, eosinophilic capsule with an inner germinal epithelium and many scoleces in the multiple daughter cysts (Fig. 13.37). The intracranial hydatid cyst usually develops in the distribution of the anterior and middle cerebral arteries and may involve the wall of the lateral ventricle. Hydatid cysts in the brain can rupture, creating an extensive inflammatory reaction. The nervous tissue around the cyst is similar to that seen in cysticercosis. Focal, chronic inflammation near the capsule with lymphocytes, plasma cells, and eosinophils are mixed with reactive astrocytes and proliferating fibroblasts. Leptomeningeal echinococcosis may extend from bone into the thickened dura and can be associated with eosinophilic leptomeningitis.

Clinical manifestations usually occur late in the disease, following the initial infection some years later. Cerebral cysts are usually single and unilocular but are quite large. All cysts within the bone tend to be multilocular. Spinal involvement in echinococ-

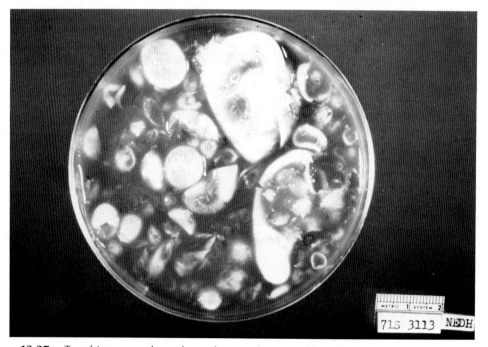

Figure 13.37. *T. echinococcus* has a larva that produces multiple daughter cysts in a single large cyst or hydatid cyst. This Petri dish possesses fluid from a large cyst with multiple smaller cysts, containing other larval cysts.

cosis occurs most often in the thoracic region (50%), followed by the lumbar (20%), sacral (20%), and cervical areas (10%). Clinical features include seizures, focal neurological deficits, and spinal cord compression, depending on the location of the cysts. Surgery is the primary form of therapy.

FILARIASIS (234)

Filariae, including adult and microfilariae, can invade the nervous tissue, its coverings, and adjacent bone. Incriminated filariae are *Acanthocheilonema perstants*, *Loa loa*, *Onchocerca volvulus*, and *Wuchereria bancrofti*. Filariae are transmitted to man by infected arthropod bites that produce slight edema with scattered petechiae. Most cases of cerebral filariasis are caused by *L. loa*. These organisms circulate in the blood and pass through cerebral vessels, causing lesions. They may be so numerous as to plug capillaries. By dying in cerebral blood vessels and disintegrating within brain parenchyma, they produce inflammatory reactions.

Granulomas can be seen microscopically around microfilariae within the neuroparenchyma and may be associated with multiple perivascular monocytes, lymphocytes, plasma cells, and microcytes involving the cerebral cortex, white matter, and brain stem. Medium-sized veins, including those in the leptomeninges, can be infected. Most perivascular lesions have central necrosis with associated inflammation, hyalinized infected veins, intravascular thrombi, and microfilariae. The cellular response to cerebral filariasis includes histiocytes, lymphocytes, reactive microglia, neutrophils, and erythrocytes. A prominent mesenchymal reaction develops around dying microfilariae, which seem more antigenically stimulating than living microfilariae. Clinical manifestations for cerebral filariasis include leptomeningeal and encephalitic features. Neuropsychiatric deficits have been associated with focal cerebrovascular and neuroparenchymal lesions. Cerebrospinal fluid examination may reveal microfilariae.

GNASTHOSTOMIASIS (222, 321)

The nematode, *Gnasthostoma spinigerum*, is found in Asia, particularly Thailand. Humans acquire this parasite by eating uncooked fresh water fish that harbor the third-stage larvae, which grow into mature adult forms. Cats and dogs are similarly infected. Involvement of the central nervous system in gnasthostomiasis may be associated with transitory seizures and leptomeningeal irritations, since the parasites usually escape spontaneously from the patient. Pleocytosis with eosinophilia may appear in the cerebrospinal fluid.

PARAGONIMIASIS (119, 242)

Paragonimus westermani primarily involves the pulmonary system and is endemic in the Far East. Man is infected by eating uncooked crabs or crayfish which are the second intermediate host. The definitive host for this lung fluke is man. The first intermediate host is the operculated snail. The parasite, which resides in the lungs, disseminates its ova through the host's sputum and feces. The expelled ova develop into free-swimming miracidia that penetrate a suitable snail, developing into a sporocyst. After several weeks, the parasite matures into cercariae that emerge from the snail and penetrate fresh water crabs or crayfish. In this second intermediate host, the larval metacercariae are encysted. After ingesting uncooked crustaceae, the human gastrointestinal tract dissolves the capsules of the metacercariae, and the parasites pass through the stomach into the peritoneal cavity. These small parasitic worms penetrate the diaphragm and pleura, infecting the lungs. Within the pulmonary parenchyma, the adult worms mature in cyst-like abscesses about 6 weeks following the initial infection. Occasionally, during migration through the body, the worms infect extrapulmonary sites. The central nervous system is the second most common infected site after the lung.

Cerebral paragonimiasis is caused by adult worms invading the brain through hematogenous routes, directly through stromal tissues, or both. After reaching the brain, larvae mature into adult worms, depositing their ova locally. The central nervous system infestation by *P. westermani* is the most common and serious extrapulmonary infection by this parasite and occurs predominantly in people under 30 yr of age. A localized cerebral mass may be associated with increased intracranial pressure (Fig. 13.38), and the adjacent tissues possess reactive astrocytosis, fibrosis, and

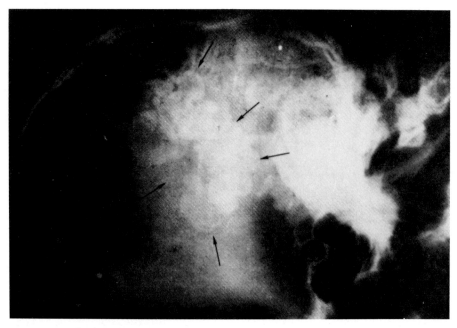

Figure 13.38. Cerebral paragonimiasis can produce intracranial calcification. (From *J Neurol Sci* 8:27, 1968.)

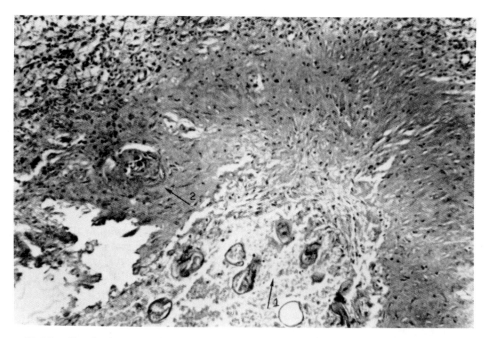

Figure 13.39. Cerebral paragonimiasis causes necrotic granulomas with eggs and an exuberant granulomatous inflammation. (From *J Neurol Sci* 8:27–48, 1968.)

chronic inflammation with lymphocytes, plasma cells, occasional eosinophils, and mononuclear phagocytes. Primary optic atrophy associated with decreased visual acuity may develop. Paragonimiasis has a predilection for the posterior cerebral hemispheres. Solid, round to oval granulomas with central necrosis contain ova, inflammatory cells, and giant cells (Fig. 13.39). Adjacent gliosis may be associated with plasma cells, lymphocytes, eosinophils, and scattered calcific debris. Intracranial calcification, which has been recognized in more than 50% of patients with cerebral paragonimiasis, is seen in chronic, long-standing infestations. Roentgenographic patterns reveal soap-bubble configurations with round or oval shapes and increased peripheral density. A poorly encapsulated abscess may possess thick yellow, purulent material with ova in the inner capsule. The adult fluke is identified rarely because of its rapid disintegration within tissues. Patients with cerebral involvement usually have pulmonary lesions that enable recognition of the disease if the parasites or their ova can be recognized in the sputum. Cerebrospinal fluid may show lymphocytic pleocytosis and occasional eosinophils.

Early pulmonary manifestations in paragonimiasis develop insidiously and affect males more often than females. Poor socioeconomic groups, children, and young adults are infected most frequently. A dry cough may become productive and blood-tinged. Rust-brown sputum can occur with fever, chest pain, and pleural effusions. Mild eosinophilia and a history of eating raw crabs or crayfish may be noted. Chest x-rays can show abnormalities suggestive of tuberculosis. Recognition of the ova in sputa, stools, or aspirated pleural fluid can make the diagnosis. Since intradermal skin tests cross-react with other metazoans, they are not helpful. Complement fixation tests are usually positive in spinal fluids. Recurrent seizures are the commonest initial neurological disturbance and may be complicated by variable neuropsychiatric deficits. An occasional patient may have meningitic episodes preceding convulsions, and chronic meningitis may be manifested by headache, vomiting, weight loss, stiff neck, and fever. A local cerebral mass can develop with papilledema. Recurrent seizures, commonly Jacksonian in type, may be followed by abrupt and persistent hemiplegia, produced by focal granulomatous cerebral lesions. Progressive dementia occurs in some patients, and mental retardation is common in children with cerebral paragonimiasis.

SCHISTOSOMIASIS (121, 307, 344)

Three species of blood flukes—*Schistosoma haematobium, Schistosoma japonicum,* and *Schistosoma mansoni*—cause human schistosomiasis. The primary host is man, whereas the secondary host is the water snail. *S. haematobium* is found primarily in Africa and resides in pelvic veins in man. *S. japonicum,* found in the Far East, resides in mesenteric veins. *S. mansoni* occurs in Africa, South America, and the West Indies and is found within mesenteric veins. The ova of these parasites are passed into venules where the miracidium develops in the egg. The latter ruptures through the venular wall and invades the urinary bladder or bowel, eventually being excreted in the urine, feces, or both. Once in water, miracidia hatch from the eggs and penetrate a snail. Fork-tailed cercariae develop and emerge from this intermediate host, swimming to contact, and enter human skin. Eventually, the cercariae invade blood vessels and finally lodge in abdominal veins to mature into adult male and female trematodes.

Factors associated with neurologial infections in schistosomiasis are not clear. Preexisting immunity and the magnitude of the initial schistosomal invasion are important. Rarely, adult female worms can migrate to cerebral intraspinal venous channels, causing mechanical venous obstruction and depositing ova which create an inflammatory response. More commonly, ova are transmitted from mesenteric or pelvic veins to nervous tissue through the valveless vertebral venous plexus of Batson or systemic channels. This embolization is related not only to size but also to the associated spines characteristic of the different *Schistosoma* species. Cerebral schistosomiasis is more common than spinal cord involvement and is caused predominantly by *S. japonicum,* which has the smallest eggs and an inconspicuous terminal spine (Fig. 13.40). The large lateral spine on the ovum of *S. mansoni* tends to inhibit its embolization, and as a result it involves the central nervous system less frequently than either *S. haematobium* or *S. japonicum.* Neurological deficits may appear 2–3 months after schistosomal exposure. The inflammatory response shows fibrosis, reactive astrocytosis, and chronic inflammation with lymphocytes, plasma cells, mononuclear phagocytes, and multinucleated giant cells. Any portion of the central nervous system and its meninges

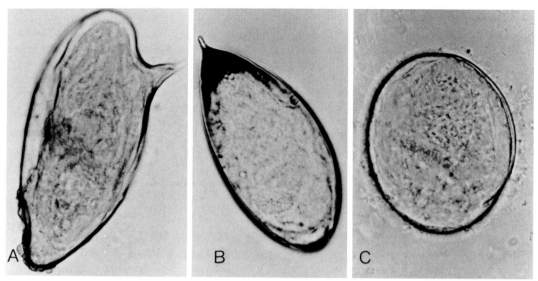

Figure 13.40.   Eggs of (A) *S. mansoni,* (B) *S. haematobium,* and (C) *S. japonicum* have characteristic spines (AFIP).

can be infected, creating variable neuropsychiatric deficits. Typical lesions in the brain include focal granulomas resembling tuberculomas and possessing schistosomal ova, adjacent gliosis, lymhoid cells, macrophages, and multinucleated giant cells. Cerebrospinal fluid shows a lymphocytic pleocytosis and elevated protein. Eosinophils may be noted in the spinal fluid.

Clinical manifestations are associated with a transient pleuritis and skin rash after the initial penetration by the cercariae. Liver invasion, recurrent urticaria, edema, respiratory distress, and eosinophilia may occur. Liver tenderness associated with hepatomegaly develops in 2–3 weeks and can be associated with fever, abdominal pain, and diarrhea. Early infestation by *S. haematobium* is associated with lesions in the bladder, genitalia, and distal intestine. Frequency and pain on micturition, as well as hematuria, develop. Bladder wall malignancies appear late in the disease. Since *S. japonicum* and *S. mansoni* are found in mesenteric veins, their eggs tend to invade the intestinal wall and can be carried through the portal system into the liver. Hepatosplenomegaly, hepatic cirrhosis, and portal hypertension with hypersplenism can be seen. Ova may be evident in the feces, urine, and biopsied tissues from the rectum and bladder. Peripheral blood leukocytosis with eosinophilia is ob-

served in most patients and is most severe early in the infection. Cerebral deficits usually appear more than 6 months after the initial infection. Focal neuropsychiatric signs resembling a space-occupying lesion have been noted. Unilateral motor or sensory deficits can complicate focal seizures and papilledema. Death from cerebral schistosomiasis is unusual, but persistent neurologic deficits are not uncommon. Spinal cord deficits can be produced by schistosomal ova that cause focal intramedullary granulomas, diffuse inflammatory myelopathy, or both. Most cases involve the low thoracic or lumbar cord. Low back discomfort may be associated with cramplike leg pains followed by paraplegia with sensory loss below the lesion. Sphincter disturbances may develop. Damage to the spinal cord is severe in most cases, and, while improvement can be expected, complete recovery of function does not usually occur.

SPARGANOSIS (13, 201, 219, 240, 258, 309, 323, 328)

Sparganosis is an infection caused by a migrating plerocercoid larva of the tapeworm *Spirometra,* referred to as a sparganum. Although human sparganosis is worldwide, it is most common in Asia. Most infections involve the subcutaneous tissues and rarely the central nervous system.

Classic sparganosis due to *Spirometra* is a nonproliferative disease in which the larvae grow slowly in man but cannot reproduce. This organism is closely related to *Diphyllobothrium latum*. On the other hand, the proliferative form of human sparganosis is caused by *Sparganum proliferum*. In this disorder, larvae grow by branching and budding, forming new organisms, and can cause death by massive proliferation throughout all host tissues, including the brain. The adult stage of this parasite is not known.

Cats and dogs are the definitive host for *Spirometra*. Eggs of this tapeworm are passed in the feces from the intestinal parasite and hatch in water producing the first larva, a coracidium. This ciliated larva is eaten by a copepod (*Cyclops* species) and develops into the procercoid larva. Vertebrate intermediate hosts include frogs, mice, raccoons, and snakes that drink water containing the infected copepods. In this animal, the procercoid larva penetrates the intestinal wall and migrates through capillaries to infect subcutaneous tissues. Eventually, the plerocercoid larva or sparganum develops. The adult tapeworm is formed about 3 weeks after the vertebrate intermediate host, with its spargana, are consumed by a dog or cat. Man is an accidental intermediate host, usually acquiring the infection by drinking contaminated water with the infected copepods, by ingesting inadequately cooked or raw meats infected with the sparganum, or by applying infected intermediate host flesh to open wounds as a poultice from which the sparganum migrates.

Sparganosis can cause circumscribed small, firm, fibrous, grey, brown, or yellow masses with hemorrhage, necrosis, and cysts. The sparganum, which may be identified grossly, is a thin white solid ribbon-like worm that measures from several millimeters to over a meter in length. Its width is variable, but usually only a few millimeters. Its anterior end is invaginated and slightly bulbous. Its body is rigid at regular intervals. Tissue response to the larvae includes a dense inflammatory reaction with lymphocytes, plasma cells, histocytes, neutrophils and, occasionally, foreign body giant cells. Eosinophils and Charcot-Leyden crystals may be seen. A sparganum must be distinguished from *Cysticercus*,

Echinococcus, and *Coenurus*. Spargana have a solid noncavitated body without bladder walls and no hooked scoleces. Most individuals with sparganosis are adults who develop slow-growing, tender, migratory subcutaneous nodules that may persist for weeks or years. Fever, chills, erythema, edema, and eosinophilia may be present, particularly when the worm migrates through tissues. The parasite has been reported throughout the body, including the intracranial contents. Cerebral sparganosis is associated with headaches, seizures, focal neurological deficits, subarachnoid hemorrhage, and sudden death. It is best treated by surgical extirpation, since no effective medical therapy is known currently.

TOXOCARIASIS (216, 256, 312, 347)

Larvae of *Toxocara canis* and *Toxocara cati* are dog and cat ascarides or round worms, respectively. The adult nematode is 7–12 cm in length and lives in the intestines of dogs and cats where eggs are excreted in the stools. After brief embryonation, the ovum contains an infective larva and may be ingested by other dogs and cats. When they hatch in the intestines of these animals, the developed larvae invade the intestinal wall, reaching portal veins and migrating to the liver and lung. Migration up the bronchial tree to the trachea is followed by reentry into the intestinal tract. Prenatal transmission to the canine fetus can cause a congenital infection. Puppies are infected more commonly with toxocariasis than adult dogs and offer a greater source for infection to children than older dogs. In man, the swallowed ova of *T. canis* produce larvae that emerge within the intestine, subsequently penetrate the bowel wall, invade portal veins, and infect the liver and lungs. These parasites do not complete their life cycle beyond the second larval stage in man. In this stage, they can survive many months in tissues, producing granulomas. Adult worms do not occur in the human intestine, and, consequently, ova are not excreted in the stool.

This nematode has been found in the eye, central nervous system, liver, and lungs. In most ocular infestations, *Toxocara* invade the eye without producing a visceral larva migrans syndrome or characteristic blood changes. Children tend to develop this intraocular infection and are usually older than those with abdominal visceral involvement. In most patients, only one eye is infected and often has altered vision and strabismus. Diffuse endophthalmitis or focal lesions with peridiscal or macular granulomas develop commonly. Peripheral retinal inflammation and optic neuritis are noted less often. Profound visual loss may be caused by vitreous inflammation and retinal detachment. Neurologic disturbances in cerebral toxocariasis are rare, but include convulsions, lethargy, and stiff neck. *Toxocara* in neural tissue are associated with granulomas possessing mononuclear phagocytes, adjacent lymphocytes, plasma cells, and reactive astrocytes. Cerebrospinal fluid may show lymphocytic pleocytosis and rare *Toxocara* larvae.

Clinical manifestations are seen primarily in children, usually between 1 and 6 yr of age. The disease is more common in boys than in girls. Intermittent contact with dogs or history of pica has been noted. Toxocariasis infects the liver, lungs, often the eye, and rarely the brain. Other infected sites include the skin, bone, bladder, and heart. Vague features like lassitude, anorexia, weight loss, and fever may be followed by cough or wheezing. Enlargement of the liver and spleen are common. Anemia may occur with eosinophilia. Visceral larva migrans develops as a consequence of the *Toxocara* larvae wandering haphazardly through the host's body. During this migration, marked inflammation occurs in the parasitic tracts as the organism passes through various tissues. If the nematode dies, the associated tissue develops a focal granuloma which encases the organism and includes lymphocytes, eosinophils, and focal foreign body giant cells. A diagnosis of toxocariasis can be suspected in any young child with hepatomegaly, hypereosinophilia, and hyperglobulinemia. A liver biopsy may demonstrate parasites with inflammatory granulomas due to its migration through the organ. An intradermal skin test for *Toxocara* has been used, although cross-reactions with other metazoans occur. Visceral larva migrans in its early stage has been treated successfully with drug therapy.

TRICHINOSIS (127)

The most prevalent helminthic or metazoal infection in man is trichinosis. Most infected individuals are asymptomatic. Over the past several decades, trichinosis in the United States has markedly declined due to reduced feeding of raw garbage to hogs and increased public awareness of the hazards of uncooked or poorly cooked pork. The causative organism, *Trichinella spiralis*, has no free-living stage in its life cycle. Lower animals and man may act as both intermediate and final hosts, harboring the adult nematode temporarily and the larvae for longer periods. Flesh that is infected with encysted larvae when eaten by another host, like the pig, other carnivorous animals, and man, can infect them. Man develops the infection by eating poorly cooked pork or other flesh containing the larvae. Older children and adults are most frequently infected. Following ingestion, encysted larvae pass into the small intestine where, after a few hours, their capsules dissolve, allowing them to invade the mucosa. Sexual maturation occurs rapidly. After mating, the male dies and is eliminated in the stools. The female worm remains buried in the intestinal wall where, 5 to 7 days later, she deposits larvae in the bowel mucosa. This larval production may continue for about 6 weeks, when the adult nematode dies and is eliminated in the intestinal tract. The larvae subsequently penetrate the intestinal lymphatics and lymph nodes and are transmitted to the thoracic duct where they enter the bloodstream, becoming disseminated throughout the body. Skeletal muscle is selectively infected with heaviest infiltrations in the diaphragm, intercostal, masseter, extraocular, biceps, and gastrocnemius muscles. Encapsulation of larvae in skeletal muscle starts after 2–3 weeks and is completed by 3 months. Mineralization of the encysted larvae begins several months later. Myocardial infiltration occurs, but encystment is rare. The brain can be infected, but symptomatic involvement is unusual.

The frequency and pathogenesis of cerebral trichinosis have not been clarified, and yet the parasites have been demonstrated in the central nervous system. Focal neurological deficits can appear 2–4 weeks after onset of systemic illness involving an area of the central nervous system. Cerebrospinal fluid may be entirely normal in patients with encephalitic trichinosis or can reveal modest lymphocytic pleocytosis, increased protein, or elevated pressure. Rarely have the larvae been identified in the cerebrospinal fluid. Neuropathologically, scattered hemorrhages may be associated with cerebral edema and granulomatous nodules, some containing the larvae. Perivascular lymphocytic infiltrates may be found in the meninges and brain.

Trichinosis has three phases, including intestinal invasion by the adult parasite, larval tissue invasion, and, finally, larval encystment in tissues, particularly skeletal muscle. The incubation period between consumption of infected meat and onset of gastroenteritis is about 2 weeks. Subsequently, abdominal pain, vomiting, or diarrhea develop and are followed by the second stage of larval migration, which varies with the severity and magnitude of the infecting dose of parasites. Mild complaints of weakness, lethargy, fever, periorbital and facial edema, headache, muscle tenderness, pain, and weakness may be evident. Local pain on extraocular movement can complicate conjunctivitis, cutaneous eruptions, and subungual splinter hemorrhages. During the second phase, most manifestations are related to the host's allergic tissue reaction to the migrating larvae. Myocardial alterations are reflected by electrocardiographic abnormalities, which have been observed in 20% of patients with trichinosis. After about 3 weeks, the systemic manifestations, including swelling and muscle pain, diminish. Neurological signs may persist or appear for the first time at this point, but, in most patients, gradual recovery ensues. Eosinophilia does not correlate with the severity of the infection. Virtually any area of the brain can be infected, giving rise to many possible deficits, including localized convulsions, hemiparesis, dysphagia, or cerebellar disturbances. Drug treatment is usually helpful.

ACKNOWLEDGMENTS

The authors gratefully acknowledge the assistance of Ms. Martha Childs and the staff of the Preston Medical Library, Ms. Jeanette Dean and Ms. Lisa Mary for their secretarial support, Ms. Lucille Simpson for word processing, and Mr. Rich McCoig for photographic assistance.

References

1. Abildgaard CF, et al: Meningococcemia associated with intravascular coagulation. *Pediatrics* 40:78–83, 1967.
2. Adams DO: The granulomatous inflammatory response. *Am J Pathol* 84:164–192, 1976.
3. Adams JH: Parasitic and fungal infections of the nervous system. In Blackwood W, Corsellis JAN (eds): *Greenfield's Neuropathology.* London, Edward Arnold Publishers, 1976, pp 269–291.
4. Agger WA, Maki DG: Mucormycosis. A complication of critical care. *Arch Intern Med* 138:925–927, 1978.
5. Agrawal S, et al: Generalized rhinosporidiosis with visceral involvement: report of a case. *Arch Dermatol* 80:22–26, 1959.
6. Ahuja GK, et al: Cerebral mycotic aneurysm of fungal origin. *J Neurosurg* 49:107–110, 1978.
7. Ajello L: The isolation of Allescheria boydii Shear, an etiologic agent of mycetomas from soil. *Am J Trop Med* 1:227–239, 1952.
8. Al-Doory Y: *Chromomycosis.* Missoula, MT, Mountain Press, 1972.
9. Alencar A: Chagas' disease. In Minckler J (ed): *Pathology of the Nervous System.* New York, McGraw-Hill, 1972, vol 3, pp 2559–2565.
10. Alexander JW: Host defense mechanisms against infection. *Surg Clin North Am* 52:1367–1378, 1972.
11. Alexander JW, Meakins JL: A physiologic basis for the development of opportunistic infections in man. *Ann Surg* 176:273–287, 1972.
12. Alture-Werber E, et al: Pulmonary infection with Allescheria boydii. *Am J Clin Pathol* 66:1019–1024, 1976.
13. Anders K, et al: Intracranial sparganosis: an uncommon infection. *J Neurosurg* 60:1282–1286, 1984.
14. Anderson P, et al: Human serum activities against *Hemophilus influenzae*, type b. *J Clin Invest* 51:31–38, 1972.
15. Arana-Iniguez R, San Julian J: Hydatid cysts of the brain. *J Neurosurg* 12:323–335, 1955.
16. Aronson SM, et al: Maduromycosis of the central nervous system. *J Neuropathol Exp Neurol* 12:158–169, 1953.
17. Baker CJ, et al: Suppurative meningitis due to streptococci of Lancefield group B: a study of 33 infants. *J Pediatr* 82:724–729, 1973.
18. Baker RD: *Human Infection with Fungi, Actinomycetes and Algae.* New York, Springer-Verlag, 1971.
19. Baker RD: Leukopenia and therapy in leukemia as factors predisposing to fatal mycoses, mucormycosis, aspergillosis, and cryptococcosis. *Am J Clin Pathol* 37:358–373, 1962.
20. Ballenger CN Jr, Goldring D: Nocardiosis in childhood. *J Pediatr* 50:145–169, 1957.
21. Banaim Pinto H: La paracoccidiodosis Brasiliensis como enfermedad sistemica. *Mycopathologia* 15:90–114, 1961.
22. Bayer AS, et al: Candida meningitis. *Medicine* 55:477–486, 1976.
23. Beal MF, et al: Aspergillosis of the nervous system. *Neurology* 32:473–479, 1982.
24. Becker BJP, Jacobson S: Infestation of the human brain with *Coenurus cerebralis*: report of a fourth case. *Lancet* 2:1202–1204, 1951.
25. Becker EL: Stimulated neutrophil locomotion. Chemokinesis and chemotaxis. *Arch Pathol Lab Med* 101:409–413, 1977.
26. Beeson PB: Cryptococcic meningitis of nearly sixteen years' duration. *Arch Intern Med* 89:797–801, 1952.
27. Beetham WP Jr, et al: A case of extensive polyarticular involvement, and discussion of certain clinical and pathologic features. *Ann Intern Med* 58:1002–1012, 1963.
28. Beisel WR, Rapoport ML: Inter-relations between adrenocortical functions and infectious illness. *N Engl J Med* 280:541–546, 596–604, 1969.
29. Bell WE, McCormick WF: *Neurological Infections in Children.* Philadelphia, WB Saunders, 1975.
30. Bell WE, McCormick WF: *Neurologic Infections in Chil-*

dren, ed 2. Philadelphia, WB Saunders, 1981, pp 551–555.

31. Bell WE, McCormick WF: Parasitic diseases. In: *Neurologic Infections in Children.* Philadelphia, WB Saunders, 1975, pp 351–384.

32. Bell WE, Myers MG: Allescheria (Petriellidium) boydii brain abscess in a child with leukemia. *Arch Neurol* 35:386–388, 1978.

33. Bellanti JA, Dayton DH: *The Phagocytic Cell and Host Resistance.* New York, Raven Press, 1975.

34. Benham RE, Georg LK: Allescheria boydii causative agent in a case of meningitis. *J Invest Dermatol* 10:99–110, 1948.

35. Bertrand I, et al: Lésions histologiques des centres nerveux dans la trypanosomiase humaine. A propos de deux cas mortels non traités. *Ann Inst Pasteur* 54:91–147, 1935.

36. Bickerstaff ER, et al: Cysticercosis of the posterior fossa. *Brain* 79:622–634, 1956.

37. Black JT: Cerebral candidiasis: case report of brain abscess secondary to *Candida albicans* and review of literature. *J Neurol Neurosurg Psychiatry* 33:854–870, 1970.

38. Blizzard RM, Gibbs JH: Candidiasis: studies pertaining to its association with endocrinopathies in pernicious anemia. *Pediatrics* 42:231–237, 1968.

39. Bobra ST: Mycotic abscess of the brain probably due to Cladosporium trichoides: report of the fifth case. *Can Med Assoc J* 79:657–659, 1958.

40. Bodey GP: Fungal infections complicating acute leukemia. *J Chronic Dis* 19:667–687, 1966.

41. Bodey GP, et al: Quantitative relationships between circulating leukocytes and infections in patients with acute leukemia. *Ann Intern Med* 64:328–340, 1966.

42. Borland DS: Mucormycosis of the central nervous system. *Am J Dis Child* 97:852–856, 1959.

43. Boxer LA, et al: Neutrophil actin dysfunction and abnormal neutrophil behavior. *N Engl J Med* 291:1093–1099, 1974.

44. Braude AI: *Medical Microbiology and Infectious Disease.* Philadelphia, WB Saunders, 1971.

45. Bredt AB, et al: Treatment of babesiosis in asplenic patients. *JAMA* 245:1938–1939, 1981.

46. Brook I: Bacteriology of intracranial abscess in children. *J Neurosurg* 54:484–488, 1981.

47. Brown HW: *Basic Clinical Parasitology,* ed 3. New York, Appleton-Century-Crofts, 1969.

48. Bryant RE, et al: Factors affecting mortality of gram-negative rod bacteremia. *Arch Intern Med* 127:120–128, 1971.

49. Buchan GC, Alvord EC Jr: Diffuse necrosis of subcortical white matter associated with bacterial meningitis. *Neurology* 19:1–9, 1969.

50. Bulova SI, et al: Hydrops fetalis and congenital syphilis. *Pediatrics* 49:285–287, 1972.

51. Butt CG: Primary amebic meningoencephalitis. *N Engl J Med* 274:1473–1476, 1966.

52. Butt CG, et al: Naegleria (sp.) identified in amebic encephalitis. *Am J Clin Pathol* 50:568–574, 1968.

53. Callicott JH Jr: Amebic meningoencephalitis due to free-living amebas of the Hartmannella (Acanthamoeba)-Naegleria group. *Am J Clin Pathol* 49:84–91, 1968.

54. Callicott JH Jr, et al: Meningoencephalitis due to pathogenic free-living amoebae. Report of two cases. *JAMA* 206:579–582, 1968.

55. Calwell HG: Pathology of brain in Rhodesian trypanosomiasis. *Trans R Soc Trop Med Hyg* 30:611–624, 1937.

56. Carmody EJ, Tappen W: Bastomycosis meningitis: report of a case successfully treated with amphotericin B. *Ann Intern Med* 51:780–791, 1959.

57. Carpenter DF, et al: Phycomycotic thrombosis of the basilar artery. *Neurology* 18:807–812, 1968.

58. Carter RF: Primary amoebic meningoencephalitis. An appraisal of present knowledge. *Trans R Soc Trop Med Hyg* 66:193–213, 1972.

59. Caudill RF, et al: Coccidioidal meningitis. A diagnostic challenge. *Am J Med* 49:360–365, 1970.

60. Chernik ML, et al: Central nervous system infections in patients with cancer. *Medicine* 52:563–581, 1973.

61. Chilcote RR, et al: Septicemia and meningitis in children splenectomized for Hodgkin's disease. *N Engl J Med* 295:798–800, 1976.

62. Christou NV, Meakins JL: Neutrophil function in surgical patients: two inhibitors of granulocyte chemotaxis associated with sepsis. *J Surg Res* 26:355–364, 1979.

63. Clancy RL, et al: Isolation and characterization of an etiologic agent in Whipple's disease. *Br Med J* 3:568–570, 1975.

64. Clark PRR, et al: Brain abscess due to Streptomyces griseus. *J Neurol Neurosurg Psychiatry* 27:553–555, 1964.

65. Clark RA, Kimball HR: Defective granulocyte chemotaxis in the Chediak-Higashi syndrome. *J Clin Invest* 50:2645–2652, 1971.

66. Clyde DF: Malaria. In Braude AI (ed): *Medical Microbiology and Infectious Diseases,* Philadelphia, WB Saunders, 1981, pp 1478–1486.

67. Conant NF: Medical mycology. In Dubos RJ, Hirsch JG (eds): *Bacterial and Mycotic Infections of Man.* Philadelphia, JB Lippincott, 1965, pp 825–885.

68. Conant NF, et al: *Manual of Clinical Mycology, ed 3.* Philadelphia, WB Saunders, 1971.

69. Coonrod JD, Dans PE: Subdural empyema. *Am J Med* 53:85–91, 1972.

70. Cooper RA Jr, Goldstein E: Histoplasmosis of the central nervous system. A report of two cases and review of the literature. *Am J Med* 35:45–57, 1963.

71. Cox GE, et al: Protothecosis: a case of disseminated algal infection. *Lancet* 2:379–382, 1974.

72. Cox F, Hughes WR: Disseminated histoplasmosis and childhood leukemia. *Cancer* 33:1127–1133, 1974.

73. Couch JR, et al: Histoplasma meningitis with hyperactive suppressor T cells in cerebrospinal fluid. *Neurology* 28:119–123, 1978.

74. Curry CR, Quie PG: Fungal septicemia in patients receiving parental hyperalimentation. *N Engl J Med* 285:1221–1225, 1971.

75. Dammin GJ, et al: The rising incidence of clinical *Babesia microti* infection. *Hum Pathol* 12:398–400, 1981.

76. Dannenberg AM Jr: Macrophages in inflammation and infection. *N Engl J Med* 293:489–493, 1975.

77. Dastur DK: Neurotuberculosis. In Minckler J (ed): *Pathology of the Nervous System.* New York, McGraw-Hill, 1972, vol 3, pp 2412–2422.

78. Dastur DK, Udani PM: Pathology and pathogenesis of tuberculous encephalopathy. *Acta Neuropathol* 6:311–326, 1966.

79. Dean DF, et al: Cranial zygomycosis caused by Saksenaea vasiformis. Case report. *J Neurosurg* 46:97–103, 1977.

80. Dennis JL, Hansen AE: Coccidioidomycosis in children. *Pediatrics* 14:481–493, 1954.

81. Denton JF, et al: Isolation of Blastomyces dermatitidis from soil. *Science* 133:1126–1127, 1961.

82. Deresinski SC, Stevens DA: Coccidioidomycosis in compromised host. Experience at Stanford University Hospital. *Medicine* 54:377–395, 1974.

83. DeVita VT, et al: Candida meningitis. *Arch Intern Med* 117:527–535, 1966.

84. Dew HR: Hydatid disease of the brain. *Surg Gynecol Obstet* 59:321–329, 1934.

85. DeWeese DD, et al: Mucormycosis of the nose and paranasal sinuses. *Laryngoscope* 75:1398–1407, 1965.

86. Dewhurst K: The neurosyphilitic psychoses today: a survey of 91 cases. *Br J Psychiatry* 115:31–38, 1969.

87. Diamond LK: Splenectomy in childhood and the hazard of overwhelming infection. *Pediatrics* 43:886–889, 1969.

88. Diamond RD, Bennett JE: Prognostic factors in cryptococcal meningitis. A study in 111 cases. *Ann Intern Med* 80:176–181, 1974.

89. Dodge PR, Swartz MN: Bacterial meningitis: a review of selected aspects. II. Special neurologic problems, post-meningitic complications and clinicopathological corre-

lations. *N Engl J Med* 272:1003–1010, 1965.

90. Dominguez A: Paracoccidioidosis del sistema nervioso central. *Gac Med Caracas* 70:377–387, 1961.

91. Duncan PG, et al: Anesthesia and the modification of response to infection in mice. *Anesth Analg (Cleve)* 55:776–781, 1976.

92. Duque O: Meningo-encephalitis and brain abscess caused by Cladosporium and Fonsecaea. Review of the literature, report of two cases, and experimental studies. *Am J Clin Pathol* 36:505–517, 1961.

93. Duttera MJ Jr, Osterhout S: North American blastomycosis. A survey of 63 cases. *South Med J* 62:295–301, 1969.

94. Eckhoff NL: Actinomycosis of the central nervous system: report of two cases. *Lancet* 1:7–8, 1941.

95. Edelson TM, et al: Candida meningitis with cerebral arteritis. *NY J Med* 75:900–904, 1975.

96. Edward PQ, Palmer CE: Nationwide histoplasmin sensitivity in histoplasmal infection. *Public Health Rep* 78:241–259, 1963.

97. Edwards VE, et al: Cryptococcosis of the central nervous system. Epidemiological, clinical, and therapeutic features. *J Neurol Neurosurg Psychiatry* 33:415–425, 1970.

98. Emmons CW: Allescheria boydii and Monosporium apiospermum. *Mycologia* 36:188–193, 1944.

99. Emmons CW, et al: *Medical Mycology*, ed 3. Philadelphia, Lea & Febiger, 1977.

100. Ende N, et al: Hodgkin's disease associated with histoplasmosis. *Cancer* 5:763–769, 1952.

101. Eng RHK, Seligman SJ: Lumbar Puncture-induced meningitis. *JAMA* 245:1456–1459, 1981.

102. Entrican JH, et al: Babesiosis in man: a case from Scotland. *Br Med J* 2:474, 1979.

103. Epstein E, et al: Intra-ocular coenurus infestation. *S Afr Med J* 33:602–604, 1959.

104. Escobar A, Nieto D: Parasitic diseases. In Minckler J, et al (eds): *Pathology of the Nervous System.* New York, McGraw-Hill, 1972, vol 3, pp 2503–2521.

105. Ewing CE, et al: Sporothrix schenckii meningitis in a farmer with Hodgkin's disease. *Am J Med* 68:455–457, 1980.

106. Farmer TW, Wise GR: Subdural empyema in infants, children and adults. *Neurology* 23:254–261, 1973.

107. Feigin RD, Dodge PR: Bacterial meningitis: newer concepts of pathophysiology and neurologic sequelae. *Pediatr Clin North Am* 23:541–556, 1976.

108. Feigin RD, et al: Prospective evaluation of treatment of *Hemophilus influenzae* meningitis. *J Pediatr* 88:542–548, 1976.

109. Feldman HA: Toxoplasmosis. *N Engl J Med* 279:1370–1375, 1431–1437, 1968.

110. Feldman WE: *Bacteroides fragilis* ventriculitis and meningitis: report of two cases. *Am J Dis Child* 130:880–883, 1976.

111. Fetter BF, et al: *Mycoses of the Central Nervous System.* Baltimore, Williams & Wilkins, 1967.

112. Finelli PF, et al: Whipple's disease with predominantly neuroophthalmic manifestations. *Ann Neurol* 1:247–252, 1977.

113. Firemark HM: Spinal cysticercosis. *Arch Neurol* 35:250–251, 1978.

114. Fiumara NJ, Lessell S: Manifestations of late congenital syphilis. *Arch Dermatol* 102:78–83, 1970.

115. Forno LS, Billingham ME: Allescheria boydii infection of the brain. *J. Pathol* 106:195–198, 1972.

116. Fraser RAR, et al: Spinal subdural empyema. *Arch Neurol* 28:235–238, 1973.

117. Freeman JW, Ziegler DK: Chronic meningitis caused by Sporotrichum schenckii. *Neurology* 27:989–992, 1977.

118. Friedman LL, Signorelli JJ: Blastomycosis: a brief review of the literature and a report of a case involving the meninges. *Ann Intern Med* 24:385–400, 1946.

119. Galatius-Jensen F, Uhm IK: Radiological aspects of cerebral paragonimiasis. *Br J Radiol* 38:494–502, 1965.

120. Gangarose EJ, et al: Botulism in the United States 1899–1969. *Am J Epidemiol* 93:93–101, 1971.

121. Garcia-Palmieri MR, Marcial-Rojas RA: The protean manifestations of schistosomiasis mansoni: a clinico-pathological correlation. *Ann Intern Med* 57:763–775, 1962.

122. Gerber HJ, et al: Chronic meningitis associated with Histoplasma endocarditis. *N Engl J Med* 275:74–76, 1966.

123. Ghatak NR, et al: Toxoplasmosis of the central nervous system in the adult: a light and electron microscopic study of three cases. *Arch Pathol* 89:337–348, 1970.

124. Gilden DH, et al: Central nervous system histoplasmosis after rhinoplasty. *Neurology* 24:874–877, 1974.

125. Gonyea EF: The spectrum of primary blastomycotic meningitis: a review of central nervous system blastomycosis. *Ann Neurol* 3:26–39, 1978.

126. Goodman JS, et al: Diagnosis of cryptococcal meningitis. Value of immunologic detection of cryptococcal antigen. *N Engl J Med* 285:434–436, 1971.

127. Gould SE, et al: Diagnostic patterns: Trichinella spiralis. *Am J Clin Pathol* 40:197–200, 1963.

128. Greenfield JG, Stern RO: Syphilitic hydrocephalus in the adult. *Brain* 55:367–390, 1932.

129. Greenwood RC, Voris HC: Systemic blastomycosis with spinal cord involvement. Case report. *J Neurosurg* 7:450–454, 1950.

130. Griponissiotis B: Hydatid cyst of the brain and its treatment. *Neurology* 7:789–792, 1957.

131. Groll A, et al: Immunological defect in Whipple's disease. *Gastroenterology* 63:943–950, 1972.

132. Gross RF, et al: Neonatal meningitis caused by *Citrobacter koseri. J Clin Pathol* 26:138–139, 1973.

133. Grossman J, Tompkins RL: Group B beta-hemolytic streptococcal meningitis in mother and infant. *N Engl J Med* 290:387–388, 1974.

134. Gruhn JG, Sanson J: Mycotic infections in leukemic patients at autopsy. *Cancer* 16:61–73, 1963.

135. Gwynn CM, George RH: Neonatal citrobacter meningitis. *Arch Dis Child* 48:455–458, 1973.

136. Haggerty RJ, Ziai M: Acute bacterial meningitis. *Adv Pediatr* 13:129–181, 1964.

137. Hale LM: Orbital-cerebral phycomycosis. Report of a case and a review of the disease in infants. *Arch Ophthalmol* 86:39–43, 1971.

138. Hameroff SB, et al: Cerebral phycomycosis in a heroin addict. *Neurology* 20:261–265, 1970.

139. Hand WL, Sanford JP: Posttraumatic bacterial meningitis. *Ann Intern Med* 72:869–874, 1970.

140. Harrell ER, Curtis AC: North American blastomycosis. *Am J Med* 27:750–766, 1959.

141. Harriman DGS: Bacterial infections of the central nervous system. In Blackwood W, Corsellis JAM (eds): *Greenfield's Neuropathology*, ed 3. London, Edward Arnold, 1976, pp 238–268.

142. Hart PD, Russell E Jr: The compromised host and infection. II. Deep fungal infection. *J Infect Dis* 120:169–191, 1969.

143. Hassin GB: Torulosis of the central nervous system. *J Neuropathol Exp Neurol* 6:44–60, 1947.

144. Hawking F, Greenfield JG: Two autopsies on Rhodesiense sleeping sickness: visceral lesions and significance of changes in cerebrospinal fluid. *Trans R Soc Trop Med Hyg* 35:155–164, 1941.

145. Healy GR: Babesia infections in man. *Hosp Pract* 14:107–111, 115–116, 1979.

146. Heathfield KWG: Neurosyphilis. *Br Med J* 1:765–766, 1968.

147. Hermos JA, et al: Fatal human cerebral coenurosis. *JAMA* 213:1461–1464, 1970.

148. Hoffman SF, Guthrie TH Jr: Cerebral cysticercosis. *South Med J* 68:105–108, 1975.

149. Hooshmand H, et al: Neurosyphilis. A study of 241 patients. *JAMA* 219:726–729, 1972.

150. Huang SN, Harris LS: Acute disseminated penicilliosis. Report of a case and review of pertinent literature. *Am J Clin Pathol* 39:167–174, 1963.

151. Hutter RV, et al: Aspergillosis in a cancer hospital.

Cancer 17:747–756, 1964.

152. Hutter RVT: Phycomycetous infection (mucormycosis) in cancer patients: a complication of therapy. *Cancer* 12:330–350, 1959.

153. Hyatt HW Sr: Coccidioidomycosis in a three-week-old infant. *Am J Dis Child* 105:93–98, 1963.

154. Ingham SD: Coccidioidal granuloma of the spine with compression of the spinal cord. *Bull Los Angeles Neurol Soc* 1:41–45, 1936.

155. Jackson IJ, et al: Solitary Aspergillus granuloma of the brain: report of 2 cases. *J Neurosurg* 12:53–61, 1955.

156. Jenkin VE, Postlewaite JC: Coccidioidal meningitis: report of four cases with necropsy findings in three cases. *Ann Intern Med* 36:1068–1084, 1951.

157. Johnson L, Diamond I: Cerebral Whipple's disease: diagnosis by brain biopsy. *Am J Clin Pathol* 74:486–490, 1980.

158. Johnstone HG, Jones OW Jr: Cerebral coenurosis in an infant. *Am J Trop Med* 30:431–441, 1950.

159. Jones SR, et al: Bacterial meningitis complicating cranial-spinal trauma. *J Trauma* 13:895–900, 1973.

160. Kaplan AM, et al: Cerebral abscesses complicating neonatal *Citrobacter freundii* meningitis. *West J Med* 127:418–422, 1977.

161. Kaplan JG, et al: Luetic meningitis with gumma: clinical, radiographic, and neuropathologic features. *Neurology* 31:464–467, 1981.

162. Karalakulasingam R, et al: Meningoencephalitis caused by Histoplasma capsulatum. Occurrence in a renal transplant recipient and a review of the literature. *Arch Intern Med* 136:217–220, 1976.

163. Kauffman CA, et al: Histoplasmosis in immunosuppressed patients. *Am J Med* 64:923–932, 1978.

164. Kaufman DM, et al: Central nervous system aspergillosis in two young adults. *Neurology* 26:484–488, 1976.

165. Kaya U, et al: Intracranial hydatid cysts: study of 17 cases. *J Neurosurg* 42:580–584, 1975.

166. Khuri-Bulos N: Meningococcal meningitis following rifampin prophylaxis. *Am J Dis Child* 126:689–691, 1972.

167. King H, Shumacker HB Jr: Splenic studies: susceptibility to infection after splenectomy performed in infancy. *Ann Surg* 136:239–242, 1952.

168. Klein RC, et al: Meningitis due to Sporotrichum schenckii. *Arch Intern Med* 118:145–148, 1966.

169. Knox DL, et al: Neurologic disease in patients with treated Whipple's disease. *Medicine* 55:467–476, 1976.

170. Kobayaski RM, et al: Cerebral vasculitis in coccidioidal meningitis. *Ann Neurol* 1:281–284, 1977.

171. Krumdieck N, Stevenson LD: Spinal epidural abscess associated with actinomycosis. *Arch Pathol* 30:1223–1226, 1940.

172. Kuberski T, Wallace GD: Clinical manifestations of eosinophilic meningitis due to *Angiostrongylus cantonensis.* *Neurology* 29:1566–1570, 1979.

173. Kuper S, et al: Internal hydrocephalus caused by parasitic cysts. *Brain* 81:235–242, 1958.

174. Lacaz CS: South American blastomycosis: a review. *Mycopathologia* 6:241–259, 1953.

175. Landells JW: Intra-medullary cyst of spinal cord due to cestode *Multiceps multiceps* in coenurus stage: report of a case. *J Clin Pathol* 2:61–63, 1949.

176. Langmaid C, Rogers L: Intracranial hydatids. *Brain* 63:184–190, 1940.

177. Latovitzki N, et al: Cerebral cysticercosis. *Neurology* 28:838–842, 1978.

178. Lavetter A, et al: Meningitis due to Listeria monocytogenes: a review of 25 cases. *N Engl J Med* 285:598–603, 1971.

179. LaVia MF, Hill RB: *Principles of Pathobiology*, ed 3. Oxford, England, Oxford University Press, 1980.

180. Leers W-D et al: Cerebellar abscess due to Blastomyces dermatitidis. *Can Med Assoc J* 107:657–660, 1972.

181. Lerner PI: Meningitis caused by *Streptococcus* in adults. *J Infect Dis* 131:S9–S16, 1975.

182. Levin S, et al: Pneumococcal meningitis: the problem of the unseen cerebrospinal fluid leak. *Am J Med Sci* 264:319–327, 1972.

183. Lewis W, Morgan AD: Actinomycosis of the brain. *J Neurol Neurosurg Psychiatry* 10:163–170, 1947.

184. Likhite VV: Immunology impairment and susceptibility to infection after splenectomy. *JAMA* 236:1376–1377, 1976.

185. Lincoln EM: Tuberculosis meningitis in children with special reference to serious meningitis. *Am Rev Tuberc* 56:75–94, 1947.

186. Littman ML, Walter JE: Cryptococcosis: current status. *Am J Med* 45:922–932, 1968.

187. Lombardo L, Mateos JH: Cerebral cysticercosis in Mexico. *Neurology* 11:824–828, 1961.

188. Long EL, Weiss DL: Cerebral mucormycosis. *Am J Med* 26:625–635, 1959.

189. Loudon RG, Lawson RA Jr: Systemic blastomycosis. Recurrent neurological relapse in a case treated with amphotericin B. *Ann Intern Med* 55:139–147, 1961.

190. Louria DB, et al: Disseminated moniliasis in the adult. *Medicine* 41:307–337, 1962.

191. Lundeberg KR: Fatal case of Chagas disease occurring in man 77 years of age. *Am J Trop Med* 18:185–196, 1938.

192. Lutwick LI, et al: Visceral fungal infections due to Petriellidium boydii (Allescheria boydii). *Am J Med* 61:632–640, 1976.

193. MacGregor RR, et al: Inhibition of granulocyte adherence by ethanol, prednisone and aspirin, measured with an assay system. *N Engl J Med* 291:642–646, 1974.

194. Macias Sanchez R, et al: Cisticercosis cerebral. Diagnóstico clínico, radiológico y de laboratorio, prognostico análisis de 186 casos. *Med Mex* 35:6–14, 1970.

195. MacLean LD, et al: Host resistance in sepsis and trauma. *Ann Surg* 182:207–217, 1975.

196. Maltby GL: Intracranial actinomycosis: report of unusual case. *J Neurosurg* 8:674–678, 1951.

197. Mangi RJ, et al: Gram-negative bacillary meningitis. *Am J Med* 59:829–836, 1975.

198. Manuelidis EE: Trypanosomal encephalitides. In Minckler J, et al (eds): *Pathology of the Nervous System.* New York, McGraw-Hill, 1972, vol 3, pp 2545–2559.

199. Manuelidis EE, et al: *Trypanosoma Rhodesiense* encephalitis: clinicopathological study of five cases of encephalitis and one of mel B hemorrhagic encephalopathy. *Acta Neuropathol* 5:176–204, 1965.

200. Margaretten W, et al: The effect of shock on the inflammatory response. A reevaluation of the role of platelets in the active arthus reaction. *Am J Pathol* 78:159–170, 1975.

201. Markell EK, Voge M: *Medical Parasitology*, ed 5. Philadelphia, WB Saunders, 1981, pp 182–183.

202. Marks MI, et al: Torulopsis glabrata—an opportunistic pathogen in man. *N Engl J Med* 283:1131–1135, 1970.

203. Martin FP, et al: Mucormycosis of the central nervous system associated with thrombosis of the internal carotid artery. *J Pediatr* 44:437–442, 1954.

204. McCracken GH Jr, Sarff LD: Current status and therapy of neonatal E. coli meningitis. *Hosp Pract* 9:57–64, 1974.

205. McCracken GH Jr, Sarff LD: Endotoxin in cerebrospinal fluid: detection in neonates with bacterial meningitis. *JAMA* 235:617–620, 1976.

206. McDonald R, et al: Cryptococcal meningitis. *Arch Dis Child* 45:417–420, 1970.

207. McDowell DE, et al: Cerebral abscess due to *Actinomyces israeli.* *South Med J* 58:227–230, 1965.

208. McKee EE: Mycotic infection of the brain with arteritis and subarachnoid hemorrhage: report of a case. *Am J Clin Pathol* 20:381–384, 1950.

209. Meinkowitz S, et al: Torulopsis glabrata septicemia. *Am J Med* 34:252–255, 1963.

210. Merriam JC Jr, Tedeschi CG: Cerebral mucormycosis. A fatal fungus infection complicating other diseases. *Neurology* 7:510–515, 1957.

211. Merritt H, et al: *Neurosyphilis.* New York, Oxford University Press, 1946.

212. Merritt HH, Springlova M: Lissauer's dementia paraly-

tica: a clinical and pathologic study. *Arch Neurol Psychiatry* 27:987–1030, 1932.

213. Meyers BR, et al: Candida endophthalmitis complicating candidemia. *Ann Intern Med* 79:647–653, 1973.

214. Meyers BR, et al: Rhinocerebral mucormycosis. Premortem diagnosis and therapy. *Arch Intern Med* 139:557–560, 1979.

215. Michal A, et al: Cerebral coenurosis. Report of a case with arteritis. *J Neurol* 216:265–272, 1977.

216. Mikhael NZ, et al: Toxocara canis infestation with encephalitis. *Can J Neurol Sci* 1:114–120, 1974.

217. Miller ME, et al: Lazy-leukocyte syndrome: a disorder of neutrophil function. *Lancet* 1:665–669, 1971.

218. Mims CA: The spread of microbes through the body. In: *The Pathogenesis of Infectious Diseases*. New York, Academic Press, 1977, pp 90–92.

219. Mineura K, Mori T: Sparganosis of the brain. Case report. *J Neurosurg* 52:588–590, 1980.

220. Mingde Q, Zhesheng H: Echinococcosis of the central nervous system. *Eur Neurol* 20:125–131, 1981.

221. Mirsky HS, Cuttner J: Fungal infection in acute leukemia. *Cancer* 30:348–352, 1972.

222. Miyazaki I: On the genus *Gnathostoma* and human gnathostomiasis with special reference to Japan. *Exp Parasitol* 9:338–370, 1960.

223. Mohandas S, et al: Aspergillosis of the central nervous system. *J Neurol Sci* 38:229–233, 1978.

224. Montgomerie JZ, Edward JE Jr: Association of infection due to Candida albicans with intravenous hyperalimentation. *J Infect Dis* 137:197–201, 1978.

225. Moore M, et al: Chronic leptomeningitis and ependymitis caused by probably U. zeae (corn smut). *Am J Pathol* 22:761–777, 1946.

226. Morningstar WA: Whipple's disease: an example of the value of the electron microscope in diagnosis, follow-up, and correlation of a pathologic process. *Hum Pathol* 6:443–454, 1975.

227. Mowat AG, Baum J: Chemotaxis of polymorphonuclear leukocytes from patients with diabetes mellitus. *N Engl J Med* 284:621–627, 1971.

228. Moxon ER, et al: The infant rat as a model of bacterial meningitis. *J Infect Dis* 136:S186–S190, 1977.

229. Moxon ER, Murphy PA: Haemophilus influenzae bacteremia and meningitis resulting from survival of a single organism. *Proc Natl Acad Sci USA* 75:1534–1536, 1978.

230. Musella RA, Collins GH: Cerebral chromoblastomycosis. Case report. *J Neurosurg* 35:219–222, 1971.

231. Myer RD, et al: Aspergillosis complicating neoplastic disease. *Am J Med* 54:6–15, 1973.

232. Myerowitz RL, et al: Disseminated candidiasis: changes in incidence, underlying diseases, and pathology. *Am J Clin Pathol* 68:29–38, 1977.

233. Nankervis GA: Bacterial meningitis. *Med Clin North Am* 58:581–592, 1974.

234. Nelson G: Current concepts in parasitology: Filariasis. *N Engl J Med* 300:1136–1139, 1979.

235. Nelson JD, et al: Histoplasma meningitis. Recovery following amphotericin B therapy. *Am J Dis Child* 102:218–223, 1961.

236. Nixon DW, Aisenberg AC: Fatal *Hemophilus influenzae* sepsis in an asymptomatic splenectomized Hodgkin's disease patient. *Ann Intern Med* 77:69–71, 1972.

237. Noguchi H, Moore JW: A demonstration of *Treponema pallidum* in the brain in cases of general paralysis. *J Exp Med* 17:232–238, 1913.

238. Norman DD, Miller ZR: Coccidioidomycosis of the central nervous system: a case of ten years' duration. *Neurology* 4:713–717, 1954.

239. Norman RM, et al: Neuropathological findings in a case of juvenile general paresis treated with penicillin. *Br J Vener Dis* 35:231–237, 1959.

240. Norman SH, Kreutner A Jr: Sparganosis: clinical and pathologic observations in ten cases. *South Med J* 73:297–300, 1980.

241. Obrador S: Cysticercosis cerebri. *Acta Neurochir* 10:320–364, 1962.

242. Oh SI: Cerebral paragonimiasis. *J Neurol Sci* 8:27–48, 1968.

243. Orr ER, Riley HD Jr: Sporotrichosis in childhood: report of ten cases. *J Pediatr* 78:951–957, 1971.

244. Ostrow PT, et al: Pathogenesis of bacterial meningitis. Studies on the route of meningeal invasion following *Hemophilus influenzae* inoculation of infant rats. *Lab Invest* 40:678–685, 1979.

245. Overall JC Jr: Neonatal bacterial meningitis. Analysis of predisposing factors and outcome compared with matched control subjects. *J Pediatr* 76:499–511, 1970.

246. Parker JC Jr, et al: Human cerebral candidosis: a postmortem evaluation of 19 patients. *Hum Pathol* 12:23–28, 1981.

247. Parker JC Jr, et al: Modifying cerebral candidiasis by altering the infectious entry route. *Arch Pathol Lab Med* 104:537–540, 1980.

248. Parker JC Jr, et al: Pathobiologic features of human candidiasis: common deep mycosis of the brain, heart, and kidney in the altered host. *Am J Clin Pathol* 65:991–1000, 1976.

249. Parker JC Jr, et al: The emergence of candidosis—the dominant postmortem cerebral mycosis. *Am J Clin Pathol* 70:31–36, 1978.

250. Pearl M, et al: Cerebral echinococcosis, a pediatric disease: report of two cases with one successful five-year follow-up. *Pediatrics* 61:915–920, 1978.

251. Perino FR, et al: Blastomicosis sudamericana: granuloma paracoccidioidico de localizacion pulmonar y cerebral. *Prensa Med Argent* 49:607–613, 1962.

252. Peter G, Smith DH: Hemophilus influenzae meningitis at the Children's Hospital Medical Center in Boston, 1958 to 1973. *Pediatrics* 55:523–526, 1975.

253. Petersdorf RG, Dale DC: Infections in the compromised host. In Thorn GW, et al (eds): *Harrison's Principles of Internal Medicine*, ed 8. New York, McGraw Hill, 1977, pp 764–770.

254. Petersdorf RG, et al: Studies on the pathogenesis of meningitis. II. Development of meningitis during pneumococcal bacteremia. *J Clin Invest* 41:320–327, 1962.

255. Phillips G: Primary cerebral hydatid cysts. *J Neurol Neurosurg Psychiatry* 11:44–52, 1948.

256. Phillips JA, et al: Letter: co-existing Guillain-Barré and visceral larva migrans syndromes. *Pediatrics* 44:142–143, 1969.

257. Pickett J, et al: Syndrome of botulism in infancy. Clinical and electrophysiologic study. *N Engl J Med* 295:770–772, 1976.

258. Pradatsundarasar A, et al: Sparganum-like parasite of the brain. *Southeast Asian J Trop Med Public Health* 2:578–579, 1971.

259. Preisler HD, et al: Serologic diagnosis of the disseminated candidiasis in patients with acute leukemia. *Ann Intern Med* 70:19–30, 1969.

260. Prockop LD, Silva-Hutner M: Cephalic mucormycosis (phycomycosis). A case with survival. *Arch Neurol* 17:379–386, 1967.

261. Rainey RL, Harris TR: Disseminated blastomycosis with meningeal involvement. Report of a patient cured by amphotericin B without resort to intrathecal administration. *Arch Intern Med* 117:744–747, 1966.

262. Rankin J, Javid M: Nocardiosis of the central nervous system. *Neurology* 5:815–820, 1955.

263. Raphael A, Pereira WC: Granuloma blastomicotico cerebral. *Rev Hosp Clin Fac Med Sao Paulo* 17:430–433, 1962.

264. Reddy PS, Satyendran OM: Ocular cysticercosis. *Am J Ophthalmol* 57:664–666, 1964.

265. Reeves DL, Baisinger CF: Primary chronic coccidioidal meningitis: a diagnostic neurosurgical problem. *J Neurosurg* 2:269–280, 1945.

266. Rich AR, McCordock HA: The pathogenesis of tuberculous meningitis. *Johns Hopkins Med J* 52:5–38, 1933.

267. Richardson PM, et al: Cerebral cryptococcosis in Malaysia. *J Neurol Neurosurg Psychiatr* 39:330–337, 1976.

268. Riley O Jr, Mann SH: Brain abscess caused by Clados-porium trichoides. Review of 3 cases and report of fourth case. *Am J Clin Pathol* 33:525–531, 1960.

269. Robinson RCV: Congenital syphilis. *Arch Dermatol* 99:599–610, 1969.

270. Robinson RG: Coenurosis of the central nervous system. *World Neurol* 3:35–42, 1962.

271. Robinson RG: Hydatid disease of the spine and its neu-rological complications. *Br J Surg* 47:301–306, 1959.

272. Roessmann U, Freide RL: Candidal infection of the brain. *Arch Pathol* 84:495–498, 1967.

273. Rose HD, Varkey B: Deep mycotic infection in the hospitalized adult: a study of 123 patients. *Medicine* 54:499–507, 1975.

274. Rosen L, et al: Eosinophilic meningoencephalitis caused by a metastrongylid lung-worm of rats. *JAMA* 179:620–624, 1962.

275. Rosen L, et al: Observations on an outbreak of eosino-philic meningitis on Tahiti, French Polynesia. *Am J Hyg* 74:26–42, 1961.

276. Rosenau W, Tsoukas CD: Lymphotoxin. A review and analysis. *Am J Pathol* 84:580–596, 1976.

277. Rosenbaum HA: Juvenile tabes dorsalis: a report of three cases. *Am J Dis Child* 35:866–871, 1928.

278. Ruebush TK II, et al: Human babesiosis on Nantucket Island: evidence for self-limited and subclinical infec-tions. *N Engl J Med* 297:825–827, 1977.

279. Ruebush TK II, et al: Neurologic complications following the treatment of human Babesia microti infection with diminazene aceturate. *Am J Trop Med Hyg* 28:184–189, 1979.

280. Ruskin J, Remington JS: Toxoplasmosis in the compro-mised host. *Ann Intern Med* 84:193–199, 1976.

281. Ruthe RC, et al: Efficacy of granulocyte transfusions in the control of systemic candidiasis in the leukopenic host. *Blood* 52:493–498, 1978.

282. Ryan GB: Inflammation and localization of infection. *Surg Clin North Am* 56:831–846, 1976.

283. Ryan GB, Majno G: Acute inflammation. A review. *Am J Pathol* 86:185–276, 1977.

284. Salles CA: Blastomyces (Paracoccidioides) brasiliensis in Africa. *Nature* 204:1211–1212, 1965.

285. Samiy E, Zadeh FA: Cranial and intracranial hydatidosis with special reference to roentgen ray diagnosis. *J Neu-rosurg* 22:425–433, 1965.

286. Sarosi GA, Davies SF: Blastomycosis. *Am Rev Respir Dis* 120:911–938, 1979.

287. Schlesinger JJ, et al: Streptococcal meningitis after mye-lography. *Arch Neurol* 39:576–577, 1982.

288. Schochet SS Jr, Lampert PW: Granulomatous enceph-alitis in Whipple's disease. Electron microscopic obser-vations. *Acta Neuropathol* 13:1–11, 1969.

289. Schulz DM: Histoplasmosis of the central nervous sys-tem. *JAMA* 151:549–551, 1953.

290. Seelig MS: Mechanism by which antibiotics increase the incidence and severity of candidiasis and alter the im-munological defenses. *Bacteriol Rev* 30:442–458, 1966.

291. Seelig MS: The role of antibiotics in the pathogenesis of Candida infections. *Am J Med* 40:887–917, 1966.

292. Selby R: Pachymeningitis secondary to Allescheria boy-dii. Case report. *J Neurosurg* 36:225–227, 1972.

293. Sell SHW, et al: Long term sequelae of Hemophilus influenzae meningitis. *Pediatrics* 49:206–211, 1972.

294. Shapiro K, Tabaddor K: Cerebral aspergillosis. *Surg Neurol* 4:465–471, 1975.

295. Shoemaker EH, et al: Leptomeningitis due to Sporotri-chum schenckii. *Arch Pathol* 64:222–227, 1957.

296. Shortland-Webb WR: Proteus and coliform meningo-encephalitis in neonates. *J Clin Pathol* 21:422–431, 1968.

297. Shuster M, et al: Brain abscess due to Nocardia. Report of a case. *Arch Intern Med* 120:610–614, 1967.

298. Siewers CMF, Cramblett HG: Cryptococcosis (torulosis) in children. A report of four cases. *Pediatrics* 34:393–400, 1964.

299. Siim JC: Acquired toxoplasmosis; report of 7 cases with strongly positive serologic reactions. *JAMA* 147:1641–1645, 1951.

300. Sinai RE, et al: Model of neonatal meningitis caused by Escherichia coli K1 in guinea pigs. *J Infect Dis* 141:193–197, 1980.

301. Singer C, et al: Bacteremia and fungemia complicating neoplastic disease: a study of 364 cases. *Am J Med* 62:731–742, 1977.

302. Sinh G, et al: The pathogenesis of unusual tuberculomas and tuberculous space-occupying lesions. *J Neurosurg* 29:149–159, 1968.

303. Smith DH, et al: Bacterial meningitis: a symposium. *Pediatrics* 52:586–600, 1973.

304. Smith ES: Purulent meningitis in infants and children: review of 409 cases. *J Pediatr* 45:425–436, 1954.

305. Smith JG Jr, et al: An epidemic of North American blastomycosis. *JAMA* 158:641–646, 1955.

306. Smith JW, Utz JP: Progressive disseminated histoplas-mosis. A prospective study of 26 patients. *Ann Intern Med* 76:557–565, 1972.

307. Smithers SR, Terry RJ: The immunology of schistoso-miasis. *Adv Parasitol* 14:399–422, 1976.

308. Snow RM, Dismukes WE: Cryptococcal meningitis. Di-agnostic value of cryptococcal antigen in cerebrospinal fluid. *Arch Intern Med* 135:1155–1157, 1975.

309. Sparks AK, et al: Sparaganosis. In Binford CH, Connor DH (eds): *Pathology of Tropical and Extraordinary Dis-eases*, ed 1. Washington, DC, Armed Forces Institute of Pathology, 1976, pp 534–538.

310. Sparling PF: Diagnosis and treatment of syphilis. *N Engl J Med* 284:642–653, 1971.

311. Spector WG: The macrophage: its origin and role in pathology. *Pathobiol Annu* 4:33–64, 1974.

312. Sprent JF: Observations on the development of Toxocara canis (Werner, 1782) in the dog. *Parasitology* 48:184–209, 1958.

313. Sproles ET III, et al: Meningitis due to Hemophilus influenzae. Long term sequelae. *J Pediatr* 75:782–788, 1969.

314. Stern WE: Neurosurgical considerations of cysticercosis of the central nervous system. *J Neurosurg* 55:382–389, 1981.

315. Stevens H: Actinomycosis of nervous system. *Neurology* 3:761–772, 1953.

316. Stone HH, et al: Candida sepsis: pathogenesis and prin-ciples of treatment. *Ann Surg* 179:697–711, 1974.

317. Stossel TP: How do phagocytes eat? *Ann Intern Med* 89:398–402, 1978.

318. Stossel TP: Phagocytosis. *N Engl J Med* 290:717–723, 774–780, 833–839, 1974.

319. Sudman NS: Prototheccosis: a critical review. *Am J Clin Pathol* 61:10–19, 1974.

320. Supena R, et al: Pulmonary alveolar proteinosis and No-cardia brain abscess. *Arch Neurol* 30:266–268, 1974.

321. Swanson VL: Gnasthostomiasis. In Marcial-Rojas RA (ed): *Pathology of Protozoal and Helminthic Diseases*. Baltimore, Williams & Wilkins, 1971, pp 871–879.

322. Swartz MN, Dodge PR: Bacterial meningitis: a review of selected aspects. I. General clinical features, special problems and unusual meningeal reactions mimicking bacterial meningitis. *N Engl J Med* 272:898–902, 1965.

323. Swartzwelder JC, et al: Sparaganosis in southern United States. *Am J Trop Med Hyg* 13:43–47, 1964.

324. Symmers WSC: A case of cerebral chromoblastomycosis (cladosporiosis) occurring in Britain as a complication of polyarteritis treated with cortisone. *Brain* 83:37–51, 1960.

325. Tandberg D, Reed WP: Blood cultures following rectal examination. *JAMA* 239:1789, 1957.

326. Tasker WG, Plotkin SA: Cerebral cysticercosis. *Pediat-rics* 63:761–763, 1979.

327. Tay CH, et al: Cryptococcal meningitis: its apparent increased incidence in the Far East. *Brain* 95:825–832, 1972.

328. Taylor RL: Sparganosis in the United States: report of

a case. *Am J Clin Pathol* 66:560–564, 1976.

329. Termini BA, Music SI: The natural history of syphilis: a review. *South Med J* 65:241–245, 1972.

330. Teutsch SM, et al: Babesiosis in post-splenectomy hosts. *Am J Trop Med Hyg* 29:738–741, 1980.

331. Todd RM, Neville JG: The sequelae of tuberculous meningitis. *Arch Dis Child* 39:213–225, 1964.

332. Torack RM: Fungus infections associated with antibiotic and steroid therapy. *Am J Med* 22:872–882, 1957.

333. Trelles JO: Cerebral cysticercosis. *World Neurol* 2:488–497, 1961.

334. White JC, et al: Cysticercosis cerebri: a diagnostic and therapeutic problem of increasing importance. *N Engl J Med* 256:479–486, 1957.

335. Truelle JL, et al: Cénurose cérébrale intraventriculaire. Etiologie rare de méningite chronique. *Nouv Presse Med* 3:1151–1153, 1974.

336. Tyler DE, et al: Disseminated protothecosis with central nervous system involvement in a dog. *J Am Vet Med Assoc* 176:987–993, 1980.

337. Udani PM, et al: Neurological and related syndromes in CNS tuberculosis. *J Neurol Sci* 14:341–357, 1971.

338. Uys CJ, et al: Endocarditis following cardiac surgery due to the fungus Paecilomyces. *S Afr Med J* 37:1276–1280, 1963.

339. van Bogaert L, Janssen P: Contribution à l'étùde de la neurologie et neuropathologie de la trypanosomiase humaine. *Ann Soc Belg Med Trop* 37:379–426, 1957.

340. Vanek J, Schwarz J: The gamut of histoplasmosis. *Am J Med* 50:89–104, 1971.

341. Wainwright J: Coenurus cerebralis and racemose cysts of the brain. *J Pathol Bacteriol* 73:347–354, 1957.

342. Ward PA: Leukotactic factors in health and disease. *Am J Pathol* 64:521–530, 1971.

343. Ward PA: Leukotaxis and leukotactic disorders: a review. *Am J Pathol* 77:520–538, 1974.

344. Warren KS: The immunopathogenesis of schistosomiasis: a multidisciplinary approach. *Trans R Soc Trop Med Hyg* 66:417–434, 1972.

345. Weinstein PP, et al: Angiostrongylus cantonensis infection in rats and rhesus monkeys, and observations on the survival of the parasite in vitro. *Am J Trop Med* 12:358–377, 1963.

345a. White JC et al: Cysticercosis cerebri: A diagnostic and therapeutic problem of increasing importance. *N Engl J Med* 256:479–486, 1957.

346. Wilbert SW, et al: Whipple's disease of the central nervous system. *Acta Neuropathol* 15:31–38, 1976.

347. Wilkinson CP, Welch RB: Intraocular toxocara. *Am J Ophthalmol* 71:921–930, 1971.

348. Wilkinson HA, et al: Central nervous system tuberculosis: a persistent disease. *J Neurosurg* 34:15–22, 1971.

349. Wilson SJ, et al: Chromoblastomycosis in Texas. *Arch Dermatol Syphilol* 27:107–122, 1933.

350. Witorsch P, Utz JP: North American blastomycosis: a study of 40 patients. *Medicine* 47:169–200, 1968.

351. Woese CR: Archaebacteria. *Sci Am* 244:98–122, 1981.

352. Wolf A, et al: Maduromycotic meningitis. *J Neuropathol Exp Neurol* 7:112–113, 1948.

353. Woodland LJ: Hydatid disease of vertebrae. *Med J Aust* 2:904–910, 1949.

354. Yardley JH, Hendrix TR: Combined electron and light microscopy in Whipple's disease. Demonstration of "bacillary bodies" in the intestine. *Bull Johns Hopkins Hosp* 109:80–98, 1961.

355. Yoshikawa T, et al: Infection and disseminated intravascular coagulation. *Medicine* 50:237–258, 1981.

356. Young LS, et al: *Nocardia asteroides* infection complicating neoplastic disease. *Am J Med* 50:356–367, 1971.

357. Young RC, et al: Aspergillosis: the spectrum of disease in 98 patients. *Medicine* 49:147–173, 1970.

358. Young RC, et al: Fungemia with compromised host resistance: a study of 70 cases. *Ann Intern Med* 80:605–612, 1974.

359. Zigmond SH, Hirsch JG: Leukocyte locomotion and chemotaxis. New methods for evaluation, and demonstration of a cell-derived chemotactic factor. *J Exp Med* 138:387–410, 1973.

360. Zweifach BW, et al: *The Inflammatory Process*, ed 2. New York, Academic Press, 1974.

CHAPTER 14

Viral Infections of the Nervous System

JAN E. LEESTMA, M.D.

INTRODUCTION

Viral infections of the nervous system form an important and diverse group of diseases, the history of which is also the history of modern virology. While diseases subsequently shown to be of viral etiology such as rabies and mumps were described clinically, often in great detail, in ancient times, it was not until 1892 that it was established by Ivanovski in Russia, that infectious agents existed which were smaller than bacteria and could pass through very fine filters. A remarkably modern concept of the virus was proposed by Beijerinck in 1898 on the basis of filtration and cultivation experiments using plant pathogens (136). It was not known at the time precisely what the infectious agents thus filtered were, although theories at the time suggested a toxic chemical or a very small bacterium (240). It became clear that viruses seemed to require living cells in which to multiply and could not be grown in simple media. Viruses, furthermore, had other strange properties, for example, the ability to form crystals when concentrated by extraction from infected tissues as in the case of polio virus. The development of the electron microscope finally allowed direct visualization of a variety of viral particles (136) and led to a system of classification still in use today, which is based largely upon viral morphology (198, 199). The development of modern nucleic acid chemistry and the advances in molecular biology catalyzed by the publication of the

structure of DNA by Watson and Crick in 1953 allowed the modern concept of the virus and its biology to be achieved.

Structure and Morphology of Animal Viruses

Viruses are now generally defined as infectious agents which contain nucleic acid of only one species, contain no organelles or a nucleus in the usual sense, do not grow by themselves or undergo fission, and lack the means of energy production or metabolism (184). The morphology of the viruses is variable, but there are many features which are basic to all viral agents regardless of type, as illustrated in typical RNA and DNA virions (Figs. 14.1 and 14.2).

All viruses contain a nucleic acid genome composed of one or more segments of double stranded RNA, "positive" or "negative" single stranded RNA, or single or double stranded DNA, but not both, which is usually associated with a small number of proteins forming a structural unit known as the nucleocapsid. The capsid, which encloses the nucleic acid, may take the form of a coiled helical structure formed by discrete complexes of proteins (capsomers), in the central spiral of which lies the nucleic acid strand, as in many of the RNA-containing viruses such as the para- and orthomyxovirus families. In others, such as the DNA-containing viruses of the *Herpesvirus* family, an icosahedral capsid is formed by hollow cylindrical capsomers which enclose a sphere of nucleic acid at its core, forming

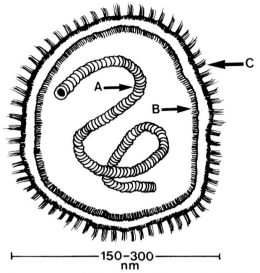

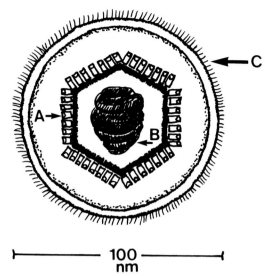

| 150–300 |
| nm |

| 100 |
| nm |

Figure 14.1. RNA virus. A virion typical of the myxoviruses (Ortho- and Paramyxoviridae families) 150–300 nm in diameter is schematically illustrated, showing (*A*) a portion of the helically wound, spaghetti-like protein capsid (composed of the so-called "P" and "NP" proteins) which enclose the RNA viral genome at its center. The entire structure is known as the nucleocapsid. The membranous envelope of the virion (*B* and *C*) encloses the nucleocapsid and contains inner envelope "M" viral proteins (*B*) and the outer envelope or outer spike "HN" and "F" glycoproteins (*C*). These various proteins have special functions during adsorption of the virus to the host cell, during the early phases of viral replication, and during budding or release of the virus from the infected cell.

Figure 14.2. DNA virus. A DNA virion typical of one of the herpesviruses (about 100 nm in diameter) is schematically illustrated, showing the capsid (*A*) composed of numerous cylindrical or prism-shaped protein capsomers arranged in an hollow, geometrical icosahedral shell which encloses the tightly compacted DNA genome of the virion (*B*). The membranous envelope (*C*) derived from the nuclear membrane of the host cell and containing several specific viral proteins encloses the particle.

the nucleocapsid unit. Some viruses may be naked or enclosed by envelopes derived from internal or external host cell membranes.

The locations of some of the more important viral proteins within the virion are illustrated in Figures 14.1 and 14.2. In some viruses, 20 or more proteins have been identified, but they generally fall into analogs of one of the following three groups: proteins associated with the nucleic acid core which form the viral capsid and may have polymerase activity; the submembranous or matrix proteins of the viral envelope which appear necessary for proper assembly and budding of the virion; or the "spike" glycoproteins associated with the external surface of the envelope (47, 55, 263). The functions of these proteins are only partly understood, but all are important in assem-

bly, release, and adsorption functions of the virion. The lack of one or more of these components may result in a modified viral particle which may behave in an unusual fashion in the host, giving rise to persistent, latent, slow, or abortive infections (112, 135, 168).

The morphology of the various classes of viruses is quite variable and when observed in whole-mount "negatively stained" or sectioned preparations under the electron microscope reveal an astonishing geometrical symmetry. Figure 14.3 illustrates some of general forms observed in the RNA viruses, and Figure 14.4 illustrates some of the forms observed in the DNA viruses.

Classification and Taxonomy of Animal Viruses

The classification of viruses is constantly changing and the subject of much scientific discussion. As an outgrowth of an early attempt to develop some standard of classification, the International Committee on

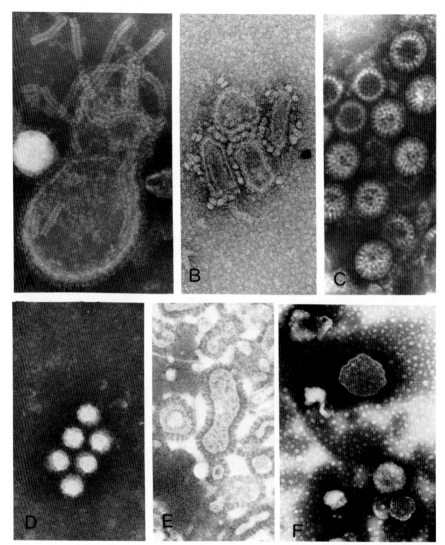

Figure 14.3. This figure depicts several RNA viruses as they appear in "negatively stained" transmission EM preparations. (*A*) A *Paramyxovirus* virion envelope is partially opened, and the helical nucleocapsid is spilling out. The appearance of this virion is also very similar to those seen in orthomyxoviruses. (Original magnification ×200,000.) (*B*) A cluster of vesicular stomatitis virus virions (*Rhabdovirus*, *Vesiculovirus* genus) displays the typical thimble-shaped particles seen in all members of this family. Sometimes tubular or extended thimble profiles are seen. (Original magnification ×150,000.) (*C*) A cluster of rotavirus virions illustrate the typical morphology of viruses of the *Reovirus* family. (Original magnification ×270,000.) (*D*) A group of six small *Enterovirus* virions illustrate the typical appearance of the picornavirus family, the smallest of the RNA viruses. (Original magnification ×256,000.) (*E*) A *Coronavirus* virion illustrates the irregular but generally rounded profile and the crown-like series of projections radiating about the outer membrane of the envelope of this family of agents. (Original magnification ×87,000.) (*F*) Lymphocytic chorio-meningitis virus, a representative of the Arenaviridiae group, illustrates the typical irregular shape and the granular or ribosome-like (sand-like) nucleocapsid from which these viruses derive their name. (Original magnification ×200,000.) (*A, C, D,* and *E,* Courtesy of Ms. Cynthia Howard. *B,* Courtesy of Dr. M. C. Dal Canto. *F,* From M. J. Buchmeier et al. (36a).)

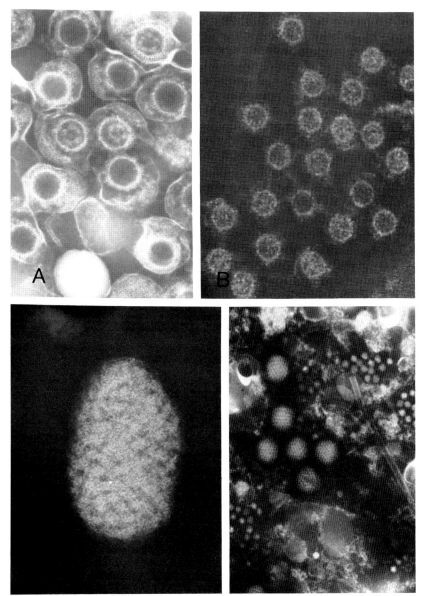

Figure 14.4. The morphology of some of the DNA viruses is illustrated in "negatively stained" transmission EM photographs. (A) Many cytomegalovirus particles within their envelopes illustrates the "spiked-ball" arrangements of capsomers about the icosahedral nucleocapsids. The images of other herpesviruses are very similar to those pictured here. (Original magnification ×118,000.) (B) A cluster of papovavirus particles illustrate the general morphology of this family of viruses. Capsomers can also be seen radiating outward from the nucleocapsid. (Original magnification ×215,000.) (C) The virus of molluscum contagiosum, a member of the *Poxvirus* family, displays many of the features of this group of very large DNA viruses. The morphology of other agents in this family, which may cause neurological diseases, varies somewhat from virus to virus, but all have many features in common. (Original magnification ×200,000.) (D) A group of *Adenovirus* virions appear amidst several much smaller but similarly shaped picornaviruses (enteroviruses) in a preparation from a stool specimen. The typical filamentous "pentons" which normally project from the facets of the adenoviruses cannot be seen in this plate. (Original magnification ×136,000.) (A–D, Courtesy of Ms. Cynthia Howard.)

Taxonomy of Viruses (ICTV) regularly holds workshops to update its scheme of classification. The results of these workshops are published regularly in the scientific journal, *Intervirology*, and in other publications (198, 199). Currently, viruses which affect vertebrates comprise 16 families and are divided into the RNA-containing viruses on the basis of those with cubic capsid symmetry, those with helical symmetry, and those with other forms of symmetry or morphology which is unknown; the DNA-containing viruses are separated into those which have cubic symmetry and a naked nucleocapsid, and those which have envelopes and/or complex coats. These groups are summarized in Tables 14.1 and 14.2. The otherwise unclassified or so-called unconventional agents do not fit well into this type of classification and will be discussed separately.

Characteristics of the Viral Infection

INITIATION AND SPREAD OF THE VIRAL INFECTION IN THE ORGANISM

Since viruses have no capacity for movement on their own they must be introduced into the host organism and ultimately to the target host cell by passive transfer in contaminated food, water, air, objects, or through traumatic introduction, as in an animal or insect bite, during a blood transfusion, injection, operation, or physical injury. For a virus to begin the process of cellular parasitism and infection it must come into contact with a living and susceptible host cell, such as the mucous membranes of the respiratory tract, gut, or urogenital tract. Once a receptive surface is reached the virus may enter the host cell

Table 14.1
The RNA Viruses[a]

Capsid symmetry	Character of virions	Capsid assembly	Site of envelopment	Diameter in nm	Family	Genus/subfamily
Cubic	Naked	Cytoplasm	None	24–30	Picornaviridae	Enterovirus Rhinovirus Cardiovirus Apthovirus
				60–80	Reoviridae	Orbivirus Reovirus Rotavirus
	Enveloped	Cytoplasm	Surface	40–70	Togaviridae	Alphavirus Rubivirus
			Cytoplasm	40–60		Pestivirus Flavivirus
Helical	Enveloped	Cytoplasm	Surface	80–120	Orthomyxoviridae	Influenzavirus
				150–300	Paramyxoviridae	Paramyxoviruses Pneumovirus Morbillivirus
				60 × 180	Rhabdoviridae	Vesiculovirus Lyssavirus
Unsym/?	Enveloped	Cytoplasm	Surface	100	Retroviridae	Lentiviruses Oncoviruses Spumaviruses
				50–300	Arenaviridae	Arenavirus
			Cytoplasm	80–130	Coronaviridae	Coronarvirus
				100	Bunyaviridae	Bunyavirus

[a] From J. L. Melnick (198).

Table 14.2
The DNA Viruses[a]

Capsid symmetry	Character of virions	Capsid assembly	Site of envelopment	Diameter in nm	Family	Genus/ subfamily
Cubic	Enveloped	Nucleus	Nuclear membrane	100	Herpesviridae	(unnamed)
		Cytoplasm	Surface	130	Iridoviridae	*Iridovirus*
Complex	Complex	Cytoplasm		230 × 300	Poxviridae	Orthopoxviruses Many others
Cubic	Naked	Nucleus	None	18–26	Parvoviridae	*Parvovirus* Adeno-associated *Densovirus*
				45–55	Papovaviridae	Papova A Papova B
				70–90	Adenoviridae	*Mastadenovirus* *Aviadenovirus*

[a] Modified from J. L. Melnick (198).

and begin the process of replication (47, 251).

There may be many phases of the viral infection, with replication occurring in several peripheral sites before a CNS infection begins. An example is poliovirus infection (28), where the primary infection probably occurs in the mucosa of the oropharynx and gut and is later spread to regional lymphoid tissues, such as the tonsils or Peyter's patches in the intestine where further replication takes place. A viremia may follow this phase of infection which then spreads the virus to other host cell tissues including the brain. During this phase, again as in poliovirus infection, virus may reach the nervous system in particulate form or within infected reticuloendothelial cells via the blood and enter the brain through the choroid plexus and the cerebrospinal fluid to be further disseminated within the brain (123). Virus particles may also enter the brain through areas in which the blood-brain barrier is incomplete or may be transported as particles across normal brain capillaries by a process of pinocytotic transfer within endothelial cells or by direct infection of endothelium and subsequent release into the interstitium of the brain (27). Infected inflammatory cells may also pass through the capillary and enter the brain interstitium and carry the infectious agent into vulnerable cells by this means (54, 270).

When viruses are traumatically introduced into the host they may infect local tissues primarily and then infect local lymphoid tissues secondarily. This leads to viremia and subsequent introduction into the central nervous system as described above. On the other hand, it has been shown in the laboratory that viruses such as rabies, herpes simplex, and vesicular stomatitis virus may enter the peripheral nervous system in a remote site and be transported into the central nervous system by passage along the peripheral nerve apparently within the perineural lymphatics, within Schwann cells, or within axoplasm by retrograde axoplasmic transport (167, 212, 247). Small branches of the trigeminal nerve in the cornea of the eye and about the mouth may also serve as a portal of entry to the CNS for viral agents such as herpes simplex (63, 167), as can the olfactory nerves in the nose for a variety of agents introduced experimentally by aerosols in the laboratory (203). Whether this latter mode is important clinically is debatable and in at least one instance, during the polio epidemics of the 1930s, led to a number of false assumptions concerning the pathogenesis of human infection (223).

Once a virus infection is established within the CNS subsequent propagation of the infection may proceed by a number of cellular mechanisms.

EXTRACELLULAR SPREAD

Infected glia or neurons may bud virions from their cell surfaces which are then released into the extracellular compartment, even though this space is very small. Whether there is significant transport of particles through this very constricted compartment is open to question, but immediate proximity to uninfected cells across the limited extracellular space undoubtedly allows spread to occur. This phenomenon has been illustrated ultrastructurally (174) for many viruses, including herpes simplex, togaviruses, and mumps viruses, and its validity supported by the fact that antibodies to a specific virus which can be found in the extracellular space can inhibit viral replication (1).

INTERCELLULAR SPREAD

Viruses may spread directly into adjacent cells in the CNS by a process of cell fusion or simple budding and immediate endocytosis in a neighboring cell perhaps via a junctional complex. This process can be observed quite distinctly in vitro where fusion of infected cells are common and cell to cell budding readily seen, as with agents such as herpes simplex and others (174).

INTRACELLULAR SPREAD

The special anatomy of the nervous system affords some unique means of viral transport within cells seen in no other organ system. Neuroplasmic transport is probably responsible for the spread of rabies virus (212), herpes viruses (63, 167), and probably other viruses within the processes of neurons to the cell soma or to a synaptic junction with an uninfected cell where the agent may bud and rapidly infect an adjacent cell (263). Transport in a similar manner within glial cells seems logical but has not been convincingly demonstrated (147).

INTRANUCLEAR SPREAD

When a primary viral genome or a DNA template of an RNA virus has been incorporated into the genome of the infected cell, as in the case of the retroviruses, the "virus" may be transmitted to progeny cells after mitosis and may later be activated or produce cytopathic effects. The importance of this process in the pathogenesis of CNS diseases is incompletely understood (147).

SPREAD BY SHEDDING AND FLUIDIC DISSEMINATION

Other means of virus spread within the CNS include propagation via the CSF, once virions are shed there from ependyma or choroidal epithelium, or via the extracellular space into the CSF (123). Secondary infection of inflammatory cells and "microglia" which are resident in the CNS may also disseminate viruses in the same manner as peripherally infected inflammatory cells (270).

The Process of Viral Replication

To begin the process of replication a viral particle must enter the host cell where the metabolic machinery of the host may be subjugated for viral synthesis. The initial process of virus-cell interaction is adsorption. So that adsorption may take place, the virus must have a surface chemistry and structure which is compatible with the host cell surface (47, 55). This compatibility implies some sort of receptor for a given virus, but it would be presumptuous to suppose that cells have specific receptors intended for viral attachment. Rather it seems probable that cell surface complexes which serve other receptor functions, such as for hormones, neurotransmitters, and other macromolecules, are coincidentally also potential sites for attachment of a virus (291).

When adsorption occurs as schematically illustrated in Figure 14.5, the virus may enter the cell by one of two processes: fusion of the viral envelope with the cell's plasma membrane followed by intrusion of the viral genome into the cytoplasm or endocytosis by the cell of the whole viral particle with subsequent transport of the virion into the cytoplasm within a vesicle (59, 82). The mechanisms which facilitate viral endocytosis and the means by which this process is induced by the enveloped myxoviruses, togaviruses, rhabdoviruses, oncornaviruses, or by the naked picornaviruses, reoviruses, papovaviruses, and adenoviruses are incompletely understood but probably involve complex interactions between the surface glycoproteins of the host cell and of the virion (47, 55, 251).

Once the virion is inside the cell a number of complex interactions between the cell

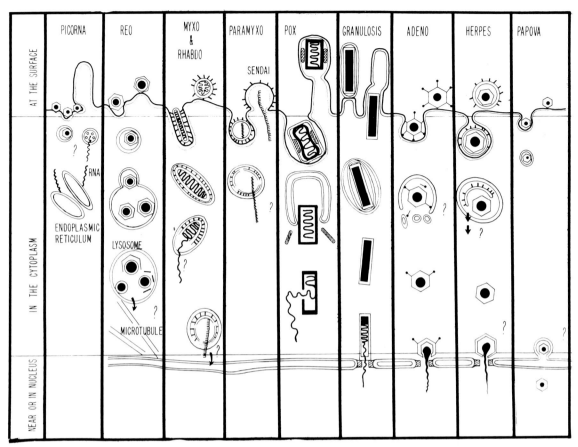

Figure 14.5. This diagram illustrates the process of adsorption, penetration, uncoating, and interaction with cellular components by several types of viruses. Some of the processes are not sufficiently well studied and hence are labeled with question marks. (From S. Dales (59).)

and virus must occur, or at any step viral replication may be interfered with. In the case of virions which enter by fusion, the viral genome is exposed and may promptly begin interaction with the synthetic machinery of the cell, but the endocytosed viruses must first be uncoated before synthetic interaction may occur. The process of uncoating may begin shortly after endocytosis by lysis of the enveloping vacuole (picorna-, toga-, myxo-, and rhabdoviruses), or by interaction of the viral envelope with the cell's vacuole membrane, or with subsequent cellular membrane interfaces during the process of transport to the cytoplasmic site of replication with RNA viruses, or to the cell's nucleus where the DNA viruses usually replicate. Reoviruses are unique, since they are transported to and uncoated by the lysosomes of the cell

where they are released into the cytoplasm (183).

Once the viral particle has been adsorbed and uncoated inside the cell, the initial events of replication occur. Depending upon the virus, the host cell's synthetic processes are partially or completely shut down by a series of mechanisms which are only partly understood.

In order for viral proteins to be synthesized, viral mRNAs must direct the process of translation, using the host cell's ribosomes to synthesize proteins. In the case of the "positive" stranded RNA viruses, such as the enteroviruses and the rhinoviruses, the viral genome may immediately interact with cellular ribosomes to translate viral proteins. Some of these proteins which are synthesized early in the infection facilitate replication of more viral RNA by initiating synthesis of "negative" or complementary RNA strands by their RNA-polymerase activity. These "negative" strands then act as templates for more "positive" or functioning viral mRNA which can further interact with cellular ribosomes or be packaged as progeny virions and released (109, 147).

Other RNA viruses, such as the picornaviruses, contain more complex RNA genomes, sometimes with RNA in several separate pieces, which perform the synthesis of "early" proteins, glycoprotein, and lipids, and facilitate synthesis of viral components in parallel with genome replication. Still other RNA viruses, such as the oncogenic RNA viruses (retroviruses), contain a double set of "positive" RNA strands as well as an RNA-dependent DNA polymerase which facilitates synthesis of a DNA copy of the viral genome (a provirus) which may become inserted into the host cell's genome and greatly modify its behavior and possibly induce neoplastic transformation (10, 147).

Some RNA viruses possess only a "negative" stranded genome, which is unable to direct translation at the ribosome until a "positive" strand is made. The rhabdovi-ruses, paramyxoviruses, and orthomyxoviruses typify this group. These viruses contain an RNA-dependent RNA transcriptase which catalyzes the formation of the required "positive" stranded RNA which can interact with the host's ribosomes to translate viral proteins (46).

Each of the RNA viral groups have developed their own sequences for virion assembly, but all generally employ typical host cell processes for synthesis and transport of viral protein, glycoprotein, and lipid components within endoplasmic reticulum or Golgi apparatus to the site of particle assembly, be it within the cytoplasm or at the cell surface where budding occurs. The process of viral assembly and release are highly complex, but some elements of the process are understood. The viral glycoproteins that interact with the lipids of the cell membrane which will ultimately form the viral envelope are crucial for alignment of other viral components and ultimate as-

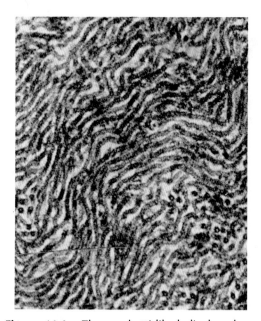

Figure 14.6. The spaghetti-like helical nucleocapsid material as yet unassembled into infectious particles in the disease, subacute sclerosing panencephalitis, lies within the infected glial cell nucleus. (Original magnification ×155,000.)

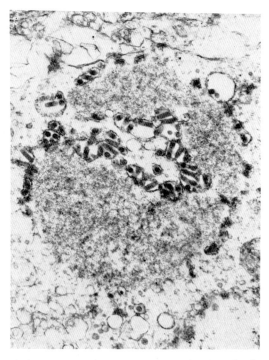

Figure 14.7. The composition of a Negri body in rabies illustrates the greater mass of unassembled viral material in the main granular mass, compared with the relatively few completed rod-like particles at the periphery in this cytoplasmic inclusion. (Original magnification ×28,000.) (From D. P. Perl (226).)

sembly and budding of the complete virion. Lack of a submembranous glycoprotein, the M protein of measles virus in SSPE, for example, appears to prevent proper transmembrane interactions with the surface or "spike" proteins. This distruption probably causes altered membrane fluidity, altered charge environment, or other dysfunctions, and prevents viral assembly (112, 263).

Viral assembly is not an efficient process and invariably results in accumulation of viral components in excess of which are ultimately released in completed form; thus, the cytoplasm or nucleus of an affected cell may contain excess amounts of RNA virus capsid material in the form of spaghetti-like masses of material, as in the paramyxoviral infections (Fig. 14.6), or in compacted masses of viral components forming cytoplasmic inclusions, as in rabies (Fig. 14.7) and VSV infections, or intranuclear inclusions, as in herpes simplex infections (Fig. 14.8). Some cells do not accumulate viral particles or components but either release completed virions as they develop (187), or cell death and lysis occurs releasing completed viruses and viral components into the environment, as in corona virus infections (241).

The DNA-containing viruses usually contain a double stranded DNA genome which replicates in the host cell nucleus to which it has been conveyed by intracellular transport after adsorption and uncoating. A sequence of events then occurs in which a number of so-called "early" proteins are synthesized from m-RNAs initially transcribed from the viral genome. Many of these "early" proteins serve to turn on host cell DNA synthesis and pave the way for viral DNA synthesis. Another family of proteins are synthesized after this initial phase of viral directed synthetic activity. These "late" proteins are mostly involved in forming the capsid of the virus, which are usualy assembled in the host cell nucleus (215). When the completed nucleocapsid approaches the nuclear membrane (Fig. 14.9) to which has been transported the envelope proteins, budding from the nuclear membrane occurs, as illustrated with herpes simplex virus (174). The complete viral particle is then usually transported within a cytoplasmic vesicle to the cell surface, where the vesicle fuses with the membrane releasing the particle by exocytosis.

This process is essentially the same for the papovaviruses, adenoviruses, and herpes viruses, all of which can show inefficient production of virions and buildup of apparently excess components in the form of intranuclear inclusion bodies which may have a paracrystalline structure (Fig. 14.8). In the course of replication, it is not uncommon for noninfectious defective particles to be produced which lack a nucleocapsid or other important structures. These defective particles may play a role in modifying the course of a viral infection and may interfere with it.

The only DNA-containing viruses which do not assemble their particles in the cell nucleus are the pox viruses, which accomplish this function in the cytoplasm after the genome has been replicated in the cell nucleus. Viral assembly occurs in zones within the cytoplasm often referred to as "viral factories." Completed particles are released periodically, but eventually the affected cell lyses, releasing all other completed particles and left-over debris (151).

INTERRUPTIONS OR ALTERATION IN VIRAL REPLICATION

Once a viral infection has occurred there are a number of events which may modify or halt the continued replication and spread of the infection. These include the formation of mutant viruses or defective interfering particles (135). As previously mentioned, the viral replicative process is inherently inefficient, with some viruses more inefficient and unstable than others. For example, herpes simplex virus infections frequently produce large numbers of noninfectious defective particles, which may be able to adsorb to an adjacent noninfected cell and interfere with subsequent entrance of an infectious virus. These are often referred to as deletion mutants, since only portions of the genome have been assembled into their nucleocapsid and thus cannot direct replication of a complete particle, resulting in a self-limited infection if sufficient numbers of these particles are produced. Sometimes this incomplete viral infection can be overcome when another "helper" virus is present, which provides the lacking genetic information and allows

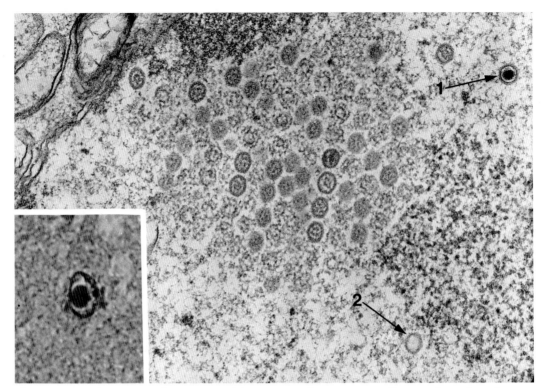

Figure 14.8. A paracrystalline array of herpes simplex virions is illustrated in this electron micrograph of an intranuclear Cowdry type A inclusion body (seen in light microscopy) (Inset, Original magnification ×5000. H&E). Virions are in various stages of assembly and are surrounded by a granular mass of viral and host cell materials near the nuclear membrane of an infected glial cell in an organized CNS tissue culture preparation. Note that some particles are empty, lacking a nucleic acid core (*arrow* 1), while some others are apparently complete (*arrow* 2), but these particles are in the minority. (Original magnification ×60,000.) (From J. E. Leestma et al. (174).)

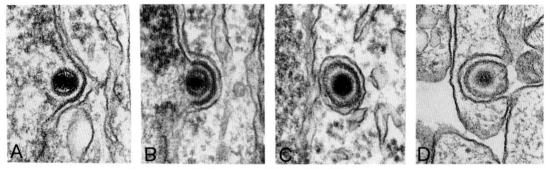

Figure 14.9. (*A–D*) Sequence of virion assembly and budding in experimental herpes simplex virus infection. A completed "naked" virion (*A*, Original magnification ×80,000) approaches the nuclear membrane, which has undergone modification and probably contains viral proteins, and begins the process of budding (*B*, Original magnification ×80,000) into the cytoplasm of the host cell (*C*, Original magnification ×75,000). At this point the virion contains two membranous envelopes as it traverses the cytoplasm. As it buds out of the cell into the extracellular space (*D*, Original magnification ×60,000), the outer membrane is incorporated into the cell surface and the particle is again enveloped by a single membrane. (From J. E. Leestma et al. (174).)

a full-blown infection to proceed as in ad-enovirus-SV 40 interactions (231) where recombination or hybridization occur. Sometimes nongenetic interactions of two viruses can occur in which viral products interact to produce a modified infection or production of virions with protein but not genetic components of the other. This same intermixing of nongenetic components can occur between viral and host proteins and resulting also in modified viral particles and possibly a modified viral infection.

Another form of mutation is the conditional lethal mutant, which is characteristically a temperature-sensitive (Ts) mutation. In this instance a mutation in the viral genome produces proteins which apparently suffer an altered conformation in a higher than normal temperature environment and fail to function. The temperature rise needed is sometimes only a degree or two Celsius above the normal or optimal replicative temperature, easily within the range of febrile responses in some animals. A number of these Ts mutants occur amongst most viral groups, especially in the herpesviruses, picornaviruses, reoviruses, rhabdoviruses, papovaviruses, parainfluenza viruses, and vesicular stomatitis virus where extensive use is made of them in experimental neurovirology as models for latency or persistence in the nervous system (57, 58), but their role in human diseases has not been proven.

VIRAL TROPISM

Tissue tropism in viral infections is a well-known phenomenon, but the mechanisms of cellular resistance and tropism are still poorly understood. It is possible to adapt an apparently nonneurotropic virus to a CNS environment by means of serial blind passage, in which usually a suckling animal is inoculated intracerebrally with a viral suspension. After some days or weeks, even though there is no evidence of viral infection in the host, its brain is homogenized and inoculated into another suckling animal. This process is repeated several times until neurotropism occurs. This process has been used to neuroadapt herpes simplex, measles virus, and other agents in the experimental laboratory (138).

Just as the brain may not be a suitable environment for natural replication of a virus, there may be some selectivity within the brain or other tissue of certain cells which will support a viral infection and others which will not (148). There may also be considerable species difference observable experimentally. The basis for this selectivity is not clear, but the importance of cellular tropism in CNS viral infection is clearly illustrated by the J-C and SV 40 viruses of progressive multifocal leukoencephalopathy (PML), which produce mostly white matter pathology by destroying oligodendrocytes (306) and by the polioviruses which affect only neurons but almost exclusively those comprising the motor system (28).

VIRAL PERSISTENCE

The phenomenon of viral persistence or "slow" expression or incubation, especially in the nervous system, has been recognized for many years, although it has been increasingly demonstrated as an important pathogenetic mechanism only in recent years (110, 261). The phenomenon is illustrated by the demonstration of an infectious agent by patient observations for long periods of time of animal inoculations, as in scrapie and kuru (182), and by sophisticated cocultivation methods which yield the viruses of PML (220) and of so-called "latent" herpes simplex virus from trigeminal ganglia obtained at autopsy from individuals who presumably had had prior herpetic infections (11).

Other examples of human disease in which a virus may be persistent with or without pathological effects on the infected cells include subacute sclerosing panencephalitis (SSPE), some infections with measles and rubella viruses in the young, cytomegalovirus infection, infectious mononucleosis (E-B virus), and herpes zoster. Jakob-Creutzfeldt disease and its variants or related conditions also certainly qualify as examples of persistent infection but with so-called unconventional agents. In animals, Sendai virus (paramyxovirus) (168), rabies (212), the arboviruses (1), visna (261), Mink encephalopathy (185), and lactic dehydrogenase-elevating virus (187) would be examples. There are certainly more examples of this phenomenon which exist or remain to be discovered in both man and animals.

Some of these infections should be considered latent or eclipsed infections, capable of reactivation, while others are chronic low-grade infections in which viral replication continues but without many symptoms, as in hepatitis B virus in man and lactic dehydrogenase-elevating virus in mice (187). Other infections are considered "slow" infections in which very long periods of time are required for the infection to show its presence or produce disease.

The importance of the latency phenomenon is that a viral agent may exist without causing obvious pathology but at some time may directly or indirectly induce degenerative changes in response to a variety of stimuli in the affected cells or their cellular extensions with or without obvious viral replication occurring. This mechanism has been hypothesized and extensively studied for multiple sclerosis and some of the degenerative neurological diseases, including Alzheimers disease, as yet without success.

There are many mechanisms of viral persistence which have been suggested and which have been demonstrated, some by processes already mentioned above, i.e., production of defective interfering particles (135), production or recombinant viral strains or hybrid viruses which are incomplete in some vital way but which remain in a dormant or nascent state (231), alterations in tissue or cellular tropisms by a variety of means, and mutation of the virus to a form which can replicate only under special conditions of temperature (58). Other possible mechanisms involve special or altered immunological interactions between host and the infected cell, which either inhibit viral release and propagation or allow some degree of continual viral production. There may be an insufficient or absent cellular or humoral immune response (166) to the virus as in scrapie or cytomegalovirus and other agents in acquired immune deficiency syndrome (AIDS) (141). On the other hand, a virus may be shielded from immune attack or even detection by direct cell-to-cell spread, as can be seen in herpes simplex virus infection (1). Furthermore, a viral agent may be capable of considerable antigenic plasticity, as in the case of enteroviruses and rhinoviruses (109), where by means of mutation and/or recombination the antigens presented to the host are constantly varying ahead of the host's abilities to inactivate them. It is also possible that the immune response generated by the host does not neutralize the infectious agent, as in the case of lactic dehydrogenase-elevating virus and hepatitis B, allowing it to continue to replicate unhindered and to possibly produce a disease caused by immune complexes (218).

There are other, nonimmunologic, host-viral interactions which may be responsible for viral persistence or latency; these include modification of viral replication by interferon (12). Such a modification may result in incomplete synthesis of key viral proteins which may cause impaired assembly, release, or blunted immune attack. Furthermore, it may be the inherent property of some viruses, for whatever reason, to fail to synthesize all the proteins needed for complete assembly of the virion. This mechanism has been suggested to explain persistence in SSPE, where there is a lack of the "M" protein as mentioned above (112). A similar lack of synthetic ability in experimental Sendai virus infection for the HN and F (hemagglutination-neuraminidase and fusion) glycoproteins at the cell surface may account for prolonged persistence in the brain of this virus (168).

Immunity and Host Defense against Viral Infection

ELEMENTS OF THE IMMUNE SYSTEM

Most immunologically competent hosts infected with a neurotropic virus will mount an immune response to one or more of the various components of the virus during the course of infection. Antibodies produced in response to a viral infection prevent subsequent viral infection and probably facilitate the clearing from the CNS of the agent by several means (284). Antibody production in connection with CNS viral infections is probably entirely systemic, since there is apparently no significant ability of lymphoid elements within the CNS to mount a separate or individual immunologic response, but controversy surrounds this point (147, 282).

Macrophages

At the initial phase of a viral infection, after early replication at some remote site, followed by an infection in the CNS, viral products may be presented to the reticuloendothelial system in the course of cell lysis and death or during a viremic episode. In tissue, macrophages, and in the blood, monocytes are the earliest and most important cellular element in the complex chain of events which follow exposure of the host for the first time to an infectious agent. In the brain, macrophages[77] play an important role in host defense and are mostly derived from blood-borne monocytes, but some undoubtedly arise from either "resting" cells in blood vessel walls or from the so-called microglial cells, the origin and nature of which are still being debated[228].

By means of an incompletely understood process, the macrophage "processes" material that has bound to its surface or been phagocytosed, concentrates this material, and eventually presents this antigenic material to lymphoid cells once it has left the CNS and has reached a regional lymph node, spleen, or other lymphoid organ. The macrophage, by its interaction with the cell surfaces of the T (thymus-derived) and B (bone marrow- or "bursa"-derived) lymphocytes, and the lymphocytes, by their interactions, determine what sort of immunological reaction will follow[245]. Each of the types of lymphoid cells involved in the immune reaction makes specific contributions to the host response (72).

Lymphocytes

T-Lymphocytes. These thymus-dependent lymphoid cells do not apparently synthesize detectable amounts of immunoglobulins and can be classified into two populations, regulators and effectors. The regulator T lymphocytes include the "helper" and the "suppressor" types which modulate the responses of other T lymphocytes, B lymphocytes, and even macrophages. The effector T lymphocytes are involved in delayed hypersensitivity reactions, mixed lymphocyte reactions, and in cytotoxic or "killer" functions (specific killer and natural killer cells) (4, 56).

B-Lymphocytes. These bone marrow-dependent cells are probably initially activated by the macrophages in concert with the regulator T cells to begin the process of proliferation and eventual differentiation to B-derived plasma cells, which account for most of the humoral antibody produced in response to infection. The precursor B cells become plasma cells and secrete one of the five forms of immunoglobulins: IgM, IgG, IgA, IgD, and IgE. The precursor B cells which will make only one of these globulins are identified as B μ, B γ, B α, B δ, and B ϵ cells, respectively. B cells have been classified into those which are precursors (as above) and those which possess a "memory" of a given antigen and are important in the rapid development of an antibody upon a second exposure to a given antigen. There may also be a class of B cells which function in a regulatory role, but these cells are not yet well understood (72).

Immunoglobulins. Immunoglobulins synthesized by B cell-derived plasma cells (292) contain at least one basic unit, or monomer, composed of four polypeptide chains: two H (heavy) chains which occur in five types, with molecular weights between 50,000 and 70,000; two L (light) chains, which occur in two types, κ and λ, both with 23,000 molecular weight. Each H and L chain has a C (constant) and V (variable) region. Within these regions are "domains," such as the so-called Fab and Fc units which constitute the active and specific sites for interaction with cell surfaces. In those immunoglobulins which are polymeric, there are two forms of "extra" polypeptide chains which interact with H and L chains to make up the immunoglobulin molecule: the J chain, with a molecular weight of 15,000 and a "secretory" component with a molecular weight of 70,000 found in IgA globulins.

IgM. These immunoglobulins constitute about 10% of serum globulins and exist normally as a pentamer of 900,000 (19S) molecular weight. They commonly bind to the surface of B cells and are important in the early immune response (20–30 h after antigenic stimulation), acting as a very efficient complement-fixing immunoglobulin. IgM has a half-life of about 5 d and a turnover rate of about 15% per day in serum.

IgG. This, the most important immuno-

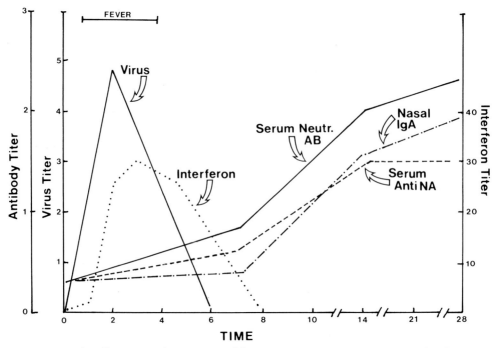

Figure 14.10. This illustration depicts typical host responses to an experimental influenza viral infection in a human volunteer, but the events are very similar to many other viral infections. There is a rise in virus production, peaking at about day 2–3 (intranasal virus titers in log units, TCID 50/ml), closely accompanied by a rise in interferon production (in units per milliliter). The febrile response roughly parallels virus production and falls at about the time serum-neutralizing antibody begins to rise by about day 6 postinfection (antibody titer in log dilutions). The intranasal antibody (most likely IgA) and serum antineuraminidase (AntiNA) all rise in a similar fashion and remain at either an increasing or static level at least a month after infection. (From S. Baron et al. (12).)

globulin, comprises 75% of serum globulin and exists as a monomer of molecular weight 150,000 (6–7S). There are four classes of IgG which have varying half-lives and rates of synthesis, as well as different abilities to fix complement, reside on the surface of "armed" macrophages, and cross the placenta to confer immunity to the developing fetus. In the CSF, IgG is present in low concentration normally (less than 0.5% of serum level) but may increase in response to infection. An illustrative example of immune responses to a model virus infection is depicted in Figure 14.10. In general, the half-life of IgG is about 21 d with a turnover rate of about 7% per day. A significant level of IgG appears in serum about 4 d after antigen exposure, falls slightly at first, then rises to a maximum at about day 8–10, where it remains for variable periods of time, even many months (12). Sometimes specific IgG titers following CNS infection may persist for protracted periods of time and actually be higher than in serum. This phenomenon may be explained by in situ IgG synthesis by a restricted "oligoclonal" population of plasma cells which migrated into the CNS preferentially or arose by transformation and differentiation from B cells resident in the CNS (282, 284).

IgA. The IgAs are dimeric molecules, with a molecular weight of 160,000 (7S) and account for 15% of the total immunoglobulins in serum. They have an important protective role in glandular secretions such as milk, sweat, nasal mucus, and saliva, where they prevent entrance of foreign antigens through epithelial surfaces. Specific IgA appears in serum at the same time as IgG. Its CSF concentration and its turnover rate are also similar.

IgD. IgD is a monomer of about 180,000 (7–8S) molecular weight and exists only in trace amounts in serum. Its turnover is very rapid, approaching 40% per day in serum, but its function is not yet clear.

IgE. IgE is a monomer of about 190,000

(8S) molecular weight, is also present in trace amounts in serum, and is very important in the mediation of allergic reactions by stimulating the release of histamine and other chemical mediators of the inflammatory response from mast cells. It has the highest turnover rate and the lowest rate of synthesis of any of the immunoglobulins. Its role in CNS infections is probably minimal.

The Complement System. An important part of the immune reaction, the complement system acts in concert with immunoglobulins at cell surfaces to lyse and inactivate infectious agents and to mobilize phagocytic and other cells. The system consists of at least 20 serum proteins designated C1, C2, ... C9, factor B and D, properdin, and by other names. The system is activated in a cascade-like sequence, much like the coagulation reactions, in order to function. There are two pathways by which this activation occurs, the "classic" pathway and the "alternate" pathway. In the "classic" pathway, IgG and IgM globulins (but not IgA, IgD, IgE, or IgG$_4$ subclass), as well as C reactive protein, DNA, and other molecules are active in binding to complement C1 and initiating the cascade of activation reactions which enable the conversion of C5 and subsequent complement factors to result in lytic reactions at a cell surface. The "alternate" or properdin pathway is activated by IgA, some IgGs, and by some polysaccharides and trypsin-like enzymes, and leads to activation of the more direct C5–C9 conversions as above and subsequent membrane interactions, usually resulting in lysis. The control of these reactions is complex and still under study (12, 230).

Lymphokines. These substances facilitate phagocytosis, migration, and attraction of both T and B cells to the site of infection and assist in cellular-antigen reactions (12). These and other substances may modulate or even prevent cytotoxicity by T cells, as well as regulate the function of B cells and macrophages (84).

Interferons. A special group of proteins which can function as lymphokines but which have many important and potent antiviral properties are the interferons, first described by Isaacs and Lindenmann in 1957 (140). These low molecular weight polypeptides, with molecular weights from at little as 2100 to 38,000, are secreted by lymphoid cells, fibroblasts, epithelial and other cells in response to polynucleotides, endotoxins, and viruses (type I interferons) and by antigens and antigen-antibody complexes (type II interferons) (127). Interferons have an inhibitory or potent antiviral action against virtually every known virus (Fig. 14.11). They act by regulating or modulating the function of specific killer T cells, natural killer T cells, and macrophages (12), and by interacting with cellular synthetic machinery to inhibit viral replication (12, 150). Proposed mechanisms of this latter action include: inhibition of viral messenger RNA but not cellular RNA translation; induction of nucleases, phosphorylases, and proteases which facilitate the hydrolysis of key viral products; and interaction with cell membranes and cisternal structures to prevent viral entry, proper assembly, or release (12, 150). While interferons have a broad spectrum of inhibition against all viruses, they are not always produced in the same quantity in response to a given viral infection. Potent inducers of interferon are the paramyxoviruses, reoviruses, herpes viruses, adenoviruses, and poxviruses.

VIRAL-IMMUNE INTERACTIONS

There are many mechanisms by which the immune system interacts with the virus itself or the virus-infected cell to limit or halt the infectious process. Most of the processes discussed below have been extensively studied in vitro but probably also operate in the tissues of living animals, including the brain.

The most important virus-host defense is the direct virus-antibody reaction between antibodies of the IgG, IgM, and IgA classes (264). In vitro and probably also in vivo, these immunoglobulins can specifically neutralize the infectivity of all known viruses and hence are referred to as *neutralizing antibodies.* The precise mechanism by which antibody neutralizes a virus is not understood, but binding between an immunoglobulin and some surface component of the virus prevents further replication of the virus, probably by interfering with subsequent adsorbtion, penetration, or intracellular uncoating of the particle (12). Some

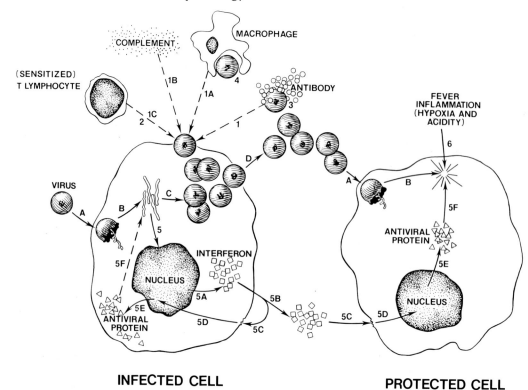

Figure 14.11. Many of the host defenses against viral infection are symbolically depicted in this illustration. Extracellular defenses include antibody (3) and macrophages (4) which may act together to inactivate a virus. Intracellular defenses which interfere with viral replication include cytolysis of infected cells by T-lymphocytes (2) acting alone or in concert with other cells or factors, such as: "armed" macrophages (1A), antibody plus complement (1B), antibody plus T-lymphocytes (1C), and antibody plus "killer" T-lymphocytes (not shown). Additional inhibition of viral replication can be affected by nonspecific defenses such as: interferon (5–5F), local pH alterations and hypoxia (6), defective interfering particles (not shown), and nonpermissive, temperature-dependent phenomena. (From S. Baron et al. (12).)

of these mechanisms are illustrated in Figure 14.11. The effects of this type of immunity may be local, in that serum IgG antibody may have no effect in preventing entrance of a virus across a mucosal surface, where a specific IgA would be most effective. Furthermore, antibodies may exist against a vital viral enzyme, such as neuraminidase which apparently functions in the release of virions from an infected cell. These antibodies apparently interfere with release and limit infection but have no neutralizing action against a virus once released (263, 264). Some instances of virus neutralization are facilitated by an interaction with complement in which viral coat lipoproteins may be sufficiently altered to interfere with subsequent replication. There may be special "complement fixing" antibodies produced in response to infection which can be employed in the laboratory for diagnosis (230).

While it has been extensively studied in vitro, complement-facilitated cell lysis in concert with immunoglobulins in vivo is less well studied, and its importance in host resistance at present is obscure. Nevertheless, complement-facilitated cell lysis probably operates by producing a small hole of submicroscopic size in the cell membrane through which water and electrolytes rush, resulting in bursting of the cell. The net result of this lysis is that cell components and viral products, complete or not, are exposed to specific immunoglobulins and may either be inactivated directly or phagocytosed (230).

Upon occasion, an antibody-viral reaction may stimulate or facilitate phagocytosis and subsequent lysosomal degradation of the viral particle by a macrophage or other phagocytic cell. This process is called opsonization and is more clearly appreciated in bacterial infections with agents like the pneumococcus (301).

In addition to, but also apart from immunoglobulin and complement-mediated immune reactions, there are a series of complex immune reactions involving T and B cells, as well as macrophages generally referred to as cell-mediated reactions. These reactions are primarily directed toward viral infected cells whose cell membranes contain viral material or viral induced "foreign" or embryonic antigens. When viral or other "foreign" antigens are presented to the surfaces of T-cells by macrophages, the antigen may act as a mitogen or it may induce other changes in T cell function, activating some cells to function as "killer" cells which can act alone or with other affector T cells (helpers or supressors) to bring about lysis of infected cells (4, 72, 245). Some T cells may also be stimulated to release lymphokines which activate and attract other lymphoid cells into the immune reaction.

GENERAL PATHOLOGICAL FEATURES OF CNS VIRAL INFECTIONS

Infections due to viral agents in the nervous system may manifest themselves in a variety of ways not always obvious in terms of classical inflammatory reactions in the affected tissues, atlhough this is usually the case. Most of the noninflammatory reactions caused by viruses have only relatively recently been appreciated and include in addition to the neoplastic reaction, apparently degenerative processes, demyelination, production of malformations, and alterations of development.

Inflammatory and Tissue Reactions

The classical viral induced inflammatory reactions in the meninges are usually referred to as meningitis, in the brain substance as encephalitis, in the spinal cord as myelitis, in nerves, as neuritis, in vessels, as vasculitis, and in the ependyma, as ependymitis or ventriculitis. Any given infection may involve one or more of the general regions of the nervous system, but may confine itself primarily to the grey matter of the spinal cord where as a generic term it is known as a poliomyelitis. When the same process occurs in the cerebrum it can be referred to as a polioencephalitis. When the white matter is primarily affected, the process is a leukoencephalitis, or if it is diffuse, panencephalitis. In fact, most viral infections are not strictly localized and generally involve both meninges and portions of the brain or spinal cord (meningoencephalitis or meningomyelitis).

The gross pathology of the classical inflammatory viral infection is highly variable, ranging from virtually no gross pathological change, as in some of the arboviral encephalitides or in rabies, to a localized necrotizing or hemorrhagic infection, as in herpes simplex encephalitis, to a rampant hemorrhagic-necrotizing, or congesting edema-producing process involving the whole brain in which the brain is congested and swollen as in some cases of herpes simplex or a few of the arboviral encephalitides. In some cases where the victim has been sustained on a respirator and associated with massive brain swelling and herniation, the "respirator brain" phenomenon may overshadow the inherent viral pathology entirely, revealing only a necrotic, nearly liquid brain. Most encephalitides, however, produce some degree of cerebral edema, congestion of meningeal vessels, possibly focal petechial hemorrhage or congestion in the grey or white matter, or other small focal lesions which may be subtle on the cut surface of the fixed specimen. Some infections show localized pathological changes, such as epidemic poliomyelitis in the acute stage where a hemorrhagic-necrotic lesion is confined to the grey matter of the cord, and herpes simplex encephalitis already mentioned, where hemorrhagic-necrotic lesions may be limited to one or both temporal lobes. These focal lesions immediately suggest the etiology, but most viral infections are not specifically diagnosable from the gross specimen.

Microscopically, there is a sameness of appearance of most viral infections, but topography of the lesions may vary with the etiologic agent. In the very early phases of infection there may be little or no inflammatory reaction in the brain or meninges, rather, only a subtle change in staining characteristics of affected cells, or an alteration in their form, be they glia or neurons. These changes can include eosinophilia, swelling, vacuolation, or fusion to form polykaryotic cells. In tissue culture cells these changes are often more easily observed than in vivo. Other changes, especially in infected neurons, may also include chromatolysis, nuclear translocation, and nucleolar specialization, all characteristics of the axon reaction. It must be remembered that some viral infections are nearly invisible histologically and may only show minimal cytopathic effects without obvious inflammation as in rabies, in which only inclusion bodies may be seen. Another ex-

ample of this phenomenon is seen in the infections with the unconventional agents of Jakob-Creutzfeldt disease, kuru, and scrapie, where inflammation is only rarely encountered and the pathology is mostly patchy neuronal loss with or without vacuolating-spongiform change and possibly amyloid plaque formation.

Usually within a day or so of infection with conventional viruses, the earliest inflammatory infiltrate will be polymorphonuclear leukocytes (PMNs) which surround vessels, infiltrate the brain substance, or cluster about affected cellular elements. This reaction may be short lived. The acute inflammatory response is espe-

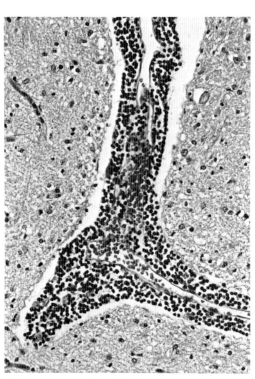

Figure 14.12. This light micrograph illustrates one of the typical features of viral infections in the nervous system, the perivascular lymphoid infiltrate, in this instance from a case of acute poliomyelitis, an RNA virus of the *Picornavirus* family. This reaction seen most often in penetrating vessels (Virchow-Robin spaces) of the cortical surface is nonspecific but in combination with inflammatory nodules and/or inclusion bodies is highly suggestive of viral or rickettsial disease. H&E. (Original magnification ×320.)

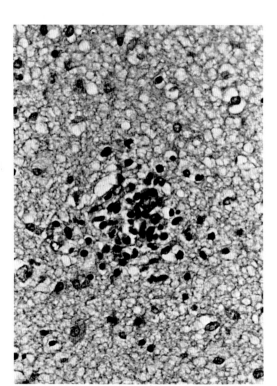

Figure 14.13. This light photomicrograph illustrates an inflammatory nodule (glial nodule, glial star, etc), another of the typical inflammatory responses to viral infections in the nervous system. In this instance the virus is cytomegalovirus, a DNA virus of the *Herpesvirus* family. Immunocytochemical staining reactions often demonstrate viral antigen in such regions, even though inclusion bodies may not be seen. The inflammatory nodule is composed of lymphoid cells, macrophages (microglia), and may include reactive astroglia and small capillaries. H&E. (Original magnification ×320.)

cially well illustrated in acute poliomyelitis, where true neuronophagia by PMNs can be observed very early.

The most common and typical inflammatory reaction appears within 4 or 5 d of infection and consists of a perivascular "cuff" of mononuclear or lymphoid cells about small vessels in the brain and within Virchow-Robin spaces (Fig. 14.12). There may be vascular congestion, dilatation, or obstruction, with capillary proliferation or prominence at this stage. Often associated with this reaction is the formation of an inflammatory nodule in the brain substance (Fig. 14.13). Synonyms include glial nodule, glial star, glial shrub, and Babes node. These focal inflammatory lesions, composed of a limited number of inflammatory cells (PMNs, monocytes, macrophages, and lymphoid cells but usually not plasma cells) are most commonly seen in the white matter or deep nuclear masses and may be associated with a very small necrotic focus. Inflammatory nodules characteristically occur in the midst of apparently normal appearing tissue and may be very widely spaced and distributed throughout the brain. Nevertheless, these "nodules" and the perivascular lymphoid cuff are probably the most typical indication of a viral or rickettsial infection in that location and in brain for that matter, but give no clue in and of themselves of the specific etiologic agent.

The phase of perivascular cuffing and inflammatory nodule formation may persist in the infected brain for years or may be overshadowed by a more destructive necrotizing or destructive process in which vascular thrombosis or capillary breakdown with edema occurs. Infected tissue may break down and a show a diffuse inflammatory process or a necrotizing process with only minimal inflammation. The determinants of this reaction depend upon not only the etiology agent, but also upon host defenses and are difficult to predict from case to case. During the more florid phase of tissue reaction, generally a week or more after infection, there may be histological features of the infection which can give a clue to the etiologic agent. The most classical of these tissue changes are the formation of inclusion bodies in infected cells which are helpful, but cannot always be depended upon for diagnosis.

Inclusion Bodies

The classical producers of intranuclear inclusions are the DNA viruses of herpes simplex, herpes zoster, and varicella; the J-C and SV 40 viruses of progressive multifocal leukoencephalopathy (PML) and cytomegalovirus (CMV); and the RNA virus of subacute sclerosing panencephalitis (SSPE). In rabies, the classical cytoplasmic inclusion bodies are the Negri and lyssa bodies.

Intranuclear inclusion bodies have been classified by Cowdry as types A and B (53). The Cowdry type A intranuclear inclusion is eosinophilic, rather glassy or amorphous, and is surrounded by a clear halo beneath the nuclear membrane beneath which granules of nucleochromatin may lie. The inclusions of herpes simplex, cytomegalovirus, and SSPE are typical type A inclusions. The type B inclusions are also eosinophilic, rounded, but smaller than the type A inclusion. They may be multiple and are not surrounded by a clear halo and resemble the paranucleolar bodies of Marinesco commonly found in the pigmented neurons of the substantia nigra (173). Type B inclusions may be seen in anterior horn cells in acute poliomyelitis. In progressive multifocal leukoencephalopathy (PML) the inclusions which affect oligodendrocytes have a unique appearance in which the nucleus is greatly enlarged and is eosinophilic, but there is no clear halo about the inclusion (238) as in the typical Cowdry type A inclusion (Fig. 14.8). Inclusion bodies may be seen in other infections, but those described above are the most commonly encountered and most widely recognized by pathologists. The light and ultrastructural characteristics of each inclusion will be discussed more fully under each infectious disease entity.

In most viral infections there is a phase, usually during the acute stage of the illness, during which inclusions, spongiform change, and other helpful histological features may be prominent, but later in the process of destruction and repair, these features may fade away and be very difficult to find. This problem often confronts the pathologist during interpretation of small biopsy specimens, where inclusions, vacuolation, and even inflammation are absent, and precise diagnosis is nearly impossible. In the autopsy specimen, however, areas of more active inflammation and reaction can usually be found where inclusions and other helpful hallmarks exist.

Viruses and CNS Tumors

The viral etiology of human brain neoplasms has been suggested by numerous clinical and pathological observations but has never been conclusively proven. Perhaps the situation which comes the closest to a virus-caused human brain tumor is in the context of PML where at least two cases of gliomas in association with the destructive-demyelinative lesions have been reported (42, 262). An apparent primary brain lymphoma has also been reported in association with PML (96). The suspicion is very high that the J-C or SV 40 viruses were causative, but rigorous proof is lacking. To be sure, there are many reports of other viruses, or virus-like particles have been reported in a variety of brain tumors, but again, rigorous proof of causation is lacking.

The most abundant literature on viral-induced brain tumors exists relative to experimental animals, in which many varieties of tumors have been produced by many viruses. One of the first viruses which was discovered to produce CNS tumors was the avian sarcoma virus (an RNA oncovirus of the Retroviridae family) described by Peyton Rous in 1911 (Rous sarcoma virus). This virus has been shown to produce gliomas in chickens, turkeys, hamsters, cats, dogs, and primates (42) and is currently a favorite of experimental neurooncologists. Other related RNA oncoviruses cause similar neoplasms.

There are a number of DNA viruses mostly of the papovavirus group, including the J-C, B-K, and SV 40 viruses, which have been used to produce experimental CNS tumors in animals. Furthermore, human adenovirus type 12 and several of the poxviruses have also produced brain neoplasms in animals (142).

Teratogenic CNS Effects of Viruses

The influence of viral infections during embryogenesis on subsequent neural development has been known for many years. Some early experiments by Hamberger and Habel (115) in the 1940's illustrated that influenza virus could produce neural tube and other defects in chick embryos. Subsequent workers have shown that several myxoviruses, some togaviruses, parvoviruses, arenaviruses, bunyaviruses, orbiviruses, reoviruses, and poxviruses could produce defects in newborn animals, ranging from neural tube defects, to cerebellar hypoplasia, porencephaly, hydranencephaly, hydrocephalus, and poor myelination (146, 147).

The role of such viruses in human neural malformations is, as expected, obscure, although neonatal hydrocephalus may be caused by intrauterine or neonatal effects of mumps virus on ventricular and aqueductal ependymal cells leading to stenosis (146). Other viral infections, such as rubella, varicella, cytomegalic inclusion disease, and probably herpes simplex, occurring during pregnancy, especially during the first trimester, may produce cardiac, ocular, skeletal, and other defects as well as damaging the brain, but no consistent pattern of defects in man have been directly ascribed to a specific virus as etiologic for CNS malformations. The crux of the problem is perhaps not so much which agent is present, but rather when it acts, disrupting some critical developmental process.

Demyelinating Diseases and Viruses

The subject of viral induced demyelination is discussed elsewhere in this volume in greater detail. The issue of a virus as a cause for multiple sclerosis confronts primarily the experimentalist but remains a tantalizing prospect for the clinical neuropathologist in the course of diagnostic studies. Viruses could be responsible either directly or indirectly through several mechanisms for diseases such as multiple sclerosis, and a number of very appealing animal-viral models exist. The subject has recently been reviewed by Dal Canto and Rabinowitz (57).

Immune Deficiency States and Viral Infections of the CNS

As more has become known about the immune system, several forms of immune deficiency have been discovered, many of which are complicated by CNS viral infections. These can basically be divided into the following: those with antibody deficiencies (congenital X-linked agammaglobulinemia, selective immunoglobulin deficiencies and subclass abnormalities, and many others); those with selective defects in cell-mediated immunity (thymic hypoplasia-DiGeorge syndrome, short-limbed dwarfism, specific T-cell defects); combined antibody, cellular immunity, and complex or combined immune deficiencies (severe combined immunodeficiency syndromes, Wiskott-Aldrich syndrome, ataxia telangiectasia, thymoma, immunodeficiencies associated with T-cell lymphoma); immune deficiency associated with inherited enzyme defects (adenosine deaminase deficiency, purine nucleoside phosphorylase deficiency, 5'-nucleotidase deficiency, Lesch-Nyhan syndrome, and others); defects in neutrophil function (actin and other cytoskeletal abnormalities), Chediak-Higashi syndrome, various neutrophil mobility defects, and glycolytic pathway defects); and secondary or acquired immune deficiency (Down's syndrome, acquired immune deficiency syndrome—AIDS, drug-associated immunosuppression therapy, malignancy, and many others) (119).

Many of these immune deficiency states have been recognized for many years to be associated with unusual or absent immune responses to viral infections, especially in children in whom the CNS may be affected directly or indirectly, as in disseminated vaccinia and encephalitis as a complication of smallpox vaccination (157). Progressive measles encephalitis and subacute sclerosing panencephalitis (SSPE) (145, 287), echovirus encephalitis (293), and herpes simplex encephalitis (147) are among other viral infections of the CNS reported in association with inherited or congenital immune deficiency in which there is hypogammaglobulinemia. A host of other virus infections sometimes involving the CNS but usually involving the gut, urinary tract, or respiratory tract are seen in children suffering from what is now known as severe combined immunodeficiency disease (SCID). In this condition not only T-cell function is abnormal but also hypogammaglobulinemia may be present. Viruses recovered include parainfluenza viruses, cytomegalovirus, adenovirus, rotaviruses, parvoviruses, reoviruses, coxsackieviruses,

and papovaviruses (143). Probably more prominent as infectious agents in all of the immune deficiency states mentioned above, are not the viruses but rather pathogens such as *Toxoplasma gondii*, *Pneumocystis carinii*, various fungi, tuberculosis, and bacterial infections.

Acquired immunodeficiency syndrome (AIDS), only recently recognized and of considerable public health concern worldwide, has been shown to be associated with unusual infections of the CNS (141). As of June 1983, a total of 1641 cases have been reported in the United States and possessions, and increasing numbers are likely to be reported in the future if past trends continue. Thirty-nine percent of these patients are now known to have died of Kaposi sarcoma with or without various opportunistic infections. The most common infection in the AIDS patients is *P. carinii* pneumonia (51% of cases). Twenty-six percent have Kaposi sarcoma without Pneumocystis pneumonia, and 8% have both. Fifteen percent of patients have another opportunistic infection, usually viral or fungal, and many of these include CNS infections (141, 211). The individuals at greatest risk for contracting AIDS are homosexual or bisexual men of any race between 20 and 29 years of age. Persons born in Haiti and living in the United States account for about 5% of cases (283), and individuals such as hemophiliacs who regularly require blood product transfusions account for about 1% of cases. Persons at lesser risk include children of affected Haitians, heterosexual partners of affected victims, intravenous drug addicts, recipients of blood transfusions, and victims of Kaposi sarcoma with apparently normal immune competence (141, 211).

Most recent experience with AIDS victims indicates a spectrum of CNS infections which includes most commonly, cytomegalovirus (CMV) encephalitis, myelitis, meningitis, and/or retinitis (7); herpes simplex encephalitis alone or in combination with CMV; papovavirus infection and progressive multifocal leukoencephalitis (PML) (202) tuberculosis and fungal infections, with probably many more to come.

The nature of the immune deficiency is still under investigation, but it appears that most AIDS patients have a more severe defect in cellular immunity than in humoral immunity. It has been found that in AIDS patients and in a population of homosexual men recently studied using immunologic surface marker methods, that there may be more suppressor and killer T-cells than helper or inducer T-cells in the blood (166). The consequence of this preponderance of suppressor and killer T-cells is that an adequate cellular immune response is interfered with before it can respond to a foreign antigen. The cause of this T-cell imbalance is not known, but there is increasing evidence to suggest that a retrovirus (human T-cell leukemia virus) which specifically infects T-lymphocytes may be involved in the pathogenesis of AIDS.

Recently, human T-cell leukemia virus antigens (81), T-cell leukemia viral DNA segments (95), and an actual recovery of a T-cell leukemia virus (92) have been reported in AIDS patients or from patients showing early symptoms of AIDS (13). Other studies suggest that the mechanism of action of this human T-cell leukemia virus, an RNA-containing retrovirus, is that in the course of replication a DNA copy of the viral genome is inserted into the host cell genome, where it can eventually transform the infected cell and interfere with its immune function. Evidence for this hypothesis has come from recent experiments with a T-cell luekemia virus in cats, feline leukemia virus (FeLV). Not all infected animals die of virus-caused leukemia, but probably more die of opportunistic infections associated with an immunodeficiency state not unlike AIDS (279). In this model, like human AIDS, it is suggested that helper T-cell function is diminished, and T-cell suppressor responses are increased directly by the viral infection, resulting in delayed B-cell triggered humoral antibody responses.

Another virus, the Epstein-Barr virus (EBV) which causes infectious mononucleosis and Burkitt's lymphoma, also has been implicated as a possible cause of AIDS. It is well known that many AIDS patients, and the homosexual population in general, have a greater than expected incidence of antibodies to EBV. Furthermore, EBV infection can produce some degree of cellular immunodeficiency during an acute infection (31). This apparently occurs when EBV infects B-cells, causing them to become activated. This activation in turn stimulates suppressor T-cells which inhibit the exaggerated B-cell response, leading to a general inhibition of a humoral antibody response to EBV and an altered suppressor/helper T-cell ratio as commonly seen in AIDS. It is not known if the presence of EBV in AIDS patients is simply another manifestation of their immune incompetence or if the agent is important in the etiology of the condition. A similar statement could probably be made for CMV, which can also infect lymphoid cells and may lead, in and of itself, to a potential immune system defect (153, 269). The possibility has also been raised that an unconventional agent may be important in the pathogenesis of AIDS, but no convincing evidence has yet been presented to justify this worrisome hypothesis.

The recent report of naturally occurring AIDS in rhesus and other monkeys (121) may offer another experimental opportunity to study this perplexing syndrome and perhaps to find its cause.

Laboratory Diagnosis of Viral Infections

The precise diagnosis of any viral disease in the nervous system by gross and histological analysis is often a very difficult and frustrating experience, and with the notable exceptions above in which rather typical inclusion bodies may be found, the only accurate means of diagnosis is by other laboratory methods which include recovery of the agent in tissue culture or by animal or embryonated egg inoculation, by serological or immunological methods.

Quite often a brain biopsy is considered for diagnoses of viral illness. When this occurs it is essential that the neuropathologist be informed in advance of the procedure so that communication can be established with the neurosurgeon as to the best region from which to obtain the specimen, how large and how deep the specimen should be, and how it will be handled after removal to achieve the best chance for diagnosis. The therapeutic issues involved in the case should also be made clear so that unnecessary delays do not occur, and the proper diagnostic methods are performed.

Preoperative consultations between all interested parties will avoid embarrassing and tragic errors later!

The widespread availability of polyclonal or monoclonal antibodies to specific viruses and the application of fluorescein isothiocyanate-tagged antibody (FITC) or peroxidase-antiperoxidase (PAP) coupled immunohistochemical reactions now allow accurate diagnosis based upon tissue analysis (66). Fluorescent methods usually require fresh frozen sections, while the immunoperoxidase methods may be performed on formalin-fixed and paraffin-embedded sections, provided fixation was prompt and not protracted and the paraffin was not excessively hot. Epoxy plastic-embedded tissues may also be used at times if the plastic is removed before immune reactions are carried out. By employing one or more of these methods, viral components or antigens can be localized in cells which otherwise would appear normal, or do not bear an inclusion body by hematoxylin and eosin (H&E) staining. This is especially evident in recent experience with brain biopsy diagnosis for herpes simplex infection.

Recent advances in in vitro nucleic acid hybridization methods may ultimately be refined to allow highly precise detection and localization of viral genome sequences in host cells by nonimmune methods using the Avidin-Biotin coupling system (172).

When tissues or fluids are to be submitted to the laboratory for virological examination care must be taken in handling and storing the specimen. The specimen, if it is tissue, should have been obtained in a sterile fashion by biopsy, aspiration, or autopsy, placed in a sterile Petri dish or other suitable sealable container, and immediately transferred to the virological laboratory, or if this is not possible directly, it should be kept cold. If storage is necessary, an ultralow temperature freezer is ideal, since most viruses are well preserved by this means but would be lost if kept at room temperature or even protracted periods in the standard refrigerator. Blood should not be frozen before it is centrifuged and the serum separated. It may be useful, when looking for viruses in buffy coat cells, to directly study heparinized or citrated blood.

It is important to note that any specimen which is contaminated with bacteria must be filtered or treated with antibiotics before inoculation into tissue culture cells, embryonated eggs, or the brains of suckling mice; otherwise, overgrowth and pathogenic effects of the contaminating organism will obscure any viral effect. The specimen should ideally be taken from an area which is known or suspected of being acutely involved in the infectious process, from the CSF, or from external lesions or body surfaces known or suspected to harbor the agent. Recovery from bronchial secretions, throat washings, enteric contents, or feces requires care to avoid bacterial contamination of the culture system, and standard handbooks of laboratory methods will usually contain the proper protocols (134, 178).

When tissues are obtained, it is often a good idea to prepare a portion for electron microscopy. This, however, requires prompt and careful selection of tissue blocks, as well as prompt and proper fixation in buffered paraformaldehyde or glutaraldehyde according to methods outlined in the many existing works of diagnostic electron microscopy. It is perhaps a saving grace, that viruses themselves are not adversely affected by routine formalin fixation insofar as their ultrastructural appearance is concerned, but the surrounding tissues may show massive and confusing artifacts. It is worthy to note that many of the first ultrastructural descriptions of CNS viral infections were made on formalin-fixed tissues, often having been stored for a long period of time. Electron microscopy can also be used for rapid diagnosis by means of negative staining on a membrane-coated grid of tissue suspensions or extracts, to look for viral particles, and to determine the classification by actual virion morphology.

When necessity prevails and all other methods have failed, it is sometimes possible to analyze by several methods for tissue concentrations of viral antigens by means of enzyme-linked immunoabsorbant assay more commonly known by the achronym, ELISA. A common enzyme employed as a link to a specific antibody is alkaline phosphatase. Using spectrophotometric and histochemical methods, enzymatic release of a coloring compound may be used to quantify a specific antigen when it is suspected. There are many commercial sources for assay kits for a variety of viruses and their various components. A similar method, not employing colorimetric determinants but rather immune precipitation in either a diffusion plate or electrophoretic assembly, in which specific antibodies are run against unfixed tissue extracts, may also be helpful in specific diagnosis of viral infection (147).

Serologic analysis of blood or CSF is one of the most commonly employed methods of viral infection identification by means of indirect techniques which imply diagnosis rather than specifically and positively provide it. In this instance one must suspect a given agent or be prepared to perform a series of time-consuming analysis with a battery of reagents. It is generally preferred to have paired sera from a given patient, from early in the infection to the convalescent period, in which rising or falling antibody titers against a given virus may be seen. The titers against the various viruses which are considered diagnostic are characteristic of each virus.

RNA VIRUS INFECTIONS OF THE NERVOUS SYSTEM

The Picornaviruses

The pico- (small) RNA viruses are the smallest of the RNA viruses, whose dimensions are in the range of 24–30 nm in diameter. They are naked virions (unenveloped nucleocapsids) which are assembled in the host cell cytoplasm, and have an icosahedral nucleocapsid as illustrated in Figure 14.3. These viruses contain a single stranded RNA genome which serves as its own messenger in host-supported viral protein translation. There are at least four genera: the enteroviruses, rhinoviruses, cardioviruses, and apthoviruses.

ENTEROVIRUSES

There are more than 70 types which are important to man and include polioviruses, which are the most important etiologic agents for poliomyelitis, the echoviruses (enteric cytopathogenic human orphan), and Coxsackieviruses which are causes of upper respiratory infections, pericarditis, pleuritis, and myocarditis, but also cause aseptic meningitis, and encephalitis, and only rarely, poliomyelitis. It has been suggested that hepatitis A virus should be in-

cluded with the enteroviruses, but there is still debate on this point. Owing to the greater number of *Enterovirus* serotypes isolated in the laboratory, there has been a tendency recently to assign numbers rather than specific names to new immunologically unique isolates (198, 199).

RHINOVIRUSES

There are hundreds of serotypes which are the major cause of the common head cold. CNS infections are practically unknown (109).

CARDIOVIRUSES

These viruses are primarily pathogens for rodents and monkeys, swine, and other domestic livestock, but some forms, encephalomyocarditis virus (EMC virus), Colombia S-K, and Mengo virus have been known to only rarely infect man (273). When this occurs, however, the illness is usually an encephalitis with no myocarditis and is much more benign than in animals who tend to suffer almost entirely from a serious myocarditis.

APTHOVIRUSES

These agents are responsible for the important disease of livestock, foot and mouth disease, but have only rarely caused disease in man (8).

Picornavirus Infections of CNS

POLIOMYELITIS (INFANTILE PARALYSIS, HEINE-MEDIN DISEASE)

Although the term, poliomyelitis, in the strict sense refers to an inflammation primarily of the grey matter of the spinal cord, it has come to be synonymous with perhaps the best known CNS viral infection in man. Acute anterior poliomyelitis probably occurred in epidemics since antiquity but rose to major public and medical consciousness during the course of epidemics after 1900 in most populated countries. The first intelligible clinical account of poliomyelitis was made by Underwood in the second edition of his *Diseases of Children* published in 1789, and in subsequent revisions of the then popular text (223). Jacob von Heine in 1840 and later in 1860, no doubt stimulated by several accounts of several cases of poliomyelitis by other workers, organized a comprehensive series of his own case descriptions in book form, which included, for the first time, the various presentations and manifestations of the disease. Some of the first pathological studies of poliomyelitis (1860–1870s) were published by the French physicians, Cornil, Prevost, Vulpian, Charcot, and Joffroy, who showed pathological changes in the anterior portion of the spinal cord (223). Important clinical and epidemiological observations were made by the Swedish physicians, Medin (223) and Wickmann (297) around the turn of the century leading to a more modern conception of the disease and its prodrome.

A major conceptual advance in the understanding of poliomyelitis occurred in 1908 with the report by Landsteiner and Popper (171) that they had transmitted the disease from a human case in which a bacteriologically sterile suspension of spinal cord was inoculated intraperitoneally into two species of monkey and that the pathology observed was very similar to the naturally occurring disease in man (223). Further work by Landsteiner in collaboration with Levaditi published in 1911 (170) showed that the virus of poliomyelitis occurred in the tonsils, mucosa of the mouth and throat, and could be found in saliva, tears, and mucus from the nose (223). The extensive work by Flexner and Lewis (87) during the period of 1909–1912 demonstrated further experimental features of the disease, characterization and isolation of the virus, and the fact that an active and passive defense against the virus infection was possible (87). The contributions of many other workers before and during this period have been reviewed by Paul (223).

In spite of the wealth of information about the disease, its pathology, and its causative agent, it was not until the middle 1940s that the mode of transmission by ingestion and the virus' initial phase of infection within the gastrointestinal tract were finally fully appreciated (28, 232, 248), and it was not before another 10 yr had elapsed that effective immunization methods were developed and put into wide clinical trials. The names of Sabin, Salk, Francis, Bodian, Enders and coworkers, and many others are well known as important contributors to development of the vaccines and the final acquisition of knowledge needed to bring this dreaded disease of childhood under control by the middle 1960s (80, 232, 248, 250).

Etiology of Poliomyelitis

Virological study of cases diagnosed clinically as poliomyelitis in the 1950s have shown that 52–57% of cases were caused by polioviruses, about 8% of ECHO and Coxsackieviruses (*Enterovirus* genera of the Picornavirus family), 3% by mumps virus (*Paramyxovirus* family and genus), 1% by herpes simplex virus (*Herpesvirus* family), 1% by a mixed viral infection, and interestingly, 30% in which no virus could be recovered (176, 177). Types identified in Coxsackievirus-caused poliomyelitis include types A7, A9, B2–B5 (60), and in echovirus-caused polio, types 1, 2, 4, 6, 7, 9, 11, 16, 18, and 30. In addition, otherwise unclassified *Enterovirus* types 70 and 71 have also been identified in cases of paralytic polio in Africa, Asia, Europe, and the Pacific islands, but not in American continents (248). In spite of the fact that other than polioviruses can cause an acute anterior poliomyelitis, these are the agents generally considered to be the most important etiologically. Three serologically distinct strains have been identified: type 1-Brunhilde strain, which has caused 85% of all permanent paralytic cases of polio; type 2-Lansing strain; and type 3-Leon strain. There appears to be little cross-immunity achievable between strains, and most modern vaccines are now polyvalent to overcome this difficulty (250). Occasional cases of live vaccine virus-caused paralytic poliomyelitis in persons who have not been vaccinated continue to be reported but must be regarded as rarities in view of the number of children receiving vaccines throughout the world (177, 250).

Pathogenesis and Clinical Features of Poliomyelitis

The disease occurs worldwide but is now largely under control following widespread immunization programs, but periodically shows itself when immunization is incomplete or has become casual. When epidemics were common until the 1950s, they usually occurred between July and September in the northern temperate regions and had longer seasons in more southerly climes. It appears that human beings are the only reservoir of the infection and that direct person to person transmission is not a major mode of infection, nor is insect transmission. There are vastly more cases of subclinical or inapparent infection than clinical cases with paralysis, and some individuals may harbor the infection for protracted periods, even years, in their intestinal tracts. Infectious virus is shed in fecal matter, which in areas of poor sanitation and hygiene may contaminate water supplies, food, eating utensils, and hands, entering the uninfected host by the oral route. Contaminated milk has been suggested as a vehicle of spread, but its importance in major epidemics has not been conclusively proven, nor has the nasal route of infection which seemed very likely at one time (129, 232).

Once the virus has entered the mouth it apparently is able to immediately infect the mucosa of the oropharynx and the lower gut. Uncoating of the virus occurs within 1 h; within 4 h completed virions already exist in infected cells, which will ultimately produce at least 500 virions each, will lyse about 6–8 h after infection, and release virions into the environment (62). Virions enter the lymphatics and bloodstream which disseminate the infection. During this phase of the disease, often referred to as the "minor illness," which is usually apparent 4–6 and sometimes as many as 35 d after exposure, there may be rather non-specific symptoms of sore throat, runny nose, fever, nausea, vomiting, or diarrhea associated with lymphadenopathy. During this phase, virus is actively shed into the stool and can spread the disease. Probably less than 10% of all infected individuals develop even this "minor illness" but rather have a clinically inapparent infection which, none the less, confers immunity to that specific virus. Of those who suffer any symptoms, 40–80% will suffer no further illness after a few days of convalescence and will also have immunity to that specific virus, but 10–20% of symptomatic individuals will develop the "major illness" of CNS poliomyelitis (129).

In those individuals who contract CNS

polio, virus has gained entrance into the CNS from the blood through the area postrema, the choroid plexus, across various capillary beds directly into the nervous system, via spinal ganglia, myenteric plexuses, sympathetic nerve and ganglia, and possibly via intraaxonal transport from the periphery. Replication then proceeds in vulnerable neurons whose distribution appears primarily in the motor system and associated neuronal groups as lucidly depicted by Bodian (Fig. 14.14). Meningeal signs, stiff neck and back, headache, muscle spasms, and cutaneous discomfort, if they are to occur, develop by 8–10 d after exposure and a few days after the "minor illness," but a small number of cases seem to bypass the prodrome and go directly to CNS symptoms. At this stage the CSF may show 25–500 and sometimes more cells, often neutrophils, protein content rises to 50–200

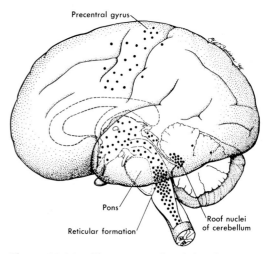

Figure 14.14. The topographical distribution of lesions in poliomyelitis is illustrated in the classic diagram of Bodian which demonstrates the motor system preponderance of the lesions. Note that while anterior horns and brain stem centers containing motor functions as well as the motor cortex host most of the lesions, motor-associated regions, such as roof nuclei in the cerebellum, and apparently nonmotor areas of the hypothalamus also may bear lesions from the viral infection. The "system" localization of this viral infection has not been satisfactorily explained in spite of the extensive information known about the polioviruses. (From D. Bodian: *Papers and Discussions Presented at the First International Poliomyelitis Conference.* Philadelphia, Lippincott, 1949.)

mg/100 ml, usually as the cell count falls, and sugar is normal. There is usually a peripheral leukocytosis. Paralysis of one or more extremities, paralysis of the muscles of respiration, and urinary bladder may develop gradually or within 24–48 h and is more likely to be severe and more widespread the older the victim, or if an infant under 1 yr of age is affected. An almost pure bulbar form of polio can occur in which severe abnormalities of cranial nerve function occur. Encephalitic forms of polio are uncommon but can occur alone or in combination with other forms of the disease. Paralysis may recede or be permanent, but generally does not progress once the fever lyses. Nonparalytic polio frequently occurs, but difficulty in recovering a virus in up to 40% of cases raises the question of correct interpretation of these cases.

Physical therapy and good general medical care provide the context in which some recovery of function in paralytic cases is possible usually over a period of months or a few years, but residua are common, especially in very young or older patients. About 2–5% of children and 15–30% of

adults with paralytic polio will die of the disease, and up to 75% of those with bulbar polio or with severe respiratory debility will die. There may be delayed effects of polio in which progressive motor deterioration resembling amyotrophic lateral sclerosis occurs in late adulthood in polio victims (2).

Pathological Appearances

In cases in which death has occurred acutely, the CNS may appear externally normal, although in severe encephalitic cases, capillary congestion may be evident. Cross-sections of the spinal cord and brain stem may show congested or frankly hemorrhagic areas (Fig. 14.15), especially in the

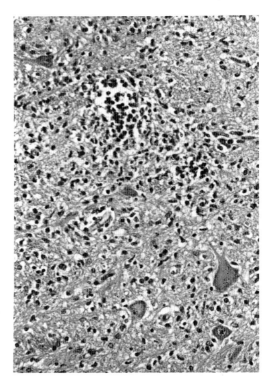

Figure 14.16. This light micrograph of the grey matter of the medulla in a case of acute poliomyelitis illustrates many coalescing inflammatory nodules, some of which appear to conform to spaces once occupied by large motor neurons (neuronophagia). Nearby large neurons appear unaffected. In the earliest phases of this disease the inflammatory infiltrate may be composed of mostly polymorphonuclear leukocytes, which are gradually replaced by mostly mononuclear cells. H&E. (Original magnification ×320.)

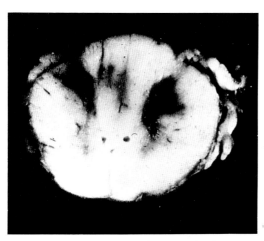

Figure 14.15. This gross photograph of a cross-section of a spinal cord illustrates the occasional phenomenon of hemorrhagic necrosis of much of the grey matter of the spinal cord including portions of the dorsal horns, where hemorrhage is more severe in this case of acute poliomyelitis. Generally, such cases have such rampant and widespread disease that survival is in jeopardy. Such a picture is seen in almost no other viral disease of the spinal cord.

anterior horns and affected bulbar nuclei. In subacute cases, affected nuclei may show a sunken, brownish discoloration, and in chronic cases, cavitation of affected nuclei may be seen in addition to secondary tract degenerations. The gross pathology of systemic organs includes lymphoid hypertrophy and congestion, splenic enlargement and congestion, myocardial congestion, and endocarditis. Atrophy and fibrosis of affected muscles is usually prominent in chronic cases.

Microscopically, the earliest changes in affected neuronal groups is infiltration by lymphoid cells, and sometimes neutrophils, development of perivascular cuffs, inflammatory nodules, and congestion or even small hemorrhages in capillaries (Fig. 14.16). Inflammatory cells begin to cluster about the larger neurons especially in the anterior horns and bases of the posterior horns of the spinal cord, where the neurons have swelled and appear acidophilic. Active neuronophagia can usually be observed, as can chromatolysis, and occasionally Cowdry type B (53) neuronal intranuclear inclusions. Meningeal inflammatory infiltrates are patchy and can persist for months or weeks after infection. Neuronophagia gradually fades after a few weeks, and some neurons which survive may contain Cowdry type B intranuclear inclusions or remain rather chromatolytic. After many weeks or months, neuronal loss is striking in affected areas, in which cystic cavities containing hemosiderin and prominent capillaries, residual inflammatory cells and macrophages, and some glial may occur (Fig. 14.17).

The most prominent lesions, acute or chronic, are to be found in grey matter of the anterior two-thirds of the spinal cord in all the cervical and lumbosacral segments of the cord, where more medial cell groups are most affected. The lower sacral levels of the cord may be spared, as are the intermediolateral columns of the thoracic cord. Clarke's column may be partially affected. The reticular formation and vestibular nuclei of the medulla, and to a lesser degree, nuclei of the pontine tegmentum and locus ceruleus, periaqueductal nuclei, red nucleus, and substantia nigra of the midbrain, the dentate nucleus and other roof nuclei and vermis of the cerebellum, as well as thalamus, hypothalamus, and

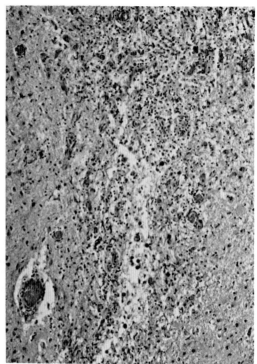

Figure 14.17.   This low power light micrograph illustrates the devastated and cavitary appearance of an anterior horn of the spinal cord from a case of poliomyelitis in the convalescent phase of the disease. Virtually no motor neurons are visible, and the anterior horn is largely a fluid-filled space occupied by various chronic inflammatory cells, and reactive astrocytes. Residual perivascular inflammatory infiltrates may persist for many weeks or even months. H & E. (Original magnification ×120.)

globus pallidus may show acute or chronic lesions. The large Betz cells of the motor cortex and similar large neurons of associated motor areas may also show loss. This "system" predilection for the virus has never been adequately explained, but appears characteristic of poliomyelitis, and most classically of the polioviruses (Fig. 14.14).

The pathology of skeletal muscles is probably mostly secondary to loss of innervation, but transient acute inflammatory changes can be observed during the active course of the disease. Once innervation is interrupted, grouped muscle fibers undergo progressive shrinkage, myofilament loss, and proliferation of subsarcolemmal nuclei. Groups which retain innervation my undergo hypertrophy. End stage muscles show fibrosis, fatty replacement, and only rare muscle fibers, but preservation of muscle spindles (41, 67, 74, 264).

ASEPTIC MENINGITIS

This is a clinical syndrome in which an abrupt febrile illness is associated with a headache out of proportion to the rest of the illness, and in which meningeal signs are variable, and no major signs of encephalitis or myelitis occur. The CSF shows pleocytosis with an early preponderance of neutrophils, which later give way to mostly a lymphocytic picture, and a slight rise in protein but no fall in glucose concentration. The CSF is sterile to bacteriologic culture. When such cases have been carefully studied, the majority have been shown to be caused by the enteroviruses (176). The most commonly isolated enteroviruses are Coxsackie B, echoviruses type 9, polioviruses, and Coxsackie A2 and A9. Viruses of other families are also commonly found and include mumps virus (Paramyxoviridae), lymphocytic choriomeningitis virus (Arenaviridae), and herpes simplex (Herpesviridae). An aseptic meningitis can be seen in association with abortive arboviral infection, measles, chickenpox, influenza, infectious hepatitis, infectious mononucleosis, atypical pneumonias, and a host of other viral illnesses. Nonviral causes of aseptic meningitis include leptospirosis and various fungal and mycobacterial infections (37). Occasionally, skin rashes associated with the syndrome can suggest meningococcal disease.

Most individuals affected are children. Transmission of the virus is most commonly fecal hand to mouth, though insect pests can also spread the agents. Most *Enterovirus*-caused cases occur during the summer months, but lymphocytic choriomeningitis virus cases occur in the winter (219). Laboratory diagnosis may be difficult but rests on either recovery of the virus from CSF or stool specimens or serological studies using paired acute and convalescent sera (176).

Since fatalities are rare and encephalitic symptoms occur in fewer than 2% of cases, pathological experience with this syndrome is very limited. Examinations of occasional fatal cases in which echoviruses (types 9, 17, and 21) and Coxsackie B5 were isolated

have been reported and showed no unique or unexpected pathological features. In other fatal cases, where autopsy studies have been made, many features typical of herpes simplex encephalitis were present, causing concern that the lesions were produced by a second infection with that virus (120).

The Togaviridae

The togaviruses resemble the picornaviruses and reoviruses in that their capsids are icosahedral, but are distinct because they are enclosed by a membranous envelope, provided by the host cell's cytoplasmic membrane during budding, or by the membranous cisternae of the host cell's cytoplasm prior to release. The genome is composed of a single stranded RNA. The group contains a number of important arboviruses (antigenic groups A and B) which cause encephalitis in man and animals: alphaviruses and flaviviruses. Other nonarboviruses in the family which are less important as human pathogens are the pestiviruses and the rubiviruses (198, 199).

Alphaviruses (Group A Arboviruses). This group contains the antigenically related agents for eastern equine encephalitis (EEE), western equine encephalitis (WEE), and Venezuelan encephalomyelitis (VEE) viruses which are all important human and animal pathogens. Other agents in this group are Chikungunya virus (113, 114), Semliki Forest virus, Sindbis virus, and other agents which have more importance in animal populations and in experimental laboratories than in human clinical neurovirology laboratories.

Flaviviruses (Group B Arboviruses). This group contains a number of important pathogens for man such as the agents for yellow fever, dengue (113), Japanese B encephalitis, Russian spring-summer, Powassan encephalitis, and St. Louis encephalitis. Other less common agents that are pathogens in man but important in animals and in the laboratory include louping ill virus and West Nile and Murray Valley encephalitis viruses.

Rubivirus. This group so far contains only the virus of rubella (German measles), an important CNS pathogen in the developing fetus.

Pestviruses. Members of this group are not human pathogens but cause hog cholera, border disease, bovine diarrhea, and other diseases which may be of interest to the experimental neurovirologist, such as the lactic dehydrogenase-elevating virus in mice (187, 218).

THE ARTHROPOD BORNE ENCEPHALITIDES

Perhaps the most common group of viral encephalitides are those which are spread by means of arthropods (mosquitos and ticks). At one time it was fashionable to classify these infections as so-called "arboviruses," but the swing in philosophy of viral taxonomy toward the morphological and biochemical and away from the epidemiological, plus the discovery of hundreds of different etiological agents in this group, has resulted in the classification of agents into three families, the togaviruses (*Alphavirus* and *Flavivirus* genera), Reoviridae (*Orbivirus* genus), and Bunyaviridae (*Bunyavirus* genus) (274). Many of these viral agents are very dangerous to handle in the laboratory, and specific suggestions and restrictions regarding them have been recently reviewed (268). The various agents will be discussed under their separate virus families below.

CNS Infections Caused by Togaviridae (*Alphavirus* Genera)

EASTERN EQUINE ENCEPHALITIS (EEE)

EEE has been the cause of epidemics of encephalitis in the eastern United States since the early 1800s and possibly before. The viral agent, a member of the togavirus group and *Alphavirus* genus was formerly classified as a group A arbovirus and was first isolated from the brain of a horse in 1933 and from human cases of EEE in 1938 (287). Periodic epidemics involving many hundreds of cases occur mostly along the eastern seaboard of the United States but have spread into the Mississippi valley, Gulf States, Great Lakes region, and even into Canada. Between 1969 and 1979, however, there have only been eight cases of EEE in man reported in the United States (206). In the past cases have been reported in the Caribbean, Central America, and South America where usually the first harbinger of a human epidemic is the loss of horses, pheasants, and other wild or domestic fowl to encephalitis. Probable isolation of EEE virus also has been reported in the Philippines, Thailand, Central Europe, and the Soviet Union (117).

The arthropod vectors for EEE are mosquitoes which usually feed on man, horses, and birds, such as the *Aedes sollicitans*, and *Aedes vexans*. Other mosquitos such as *Culex melanura*, as well as other *Culex* species, and *Coquillettidia perturbans* may serve as reservoirs of infection but sustain endemic rather than epidemic infections (118). These mosquitoes usually inhabit fresh water swamps and stagnant ground water areas. Animal reservoirs of infection include the common sparrow and other small flock birds in which the infection is usually inapparent. Pheasants and domesticated fowl, such as chickens and ducks, may also harbor the infection which can be spread by pecking, but these infected animals may die from the infection (118). Most outbreaks of EEE in humans occur between late August and the first killing frost of the fall, but animal cases usually precede the human cases by 1–2 weeks.

Infants, children, and adults over 55 yr of age are the age groups most commonly affected. The clinical appearance of EEE in man is usually abrupt, with headache, high fever, and evolution of meningeal signs over 2 or 3 d. Photophobia and myalgia may also be present. Behavioral symptoms may also occur. All symptoms may subside or worsen, leading to a more severe headache, nausea and vomiting, lethargy, stupor, and seizures which may precede a comatose state. In children especially, the presenting symptoms must be differentiated from bacterial meningitis and gastrointestinal viral infections with dehydration. In the 15- to 55-yr age group, infection may be very mild or inapparent and may be passed off as a flu-like illness. Probably there are many more times the number of inapparent cases than overt and serious cases of EEE. In ill patients, lumbar puncture reveals CSF pleocytosis in which cell counts range from 100 to 1000 cells, most of which are lymphoid. The CSF protein is elevated, but the glucose concentration is usually normal. The peripheral hemogram may be normal or show leukocytosis (85). Serological methods for hemagglutination inhibition and neutralization but not complement fixation studies are helpful in diagnosis when acute and convalescent sera are compared.

Those most likely to develop clinical disease are those over 50 yr of age, and the mortality rate of those who have clinically evident and diagnosed disease is between 50 and 80%, with most victims dying within the first 5 d of the infection. The usual survivors are children under 10 yr of age, but most will bear the sequelae of the infection manifested as mental retardation, epilepsy, emotional disorders, deafness, blindness, and perceptual and motor difficulties.

Horses suffering from EEE show staggering, aimless wandering or circling behavior, stupor, seizures, and coma. More than 80% of sick animals die within a few days of the onset of encephalitis, but some show less severe symptoms. In infected and ill birds, trembling, ataxia, leg paralysis, and generalized weakness are usually seen (161, 162).

Pathological Appearances

The gross appearance of the brain in patients not maintained on a respirator is that of a swollen, congested surface. There is no obvious exudate in the leptomeninges which may appear cloudy (15). The brain stem may appear more swollen and softened than other portions of the brain. Symmetrical uncal and tonsillar herniations are common. The gross appearance of the brain is not diagnostic for EEE, or any other encephalitis for that matter, and could be mimicked by many other conditions. If the victim had been maintained on a respirator, the changes of the so-called "respirator" brain may be evident and overshadow any pathological changes directly ascribable to the encephalitis.

Microscopically, there is little to differentiate EEE from any other encephalitis, since there are no inclusion bodies in infected cells, no special form of exudation, and apart from a tendency to show more intensity of perivascular inflammation, and inflammatory nodule formation in the brain stem and basal ganglion regions, there is no special regional pathology. Depending upon the age of the infection, the pathology may show more or less lymphoid infiltrate about vessels. The more acute the death, the more likelihood to note PMNs in the exudate. There may be an obvious vasculitis in EEE, with thrombosis and congestion of small arterioles, venules, and capillaries. Edema about these vessels may be severe. In areas of active inflammation in the cortex or in deep nuclear masses, neuronophagia may be evident. There is no predilection for grey or white matter localization of the lesions. In cases where survival has been prolonged, there is obvious evidence of repair and resolution, with areas of demyelination and axonal loss in white matter, glial replacement, and scarring in damaged cortical and deep nuclear regions. Patchy areas of demyelination may be seen in white matter where inflammatory nodules once existed (15). A perivascular lymphoid cuff and the occasional inflammatory nodule may persist many months after infection, but in cases coming to autopsy years after infection, only old, rather nonspecific changes of scarring and neuronal or myelin loss remain. The leptomeninges may in such cases be somewhat thicker than normal, and some difficulty may be encountered in dissecting individual cranial nerves at the base of the brain.

The pathological changes observed in horses dying with EEE are similar to those observed in man. The tendency for localization of inflammatory and necrotizing lesions to the basal ganglia, thalamus, and brain stem is also noted. Inflammatory nodules and perivascular cuffing, as well as other histological reactions, are identical with man (139).

WESTERN EQUINE ENCEPHALITIS (WEE)

The history of western equine encephalitis, WEE, is similar to that of EEE. The disease first became recognized in 1930 in California during an equine encephalitis epidemic in which nearly 6000 horses were stricken, of which almost 50% died. In 1933 the agent responsible was isolated and transmitted to guinea pigs. In 1938 the first human isolation of WEE from a human case was accomplished. The disease has a geographic distribution different from EEE, having been reported most often in

Arizona, California, Colorado, and other western and southwestern states, as well as in some midwestern states in America. The disease has been found also in Mexico, Canada, and South America, and sporadically in the eastern and gulf areas of the United States. Major epidemics in the past involved thousands of individuals, but fortunately such epidemics are only sporadic. Like EEE, WEE is caused by *Alphavirus* genera of the Togaviridae family (274). There are a number of strains characterized, and it has been possible to discriminate immunologically between WEE viruses isolated in the western United States from isolates in the eastern areas (117).

As with EEE, WEE exists in a reservoir of infected wild birds upon which mosquitos feed, but domestic fowl may also harbor the infection and show little or no disease. Interestingly, it has been shown that reptiles and amphibia may also harbor the disease, even through hibernation, and may be able to pass it on the following spring, should the animal be bitten by a suitable mosquito. The disease is epidemic in horses and can also affect swine. The mosquito vector for WEE is usually *Culex tarsalis* or *Culiseta melanura*, although the virus can infect and be transmitted by other mosquitos such as species of *Aedes*, *Anopheles*, and *Psorophila*. Those factors which affect mosquito populations such as high rainfall, availability of standing water, and warm spring and fall weather also have impact upon the likelihood of a WEE epidemic occurring. Epidemics usually occur in June or early July, before epidemics of EEE are seen, and taper off as cooler weather develops. The first killing frost terminates most endemic and epidemic infection. Prediction of epidemics can usually be accomplished by virological studies on vectorial mosquitos or reservoir populations when climatic conditions are especially favorable for mosquito breeding (117).

Clinical features of WEE are similar to EEE, but with a more decided incidence in infants under 1 yr of age (165). The severity, morbidity, and mortality of the disease are inversely related to the age of the victim. Young victims suffer from abrupt onset of headache, high fever, nausea and vomiting, photophobia, restlessness or lethargy and stupor, and sometimes seizures.

Older victims generally have milder symptoms which include in addition to the above, myalgia, stiff neck, and back pains, vertigo, and tremors. Symptoms evolve over 3 or 4 d after infection and then gradually decline in nonfatal cases. Fatality may reach 60% in very young victims but falls to 3% in adults. During the convalescent period which may last for 6 months or more, patients may complain of nervousness, tremors, irritability, malaise, and easy fatigability, as well as inability to perform challenging intellectual functions. Long-term sequelae are more common for those affected before 1 yr of age (12–50%) and less likely in adults (5% or less).

WEE in horses is more mild than with EEE, in spite of the fact that in some animal epidemics mortality has been as high as 50%, but generally averages between 20 and 30%. After being bitten by an infected mosquito, the incubation period varies from 1–3 weeks after which the affected animals show fatigue, sleepiness, and incoordination, and less commonly inability to eat or drink and falling (117, 139).

Pathological Appearances

The gross appearance of the brain at autopsy is similar to that observed in EEE and may appear normal externally. Microscopically, the reactions are usually more mild than seen in EEE, and there is a tendency for less of a PMN infiltrate in the acute phase of the disease. Perivascular cuffing and inflammatory nodules are present diffusely in the same distribution as in EEE, but there is likely to be more white matter inflammation and destruction, and cerebellar Purkinje cell loss may be prominent. In some cases extensive white matter lesions may coalesce into cystic spaces. When the infection has abated the brain will show the effects of neuronal loss by glial proliferation. Damaged white matter areas will show patchy demyelination (Fig. 14.18) or cyst formation, and the cerebellum, if severely affected, may be smaller than normal (236, 244, 289).

VENEZUELAN EQUINE ENCEPHALITIS (VEE)

Venezuelan equine encephalitis has a history similar to that of EEE and WEE.

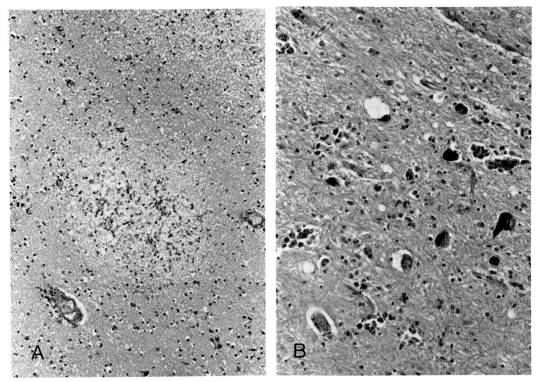

Figure 14.18. (*A*) This light micrograph illustrates some of the residual lytic areas in the white matter remaining after an infection with western equine encephalitis virus. (*B*) The multiple demyelinated areas are populated by reactive astrocytes and an occasional inflammatory cells. A residual inflammatory infiltrate may be found about some vessels. H&E. (*A*, Original magnification ×200; *B*, Original magnification ×350.)

The agent is an *Alphavirus* of the Togaviridae family with many subtypes, having been isolated since the 1930s (198, 199, 274). Outbreaks of VEE have been sporadic usually in Central and South America, but since 1961 the virus has moved into the southern border regions of the United States, causing occasional epidemics in Texas, Colorado, and Florida (205). Reservoirs of infection may be quite wide, with more than 150 animal species known to harbor the virus of VEE. In contrast to EEE and WEE where birds are the major reservoir, dogs, cats, rodents, bats, horses, cattle, sheep, goats, and to a lesser extent, birds appear to be maintaining hosts for VEE. The host becomes infected after an incubation period of 12–24 h after being bitten by a vector and may be viremic for several days thereafter. The vectors in VEE are mosquitos of the *Culex, Aedes, Anopheles,* and other species, and may include black flies and other insects as well (206).

Vampire bats have also been suspected to spread the disease in South America. In the mosquito, the incubation period for the virus may be as long as 3 weeks before it is capable of transmitting the agent to an animal host. Outbreaks of VEE in the United States are uncommon but seem to occur in April, May, or June.

The clinical features of human VEE are that of a rather mild infectious syndrome beginning as a respiratory illness with frontal headache, myalgia, and fever which may be high. Nausea, vomiting, and diarrhea, sore throat, and lethargy may also be seen. The incubation period is 1–4 d (69). The picture of an encephalitis is not usually seen and occurs in only 0.4% of cases in adults and 4% in young children. Most patients recover in 5 d, but in the rare fatalities, most are young children.

VEE in animals is more severe than in man and is clinically indistinguishable from EEE or WEE.

Pathological Appearances

Pathological descriptions of VEE in man are sparse (144), and there are few characteristics which would be considered unique for this disease when compared with the other equine encephalitides in man. Perivascular lymphoid cuffing, inflammatory nodules, and focal necrotizing lesions are the typical picture. The viscera show: bronchopneumonia, congestion, hemorrhagic infarction in lungs, fatty change, and inflammation in the liver. In animals (242), the disease is more severe, and the brain, grossly, may be severely swollen and showing hemorrhagic and necrotic foci or appear entirely normal. Microscopically, the spectrum of severity is also wide ranging, from minimal inflammation to a diffuse necrotizing and hemorrhagic meningoencephalitis with prominent vasculitis and thrombosis. Systemic pathology may include a curious tendency to destruction of bone marrow, lymph nodes, and spleen.

CNS Infections Caused by Togaviridae (*Flavivirus* Genera)

ST. LOUIS ENCEPHALITIS (SLE)

St. Louis encephalitis was first recognized in 1932 and 1933 in southern Illinois and in St. Louis, Missouri during summertime epidemics of encephalitis affecting more than 1000 individuals. Subsequent epidemics over the intervening years have occurred in virtually all parts of the United States with major concentrations along the Mississippi valley and Gulf states, making this form of encephalitis by far the most prevalent and most common in the United States. Epidemics also have been reported in Canada and Mexico, the Caribbean, and Central America (156). The last major epidemic was in 1975 when more than 1000 cases were reported (237). The disease is caused by a *Flavivirus* of the Togaviridae family which also includes several other arboviral encephalitis-producing agents, as well as the viruses of yellow fever and dengue. Outbreaks generally occur in midsummer or early fall and in the western United States may coexist with epidemics of WEE. Wild birds, including sparrows, pigeons, as well as domesticated fowl are the natural reservoir of the infection, and mosquitos, such as *Culex pipiens* and *Culex quinequefaciatus*, are the usual vectors. These mosquitos are known as "dirty water" mosquitos, residing in polluted, standing water mostly in urban areas. In rural areas, *Culex tarsalis* and other mosquitos are responsible vectors and tend to inhabit irrigation ditches and other "clean" water areas. The amount of rain and drainage conditions govern whether an epidemic will be possible.

St. Louis encephalitis in man is characterized clinically as a relatively mild illness beginning with fever and headache (33). This rather nonspecific illness may evolve into a mild encephalitis (75% of cases) or a mild aseptic meningitis (20% of cases). Most affected individuals are adults; hence the diagnosis of SLE should be considered when an individual over the age of 35 develops febrile aseptic meningitis or encephalitis with CSF pleocytosis between June and September in the United States. Laboratory diagnosis may be difficult, since SLE virus is only rarely recovered from CSF or blood, and antibodies may cross-react with other flaviviruses, notably dengue. Comparison of paired acute and convalescent sera by hemagglutination-inhibition or complement fixation reactions can usually confirm the disease. Neutralization tests may also be useful (177). Mortality in SLE is between 2 and 12%, but recent epidemics seem to show a lower mortality rate compared with those in years past. Children may have a clinically inapparent infection with no residue. Sequelae are seen in 5% or fewer of survivors and consist of nervousness, irritability, headaches, fatigability, and more rarely motor, perceptual, or speech difficulties.

Pathological Appearances

The gross pathology of the brain may be minimal and resembles any of the equine encephalitides. Microscopically, the changes of encephalitis are diffuse but are most prominent in the substantia nigra, midbrain, thalamus, spinal cord grey matter, pons, and medulla, cerebellum, and to a lesser extent in the hypothalamus, cerebral cortex, and white matter (237, 271). The meninges may show considerable inflammation, but it may be focal and localized to the sulci rather over the gyral surface.

Pathological changes of SLE in the reservoir animal are probably minimal, but in mice inoculated intracerebrally, after 3 to 4 d they become ataxic, show ruffled fur, and may have seizures. After becoming ill, the mice die in 1–5 d and show an obvious diffuse meningoencephalomyelitis pathologically (156).

JAPANESE ENCEPHALITIS (JBE)

Japanese encephalitis, at one time called Japanese B encephalitis to distinguish it from "A" encephalitis of von Economo, is also known by other names, Russian autumnal encephalitis and summer encephalitis. Though it was not isolated until 1935, it has probably been responsible for sporadic late summer epidemics of encephalitis in Japan since the 1870s (94). It has also caused epidemics of encephalitis in Korea, the Ryukyu islands (Okinawa), Taiwan, Asian USSR, China, several southeast Asian countries, and Guam. The JBE virus is a *Flavivirus* of the Togaviridae family. The mosquito vectors for JBE are *Culex pipiens*, *Culex tritaeniorhynchus*, and other *Culex* species, *Aedes vexans*, and *Anopheles* species. The reservoir animals for JBE include snakes, swine, horses, birds, and probably other animals who, after being bitten with infected mosquitos, maintain a viremia sufficient to reinfect other mosquitos. Infected animals generally do not become ill. Outbreaks of the disease rise with the peaking of the monsoon seasons and when the rice paddies are flooded. Since many of the vectorial mosquitos feed in open areas after dark, man becomes infected only when mosquito populations become very large and invade living areas (181).

The pattern of infection in the human population is similar to EEE, where children and adults over 60 yr of age are the usual victims of the disease. Other individuals may have a clinically inapparent infection. The incubation period is 6–16 d, and the prodrome is similar to any other encephalitis, but shaking chills and spasms may characterize the early phase which develops in 2–4 d. Deterioration of the sensorium with loss of facial affect and localized motor paresis are also rather typical for JBE infections. With resolution of the high fever (7–10 d), motor deficits and exaggerated deep tendon reflexes return to normal over a period of 4–7 weeks (94). Pleocytosis with levels up to 1000 cells/cu mm and moderate elevation in protein, as well as increased levels of glucose in the CSF, may persist for a month or more. A peripheral neutrophilic leukocytosis is common. Virus isolation from infected brain tissue is possible during the 1st week of the illness but is uncommon later. Hemagglutination inhibition, neutralizing, and complement fixation antibody analyses can be employed, using paired acute and convalescent sera to aid in diagnosis. Long-term residua, such as confusion, psychosis, seizures, and mental deficiency are commonly seen. The usual incidence of neurological residua is between 3 and 14%, varying inversely with the mortality rate in any given epidemic. The mortality rate may be as high as 50% in infants and children, but from from 7 to 33% in adults (94).

Pathological Appearances

The gross pathology of JBE is usually minimal, showing only congestion and swelling of the brain in acute cases. But in chronic cases, there may be areas of cerebral softening and deposition of mineral within the brain, perhaps so prominent that a gritty sensation can be perceived upon cutting with a knife. Massive mineralization has been reported (305).

Microscopically, perivascular lymphoid cuffing is common, especially in the subcortical white matter, and inflammatory nodules are found diffusely throughout the brain, basal ganglia, brain stem, cerebellum, and spinal cord. Early in the infection PMNs may be prominent in any inflammatory focus, but these later give way to mononuclear cells and lymphocytes. In necrotic areas, macrophages are prominent. Neuronal loss may be severe in any area affected, and there may be some association of inflammatory nodules in the cerebellum with Purkinje cell dendrites. Neuronophagia can be prominent in the grey matter of the spinal cord. Perhaps because small vessels are damaged in JBE, transudation of proteinaceous fluid into the interstitium or into vessel walls occurs, which becomes a focus for subsequent mineralization. Mineral deposits may be localized in vessel walls, in a pseudolaminar fashion in cortex, or in other damaged areas in chronic cases.

MURRAY VALLEY ENCEPHALITIS

Murray Valley encephalitis (70), once known as Australian X disease, is a disease caused by a *Flavivirus* (Togaviridae family) very similar to that of Japanese encephalitis. Epidemics of encephalitis due to MVE have been recorded since 1917 in the Murray-Darling river basins of New South Wales, Queensland, Northern and Northwestern Australia, and more recently in Papua-New Guinea. Like JBE, the vector is a mosquito, usually *Culex annulirostris* or *Aedes* species, and the reservoir hosts are thought to be water birds. The epidemics occur in summer and fall during times when rainfall is high. Like JBE and EEE, children and older adults are most likely to be affected, but inapparent or minor infections are probably very common in young and middle aged groups. In full blown cases, MVE closely resembles JBE with spasms, rigidity, motor paralysis especially in muscles of swallowing or breathing, as well as all the usual symptoms of encephalitis. Mortality rates are highest in young children where they approximate 20%. Sequelae are common in survivors (21). The virus can be isolated from infected tissue but not from CSF or blood. Hemagglutination inhibition, complement fixation, and neutralization antibodies in paired acute and convalescent sera aid in the diagnosis. The pathology of MVE is little different from JBE, but mineralizations apparently are not prominent (243).

WEST NILE FEVER (WN)

West Nile fever is a relatively mild mosquito-borne encephalitis very closely related to St. Louis encephalitis and Japanese encephalitis and is caused by a *Flavivirus* of the Togaviridae family. It has caused epidemics in East Africa, Egypt, Israel, and South Africa. The mosquito vectors are usually *Culex* species and the reservoir hosts are usually birds. Clinically, the disease presents with sore throat, fever, headache, myalgia, nausea and vomiting, lymphadenopathy, and sometimes a skin rash. Usually the symptoms subside within a week. Children seem to be less affected by the disease than adults who may suffer more prolonged symptoms. Fatalities are not common, and sequelae, if they occur, include weakness and fatigability (194). The pathology of WN has not been extensively described, but is probably rather mild, showing no distinctive features which would allow specific histopathological diagnosis.

Tick-Borne Encephalitides (TBE)

There are a variety of encephalitides which are spread by ticks rather than mosquitos which are important in several regions of the world, chiefly the northern woodlands of the northern North American continent, northern Great Britain, northern Europe and Scandinavia, Soviet Union, and Japan. Most of these illnesses are caused by flaviviruses of the Togaviridae family and include such diseases as Russian spring-summer encephalitis (Far Eastern and Central European encephalitis), Powassan (299) encephalitis, and Louping-ill (36), as well as other diseases in which encephalitis may be a less prominent feature of the illnesses. Colorado tick fever is caused by an *Orbivirus* of the Reoviridae family and is discussed with the Reoviridae.

Most of the TBE viruses are spread by ticks of the Ixodidae family and harbored in reservoir animals which are usually rodents, hedgehogs, shrews, bats, and moles, but domesticated animals and water birds may also support the infection (106). In the larger hosts of convenience, fatal illness can occur. This is especially so with Louping-ill, primarily a disease of sheep which can occasionally affect man (36, 285).

Most cases of TBE in man or animals follow a biphasic form in which there is a 1- or 2-week incubation period after a tick bite or consumption of milk from an infected domestic animal, followed by an influenza-like illness for about a week, after which there is clinical improvement. An abrupt severe illness may then follow, in which meningoencephalitis, encephalitis, or myelitis may be seen. In this phase, all the signs of a viral encephalitis may be seen and include disturbances of perception and sensation, paralysis which can resemble epidemic poliomyelitis, and seizures. Usually within 7–10 d recovery is well underway, and most fatalities have occurred by day 7. In some cases one or the other phases of the illness may be inapparent. The mortality rate is variable with each form of the TBE and ranges from as little as 1% (Central European TBE) to about 20% (Far Eastern-Russian spring-summer TBE). In the more severe forms, residua are common and resemble those of poliomyelitis (106) or of herpes simplex encephalitis (78). Laboratory diagnosis relies upon animal inoculations and serological methods.

Pathological Appearances

The gross and microscopic pathology in each form of TBE is dependent upon its clinical forms, e.g., meningitic, encephalitic, or myelitic. The gross pathology is rather nonspecific, and like any other viral encephalitis, with the exception of the fulminant myelitic form in which patchy necrosis of the bulbar region and extensive necrosis of the grey matter of the spinal cord, like acute poliomyelitis, is seen. Microscopially, there is little to distinguish TBE from any other encephalitis, but inflammatory nodules and perivascular infiltrates may be found more prominently in the brain stem and spinal cord, as well as in the spinal and cranial nerve ganglia (104). In other types of tick-borne arboviral infections, as with corresponding mosquitoborne arbovirus infections, where encephalitis is not the major component of the diseases but can be a part of the illness, the precise basis for the symptomatology could be direct viral infection in CNS or due to extension of the systemic hemorrhagic diathesis to the CNS which is the most obvious effect of the diseases. This is the case with the Tick-borne Crimean-Congo hemorrhagic fever group of diseases (125).

CNS Infections Caused by Togaviridae (*Rubivirus* Genus)

RUBELLA (GERMAN MEASLES)

Rubella has been well known as an ubiquitous exanthem of childhood probably for centuries, but its importance to the developing fetus and as a cause of congenital disease was not recognized until 1941 when Gregg et al. (105) reported that congenital cataracts and probably cardiac and neurological defects could be caused by maternal rubella infection which presumably crossed the placental barrier to the fetus. The role of rubella virus in occasional cases of encephalitis in children and in many congenital systemic and CNS diseases has since been well established. The viral etiology of rubella had been suspected well before the virus was finally isolated and cultivated in tissue culture in 1962 (222). Development of the first of the vaccines against the virus soon followed.

The classic rubella infection is a highly contagious epidemic infection usually affecting older children and young adults. The incubation period is 12–21 d after exposure and usually has almost no prodrome. Early symptoms are postauricular, occipital, and cervical nontender nodal enlargement. A macular or maculopapular nonitching rash generally appears first over the face and neck and rapidly spreads over the body but spares the palms of the hands and soles of the feet. The rash may become confluent before it recedes about 4 or 5 d after it began. There may be a minimal fever, slight malaise, or sore throat which accompanies the rash. In adults, other systemic symptoms may include joint pain, headache, and occasionally more severe CNS symptoms which are rarely serious or fatal. Laboratory studies may indicate a leukopenia and/or thrombocytopenia. Usually within a week of the onset the rash disappears, and all symptoms resolve. Rubella virus is shed from the mucosa of the nasopharynx before symptoms and signs of the disease appear and persist until the rash disappears. Prior to the advent of prophylactic immunization, 80% of individuals 17–22 yr of age and more than 85% of pregnant women in most countries had antibodies against the virus. This still left about 15% of women who might become pregnant able to contract the disease during pregnancy.

CONGENITAL RUBELLA SYNDROME

While childhood or adult rubella is a self-limited disease, when contracted prenatally, it may have devastating effects on the developing fetus or infant, and the virus may persist for protracted periods of time. In most series (116) the majority of intrauterine rubella exposures appear to occur within the first trimester of pregnancy, and it is during the first 8 weeks of gestation that the virus appears able to cause most of its pathology (52). The virus apparently replicates in and kills rapidly developing cells at the time of its entry or alters the mitotic rate of affected cells which later causes disorders of organ development and may even produce an infant of smaller than normal size (213). There is also an increased likelihood of fetal and perinatal mortality, infantile failure to thrive, and subsequent growth retardation.

Pathological Appearances

Ocular defects were one of the first recognized effects of congenital rubella infection and include cataracts, pigmentary retinopathy, glaucoma, microphthalmos, and other problems. The cardiovascular lesions seen include: complex defects such as tetralogy of Fallot, transpositions of vessels, atretic valves and major vessels, and combinations of these; patent ductus arteriosus; septal defects; valvular stenoses; myocarditis and fibrosis. The liver and/or the spleen may be enlarged, and neonatal jaundice may be present on the basis of liver disease, as well as cardiac failure. Metaphyseal abnormalities of extremity bones and of the skull result in abnormal bone development and deformities. Hematological abnormalities seen at birth include thrombocytopenia and purpura, anemia.

Pathological changes in the nervous system include nerve and cochlear damage (which may account for more than 25% of all congenital forms of deafness), and microcephaly, hydrocephalus, agenesis of corpus callosum, cerebral cortical anomalies, and subcortical cavitation-mineralization (clinically associated with autism, profound retardation, seizures, hypotonia and paresis, and severe perceptive disorders). The prevalence of all these abnormalities is probably related to how early in the first trimester the infection occurred (52) but translates graphically into the fact that 68% of 57 fetuses aborted because of maternal rubella infection showed one or more organ system to be damaged by the infection (277).

Microscopic changes in the nervous system in congenital rubella syndrome are varied and related to the overlying malformation (see also CNS malformation chapter). Those aspects of the disease which are unique to rubella, however, are focal or

massive neuronal loss, and generally fine, intraparenchymal, or perivascular deposits of mineral (which contain iron and calcium and associated anions (175). These deposits may appear powdery and confluent or fine and localized to one or more areas (Fig. 14.19), but are seldom as obvious or dense as in congenital cytomegalovirus or *Toxoplasma* infections where the mineralizations may be appreciated grossly. The subtlety of the deposits is suggestive in itself of rubella. There may be perivascular lymphoid infiltrates in the leptomeninges, cerebral cortex, or deeper structures. When fetuses are examined there is a preponder-

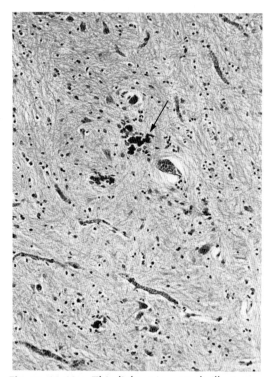

Figure 14.19. This light micrograph illustrates one of the common findings in congenital rubella syndrome, that of small punctate deposits of mineral (*arrow*) in basal ganglia-thalamic and subcortical locations. Many of these small spherical concretions which contain calcium, iron, phosphorus, and other elements appear associated with small capillaries and probably arose as a consequence of protein transudation into the neuropil by virus-damaged endothelium in utero. Inflammatory infiltrates may be entirely absent in such cases, and mineralization is seldom as obvious or extensive as in perinatal cytomegalovirus or toxoplasmosis infections. H&E. (Original magnification ×320.)

ance of destruction of neuroblastic elements within the periventricular germinal plate (255).

PERINATAL RUBELLA AND PROGRESSIVE RUBELLA SYNDROME

Some infants apparently contract rubella shortly before or after birth or within the first month or so of life and thus escape much of the developmental pathology described above, but they nevertheless suffer the effects of a more serious infection than at a later age. These infants show leukopenia and thrombocytopenia sometimes with purpura, immune deficiency, hepatosplenomegaly, pulmonary insufficiency, and evidence of CNS infection along with a rash which may persist for weeks or months. These infants show failure to thrive and developmental retardation, including sensory and perceptual deficits including deafness. Growth disorders and endocrine abnormalities may characterize their later development. In slightly older children more of these latter defects are seen. Pathological changes in the CNS are those of a nonspecific encephalitis without the mineral deposits seen free in the neuropil in the congenital cases. Perivascular mineralization may sometimes be seen, however. Rarely, a progressive, persistent form of rubella occurs either in postnatal or congenital rubella cases, often after a period of months or years of delay, which closely resembles the clinical and pathological appearance of SSPE, except that intranuclear inclusions are not seen in infected cells (278).

THE REOVIRIDAE

These viruses resemble the picornaviruses in form but are about twice as large. They are naked virions assembled in the host cell cytoplasm and have a unique form of double stranded RNA genome divided into 10 or more linear segments. The *Reovirus* (respiratory enteric orphan viruses) family contains three genera: orbiviruses, reoviruses (orthoreoviruses), and rotaviruses.

Orbiviruses. This genus contains at least two human arthropod-borne (arbovirus) pathogens, Colorado tick fever, and the so-called tick-borne (Kemerovo) encephalitis virus group seen in central Europe and the Soviet Union. An important animal disease caused by another agent in this group is blue tongue disease in sheep.

(Ortho)Reoviruses. In man, viruses of this genus are usually carried without symptoms in the gut or respiratory tract but may produce a mild illness in these systems. Only rarely may encephalitis, meningitis, or coexistent hepatic and CNS infections be caused by viruses of this group. Reoviruses have been used experimentally to produce congenital hydrocephalus in experimental animals (188).

Rotaviruses. These are not known to be neural pathogens but are a major cause of nonbacterial infantile diarrhea and common upper gastroenteritis in man and many animals. Infections are rarely fatal (303).

CNS Infections Caused by Reoviridae (*Orbivirus* Genera)

COLORADO TICK FEVER

While fatal encephalitis is not a prominent part of this disease caused by an *Orbivirus* of the Reoviridae family and spread by a common rocky mountain tick, *Dermacentor andersoni*, meningitic and mild encephalitic symptoms are common. These include headache, photophobia, stiff neck, and obtundation. Other more severe CNS symptoms are most commonly seen in affected children (73, 79). Pathological examination of the rare fatal human cases disclosed disseminated intravascular coagulopathy, hepatic, pericardial, myocardial, gastrointestinal, and focal CNS necrosis in which sparse intracytoplasmic inclusions could be seen (79).

So-called "tick" paralysis is sometimes confused with tick-borne encephalitis, but is not of viral etiology; rather, it is a toxic phenomenon, occurring very rarely with *D. andersoni* and other tick bites (257).

THE ORTHOMYXOVIRIDAE

These viruses are the major cause of influenza in man and animals and have a spherical or filamentous structure containing a helical single stranded RNA genome in several segments. Influenza viruses can be classified as types A, B, or C. The most important pathogens, which include human, equine, and swine influenza reside in group A. Groups B and C apparently only cause disease in man. All of these viruses are well known for their ability to undergo recombination and to produce periodic epidemics in man (302). A particularly important influenza pandemic, that of 1914–1918, killed thousands of persons in Europe and America and was ascribed at one time to have caused delayed tragic consequences, such as encephalitis lethargica (von Economo's encephalitis) and subsequent postencephalitic Parkinson's disease, although it is now thought that von Economo's encephalitis was a separate but coincident infection which produced Parkinson's disease and occasionally an ALS-like syndrome in some persons (32, 147).

Influenza viruses have been also implicated by their frequent association and isolation from CNS tissue or CSF in cases of Reye's syndrome, but many other viruses of several groups have also been similarly associated. It is far from clear what, if any, relationship influenza viruses have with the pathogenesis of this perplexing and feared syndrome of childhood, and for the time being, its viral etiology must remain unproven (147).

THE PARAMYXOVIRIDAE

This group contains some of the most intensively studied and important viruses to experimental neurovirologists, since many of them display latency and persistence in the nervous system (57, 149, 168). The paramyxoviruses viruses are usually spherical in shape and contain a linear single stranded, "negative" RNA genome enclosed within a helical nucleocapsid. This "negative" RNA cannot directly code for mRNA, so a funtioning "positive" RNA strand must be made using a viral RNA-dependent RNA transcriptase (198, 199). The resulting intermediate genome can then direct synthesis of viral mRNAs and then viral proteins. Glycoproteins migrate to the cell surface where final virion assembly occurs, and completed virions bud from the surface (46, 263). There are three genera: paramyxoviruses, pneumoviruses, and morbilliviruses.

Paramyxoviruses (Parainfluenza Viruses)

This group includes a number of important viruses pathogenic to man and important in the experimental laboratory (134): the so-called parainfluenza viruses, types 1 to 4 which produce croup or symptoms of the common cold in children, and Sendai virus, which is endemic and occasionally epidemic in mouse and other rodent colonies, where it causes a chronic respiratory tract infection and occasionally kills many animals (203). It can also produce hydrocephalus and a persistent infection in mouse CNS (168); mumps virus (epidemic parotitis), which may be important in the etiology of neonatal hydrocephalus in man (146); Newcastle disease virus, which causes a devastating disease of chickens but can cause a mild flu-like disease or conjunctivitis in man (61); and includes other, primarily avian, agents.

Pneumoviruses. These paramyxoviridae are sometimes referred to as the respiratory syncytial viruses, since they produce pulmonary infections in man and animals. There are a number of poorly characterized agents tentatively assigned to this genus which are so-called "foamy" agents resembling some of the RNA tumor viruses (127).

Morbilliviruses. Viruses of this genus are responsible for measles, subacute sclerosing panencephalitis (SSPE) in man, and canine distemper in dogs, as well as rinderpest virus in cattle. All are agents of great interest to the experimental neurovirologist (57).

CNS Infections Caused by Paramyxoviridae (*Morbillivirus* Genera)

SUBACUTE SCLEROSING PANENCEPHALITIS (SSPE)

SSPE is a viral infection of the CNS caused by a measles virus which is of insidious onset producing confusion, failure in intellectual functioning, personality and behavioral deterioration, perceptual difficulties, weakness and paralysis, stupor, and ultimately death in a vegitative state. The CSF shows minimal or no pleocytosis, no alteration in glucose, little or no elevation of protein, but there is more IgG present than normal, and there may be oligoclonal IgG bands by electrophoresis. CSF antibody titers against measles virus are usually high and may show greater titers than in the serum, probably indicating some preferential local antibody synthesis. The EEG may show a typical burst suppression activity, sometimes with myoclonic jerks (254).

SSPE occurs in apparently healthy individuals between 2 and 40 yr of age, but usually in children, where the mean age of onset of 10.9 yr. Most victims have had measles prior to age two. Males are affected three times as frequently as females, whites are affected nearly 20 times more frequently than blacks, and rural rather than urban children are more likely to contract the disease. The course of the disease is generally progressive, causing death in 1 or 2 yr in a majority of cases. A fulminant form of the disease occurs in 10% of cases, and very protracted course lasting years is seen in 10% of cases (254).

The first cases of what is now known as SSPE were described by Dawson in 1933–1934 (64) as subacute inclusion body encephalitis in which Cowdry type A inclusion bodies were seen in neurons, and which were originally thought to be typical of herpes simplex, but all efforts to recover the virus by animal inoculations were unsuccessful. Later important case descriptions by Pette and Döring in 1939 (229) and van Bogaert in 1945 (281), as well as a host of other case studies eventually clarified the entity and showed the pathological spectrum of SSPE to be quite broad, encompassing adult and childhood cases. Some of the early confusion about the spectrum of pathological change was alleviated when it was realized that the acute and fulminant cases often showed mostly cortical pathology, while chronic cases tended to show prominent white matter lesions.

A basis for the viral etiology of SSPE initially was laid by the demonstration of herpes simplex virus antigen in one apparently typical fulminant case, similar to those of Dawson (256), and by a report of transmission of a neurological disease to ferrets, by inoculation of a brain suspension from cases of SSPE with no recovery of a viral agent (154). Recovery of the actual etiological agent did not occur until cocultivation tissue culture techniques were applied successfully by Horta-Barbosa et al. (130) and simultaneously by Payne et al. in 1969 (224). These studies showed the agent of SSPE to be virtually identical to measles virus. Subsequent studies have suggested subtle differences between wild type measles virus and the SSPE virus (288).

It is still unknown how measles virus produces a chronic persistent infection in the CNS in which viral products appear to remain within cells for protracted periods of time in the apparent absence of viral release. Explanations for this enigmatic phenomenon have been reviewed by Johnson et al. (149) and include the possibility that there is an altered host immune response perhaps involving a suppressed T cell response or a process by which key viral components are segregated at the cell surface and removed before a complete particle can be assembled. Other possibilities include a synergistic or recombinant interaction between measles virus and another agent which either alters the host cell response or the replication processes of the original virus. In any case, it has been shown that a key viral protein, the M protein, which should be associated with the inner surface of the cytoplasmic membrane in infected cells is lacking in SSPE, and that it is probable that this deficiency inhibits assembly and release of the agent (46, 47, 75, 145). How the lack of M protein occurs is not known.

Pathological Appearances

The external gross pathological appearance of SSPE is not specific and rather bland, showing only occasionally slight convolutional atrophy and focal softening of the cerebral cortex. More consistently, coronal sections of the fixed brain are firm or rubbery (Fig. 14.20). The white matter in chronic cases may appear to be motheaten and to have a spotty grey discoloration suggesting demyelination in a diffuse pattern as in early or mild cases of a leukodystrophy. Symmetrical enlargement of the ventricles may be seen. Gross pathological differential diagnosis includes the leukodystrophies, unusual cases of multiple sclerosis (so-called transitional sclerosis), progressive multifocal leukoencephalopathy (PML), lipid storage diseases, such as Tay-Sachs disease, and possibly infantile

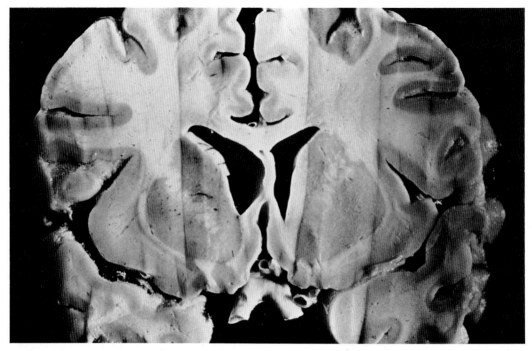

Figure 14.20. This gross photograph of a chronic case of SSPE illustrates slight cortical atrophy (widening of sulci) and possibly minimally enlarged ventricles. This fixed brain had a particularly "rubbery" consistency, no doubt accounting for some difficulty in cutting the specimen and the artifactual knife marks on the specimen. The tough consistency was probably caused by the intense gliosis in both grey and white matter in this case.

or juvenile variants of Jakob-Creutzfeldt disease (Heidenhain's disease) or Alper's disease.

Microscopic pathologial changes are usually diffuse, involving neuronal populations to a lesser degree than the white matter areas, although in some cases the topography of the lesions is mostly confined to the cerebral cortex, basal ganglia, and thalamus. Occasionally, the spinal cord may be involved, showing inclusion bodies in neurons of the ventral and dorsal horns. The more usual circumstance, however, shows the most severe lesions to be patchy demyelinating and degenerative lesions in the centrum ovale, which on myelin strains resemble adrenoleukodystrophy where the "U" fibers may be spared and the deeper regions show diffuse damage but not discrete plaques. Inflammation is usually minimal, but perivascular lymphoid cuffs may be seen as well as a minimal leptomeningeal infiltrate. Inflammatory nodules are uncommon. Astroglial proliferation and hypertrophy may be very striking in damaged areas of grey or white matter where little else remains (Figs. 14.21 and 14.22). Necrosis and cavitation can be seen but are not usually the most prominent lesions, although macrophages are a prominent part of the early lesions and contain abundant sudanophilic myelin breakdown products. Neuronal loss may be so prominent that affected gyri may appear ulegyric, and white matter loss so significant, that hydrocephalus ex vacuo becomes very prominent. Secondary degeneration of the pyramidal tract may occasionally be seen due to loss of axons in the white matter. The topography of the lesions from case to case is probably not so constant as some observers would indicate, but may correlate with predominant symptoms at times.

The most striking change, which suggests the diagnosis, is the presence of Cowdry type A intranuclear inclusions (Fig. 14.23). In the predominantly cortical-neuronal cases, these are in neurons, but in most cases these are in oligodendroglia and occasionally in astroglial cells. The search for

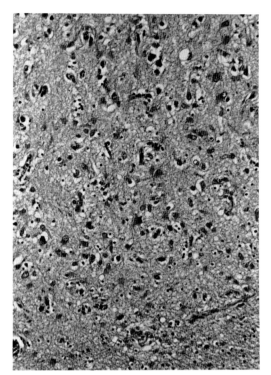

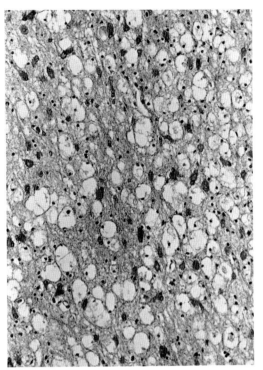

Figure 14.21. This light micrograph of the cerebral cortex from a chronic case of SSPE illustrates profound neuronal loss and reactive astroglial replacement. This section includes a portion of the subcortical white matter at the bottom of the photograph which is much less affected than the grey matter in this case. No obvious intranuclear inclusion bodies are seen in this section perhaps due to the chronicity of the case, but in other portions of the brain typical inclusions were found. H&E. (Original magnification ×320.)

Figure 14.22.   This light micrograph from a case of SSPE illustrates a predominance of white matter pathology. Here the white matter is devastated, replaced by vacuoles (which may be somewhat artifactually enhanced here), many hypertrophied reactive astroglial cells, and glial fibers. In this case, there was comparatively little grey matter disease. While intranuclear inclusions were not obvious in this section, they were found in other sections after careful searching. H&E. (Original magnification ×320.)

inclusions may be frustrating if the case is very chronic, since it appears that inclusions represent evidence for replicative activity and therefore probably acuteness of infection (182). Sometimes, both nuclear and cytoplasmic inclusions are noted, in which it appears that heavily infected cells have been transformed into so-called virus factories. SSPE must be differentiated from the storage diseases where large gemistocytic astrocytes may be mistaken for neurons filled with stored lipid material. In Jakob-Creutzfeldt disease, where astrocytic proliferation is very prominent in areas of neuronal loss, the gliosis may resemble SSPE, but the lack of inclusions and white matter pathology are important differentiating features. In PML, the differentia-

tion may be very difficult at times, unless the characteristic viral inclusions are found, but the tendency toward more bizarre astroglial forms in PML may be helpful, as is the tendency for multifocal necrotizing or demyelinating lesions to be seen. The leukodystrophies are characteristics for their lack of inclusion bodies, characteristic phagocytic cells (globoid cells), metachromasia, and other features, but when inclusions are rare, interpretation may be challenging. In cases involving very young patients in whom a white matter disease is suspected, bizarre, often swollen "myelination" glia in immature unmyelinated white matter may also be confusing, but again lack of inclusions and inflammation may be helpful. Antibodies against the SSPE agent (or measles virus) and other viruses

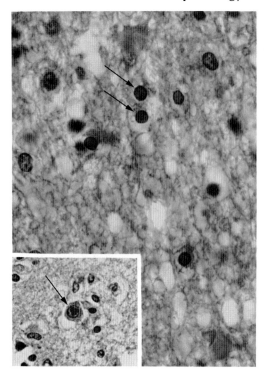

Figure 14.23. The typical intranuclear inclusions in SSPE are illustrated in several oligodendrocytes (*arrows*). Here the inclusions have a different optical texture than nearby unaffected astroglial nuclei, and the inclusion fills the center of the nuclei. H&E. (Original magnification ×500.) These are the most typical forms of the inclusions found in SSPE. In the *inset*, an intranuclear inclusion more typical of a Cowdry type A inclusion is illustrated in a cortical neuron from another area of the same case (*arrow*). H&E. (Original magnification ×320.)

in the differential diagnosis (PML, herpes simplex, and cytomegalovirus) can be used immunohistochemically to differentiate the causative agent and show antigen in cells, even though no inclusions are seen.

Electron microscopic study of SSPE inclusions, first published by Bouteille et al. (30) in 1965, and later by many others, illustrate a tangled mass of hollow, spaghetti-like helical nucleocapsids with an inside diameter of about 17 nM and an inner diameter of about 7 nM (Fig. 14.6) which may fill the center of the nucleus or be associated with altered nucleoli. In some cells, nucleocapsid material may be found in the cytoplasm within occasional viral particles (99). It was these observations of nucleocapsids typical for paramyxoviruses

in SSPE that served as the driving force for continued attempts to recover the infectious agent which morphologically and serologically is now known to be identical with measles virus.

MEASLES ENCEPHALITIS

Prior to widespread use of measles vaccine measles encephalitis as a complication of measles occurred 7.3 times per 10,000 cases between 1962 and 1979 in the United States. Since 1979, clinical measles is greatly reduced, and measles encephalitis is only very rarely seen in apparently normal children but more commonly affects children who have an immunodeficiency disease or who have been immunosuppressed by treatment for lymphomas or leukemias. Such children have been exposed to measles or have had the disease within a few months of appearance of the encephalitis and develop a fulminant syndrome characterized by seizures, coma, and death usually within a few days or weeks. Measles encephalitis resembles SSPE pathologically, but in contradistinction to SSPE, there is a systemic infection with a pneumonitis showing typical Warthin-Finkeldy giant cells and other systemic pathology. The CNS pathology consists of typical intranuclear and occasionally cytoplasmic inclusions, necrosis of affected tissues, but minimal inflammation (294).

THE RHABDOVIRIDAE

These rather large viruses have a unique bullet shape as illustrated in Figure 14.3. Their unsegmented single stranded genome of "negative" stranded RNA exists in the form of a tubular helix inside the membranous envelope of the virus. The virus possesses an RNA-dependent RNA transcriptase which catalyzes the formation of a "positive" RNA strand which is able to direct synthesis of specific viral proteins in much the same manner as is seen in the paramyxoviruses. Cytoplasmic inclusion bodies in many of these infections are common. There are two genera: vesiculoviruses and lyssaviruses (198, 199). Included provisionally in this family are at least two agents, Marburg and Ebola viruses, which produce davastating human illnesses, which are usually in the form of hemorrhagic fevers but may present with encephalitis (16). The agents may be different enough from the other rhabdoviruses that they will one day occupy their own group, the so-called toroviruses (265).

Vesiculoviruses. The most important of the animal viruses in this genus is the vesicular stomatitis virus (VSV), a useful and much studied virus by neurovirologists (57, 58). The Chandipura virus and several other vesiculoviruses cause diseases mostly in insects and animals.

Lyssaviruses. These viruses are responsible for rabies in animals and man, but include a number of other related agents such as Duvenhage and Mokola viruses which may affect man, and a number of other serologically similar viruses of animals.

CNS Infections Caused by Rhabdoviridae (*Vesiculovirus* Genus)

VESICULAR STOMATITIS

Vesicular stomatitis is primarily a disease of cattle, swine, horses, and other farm animals in which there are vesiculating sores about the muzzle (clinically resembling foot and mouth disease). Sores may also affect the teats and cause mastitis. Most infected animals recover, but when the virus is inoculated experimentally it may produce a fatal neurological disease in which demyelination may be seen. In man, VSV is usually contracted by contact with infected animals or in the laboratory. The symptoms of human VSV infection include a flu-like syndrome with headache and myalgia. Mucosal sores are not common, and most cases recover with little or no residual pathology. The neuropathology of VSV infection in man has apparently not been studied, owing to the lack of fatal cases (272, 304).

CNS Infections Caused by Rhabdoviridae (*Lyssavirus* Genus)

RABIES

Rabies is a disease known and feared since antiquity in virtually all regions of the world and is known by a variety of names in various languages: die Tollwut (German); La Rage (French); La Rabbia (Italian); Lyssa (Greek); and Beshenstva (Russian). One of the first accounts of rabies is found in the Sumerian code (19th century B.C.) where a penalty was stipulated for the owner of a rabid dog which was allowed to bite and cause the death by rabies of a man. Clearly, the bites of carnivorous animals were known to cause rabies, and cautery or surgical excision of the bite area was advised as a preventative by Celsus (100 A.D.) and by Galen (200 A.D.). Experimental transmission of rabies by inoculation of the saliva from an infected animal was demonstrated by Zinke in 1804, and the "filterability" of the infectious agent was noted by Remlinger (1903) and its dimensions postulated by Levaditi in 1936. Pasteur was the first to develop an effective postbite preventative vaccine in 1883. Early histological studies of rabies in man and animals were published by Gowers (1877), Babes (1892), by Negri and by Bosc in 1903, both of whom described the characteristic cytoplasmic inclusion body, perhaps wrongly named after Negri (22, 104).

Rabies is caused by a *Lyssavirus* of the Rhabdoviridae family as described above. The reservoir animals are mostly carnivores and include most prominently, dogs, wolves, foxes, raccoons, and skunks, but in Central and South America and some other parts of the world, bats maintain and spread the disease. Occasionally domesticated livestock animals such as swine, goats, horses, and cattle may harbor the infection and transmit it to man (22). Most human cases are caused by bites from infected animals, most commonly the dog. During the 12-yr period from 1970–1981 there were 25 cases of human rabies in the United States, 15 of which were caused by known animal bites, 8 by dogs, but 7 of the 8 dog bites occurred outside the United States (210). In a unique instance, rabies was contracted, presumably by the pulmonary route, by explorers in a bat-infested cave where the guano on the floor of the cave was heavily contaminated by rabies virus (51). Laboratory-acquired infections have been reported, and most workers, veterinarians, and other health care personnel who anticipate possible contact with the virus should be preimmunized with one of the current vaccines (209).

Rabies is found in virtually every country

of the world except Australia, New Zealand, Papua-New Guinea, and most of the islands of the Pacific, Atlantic, and Caribbean. When rabies has been introduced into previously rabies-free regions usually by the careless importing of infected dogs, the virus rapidly becomes endemic in wildlife and is extremely difficult to eradicate (22).

In the dog, the incubation period after infection is 3–8 weeks but may be shorter or longer depending upon the site of the infecting bite. The first signs of the disease are usually behavioral. An otherwise friendly dog may become withdrawn and hostile, or paradoxically, a normally suspicious and hostile dog may become friendly and approach strangers, licking them. It is at this phase that saliva is infectious, and the disease may first be transmitted. This prodromal phase may last a few days to a week and then evolves into usually an excited state in which the animal may wander widely, attacking animals and man indiscriminantly, biting inanimate objects or imaginary enemies. Dogs and wolves in this phase have been known to attack and bite literally scores of persons and animals before being killed or captured (10, 22). The excited dog may lose its appetite or may be stimulated to eat voraciously, even inedible objects, and may attempt to drink water but be frustrated owing to an inability to swallow. At this time the dog may drool or foam at the mouth. Some animals never display an excited phase and pass into what is sometimes referred to as "dumb" rabies. Such an animal may stagger about in a stuporous and delirious state until it collapses and passes into coma and death. This or the excited stage may last up to a week after which progressive obtundation and paralysis usually leads to death in a few days. Although not thought to occur commonly in Europe or America and reported mostly in Africa and Asia, some dogs and other animals may show little or no symptoms of rabies but can be carriers of the disease and capable of infecting other animals or man. In domesticated livestock, the clinical appearance of rabies may be different, and the excitatory phase may be abbreviated, leading to a more subdued infection more typical of "dumb" rabies. The pathological appearance of rabies in animals is virtually the same as in man, described below (139).

In man, infection usually follows a dog bite into which contaminated saliva bearing the virus has been introduced. Rabies virus can be recovered from the general area of the bite for up to 24 h, and after this it has either been inactivated, undergone eclipse, or has been taken up by local muscle where some replication may occur. Rabies virus gains entrance to peripheral motor nerves either via infected muscle or via local sensory fibers which transport the virus centripetally by propagation in the nerve sheath or by retrograde axonal transport to sensory ganglia or to the spinal cord (212). This retrograde transport may proceed at a rate of 3 mm/h or slower (9, 226).

The incubation period, during which transport of the virus is occurring, lasts between 3 and 8 weeks, sometimes shorter or longer depending upon many factors, including the proximity of the bite to the CNS and the age of the victim. When symptoms appear there may be a tingling or painful sensation, itching, or paresthesia along the affected extremity or at the bite site. After appearance of the first symptoms there may be a prodromal phase, lasting up to 48 h, in which there is a feeling of malaise or dread, headache, low grade fever, myalgia, or a flu-like syndrome with sore throat, and gastrointestinal irritation.

Somewhat like the infection in the dog, in man there is an encephalitic phase in which excitability is seen. This takes the form of irritability, agitation, confusion, hallucinations, spasms, bizarre behavior, seizures, and paralysis which may be initiated by minimal stimuli. Painful spasms of the throat and neck may accompany attempts to drink (hydrophobia), and vocal paralysis is common. Periods of delirium and agitation may alternate with calm lucid intervals. At this phase the temperature may be high, there is usually a peripheral leukocytosis, the CSF is under normal pressure but shows a 100 cells or less (mostly lymphoid cells), normal glucose, and elevated protein (60–80 mg%). Increased salivation and lachrymation may be evident, and virus can usually be isolated from the saliva. The deep tendon reflexes are brisk and may be pathological. Cranial nerve paralysis and other brain stem dysfunctions are common. With progressive brain stem involvement, the patient lapses into coma, has difficulty handling secretions, may aspirate, and die a respiratory death (22).

Pathological Appearances

The gross appearance of the brain and spinal cord are that of congestion, edema, and occasionally subarachnoid hemorrhage (226). The principal findings are microscopic and are basically the picture of a polioencephalomyelitis where foci of lymphoid infiltration occurs about penetrating vessels in the Virchow-Robin spaces, and other smaller vessels, in the leptomeninges, and in the major cranial nerve ganglia, dorsal root ganglia, and peripheral nerves. In ganglia, there may be considerable neutrophilic inflammation, proliferation of satellite cells, and a spectrum of chromatolysis and neuronal eosinophilia. In the cervical-medullary region (dorsal grey horns), substantia nigra of the midbrain, hypothalamus, spinal cord, cerebral hemispheres, and cerebellum in roughly descending order, diffuse inflammation and inflammatory nodules (Babes nodes) may be noted. In cases which have had a long course, for unexplained reasons, there may be little if any inflammation. In most cases, however, neuronophagia may be seen focally, but the predominant involvement of neurons in the above and other locations is the formation of cytoplasmic inclusions. The most typical are the Negri bodies (Fig. 14.24), which are round or ovoid, single or multiple eosinophilic rather hyaline bodies, which may have small internal or peripherally arranged basophilic granules. These affect the larger neurons, characteristically of the hippocampal formation, Purkinje cells of

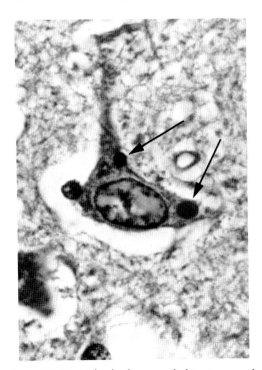

Figure 14.24. This high power light micrograph illustrates an Ammon's horn neuron containing two Negri bodies (*arrows*). The structure of the neuron appears otherwise normal, and in the surrounding neuropil there is little evidence of inflammation or other pathology. The Negri bodies may be of varying size and number but are generally eosinophilic with slight basophilia peripherally. Sometimes they may appear granular. When there are many small cytoplasmic inclusions they may be referred to as lyssa bodies. H&E. (Original magnification ×800.)

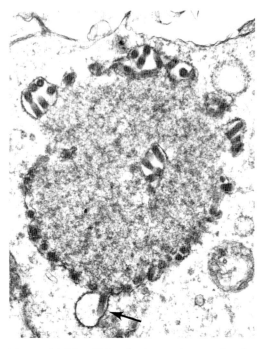

Figure 14.25. This electron micrograph of a Negri body illustrates the granular or filamentous character of most of the body and the peripherally budding capsids of rabies virus into vesicles of endoplasmic reticulum (*arrow*). (Original magnification ×35,000.) (From D. P. Perl (226).)

the cerebellum, and brain stem nuclei. Other rather homogeneous eosinophilic bodies without internal structures, lyssa bodies, may also occur in the cytoplasm. In areas where Negri bodies inhabit neurons, there is usually no inflammatory infiltrate and no apparent change in the neuropil. The white matter is usually unaffected (22, 104, 226).

Ultrastructural studies of the negri body (226) reveal that in most cases, the bullet-shaped *Lyssavirus* nucleocapsids are arranged about the periphery of a nondescript granular body composed of viral proteins. These findings confirm the elegant descriptions of Negri and lyssa bodies made with the light microscope in the 1930s by Marinesco and Stroesco (104) (Fig. 14.25).

Rabies Treatment and Its Complications

Since the time of Pasteur, who developed the first antirabies vaccine using homogenized CNS tissue previously infected with a killed attenuated ("fixed") virus, there were complications resulting from the components of the vaccine. The most common reaction observed was an ascending paralysis similar to Landry-Guillain-Barré syndrome in which 50–70% of affected individuals recovered but suffered residual paralysis of one or more limbs. Postvaccinial encephalomyelitis was a serious, but less common complication (259). Between 25 and 57% of persons who suffered reactions died, no doubt from complications similar to experimntal allergic encephalitis or neuritis (EAE or EAN). The problem of postinfectious or postvaccinial encephalomyelitis is discussed in greater detail elsewhere in this volume. The incidence of such complications with brain tissue-derived vaccines has been reported to be about 0.01%. With the development of vaccines which were raised in embryonated eggs, suckling mouse brain, or tissue culture cells, the incidence of complications has fallen considerably. The most recent vaccines prepared in human cell cultures have shown themselves to be virtually complication-free (22, 209). The effectiveness of vaccination is always raised, when previously vaccinated individuals develop rabies, but such cases always seem to be complicated by either incomplete programs of vaccination, unusual circumstances, delays in postbite immunization, or extremely heavy exposure to a rabies agent.

THE RETROVIRIDAE

The classification of these viruses is still in a state of flux, but they appear to fall into three main subfamilies: lentiviruses, oncoviruses, and spumaviruses. Most of these viruses have icosahedral capsids, contain a single segment of single stranded RNA genoma, and are enclosed in a membranous envelope. They possess an RNA-dependent DNA polymerase (reverse transcriptase) which creates a DNA provirus during replication that is inserted into the host cell DNA (198, 199).

Lentiviruses. This group includes agents which are of primary interest to the neurovirologist and experimental neuropathologist, such as the maedi/visna group, and produce diseases mostly in sheep (261).

Oncoviruses. These viruses, sometimes also known as oncornaviruses or leukoviruses, may be oncogenic, can produce leukemias, lymphomas, sarcomas, mammary tumors, and have produced a viral induced motor neuron disease (5) in experimental animals and have been divided into four categories, designated A, B, C, and D (23). "A" particles have a double envelope and appear empty; "B" particles appear similar but have eccentric cores; "C" particles, on the other hand, have central cores, while "D" particles have either a tubular or cylindrical core. Recently viruses of this group have been implicated in the possible etiology of acquired immune deficiency syndrome (AIDS) in man (92).

Spumaviruses. These agents, named for their ability to produce a vacuolating change (foamy cytopathic effect) in tissue culture cells, are poorly characterized and are not associated with an obvious human disease.

THE ARENAVIRIDAE

The arenaviruses fall into only one genus, are small, spherical, or pleomorphic particles with a dense envelope. The genome is composed of a single stranded clumped, ribosome-like RNA. The form of the RNA evokes the name of the family (Arena—from the Latin meaning sandy)

(Fig. 14.3F). Many of these agents produce a persistent infection, and one of them, lymphocytic choriomeningitis (LCM) virus, has been extensively studied experimentally (219). This and other members of the family can infect man, sometimes with devastating and tragic results. The latter include the virulent Lassa, Junin, and Machupo hemorrhagic fever viruses, which are not primary CNS pathogens but may cause focal hemorrhagic lesions in the brain. Other agents include the Tacaribe and Pichinde-Tamiami viruses about which much needs to be learned (132).

Lymphocytic Choriomeningitis

LCM is commonly harbored by rodents including those often kept as pets, such as the hamster. The virus may cause no obvious disease in the animal and is shed in the urine. When humans are affected by LCM, it is usually in the young, between the ages of 15 and 40 yr of age, although intrauterine infection can also occur. The illness may take one of four forms: a subclinical or inapparent infection; a flu-like syndrome; aseptic meningitis; and meningoencephalitis. In the latter two syndromes, there is little that is distinguishing or diagnostic about LCM-caused infections. The infection is not common, but between 1973 and 1974 181 cases of LCM infection came to the attention of authorities. Of these, 46 had to be hospitalized, but there were no fatalities (219).

PATHOLOGICAL APPEARANCES

Few studies have been made in man since the disease is only rarely fatal, but it appears that the pathology is very similar to that in animals. When aseptic meningitis or meningoencephalitis is found, it usually takes the form of a mild lymphoid infiltrate in meninges and about vessels superficially. There is little evidence of involvement in the brain, with only rare inflammatory nodules or evidence of neuronal damage seen. The systemic pathology may be more substantial, showing foci of necrosis and inflammation in liver, kidney, lungs, heart, and adrenals. Diagnosis cannot definitely be made histologically, unless immunohistochemical methods are used. Recovery of the agent or serological evidence of its presence are usually diagnostic (219).

THE CORONAVIRIDAE

Coronaviruses are occasional human, but more commonly animal, pathogens which have been employed by experimental neurovirologists studying viral induced demyelination and viral persistence (57, 260). The viruses have a unique morphology illustrated in Figure 14.3. The genome is a single molecule of a single stranded RNA. The viruses most commonly produce mild, cold-like upper respiratory illness in man, and a variety of respiratory and gastrointestinal diseases in animals. Occasional cases of aseptic meningitis in man caused by coronaviruses have been reported, but fatal cases have thus far occurred, and thus no pathological information exists about the diseases in the CNS (239).

THE BUNYAVIRIDAE

This is a large family of viruses which are essentially all arthropod-borne (arboviruses), mostly spread by the mosquito, but a few are tick-borne. The viral particles are variable, but most show a spherical shape, sometimes with surface structures that show icosahedral symmetry. The genome is a single stranded RNA which may exist in two or more units, circular in form, within the nucleocapsid. Bunyaviruses produce a number of CNS infections in man and animals which include California encephalitis, Rift Valley fever, and a number of hemorrhagic fevers in tropical parts of the world (198, 199).

California Group Encephalitides

The California group viral encephalitides are a group of arthropod-borne viral infections of the Bunyaviridae family which exist in 12 serotypic groups of the Bunyawera subgroup, most of which occur in the United States (40). Although the first, and naming, member of the group was isolated from mosquitoes in California in 1943, and later confirmed to have caused human encephalitis in that area, the most prominent and prevalent virus of the group was isolated in 1960 from a fatal case of encephalitis in La Crosse, Wisconsin, from which this virus derives its name. La Crosse encephalitis is now generally considered to be synonymous with California encephalitis, since most cases of what had been called

California encephalitis are serologically identical with cases of La Crosse encephalitis. Other related viruses which generally bear the names of the places from which they were isolated are the San Angelo, Jamestown Canyon, Jerry Slough, South River, and Snowshoe Hare viruses. The Tahyna virus from Europe and Africa as well as the Inkoo virus of Finland are other examples.

California (La Crosse) encephalitis is spread by *Aedes triseriatus* mosquitoes which live in a very restricted sylvan environment, apparently breeding in water left standing in holes in trees and stumps, and only infecting those who hike or camp in areas infested with the appropriate mosquito. In Canada other *Aedes* species are the vector (119). Infected mosquitoes can infect other mosquitoes during breeding, which perpetuate the infection. Possible reservoirs are small mammals, such as foxes and raccoons, but not birds, living in the forest, a considerable difference from other arbovirus caused encephalitides (3, 275).

California (La Crosse) encephalitis may be responsible for 5–6% of all viral CNS infections in the United States and is most common in Wisconsin, northern Illinois, Ohio, and Minnesota, where each year in each state a dozen or more cases occur (49). Related strains have been isolated from cases in several parts of Canada, including far northwest areas (195). These agents produce a disease usually of children, varying from a mild viral meningitis to a full-blown encephalitis, which is happily uncommon. The most common presentation is a 2- to 3-d period of fever, headache, malaise, nausea and vomiting, after which signs of meningitis develop. All signs gradually resolve after about a week. The less common presentation is more typical for any of the equine encephalitides, with abrupt onset of fever, disorientation, seizures, focal flaccid paralysis, Babinski signs, tremors, papilledema, and coma. The CSF may contain up to 500 cells/cu mm (mostly mononuclear), protein levels up to 100 mg%, but with normal glucose concentrations. There may be a peripheral neutrophilic leukocytosis. Fortunately, most patients recover to normal within 2 weeks, but some suffer residua like that in any other encephalitis (275). The usual serological methods are helpful in diagnosis of the condition.

PATHOLOGICAL APPEARANCES

Because there have been few fatal cases, case reports with complete neuropathological examinations are few, but the gross and microscopic pathology are reported to be little different from any other arbovirus encephalitis, with perivascular cuffing, inflammatory nodules, and focal necrosis observed. These changes are said to be most common in the cerebral cortex and basal ganglia, in keeping with some of the typical clinical findings in the cases (276).

DNA VIRUS INFECTIONS OF THE NERVOUS SYSTEM

The Herpesviridae

The herpesviruses are well-known as CNS pathogens in man and animals. All members of this family have a similar, if not identical morphology. They are icosahedral and enveloped viruses which are assembled in the host cell nucleus from which they bud, then pass through the cytoplasm to be released by another budding process at the cytoplasmic membrane surface. Viral replication is inefficient, with almost 90% of viral DNA not incorporated into infectious particles, and mostly remaining as viral inclusions in infected cells (198, 199, 214). The large genome is composed of double stranded DNA which can code for a hundred or more viral proteins. All the herpesviruses have the property of persistence and latency in the infected host and can reactivate even after very long dormant periods. The members of this family which can infect man include *herpes simplex virus (types I and II), cytomegalovirus, varicella-zoster virus, B virus (simian herpes virus), and the Epstein-Barr (EB) virus.* Herpes simplex viruses produce "cold sores" and encephalitis (usually type I), genital lesions (usually type II), and encephalitis in the newborn. The varicella-zoster group is well known as the cause of "chickenpox," "shingles," and occasional neural infections. Cytomegalovirus is an important intrauterine pathogen for the developing fetus and is harbinger of the immunosuppressed or depressed state as in organ transplant recipients and victims of acquired immune deficiency syndrome (AIDS) (141, 153). The B virus of monkeys is a serious and often fatal disease usually contracted following laboratory-acquired monkey bites. The E-B virus is the cause of infectious mononucleosis and is associated with Burkitt's lymphoma and nasopharyngeal carcinomas in man. An important animal herpes virus pathogen is Marek's disease, which may devastate poultry flocks (198, 199, 214).

Infections Caused by Herpes Simplex Types I and II

Herpes simplex type I (HSV-I) is a very prevalent virus to which nearly every adult has had exposure and against which has maintained significant antibody titers. It usually produces "cold sores" about the lips, but may cause oral, pharyngeal, respiratory, or ocular infections, and is the primary agent responsible in nonepidemic viral encephalitis. The agent is spread by physical contact or by saliva-contaminated hands, objects, or via aerosol.

Herpes simplex type II (HSV-II) is less prevalent than type I, as evidenced by the fact that perhaps 30% of the population has antibodies to this virus. This form of herpes simplex affects the genital regions, where it produces painful, vesicular and ulcerating lesions, and is mostly spread through sexual contact. It can cause a diffuse encephalitis imparted to the newborn during birth, or sporadic, rather benign forms of neuritis, myelitis, meningitis, or encephalitis in adults (54). It may produce a devastating illness in immunosuppressed individuals.

During the course of primary infection with either HSV-I or HSV-II, virions are apparently conducted by retrograde axonal transport in peripheral nerves to the sensory ganglia serving the infected region (167), where a persistent and usually latent infection is established (164). Viral infection of and transport by infected leukocytes as well as frank viremia may also be important in the spread of HS-II (54). The prevalence of this phenomenon is illustrated by the fact that it has been possible to recover herpes simplex virions from dorsal root ganglia, trigeminal, or other sensory ganglia from a very high percentage of unselected individuals at autopsy (11). The mechanisms for HSV latency are poorly understood, but viral mRNA and protein antigens can be detected in the cells during the latent or eclipsed phase, and *Herpesvirus* genome is probably incorporated in neuronal nuclei, but does not exist as a viral particle as has been shown by nucleic acid hybridization experiments (235).

Following exposure to the virus for the first time, the immune response is similar to that for other agents: IgM appears in serum first but begins to fall at about a week; IgA and IgG neutralizing antibodies follow at about 1 week but remain for years; complement-fixing IgG appears by about 2 weeks but falls within a few months (179).

Reactivation of the latent infection in both HSV-I and II can occur in response to illness, physical or emotional stress, exposure of the skin to ultraviolet light, X-rays, and many other circumstances in up to 25% of previously infected persons. Reactivation does not always involve the appearance of lesions, but can result in viral shedding from oral, pharyngeal, or genital mucosae. It appears that when a neuron bearing HSV is reactivated, it may perish during the process of releasing its virions and forming a new infection (196).

Clinically, the primary herpetic lesion (HSV-I) is usually a painful papular or vesicular, weeping, ulcerating lesion on the lips, a diffuse painful often necrotizing rash which may bleed or exude serum, or less commonly a diffuse systemic illness with respiratory symptoms. When the eye is affected, there is great danger of corneal ulceration and loss of vision. HSV-II lesions are similar, except that they occur in or about the genitals. Reactivation herpes lesions may follow the distribution of nerves, classically mandibular, maxillary, or ophthalmic branches of the trigeminal nerve for HSV-I, and sacral dermatomes for HSV-II.

The most serious form of herpes simplex infection is encephalitis, which in the neonate (HSV-II), naive, or immunoincompetent host (215) is a diffuse process (HSV-I or HSV-II), but in adults, who have presumably had prior exposure to HSV-I, the CNS infection is curiously localized to the basal frontal-temporal regions, often on one side only. It has been suggested that virus reaches the basal portions of the brain during reactivated infection in the trigeminal ganglia via branches of its nerves which innervate the meninges of the middle and anterior fossae. Virions transported in this mode escape immune attack, since they are intracellular (63).

The clinical presentation of herpes encephalitis (HSV-I) is a prodrome of a few days consisting of fever, headache, a flulike illness with sore throat, and in some patients, recurrence of dermal herpetic lesions. The neurological illness then appears with symptoms, which may take several days to evolve, including disorientation, personality and behavioral changes, hallucinations, memory disturbances, weakness, paralysis, seizures, and bladder-bowel dysfunctions. The behavioral features of herpes encephalitis are rather more pronounced than in other encephalitides, and the illness may be misinterpreted as a primary psychiatric illness. Because of occasional bilateral destruction of the hippocampal formations, all or some of the features of the Klüver-Bucy syndrome may be seen. There may be a peripheral neutrophilic leukocytosis, and the CSF may be normal or show up to 1000 neutrophils or mononuclear cells. The protein may rise to 200 mg% or higher; glucose concentration may be low. If bloody fluid is noted and the tap is atraumatic, the prognosis is grave. EEG studies may show slow-wave focality, and CT scans may localize several basal lesions. By the time CNS symptoms have appeared, most patients will have significantly elevated neutralizing antibodies compared with complement-fixing antibodies (179), considered by some to be diagnostic, but often precise diagnosis requires open brain biopsy of an affected area. Attempts at recovery of the virus by culture of CSF or tissue are unreliable, and immunocytochemical study of biopsied brain tissue has shown itself to be rapid, accurate, and reliable. The treatment of herpes simplex encephalitis with cytosine and adenine arabinoside and other nucleic acid analogs is currently showing promise (295, 296).

The prognosis of herpes simplex encephalitis without antiviral treatment is grave, with up to 80% of cases dying. Current unselected survival figures indicate that up to 90% of patients who do not become comatose during the illness can now survive with appropriate antiviral therapy, but 60% of those who are comatose die (295).

When, in rare instances, HSV-II involves the CNS, it can present as an aseptic meningitis, radiculitis, or neuritis which can be mistaken for lumbosacral disc disease, a mild or severe encephalitis or encephalomyelitis, which is usually diffuse rather than focal. The latter two forms of the disease are especially likely to occur in immunosuppressed individuals, and recently in acquired immunodeficiency syndrome (AIDS), in which the prognosis was complicated by the coexistence of other infectious diseases including other viral diseases (141).

PATHOLOGICAL APPEARANCES

The gross pathological appearance of typical acute herpes simplex (HSV-I) encephalitis is that of a hemorrhagic, necrotizing, focal encephalitis of the inferior portions of one or both frontal or temporal lobes (Fig. 14.26). Occasionally foci of involvement may occur over the hemispheres or in the cerebellum, and rarely the involvement may be localized in the brain stem. The leptomeninges are not prominently involved, although there may be staining or even thickening of them over the areas of cortical pathology. Occasionally the lesions may be so hemorrhagic and destructive that they resemble cortical contusions or hemorrhagic infarcts. After fixation and coronal sectioning, the hemorrhagic and necrotizing lesions appear confined to the cortical regions of the frontal, temporal, or hippocampal regions, and still may resemble traumatic lesions or infarctions, except that deep white matter changes are most uncommon. In diffuse HSV-II encephalitis, lesions are not focal, often much less grossly necrotizing and hemorrhagic than HSV-I encephalitis, or the brain may appear essentially normal. In newborn cases, the brain may be very congested, showing focal cortical petechiae.

Microscopically, the necrotizing character of the lesions is evident (Fig. 14.27), as is a prominent inflammatory infiltrate in the leptomeninges, neuropil, about vessels, and surrounding some nerve cells which can display neuronophagia. Macrophages are prominent and contain sudanophilic

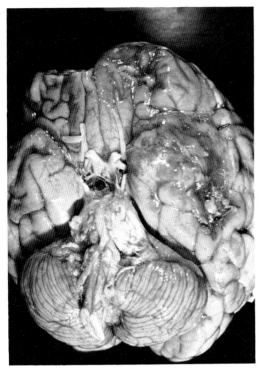

Figure 14.26. The focal and often lobar topography of acute herpes simplex encephalitis is illustrated in this gross photograph of the base of the brain. Here, hemorrhagic and necrotizing lesions are seen in the left temporal and inferior frontal lobes. The right frontal lobe tip had been removed for virus culture studies prior to photography. The attempt to recover the virus by culture of the right frontal lobe was unsuccessful, in spite of the clear demonstration by electron microscopy of herpes virions in many cells from other regions of the brain. This underscores the necessity of culturing tissue which is in or near an active lesion.

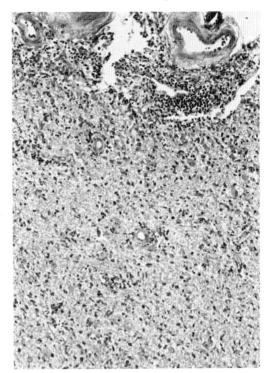

Figure 14.27. This light micrograph illustrates the intense meningoencephalitis typical for herpes simplex virus infection of the nervous system. Here the subarachnoid space and pia are suffused with lymphoid and polymorphonuclear inflammatory cells and blood. The underlying cerebral cortex is heavily infiltrated by inflammatory cells, and a glial proliferative response is already evident. Cowdry type A intranuclear inclusion bodies are not obvious in this section, and in fact had to be diligently searched for in this case. H&E. (Original magnification ×180.)

lipid material. The subcortical white matter may also be necrotic but is seldom deeply involved. There is astroglial swelling and reaction appropriate for the duration of the process, and in active lesions, Cowdry type A intranuclear inclusions (Fig. 14.28) may be found in neurons, astrocytes, or oligodendroglial cells. Sometimes, cytoplasmic inclusions ("viral factories") can be found.

Ultrastructural features of the infection include intranuclear paracrystalline arrays of virions (Fig. 14.8), in various stages of completion, with many lacking some component. There is usually abundant fibrillary or granular electron-dense material intermixed with spherical virions, reflecting the

inefficient production of viral components in the infected cell (Fig. 14.29). Virions may be found budding from the nucleus, enveloped by endoplasmic reticulum in the cytoplasm, or being extruded from the cell surface (Fig. 14.9). Electron microscopy as a diagnostic tool in herpes simplex infection is limited because virus-like particles are common in nervous tissues, areas which can be covered are very small, and the "track record" of this method of diagnosis has not been encouraging.

In chronic cases or areas in which inflammation is scant, inclusions may be scarce or absent entirely, which can complicate histological diagnosis in a small biopsy. It is for this reason that an immunocytochem-

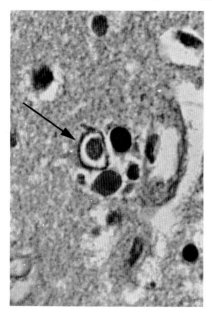

Figure 14.28. A high power light micrograph illustrates typical Cowdry type A intranuclear influsion bodies in glial cells in a case of herpes simplex encephalitis. Such inclusions are not always obvious and may have to be carefully searched for. H&E. (Original magnification × 450.)

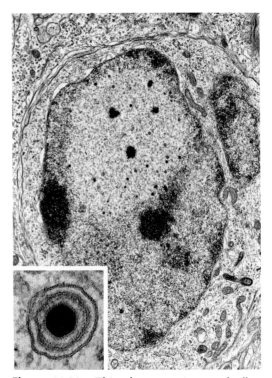

Figure 14.29. This electron micrograph illustrates a small intranuclear inclusion body in a glial cell in experimental herpes simplex virus infection studied in an organized tissue culture preparation. Here, the nuclear chromatin is pushed aside by amorphous and granular material containing scattered virions, some empty, others containing nucleoid material. (Original magnification ×10,000.) Not all inclusions are composed of viral crystals or compact masses of virions, and probably the majority are simply masses of viral products in an unassembled state. An enveloped herpes virion is illustrated in the *inset* and is enclosed by two membranes, the outer of which will be lost when the virion is budded from the cell surface. (Original magnification ×180,000.) (From J. E. Leestma et al. (1974).)

ical method applied to paraffin-embedded formalin-fixed tissues employing the peroxidase-antiperoxidase coupled antibody reaction is so useful, since it can detect very small amounts of viral antigen even in non-inclusion-bearing cells (Fig. 14.30). Fluorescent antibody methods which require unfixed tissues are often unreliable, as are attempts to localize virus blindly in tissue blocks prepared for electron microscopy.

In cases coming to autopsy many weeks or months, following infection, specific diagnosis of herpes simplex encephalitis may be difficult and circumstantial based mostly on the topography, except where viral antigen can be detected immunocytochemically. Devastated areas are microcystic and gliotic, resembling old infarctions or contusions, but lymphoid perivascular inflammation may persist for extended periods of time. It must be remembered that in some individuals herpes simplex may behave in a nontypical, progressive, chronic manner and be confused with SSPE, PML, and other diseases (256), and that it can cause a low grade encephalitis involving the brain stem or a myelitis primarily (possibly HSV-II). Such cases, unless suspected as being due to herpes, may be wrongly diagnosed as due to arboviruses or poliomyelitis. Many such cases have been reported.

In the unusual diffuse herpetic encephalitis cases, usually due to HSV-II in the newborn, the picture is similar to any diffuse viral fatal encephalitis, but typical herpes inclusions may be seen in neurons and in glial cells, and pathological alterations are more in the grey than in the white matter.

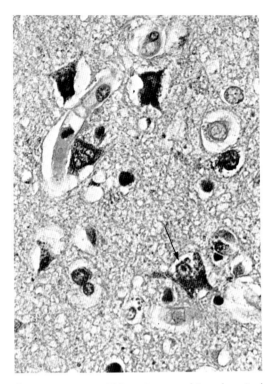

Figure 14.30. This immunohistochemical preparation made using the peroxidase-antiperoxidase coupled immunological reaction with anti-herpes simplex antibody applied to a paraffin-embedded section from a case of herpes simplex encephalitis illustrates the dark reaction product precipitated upon several neurons and a few glial cells. One of the neurons appears to contain a small intranuclear inclusion showing specific reaction product (*arrow*), but most cells appear entirely normal even though they clearly contain viral antigen. This picture is typical for brain biopsies taken in suspected herpes encephalitis cases and illustrates the difficulty of diagnosis based solely on visualization of inclusion bodies by H&E staining. Lightly counterstained PAP-antiherpes stain. (Original magnification ×800.)

Infections Caused by Cytomegalovirus

Cytomegalovirus (CMV) is probably as ubiquitous as herpes simplex in the population, as nearly 90% of adults have antibodies against it. Although it is not known how most individuals are exposed to the agent, 10% or more of females harbor the agent in their cervix, and probably 1–2% of newborns had initial exposure probably during birth as evidenced by serological studies. The remainder of individuals prob- ably acquire the infection, which is usually asymptomatic, through oral or respiratory routes. Infection via blood transfusion may also occur. Many individuals harbor the virus and shed it in the urine, semen, breast milk, and other secretions. Viral persistence and latency probably occur in many organs including hematopoietic cells (153). An excellent animal model of CMV infection showing many of the features of the human infection has been developed in the guinea pig (25).

Cytomegalic inclusion disease takes many forms, ranging from a flu-like illness, gastroenteritis, and an infectious mononucleosis-like syndrome, with an exanthematous skin rash, hepatitis, and myocarditis-pericarditis, and finally a spectrum of nervous system illnesses, which include polyneuritis, meningitis, and encephalitis (71).

CMV infection in the newborn is the commonest cause of neonatal viral infection and accounts for a signifiant number of fetal deaths and lasting debility in infants each year. Most infants born with CMV infections appear normal at first but may suffer from microcephaly and other gyral abnormalities of the brain with mineralizations (10–30% of cases); from seizures and mental retardation; chorioretinitis, strabismus, and blindness; and deafness and other sensory defects. Cardiovascular, skeletal, visceral, and hematologic malformations and dysfunctions can also occur (269). About 5% of infants die either at birth or some time later; 70% carry some debility because of the disease, and only 15% are apparently normal.

PATHOLOGICAL APPEARANCES OF NEONATAL CMV INFECTION

The infant dying acutely shows hepatosplenomegaly, jaundice, and purpura with evidence of inflammation and huge, enlarged inclusion-bearing cells in most viscera as well as extensive extramedullary hematopoiesis. The brain, in intrauterine-acquired infections, is small or represented only by a shrunken walnut-like mass, which is more characteristic of intrauterine toxoplasmosis than of CMV. There may be abnormalities of cortical architecture, and development such as micropolygyria in cerebrum and cerebellum, mineralization of periventricular structures, and granular ependymitis with hydrocephalus. Neuronal heterotopias may be found. Cystic, mineralized areas of tissue destruction may also be seen but are generally less severe than with toxoplasmosis.

Microscopically there may be an active meningoencephalitis in which typical large cells contain Cowdry type A intranuclear inclusion bodies are found (Fig. 14.31). There are focal mineralized lesions in grey and white matter (Fig. 14.32) where perivascular cuffing and inflammatory nodules, and inclusion bearing cells are seen which can be neurons, glial cells, endothelial cells, or inflammatory cells. Glial scarring may occur where lesions appear burned out. the ependymal surface may be destroyed, show

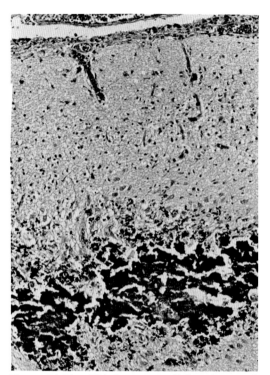

Figure 14.32. This low power light micrograph illustrates the subcortical and subependymal band of calcification which is commonly seen grossly in neonatal victims of intrauterine CMV infection of the brain. The mineralization has clearly been present for some time, as evidenced by the well developed astroglial scarring about its margins. An inflammatory infiltrate is still present in the brain and in the leptomeninges in this case. H&E. (Original magnification ×150.)

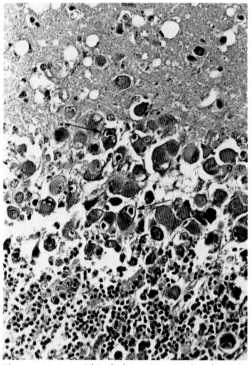

Figure 14.31. This light micrograph of a portion of the cerebellar cortex from a victim of acquired immune deficiency syndrome (AIDS) and cytomegalovirus infection illustrates the huge, distorted Cowdry type A inclusion-bearing cells typical for this disease (*arrows*). Note also the lack of inflammation amidst the distorted and obvious infected cells. It should be noted that immunocytochemical studies, as in herpes simplex infections, show viral antigen in apparently unaffected cells much more frequently than typical inclusions are found. H&E. (Original magnification ×320.)

glial proliferation and scarring, or active lesions. The choroid plexus may be involved. Obstruction to the cerebral aqueduct by glial scarring and active inflammation can occur. Somewhat less commonly the brain stem and spinal cord can show lesions as described above. In very chronic cases, actual evidence of viral infection may be minimal, only the destructive effects of the past infection, cystic and mineralized or gliotic areas remain, but some perivascular inflammation may still be present focally, and rarely inclusion bearing cells may be found.

CMV INFECTIONS IN CHILDREN AND ADULTS

In children and adults, CMV can rarely produce a meningoencephalitis with a clinical picture, in no way suggestive of CMV infection, except that high antibody titers and recovery of CMV from urine or other fluids may suggest but not be specific for the diagnosis. In the rare instances in which these cases have been examined pathologically, the gross pathological appearance is of a diffuse meningoencephalitis showing cortical petechial hemorrhages and brain swelling (Figs. 14.33 and 14.34). Microscopically, there is perivascular cuffing, inflammatory nodules, neuronophagia, focal necrosis, and many inclusion-bearing cells, which suggest the diagnosis.

Recently, it has been shown that CMV is a common cause for viral encephalitis and myelitis in victims of acquired immune deficiency syndrome (AIDS) (141) and in transplant patients. In these cases, the tissue response to injury appears attenuated, and necrotic lesions may contain many inclusion-bearing cells in cerebral cortex, cerebellar cortex, brain stem, spinal cord, and eye, as well as in visceral organs. At times no inclusions are obvious, and the only lesions are either necrotic or focal inflammatory nodules. Immunocytochemical study may be required to demonstrate CMV etiology for the subtle and diffuse pathology seen. There may be coexistent viral infestation by herpes simplex and other viruses as well, as many neuropathologists are encountering in AIDS victims coming to autopsy.

CMV has been implicated in the pathogenesis of Landry-Guillain-Barré syndrome, since some patients appear to have high levels of viral specific IgM in the sera, but conclusive proof that the CMV is directly responsible is lacking (252).

Infections Caused by Varicella-Zoster Viruses

The two diseases, varicella or chickenpox and herpes zoster, appear clinically as distinct entities, but the viral agent, a *Herpesvirus*, is identical and is morphologically indistinguishable from herpes simplex virus. However, this agent is immunologically distinct, even though there are some shared antigens (107).

Varicella is typically an epidemic vesiculating cutaneous disease of childhood spread by the respiratory route which usually causes only mild systemic symptoms and is commonly complicated by bacterial superinfection with some scarring of the itchy lesions. In some apparently otherwise healthy children, the virus causes a severe pneumonia which is the most common cause of death in the rare fatal cases in childhood. Even more rarely, there can be an acute viral meningoencephalomyelitis, Landry-Guillain-Barre syndrome, or a delayed postinfectious encephalomyelitis. Other children, who are immunosuppressed in connection with treatment of neoplasms or organ transplants, may acquire CNS or systemic varicella infection indistinguishable from the infection in normal children.

PATHOLOGICAL APPEARANCES

In the systemic infections, focal necrotic lesions in which Cowdry type A intranuclear inclusion bodies are exhibited are seen in viscera and in the brain where the infection is reminiscent of herpes simplex or acute cytomegalovirus encephalitis in its acute diffuse form. In those infants who have acquired the infection in utero, the CNS damage is much like that seen with perinatal CMV infection, except mineralization is not as common. There may be chorioretinitis, destructive and necrotizing lesions in the brain, spinal cord, and peripheral nerves associated with dermatome-distributed necrotic skin lesions.

Herpes zoster or shingles is usually a disease of older adults in which a painful vesiculating eruption of the skin occurs within the distribution of several dermatomes in the lumbar, cervical, or sacral regions and which heals slowly, causing great discomfort. The disease is more likely to occur in immunosuppressed individuals or those with systemic malignancies or diabetes. The lesions may recur many times, in the same or different regions, and may be precipitated by stress, trauma, or illness. When lesions occur in the distribution of a cranial nerve, with vesicles in the mouth, pharynx, or face, there may be concomitant symptoms of headache, ptosis, Bell's palsy, ocular symptoms, deafness, vertigo, and lingual paralysis. There may be meningeal signs and rarely, symptoms of encephalitis, or myelitis (107).

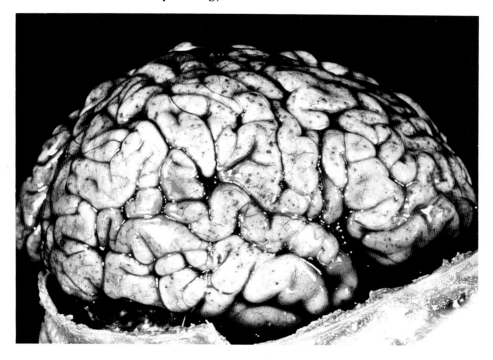

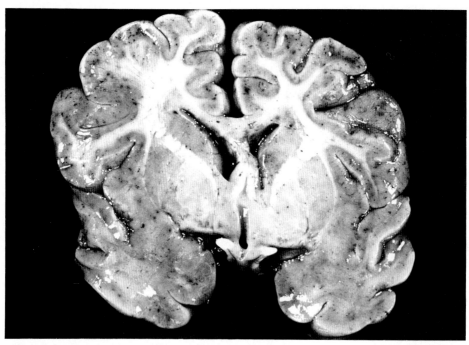

Figures 14.33 (*Top*) and 14.34 (*Bottom*). In these figures the external gross appearance of active, CMV infection of the brain in an infant is illustrated. Note here the congested vessels and numerous punctate hemorrhages on and within the cerebral cortex. This form of CMV infection is rare. There is nothing grossly about this brain that would immediately suggest CMV, but the appearance is suggestive of viral encephalitis. Differential diagnosis would also include leukemia and purpuric disseminated coagulation disorders.

PATHOLOGICAL APPEARANCES

When the CNS is involved directly by herpes zoster, the pathology may be very similar to that seen in varicella, except that lesions tend to be more localized in dorsal root ganglia or cranial nerve ganglia of affected segments. Here one encounters varying degrees of lymphoid infiltration of the tissues, depending upon the ability of the patient to respond with inflammation. Perivascular lymphoid cuffing is typical. Ganglion cells may bear inclusions, but most typically the satellite cells show prominent Cowdry type A inclusions. Destruction of ganglion cells and necrosis of ganglia may occur. Affected portions of peripheral nerve may show little inflammation or focal lymphoid infiltrates, variable pathology of Schwann cells, with bubbling disintegration or loss of myelin and variable disruption of nerve fibers. Affected areas of the CNS are often necrotic and typical for necrotizing lesions seen with any of the herpesviruses, but can resemble PML (131, 193).

Infections Caused by Epstein-Barr Virus (EBV)

The EB virus is the cause of infectious mononucleosis and probably also is the etiologic agent for Burkitt's lymphoma and some nasopharyngeal carcinomas. The EB virus is widely distributed throughout the world, and about 50% of individuals by the time they are 18 hr of age have antibodies to the virus. During the teen years are when most clinically significant infections due to the virus occur, and evidence is that the infection persists for life in the body (101). The disease is traditionally thought to be spread via kissing, but blood transfusions may also spread the virus. After an incubation period of 4–6 weeks after exposure, and less in children, there may be a prodrome of a few days in which there is fatigue, malaise, and headache which worsen over the next 1–3 weeks to include fever, sore throat, profound tiredness, enlargement of cervical and other nodal groups. The spleen and liver may be enlarged and tender. There may be a maculopapular eruption over the trunk, and there may be petechiae on the hard palate. Serious neurological involvement is not common, but is more likely to occur in severe cases of infectious mononucleosis and can include aseptic meningitis, or encephalitis, cerebellar ataxia, mononeuritis, including Bell's palsy, a myelopathy, and Landry-Guillain-Barré syndrome (18, 101). Most cases recover completely, but some neurological residua may remain.

Neurological disease due to EB virus is difficult to prove, since the virus is rarely recovered, and evidence of infection is often implied by serological studies. Fatalities are uncommon, and few have been carefully studied (225). The pathological changes in brain in meningoencephalitic cases is of a diffuse lymphoid inflammation of meninges and brain, with few features that would be considered specific or helpful in a diagnosis.

THE IRIDOVIRIDAE

These are insect, amphibian, and fish viruses which have not been shown pathogenic for man (198, 199).

THE POXYVIRIDAE

These are large block-shaped viruses illustrated in Figure 14.3B. They have a complex lipid-protein coat with a central core containing the double stranded DNA genome. There are two subfamilies, those affecting insects and those affecting vertebrates. The latter subfamily contains six genera, the most important to man being the smallpox virus. Poxviridae contain many proteins, and there is immunological overlap between all of the them, a most fortunate phenomenon, which enabled the development of a very effective vaccine against smallpox and near irradication of that disease worldwide (198, 199). Vaccinia virus (cowpox) used in vaccinations against smallpox in man may rarely result in generalized vaccinia with CNS involvement in children who are presumably immunologically incompetent (157).

THE PARVOVIRIDAE

These viruses are very small, naked icosahedral particles which replicate in the host cell nucleus. Their genome is unique, since it is composed of single stranded DNA, while all other DNA viruses have a double stranded DNA. They produce no known disease of man but are the object of study, since they produce persistent and latent infections in mice, rats, cats, and other animals. There are three genera: parvoviruses, adeno-associated viruses, and densoviruses (198, 199).

Parvoviruses. These agents are an interesting group from the experimental point of view, since they appear to replicate only in rapidly dividing cells. One type, the Kilham virus (159), can pass the placental barrier and induce necrosis of selected populations of neuroblasts in the fetus, especially in the developing cerebellum, and has been utilized to study congenital cerebellar atrophy in the cat. It is possible that the so-called Dane particle found in the serum of hepatitis B victims is a form of *Parvovirus*, and that this disease will ultimately be classified under this family (198, 199).

Adeno-associated virus. These viruses are unique in that they cannot replicate except in the presence of a replicating "helper" adenovirus or *Herpesvirus* (231). The phenomenon illustrated by these viruses holds considerable interest for those studying virus-induced demyelination and experimental model for multiple sclerosis (57).

Densoviruses. These viruses are principally insect viruses, and as yet not important to man or the experimental laboratory.

THE PAPOVAVIRIDAE

The name of these viruses is an acronym (PApilloma-POlyoma-VAcuolating agents) for a group of related agents which are small, naked, icosahedral virions with double stranded DNA genomes. Replication, like most of the other DNA viruses, occurs in the host cell nucleus. They are divided into two genera, papova A and papova B, both of which are tumorigenic in some but not all species of animals (142, 198, 199).

Papovavirus, Group A. This group contains the Shope papilloma virus of rabbits and papilloma viruses of man and other animals. CNS infections are not an important area of activity for these viruses.

Papovavirus, Group B. This group contains the simian vacuolating agents (SV 40), polyoma virus in mice, and the JC virus which have been isolated from immunosuppressed patients and in cases of progressive multifocal leukoencephalopathy (PML) (220, 290). All of these viruses have been extensively studied, and a curious phenom-

enon similar to the adenovirus-associated agents has been discovered. When SV 40 and adenovirus are replicating in the same cell, a hybrid virus is formed which displays some intriguing properties of current interest to virologists (231).

Papovavirus Infections of the CNS

PROGRESSIVE MULTIFOCAL LEUKOENCEPHALOPATHY (PML)

This disease, as the name implies, is a progressively destructive, patchy process, principally affecting white matter in all areas of the nervous system, although it cannot be considered strictly a demyelinating process. It is caused by two known viral agents belonging to the papovavirus group B (JC and SV 40 viruses). The disease was first formulated conceptually and named by Åström et al. (6) who reported three cases, but drew attention to five previously published case reports, beginning with the two cases of Hallervorden (1930) which probably represented the same entity. The disease is now viewed as an opportunistic infection affecting in the vast majority of cases immunologically incompetent individuals who are generally suffering from chronic leukemias, Hodgkin's or other lymphomas. Other disease states reported in conjunction with PML include tuberculosis, sarcoidosis, nonlymphomatous neoplasms, and in connection with immunosuppressive therapy in lupus erythematosus, rheumatoid disease, organ transplants, and occasionally other diseases (86, 202). A number of cases have also been reported in apparently healthy individuals (86). Most cases occur in adults but occasionally appear in childhood.

The onset of PML is insidious and can occur at any time during the course of the underlying major disease. The symptoms include mental deterioration and dementia, behavioral abnormalities, cortical blindness and apraxias, sensory disturbances, ataxia, paralysis, and occasionally, seizures. Sometimes the symptoms are suggestive of a brain tumor, but usually headaches and signs of increased intracranial pressure are absent. There is usually no fever, and the CSF is normal. Serological studies are complicated by the fact that most adults normally carry antibodies to the virus which must be ubiquitous. Computerized tomography may show multifocal lesions in the white matter of the brain. The premortem diagnosis of PML is occasionally made, since there is a general awareness of PML as a remote effect of neoplasia and immune deficiency states, but most cases are still diagnosed at autopsy.

The viral etiology of PML was suggested by Cavanagh et al. (43) and by Richardson (238), but Zu Rhein and Chou (306) studied the brains of two cases which had been in formalin for 2 yr and reported the appearance of PML and its viral agent with electron microscopy in 1965. Further studies indicated that within the inclusions of oligodendrocytes, described below, regular paracrystalline arrays of virus-like particles typical for polyoma group virions were seen.

Initial attempts to recover the virus by ordinary methods were not successful, but Padgett et al. (220) in 1971 was able to cultivate SV 40 virus using human fetal brain cultures exposed to extracts of brain from a PML case. Weiner and Narayan (290) recovered a similar agent from a case using cell fusion methods, but this virus proved to be different from Padgett's JC virus. Subsequently, other laboratories isolated viruses from cases of PML and discovered that most cases were caused by JC virus. Another papovavirus, the BK virus, was isolated from the urine of an immunosuppressed patient who did not show PML (93). The JC and other related viruses which cause PML are oncogenic in experimental animals and can produce CNS tumors, but in man only two instances have been reported where primary glial tumors of the brain may have been related to PML viruses (42, 262). Otherwise, these agents, even though virtually everyone has been exposed to them probably during childhood, do not apparently cause other diseases and are not normally found in the brain. Experimentally produced PML in animals has not been possible, but a naturally occurring version of PML has been observed in monkeys, caused by SV 40 virus (124).

The pathogenesis of PML is not well understood, in spite of the isolation of the viral agent which causes the disease. It is not known when or how the virus enters the CNS, how long it takes to produce the disease, and why there are certain characteristics of a persistent, even latent infection. The agents apparently do not infect neurons, but show predilection for oligodendrocytes (which show characteristic nuclear inclusions), and for astrocytes (which show bizarre anaplastic reactive changes). The basis for the demyelinating character of the lesions is that oligodendroglia are uniquely affected by the virus because they lack a well developed lysosomal system in the cytoplasm (147).

PATHOLOGICAL APPEARANCES

The gross lesions of PML cannot be appreciated from an external examination of the brain. Only when it has been sectioned can the characteristic moth-eaten, crumbly, areas of white matter destruction be appreciated (Fig. 14.35). These areas, which can be very small or involve the entire centrum ovale, occur in multiple foci through the brain but tend to reside more posteriorly. The basal ganglia and thalamus may show lesions, but lesions in cerebellum, brain stem, and spinal cord are less common. Long-standing lesions may become cavitary.

The microscopic appearance of PML is primarily one of white matter destruction in which inflammation is not very prominent. Occasionally there will be perivascular lymphoid cuffing and a mild leptomeningeal infiltrate, but inflammatory nodules are rare. The main cellular reaction is one of a bizarre, almost neoplastic transformation of reactive astroglial cells (Fig. 14.37) without greatly increased cellular density, distortion, and enlargement of some oligodendroglia with huge eosinophilic or basophilic nuclear inclusions not of the Cowdry types (Fig. 14.38). In the areas which show major patchy myelin loss (Fig. 14.36) as observed with myelin stains, and apparent activity of the lesion has diminished, most oligodendrocytes are gone, as are the inclusion-filled cells, which tend to be found in more cellular and active regions. Macrophages in areas of activity may be prominent and contain sudanophilic material.

The differential microscopic diagnosis of PML may be difficult at times and is easily confused with SSPE, adrenoleukodystrophy, and other white matter degenerative

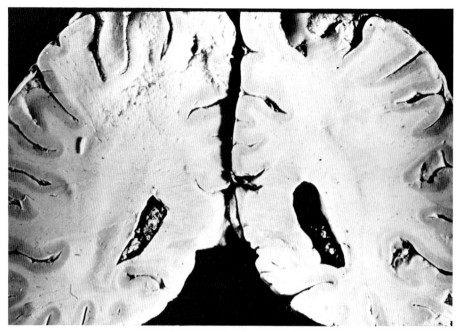

Figure 14.35. This gross photograph of a brain with extensive lesions of progressive multifocal leukoencephalopathy (PML) in the left hemisphere illustrates the moth-eaten or crumbly appearance of the lesions in the white matter. The destructive process results in major interruption of axons in the white matter and is thus the basis for the dementia often associated with the condition.

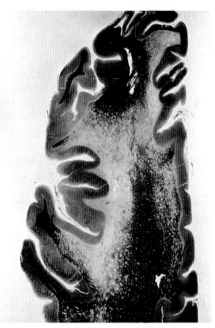

Figure 14.36. This large myelin-stained whole brain section from a case of PML illustrates the macroscopic appearance of moth-eaten myelin in many areas throughout the centrum ovale. Such myelin and axon loss is irreparable and may progress to cavitation if the individual survives long enough (Woelcke myelin section). (Courtesy of Dr. William C. Schoene.)

diseases. Occasionally, radiation necrosis of white matter may appear identical with PML, except that inclusion-filled cells are never seen. In the rare instances in which PML presents unexpectedly in a normal individual as a suspected mass lesion, interpretation of the frozen section taken at biopsy may be very challenging, since the astroglial anaplasia is not in keeping with the sparse cellularity of the biopsy. Ultrastructural examination of the specimen or immunocytochemical staining for JC viral antigens can aid in diagnosis.

ELECTRON MICROSCOPIC APPEARANCES

The intranuclear inclusions are usually composed of paracrystalline arrays of regular spherical particles 35–40 nM in diameter, but may be interlaced with filamentous material of somewhat smaller dimension. Occasionally paracrystalline arrays and masses of the filamentous material can be found in the cytoplasm of some glial cells (Figs. 14.39 and 14.40). Chains or groups of particles may be found in astroglial or oligodendroglial cytoplasm and rarely free in the neuropil.

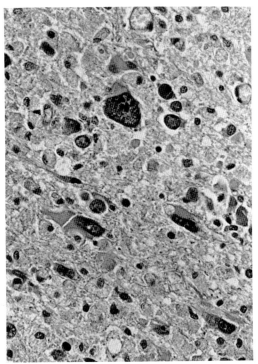

Figure 14.37. This light micrograph illustrates the striking glial reaction, which is almost neoplastic appearing, the loss of normal white matter architecture, and many inclusion-filled oligodendrocytes in an affected area of white matter from a case of PML. Inflammation may be prominent or entirely absent. H&E. (Original magnification ×320.)

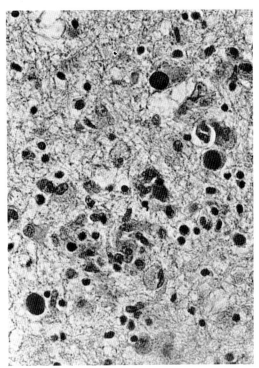

Figure 14.38. This high power light micrograph illustrates the grossly enlarged and swollen oligodendroglial nuclei which contain typical inclusions of PML. These inclusions are not the typical Cowdry type A inclusions as seen in *Herpesvirus* infections or in SSPE, but rather produce enlargement of the nucleus and rarely show a clear space beneath the thin nuclear membrane. Rarely the inclusion may even appear crystalline under light microscopy. H&E. (Original magnification ×500.)

THE ADENOVIRIDAE

Adenoviruses are naked, icosahedral particles which possess filamentous projections from the vertices of the particle. There are two genera: mastadenoviruses and aviadenoviruses.

Mastadenoviruses. At least 33 different human serotypes exist within the genus. These viruses inhabit the mucosal and respiratory membranes and produce upper respiratory infections, pharyngitis, and conjunctivitis. Long latency of this virus in lymphoid tissue has been reported. While this virus may produce a nonfatal aseptic meningitis, it is rarely isolated from the CNS and as such is not an important pathogen for the CNS in man. Some human adenoviruses (types 12 and 18) have been employed as neurooncogens in animals but apparently have no role in human brain tumors (142).

Aviadenoviruses. These agents do not infect man or other mammals and as yet are not of interest to neurovirologists.

ATYPICAL AND UNCONVENTIONAL AGENTS

The concept of the "unconventional" infectious agent arose in the course of laboratory investigation of several unusual plant, animal, and human diseases at first thought to be degenerative diseases, but which were shown to be transmissible. The many puzzling aspects of these diseases and their etiologic agents have necessitated a special category within the catalog of infectious agents, referred to by many names which include viroids, virinos, prions, unconventional agents, and "slow" viruses. Examples of the diseases are scrapie, a CNS

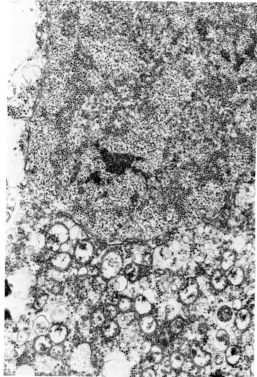

Figure 14.39. This electron micrograph illustrates an oligodendrocyte which is almost entirely filled with small viral particles typical for papovavirus virions. Note that while the nucleus contains more virions, many can also be found in the cytoplasm as well. (Original magnification ×19,250.) (From Dr. Garielle Zu Rhein.)

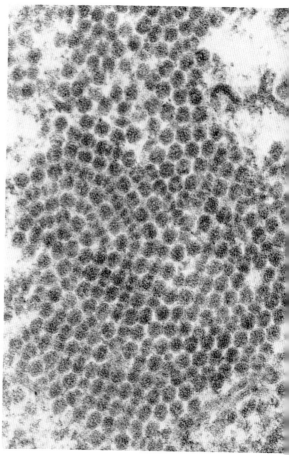

Figure 14.40. This high power electron micrograph illustrates a paracrystalline array of papovavirus virions (J-C virus) from a case of PML. (Original magnifiation × 108,150.) (Courtesy of Dr. Gabrielle Zu Rhein.)

degeneration in sheep and goats, transmissible mink encephalopathy (now thought actually to be scrapie in mink) (189), Jakob-Creutzfeldt disease and kuru, diseases in man, and potato spindle tuber and other diseases in plants (232).

These diseases and their agents have many characteristics of viral infections but are clearly very different from them in that incubation periods may be very long (233), there is no immunological or inflammatory response to the infection, and their agents have eluded persistent attempts at isolation and precise characterization. No actual infectious particles have yet been demonstrated by electron micrographs of infected tissues or tissue extracts. Studies by many investigators indicate that the unconventional infectious agents of scrapie, Jakob-Creutzfeldt disease, and kuru may be proteins of low molecular weight (60,000 to 100,000) and of very small size. They may contain a small DNA genome which could be highly protected by a protein coat, but some have suggested that there is no nucleic acid component present at all and that one report of DNA-ase inactivation of infectivity in scrapie may be incorrect, since it has not been reproduced (189, 234). Such a suggestion, which implies that a nonnucleic acid molecule can direct self-replication in vivo, has immense theoretical implications for molecular biology, genetics, and evolutionary biology.

The pathology of most of the unconventional agents is similar and tends to be that of a spongiform encephalopathy in which deposition of amyloid material is often seen. There is also the rather worrisome property these agents possess of being resistant to normal sterilization methods, to organic solvents, and to formalin fixation, irradiation, and heat which instills considerable fear in laboratory workers and health care personnel in contact with affected animals or patients. It is, however, possible to inactivate infectivity by hypochlorite solutions and prolonged high temperature sterilization of instruments and tissues. Several recommendations have been made concerning the proper handling, disposal, and sterilization of contaminated instruments, excreta, dressings, and tissues of persons with these diseases, and it appears that their use as well as reasonable caution as would be applied in any communicable disease is adequate to protect persons in contact with such patients (34).

Kuru

Kuru is a progressive degenerative disease of the nervous system of infectious etiology which is apparently limited to the Fore linguistic group of about 15,000 persons who reside in the eastern highlands of Papua-New Guinea (91, 102). In the Fore language, kuru means to tremble or shake and graphically describes one of the main symptoms of the disease. Acting on reports of a peculiar neurological disease, thought at first to be encephalitis, Dr. Vincent Zigas, the local medical officer of the region, went to the area in 1956, examined several afflicted persons, and reported his findings to his superiors. In 1957, D. Carleton Gajdusek visited Papua-New Guinea intending to pursue his interest in child growth and development and disease patterns within primitive societies, learned of the existence of kuru, and went to the remote region where the disease was epidemic. There, for the next 10 months Gajdusek, Zigas, and others examined hundreds of victims of kuru, delineated the geographical boundaries of the disease, followed the course of the illness, attempted to treat it, and began extensive studies in cooperation with both Australian and American laboratories to find the etiology of the disease. Gajdusek and his coworkers found that the disease appeared to affect adult females, infants, and children of both sexes, but uncommonly, men. The disease was apparently unknown to the Fore people prior to 1920

but occurred about the time of entry of Europeans to the region and after cannibalism was introduced in the early 1900s from other peoples in the north (83).

Kuru is characterized by the insidious onset of muscular aches and pains, headache, and other nonspecific complaints which give way to a progressive ataxia, with eventual choreiform or athetoid movements and myoclonic jerks which are not seen at rest. Fairly early in the course walking is difficult without support of a walking staff. There is no fever, sign of inflammation of the CNS, and no somatic symptom. Dementia, muscular weakness, and paralysis eventually occur and lead to death within 3 to 24 months after the onset of symptoms (91).

The etiology of kuru was originally suspected to be infectious, but upon examination of many patients and scrutiny of their history it seemed that the etiology was more likely to be nutritional, toxic, parainfectious, or heredofamilial and degenerative (83). However, no support for these causes could be found. The clue to the eventual discovery of the infectious etiology of kuru was found in the pathological examination of the brains of kuru victims (163), which showed similarities to the findings in Jakob-Creutzfeldt disease and to the animal disease, scrapie, which had been previously suggested to be of infectious etiology, and prompted the experimental approach (110) which eventually lead to the demonstration of transmissibility of both kuru (90) and Jakob-Creutzfeldt disease (97) in monkeys.

The experimental approach developed by Gajdusek, Gibbs, and their co-workers involved inoculating homogenized samples of kuru brains intracerebrally in young chimpanzees. After an incubation period of 14–82 months, the animals showed symptoms quite similar to those of the original kuru victims, although the pathology was somewhat different, that of a subacute spongiform encephalopathy (17). Subsequent passages from animal to animal were accomplished in a shorter time and infectivity of various tissues determined (98). Oral transmission of kuru was found possible in experimental animals and to produce a shorter incubation period than if infectious material was introduced through cuts or abrasions in the extremities. It now seems very likely that ritual cannibalism practiced by the Fore people on the bodies of victims of kuru, as a part of the mourning rite for the victim, ironically resulted in frequent transmission of the disease to the mourners, mostly the women and children. As a result of these studies, the Fore people were encouraged to discontinue the practice of ritual cannibalism with the gratifying result that kuru is now a very rare disease in Papua-New Guinea, with only about 20–25 cases in existence, where once it affected more than 1% of the Fore people. Those currently affected by the disease live in villages where cannibalism ceased more than 20 yr ago and probably represent individuals whose exposure to the agent as children was not via the oral route, and in whom the incubation period may exceed 20 yr (233).

PATHOLOGICAL APPEARANCES

Grossly the brain appears normal with the exception of cerebellar folial atrophy which is most severe in the vermis and flocculonodular lobe (163). The microscopic lesions are strikingly uniform from case to case and consist most prominently of loss of Purkinje and granule cells in the paleocerebellum. Here there are numerous torpedo fibers, deformed and altered Purkinje cell dendrites, empty baskets, hypertrophy of Bergmann glia, increased numbers of rod cells and astrocytes in the molecular layer, and so-called kuru amyloid plaques. These characteristic deposits consist of a core of amyloid surrounded by a paler granular or fibrillary halo (Fig. 14.41). The plaque is not neuritic as in the senile plaque of Alzheimer's disease and is not

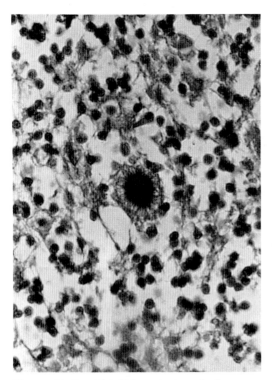

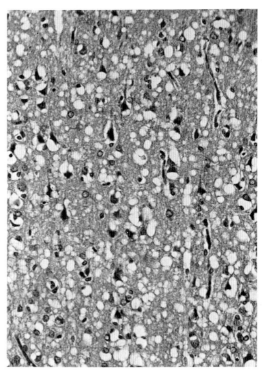

Figure 14.41. This light micrograph illustrates the typical appearance of a kuru plaque from a case of kuru. Note the characteristic "spiked ball" appearance of the material within a Purkinje cell from the cerebellar cortex. Such kuru plaques may be seen in dementing illnesses of uncertain classification in apparently otherwise typical Jakob-Creutzfeldt disease. (Original magnification ×640.) (Courtesy of Dr. Dikran Horoupian.)

Figure 14.42. This light micrograph illustrates the pathology seen in the cerebral cortex of a capuchin monkey inoculated intracerebrally with an extract of the brain from a case of human kuru. The typical vacuolated appearance of many of the subacute spongiform encephalopathies is well shown here. There would be little to distinguish this picture from scrapie or experimental Jakob-Creutzfeldt disease in any of the animals. H&E. (Original magnification ×320.)

seen in the cerebral cortex. There is neuronal loss and gliosis in pontine nuclei, olives, and other nuclei concerned with coordination and modulation of motor responses. There is degeneration and demyelination of the corticospinal and spinocerebellar tracts in the spinal cord. Some degree of spongiosis can be found in many cases in the corpus striatum and in scattered locations in the cerebral cortex, where neuronal swelling, shrinkage, chromatolysis, and replacement gliosis can also be noted. The anterior nuclei of the thalamus and other associated limbic structures may show neuronal loss, gliosis, and occasionally spongiosis as well (163). Kuru-like neuropathological changes have been reported in occasional cases of dementing illnesses outside of Papua-New Guinea (91), and in some cases of Jakob-Creutzfeldt disease (128), raising the question of the exclusiveness of the pathology of kuru and the relationship of this unusual disease with other diseases caused by unconventional agents.

Kuru in the experimental animal has a different picture and like animal-transmitted J-C disease, appears more like scrapie than the original pathology in man. The picture is one of a diffuse spongiform encephalopathy (Fig. 14.42), with severe neuronal loss and gliosis. Purkinje cell changes and torpedoes are common, but kuru plaques are not seen (17, 18).

Jakob-Creutzfeldt (J-C) Disease

In 1921 Alfons Maria Jakob published a paper entitled: "About Peculiar Diseases of the Central Nervous System with Remarkable Anatomical Findings (spastic pseudosclerosis-encephalomyelopathy with disseminated foci of degeneration)," based upon the clinical and pathological study of three cases he had collected over the previous 2 yr and a review of a number of possibly related cases reported previously by Alzheimer, von Economo and Schilder, van Woerkom, and by Creutzfeldt (160). In the minds of some students of the disease, it is Jakob who deserves the credit for formulating the concept of the disease and differentiating it from other conditions (160). Jakob later published details on a fourth case the same year and a fifth case in 1923. Several other reports of similar or related cases under various names followed and include the descriptions by Spielmeyer (267), who in 1922 suggested the name Creutzfeldt-Jakob disease, and Kirschbaum (160), who reported the first of the Backer (or Becker) family members to die of this disease. Through the 1930s and 1940s several additional cases were added, most of which have been reviewed by Kirschbaum (160). In 1954 Jones and Nevin (152) and in 1955 McMenemey and Nevin (160) described additional cases and proposed a vascular etiology for the disease. They also stressed the microscopic spongiform changes in the grey matter which now are accepted as an important feature of the disease. Spongiform change, however, was not described in the earliest cases, but was reported in the 5th case (Hoffert) of Jakob's in 1923 and in several subsequent cases, although it appears that major emphasis on this change was not made until much later (160). It is curious that spongiform change seems to have become more prevalent after about 1940 as more cases were described and now seems to be accepted by many as the sine qua non of the disease, even though occasional cases of otherwise classical J-C cases coming to postmortem study today lack significant spongiform changes. The lack of spongiosis in some cases should not rule out the diagnosis of J-C disease, even though it complicates the histological diagnosis by its absence.

The first ultrastructural studies on J-C disease were published by Gonatas et al. in 1965 (100), and transmission of the disease to a chimpanzee via intracerebral inoculation of a human brain homogenate was accomplished by Gibbs et al. in 1968 (97), using their method which was so successful in demonstrating the transmissibility of kuru 2 yr previously (90). Subsequent workers have been able to transmit the disease from man to several species of primates, to other animals, and to rodents, through several serial passages, and to significantly shorten the incubation period in the process (185, 186). In experimental J-C disease in rodents it has been shown that following intracerebral inoculation of infected material there is eventual spread of infectivity to the viscera and that the reverse is also possible. These and other observations suggest that viremia may be important in the pathogenesis of the disease and that replication of the agent in some intermediate tissue such as the reticuloendothelial system may occur at some point in the disease in a manner analogous to poliomyelitis (185).

The actual agent responsible for Jakob-Creutzfeldt disease has not been isolated and precisely characterized morphologically, although there are many compelling reasons to suspect that it is very similar to the agent for scrapie (189). Ultrastructural studies by a number of workers (48, 100, 192) have shown a variety of virus-like particles and other forms suggestive of plant viruses or other unusual agents in J-C material, but etiologic connections between the observed structures and the disease have not been proven (14).

The clinical characteristics of J-C disease are varied, and there are several recognized variants of the disease. The usual case occurs in a middle aged individual of either sex but may occur in childhood, adolescence, or in aged persons. Ten–fifteen percent of cases seem to have a familial pattern, suggestive of a dominant mode of inheritance (190). There is no occupational predisposition, although some have suggested that meat handlers and butchers may have a disproportionate incidence. Recently it has been suggested that persons with J-C disease have a greater than expected likelihood of having had a neurosurgical procedure (298). The concern in this observation is no doubt motivated by the several reports of passage of the disease from person to person via corneal transplantation and apparently inadequately sterilized neurosurgical instruments (24, 76, 298). With the exception of the above rare cases, the mode of transmission of the disease is unknown, and no animal transmission of J-C disease has ever been demonstrated using external secretions, hair, skin, or excreta from victims as an inoculum (189). There is no evidence that medical or paramedical personnel, morticians, and morgue workers are any more likely to contract the disease than anyone in the general population. In view of the transmissibility of the disease, however, proper procedures for handling tissue from J-C patients have been formulated and recently reviewed (45).

The onset of the classical form of the disease is usually insidious with a "prodro-mal" period in which fatigue, dizziness, anxiety, vague memory defects, weakness, or slight locomotion problems may occur. These symptoms may persist and get worse over several months and be attended by an increasingly apparent failure of high order mental functioning characterized by disturbances of calculation, abstract thought, reasoning, and judgment. In some patients visual difficulty, aphasia, apraxia, ataxia, choreiform-athetotic movements, and pyramidal tract signs with amyotrophy may be associated with the progressive mental deterioration. J-C disease has been divided into several variants by some workers based upon the clinical presentation and the pathology of the disease at autopsy. Heidenhain's variant is characterized by predominantly occipital lobe degeneration and visual impairment (201), an amyotrophic form in which pyramidal signs predominate (189), and a cerebellar form sometimes referred to as the Brownell-Oppenheimer variant occurs, in which ataxia and cerebellar signs are prominent (35). An ophthalmoplegic variant has also been described (246). Another variant or related condition is the Gerstmann-Sträussler syndrome which in some ways resembles kuru with ataxia, slurred speech, pyramidal tract signs, and ophthalmoplegias with a relapsing downhill course including dementia (29, 191).

In the usual case of Jakob-Creutzfeldt disease, about 6 months from the onset of whatever constellation of symptoms present themselves, the dementia is profound, and myoclonic jerking is evident; the victim becomes vegetative, mute, and bedfast. Death usually occurs within 12 months of the onset but may be delayed for up to several years (160). Laboratory studies are usually noncontributory, the EEG shows diffuse slowing, with periodic sharp spike and wave complexes which are considered by some to be highly suggestive of the J-C disease. The CSF is usually normal but may show slight elevation of protein content. Death is usually due to intercurrent infection and cachexia.

PATHOLOGICAL APPEARANCES

As is true for the variable clinical presentations of J-C disease, the range of pathological expression is also broad and shows considerable topographic and indi-

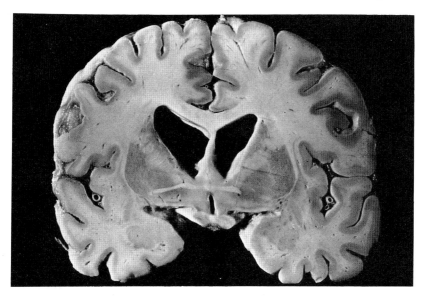

Figure 14.43. This gross photograph of the brain of 40-yr-old female who died about a year after the onset of progressive and rapid dementing illness characterized eventually by myoclonic jerking illustrates the common appearance of Jakob-Creutzfeldt disease. There is a slight suggestion of cortical atrophy, the ventricles are enlarged, and the head and body of the caudate nuclei are shrunken. A brain biopsy from this case was inoculated into a monkey in the laboratory of Dr. J. C. Gibbs, Jr. The monkey died of a neurological illness and showed typical spongiform encephalopathy at its autopsy.

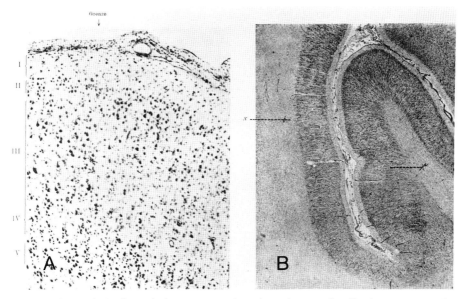

Figure 14.44. (*A* and *B*) These light micrographs of Nissl-stained celloidin sections of cerebral cortex of one of Creutzfeldt's early cases of Jakob-Creutzfeldt disease illustrate the subtle focal loss of nerve cells with little gliosis and no inflammation which characterized many of the early reported cases. Some focal areas of neuron loss are labeled by *dashed lines* and *x*'s. (From W. R. Kirschbaum (160).)

vidual histological variations from case to case. This variation is exhaustively reviewed by Kirschbaum (160). In general, the gross appearance of the usual J-C brain may be entirely normal or show slight diffuse convolutional atrophy and slight ventricular dilatation (Fig. 14.43). In cases which correspond to the corticostriatospinal degenerative pattern described by Wilson (300), there may be some atrophy of the caudate and putamen associated with slight brownish discoloration, slight cortical atrophy, and grossly visible lateral corticospinal tract degeneration in the spinal cord. In some cases the cerebellum may appear slightly atrophic. At times, the cortical ribbon thickness may be diminished.

The outstanding changes are microscopic and usually take the form of tremendous neuronal loss, replacement gliosis, and status spongiosis of cerebral cortex (frontal and temporal lobes more affected) where the deeper lamellae show the greatest change (Figs. 14.44 and 14.45). The corpus striatum (caudate and putamen), thalamus, upper brain stem tegmentum, and superficial layers of the cerebellar cortex also show these changes. The spongiform change (189, 192), a dynamic process which is not always obvious by light microscopy in brain biopsy specimens but can usually be seen ultrastructurally, waxes and wanes with time. Often inapparent in an early biopsy, it will be obvious on a later one from the same region and again be nearly absent in the autopsy specimen, however; regional differences and the speed of progression of the case are important variables. It should be remembered that spongiform changes can be mimicked by anoxic or ischemic damage and can be seen in conjunction with a variety of inflammatory and toxic conditions, inborn and acquired metabolic encephalopathies, and can be confused with cerebral edema or preparation artifacts. To properly interpret spongiform change requires cognizance of its context in each case and its relation to other pathological findings (192).

Ultrastructurally, the spongiform change in J-C disease consists of intraneuronal, complex, clear vacuoles with membranous septa (Fig. 14.46), curled membranous profiles within the vacuoles (Fig. 14.47), and sometimes ill defined particles or granular debris (48, 100, 169). These spongiform changes are similar, if not identical, to those seen in scrapie, both natural and experimental, and in experimentally transmitted kuru and J-C disease.

Individual neurons may appear swollen or shrunken and may contain excess lipofuscin pigment. Neuronophagia can be seen but is probably harder to visualize in standard 6-μm H&E-stained slides than in much thicker Nissl-stained celloidin or paraffin sections. When a given gyrus has not already been decimated, neuronal loss may be patchy and difficult to appreciate unless thicker sections are made. This is especially true in those cases in which spongiform change is limited or absent (Fig. 14.44).

Lymphoid infiltration in the brain is rarely seen, inflammatory nodules (glial nodules) may occasionally be found, and the white matter appears preserved until late, when, if large myelin-stained histological sections are prepared, they may show pallor of the deep portions of the centrum ovale. Recently it has been suggested that white matter pathology is more prevalent than appreciated. Often the degree of gliosis in an affected region is not appreciated unless specifically stained for by the Holzer method or the newer immunocytochemical methods for glial fibrillary acidic protein (GFAP).

Neuronal loss and spongiform changes in some cases of J-C disease have been reported in the autonomic nervous system (158) and in the eye where optic atrophy has been seen (180). In the spinal cord, as previously mentioned, degeneration and demyelination of the lateral corticospinal tract and sometimes other tracts may be seen, but not in every case. Varying amounts of brain stem pathology may be seen, including degeneration of pons and medulla reminiscent of the olivopontocerebellar degenerations (189).

Some cases of J-C disease show kuru-like amyloid plaques in the cerebellum (128); likewise, there are cases which are otherwise typical for Alzheimer's disease (especially familial cases) which show some spongiform change. Furthermore, there are cases in which the clinical course suggested Steel-Richardson-Olszewski syndrome, but the pathology was spongiform in a subcortical pattern without neurofibrillary tangles (189). In cases of the so-called Gerstmann-Sträussler syndrome (discussed above)

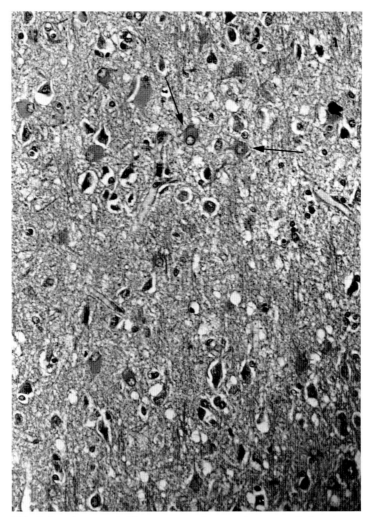

Figure 14.45. This light micrograph illustrates moderate microvacuolating (spongiform) changes, neuronal loss, and reactive astroglial replacement (*arrows*) without inflammation in the cerebral cortex of a case of Jakob-Creutzfeldt disease. The distribution and degree of spongiform change is quite variable and may be so subtle that it is only visible in electron micrographs of biopsy specimens. Histochemical stains which highlight the reactive gliosis are sometimes helpful in locating regions of neuronal loss in cases where spongiform changes are minimal or very subtle. It is often difficult to appreciate the degree of neuronal loss in H&E sections of normal thickness. H&E. (Original magnification ×320.)

where probably unique forms of amyloid plaques are found (29, 191), there are many clinical and pathological parallels to otherwise classical J-C disease, and to some, this syndrome is only another variant of J-C disease.

The appearance of J-C disease in the experimental animal both clinically and pathologically is similar to that in man, although the neuropathology of the disease is always spongiform and without added information would be difficult to differen-

tiate from experimental kuru, or scrapie for that matter. Diffuse neuronal loss, gliosis, and spongiosis without amyloid plaques are the usual pathology. These changes are very similar in all the animals inoculated and studied (17–19, 185, 186).

Scrapie

Scrapie is a disease of domesticated sheep and goats known since the 1700s in England. Since that time it has occurred worldwide, no doubt having been transmit-

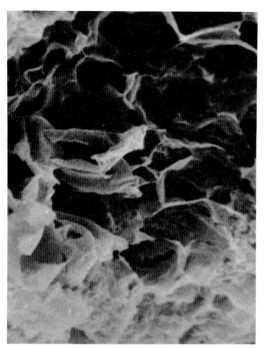

Figure 14.46. This scanning electron micrograph of a portion of cerebral cortex from a case of Jakob-Creutzfeldt disease, illustrates the nearly three-dimensional character of the vacuolating process within a neuron. (Original magnification ×10,000.) (From S. M. Chou et al. (48).)

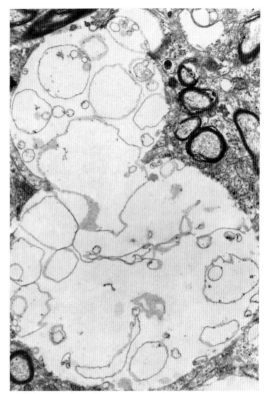

Figure 14.47. This transmission electron micrograph illustrates the intracellular vacuoles in Jakob-Creutzfeldt disease and shows the numerous membranous septae with often curled edges. (Original magnification ×25,000.) (From S. M. Chou et al. (48).)

ted unknowingly by breeding animals who were asymptomatic and in the latent phase of the disease when they were exported. The disease was shown to be transmissible by inoculation by Cuille and and Chelle in 1936 (88). Since that time a huge body of literature has accumulated on the clinical, pathological, and biological aspects of the disease and its causative agent.

The importance to human neuropathology of scrapie is that it seems to qualify as the prototype for all of the other unconventional agents mentioned above and has even been suggested as the etiological agent for diseases such as kuru and Jakob-Creutzfeldt disease (189), even though there has never been a documented laboratory-acquired human infection of scrapie (45). It has been shown to probably cause transmissible mink encephalopathy, which is transmitted by feeding contaminated carcasses of sheep and goats to farm-raised mink (189). The agent is small, probably on the order of 20–40 nm. It is resistant to

heat, ultraviolet, and ionizing irradiation, formalin fixation, ether and alcohol treatment, but can be neutralized with a 2% hypochlorite solution and shares these properties with the agent of Jakob-Creutzfeldt disease. Attempts to isolate and purify the agent have been thus far frustrated (232, 234), but recent work by Merz et al. (200) point to possible association of the agent with a fibrillary protein extract from scrapie brains known as scrapie-associated fibrils (SAFs) illustrated in Figure 14.48.

The clinical features of scrapie are that affected animals do not thrive, seem excessively skittish and excitable, have a change in their vocalization, and may present with a clear nasal discharge. Tremor, jerking of the head, and chewing movements appear and lead to disorders of gait and ataxia. Weakness, spasticity, and ataxia are usually seen later in the disease when an apparent pruritus causes the animal to nibble

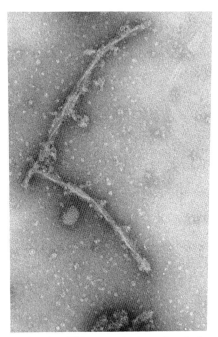

Figure 14.48. This negatively stained electron micrograph of so-called scrapie-associated fibrils (SAF's) illustrates the fibrillary material originally isolated from the brains of scrapie-infected animals, and now also isolated from hamster brains inoculated with extracts of human Jakob-Creutzfeldt disease and from primary cases of Jakob-Creutzfeldt disease. These protein extracts possess infectivity in experimental animals and may represent an unusual fibrous protein produced in response to the infectious agent or may represent the infectious agent itself. (Original magnification ×86,000.) (From P. A. Merz et al. (200).)

or bite, scratch, or scrape against objects and denude most of the wool or fur from large areas of the skin. The animal may live several months with obvious symptoms and die of poor nutriton and wasting (139).

PATHOLOGICAL APPEARANCES

The gross appearance of the brain is usually normal. Microscopically, the most prominent lesion is degenerative vacuolating changes (Fig. 14.42) in grey and to a lesser degree in white matter of the cerebellum, brain stem, deep nuclear masses and cerebral cortx without any inflammation. There is usually gliosis in affected regions and Alzheimer-like amyloid plaques in the cerebral cortex. Distribution of the vocauolating changes, gliosis, and amyloid plaques is diffuse and usually symmetrical, but differences are noted between the various "strains" of scrapie agent encountered, and in the experimental situation, the animal and mode of inoculation (88).

Ultrastructural examination of naturally occurring and experimental scrapie has been reported in numerous publications and consists of intraneuronal, perikaryal, and neuritic vacuoles with numerous blebs and curled membranous profiles within the vacuoles, much as has been described in Jakob-Creutzfeldt disease (196). Biochemical extracts of infected brains have repeatedly yielded a "sticky" fibrous protein (so-called scrapie associated fibrils) (200) seen in negatively stained preparations under electron microscopy as filaments composed of two to four fibrils 4–6 nm in diameter sometimes with a beaded appearance in segments usually 100–500 nm long (Fig. 14.48). These filaments which resemble amyloid filaments appear at about 60 d after inoculation in mice and before clinical signs of scrapie appear. They are apparently seen in no other condition and only in scrapie-infected brains (200).

ATYPICAL VIRUS-LIKE AGENTS OR PARTICLES

Pseudovirions

Pseudovirions result during the course of a viral infection where a capsid contains host cell rather than viral genome. These virus-like particles, which can be visualized ultrastructurally and even physically isolated at times, are probably not replicable but could lead to naturally occurring recombinations of DNA.

Viroids

The viroids are plant pathogens which are unique in that they are very small infectious agents which contain circular RNA genomes composed of only a few hundred nucleotides. These agents are highly resistant to heat, ionizing and ultraviolet radiation, as are most of the other so-called unconventional agents described above. They cause diseases in plants which could probably be considered as degenerative processes mostly involving membranous structures (253). The relevance to human neuropathology is obscure, but parallels have been drawn between these agents and the scrapie agent, not to mention suggestions that particles like the viroids, other plant pathogens, and other organisms strange to neuropathologists have been found in Jakob-Creutzfeldt brain tissue (14).

DISEASES WHICH MAY BE OF VIRAL ORIGIN

Von Economo's Encephalitis (Encephalitis Lethargica)

Encephalitis lethargica first appeared in Austria in the winter of 1916–1917 but spread throughout Europe and the North American continent, producing epidemics until the late 1920s after which it apparently disappeared. Clinically, the disease began with influenza-like symptoms which progressed into signs of meningeal irritation, headache, vertigo, and a peculiar lethargic-somnolent state from which the patient could easily be aroused to full consciousness, but after a short while, would return, become drowsy, and sleep. Ophthalmoplegia and other cranial nerve palsies often accompanied this symptom. Some patients experienced oculogyric crises, hyperkinesias, involuntary movements, and athetotic or dystonic posturing (26). The disease varied in severity but tended to be more severe and to produce more severe sequelae in children than in adults. The lethargic state generally abated after a few days, but occasionally lasted for weeks or months. Most victims survived.

Laboratory examination of CSF in encephalitis lethargica showed a mild pleocytosis (usually fewer than 20 mononuclear cells/cu mm), minimal rise in protein, and occasionally a rise in CSF glucose levels not associated with any peripheral leukocytosis. Pathologically the cases appeared to be consistent with a viral infection, although no viral isolation has ever been accomplished. There is a mild gross hyperemia in the leptomeninges, and there may be brain swelling. Microscopically (39, 104), there is a diffuse lymphoid perivascular cuffing, sometimes including a few plasma cells, a rather diffuse inflammatory infiltrate, inflammatory nodules, focal meningeal infil-

tration, and a propensity for focal neuronophagia and neuronal loss with release of neuromelanin pigment into the neuropil in the zona compacta of the substantia nigra and locus ceruleus. Cerebellar Purkinje cells and neurons of the oculomotor nuclei may also be lost. There may be destruction of venules and other small vessels leading to focal hemorrhages. In chronic cases, replacement gliosis of affected regions, a persistence of lymphoid perivascular infiltrates, and perivascular or intraparenchymal mineralization in the striatum, hippocampus, and thalamus have been reported (39, 104).

The most striking feature of encephalitis lethargica, and perhaps the one which established a place in posterity for this extinct disease, was the frequent sequel of postencephalitic parkinsonism. After a symptom-free interval of weeks to months, and sometimes many years, parkinsonian symptoms would appear, often accompanied by oculogyric crises and mental deterioration. Pathologically, loss of pigmented neurons and the occurrence of complex neurofibrillary tangles in the substantia nigra and locus ceruleus are striking. The neuronal loss may be asymmetric and may be greatest on the side opposite to the greatest neurological abnormality (39, 104).

Although less commonly recognized, another apparent later complication of encephalitis lethargica was progressive motor neuron disease with many features of amyotrophic lateral sclerosis alone or in combination with Parkinsonian symptoms and occasionally dementia. These correlations raise intriguing parallels between these clinical appearances and the Parkinson-ALS-dementia complex occurring amongst the Chamorro people on Guam (32).

Encephalitis lethargica itself has remained an enigma, since no virus was ever recovered from affected cases, but has been assumed to be due to a virus, probably not transmitted by any vector, but rather contracted by contact with infected persons. The relationship of encephalitis lethargica to the influenza epidemics occurring roughly during the same time is probably serendipitous. In spite of many papers in the literature which attempt to link influenza or even herpes simplex virus infections to postencephalitic Parkinson disease, there is no conclusive evidence of such a link, and the attempts to identify the agent responsible have remained unsuccessful (147).

Borna Disease

This disease, which affects horses and sheep in parts of Germany and Switzerland, and which has been transmitted into experimental animals produces either a rapidly fatal encephalitis or a more chronic disease characterized by behavioral abnormalities, not unlike those seen in rabies. These affective disturbances range from frenzied activity, jumping, running, agressive behavior, ravenous eating patterns, and sexual hyperactivity. The pathology of the disease is that of a rather typical neurotropic viral meningoencephalitis which is most concentrated in the limbic structures. The pathological changes can be modulated by the immune response of the animal, like lymphocytic choriomeningitis, where the immune response is responsible for most of the destructive lesions. There is a curious late immunological tolerance for this virus which occurs and allows a persistent infection with little or no inflammation. Although the virus is poorly characterized and not presently classified, it may be a most interesting model of behavioral disorders in higher animals. No conclusive evidence exists that this agent can infect man, but a human disease which has some similarities and includes an acute and then chronic phase of encephalitis with hydrocephalus and dementia has been reported in the Soviet Union (216).

Acute Hemorrhagic Leucoencephalitis

The entity was defined by Hurst in 1941, but cases undoubtedly representing this condition include a report by Strümpell in 1891 and others since that time (137). The condition is characterized by a devastating CNS disease which may follow a mild upper respiratory tract infection, mild, presumably viral, enteritis, an attack of ulcerative colitis, acute glomerulonephritis, a reaction to sulfa or other drugs, or follow an immunization. After an interval of a few days after one of the above there is the abrupt onset of fever, lethargy, progressing to unconsciousness and coma. Sometimes there

is hemiparesis, aphasia, or seizures. Death in coma usually occurs within a week of the onset of symptoms.

At first thought to be causd by a viral infection of the nervous system, the condition is now regarded as a CNS manifestation of the generalized Schwartzman reaction. This reaction is classically produced in rabbits by injection of bacterial endotoxins 24 h apart, which leads to pronounced intravascular coagulation and thrombosis of small vessels with endothelial necrosis. Apparently the reaction is the result of activation of the complement pathway by endotoxin with localized action upon endothelium (103). Some regard the disease as a particularly violent form of postinfectious encephalomyelitis in which some unknown factor has potentiated the local brain vessel response to a sensitizing agent, perhaps somewhat analogous to the experimental situation produced by manipulation of the adjuvant which produces hyperacute experimental allergic encephalomyelitis with similar features in the experimental animal (20).

Mollaret's Meningitis

The original description of this rare form of recurrent benign meningitis of unknown etiology was made in 1944 by Mollaret, and since that time until 1972 only about 30 cases have been reported (122). The syndrome involves all ages and both sexes equally and has no apparent predisposing cause. Most cases have several bouts of aseptic meningitis over a period of a few years, but occasionally recurrences may occur over more than 20 yr (280). The clinical examinations are typical for aseptic meningitis, and the CSF examination shows low or normal glucose concentrations, mild elevation of protein, mild to moderate elevation of IgG in the CSF, and sometimes there is oligoclonal banding. The cytology of the CSF includes polymorphonuclear leukocytes early, and later more lymphoid cells. In addition there may be large peculiar appearing mononuclear cells which Mollaret thought were endothelial cells but have subsequently been shown to be macrophages. The pathological basis for this clinical syndrome is variable and has been shown in some cases to be viral (Coxsackie B5 and B2, echovirus 9 and 7, herpes simplex type 2), to be associated with lupus erythematosus, epidermoid cyst, and chemical meningitis, but the majority of cases remain of unknown etiology. The treatment for the condition has included steroid therapy, antihistamines, and systemic colchicine, all of which have been of benefit for some but not all victims (122, 207, 280).

The condition is probably more of a clinical syndrome than a pathological entity, and no consistent viral etiology has been established.

Behçet's Disease

Behçet's disease is a syndrome characterized by recurring oral and genital mucosal ulcerations, arthritis, migratory thrombophlebitis, uveitis and conjunctivitis, skin lesions, myositis, and neurological symptoms. Some of the features of the disease resemble Reiter's syndrome. Men in their 30s are most commonly affected, and the disease is more prevalent in the middle and far east than other parts of the world (44, 258). About one-fourth of all victims suffer neurological symptoms which include meningoencephalitis or myelitis, cranial and/or peripheral neuropathies, increased intracranial pressure, and behavioral symptoms. Rarely hemiplegia, hemiparesis, or quadriplegia are seen, and even more rarely death from encephalitis and major neurological dysfunction may occur. Pathologically the disease is primarily a vasculitis, sharing some features of polyarteritis and the other collagen-vascular diseases. Like Mollaret's meningitis, no specific etiology has been determined, although a viral etiology and an autoimmune basis have been suggested repeatedly over the years (258). Treatment has been disappointing but has included systemic steroid therapy and immunosuppression (221). Pathological reports on the CNS forms of the disease are scanty.

ACKNOWLEDGMENTS

I would like to acknowledge the assistance of the following individuals and organizations in the preparation of this chapter.

Drs. Samuel Baron, Samuel Chou, Elizabeth Cochran, Mauro C. Dal Canto, Samuel Dales, C. J. Gibbs, Jr., M. B. A. Oldstone, Daniel Perl, Cedric Raine, William C. Schoene, Katsushi Taomoto, Gabriele ZuRhein, M. J. Buchmeier, F. O. Bastian, Walter Kirschbaum (deceased), D. S. Horoupian, P. A. Merz, H. M. Wisniewski, Cedric Raine, Ms. Cynthia Howard, Albert Einstein College of Medicine (Neuropathology Laboratory), Armed Forces Institute of Pathology (Neuropathology Branch), Northwestern University School of Medicine Department of Pathology, and Children's Memorial Hospital Department of Pathology and the John Radcliffe Hospital, Virology and Public Health Laboratory, Oxford, England.

References

1. Albrecht P: Pathogenesis of neurotropic arbovirus infections. *Curr Top Microbiol Immunol* 43:44, 1968.
2. Alter M, Kurland LT, Mulgaard CA: Late progressive muscular atrophy and antecendent poliomyelitis. In Rowland LP (ed): *Human Motor Neuron Diseases.* New York, Raven Press, 1982, p. 303–310.
3. Amundson TE, Yuill TM: Natural LaCrosse virus infection in the red fox (Vulpes fulva), gray fox (Urocyon cinereoargenteus), raccoon (Procyon lotor) and opossum (Didelphis virginiana). *Am J Trop Med Hyg* 30:706, 1981.
4. Andersson U, Bird AG, Britton S, Palacios R: Humoral and cellular immunity in humans studied at the cell level from birth to two years old. *Immunol Rev* 57:5, 1981.
5. Andrews JM, Gardner MB: Lower motor neuron degeneration associated with type C RNA virus infection in mice. Neuropathologic features. *J Neuropathol Exp Neurol* 33:285, 1974.
6. Åström KE, Mancall EL, Richardson EP Jr: Progressive multifocal leukoencephalopathy. *Brain* 81:93, 1958.
7. Bachmann DM, Rodrigues MM, Marshall WC, Cogan DG, Macher AM: Culture proven cytomegalovirus retinitis in homosexual man with the acquired immunodeficiency syndrome. *Ophthalmologica* 89:797, 1982.
8. Bachrach HL: Foot-and-mouth disease. *Ann Rev Microbiol* 22:201, 1968.
9. Baer GM, Shantnaveerapa TR, Bourne G: The pathogenesis of street rabies virus in rats. *Bull WHO* 38:119, 1968.
10. Baltimore D: Expression of animal virus genomes. *Bacteriol Rev* 35:235, 1971.
11. Baringer JR: Herpes simplex virus infection of nervous tissue in animals and man. *Prog Med Virol* 20:1, 1975.
12. Baron S, Dianzani F, Stanton GJ: General considerations of the interferon system. The interferon system: a review to 1982. *Tex Rep Biol Med* 41(1):1, 1982.
13. Barre-Sinoussi F, Chermann JC, Rey F, Nugeyre MT, Chamaret S, Gruest J, Dauguet, C, Axler-Blin, Vezinet-Brun F, Rouzioux C, Rozenbaum W, Montagnier L: Isolation of a T-lymphotropic retrovirus from a patient at risk for acquired immune deficiency syndrome (AIDS). *Science* 220:868, 1983.
14. Bastian FO, Hart MN, Cancilla PA: Additional evidence of spiroplasma in Creutzfeldt-Jakob disease. *Lancet* 1:660, 1981.
15. Bastian FO, Wende RD, Singer DB, Zeller RS: Eastern equine encephalomyelitis. Histopathologic and ultrastructural changes with isolation of the virus in a human case. *Am J Clin Pathol* 64:10, 1975.
16. Bechtelsheimer H, Jakob H, Solcher H: Zur Neuropathologie der durch Grüne Meerkatzen ubertragenen Infecktionskrankheiten in Marburg. *Dtsch Med Wochenschr* 93:602, 1968.

17. Beck E, Daniel PM, Alpers M, Gajdusek DC, Gibbs CJ Jr: Experimental "kuru" in chimpanzees. A pathological report. *Lancet* 2:1056, 1966.
18. Beck E, Daniel PM, Asher DM, Gajdusek DC, Gibbs CJ Jr: Experimental kuru in the chimpanzee. A neuropathological study. *Brain* 96:33, 1973.
19. Beck E, Daniel PM, Matthews WB, Stevens DL, Alpers MP, Asher DM, Gajdusek DC, Gibbs CJ Jr: Creutzfeldt-Jakob disease. The neuropathology of a transmission experiment. *Brain* 92:699, 1969.
20. Behan PO, Behan WMH, Feldman RG, Kies MW: Cell-mediated hypersensitivity to neural antigens. Occurrence in humans and non-human primates with neurological diseases. *Arch Neurol Psychiatry* 27:145, 1972.
21. Bennett N McK: Murray valley encephalitis, 1974: clinical features. *Med J Aust* 2:446, 1976.
22. Beran GW: Rabies and infectious rabies-related viruses. In Beran GW (ed): Section B: Viral Zoonoses. In Steele JH (ed): *CRC Handbook Series in Zoonoses*. Boca Raton, FL, CRC Press, 1981, Vol 2, pp 57–135.
23. Bernhard W: Electron microscopy of tumor cells and tumor viruses. *Cancer* 18:491, 1958.
24. Bernoulli C, Siegfried J, Baumgartner G, Regli F, Rabinowicz T, Gajdusek DC, Gibbs CJ Jr: Danger of accidental person-to-person transmission of Creutzfeldt-Jakob disease by surgery. *Lancet* 1:478, 1977.
25. Bia FJ, Griffith BP, Fong CKY, Hsiung GD: Cytomegalovirus infections in the guinea pig: experimental models for human disease. *Rev Infect Dis* 5:177, 1983.
26. Biemond A: *Brain Diseases*. Amsterdam, Elsevier, 1970, p 588.
27. Blinzinger K, Muller W: The intercellular gaps of the neuropil as pathways for virus spread in viral encephalomyelitis. *Acta Neuropathol* 17:37, 1971.
28. Bodian D: Emerging concept of poliomyelitis infection. *Science* 122:105, 1955.
29. Boellaard JW, Schlote W: Subakute spongiforme Encephalopathie mit multiformer Plaquebildung. *Acta Neuropathol* 49:205, 1980.
30. Bouteille M, Fontaine C, Vedrenne CL, Delarue J: Sur un cas de' encéphalite subaiguë à inclusions. Etude anatomo-clinique et ultrastructurale. *Rev Neurol* 113:454, 1965.
31. Bowen TJ, Wedgwood RJ, Ochs HD, Henle W: Transient immunodeficiency during asymptomatic Epstein-Barr virus infection. *Pediatrics* 71:964, 1983.
32. Brait K, Fahn S, Schwarz GA: Sporadic and familial Parkinsonism and motor neuron disease. *Neurology* 23:990, 1973.
33. Brinker KR, Monath TP: The human disease: acute central nervous system infection. In Monath TP (ed): *St Louis Encephalitis*. Amer Pub Health Assoc, Washington DC, 1980, p 503.
34. Brown P, Gibbs CJ Jr, Amyx HL, Kingsbury DT, Rohwer RG, Sulima MP, Gajdusek DC: Chemical disinfection of Creutzfeldt-Jakob disease virus. *N Engl J Med* 306:1279, 1982.
35. Brownell B, Oppenheimer DR: An ataxic form of subacute presenile polioencephalopathy (Creutzfeldt-Jakob disease). *J Neurol Neurosurg Psychiatry* 28:350, 1965.
36. Brownlee A, Wilson DR: Studies in the histopathology of Louping-ill. *J Comp Pathol* 45:67, 1932.
36a.Buchmeier MJ, Welsh RM, Dutko FJ, Oldstone MBA: The virology and immunobiology of lymphocytic choriomeningitis virus infection. *Adv. Immunol.* 30:275, 1981.
37. Buescher EL, Artenstein MS, Olson LC: Central nervous system infections of viral etiology. The changing pattern. *Res Publ Assoc Nerv Ment Dis* 44:147, 1968.
38 Burakoff SJ, Reiss CS, Finberg R, Mescher MF: Cell-mediated immunity to viral glycoproteins. *Rev Infect Dis* 2:62, 1980.
39. Buzzard EF, Greenfield JG: Lethargic encephalitis: its sequelae and morbid anatomy. *Brain* 13:305, 1919.
40. Calisher CH, Thompson WH: *California Serogroup Viruses*. New York, Alan R Liss, 1983.
41. Carey EJ, Massopust LC, Zeit W, Haushalter E: Ana-

42. Castaigne P, Rondot P, Escourolle R, Dumas JLR, Cathala F, Hauw JJ: Leucoencephalopathie multifocale progressive et "gliomes" multiples. *Rev Neurol* 130:379, 1974.
43. Cavanagh JB, Greenbaum D, Marshall AHE, Rubenstein LJ: Cerebral degeneration associated with disorders of the reticuloendothelial system. *Lancet* 2:525, 1959.
44. Chajek T, Fainaru M: Behcet's disease. A report of 41 cases and a review of the literature. *Medicine* 54:179, 1975.
45. Chatigny MA, Prusiner SB: Biohazards of investigations on the transmissible spongiform encephalopathies. *Rev Infect Dis* 57:391, 1980.
46. Choppin PW, Compans RW: Reproduction of paramyxoviruses. In Fraenkel-Conrat H, Wagner RR (eds): *Comprehensive Virology*. New York, Plenum, 1975, p 95.
47. Choppin PW, Scheid A: The role of viral glycoproteins in adsorption, penetration, and pathogenecity of viruses. *Rev Infect Dis* 2:40, 1980.
48. Chou SM, Payne WN, Gibbs CJ Jr, Gajdusek DC: Transmission and scanning electron microscopy of spongiform change in Creutzfeldt-Jakob disease. *Brain* 103:885, 1980.
49. Clark GG, Pretula HL, Rohrer WH, Harcroft RN, Jakubowski T: Persistence of LaCrosse virus (California encephalitis serogroup) in north-central Illinois. *Am J Trop Med Hyg* 32:175, 1983.
50. Connolly JH, Allen IV, Hurwitz LJ, Millar JHD: Measles-virus antibody and antigen in subacute sclerosing panencephalitis. *Lancet* 1:542, 1967.
51. Constantine DG: Rabies transmitted by the non-bite route. *Pub Health Rep* 77:287, 1962.
52. Cooper LZ, Ziring PR, Ockerse AB, Keily B, Krugman S: Rubella: clinical manifestations and management. *Am J Dis Child* 118:18, 1969.
53. Cowdry EV: The problem of intranuclear inclusions in virus diseases. *Arch Pathol* 18:527, 1934.
54. Craig CP, Nahmias AJ: Different patterns of neurologic involvement with herpes simplex virus types 1 and 2: isolation of herpes simplex virus type 2 from the buffy coat of two adults with meningitis. *J Infect Dis* 127:365, 1973.
55. Crumpacher CS II: Viral glycoproteins in infectious disease processes. *Rev Infect Dis* 2:78, 1980.
56. Cudkowicz G, Hochman PS: Do natural killer cells engage in regulated reactions against self to ensure homeostasis? *Immunol Rev* 44:11, 1979.
57. Dal Canto MC, Rabinowitz SG: Experimental models of virus-induced demyelintation of the central nervous system. *Ann Neurol* 11:109, 1981.
58. Dal Canto MC, Rabinowitz SG: Murine central nervous system infection by a viral temperature-sensitive mutant. *Am J Pathol* 102:412, 1981.
59. Dales S: Early events in cell-animal virus interaction. *Bacteriol Rev.* 37:103, 1973.
60. Dalldorf G, Melnick JL: Coxsackie viruses. In Horsfall FL Jr, Tamm I (eds): *Viral and Rickettsial Infections of Man*, ed 4. Philadelphia, Lippincott, 1965, pp 492–494.
61. Dardiri AH, Yates VJ, Flanagan TD: The reaction to infection with the B1 strain of Newcastle disease virus in man. *Am J Vet Res* 23:918, 1962.
62. Darnell JE Jr, Levintow L, Thoren MM, Hooper JL: The time course of synthesis of poliovirus RNA. *Virology* 13:271, 1961.
63. Davis LE, Johnson RT: An explanation for the localization of herpes simplex encephalitis? *Ann Neurol* 5:2, 1979.
64. Dawson JR: Cellular inclusions in cerebral lesions of epidemic encephalitis. *Arch Neurol Psychiatry* 31:685, 1934.
65. Dean DJ, Evans W, McClure R: Pathogenesis of rabies. *Bull WHO* 29:803, 1963.
66. De Lellis RA: *Diagnostic Immunohistochemistry*. New

York, Masson, 1981.

67. Denst J, Neuberger KT: A histologic study of muscles and nerves in poliomyelitis. *Am J Pathol* 26:867, 1950.

68. DeSimone PA, Snyder D: Hypoglossal nerve palsy in infectious mononucleosis. *Neurology* 28:844, 1978.

69. Dietz HW Jr, Peralta PH, Johnson KM: Ten clinical cases of human infection with Venezuelan equine encephalomyelitis virus subtype I-D. *Am J Trop Med Hyg* 28:329, 1979.

70. Doherty RL: Arboviral zoonoses in Australasia. Murray Valley encephalitis. In Beran GW (ed): *Section B: Viral Zoonoses.* In Steele JH (ed): *CRC Handbook Series in Zoonoses.* Boca Raton, FL, CRC Press, 1981, vol 1, pp 467–472.

71. Dorfman LJ: Cytomegalovirus encephalitis in adults. *Neurology* 23:146, 1973.

72. Douglas SD, Ackerman SK: Anatomy of the immune system. *Clin Hematol* 6:299, 1977.

73. Draughn EE, Sieber OE Jr, Umlauf HJ Jr: Colorado tick fever encephalitis. *Clin Pediatr* 4:626, 1965.

74. Drachman DB, Murphy SR, Nigam MD, Hills JR: "Myopathic" changes in chronically denervated muscle. *Arch Neurol* 16:14, 1967.

75. Dubois-Dalcq M, Barbosa LH, Hamilton R, Sever JL: Comparison between productive and latent subacute sclerosing panencephalitis viral infection in vitro. *Lab Invest* 30:241, 1974.

76. Duffy P, Wolf J, Collins G, DeVoe A, Streeten B, Cowen D: Possible person-to-person transmission by Creutzfeldt-Jakob disease. *N Engl J Med* 290:692, 1974.

77. Elsbach R: Degradation of microorganisms by phagocytic cells. *Rev Infect Dis* 2:106, 1980.

78. Embil JA, Camfield P, Artsob H, Chase DP: Powassan virus encephalitis resembling herpes simplex encephalitis. *Arch Intern Med* 143:341, 1983.

79. Emmons RW: Colorado tick fever. In Beran GW (ed): *Section B: Viral Zoonoses.* In Steele, JH (ed): *CRC Handbook Series in Zoonoses.* Boca Raton, FL, CRC Press, 1981, vol 1, pp 113–124.

80. Enders JF, Weller TH, Robbins FC: Cultivation of the Lansing strain of poliomyelitis in cultures of various human embryonic tissues. *Science* 109:85, 1949.

81. Essex M, McLane MF, Lee TH, Falk L, Howe CWS, Mullins JI, Cabradilla C, Francis DP: Antibodies to cell membrane antigens associated with human T-cell leukemia virus in patients with AIDS. *Science* 220:859, 1983.

82. Fan DP, Sefton BM: The entry into host cells of sindbis virus, vesicular stomatitis virus, and sendai virus. *Cell* 15:985, 1978.

83. Farquahar J, Gajdusek DC: *Kuru. Early Letters and Field Notes from the Collection of D. Carleton Gajdusek.* New York, Raven Press, 1981.

84. Farrar JJ, Benjamin WR, Hilfiker ML, Howard M, Farrar WL, Fuller-Farrar J: The biochemistry, biology, and role of interleukin 2 in the induction of cytotoxic T cell and antibody-forming B cell responses. *Immunol Rev* 63:127, 1982.

85. Feemster RF, Haymaker W: Eastern equine encephalitis. *Neurology* 8:882, 1958.

86. Fermaglich J, Hardman JM, Earle KM: Spontaneous progressive multifocal leukoencephalopathy. *Neurology* 20:479, 1970.

87. Flexner S, Lewis PA: Experimental poliomyelitis in monkeys; active immunization and passive serum protection. *JAMA* 54:1780, 1910.

88. Fraser H: Neuropathology of Scrapie: The precision of the lesions and their diversity. In Prusiner SB, Hadlow WJ (eds): *Clinical, Epidemiological, Genetic, and Pathological Aspects of the Spongiform Encephalopathies. Slow Transmissible Diseases of the Nervous System.* New York, Raven Press, 1979, vol 1, pp 387–406.

89. Freeman JM, Magoffin RL, Lennette EH, Herndon RM: Additional evidence of the relation between subacute inclusion-body encephalitis and measles virus. *Lancet* 2:129, 1967.

90. Gajdusek DC, Gibbs CJ Jr., Alpers M: Experimental transmission of a kuru-like syndrome to chimpanzees. *Nature* 209:794, 1966.

91. Gajdusek DC, Zigas V: Degenerative disease of the central nervous system in New Guinea. The epidemic occurrence of "kuru" in the native population. *N Engl J Med* 257:974, 1957.

92. Gallo RC, Sarin PS, Gelmann EP, Robert-Guroff M, Richardson E, Kalyanaraman VS, Mann D, Sidhu GD, Stahl RE, Zolla-Pazner S, Liebowitch J, Popovic M: Isolation of human T-cell leukemia virus in acquired immune deficiency syndroms (AIDS). *Science* 220:865, 1983.

93. Gardner SD, Field AM, Coleman DV, Hulme B: New human papovavirus (BK) isolated from urine after renal transplantation. *Lancet* 1:1253, 1971.

94. Gatus BJ, Rose MR: Japanese B encephalitis: epidemiological, clinical and pathological aspects. *J Infect* 6:213, 1983.

95. Gelmann EP, Popovic M, Blayney D, Masur H, Sidhu G, Stahl RE, Gallo RC: Proviral DNA of a retrovirus, human T-cell leukemia virus, in two patients with AIDS. *Science* 220:862, 1983.

96. GiaRusso MH, Koeppen AH: Atypical progressive multifocal leukoencephalopathy and primary malignant lymphoma. *J Neurol Sci* 35:391, 1978.

97. Gibbs CJ, Gajdusek DC, Asher DM, Alpers MP, Beck E, Daniel PM, Matthews WB: Creutzfeldt-Jakob disease (spongiform encephalopathy): transmission to the chimpanzee. *Science* 161:388, 1968.

98. Gibbs CJ Jr, Gajdusek DC: IV. Kuru: pathogenesis and characterization of virus. *Am J Trop Med Hyg* 19:138, 1970.

99. Gonatas NK: Subacute sclerosing leukoencephalitis: electron microscopic and cytochemical observations on a cerebral biopsy. *J Neuropathol Exp Neurol* 25:177, 1966.

100. Gonatas NK, Terry RD, Weiss M: Electron microscopy study in two cases of Jakob-Creutzfeldt disease. *J Neuropathol Exp Neurol* 24:575, 1965.

101. Gotlieb-Stematsky T: Association of Epstein-Barr virus with neurologic diseases. In Glaser R, Gotlieb-Stematsky T (eds): *Human Herpesvirus Infections. Clinical Aspects.* New York, Dekker, 1982, ch 5, pp 169–203.

102. Grabow JD, Campbell RJ, Okazaki H, Schut L, Zollman PE, Kurland L: A transmissible subacute spongiform encephalopathy in a visitor to the eastern highlands of New Guinea. *Brain* 99:637, 1976.

103. Graham DI, Behan PO, More IAR: Brain damage complicating septic shock. Acute hemorrhagic leucoencephalitis as a complication of the generalized Schwartzman reaction. *J Neurol Neurosurg Psychiatry* 42:19, 1979.

104. Greenfield JG: Infectious diseases of the nervous system. In Greenfield JG, Blackwood W, McMenemey WH, Meyer A, Norman RM (eds): *Neuropathology.* London, Arnold, 1958, ch 3, pp 194.

105. Gregg NM, Beavis WR, Heseltine M, Macklin AE, Vickery D: Occurrence of congenital defects in children following maternal rubella during pregnancy. *Med J Aust* 2:122, 1945.

106. Gresikova M, Beran GW: Arboviral zoonoses in central Europe. Tick-borne encephalitis (TBE). In Beran GW (ed): *Section B: Viral Zooneses.* In Steele JH (ed): *CRC Handbook Series in Zooneses.* Boca Raton, FL, CRC Press, 1981, vol 1, pp 201–213.

107. Grose C: Varicella-Zoster virus infections: chicken pox (varicella) and shingles (zoster). In Glaser R, Gotlieb-Sematsky T (eds): *Human Herpesvirus Infections. Clinical Aspects.* New York, Dekker, 1982, ch 3, pp 85–150.

108. Grose C, Henle W, Henle G, Feorino PM, Primary Epstein-Barr virus infections in acute neurological diseases. *N Engl J Med* 292:392, 1975.

109. Gwaltney JM Jr: Rhinoviruses. In Evans AS (ed): *Viral Infections in Humans.* New York, Plenum, 1976, pp 383–408.

110. Hadlow WJ: Scrapie and kuru. *Lancet* 2:289, 1959.

111. Hadlow WJ, Prusiner SB, Kennedy RC, Race RE: Brain tissue from persons dying of Creutzfeldt-Jakob disease causes scrapie-like encephalopathy in goats. *Ann Neurol* 8:628, 1980.

112. Hall WW, Choppin PW: Measels virus proteins in the brain tissue of patients with subacute sclerosing panencephalitis: absence of M protein. *N Engl J Med* 304:1152, 1981.

113. Halstead SB: Dengue and dengue hemorrhagic fever. In Beran GW (ed): *Section B: Viral Zoonoses*. In Steele JH (ed): *CRC Handbook Series in Zoonoses*. Boca Raton, FL, CRC Press, 1981, vol 1, pp 421–443.

114. Halstead SB: Chikungunya fever. In Beran GW (ed): *Section B: Viral Zoonoses*. In Steele JH (ed): *CRC Handbook Series in Zoonoses*. Boca Raton, FL, CRC Press, 1981, vol 1, pp 437–447.

115. Hamberger V, Habel K: Teratogenic and lethal effects of influenza A and mumps viruses on early chick embryos. *Proc Soc Exp Biol* 66:608, 1947.

116. Hanshaw JB, Dudgeon JA: *Viral Diseases of the Fetus and Newborn*. Philadelphia, Saunders, 1978.

117. Hayes RO: Eastern and western equine encephalitis. In Beran GW (ed): *Section B: Viral Zoonoses*. In Steele JH (ed): *CRC Handbook in Zoonoses*. Boca Raton, FL, CRC Press, 1981, vol 1, pp 29–57.

118. Hayes RO, Beadle LD, Hess AD, Sussman O, Bonese MJ: Entomological aspects of the 1959 outbreak of eastern encephalitis in New Jersey. *Am J Trop Med Hyg* 11:115, 1962.

119. Hayward A: Immunodeficiency. In Lachmann PJ, Peters DK, (eds): *Clinical Aspects of Immunology*. Oxford, England, Blackwell Scientific, 1982, vol 2, pp 1658–1712.

120. Heathfield KWG, Pilsworth R, Wall J, Corsellis JAN: Coxsackie B5 infections in Essex, 1965, with particular preference to the nervous system. *Q J Med* 36:579, 1967.

121. Henrickson RV, Maul DH, Osborn KG, Sever JL, Madden DL, Ellingsworth LR, Anderson JH, Lowenstine LJ, Gardner MB: Epidemic of acquired immunodeficiency in rhesus monkeys. *Lancet* 1:388, 1983.

122. Hermans P, Goldstein N, Wellman W: Mollaret's meningitis and differential diagnosis of recurrent meningitis. *Am J Med* 52:128, 1972.

123. Herndon RM, Johnson RT, Davis LE, Descalzi LR: Ependymitis in mumps virus meningitis. Electron microscopical studies of cerebrospinal fluid. *Arch Neurol* 30:475, 1974.

124. Holmberg CA, Gribble DH, Takemoto KK, Howley PM, Espana C, Osburn BI: Isolation of simian virus 40 from rhesus monkeys (Macaca mulatta) with spontaneous progressive multifocal leukoencephalopathy. *J Infect Dis* 136:593, 1977.

125. Hoogstraal H: Tick-borne crimean-congo hemorrhagic fever. In Beran GW (ed): *Section B: Viral Zoonoses*. In Steele JH (ed): *CRC Handbook Series in Zoonoses*. Boca Raton, FL, CRC Press, 1981, vol 1, pp 267–402.

126. Hooks JJ, Gibbs CJ Jr: The foamy viruses. *Bacteriol Rev* 39:169, 1975.

127. Hooks JJ, Montsoupoulos HM, Notkins AL: The role of interferon in immediate hypersensitivity and autoimmune diseases. Regulatory functions of interferons. *Ann NY Acad Sci* 350:201, 1980.

128. Horoupian DS, Powers JM, Schaumberg HH: Kuru-like neuropathological changes in a North American. *Arch Neurol* 27:555, 1972.

129. Horstmann DM: Epidemiology of poliomyelitis and allied diseases. *Yale J Biol Med* 36:5, 1963.

130. Horta-Barbosa L, Fuccillo DA, London WT, Jabbour JT, Zeman W, Sever JL: Isolation of measles virus from brain cell cultures of two patients with subacute sclerosing panencephalitis. *Proc Soc Biol Med* 132:272, 1969.

131. Horten B, Price RW, Jimenez D: Multifocal varicella-zoster virus leukoencephalitis temporally remote from herpes zoster. *Ann Neurol* 9:251, 1981.

132. Howard CR, Simpson DIH: Review article. The biology of the arena viruses. *J Gen Virol* 51:1, 1980.

133. Hsiung GD: Parainfluenza virus infections. In Beran

134. Hsiung GD, Fong CKY: *Diagnostic Virology Illustrated by Light and Electron Microscopy*, ed 3. New Haven, CT, Yale Univ. Press, 1982.

135. Huang AS, Baltimore D: *Defective Interfering Animal Viruses*. New York, Plenum, 1977.

136. Hughes SS: *The Virus. A History of the Concept*. New York, Heinemann/Science History Books, 1977.

137. Hurst EW: Acute hemorrhagic leucoencephalitis: a previously undefined entity. *Med J Aust* 2:1, 1941.

138. Imagawa DT, Adams JM: Propagation of measels virus in suckling mice. *Proc Soc Exp Biol Med* 98:567, 1958.

139. Innes JRM, Saunders LZ: *Comparative Neuropathology*. New York, Academic Press, 1962.

140. Isaacs A, Lindenmann J: Virus interference. I. The Interferon. *Proc R Soc Lond [Biol]* 147:258, 1957.

141. Jaffe HW, Bregman DJ, Selik RM: Acquired immune deficiency syndrome in the United States: the first 1000 cases. *J Infect Dis* 148:339, 1983.

142. Jänisch W, Schreiber D: In Bigner DD, Swenberg JA (eds): *Experimental Tumors of the Central Nervous System. First English Edition*. Kalamazoo, MI, Upjohn Co., 1977.

143. Jarvis WR, Middleton PJ, Gelfand EW: Significance of viral infections in severe combined immunodeficiency disease. *Pediatr Infect Dis* 2:187, 1983.

144. Johnson KM, Shelokov A, Peralta PH, Dammin GJ, Young NA: Recovery of venezuelan equine encephalomyelitis virus in Panama. A fatal case in man. *Am J Trop Med Hyg* 17:432, 1968.

145. Johnson KP, Norrby E, Swoveland P, Carrigan DR: Experimental subacute sclerosing panencephalitis: selective disappearance of measles virus matrix protein from the central nervous system. *J Infect Dis* 144:161, 1981.

146. Johnson RT: Hydrocephalus and virus infection. *Dev Med Child Neurol* 17:807, 1975.

147. Johnson RT: *Viral Infections of the Nervous System*. New York, Raven Press, 1982.

148. Johnston RT: Selective vulnerability of neural cells to viral infection. *Brain* 103:447, 1980.

149. Johnston RT, Lazzarini RA, Waksman BH: Mechanisms of viral persistence. *Ann Neurol* 9:616, 1981.

150. Joklik WK: The molecular basis of the antiviral activity of interferons. Introductory remarks. Regulatory function of interferons. *Ann NY Acad Sci* 350:432, 1980.

151. Joklik WK: The poxviruses. *Bacteriol Rev* 30:1, 1966.

152. Jones DP, Nevin S: Rapidly progressive cerebral degeneration (subacute vascular encephalopathy) with mental disorder, focal disturbances and myoclonic epilepsy. *J Neurol Neurosurg Psychiatry* 17:148, 1954.

153. Jordan MC: Latent infection and the elusive cytomegalovirus. *Rev Infect Dis* 5:205, 1983.

154. Katz M, Rorke LB, Masland WS, Koprowski H, Tucker SH: Transmission of an encephalitogenic agent from brains of patients with subacute sclerosing panencephalitis to ferrets. Preliminary report. *N Engl J Med* 279:793, 1968.

155. Kelsey DS: Adenovirus meningoencephalitis. *Pediatrics* 61:291, 1978.

156. Kemp GE: St. Louis encephalitis. In Beran GW (ed): *Section B: Viral Zoonoses*. In: Steele JH (ed): *CRC Handbook Series in Zoonoses*. Boca Raton, LA, CRC Press, 1981, vol 1, pp 71–83.

157. Kempe CH: Studies on small pox and complications of small pox vaccination. *Pediatrics* 26:176, 1960.

158. Khurana RK, Garcia JH: Autonomic dysfunction in subacute spongiform encephalopathy. *Arch Neurol* 38:114, 1981.

159. Kilham L, Margolis G: Viral etiology of spontaneous ataxia of cats. *Am J Pathol* 48:991, 1966.

160. Kirschbaum WR: *Jakob-Creutzfeldt Disease*. New York, Elsevier, 1968.

161. Kissling RE, Chamberlain RW, Eidson ME, Bucca MA: Studies on the North American arthropod-borne ence-

phalitides. II. Eastern equine encephalitis in horses. *Am J Hyg* 60:237, 1954.

162. Kissling RE, Chamberlain RW, Sikes RK, Eidson ME: Studies on the North American arthropod-borne encephalitides. III. Eastern equine encephalitis in wild birds. *Am J Hyg* 60:251, 1954.

163. Klatzo I, Gajdusek DC, Zigas V: Pathology of kuru. *Lab Invest* 8:799, 1959.

164. Klein RJ: The pathogenesis of acute, latent, and recurrent herpes simplex infections. *Arch Virol* 72:143, 1982.

165. Kokernot RH, Shinefield HR, Longshore WA Jr: The 1952 outbreak of encephalitis in California. Differential diagnosis. *Calif Med* 79:73, 1953.

166. Kornfeld H, Vande Stouwe RA, Lang M, Reddy MM, Grieco MH: T-lymphocyte subpopulations in hemosexual men. *N Engl J Med* 307:729, 1982.

167. Kristensson K, Vahlne A, Persson LA, Lycke E: Neuronal spread of herpes simplex virus types 1 and 2 in mice after corneal or subcutaneous (footpad) inoculation. *J Neurol Sci* 35:331, 1978.

168. Kristensson K, Örvell C, Leestma JE, Norrby E: Sendai virus infection in the brains of mice: distribution of viral antigens studied with monoclonal antibodies. *J Infect Dis* 147:297, 1983.

169. Lampert PW, Gajdusek DC, Gibbs CJ Jr: Subacute spongiform virus encephalopathies. *Am J Pathol* 68:626, 1972.

170. Landsteiner K, Levaditi C, Pastia C: Etude experimentale de la poliomyelite aigue (maladie de Heine-Medin). *Ann Inst Pasteur (Paris)* 25:805, 1911.

171. Landsteiner K, Popper E: Mikroscopische Präparate von einem menschlichen und zwei Affenrückenmarken. *Wien Klin Wochenschr* 21:1830, 1908.

172. Langer PR, Waldrop AA, Ward DC: Enzymatic synthesis of biotin-labeled polynucleotides: novel nucleic acid affinity probes. *Proc Natl Acad Sci USA* 78:6633, 1981.

173. Leestma JE, Andrews JM: The fine structure of the Marinesco body. *Arch Pathol* 88:431, 1969.

174. Leestma JE, Bornstein MB, Sheppard RD, Feldman LA: Herpes simplex virus infection in organized cultures of mammalian nervous tissue. *Lab Invest* 20:70, 1969.

175. Leestma JE, Wisniewska K, Martin E: Electron probe analysis of mineral deposits in the central nervous system. *J Neuropathol Exp Neurol* 28:157, 1969.

176. Lennette EH, Magoffin RL, Knouf EG: Viral central nervous system disease. An etiologic study conducted at the Los Angeles County General Hospital. *J Am Med Assoc* 179:687, 1962.

177. Lennette EH, Magoffin RL, Schmidt NJ, Hollister AC Jr: Viral disease of the central nervous system; influence of poliomyelitis vaccination on etiology. *J Am Med Assoc* 171:1456, 1959.

178. Lennette EH, Schmidt NJ: *Diagnostic Proceedures for Viral, Rickettsial and Chlamydial infections*, ed 5. Washington DC, Am Pub Health Assoc, 1979.

179. Lerner AM, Shippey MJ, Crane LR: Serologic responses to herpes simplex virus in rabbits: complement-requiring neutralizing conventional neutralizing and passive hemagglutinating antibodies. *J Infect Dis* 129:623, 1974.

180. Lesser RL, Albert OM, Bobwick AR, O'Brien FH: Creutzfeldt-Jakob disease and optic atrophy. *Am J Ophthalmol* 87:317, 1979.

181. Lim TW, Beran GW: Japanese encephalitis. In Beran GW (ed): *Section B: Viral Zoonoses.* In Steele JH (ed): *CRC Handbook Series in Zoonoses.* Boca Raton, FL, CRC Press, 1981, vol 1, pp 449–456.

182. Lorand B, Nagy T, Tariska S: Subacute progressive panencephalitis. *World Neurol* 3:376, 1962.

183. Lonberg-Holm K, Philipson L: Early interaction between animal viruses and cells. *Monogr Virol* 9:1, 1974.

184. Lwoff A: The concept of virus. *J Gen Virol* 17:239, 1957.

185. Manuelidis EE, Manuelidis L: Observations on Creutzfeldt-Jakob disease propagated in small rodents. In Prusiner SB, Hadlow WJ (eds): *Pathogenesis, Immunology, Virology, and Molecular Biology of the Spongiform Encephalopathies. Slow Transmissible Diseases of the Nervous System.* New York, Academic Press, 1979, pp 147–173.

186. Manuelidis EE, Gorgacz EJ, Manuelidis L: Interspecies transmission of Creutzfeldt-Jakob disease to syrian hamsters with reference to clinical syndromes and strains of agent. *Proc Natl Acad Sci* 75:3432, 1978.

187. Martinez D, Brinton MA, Tachovsky TG, Phelps AH: Indentification of lactic dehydrogenase-elevating virus as the etiologic agent of genetically restricted, age-dependent polioencephalomyelitis of mice. *Infect Immun* 27:979, 1980.

188. Margolis G, Kilham L: Hydrocephalus in hamsters, ferrets, rats and mice following inoculations with reovirus type 1. II. Pathologic studies. *Lab Invest* 21:189, 1969.

189. Masters CL, Gajdusek DC: The spectrum of Creutzfeldt-Jakob disease and the virus induced subacute spongiform encephalopathies. In Smith T, Cavanagh JB (eds): *Recent Advances in Neuropathology.* New York, Churchill-Livingston, 1982, vol 2, pp 139–163.

190. Masters CL, Gajdusek DC, Gibbs CJ Jr: The familial occurrence of Creutzfeld-Jakob disease and Alzheimer's disease. *Brain* 104:535, 1981.

191. Masters CL, Gajdusek DC, Gibbs CJ Jr: Creutzfeldt-Jakob disease virus isolations from the Gerstmann-Sträussler syndrome with an analysis of the various forms of amyloid plaque deposition in the virus induced spongiform encephalopathies. *Brain* 104:559, 1981.

192. Masters CL, Richardson EP Jr: Subacute spongiform encephalopathy (Creutzfeldt-Jakob disease). The nature and progression of spongiform change. *Brain* 101:333, 1978.

193. McCormick WF, Rodnitzkey RL, Schochet SS, McKee AP: Varicella-zoster encephalomyelitis. *Arch Neurol* 21:559, 1969.

194. McIntosh BM, Gear JHS: West Nile fever. In Beran GW (ed): *Section B: Viral Zoonoses.* In Steele JH (ed): *CRC Handbook Series in Zoonoses.* Boca Raton, FL, 1981, vol 1, pp 227–230.

195. McLean DM: California group viral infections of Canada. In Beran GW (ed): *Section B: Viral Zoonoses.* In Steele JH (ed): *CRC Handbook Series in Zoonoses.* Boca Raton, FL, CRC Press, 1981, vol 1, pp 107–111.

196. McLennan JL, Darby G: Herpes simplex virus latency: the cellular location of virus in dorsal root ganglia and the fate of the infected cell following virus activation. *J Gen Virol* 51:233, 1980.

197. Mellor DH: Virus infection of the central nervous system in children with primary immune deficiency disorders. *Dev Med Child Neurol* 23:807, 1981.

198. Melnick JL: Taxonomy and nomenclature of viruses. In Beran GW (ed): Section B, *Viral Zoonoses.* In Steele JH (ed): *CRC Handbook Series in Zoonoses.* Boca Raton, FL, CRC Press, 1981, vol 1, pp 5–9.

199. Melnick JL: Classification of viruses. In Braude AI, Davis DE, Fierer J (eds): *Medical Microbiology and Infectious Diseases.* Philadelphia, WB Saunders, 1981, pp 83–93.

200. Merz PA, Sommerville RA, Wisniewski HM, Manuelidis L, Manuelidis EE: Scrapie-associated fibrils in Creutzfeldt-Jakob disease. *Nature* 306:474, 1983.

201. Meyer A, Leigh D, Bagg CE: a rare presenile dementia associated with cortical blindness (Heidenhain's syndrome). *J Neurol Neurosurg Psychiatry* 17:129, 1954.

202. Miller JR, Barrett RE, Britton CB, Tapper ML, Bahr GS, Bruno PJ, Marquardt MD, Hays AP, McMurtry JG III, Weissman JB, Bruno MS: Progressive multifocal leukoencephalopathy in a male homosexual with T-cell immune deficiency. *N Engl J Med* 307:1436, 1982.

203. Mims CA, Murphy FA: Parainfluenza virus Sendai infection in macrophages, ependyma, choroid plexus, vascular endothelium and respiratory tract of mice. *Am J Pathol* 70:315, 1973.

204. Mittelbach F: Die Begleitmyopathie bei Neurogenen Atrophien. *Monographien auf dem gesamt gebiet der Neurologie und Psychiatrie.* Berlin, Springer-Verlag, 1966, vol 113.

205. Monath TP: Arthropod-borne encephalitides in the Americas. *Bull WHO* 57:513, 1979.

206. Monath TP, Lazvick JS, Cropp CB, Rush WAS, Calisher CH, Kinney RM, Trent DW, Kemp GE, Bowen GS, Francy DB: Recovery of tonate virus ("Bijou Bridge" strain), a member of the Venezuelan equine encephalomyelitis virus complex, from cliff swallow nest bugs (Oeciacus vicarius) and nestling birds in North America. *Am J Trop Med Hyg* 29:969, 1980.

207. Mora JG, Gimeno A: Mollaret meningitis: report of a case with recovery after colchicine. *Ann Neurol* 8:631, 1980.

208. Morbidity and Mortality Weekly Report (MMWR): Measles encephalitis-United States, 1962–1979. *MMWR* 30:362, 1981.

209. Morbidity and Mortality Weekly Report: Rabies. Current Trends: compendium of animal rabies vaccines, 1981. *MMWR* 30:161, 1981.

210. Morbidity and Mortality Weekly Report: Epidemiologic notes and reports. Human rabies acquired outside the United States from a dog bite. *MMWR* 30:537, 1981.

211. Morbidity and Mortality Weekly Report: Leads from MMWR. *JAMA* 250:335, 1983.

212. Murphy FA: Rabies pathogenesis. Brief review. *Arch Virol* 54:279, 1977.

213. Naeye RL, Blanc W: Pathogenesis of congenital rubella. *J Am Med Assoc* 194:1277, 1965.

214. Nahmias AJ, Dowdle WR, Schinazi RF: *The Human Herpesviruses: An Interdisciplinary Perspective.* New York, Elsevier, 1981.

215. Nahmias AJ, Shore SL, Kohl S, Starr SE, Ashwamn RB: Immunology of herpes simplex virus infection: relevance to herpes simplex vaccines and clinical course. *Cancer Res* 36:836, 1976.

216. Narayan O, Herzog S, Frese K, Scheefers H, Rott R: Behavioral disease in rats caused by immunopathological responses to persistent Borna virus in brain. *Science* 220:1401, 1983.

217. Nathanson N, Stolley PD, Boolukos PJ: Easter equine encephalitis. Distribution of central nervous system lesion in man and rhesus monkey. *J Comp Pathol* 79:109, 1969.

218. Oldstone MBA, Dixon FJ: Lactic dehydrogenase virus-induced immune complex type of glomerulonephritis. *J Immunol* 106:1260, 1971.

219. Oldstone MBA, Peters CJ: Arenavirus infections of the nervous system. In Vinken PJ, Bruyn GW, Klawans HL (eds): *Handbook of Clinical Neurology*, part 2. Amsterdam, Elsevier-North Holland, 1978, vol 24, pp 193–207.

220. Padgett BL, Walker DL, Zu Rhein GM, Eckrode RJ: Cultivation of papova-like virus from human brain with progressive multifocal leukoencephalopathy. *Lancet* 1:1257, 1971.

221. Palmeris G, Koliopoulos J, Theodossiadis G, Roussos J, Tsimbidas P: The Adamantidis-Behcet syndrome. Clinical and immunological observations. *Trans Ophthalmol Soc UK* 100:527, 1980.

222. Parkman PO, Buercher EL, Artenitein MS: Recovery of rubella virus from army recruits. *Proc Soc Exp Biol Med* 111:225, 1962.

223. Paul JR: *A History of Poliomyelitis.* New Haven, CT, Yale Univ Press, 1971.

224. Payne FE, Baublis JV, Itabashi HH: Isolation of measles virus from cell cultures of brain from a patient with subacute sclerosing panencephalitis. *N Engl J Med* 281:585, 1969.

225. Penman HG: Fatal infectious mononucleosis; a clinical review. *J Clin Pathol* 2:765, 1970.

226. Perl DP: The pathology of rabies in the central nervous system. In Baer GM (ed): *The Natural History of Rabies.* New York, Academic Press, 1975, vol 1.

227. Peters CJ, Meegan JM: Rift valley fever. In Beran GW (ed): *Section B: Viral Zoonoses.* In Steele JH (ed): *CRC Handbook Series in Zoonoses.* Boca Raton, FL, CRC Press, 1981, vol 1, pp 403–420.

228. Peters A, Palay SL, Webster HDeF: *The Fine Structure of the Nervous System: The Neurons; and Supporting Cells.* Philadelphia, WB Saunders, 1976, pp 262–263.

229. Pette H, Döring G: Über einhemishce Panencephalomyelitis von Charakter der Encephalitis japonica. *Dtsch Z Nervenheilk* 149:7, 1939.

230. Porter RR, Ried KBM: The biochemistry of complement. *Nature* 275:699, 1978.

231. Pringle DR: The genetics of viruses. In Braude AI, Davis CE, Fierer J (eds): *Medical Microbiology and Infectious Disease.* Philadelphia, WB Saunders, 1981, pp 110–120.

232. Prusiner SB: Novel proteinaceous infectious particles cause scrapie. *Science* 216:136, 1981.

233. Prusiner SB, Gajdusek DC, Alpers MP: Kuru with incubation periods exceeding two decades. *Ann Neurol* 12:1, 1982.

234. Prusiner SB, Groth DF, Cochran SP, McKinley MP, Masiarz FR: Gel electrophoresis and glass permeation chromatography of the hamster scrapie agent after enzymatic digestion and detergent extraction. *Biochemistry* 19:4892, 1980.

235. Puga A, Rosenthal JD, Openshaw N, Notkins AL: Herpes simplex virus DNA and mRNA sequences in acutely and chronically infected trigeminal ganglia of mice. *Virology* 89:102, 1978.

236. Quong TL: The pathology of western equine encephalomyelitis. *Can J Public Health* 33:300, 1942.

237. Reyes MG, Gardner JJ, Poland JD, Monath TP: St. Louis encephalitis. Quantitative histological and immunofluorescent studies. *Arch Neurol* 38:329, 1981.

238. Richardson EP Jr: Progressive multifocal leukoencephalopathy. *N Engl J Med* 265:815, 1961.

239. Riski H, Hovi T: Coronavirus infections of man associated with diseases other than the common cold. *J Med Virol* 6:259, 1980.

240. Rivers TM: Some general aspects of pathological conditions caused by filterable viruses. *Am J Pathol* 4:91, 1928.

241. Robb JA, Bond CW: Pathogenic murine coronaviruses. I. Characterization of biological behavior in vitro and virus specific intracellular RNA of strongly neurotropic JHMV and weakly neurotropic A59v virus. *Virology* 94:352, 1979.

242. Roberts ED, San Martin C, Payan J, Mackenzie RB: Neuropathologic changes in 15 horses with naturally occurring Venezuelan equine encephalitis. *Am J Vet Res* 21:1223, 1970.

243. Robertson EG: Murray Valley encephalitis: pathological aspects. *Med J Aust* 1:103, 1952.

244. Rozdilsky B, Robertson HE, Chorney J: Western encephalitis: report of eight fatal cases: Saskatechewan epidemic, 1965. *Can Med Assoc J* 98:79, 1968.

245. Rosenstreich DL, Mizel SB: The participation of macrophages and macrophage cell lines in the activation of T lymphocytes by mitogens. *Immunol Rev* 40:102, 1978.

246. Russell RWR: Supranuclear palsy of eyelid closure. *Brain* 103:71, 1980.

247. Sabin AB: The nature and rate of centripetal progression of certain neurotropic viruses along peripheral nerves. *Am J Pathol* 13:615, 1937.

248. Sabin AB: Pathogenesis of poliomyelitis. Reappraisal in light of new data. *Science* 123:1151, 1956.

249. Sabin AB: Oral poliovirus vaccine. History of its development and prospects for eradication of poliomyelitis. *J Am Med Assoc* 194:872, 1965.

250. Salk D: Eradication of poliomyelitis in the United States. I. Live virus vaccine-associated with wild polio virus disease. *Rev Infect Dis* 2:228, 1980.

251. Scheid A, Choppin PW: Identification of the biological activities of paramyxovirus glycoproteins. Activation of cell fusion, hemolysis and infectivity by proteolytic cleavage of an inactive precursor portion of the Sendai virus. *Virology* 57:475, 1974.

252. Schmitz H, Enders G: Cytomegalovirus as a frequent cause of Guillian-Barre syndrome. *J Med Virol* 1:21, 1977.

253. Semancik JS: Pathogenesis and replication of plant vi-

roids. In Prusiner SB, Hadlow WJ (eds): *Pathogenesis, Immunology, Virology, and Molecular Biology of the Spongiform Encephalopathies. Slow Transmissible Diseases of the Nervous System*, New York, Academic Press, 1979, vol 2, pp 343–362.

254. Sever JL: Persistent measels infection of the central nervous system: subacute sclerosing panencephalitis. *Rev Infect Dis* 5:467, 1983.

255. Shaw CM, Alvord EC Jr: Subependymal germinolysis. *Arch Neurol* 31:374, 1974.

256. Sherman FE, Davis RL, Haymaker W: Subacute inclusion encephalitis. Report of a case with observations on the fluorescent anti-herpes simplex antibody reaction. *Acta Neuropathol* 1:271, 1961.

257. Sherrington M, Snyder RD: Tick paralysis: neurophysiologic studies. *N Engl J Med* 278:95, 1968.

258. Shimizu T, Ehrlich GE, Inaba G, Hayashi K: Behcet's disease (Behcet syndrome). *Semin Arthritis Rheum* 8:223, 1979.

259. Shiraki H, Otani S: Clinical and pathological features of rabies postvaccinial encephalomyelitis in man. Relationships to multiple sclerosis and to experimental "allergic" encephalomyelitis in animals. In Kies MW, Alvord EC (eds): *"Allergic" Encephalomyelitis*. Springfield, IL, Thomas, 1959, p 58.

260. Siddell S, Wege H, Ter Meulen V: Review article: the biology of coronaviruses. *J Gen Virol* 64:71, 1983.

261. Sigurdsson B: Rida A: Chronic encephalitis of sheep. With general remarks on infections which develop slowly and some of their special characteristics. *Br Vet J* 110:341, 1954.

262. Sima AAF, Finkelstein SD, McLachlan DR: Multiple malignant astrocytomas in patient with spontaneous progressive multifocal leukocencephalopathy. *Ann Neurol* 14:183, 1983.

263. Simons K, Garoff H: Review article. The budding mechanisms of enveloped animal viruses. *J Gen Virol* 50:1, 1980.

264. Sissons JGP, Oldstone MBA: Antibody-mediated destruction of virus infected cells. *Adv Immunol* 29:209, 1980.

265. Slenczka W: Marburg virus disease. In Beran GW (ed): *Section A: Viral Zoonoses*. In Steele JH (ed): *CRC Handbook Series in Zoonoses*. Boca Raton, LA, CRC Press, 1981, vol 2, pp 41–51.

266. Spalke G, Eschenbach C: Infantile cortical measles inclusion body encephalitis during combined treatment of acute lymphocytic leukemia. *J Neurol* 220:269, 1979.

267. Spielmeyer W: *Histopathologie des Nervensystems*, Berlin, Springer Verlag, 1922.

268. Subcommittee on Arbovirus Laboratory Safety of the American Committee on Arthropod-borne Viruses (W. F. Scherer, Chairman): Laboratory safety for arboviruses and certain other viruses of vertebrates. *Am J Trop Med Hyg* 29:1359, 1980.

269. Sullivan JL, Hanshaw JB: Human cytomegalovirus infections. In Glaser R, Gotlieb-Stematsky T (eds): *Human Herpesvirus Infection. Clinical Aspects*. New York, Dekker, 1982, ch 2, pp 57–83.

270. Summers BA, Griesen HA, Appel MJG: Possible initiation of viral encephalomyelitis in dogs by migrating lymphocytes infected with distemper. *Lancet* 1:187, 1978.

271. Suzuki M, Phillips CA: St. Louis encephalitis. A histopathologic study of the fatal cases from the Houston epidemic in 1964. *Arch Pathol* 81:47, 1966.

272. Tesh RB, Peralta PH, Johnson KM: Ecologic studies of vesicular stomatitis virus. I. Prevalence of infection among animals and humans living in an area of endemic VSV activity. *Am J Epidemiol* 90:255, 1969.

273. Tesh RB, Wallace GD: Observations on the natural history of encephalomyocarditis virus. *Am J Trop Med Hyg* 27:133, 1978.

274. Theiler M, Downs WG: *The Arthropod-Borne Viruses of Vertebrates*, New Haven, CT, Yale Univ Press, 1973.

275. Thompson WH: California group viral infections in the

United States. In Beran GW (ed): *Section B: Viral Zoonoses*. In Steele JH (ed): *CRC Handbook Series in Zoonoses*. Boca Raton, FL, CRC Press, 1981, vol 1, pp 97–106.

276. Thompson WH, Kallayan B, Anslow RO: Isolation of California encephalitis group virus from a fatal human illness. *Am J Trop Med Hyg* 81:245, 1965.

277. Töndury G, Smith DW: Fetal rubella pathology. *J Pediatr* 68:867, 1966.

278. Townsend JJ, Baringer JR, Wolinsky JA, Malamud N, Mednick JP, Panitch HS, Scott RAT, Oshiro LA, Cremer NE: Progressive rubella panencephalitis. Late onset after congenital rubella. *N Engl J Med* 292:990, 1975.

279. Trainin Z, Wernicke D, Ungar-Waron, Essex M: Antibodies to cell membrane antigens associated with human T-cell leukemia virus in patients with AIDS. *Science* 220:859, 1983.

280. Tyler KL, Adler D: Twenty eight years of benign recurring Mollaret meningitis. *Arch Neurol* 40:42, 1983.

281. Van Bogaert L: Die klinische Einheit und pathologische Varionsbreite der subacuten sklerosierenden Lauko-encephalitis. *Wien Z Nervenheilkd* 13:185, 1957.

282. Vandvik B, Nordal H: Local synthesis in the central nervous system of diclonal IgM-kappa and homogeneous free kappa light chain proteins in a case of chronic meningoencephalitis. *Eur Neurol* 17:23, 1978.

283. Vieira J, Frank E, Spira TJ, Landesman SH: Acquired immune deficiency in Haitians: opportunistic infections in previously healthy Haitian immigrants. *N Engl J Med* 308:125, 1983.

284. Waksman BH: Immunity and the nervous system: basic tenets. *Ann Neurol* 13:587, 1983.

285. Webb HE, Connolly JH, Kane FF, O'Reilly KJ, Simpson DIH: Laboratory infection with louping-ill with associated encephalitis. *Lancet* 2:255, 1968.

286. Webster AD, Tripp JH, Hayward AR, Dayan AD, Doshi R, MacIntyre EH, Tyrell DA: Echovirus encephalitis and myositis in primary immunoglobulin deficiency. *Arch Dis Child* 53:33, 1978.

287. Webster LT, Wright FH: Recovery of eastern equine encepohalomyelitis virus from brain tissue of human cases of encephalitis in Massachusetts. *Science* 88:305, 1938.

288. Wechsler SL, Fields BN: Differences between the intracellular polypeptides of measels and subacute sclerosing panencephalitis virus. *Nature* 272:458, 1978.

289. Weil A, Breslich PJ: Histopathology of the central nervous system in the North Dakota epidemic encephalitis. *J Neuropathol Exp Neurol* 1:49, 1942.

290. Weiner LP, Narayan O: A papovirus isolated from patients with progressive multifocal leukoencephalopathy. *Ann Clin Res* 5:279, 1973.

291. Weiss RA: Receptors for RNA tumor viruses. In Beers RF Jr, Bassett EG (eds): *Cell Membrane Receptors for Viruses, Antigens, and Antibodies, Peptide Hormones, and Small Molecules*. New York, Raven Press, 1976, pp 237–251.

292. Wells JV: Immunoglobulin biosynthesis and metabolism. In Fudenberg HH, Stites DP, Caldwell JL, Wells JV (eds): *Basic and Clinical Immunology*. Los Altos, CA, Lange, 1980, pp 64–78.

293. Whillis D, Hawkey CJ, Toghill PJ: Neurological illness in patient with no immunological response to mumps. *Lancet* 2:1214, 1982.

294. White HH, Kepes JH, Kirkpatrick CH, Schimke RN: Subacute encephalitis and congenital hypogenital hypogammaglobulinemia. *Arch Neurol* 26:359, 1972.

295. Whitley RJ, Soong SJ, Dolin R, Galasso GJ, Ch'ien LT, Alford CA, The Collaboratory Study Group: Adenine arabinoside therapy of biopsy proved herpes simplex encephalitis. National Institute of Allergy and Infectious Disease Collaborative Antiviral Study. *N Engl J Med* 297:289, 1977.

296. Whitley RJ, Soong SJ, Hirsch MS, Karchner AW, Dolin R, Galasso G, Dunnick J, Alford CA, NIAID Collabora-

tive Antiviral Study Group: Herpes simplex encephalitis: Vidarabine therapy and diagnostic problems. *N Engl J Med* 304:313, 1981.

297. Wickmann I: Classics in infectious disease: On the epidemiology of Heine-Medin's disease. *Rev Infect Dis* 2:319, 1980.

298. Will RG, Matthews WB: Evidence for case-to-case transmission of Creutzfeldt-Jakob disease. *J Neurol Neurosurg Psychiatry* 45:235, 1982.

299. Wilson MS, Wherett BA, Mahdy MS: Powassan virus meningoencephalitis: a case report. *Can Med Assoc J* 121:320, 1979.

300. Wilson SAK: Syndrome of Jakob; cortico-striato-spinal degeneration. In Bruce AN (ed): *Neurology.* Baltimore, Williams & Wilkins, 1955, p 1044.

301. Winkelstein JA: Opsonins: their function, identity, and clinical significance. *J Pediatr* 82:747, 1973.

302. World Health Organization: The ecology of influenza virus: a WHO memorandum. *Bull WHO* 59:869, 1981.

303. Wyatt et al: Rotaviruses. *Perspect Virol* 10:121, 1978.

304. Yuill TM: Vesicular stomatitis. In Beran GW (ed): *Section B: Viral Zoonoses.* In Steele JH (ed): *CRC Handbook Series in Zoonoses.* Boca Raton, FL, CRC Press, 1981, vol 1, pp 125–142.

305. Zimmerman HM: The pathology of Japanese B encephalitis. *J Neuropathol Exp Neurol* 7:106, 1948.

306. Zu Rhein GM, Chou SM: Particles resembling papova virus in human cerebral demyelinating disease. *Science* 148:1477, 1965.

CHAPTER 15

Degenerative Diseases of the Central Nervous System

WILLIAM C. SCHOENE, M.D.

When diseases of the nervous system are classified according to etiology, there remains a group of heterogeneous conditions called the "degenerative diseases of the nervous system," about which virtually nothing is known as to cause or pathogenesis. Some conditions have been shifted out of this idiopathic group into other categories, following understanding of their nature, e.g., metabolic diseases as in Wilson's disease.

Most degenerative diseases are inherited, e.g., Huntington's chorea; some are sporadic, e.g., idiopathic Parkinson's disease; and a few with identical clinical and pathological features may be inherited or sporadic, e.g., cerebello-olivary degeneration.

Pathologically, these conditions result from the progressive degeneration of neurons and their processes within an anatomical region or system(s) of related neurons with atrophy of the structure(s) they involve, e.g., caudate nucleus in Huntington's disease. In some conditions, neuronal disappearance is accompanied by an intracellular derangement, e.g., neurofibrillary tangles, while in others, neurons vanish without a trace (simple atrophy), e.g., amyotrophic lateral sclerosis. Inflammation, stored material in neurons, and other changes which occur in conditions with a known cause or pathogenesis such as infections and lipoidosis, are minimal or absent.

Present classification of these heterogeneous conditions is confusing and imprecise. Nosologic separation of these entities currently rests on clinicopathological correlation, as neither the clinical manifestations, e.g., dementia, nor pathological features, e.g., neurofibrillary tangles, alone are specific to a single disease. Clinically similar cases, e.g., slowly developing dementia, may have different histopathological substrates, e.g., neurofibrillary tangles in Alzheimer's disease and Pick bodies in Pick's disease. Conversely, similar histological abnormalities, such as neurofibrillary tangles, may be associated with different clinical conditions, e.g., Alzheimer's disease, and postencephalitic parkinsonism.

The etiology of specific conditions is probably different, and there is little to suggest a common cause among the degenerative diseases. Metabolic defects, enzyme deficiencies, viruses and other transmissible agents, and neurotoxins have been looked for in many of these conditions without success. Specific genetic flaws and/or acquired inability of neurons to deal with external toxins, infections, or age-related failure of biological mechanisms have yet to be elucidated. Hopefully, newer techniques of investigation will provide etiological clues which will lead to curative or preventive therapy.

DISEASES INVOLVING THE CORTEX

Diffuse dysfunction or injury to cerebral cortical neurons secondary to idiopathic cortical degeneration, e.g., Alzheimer's disease, results in dementia characterized by loss of intellect and often memory, usually without focal signs. The known causes of dementia are many, such as multiple infarcts, hydrocephalus, encephalitis, neoplasm, trauma, and metabolic abnormalities. In these conditions, focal deficits, e.g., paralysis, frequently are present in addition to dementia. Idiopathic dementias classically have been divided by their age of onset into presenile or senile dementia, depending on whether clinical signs begin before or after the age of 65. The idiopathic presenile dementias include Alzheimer's, Pick's, and formerly Creutzfeldt-Jakob disease, which now is known to be caused by a transmissible agent (Chapter 14).

Alzheimer's Disease and Senile Dementia of the Alzheimer Type

The relationship of presenile Alzheimer's disease and senile dementia of the Alzheimer type is controversial (76, 182). There is a difference of opinion as to whether these clinical entities with identical histological features are the same disease with a different age of onset or whether they represent distinct diseases with separate etiologies. It has been estimated that over 1,300,000 people in the general population of the United States suffer from severe dementia, of which 50–60% is of the Alzheimer type (183). Since Alzheimer's disease and senile dementia of the Alzheimer type are currently topics of intense investigation, an entire chapter (Chapter 16) has been devoted to their review.

Pick's Disease (Lobar Atrophy)

Of the idiopathic cortical dementias, Pick's disease is the rarest. It usually is sporadic, progressive, and more common in women. The average course to death is between 2 and 5 years, with some cases living 10 years or more. One or more lobes of the cerebrum are involved, which has resulted in the synonym "lobar atrophy." Pick's disease clinically is often indistinguishable from Alzheimer's disease. The usual case begins insidiously with decline of intellect, often accompanied by intermittent restlessness and loss of inhibition with inappropriate social behavior and sloppiness of dress. Two-thirds of the patients

have speech disturbances, usually beginning with incorrect use of words which may progress to bursts of incomprehensible jargon (4). Patients frequently show lack of awareness. Memory, orientation, and attention may be relatively unaffected when the temporal lobe is spared. This is in contrast to Alzheimer's disease, in which both the frontal and temporal lobes usually are affected, with early deterioration of recent memory. Shuffling gait and ataxia may be present. Seizures, rigidity, and abnormal movements are uncommon. Later, patients may evolve into a vegetative stage with inanition and may die from infection. No effective treatment is known.

Of the various clinical and pathological features associated with Pick's disease, the pattern of gyral atrophy characterized grossly by sparing of the posterior two-thirds of the superior temporal gyrus is perhaps the most characteristic (Fig. 15.1). Atrophy may be so extreme as to reduce the affect gyri to a thin edge referred to as "knife blade atrophy." In the most extreme state the brain has the appearance of a desiccated walnut. The subcortical white matter may be involved in addition to the cortex. Cortical atrophy occurs most commonly in the frontoparietal region, although it may be confined to the frontal or temporal lobes and, in rare cases, to the parietal and, even less commonly, the occipital lobes. In the most authoritative study, cerebral atrophy was symmetrically distributed in about one-third of the cases, while in two-thirds of the cases it was asymmetrical, distributed to the left hemisphere in half the cases and to the right in one-fifth of the brains examined (118). Various authorities have suggested that vulnerable regions for atrophy are phylogenetically newer parts of the brain (48). Atrophy of the caudate nucleus may be extensive and may resemble that seen in Huntington's chorea, although the putamen is never as severely involved. Changes in the thalamus, globus pallidus, subthalamic nucleus, and substantia nigra have been described (4, 125).

Neuronal loss in the outer three layers of the cortex is severe, although all layers may be involved. Remaining neurons may show round-oval cytoplasmic swellings, or Pick bodies (Fig. 15.2). In a topographic analysis

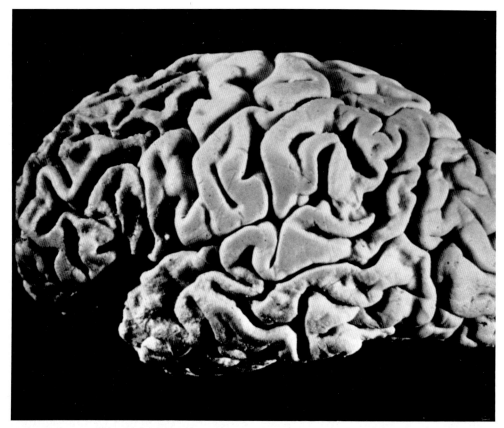

Figure 15.1.   Pick's disease. Atrophy of the frontal and temporal lobes with sparing of the posterior two-thirds of the superior temporal gyrus.

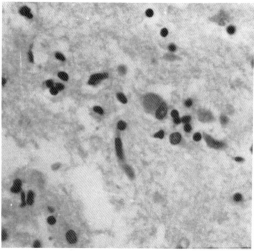

Figure 15.2.   Pick body. Round homogenous structure in the cytoplasm of a neuron. H&E. (Original magnification ×500.)

of the hippocampi from two patients, Pick bodies were found to be most prevalent in Rose's H_1 field, with adjacent subiculum and entorhinal cortex in comparison to the H_2 field and presubiculum. The end plate was least affected (10). Some brains show extensive loss of subcortical white matter. Gliosis in the cortex and adjacent white matter usually are extensive. There is a difference of opinion as to whether subcortical white matter loss is secondary to cortical neuronal loss or is the result of primary involvement of the proximal axons near and in the subcortical white matter. Electron microscopic studies of Pick bodies have shown variable findings (147, 161, 184, 195). They apparently can be composed of normal appearing straight 10-nm neurofilaments, straight 15-nm filaments, paired helical 20–24-nm filaments, vesiculated endoplasmic reticulum, or a combination of these elements. Positive staining with antiserum to neurofilaments and neurofilament polypeptides using a peroxidase-antiperoxidase technique has been found in Pick bodies from two cases (71). The formation of Pick bodies may be the result of retrograde or transynaptic degeneration (195) or may be subsequent to recent axonal damage near the cell of origin, possibly representing a form of chromatolysis (194). Pick bodies are not diagnostic of Pick's disease, as neurons with an identical appearance have been found in various conditions, e.g., syphilis, infarcts, and near tumors (194). Neurofibrillary tangles, senile plaques, granulovacuolar degeneration, lipofuscin, and Hirano bodies common to other conditions such as Alzheimer's disease may be seen in cases of Pick's disease. Widespread loss of dendritic spines, in addition to thinning of the major basilar shaft of dendrites with essentially no tertiary branching, has been reported (190), using a rapid Golgi staining method. The significance of these findings has to be evaluated. In a recent study of two cases of Pick's disease, loss of neurons in the basal nucleus of Meynert was noted (186). This abnormality was not found in an earlier study (145). The reason for this discrepancy may be methodological, although it probably suggests that neuronal loss is variable in individual cases. In one preliminary study, the muscarinic receptor binding sites in the temporal lobe were reduced (191). Diagnosis of Pick's disease does not rest solely on microscopic features but rather depends on a constellation of clinical, gross, and microscopic findings.

Creutzfeldt-Jakob Disease

Among the presenile dementias this disorder is associated with the most rapid course, usually ending in death between 6 months and 2 years of age. Since this condition can be passed from man to monkey or from monkey to monkey by a so-called transmissible agent or unconventional "slow" virus, it seems more appropriate to consider it under the viral diseases.

DISEASES OF THE BASAL GANGLIA AND MESENCEPHALON

The basal ganglia is a broad term which encompasses deep gray matter nuclei situated at the base of the forebrain bounded by the extreme and internal capsule and including the caudate and putamen, globus pallidus, subthalamic nucleus, substantia nigra, red nucleus, and some thalamic nuclei. This term is imprecise, as these structures do not make up a unified "system." The caudate and putamen together, called the corpus striatum, are histologically identical, composed of a mixed population of large and small neurons in a ratio of about 1:60 (121). Small neurons have spiny dendrites, in contrast to the larger neurons with smooth dendrites (121), and are believed to be cholinergic. Intrafascicular oligodendrocytes are arranged in such a way as to give these structures a striated appearance. The putamen and globus pallidus, because of their lense shape, are called the lenticular nucleus. The globus pallidus histologically does not resemble the putamen, as it contains large neurons scattered among distinct myelinated pencil-shaped bundles of fibers. The primary connections of these nuclei consist of topographically arranged fibers from a variety of structures which include the cerebral cortex, thalamus, and substantia nigra. Briefly, the major input to the striatum is from the motor cortex, some thalamic nuclei, zona compacta of the substantia nigra, and the raphe nuclei of the midbrain. Neurotransmitters linked with input structures include glutamate in the corticostriate, choline in the thalamostriate, dopamine in the nigrostriate, and ventral tegmental pathways. 5-Hydroxytryptamine is associated with the raphe nuclei's projection to the striatum, and a small noradrenaline pathway from the locus ceruleus to the nucleus accumbens also exists. The major projection of the striatum is to the globus pallidus and the zone reticulata of the substantia nigra. The external segment of the globus pallidus sends its efferents to the subthalamic nucleus and to ventral and medial nuclei of the thalamus. The zone reticulata also projects to the ventral nucleus of the thalamus, superior colliculus, and some regions of the reticular formation. γ-Aminobutyric acid (GABA) is the neurotransmitter utilized in the major output of the striatum to the globus pallidus and substantia nigra. Other striatonigral and striapallidal pathways are associated with substance P and Met-enkephalin. The major outflows of the internal segment of the globus pallidus and the zone reticulata to the thalamus are GABA-ergic. For detailed anatomical and biochemical aspects of the basal ganglia, the reader is referred to the following references (29, 121, 122). Structures of the basal ganglia are involved with mediation and control of motor function comprise, the so-called "extrapyramidal system." Disorders of the extrapyramidal system result in akinesia, abnormalities of posture and disequilibrium, disturbances of muscle tone (rigidity), and involuntary movements such as chorea, athetosis, and dystonia. This system consists of motor pathways not included in corticospinal pathways, or the "pyramidal system." Broadly speaking, the extrapyramidal system includes the striatopallidonigral connections and the cerebellum. For a detailed analysis of the functional derangement resulting from injury to the basal ganglia, the reader is referred to the work of Adams and Victor (5).

Before considering individual entities, it is helpful to realize that they consist of heterogeneous conditions with little morphological similarity in the pattern of their neuronal loss. They are grouped together only because the structures they principally affect are located within the basal ganglia. Most of these conditions also involve contiguous structures such as the cortex or brainstem. They do not appear to have a common etiology.

Huntington's Disease

This disease was first described by George Huntington in 1872. It's course is variable, lasting a decade or so, although some patients die within 5 years and others survive for many years. The usual age of onset is in the fourth or fifth decade; however, 5–10% start before the second decade, and a few cases begin either in early childhood or late in life. The condition is dominantly inherited, although sporadic cases possibly occur. Death can result from cardiovascular disease, pneumonia or, sometimes, suicide.

The clinical onset is insidious and progressive, beginning in a previously well patient. Early signs include abnormalities of movement and mentation. The age of onset, the sequence of their appearance, and progression is unpredictable. Most patients begin with a disorder of movement while others first show a decline of cognitive function. Initially, clinical signs are slight with the subsequent development of restlessness, grimacing, writhing motions, and chorea. Early evidence of mental and emotional deterioration include change in character and emotional lability, indifference to the environment, and loss of memory, leading to dementia. Young patients occasionally have seizures and frequently show rigidity rather than chorea, the Wesphal variant. Adult cases with the rigid form of the disease also occur. Abnormalities of saccadic eye movements and ocular fixation occur in some patients. Deep tendon reflexes are brisk, and the limbs may be hypotonic.

Gross atrophy of the caudate and putamenal nuclei is striking. Loss of the caudate nuclei is accompanied by a compensating enlargement of the anterior lateral ventricle. Atrophy of the cerebral gyri, especially in the frontal and temporal lobes and rarely of the entire cortex, may be present (Fig. 15.3). In life these anatomic alterations may be demonstrated by a CT scan. Coronal sections of the brain show shrunken yellow structures in place of the normal caudate and putamen.

A variable loss of small neurons and gliosis occurs in the corpus striatum. Remaining neurons may appear normal, although satellitosis and neuronophagia have been seen (151). In later and more devastating stages of the disease large neurons disappear, and the neurophil may even appear spongy. The site of neuronal loss is variable. In some cases, both the caudate and striatum may be affected while in others either the caudate or putamen may selectively be more involved (48). Some investigators have found neuronal loss to be more severe in the anterior regions of the corpus striatum (4) while others have found it to be more severe posteriorly (60). Myelinated fibers in these nuclei are sometimes lost. Variable and inconsistent nerve cell loss has been reported in other regions of the brain, such as the globus pallidus, hypothalamus, dentate nucleus, and the Purkinje neurons of the cerebellum, and brainstem. The distribution and degree of this loss differs considerably between reports and probably represents true variation in individual cases (48). Cortical neuronal loss is present in patients with profound dementia, although the intensity and distribution

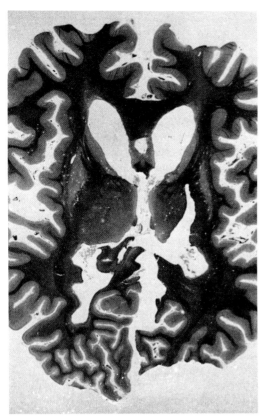

Figure 15.3. Huntington's chorea. Severe atrophy of the caudate and putamen and enlarged lateral ventricles. Giant paraffin section (H&E stain).

of loss is variable. It may be diffuse or circumscribed. Some cases seem to have more loss in the middle cortical layers while others show a predilection for the deeper layers. Loss of myelinated fibers in the subcortical regions may be quite severe. An important morphological study of 139 cases of clinically diagnosed Huntington's disease has attempted to grade the gross and histological changes (188). These investigators, using a grading system which ranged from 0 to 4 (five grades), evaluated neuronal loss and accompanying fibrillary gliosis. At death, most cases fell into grades 3–4, characterized by extreme atrophy of the caudate nucleus, which was reduced to a yellow-brown concave thin ribbon of tissue with enlargement of the adjacent anterior lateral ventricle. The internal capsule was reduced to a thin strip. Grey matter bridges to the putamen showed similar changes, and the putamen and lateral portion of the globus pallidus were reduced in size. At the other extreme were three patients (grade 0) with clinically diagnosed Huntington's disease who showed no morphological changes in their deep gray structures. Investigation of the cortex in all five categories showed no appreciable loss of neurons or gliosis. It was suggested that the anatomical changes in Huntington's disease probably lag behind the clinical manifestations and that diagnosis of these early cases using a CT scan might be missed. This study points out that the great morphological variation occurring in Huntington's disease and raises questions as to the nature and extent of reported changes in the cortex. Cases of Huntington's and Pick's disease may be confused with each other when involvement of the cortex, subcortical white matter, and caudate nucleus is severe. About 7% of cases diagnosed clinically as Huntington's disease at postmortem have other conditions, e.g., Alzheimer's disease, less commonly a dominantly inherited cerebellar ataxia, and rarely Creutzfeldt-Jakob disease (21). Ultrastructural changes within neurons include abnormalities of nuclear membranes with intranuclear and intranucleolar clumps of osmiophilic granules. Cytoplasmic variations occurred with increased numbers of organelles and lipofuscin: the cisternae of the endoplasmic reticulum may be dilated with loss of ribosomes; canals of the Golgi apparatus are variable in dimension; and mitochondria and lysosomes of various sizes and numbers accumulate. Some axons have reduced numbers of presynaptic vesicles (151). Histochemical studies suggested a possible abnormality of lysosomal enzymes which results in excessive accumulation of lipofuscin. Biochemical studies have shown decreased GABA and glutamic acid decarboxylase in the basal ganglia. A decrease in choline acetyltransferase, substance P, angiotensin-converting enzyme, and Met-enkephalin also has been reported. These findings have been well reviewed by Bird and Spokes (21) and Marsden (122). The etiology of these biochemical abnormalities is unknown and is likely to be secondary to neuronal degeneration. Injection of kainic acid, a neurotoxin, into the striatum of laboratory animals produces tissue and biochemical alterations reminiscent of Huntington's disease. Search for such an agent in man has been unrewarding (122). Recently, a new and very exciting development in unraveling Huntington's disease has appeared, reporting a restriction enzyme marker which indicates that a "Huntington's disease gene" is located on chromosome 4 (77). This discovery has great importance in determining whether a person at risk will develop the disease. Hopefully, it will not be long before the offending gene(s) will be isolated and progress will be made in altering the expression of Huntington's chorea.

Hallervorden-Spatz Disease

This exceedingly rare condition was first described in 1922 by Hallervorden and Spatz (79) in 5 sisters in a family of 12 children. At postmortem there was a striking yellow-brown discoloration of the globus pallidus and substantia nigra. Following this clearly defined description, some cases were reported which differed considerably from those of the 1922 report and resulted in blurring of the criteria necessary to make the diagnosis of Hallervorden-Spatz disease. In 1974, Dooling et al. (54) summarized all previous pathologically verified cases in the literature, along with their own material. Cases varied considerably from one to another in their clinical expression and pathological findings; some were identical to those classically described cases in 1922, whereas others were not familial but had typical clinical and pathological features. A third group of cases were without nigral lesions. This study resulted in the conclusion that a group of patients does exist, if strict criteria are observed, which constitutes a clinicopathological entity that can be designated as having Hallervorden-Spatz disease.

Cases which do not adhere to classic criteria should not be lumped into the restricted category of Hallervorden-Spatz disease but rather should remain unclassified or be placed in a broad category, such as spheroid pigmentary degeneration of the pallidonigral region. It may turn out that spheroid pigmentary degeneration affecting the globus pallidus and sometimes the substantia nigra will encompass a spectrum of clinicopathological entities which have a common metabolic error. Until this is known, we prefer to separate the classic cases of Hallervorden-Spatz disease from the atypical cases by their clinicopathologic features.

Patients have a normal early life with an onset generally after childhood; a progressive motor disorder predominantly extrapyramidal in expression develops. Abnormalities of posture, often impeding walking, are the presenting signs in many cases. Rare cases begin with mental changes. As the disease advances, rigidity of the musculature with involuntary movements of the chorioathetoid or tremulous type, along with dystonia, may appear. Spasticity and an extensor plantar response are present in some patients. Dysarthria occurs in most cases. Progressive failure of intellect leading to dementia develops in the majority of patients; ocular abnormalities, e.g., retinal degeneration, may develop. A blood smear may show acanthocytosis. Most laboratory tests are normal, except for the electroencephalogram, which in some cases has been abnormal. The course extends for about two decades and ends in death in early adulthood. The disease is not known to have affected more than one generation in a family.

Externally, the brain is normal while on cut section the globus pallidus, especially in its medial segment, and the substantia nigra show a rust-brown discoloration (Fig. 15.4). These regions contain axonal spheroids, loss of neurons, gliosis, and the deposition of a brown-yellow pigment variably positive for iron (Figs. 15.5A and B). Granules and conglomerates of pigment may be lying free or encrusted on remaining neurons or astrocytes, or may be in macrophages, especially around blood vessels. Calcifications may be present in tissue or in the walls of the blood vessels. Some cases show hyaline eosinophilic structures adjacent to neurons in the cortex that are identical to axonal spheroids, although overall morphological changes are essentially limited to the pallidonigral system. Electron microscopy shows axonal spheroids typical of dystrophic axons (100). In one study, CT scans in a patient with advanced disease and with long survival whose sister at autopsy had proven Hallervorden-Spatz disease have shown enlarged lateral ventricles

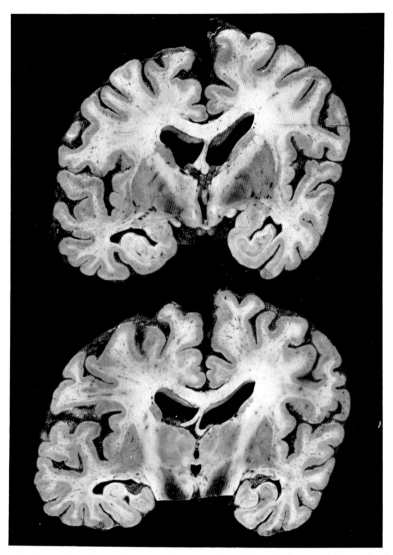

Figure 15.4. Hallervorden-Spatz disease. Pigmentation of the globus pallidus and substantia nigra.

with increased ratios between the intercaudate distance and the width of the frontal horns. It must be pointed out that these CT changes are not diagnostic but, in association with a typical clinical history, are suggestive of Hallervorden-Spatz disease (55). Two recent reports without pathologic studies based on CT evidence and an increased iron uptake in the basal ganglia suggest that patients with presumed Hallervorden-Spatz disease may show abnormalities outside the central nervous system (175, 179). In one study, electron microscopy of skin biopsies from three patients have demonstrated unusual electron-dense,

membrane-bound, and mostly intracellular material (175). In the other study of a brother and sister, the boy had sea blue histiocytes in his bone marrow, and electron microscopy of his circulating lymphocytes revealed cytoplasmic vacuolation, fingerprint profiles, multilaminar profiles, granular osmophilic deposits, and curvilinear bodies. His sister's lymphocytes contained vacuoles and ultrastructurally showed granular osmophilic deposits (179). Similar studies in patients who eventually have postmortem confirmation of Hallervorden-Spatz disease will be necessary to substantiate these preliminary but inter-

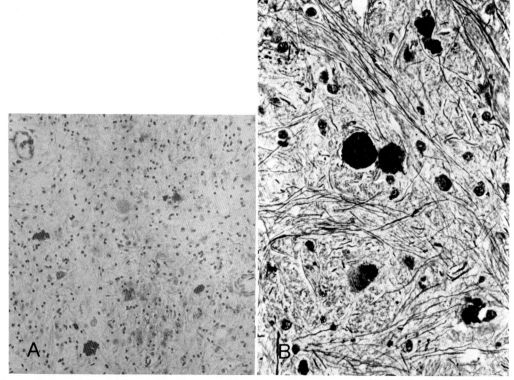

Figure 15.5. Hallervorden-Spatz disease. (*A*) Spheroids, neuronal loss, pigment deposition, and gliosis in the globus pallidus. H&E stain. (Original magnification ×100.) (*B*) Spheroids in globus pallidus. Silver stain. (Original magnification ×600.)

esting findings. Gross and microscopic findings identical to those in Hallervorden-Spatz disease in man have been found in apparently asymptomatic old monkeys (30). The significance of spontaneous pallidonigral spheroid pigmentary degeneration in these animals and its possible relation to Hallervorden-Spatz disease in man is unknown. The pathogenesis of the human disease is an enigma.

Effective treatment is not available. Levodopa has been given with transient improvement of rigidity. The presence of iron-containing deposits has suggested that iron-chelating agents might be of some benefit; several attempts at using this treatment have not appeared to affect the course of the disease (54, 115). Spheroids are a prominent feature in both vitamin E deficiency and Hallervorden-Spatz disease. Unfortunately, treatment of Hallervorden-Spatz disease with vitamin E has not been helpful (115).

Neuroaxonal Dystrophy

This rare autosomal recessively transmitted disease was first described in 1952 by Seitelberger and is characterized by a widespread accumulation of axonal spheroids in the spinal cord, brainstem, mesencephalon, basal ganglia, and cortex. It usually begins in the second year of life. Weakness, difficulty standing, hypotonia, and diminished deep tendon reflexes develop. Rigidity and corticospinal tract signs may become prominent. Diminished pain sensation, loss of vision, and optic atrophy may appear. Mental impairment develops. The EMG may confirm denervation. This condition clinically must be differentiated from metachromatic leukodystrophy, as these two conditions may show almost identical clinical manifestations (6). The nervous system progressively is involved, with the usual course lasting between 5 and 10 years.

Externally and on cut section the brain and spinal cord are grossly normal. Spheroids are scattered throughout the central nervous system, especially in its caudal regions, e.g., brainstem and spinal cord (50). The peripheral and autonomic nervous systems (59), conjunctiva, and dental pulp of deciduous teeth can contain spheroids (8, 38). Ultrastructurally, spheroids are composed of membrane whorls, increased numbers of various-sized mitochondria, vesicles, and increased neurofilaments, along with tubular and cisternal profiles (100, 110). Spheroids with an identical appearance have been seen in a variety of pathological and experimental conditions and *per se* represent a nonspecific reaction to injury (100). Neuroaxonal dystrophy and Hallervorden-Spatz disease have been considered to be a spectrum of the same condition (166). We, however, prefer to separate these conditions on clinicopathological grounds. Attempts at treatment have not altered the fatal outcome of this condition.

FAMILIAL MYOCLONIC EPILEPSY

Myoclonus is characterized by asymmetric, random, very brief, shock-like contractions of a portion of a muscle, an entire muscle, or a group of muscles. The abnormality underlying myoclonus is not understood. It is due, presumably, to inappropriate discharge of motor units. Myoclonus occurs in both acquired and familial disorders (26, 109). Meningitis, encephalitis, general paresis, advanced Alzheimer's disease, and some intoxications, e.g., uremia, are examples of acquired conditions associated with myoclonus. Nongenetic diseases such as subacute sclerosing panencephalitis and Creutzfeldt-Jakob disease may develop myoclonus as a prominent feature. Familial or inherited myoclonic epilepsy can be divided into: (*a*) progressive familial myoclonic epilepsy; (*b*) benign familial polymyoclonia; and (*c*) myoclonic epilepsy associated with the lipidoses (6).

PROGRESSIVE FAMILIAL MYOCLONIC EPILEPSY

Unverricht (187) in 1891 first reported a distinctive form of progressive familial myoclonic epilepsy with dementia which had an onset beginning in late childhood or teenage years. Similar cases were added to the literature by Lundborg (114) in 1903. In 1911, Lafora et al. (106, 107) described the pathological features of intraneuronal inclusions (Lafora bodies) in patients clinically similar to those patients described by Unverricht and Lundborg. Subsequent reports of patients with progressive familial myoclonic epilepsy have shown that Lafora bodies are not present in all clinical cases. The syndrome in one family may vary as to anatomic involvement and consequent neurological impairment. Some cases have shown choreoathetosis while others have had signs referable to the cerebellum and spinal cord. Whether these cases are the result of different etiologies or incomplete manifestations of the same disease is unknown.

Familial myoclonic epilepsy with Lafora bodies typically affect more than one child in a family. The onset between childhood and early adulthood in an apparently normal individual is initiated by convulsions, frequently grand mal in type, with or without myoclonic jerks. As the disease progresses, shock-like myoclonic contractions develop in one part of the body, eventually involving most if not all of the body. A series of myoclonic jerks may precede a generalized seizure. Patients become incapacitated, and a progressive dementia develops. Seizures appear to become less frequent later, although myoclonus continues. Rigidity, hypotonia, impaired tendon reflexes and, sometimes, later corticospinal tract signs are seen (6). Patients eventually become helpless and cachectic, and die of infection. The course is usually 5–10 years, with most patients dying by the age of 30. Laboratory tests of CSF, urine, and blood are normal.

The brain may show some atrophy. The diagnosis of this disease rests on finding Lafora bodies in the cytoplasm or processes of neurons. These bodies are round and concentric, sometimes homogeneous, with dense irregular cores surrounded by paler rings with radial striations (Fig. 15.6). They are basophilic in all of the usual preparations, do not stain with Congo red, and vary in size between 1 and 20 μm. More than one body may be present in a neuron. They rarely have been found extracellularly free in tissue (45). Electron microscopy of La-

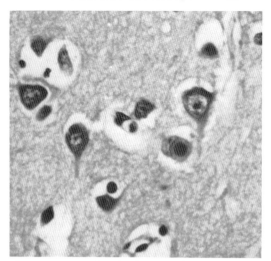

Figure 15.6. Lafora body. Round structure with dense core surrounded by a lighter rim with spicules in the cytoplasm of a neuron. H&E stain. (Original magnification ×600.)

fora bodies shows fibrillary elements, sometimes branched, which appear as tubules that are often associated with endoplasmic reticulum and ribosomes (45). Biochemically, they consist of an unusual polyglycosan material. Lafora bodies are found throughout the central nervous system, especially in the dentate nucleus, thalamus, inferior olive and substantia nigra, and the cerebral cortex. The work of Austin and Sakai (9) is an excellent review of the structural and biochemical features of Lafora bodies. In some cases, inclusions somewhat resembling Lafora bodies have been seen in the liver (134), myocardium (80), and in muscle (40).

Treatment is limited to control of epilepsy and myoclonus.

BENIGN FAMILIAL POLYMYOCLONIA

This probably heterogeneous entity is separated from progressive familial myoclonic epilepsy on the basis of its clinicopathological features. The main differences are: patients with myoclonus may have features of an hereditary cerebellar ataxia or spinocerebellar degeneration (dysynergia cerebellaris myoclonica) (95); epilepsy is not as consistent and is often less prominent; progressive dementia may or may not develop, and when it does it is often late in

the illness; and the course is more unpredictable. While some patients have myoclonus, others may show localized neurological signs of cerebellar dysfunction. Nerve deafness may occur. The disease does not appear to progress in some patients whereas in others, there may be a long period of quiescence before symptomatology recurs. In most patients the course is more benign than progressive familial myoclonic epilepsy.

The neuropathological findings of this benign condition(s) are inconsistent and are not understood. Primary atrophy of the dentate nucleus, with thinning of the superior cerebellar penduncles along with degeneration of the posterior columns and spinocerebellar tracts, was described by Hunt (95) in one of his patients. Lafora bodies are not present in most published reports.

MYOCLONIC EPILEPSY ASSOCIATED WITH THE LIPIDOSES

This group of cases associated with the lipidoses do not have Lafora bodies and are quite different from progressive familial myoclonic epilepsy and benign familial polymyoclonia. They are only mentioned here to include them as conditions which manifest prominent familial myoclonic epilepsy as part of their clinical expression.

DISEASES OF THE MESENCEPHALON INVOLVING THE SUBSTANTIA NIGRA AND RELATED SYSTEMS OF NEURONS

Parkinson's Syndrome: (Parkinsonism)

The first comprehensive neurological description was given by James Parkinson (138), who in 1817 stated that patients show "involuntary tremulous motion, with lessened muscular power in parts not in action and even when supported; with a propensity to bend the trunk forward, and to pass from a walking to a running pace; the senses and intellect being uninjured". Parkinsonism is produced or brought about by damage to or malfunction of the nigral system. Conditions associated with this syndrome are numerous, e.g., sequelae of a viral infection, a reaction to drugs, and intoxication or poisoning. The majority of cases are spontaneous and idiopathic. Parkinsonism, or Parkinson's syndrome, is a clinical term which refers to a constellation of clinical manifestations which include all or fragments of the neurological abnormalities which James Parkinson elucidated. It does not imply specific pathological change or etiology. Parkinson's syndrome is not synonymous with Parkinson's disease. The term Parkinson's disease, as used in this chapter, is restricted to paralysis agitans, or idiopathic parkinsonism, which is the idiopathic form of parkinsonism associated with the formation of Lewy bodies and the loss of neurons in the substantia nigra and locus ceruleus.

Parkinson's Disease (Idiopathic Parkinsonism, Paralysis Agitans)

Parkinson's disease is well known to every neurologist, although its exact incidence is difficult to determine. It has been suggested that this disease is increasing in the population, although not all authorities agree with that assessment (167). The age of onset in most cases is around the fifth to the sixth decade of life. Apparently, there is no increased prevalence in any country, race, or class. Recent epidemiological studies have reported a decreased incidence of idiopathic Parkinsonism in cigarette smokers (13). A hereditary thread has not been demonstrated (189). The onset is insidious and may vary considerably, appearing with such signs as reduced blinking, masked facies, development of stiffness and slowness of movements, and a coarse "pill-rolling" tremor of the thumb and fingers at rest. Frequently the tremor begins in one hand, then becomes bilateral. The fully developed state in addition shows cogwheel rigidity, bradykinesia, stooped posture, and a shuffling gait which may advance from walking to a running pace (festinating gait). Speech in some patients may be reduced to a whisper. The sensory system is spared and the intellect generally remains intact, although dementia can occur. The course is always progressive, generally over a decade or so and eventually leading to helplessness.

Externally, the brain generally is within normal limits, except in very old patients, who may show coincidental senile changes. The brainstem shows a striking depigmentation of the substantia nigra and the locus ceruleus (Fig. 15.7). Loss of pigmented neurons and gliosis in the substantia nigra, particularly in the zona compacta, in the substantia innominata, and in the locus ceruleus, are present. Remaining neurons often contain intracytoplasmic eosinophilic bodies with a halo, Lewy bodies, which vary in shape from round to elongated (Fig. 15.8). Neuronal loss has been reported in other locations such as the hypothalamus, globus pallidus, and cerebral cortex; however, studies revealing the loss have been inconsistent. The core of Lewy bodies, ultrastructurally, is composed of filaments and granular material, with the rim or halo containing a looser arrangement of filaments (58, 156). These filaments are consistent with intermediate-type filaments having a diameter of 7 to 8 nm (73). Using a peroxidase-antiperoxidase technique, immunocytochemical reactions of Lewy bodies examined with antisera to several filamentous proteins of the nervous system are positive against neurofilaments (73).

The biochemical makeup and interrelationships of the anatomical regions involved in idiopathic parkinsonism and postencephalitic parkinsonism are impossible to include in a chapter such as this, and the reader is referred to the work of

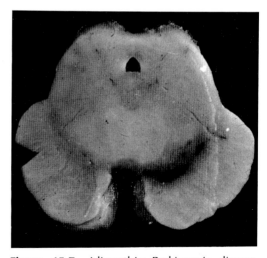

Figure 15.7. Idiopathic Parkinson's disease. Unilateral loss of pigment (*left*) in the substantia nigra. Rare occurrence; most cases show bilateral depigmentation. (From W. C. Schoene: The nervous system. In Robbins, Cotran (eds): *Pathology of the Central Nervous System*, ed 2. Philadelphia, WB Saunders, 1979.)

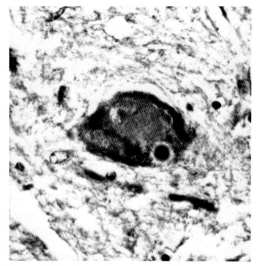

Figure 15.8. Lewy body. Round structure surrounded by a halo in the cytoplasm of a neuron. H&E. (Original magnification ×400.)

Marsden (121, 122) for specific information. Briefly, the principle abnormality appears to be a depletion of dopamine in the corpus striatum and in some other structures. There is moderate loss of noradrenaline in the nucleus accumbens and hypothalamus. Brain serotonin is somewhat reduced; glumatic acid decarboxylase is decreased, especially in the substantia nigra; and Met-enkephalin, although normal in the striatum, is decreased in the substantia nigra. The significance of these findings and variations in substance P is not understood. The severity of the illness can be correlated with dopamine deficiency and probably noradrenaline depletion associated with loss of pigmented cells in the zona compacta of the substantia nigra and locus ceruleus.

Treatment of this disease does not appear to alter the progressive degeneration of neurons. Various drug combinations are used. Levodopa appears to be the most effective drug in relieving motor abnormalities. The side effects of dopamine therapy, which include dyskinesias, gastrointestinal complications, anemia, and/or psychiatric disturbances, may be serious and may limit its use. Regardless of the therapy, patients eventually become refractory to long-term treatment, and their old disabilities return, and progress to incapacity.

Idiopathic Parkinson's Disease Associated with Dementia

There seems to be clinical agreement that patients with idiopathic parkinsonism are more likely to develop dementia than the general population, although the frequency is difficult to determine (129). Two recent studies suggest it to be about 56% (25, 78). Dementia in idiopathic parkinsonian patients appears to be about 6 times more common than in age-matched controls (25, 78). Severity of the dementia varies from mild to severe, with a duration between months and years prior to death. Postmortem examination reveals a brain weight less than that in age-matched controls. The pathological findings in most cases consisted of a variable number of neurofibrillary tangles, senile plaques, granulovacuolar degeneration, and neuronal cell loss in the cerebral cortex. The substantia nigra and locus ceruleus are pale and show loss of pigmented neurons and Lewy bodies. Neurofibrillary tangles are not present in the brainstem. The changes in the cortex are indistinguishable from those in Alzheimer's disease, and changes in the brainstem are identical to idiopathic parkinsonism. The nature of these cases is unknown. They may represent the association of two separate diseases, Alzheimer's disease and idiopathic parkinsonism, or some unknown common interlinking etiological factor which can cause these findings in the same patient. The occurrence of Lewy bodies in the brainstem with the absence of neurofibrillary tangles eliminates other conditions associated with dementia and parkinsonism, such as Parkinson's dementia complex of Guam or progressive supranuclear palsy. There are, however, a small number of idiopathic parkinsonian patients with clinical dementia who at postmortem do not have neurofibrillary tangles and senile plaques (25). The origin of the dementia in these cases is unclear. A few cases in addition to senile changes in their cortex also have scattered Lewy bodies in some of their cortical neurons. Diffuse occurrence of Lewy bodies is discussed in the following paper (199).

Recently, several reports of idiopathic parkinsonism (37, 193) and the Parkinson-dementia complex of Guam have suggested neuronal loss in the nucleus basalis of Meynert. One study of 12 patients consisting of 4 cases of idiopathic Parkinsonism without dementia, 5 cases of idiopathic parkinsonism with dementia, and 3 cases of postencephalitic parkinsonism showed neuronal loss in the nucleus basalis in demented patients. Results were difficult to interpret in the nondemented patients, and no neuronal loss in the nucleus basalis was seen in the three postencephalitic cases. Although the presence of neurofibrillary tangles and senile plaques in the material available was difficult to evaluate, neurofibrillary tangles appeared to be present in some cases (193). Another study of three patients with idiopathic parkinsonism showed neuronal loss in the nucleus basalis (37); some senile plaques, although no neurofibrillary tangles, were found in samples of their cortex. These initial studies bring up the question as to what the relationship is between neuronal loss in the nucleus basalis and idiopathic parkinsonism. It seems reasonably well established that there is loss of neurons in the nucleus basalis in Alzheimer's disease (192), but whether this loss can be caused by the etiology responsible for idiopathic parkinsonism or is dependent upon the coexistence of Alzheimer's disease has yet to be determined.

Postencephalitic Parkinsonism

This condition is the sequela of the great pandemic of encephalitis lethargica which occurred around 1916. Techniques for viral isolation were not available, and the causal agent was never identified. Pathological material from patients with the acute illness in the 1920s showed perivascular cuffing and infiltration of meninges, with lymphocytes and mononuclear cells typical of a viral encephalitis. Some patients died; others recovered from the encephalitis; still others survived and later developed postencephalitic parkinsonism. Postencephalitic parkinsonism, once well established, does not progress. It has been suggested that postencephalitic parkinsonism will eventually disappear (146).

At autopsy, postencephalitic parkinson's patients have depigmentation of their substantia nigra and locus ceruleus, with loss of the pigmented neurons and gliosis. Neu-

rofibrillary tangles may be present in the remaining neurons (Fig. 15.9), similar to those seen in Alzheimer's disease and composed principally of paired helical filaments and some straight filaments (96). In a recent study of three cases of postencephalitic parkinsonism, neurofibrillary tangles stained with the antiperoxidase-peroxidase technique, using an antiserum known to react with normal neurofilaments and neurofilament polypeptide, showed positive staining (71). In another group cases of postencephalitic parkinsonism showed positive staining, with an antiserum raised against a two cycle-purified human brain microtubular fraction, using the antiperoxidase-peroxidase technique (198).

As far as is known, postencephalic parkinsonism has not resulted from any other viral infection, except for that responsible for the 1914–1918 pandemic of encephalitis lethargica. Treatment of this condition consists of drug therapy, e.g., levodopa.

Parkinson Dementia Complex of Guam (PD Guam)

This condition occurs in the Chamorro population of Guam, in which parkinsonism is associated with dementia (83, 84). Many of these cases are seen in conjunction with a Guamanian variant of amyotrophic lateral sclerosis (PD Guam-ALS). This constellation of conditions may represent the same disease (86). The onset of PD

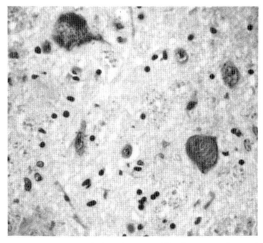

Figure 15.9. Globoid neurofibrillary tangle and a pigmented neuron in the locus ceruleus. H&E. (Original magnification ×300.)

Guam is between the fifth and sixth decades. Patients show features of parkinsonism in association with dementia and loss of corticospinal function. Males are affected three times as often as females. The course is progressive to death in about 4 years. Pathological findings include cortical atrophy, especially of the frontal and temporal lobes, and depigmentation of the substantia nigra and the locus ceruleus. Diffuse neuronal loss with fibrillary gliosis and neurofibrillary tangles occur in the hippocampus, cerebral cortex, amygdala, hypothalamus, globus pallidus, thalamus, substantia nigra, and periaqueductal grey and tegmentum of the brainstem (84). Recently, neuron loss has been reported in the nucleus basalis of Meynert in two cases with Guamanian Parkinson's dementia (132). Neither senile nor neuritic plaques nor Lewy bodies are present. Ultrastructurally, neurofibrillary tangles in Guamanian Parkinson's dementia are similar to those seen in Alzheimer's disease, consisting of paired helical filaments and some straight filaments (84). In cases, eosinophilic paracrystalline "silver-shaped" neuronal cytoplasmic inclusion bodies (Hirano bodies) are seen in neurons, especially in the hippocampus (85). Ultrastructurally, they are composed of approximately 10-nm filaments which run in alternating perpendicular sheets (88, 162). Hirano bodies are nonspecific and have been found also in Alzheimer's and Pick's disease. As Lewy bodies are not present in PD Guam cases, it seems reasonable at this point in our understanding to consider idiopathic parkinsonism with dementia and PD Guam as separate entities with different etiologies.

Other Known Conditions Associated with Parkinsonism

The relationship of a wide range of conditions linked with the clinical features of parkinsonism is controversial. The subject has been reviewed in detail by Schwab and England (163). They include: emotional trauma; cerebroatherosclerosis; trauma; electroshock; brain tumors; insect bites; malaria; poliomyelitis; endocrine abnormalities; drug reactions; toxins; and poisons. Many reports in the literature are merely clinical descriptions, and loss of nigral neurons has not been verified pathologically. Frequently, patients, in addition to their parkinsonian features, have atypical features not associated with idiopathic parkinsonism, such as choreoathetosis or corticospinal tract signs. Often these patients manifest only a part of the classic symptom complex of parkinsonism, such as masked facies without rigidity. Most of these conditions can be dismissed as coincidental or, at most, aggravating subclinical parkinsonism.

Drug-induced parkinsonism has been encountered with the use of reserpine, phenothiazines, and butyrophenones.

Various toxins and poisons, e.g., manganese, carbon monoxide, carbon disulfide, and mercury, have been associated with parkinsonism, generally with atypical features. Pathological examination in many of these cases has shown sparing of nigral neurons. Recently, several reports have described a parkinsonian syndrome in patients exposed to meperidine analogues, e.g., 1-methyl-4-phenyl-1,2,5,6-tetrahydropyridine (36, 52, 111). One of these patients, a drug addict, died and at postmortem showed selective loss of neurons in the substantia nigra. Classic Lewy bodies were not found, although an eosinophilic cytoplasmic inclusion was seen in one neuron. The locus ceruleus was not involved. Intravenous administration of N-methyl-4-phenyl-1,2,3,6-tetrahydropyridine in rhesus monkeys has produced selective loss of the neurons in the zona compacta of the substantia nigra (35). Lewy bodies were not present. The observation that a chemical can selectively damage neurons in the substantia nigra encourages further study into the possibility that a toxic factor may contribute to or cause idiopathic Parkinson's disease.

Striatonigral Degeneration

This rare idiopathic sporadic condition, described in 1961 by Adams et al. (1), is so similar clinically to paralysis agitans that in life it usually is misdiagnosed as Parkinson's disease. Striatonigral degeneration, however, differs from idiopathic Parkinson's disease and postencephalitic parkinsonism pathologically.

The onset of this condition is between 50

and 60 years of age, with a slow progression of symptoms ending in death within 5–7 years and patients usually succumbing to some intercurrent infection. Clinical features include restlessness, development of rigidity, stiffness, akinesia, and flexion dystonia of the trunk and limbs in association with a normal intellect (1, 2). Orthostatic hypotension may be a prominent initial symptom. Changes in speech, slowness of chewing and swallowing, masked facies, and decreased eye blinking can occur. A stooped posture may develop, along with a festinating gait. Dystonia, athetosis, and chorea usually are not present. Rare patients have clinical signs and symptoms indicative of olivopontocerebellar degeneration. In these cases, cerebellar ataxia seems to precede the parkinsonian symptoms.

Prominent features consist of atrophy of the putamen and caudate nuclei, with the putamen generally more involved, accompanied by paleness of the substantia nigra and locus ceruleus, sometimes asymmetrical in distribution (Fig. 15.10). Loss of striatal neurons is extensive, with virtual disappearance of small neurons. Neurons eventually disappear with an accompanying gliosis. Neither Lewy bodies nor neu-

rofibrillary tangles are present. Patients who have a prominent cerebellar ataxia pathologically show changes similar to those in olivopontocerebellar degeneration. The etiology of this rare condition and its relationship to the other neuronal atrophies are unknown. Anticholinergic drugs have been used in some cases with transient improvement.

Progressive Supranuclear Palsy

This condition, described by Steele (174), Richardson et al. (148), and Olszewski (173), combines the clinical features of Parkinsonism with a supranuclear ophthalmoplegia. The onset is gradual, usually beginning between the fifth and seventh decades. Men are affected more than twice as often as women. Initially, patients begin to loose their ability to look down, which may progress to complete loss of vertical and sometimes horizontal eye movements. Oculocephalic and vestibular reflexes early on may be increased, although they may disappear later in the disease. Axial rigidity, particularly of the neck, paroxysmal dysequilibrium, expressionless facies, pseudobulbar palsy, and personality changes frequently follow. Walking becomes impaired, with a propensity to fall forward. The dis-

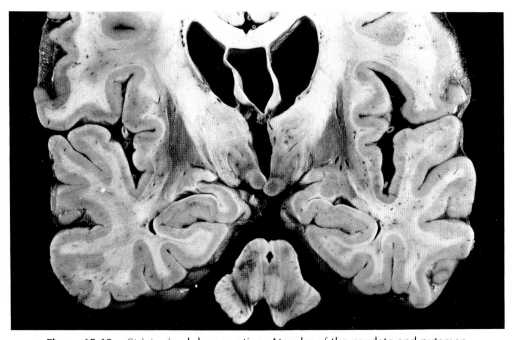

Figure 15.10.   Striatonigral degeneration. Atrophy of the caudate and putamen.

ease is progressive, leading to helplessness with some degree of dementia, and ends in death within 5–10 years.

The substantia nigra and locus ceruleus grossly are pale. Widespread loss of neurons is accompanied by fibrillary gliosis; remaining neurons often contain neurofibrillary tangles. Affected regions include the globus pallidus, subthalamic nucleus, red nucleus, substantia nigra, tectum, periaqueductal grey matter, and dentate nuclei. The neurons of the cerebrum and cerebellum usually are uninvolved. The ultrastructural features of neurofibrillary tangles in this condition recently have been reviewed (71). They generally contain 15-nm-wide straight filaments. Some cases have shown paired helical filaments of the Alzheimer type; others have contained 15-nm-wide filaments; still other cases have had both straight and paired helical filaments in the same tangle. Recent peroxidase-immunoperoxidase studies using an antiserum against normal neurofilaments and their polypeptides demonstrated positive staining (71). Another team of investigators using an antiserum against a two cycle-purified human brain microtubule fraction have shown positive staining against straight filaments (198).

The etiology of this condition is unknown. Treatment with levodopa has been disappointing.

DISEASES OF THE CEREBELLUM, BRAINSTEM, AND SPINAL CORD

Diseases classified under the broad term *spinocerebellar degenerations* or the spinocerebellar ataxias generally are inherited and are characterized by simple disappearance of neurons (abiotrophy) in groups or systems of neurons in the brainstem, cerebellum, and spinal cord. Within a single family, the expression of these diseases is vaguely similar, although between families there are *many overlaps* and *inconsistencies* in clinical expression and anatomy involved.

Signs and symptoms depend on the specific CNS structures affected, e.g., brainstem, cerebellum, and/or spinal cord. A parkinsonian picture with rigidity and tremor may occur when the brainstem is involved. Unsteadiness, abnormal gait, and intention tremor can be found in cerebellar involvement. Loss of deep tendon reflexes, vibration, and pain sensation, with spasticity and amyotrophy, can result when the spinal cord and peripheral nerves are affected. Nowhere in neuropathology is nosology more confusing than in these diseases (75). The spinocerebellar degenerations anatomically can be viewed as a spectrum of involvement along the neuroaxis between the cerebellum, e.g., cerebello-olivary degeneration of Holmes and the spinal cord, e.g., Friedreich's ataxia (see Table 15.1). Most of these conditions are extremely rare, and postmortem examinations are few and frequently fragmentary. An ultimate classification must await knowledge of the etiologies responsible for these conditions. Various biochemical abnormalities have been reported in the spinocerebellar degeneration and are reviewed in Kark et al. (102). These studies are preliminary, and in many of them a postmortem examination is not available.

Table 15.1
Spinocerebellar Degenerations

Conditions centered around the cerebellum
  Inherited cerebello-olivary degeneration of Holmes
  Sporadic cerebello-olivary degeneration of Marie, Foix, and Alajouanine
Conditions centered around the brainstem and cerebellum
  Inherited olivopontocerebellar degeneration of Menzel
  Sporadic olivopontocerebellar degeneration of Dejerine and Thomas
Conditions centered around the brainstem, spinal cord, and cerebellum
  Machado-Joseph disease
  Hereditary spinopontine atrophy
  Other rare conditions
    Family of Klippel and Durante
    Family of Fraser
    Family of Nonne
    Family of Sanger-Brown (hereditary spastic ataxia)
Conditions centered around the spinal cord
  Hereditary spastic paraplegia (Strümpell's disease)
  Hereditary posterior column ataxia (Biemond's disease)
  Friedreich's ataxia

Cerebello-olivary Degeneration of Holmes

This rather steroteyped familial condition of unknown cause appears to be a relatively pure cerebellar degeneration, with secondary loss of neurons in the olivary nucleus (90). The work of Eadie (65) is an excellent review.

Cerebello-olivary degeneration is autosomally inherited and extremely rare. There is an almost equal division between the sexes in family members, although there has been a male predominance in autopsy cases. Two-thirds of the cases begin at about 35 years of age, although its onset can occur between infancy and old age. Duration of the cases varies, most between 10 and 25 years. Rare cases have had a course of 5 years while others have lived 35 years. A progressive cerebellar ataxia forms the core of cerebello-olivary degeneration symptomatology. Abnormalities of gait, an ataxia of the extremities, especially in the arms, and difficulties of speech first develop. Later, some cases show nystagmus, dysphagia, dementia, and impairment of sphincter function. The sensory system is not involved.

At postmortem, atrophy of the cerebellum and olives is pronounced. Absence of the Purkinje cells, most severe in the superior portion of the vermis and the cerebellar hemispheres, is characteristic. Remaining Purkinje cells may be shrunken or swollen and sometimes contain vacuoles. Empty basket cells, astrocytosis in the Bergman cell layer, torpedoes in the granule cell layer, and loss of granule cells may occur (Fig. 15.11). The olive shows loss of neurons and gliosis with loss of olivocerebellar fibers. The dentate nucleus may show neuronal depletion. Senile plaques, neurofibrillary tangles, neuronal loss with neuronophagia, and degeneration of the long tracts have been seen in a few cases. Their significance is unknown and is probably coincidental. Cerebello-olivary degeneration probably represents a disorder of the cerebellar cortex with retrograde transsynaptic degeneration in the neurons of the olive. Differential diagnosis includes other inherited progressive, spinocerebellar atrophies, e.g., olivopontocerebellar atrophy of Menzel, idiopathic sporadic cerebello-olivary degeneration, and acquired cerebellar degeneration such as that associated with alcohol, diphenylhydantoin, and malignancy.

Marie et al (120) described idiopathic sporadic cerebello-olivary degeneration, a condition pathologically and clinically almost identical to Holmes' inherited cerebello-olivary degeneration, except that the cerebellar atrophy is perhaps more restricted to the lobulus quadrangulars, su-

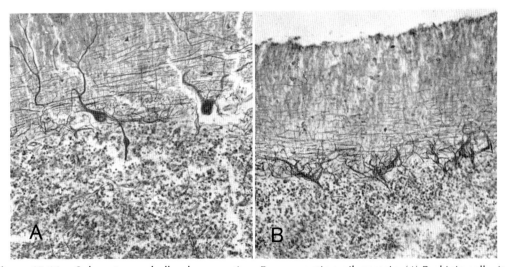

Figure 15.11. Subacute cerebellar degeneration. Frozen section, silver stain. (*A*) Purkinje cell with swollen axon or torpedo. (Original magnification × 200.) (*B*) Empty basket cells. (Original magnification ×200.)

perior vermis, and flocculus. The age of onset in this very rare condition is 10 or 20 years later than that of the inherited cerebello-olivary atrophy of Holmes (120). Some authorities view these conditions as being the same clinicopathological entity, except that one is inherited, the other sporadic. Whether they have the same etiology remains to be seen.

Olivopontocerebellar Degeneration

In contrast to cerebello-olivary atrophy, which is relatively constant in affected family members, inherited olivopontocerebellar degeneration is inconsistent and varied in its expression. This condition was described by Menzel (127) and recently well reviewed by Eadie (66). No two cases are identical. Overall loss of neurons is centered around the olive and pons with involvement of the cerebellum and, in some cases, the basal ganglia and spinal cord.

Olivopontocerebellar degeneration appears to be dominantly inherited. There is some disagreement as to whether one sex is affected more than the other. The onset varies between early childhood and old age, with most cases evenly spread from the first through fifth decades. The duration of the illness is between 10 and 20 years. Early in the course, gait abnormalities dominate and progress to a bedridden patient. Dysphagia, dysarthria, various involuntary movements, features of parkinsonism,

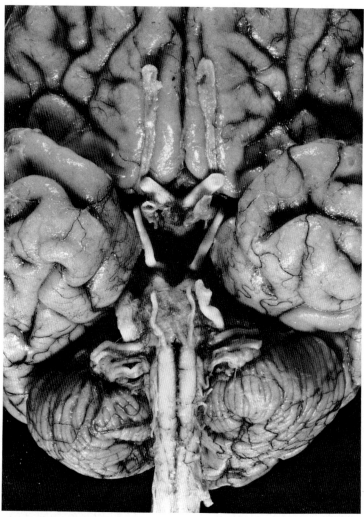

Figure 15.12. Olivopontocerebellar degeneration. Shrinkage of the pons. Loss of olivary bulge. Moderate atrophy of cerebellum.

spasticity, cranial nerve deficits, muscular wasting, nystagmus and, rarely, dementia have been seen. Abnormalities of sensation, e.g., impaired vibration and position sense, are uncommon. Death usually results from some intercurrent condition such as pneumonia. Effective treatment is unknown.

Shrinkage of the pons and loss of the olivary bulge with moderate cerebellar atrophy, especially in the lateral portions of the hemispheres, is striking (Fig. 15.12). Gross changes of the spinal cord and roots are uncommon. Neurons disappear, focally or diffusely, accompanied by a delicate fibrillary gliosis. Remaining neurons may be shrunken or swollen. The medulla shows loss of neurons in the inferior olivary nucleus, with degeneration of the olivocerebellar fibers running through the inferior cerebellar penduncle. There usually is severe reduction of neurons in the basis pontis and loss of the transverse pontocerebellar fibers with preservation of longitudinal fibers. Loss of Purkinje cells is seen in the lateral portions of the cerebellar hemisphere, with sparing of the vermis and flocculus. Empty basket cells, torpedoes in the granular cell layer, and hypertrophy of the Bergman cell layer are common (Fig. 15.11). Granule cells and neurons in the dentate nucleus may be lost with fibrillary gliosis. The white matter of the cerebellum often is pale as a result of nerve fiber and myelin sheath loss. Microscopic changes in the spinal cord are frequent, e.g., loss of fibers in the posterior columns and spinocerebellar tracts. Corticospinal tract involvement, loss of neurons in Clarke's column, and anterior horn cells have been reported. Variable cell loss has been seen in the substantia nigra, red nucleus, thalamus, and basal ganglia. Swelling of neurons and some cell loss have been noted, rarely, in the cortex. It appears that the primary degeneration in this condition centers on the olivary and pontine nuclei, with a later progressive anterograde transsynaptic atrophy of the cerebellar cortex. In the last few years a mutant gene on chromosome 6 has been reported (99) in an individual (on whom autopsy information is unavailable) from a family in which other members have autopsy findings consistent with olivopontocerebellar degeneration (144). The significance of this finding is difficult to evaluate. Biochemical and genetic studies of patients who have had a postmortem examination are few, and are preliminary. Analogous to the inherited form of olivopontocerebellar degeneration is a sporadic type of olivopontocerebellar degeneration described by Dejerine and Thomas (53). This sporadic condition is almost identical to inherited olivopontocerebellar degeneration of Menzel, except that the sporadic form tends to occur later in life and runs a shorter course. The Menzel form usually is more varied in its extrapyramidal manifestations, as compared to the Dejerine-Thomas form. Effective treatment is unknown. The reader is directed to the review by Eadie (64) for detailed information.

Other sporadic and inherited conditions have been reported which have morphological changes in the olive, pons, and cerebellum similar to those just described in the Menzel and Dejerine-Thomas types of olivopontocerebellar degeneration, but which differ considerably from a clinicopathological standpoint. These cases are associated with optic atrophy, profound dementia, unilateral olivopontocerebellar atrophy, and amyotrophy. These cases seem to differ sufficiently from the Menzel and Dejerine-Thomas forms of olivopontocerebellar atrophy to put them in a separate miscellaneous category. Probably these conditions will be found to have multiple etiologies. This subject is particularly well discussed in the *Handbook of Clinical Neurology* (63).

Machado-Joseph Disease

This rare autosomal, dominantly inherited, multisystem degeneration particularly affects Portuguese families with ties to the Azores. Two black families (46, 82) and a Japanese family (159) who apparently had no connection with the Azores have been reported with a similar disorder. Studies of affected families revealed three variants: Type I with extrapyramidal and pyramidal manifestations; Type II with pyramidal and cerebellar deficits; and Type III, which is associated with a cerebellar ataxia and a motor polyneuropathy with symmetric distal atrophy (49, 154). Progressive opthalamoplegia may be present. Patients show marked clinical variation, and even within a single family more than one of the three clinical variants may be present.

Neuropathological studies reveal variations in findings (131, 133, 152, 153, 158, 196, 197). This nosological entity appears to be a multisystem degeneration of neurons accompanied by reactive astrocytosis. Degeneration is prominent in the substantia nigra, the anterior horn cells, Clarke's column, and spinocerebellar tracts of the spinal cord. *The olivary nuclei are normal.* Changes have been described in the basal ganglia, subthalamic nuclei, brainstem, and cerebellum, especially the dentate nuclei.

Biochemical studies are preliminary (154), and their significance awaits further understanding.

Spino-Pontine Degeneration

Boller and Segarra (23, 24) described a disorder called hereditary spinopontine atrophy. Taniguchi and Konigsmark (181) described a second family with similar features. The onset is between the third and fifth decades, with a slow progressive course. Ataxia of extremities and gait disturbances were prominent. A Babinski sign and increased deep tendon reflexes were present, although ankle jerks usually were absent. The sensory system generally was unimpaired. Abnormal movements and rigidity were not observed, except for a slight intention tremor. The intellect in almost all cases was not affected. The pons and cerebellar peduncles grossly were markedly atrophied. Neuronal loss was seen in the pontine nuclei and Clarke's column, and degeneration was observed in the spinocerebellar and pontocerebellar tracts. The cerebellum, inferior olives, and cerebral hemispheres were unaffected.

Ishino et al. (97) described a third family who suffered from a condition similar to that described by Boller and Segarra. The only difference was the severe loss of anterior horn cells and neurons of the substantia nigra. This disorder appears to be dominantly inherited.

Other Rare Conditions

Marie (119) described the classical manifestations of l'hérédo-ataxie cérébelleuse (Marie's ataxia) based on the descriptions of four families (31, 68, 104, 135). This has been reviewed in the *Handbook of Clinical Neurology* (62). Cases of hereditary ataxia were separated from Friedreich's ataxia on the basis of anatomical involvement. Marie

thought the cerebellum was the principle region involved in these four families as compared to the spinal cord in Friedreich's ataxia (113). Later postmortem examinations, however, showed some of these cases inconsistently involved the cerebellum, with spinal cord lesions similar to those found in Friedreich's ataxia (113). Holmes (91) pointed out that Marie's ataxia represented a heterogeneous group of conditions rather than one entity.

In 1892, Klippel and Durante (104) described a family which was further reported in a number of studies. This disorder was inherited in an autosomal dominant way, with an onset in the fourth decade and a course of about 20 years. Cramps of the leg which progressed to disturbances of gait were early signs. Abnormalities of speech and lack of control in moving the arms developed. Nystagmus and pes equinus occurred in several patients. Some patients had abnormal tendon reflexes. At autopsy, the brainstem and spinal cord were small; both spinal roots were thin; loss of neurons was seen in the anterior horns and in Clarke's column; the spinocerebellar tracts and posterior columns were degenerated. The transverse fibers of the pons were pale; the granule cells of the cerebellum were lost; paleness was seen in the cerebellar white matter and superior cerebellar peduncle; the dentate nuclei and the substantia nigra showed some loss of neurons.

Fraser (68) in 1880 described a brother and sister with a progressive loss of cerebellar function and strabismus. Choreic movements were present in the brother, and both children had pale optic discs. The cerebellar cortex apparently was thin. The pathological details are somewhat vague, and the spinal cord was not examined well.

Nonne (135) in 1891 reported a family of three brothers who showed gait abnormalities, ataxia of the arms, nystagmus and, later, deterioration of mental function. Corticospinal tract signs and abnormalities of sensation were absent. At postmortem, the central nervous system, especially the cerebellum, was small. Optic atrophy and loss of large nerve fibers in the spinal nerve roots were found; however, the spinal cord apparently was normal (62).

In 1892, Sanger Brown (31) reviewed the clinical details of 21 members of a family with an hereditary ataxia associated with spasticity in the legs. Autopsy findings were provided in one case by Meyer in 1897 (128) and in two cases by Barker (14) in 1903. The clinical presentation and course varied between generations and in members of the same generation. The mode of inheritance appeared to be autosomal dominant. Ten men and twelve women were affected. The age of onset in different generations varied between 11 and 45 years, the mean being about 28 years. The disease ran an average course of 15 years, with a range between 2 and 27 years. Abnormality of gait and an ataxia of the arms were the most common presenting manifestations. Patients eventually had difficulty walking, and some became helpless. Most patients developed corticospinal tract signs in their legs; some had increased deep tendon reflexes and, rarely, ankle clonus. Dysarthria developed in many patients, and dysphagia occurred occasionally. As the course advanced, abnormal movements of the face and body resembling chorea evolved. Disturbance of the visual system was common. Sensation appeared to be intact.

On postmortem study, the spinal cord, brainstem, and cerebellum appeared to be small. Axons and myelin sheaths were lost, accompanied by gliosis in the posterior columns and dorsal spinocerebellar tracts. This degeneration was more severe in the cervical cord and medulla. Loss of neurons was seen in Clarke's column. One of the three cases showed some loss of anterior horn cells, and the ventral roots were described as being thin. Examination of the cerebellum, brainstem, and optic nerves revealed only minimal changes.

The clincopathological correlation in these cases is poor, as the clinically presumed corticospinal tract dysfunction was not found pathologically, and the prominent posterior column degeneration seen on microscopic sections was not manifested clinically.

Hereditary Spastic Paraplegia

Strümpell (176–178), in three papers, delineated an idiopathic entity occurring in two separate families who developed leg weakness which progressed to a spastic paraplegia. Degeneration of the lateral corticospinal tracts, especially at the lumbar level; moderate involvement of the anterior corticospinal tracts; degeneration of the posterior columns, notably in the thoracic and cervical region; severe involvement of the gracile fasciculus; and some degeneration of the spinocerebellar tracts were reported.

Following these reports, various additions appeared in the literature describing other families with neuronal degeneration, in whom a progressive, spastic paraplegia was associated with a wide range of miscellaneous neurological manifestations, e.g., amyotrophy, ataxia of gait, extrapyramidal signs, mental deterioration, retinal degeneration, etc. This led to a muddy definition as to what should be included under the term hereditary spastic paraplegia. Various reviewers have examined these cases in the light of the original crisply described cases and are of the opinion that the clinicopathological entity which Strümpell described does exist in a relatively pure form (16). They suggested that the term "Strümpell's hereditary spastic paraplegia" should be restricted to cases which clinically and pathologically conform to a rather sterotyped picture and should not include cases with a spastic paraplegia associated with other neurological defects.

The incidence of Strümpell's hereditary spastic paraplegia is difficult to determine since it does not significantly shorten life, and few patients die in hospital and have subsequent postmortem examinations.

The mode of inheritance usually is autosomal dominant, less frequently autosomal recessive and, in rare cases, is x-linked. The autosomal recessive group seem to have an earlier onset and a more rapid course. The onset in most cases is before the age of 10, in contrast to the dominant form, which begins between the third and fifth decades. Men seem to be affected more than women. Patients with leg weakness progress to a spastic paraplegia. Much later weakness may spread to the arms. Ataxia, amyotrophy, extrapyramidal signs, and dementia are absent. A Babinski sign is present, and abdominal reflexes are absent in some patients. As the disease progresses, loss of deep sensation in the legs and corticospinal tract signs appear in the arms. The progression of the disease differs between families but is similar in members of a single family. Patients become quite helpless.

Gross changes of the brain and spinal

cord are not conspicuous. Degeneration of the lateral corticospinal tracts, most severe at the lumbar level, is present, along with some degeneration of the anterior corticospinal tracts. Dorsal column degeneration is most severe in the upper thoracic and cervical levels, with severe involvement of the gracile fasciculus and some degeneration of the spinocerebellar tracts. Loss of Betz cells has been reported. Neurons in the dorsal root do not appear to be affected. The pathogenesis of this condition is unknown. The basic morphological change appears to be a dying back of axons. Transsynaptic degeneration is not present.

Hereditary Posterior Column Ataxia

This exceedingly rare and apparently distinct entity was first described and was recently reviewed by Biemond (18–20). Only one family has appeared in the literature for whom postmortem material is available. Affected members occurred in two generations. The first generation contained seven children, five normal girls and two affected boys. One of the boys married his cousin and had four affected children, three boys and one girl. Neuropathological studies are available from the father and one son. The inheritance appears to be autosomal dominant. The clinical progression of this disease is very slow and may appear to halt, although in several patients acceleration was seen. In the two most advanced cases, numbness of the hands and feet developed which later progressed to total absence of posterior column sensation. Arms and legs become ataxic, especially when the eyes were closed. All deep tendon reflexes were lost. Oral sensation disappeared, and there was decreased appreciation of touch on the fact. Pain and temperature sensation remained intact. Two patients showed optic atrophy.

The spinal cord appeared thin. There was complete degeneration of the posterior columns, partial degeneration of the posterior roots, demyelination of the trigeminal roots bilaterally, and some loss of Purkinje cells in some folia of the neocerebellum. Loss of granule cells was not seen.

Friedreich's Ataxia

Friedreich (68, 70) in the 1860s described a form of spastic hereditary ataxia now known as Friedreich's ataxia. Among diseases of the nervous system, this ataxia is uncommon; however, it is the most frequently encountered of all of the hereditary ataxias. It is set apart from the other herediatry ataxias by its combined degenerations of the posterior columns and corticospinal and spinocerebellar tracts. Some authorities believe that its core manifestations are more constant, as compared to many of the other spinocerebellar degenerations, e.g., olivopontocerebellar degeneration of Menzel. There are, however, variations in a family, and Friedrich's ataxia has been associated with other conditions, such as olivopontocerebellar degeneration, Roussy-Levy syndrome, and Charcot-Marie-Tooth disease, which involve structures adjacent to the spinal cord, such as the cerebellum, brainstem, or peripheral nerves. It is our position that these mixed or combined conditions form separate clinicopathological entities. Space does not permit their inclusion here, and the reader is directed to other accounts for detailed information (4, 185).

The sex incidence is controversial (185). Onset is almost always before the 20th year. Two modes of inheritance have been identified: a recessive form with an average age of onset around 11 years and a dominant form with a later onset of about 20 years of age. Some cases are sporadic. The course of the disease lasts between 20 and 30 years in both groups. Difficulty with balance, incoordination, and problems with running are early signs. There may be some asymmetry, although both legs are affected eventually. Cramps, lightening pains, aching in the legs, and fatigability occasionally have been reported. Years later the hands become clumsy, and dysarthria develops. Kyphoscoliosis may appear. The foot is usually deformed, with a high plantar arch and pes cavus, and there is extension of the toes at the metatarsophalangeal joint and flexion at the interphalangeal joints. As the gait abnormality progresses, it shows mixed sensory and cerebellar components. Patients sway and teeter in an effort to maintain balance. A positive Romberg sign usually is present. Incoordination of movement is profound, with ineffective wild oscillating motions when a patient tries to regain balance. Titubation of the head is sometimes observed. The arms become ataxic, and an intention tremor may be present. As incoordination increases, speech may become slurred, and breathing becomes incoordinated. Higher cortical function is unaltered, although some patients may show emotional lability. Horizontal nystagmus and deafness have been described. More rarely, blindness and optic atrophy occur. Ocular movements remain normal. Slight wasting of muscle may occur late in the illness, and deep tendon reflexes by this time are lost in almost every case. Plantar reflexes are extensor, and flexor spasms may be present. Vibration and position sense are lost early in the illness. Later, decrease of touch, pain, and temperature sensation occur. Cardiac abnormalities frequently develop, usually well after neurological manifestations are present. Clinical examination, chest films, and electrocardiograms have been unreliable in evaluating early cardiac disease. A recent study of 17 patients using more sophisticated methods of evaluation, e.g., continuous ambulatory electrocardiographic monitoring, echocardiography, and isotope ventriculography, showed cardiac abnormalities even when neurological signs in the patients were minimal (143). Eventually, patients are reduced to spending a helpless existence

in bed and die from a cardiac arrythmia, congestive heart failure, and/or respiratory failure.

The spinal cord is small. Degeneration of the posterior columns and roots and spinocerebellar and corticospinal tracts, and loss of neurons in Clarke's columns, occurs (Fig. 15.13). Degeneration of the direct spinocerebellar tracts usually is complete, in contrast to the indirect spinocerebellar tracts which show variation in their involvement (75). Affected neurons die back and eventually are lost. Long tract degeneration is most complete in the lower spinal cord. Betz cells are diminished in some cases. Neurons in the nuclei of cranial nerves VIII, X, and XII show some loss. Degeneration of the large neurons and their myelinated axons in the posterior root ganglia is seen. Unmyelinated fibers in the sensory roots and peripheral sensory nerves are uninvolved. Neuronal loss of varying degrees in the dentate nucleus and fiber loss in the superior cerebellar peduncle can be seen. Purkinje cell depletion may be found, especially in the superior vermis, with cell loss in corresponding regions of the inferior olivary nucleus. Pathological changes in the heart consist of cardiac hypertrophy with a chronic interstitial myo-

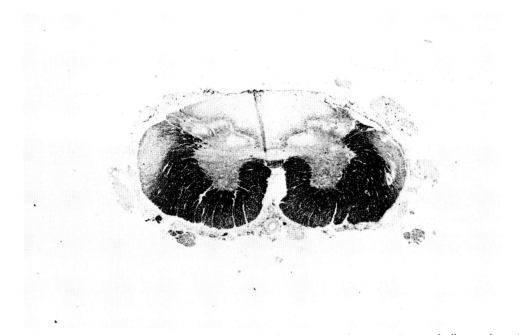

Figure 15.13.   Friedreich's ataxia. Degeneration of posterior columns, spinocerebellar, and corticospinal tracts-spinal cord. Myelin stain.

carditis (157, 185). Cardiac muscle fibers become hypertrophied, developing hyperchromatic, large, sometimes vacuolated nuclei. The cytoplasm becomes granular; lipofuscin may be deposited, striations are lost with swelling and vacuolation of the fiber; and interstitial fibrosis develops. It is unclear as to whether the conduction system of the heart is involved. Tests of the blood and cerebrospinal fluid are normal. Deficient lipoamide dehydrogenase have been found in some patients with Friedreich's ataxia (101). It has been suggested that abnormalities in membrane lipids or protein constituents may play a role in the pathogenesis of Friedreich's ataxia (12). No treatment halts the progression of this disease. Supportive treatment, especially in regard to the heart disease, may help to prolong life. The reader is directed to Adams and Victor (4) and Tyler (185) for a good review of the subject.

DISEASES OF THE "MOTOR SYSTEM"

There is a group of sporadic and familial conditions which results in degeneration of the corticospinal tract and/or the lower motor neuron, with wasting, weakness, and eventual paralysis of the muscles of the body. Some authors regard these conditions as a spectrum of the same process while others view them as separate entities. Cortical motor neurons, including the Betz cells, comprise the cell of origin of the upper motor neuron, whose axon descends through the posterior limb of the internal capsule through the brainstem, where it runs in the lateral and anterior corticospinal tract. These axons synapse, with cell body of the lower motor neurons, located either in the motor nuclei of the brainstem, whose processes form the motor cranial nerves, or with the anterior horn cells, whose axons run out through the spinal ventral root and into the peripheral nerves to the end organ muscle.

One of the celebrated events in clinical neurology was delineation of the muscular atrophies. Duchenne (57) and Aran (7) in the mid-1800s identified a heterogeneous condition which came to be known as "progressive muscular atrophy." Subsequently, Charcot et al. (41, 42) defined and named the entity of amyotrophic lateral sclerosis.

Amyotrophic Lateral Sclerosis (ALS); Motor Neuron Disease

The amyotrophic lateral sclerosis complex or motor neuron disease includes the subtypes amyotrophic lateral sclerosis, progressive muscular atrophy, progressive bulbar paralysis, and primary lateral sclerosis. Not all authorities approve of the term motor neuron disease since degeneration of the nervous system may not be restricted to the "motor" system. There has been a dispute from the time of their clinical delineation as to whether these conditions are variants caused by the same etiology or different diseases. Today, there is general agreement that at least the first three subtypes are variants of the same pathological processes as most patients, regardless of how they present, evolve into a clinical state with similar pathologic changes at autopsy. The most frequent form of the amyotrophic lateral sclerosis complex consists of wasting of muscles (amyotrophy), along with corticospinal tract signs. Less common is progressive muscular atrophy, in which weakness and atrophy occur without corticospinal tract dysfunction. Still less frequent is progressive bulbar palsy, characterized by weakness of muscles innervated by cranial motor nerves originating in the medulla. The intellect is preserved in all forms.

Sporadic amyotrophic lateral sclerosis usually begins with impairment of fine finger movement, weakness, and wasting of the muscles of the hand which later spreads to other limbs. Cramping and fasciculations advance to the upper arms and hyperreflexia develops as the disease progresses. Weakness and atrophy occur in the muscles of the back of the neck, tongue, pharynx, and largnx. Eventually, muscles in the lower extremity become weak and wasted, and spasticity appears. Bowel and bladder function usually are normal. Abdominal reflexes are variable. The course lasts about 2–6 years, with eventual involvement of brainstem motor nuclei which results in dysphagia, inanition, and aspiration pneumonia. The respiratory muscles may also be paralyzed.

Progressive muscular atrophy frequently starts with wasting of the hand muscles and usually ascends to the upper arm and shoulder. The lower extremities generally are affected later in the illness. Less commonly, atrophy may begin in the legs and later may involve the upper extremities. Signs of corticospinal tract involvement are absent, and deep tendon reflexes are decreased or lost. Patients with progressive muscular atrophy tend to have a longer course than those with the amyotrophic lateral sclerosis form.

Progressive bulbar palsy usually presents with dysarthria and dysphagia; paralysis of the palate and vocal cords develops, and the tongue shows fasiculations and becomes atrophic and paralyzed. Movement of the chin and lips becomes impaired. Spasticity may be so great that a tap on the jaw will produce clonus. Inappropriate laughing and crying may appear. Ocular muscles are not involved. Muscles of respiration eventually fail, and patients cannot swallow, and thus they die of malnutrition and aspiration pneumonia. The course is usually 2–3 years. Most patients who begin with bulbar signs soon show other manifestations indicative of spinal involvement. The earlier the onset of bulbar symptomatology, the more rapid the course. Neurophysiologic tests indicate slow motor nerve conduction. The amplitude of sensory action potential usually is normal.

Electromyography frequently shows signs of acute and chronic denervation in more than one limb.

Classical amyotrophic lateral sclerosis complex is almost always sporadic. This complex is distributed uniformly throughout the world. There seems to be a male predominance in most series. The mean age of onset is about 60 years of age. Cases with some clinical similarities to sporadic amyotrophic lateral sclerosis cluster on Guam, on other Pacific islands, and in the Kii peninsula of Japan. This Guamanian form of amyotrophic lateral sclerosis with distinctive pathological finding is discussed elsewhere in this chapter.

The spinal cord shows thin anterior (motor) roots and normal posterior (sensory) roots (Fig. 15.14). The hypoglossal nerve may be thin, and the precentral gyrus, rarely, may show some atrophy. On cut section of the spinal cord, a white appearance can often be seen in the region of the corticospinal tracts. A progressive degeneration, with loss of somatic motor neurons, especially the anterior horn cells, along with degeneration of the corticospinal tracts is present (Fig. 15.15). Neuronal loss ranges from complete to partial and varies along the neural axis, generally being most

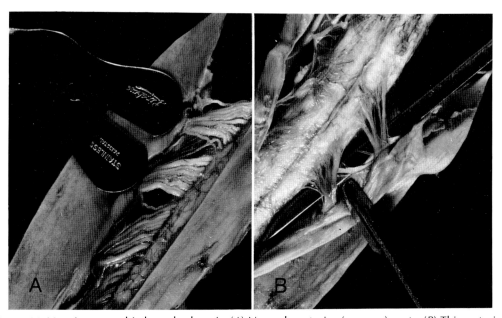

Figure 15.14.   Amyotrophic lateral sclerosis. (*A*) Normal posterior (sensory) roots. (*B*) Thin anterior (motor) roots.

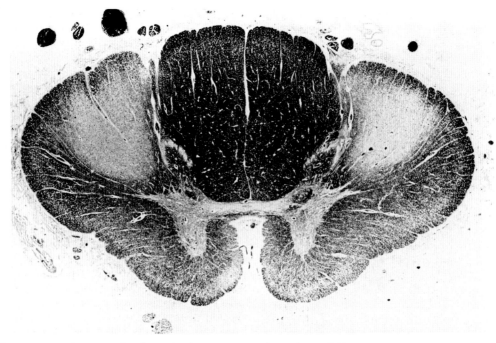

Figure 15.15. Amyotrophic lateral sclerosis. Loss of myelinated fibers in the corticospinal tracts-spinal cord. Myelin stain. (From W.C. Schoene: The nervous system. In Robbins, Cotran (eds): *Pathology of the Central Nervous System*, ed 2. Philadelphia, WB Saunders, 1979.)

severe in the cervical enlargement of the spinal cord, less but substantial in the lumbosacral region, and least and most varied in the thoracic segments. Remaining motor neurons show a variety of changes. They may be completely normal in appearance; others may be shrunken; some may undergo neuronophagia; and still others become ghost cells, degenerating without eliciting a microglial reaction. Lost neurons are replaced by a variable degree of gliosis. Shrunken and diffusely rarefied anterior horns in the cervical and lumbar regions of the spinal cord can occur which suggest the loss of afferent fibers. Empty cell beds may be present (98). Spheroids may form within the proximal axon of motor cells (39). Ultrastructurally, spheroids are composed of irregularly arranged 10-nm filaments, intermingled with smooth endoplasmic reticulum and mitochondria. Ribosomes and lipofuscin granules are absent (89). These structures are not specific to sporadic amyotrophic lateral sclerosis, as similar structures have been found in familial and Guamanian forms of amyotrophic lateral sclerosis (43). Similar accumulations of 10-nm filaments have been described within the cytoplasm of motor neurons. It has been

suggested that spheroids and cytoplasmic accumulations may occur early in the course of amyotrophic lateral sclerosis (89). Neurons with accumulations are swollen, with varying degrees of argentophilia within their cytoplasm. This change has been called chromatolysis, as there is a loss of Nissl substance in standard staining which may appear similar to that from axonal reactions or central chromatolysis. In distinction to this change, classic axonal reaction or central chromatolysis resulting from axotomy do not show argyrophilia of neuronal cytoplasm, and their cytoplasm contains swollen mitochondria and cisternae of rough endoplasmic reticulum, rather than a mass of 10-nm filaments. Classic central chromatolysis also has been seen in cases of amyotrophic lateral sclerosis with a rapid course (89). Neurons may contain small eosinophilic cytoplasmic bodies or Bunino bodies composed of granular material surrounded by a less dense region sometimes containing 10-nm filaments identical to normal neurofilaments. Mitochondria, rough endoplasmic reticulum, smooth membrane-bound vesicles, and lipofuscin granules surround these bodies (89). Bunino bodies are not found in all cases of amyotrophic lateral sclerosis and are not specific to this condition. Intracytoplasmic hyaline inclusions have been reported in rare cases of sporadic amyotrophic lateral sclerosis (43, 89), identical to those seen in familial amyotrophic lateral sclerosis.

Loss, especially of large axons, occurs in the ventral roots, which is reflected as neurogenic atrophy in muscle. The dorsal roots are normal. Routine paraffin sections of peripheral nerve usually show few if any changes. Recent studies of peripheral nerve, using light and electron microscopy and biochemical techniques, suggest that degeneration of large myelinated axons and possibly of unmyelinated fibers does occur with a small degree of dying back superimposed on the degeneration of motor neuron cell bodies (28).

Degeneration of the corticospinal tracts, direct and indirect, is dramatic, particularly in myelin-stained preparations. Nerve fibers degenerate at different rates, and all stages of myelin breakdown and axonal degeneration can be seen in the same fascicle. Macrophages may be present where degeneration is intense and there is a variable degree of gliosis. Corticospinal tract degeneration is generally most apparent in the lower portions of the spinal cord, and it can be traced up through the medulla, where it disappears in standardly stained preparations. Special stains, e.g., Marchi, have shown degeneration of motor fibers to proceed upward through the posterior part of the posterior limb of the internal capsule and corona radiata (93, 170). Although corticospinal tract degeneration is the principle tract involved in amyotrophic lateral sclerosis, adjacent tracts, particularly the spinocerebellar, the rubrospinal, and vestibulospinal tracts, may be found. Their degeneration is never as complete as in the corticospinal tracts, and the degeneration may be segmental. Posterior column degeneration, although very rare, has been reported (32). Variable loss of motor neurons is seen in brainstem nuclei. The nucleus and fibers of the hypoglossal nerve usually are the most conspicuous; other nuclei, such as dorsal medial nucleus of the vagus, nucleus ambiguus, or the Vth nerve motor nucleus, may show some changes. Loss of Betz cells can be seen in some cases. Pathological changes in other structures, such as the thalamus, striatum, globus pallidus, subthalamic nucleus, and the substantia nigra, have been described. The significance of these changes is unknown. At postmortem, loss of anterior horn cells and degeneration of corticospinal tracts occur, regardless of whether they begin clinically as amyotrophic lateral sclerosis, progressive bulbar palsy, or progressive muscular atrophy.

Unfortunately, no effective treatment is available for amyotrophic lateral sclerosis. The reader is directed to three recent reviews for a more detailed account of amyotrophic lateral sclerosis (27, 92, 155).

The existence and relationship of primary lateral sclerosis to classical amyotrophic lateral sclerosis complex has recently been debated and well discussed (15). Modern pathological documentations are contained in two case reports (15, 67). The case described by Fisher (67) was complicated by a pontine infarct. Both cases showed degeneration of the corticospinal tracts with relative preservation of anterior horn cells, and cytoplasmic hyaline inclusions were present in some of the anterior horn cells in the case described by Beal (15). Death occurred 5 years after the onset in the Fisher case and 3½ years in the Beal case.

Down through the decades there has been a question as to whether patients with amyotrophic lateral sclerosis ever have involvement of their sensory system. Clinically, rare patients with otherwise typical amyotrophic lateral sclerosis have had sensory symptoms such as paresthesias, burning, tightness, and pain. Recent studies using modern methods have suggested that some patients may have raised vibratory thresholds (130), abnormalities of touch-pressure sensation of the toe, abnormalities of the superficial sensory branch of the peroneal nerve (61), and acute axonal degeneration in the sural nerve (28), reflecting dysfunction of the peripheral sensory nerves. Abnormalities of semotosensory evoked potentials have been described which probably reflect dysfunction of central sensory pathways (123). The relationship of these patients to those with a typical pure motor disability has yet to be determined. Although damage to the motor system is the major manifestation of amyotrophic lateral sclerosis, it has been suggested that involvement of other parts of the nervous system in some patients can occur (28). Until the etiology of amyotrophic lateral sclerosis is better understood, there will be uncertainty as to the range of manifestations which this disease can produce.

Familial Amyotrophic Lateral Sclerosis

According to a recent review (92), 61 families with amyotrophic lateral sclerosis have been reported. Forty-eight families showed typical clinical features of amyotrophic lateral sclerosis. Three families had members with an onset of amyotrophic lateral sclerosis in childhood, and 10 families had associated dementia and/or parkinsonism. Twelve of the families with features typical of amyotrophic lateral sclerosis had a pathological examination of their nervous system. Findings varied; however, degeneration in the middle zones of the fasciculus cuneatus or gracilis was seen in at least one family member in 10 families. Posterior column degeneration appears to be more prevalent in familial cases of amyotrophic lateral sclerosis. Degeneration of Clarke's column in six and spinocerebellar tract degeneration in four families was present. Three families had a member with variable degeneration of neurons in the cortex, basal ganglia, brainstem, cerebellum, and posterior horns of the spinal cord. Three families contained members with dementia. At autopsy, neuronal degeneration, status spongiosus, and gliosis in the upper cortical layers were the main features. One case with amyotrophic lateral sclerosis, dementia, and extrapyramidal signs, pathologically studied, showed degeneration of the cerebral cortex, caudate nucleus, and putamen. Some cases, particularly those with posterior column degeneration, have ,intracytoplasmic hyaline inclusions in their neurons (86) which ultrastructurally are quite similar to Lewy bodies (180). Similar inclusions have been seen rarely in sporadic amyotrophic lateral sclerosis (44, 98). The etiologic relationship between sporadic amyotrophic lateral sclerosis and familial forms of amyotrophic lateral sclerosis is not understood.

Juvenile Amyotrophic Sclerosis

Amyotrophic lateral sclerosis starting in childhood is exceedingly rare and may be sporadic or familial. The subject is well reviewed in the following publication (92). The sporadic form is quite similar to the adult form. Degeneration of the corticospinal tract and lower motor neuron occurs. Neurons with cytoplasmic inclusion bodies have been seen in the cortex, subcortical and brainstem nuclei, and anterior horn cells of the spinal cord. Only one autopsied case of "familial juvenile amyotrophic lateral sclerosis" has been recorded which showed degeneration of the corticospinal tracts with some loss of the spinocerebellar tracts and loss of the anterior horn cells of the spinal cord. There were also changes in the white matter, basal ganglia, and cerebellum (172). The relationship of the etiology of juvenile amyotrophic lateral sclerosis to the etiology of sporadic amyotrophic lateral sclerosis is unknown.

Guamanian Amyotrophic Lateral Sclerosis

Earlier in the chapter reference was made to a Parkinson's dementia complex which occurs on Guam, some Pacific islands, and the Kii peninsula of Japan and is characterized by diffuse neuronal loss with neurofibrillary tangles in the cortex, deep grey structures, substantia nigra, and brainstem. Guamanian Parkinson's dementia complex associated with Guamanian ALS appears to be quite different from idiopathic parkinsonism associated with dementia. The incidence of Guamanian amyotrophic lateral sclerosis and Parkinson's dementia complex appears to be decreasing. In common with sporadic amyotrophic lateral sclerosis is degeneration of the corticospinal tracts and loss of anterior horn cells of the spinal cord. In contrast to the sporadic form, however, there are the widespread loss of neurons and the formation of neurofibrillary tangles in the brain, brainstem, and spinal cord. Some authorities suggest that Guamanian forms of amyotrophic lateral sclerosis and Parkinson's dementia complex constitute a spectrum of the same disease process (86). The etiology of Guamanian ALS and sporadic amyotrophic lateral sclerosis is probably different.

The relationship of familial, juvenile, and Guamanian ALS to sporadic amyotrophic lateral sclerosis is controversial. The reader is referred to an excellent review of the subject for detailed information and a list of authoritative references (92).

Familial Spinal Muscular Atrophy

The term "progressive spinal muscular atrophy" is used to describe an inherited motor system degeneration which involves the lower motor neuron. It is unknown as to whether this category of disease represents a heterogenous group of inherited diseases or a single genetic abnormality with variation in its clinical expression. Inheritance is autosomal recessive. Delay in motor development, weakness, and hypotonia begins at or shortly after birth. The principal clinical concern is to distinguish progressive spinal muscular atrophy from other forms of infantile hypotonia gathered under the term benign congenital hypotonia that generally do not progress.

Inherited progressive spinal muscular atrophy can be separated into severe, intermediate, and mild forms. The most severe form, *infantile spinal muscular atrophy* or *Werdnig-Hoffmann disease*, begins within a few months after birth. Some mothers report a lack of fetal movement, which suggests the onset may begin *in utero*. Pregnancy and birth are normal. From the beginning, muscular weakness is associated with hypotonia. Infants have a "floppy" appearance. Deep tendon reflexes usually are absent, and there is atrophy of muscle. Fasciculations are not present, except occasionally in the tongue. The sensory system appears to be unaffected, and the child is alert and bright without any sign of cortical involvement. As the disease progresses all skeletal muscles become affected, except for the eye muscles, and the patient frequently assumes a "frog position" with external rotation and abduction of the hips and flexion at the hips and knees (3). Difficulty sucking and swallowing may appear, indicating bulbar involvement. Intercostal muscles eventually fail, the chest collapses, and diaphragmatic breathing with paradoxical respiratory movements occurs. Respiratory infections ensue, and death usually follows within the first year.

At the other end of the clinical spectrum are those cases which do not threaten life, subclassified as chronic proximal spinal muscular atrophy or Wolfart-Kugelberg-Welander syndrome. Children affected initially have normal motor development but later develop weakness, waddling gait, and difficulty climbing stairs, and they often walk "flat-footed" with eversion of the foot (56). The muscles of the pelvic girdle are especially vulnerable; arms are frequently affected; and a tremor in the hands develops. The prognosis is good, with slow or no progression over the years, and the respiratory system is not affected.

Between severe and mild forms of familial spinal muscular atrophy is an intermediate group of cases with a variable course and prognosis. The time of onset is not reliable in predicting outcome. Some cases with an early onset may develop a more benign form of the disease. The only guide to severity is watchful waiting (56). Prognosis depends upon the degree of respiratory muscle impairment. Contractures and deformities such as scoliosis frequently develop. Serum enzymes, e.g., creatine phosphokinase, are normal. Electromyographic studies are useful in substantiating neurogenic atrophy. Numerous fibrillation potentials occur. There may be polyphasic motor unit potentials; the interference pattern is reduced; and rhythmic firing of motor units at 5–15 Hz may be present (33). Motor nerve conduction can be normal but slow in some cases (56). Unfortunately, it is impossible to distinguish the severe and intermediate forms of familial spinal muscular atrophy from a muscle biopsy, as the histological features are almost identical (56). There are, however, some differences between the severe form, Werdnig-Hoffmann disease, and the mild Wolfart-Kugelberg-Welander type of disorder.

In Werdnig-Hoffmann disease, muscle atrophy is characterized by groups of contiguous atrophic muscle fibers interspersed with groups of normal or, more commonly, hypertrophied muscle fibers. Groups may be large, with the fibers of a whole fascicle atrophied or hypertrophied. Hypertrophied groups of fibers usually are of a single enzyme type, suggesting that they represent reinnervated fibers, whereas atrophic fibers contain both Type I and Type II varieties. Atrophic muscle fibers in Werdnig-Hoffmann disease are round rather than angular, as seen in neurogenic atrophy secondary to the peripheral neuropathies. Degenerative changes in muscle fibers are uncommon; target fibers are often present; and muscle spindles frequently are prominent and may even be increased in number.

Patients with Wolfart-Kugelberg-Welander disease usually have small groups of atrophic and hypertrophic fibers. Huge hypertrophic fibers are uncommon, and atrophic fibers frequently show a type II predominance. Myopathic changes, e.g., fiber splitting and internalization of sarcolemmal nucleic and/or degeneration of muscle fibers, sometimes are seen.

At autopsy, patients with Werding-Hoffmann disease have thin anterior spinal roots. There is loss of neurons in the anterior horns and hypoglossal nuclei. Similar loss can occur in the nucleus ambiguus, facial, abducens, trochlear, oculomotor, and trigeminal nuclei (136). Remaining cell bodies may show swelling and chromatolysis, while others are shrunken or undergo neuronophagia. Loss of neurons results in empty cell beds with little change in the neurophil. Spheroids in the anterior roots and cytoplasmic Bunina bodies in the anterior horn cells, as described in amyotrophic lateral sclerosis, are not found in the familial spinal muscular atrophies (98). Glial bundles which consist of closely packed astrocytic processes located in the proximal portion of the anterior roots are seen in some cases. Although these structures are closely linked with Werdnig-Hoffman disease, they are not specific, as they have been found in atrophied anterior roots of healed anterior poliomyelitis (98) and have been reproduced experimentally by sectioning and suturing of spinal nerve roots (126). Active degeneration of fibers in the peripheral nerve is usual in routine sections. Special techniques, e.g., intravital dyes, however, have demonstrated dying back of axons. Postmortem changes in muscle are similar to those in biopsied muscle.

Differential diagnosis includes congenital muscular dystrophy, congenital myopathies, congenital fiber disproportion, and injury associated with breech deliveries (56).

Treatment of inherited spinal muscular atrophy is supportive. Contractures must be prevented by physical therapy; scoliosis must be inhibited by bracing; and intercurrent respiratory tract infections must be treated. The reader is referred to the work of Dubowitz (56) and Hausmanowa-Petrusewicz for a detailed review.

DISEASES OF THE AUTONOMIC NERVOUS SYSTEM

A detailed account of progressive autonomic dysfunction is far beyond the breadth of this chapter; the subject recently has been covered in a textbook of clinical disorders of the autonomic nervous system (11).

Familial Dysautonomia (Riley-Day)

Riley et al. (149) described a rare condition called "central autonomic dysfunction with defective lacrimation." This recessively inherited condition almost exclusively affects Ashkenazic Jewish children. The sexes appear to be affected equally. Clinical features are distinctive and include abnormalities of the peripheral sensory and autonomic nervous system. Soon after birth, infants may have difficulty feeding and may fail to thrive. Episodes of vomiting may be severe. Hyperpyrexia and bouts of pneumonia occur. Pain and temperature sensation, along with reflexes, are lost in association with relative preservation of touch and pressure. Overflow of tears (alacrima), absence of fungiform papillae of the tongue, blotching of the skin, excessive sweating, lability of blood pressure, disturbances of gastrointestinal motility, and difficulty swallowing are often present. Wasting and prominent motor weakness are not features of this condition, and higher cortical functions are normal. Motor nerve conduction velocities may be slowed. Sensory nerve action potentials generally are diminished. A screening test for this condition consists of putting 2.5% solution of methacholine into the cornea, which results in miosis (169). Most patients die in infancy or early childhood from repeated respiratory tract infection. Manifestation of this disease appears to be the functional denervation of the autonomic nervous system.

Pathological studies of the central nervous system have not shown consistent changes (34, 51), whereas in the peripheral nervous system, findings have been more repetitive (51). Loss of small myelinated and nonmyelinated axons has been described in the sural nerve (141), in reduction of the dorsal root ganglia and its neurons with neuronophagia and residual nodules of Nageotte, and in reduction of neurons in the sympathetic ganglia (51, 140, 142). Neurons thought to be of parasympathetic origin are decreased (51). Loss of neurons in the nucleus of Onufrowicz has been reported (116).

A specific biochemical abnormality, presumably a defect in the production or release of a neurohumoral transmitter agent, is suspected but so far has not been demonstrated. Absence of a trophic factor, e.g., nerve growth factor, during development of the fetus has been postulated; however, difficulty in assaying this factor in man has prevented any meaningful study (141). The reader is referred to good reviews of this condition by Brunt and McKusick (34) and for detailed information.

Idiopathic Orthostatic Hypotension (Shy-Drager Syndrome)

Orthostatic hypotension is a well-known clinical phenomenon associated with many disorders, such as emotional stress, vasovagal instability, drugs (especially ganglion blockers), tabes dorsalis, some polyneuropathies, Holmes-Adie syndrome, and others (94, 164). In addition to these forms of postural hypotension, a distinct type of orthostatic hypotension results from an idiopathic degeneration of neurons in many parts of the nervous system, especially those in the intermediolateral cell column of the spinal cord. This clinical entity was well described pathologically in 1960 and has subsequently become known as the Shy-Drager syndrome (168).

Clinically, this disorder appears to have a prevalence for men, with an average age of onset in the sixth decade, although it can begin from the second to eighth decades. The onset is usually subtle, and the course varies in length, from a few years to a decade or more. Some patients initially show postural hypotension, atonic bladder, loss of sphincter tone, and loss of sweating; others first develop neurologic abnormalities suggestive of a widespread multisystem disorder, as manifested by incoordination, ocular palsies, atrophy of the iris, rigidity, tremors, weakness, ataxia, fasciculations, and amyotrophy. Most cases are associated with either Lewy bodies or changes similar

to olivo-ponto degeneration and striatonigral degeneration (74, 137). Patients usually develop syncope some time in the course of their illness. The sensory system generally is spared. Routine laboratory tests are of little help in diagnosing this condition. A negative Valsalva test, fall of blood pressure with no increase in the pulse rate, failure to produce sweating with heat, and other tests which evaluate the autonomic nervous system may be of help in confirming the diagnosis. It is important to exclude other forms of postural hypotension associated with heart valve disease or diabetic neuropathy. Progression of this disease is slow but may lead to severe disability.

The pathologic features are somewhat variable but consist principally in loss of the neurons from the intermediolateral column of the spinal cord. Neurons disappear simply, accompanied by a fibrillary astrocytic gliosis (74, 94, 164). Pathological changes in the putamen, globus pallidus, substantia nigra, locus ceruleus, pontocerebellar tracts, cerebellar cortex, dorsal vagal nucleus, inferior olivary nucleus, anterior horn cells, sympathetic ganglia, and striated muscle (164) can occur. Some cases have shown Lewy bodies in pigmented nuclei and elsewhere (74). The relationship of these cases to each other and their etiologie(s) remains to be worked out. For a particularly good account of this condition, the reader is directed to reviews of the subject by Oppenheimer (137) and Schwartz (164). Treatment is directed at trying to control the blood pressure. Elastic bandages, support stockings, and various drugs have been used which become less and less effective as the disease progresses.

ACKNOWLEDGMENTS

The author is grateful to Hugh Harrington, M.B., M.R.C.P., for his unfailing help; to Ms. D.M. Jackson for her patience and suggestions in preparing this chapter; and to Ms. E. DeFigueiredo for her help with the bibliography.

References

1. Adams RD et al: Dégénérescences nigro-striées et cerebello-nigro-striées. *Psychiatr Neurol* 142:219, 1961.
2. Adams RD et al: Striato-nigral degeneration. *J Neuropathol Exp Neurol* 23:584, 1964.
3. Adams RD, Victor M: Congenital neuromuscular disorders. In *Principles of Neurology.* New York, McGraw-

Hill, 1981.

4. Adams RD, Victor M: Degenerative diseases of the nervous system In *Principles of Neurology.* New York, McGraw-Hill, 1981.

5. Adams RD, Victor M: Abnormalities of movement and posture due to disease of the extrapyramidal motor system. In *Principles of Neurology,* New York, McGraw-Hill, 1981.

6. Adams RD, Victor M: The inherited metabolic diseases of the nervous system. In *Principles of Neurology.* New York, McGraw-Hill, 1981.

7. Aran FA: Recherches sur une maladie non encore décrite du système musculaire (atrophie musculaire progressive). *Arch Générales Med* 24:172, 1850.

8. Arsenio-Nunes ML, Goutières F: Diagnosis of infantile neuroaxonal dystrophy by conjunctival biopsy. *J Neurol Neurosurg Psychiatry* 41:511, 1978.

9. Austin J, Sakai, M: Disorders of glycogen and related macromolecules in the nervous system. In Vinken PJ, Bruyn GW (eds): *Metabolic and Deficiency Diseases of the Nervous System, Handbook of Clinical Neurology.* Amsterdam, North-Holland, 1976, part 1.

10. Ball MJ: Topography of Pick inclusion bodies in hippocampi of demented patients. *J Neuropathol Exp Neurol* 38:614, 1979.

11. Bannister R: Autonomic failure. In Bannister R: *A Textbook of Clinical Disorders of the Autonomic Nervous System.* Oxford, Oxford University Press, 1983.

12. Barbeau A: Biochemistry of Friedreich's ataxia. In Sobrie I (ed): *Spinocerebellar Degenerations.* Proceedings of the International Symposium on Spinocerebellar Degenerations, October 12–14, Tokyo. Baltimore, University Park Press, 1978.

13. Baumann RJ, et al: Cigarette smoking and Parkinson's disease. A comparison of cases with matched neighbours. *Neurology* 30:839, 1980.

14. Barker LF: A description of the brains and spinal cords of two brothers dead of hereditary ataxia: Cases XVIII and XX of the series of the family described by Sanger Brown, with a clinical introduction by Dr. Sanger Brown. Decennial Publications of the University of Chicago, Chicago, *University of Chicago Press* 10:349, 1903; or *Trans Assoc Am Phys* 18:637, 1903.

15. Beal MF, Richardson EP Jr: Primary lateral sclerosis. *Arch Neurol* 38:630, 1981.

16. Behan WMH, Maia M: Strümpell's familial spastic paraplegia: genetics and neuropathology. *J Neurol Neurosurg Psychiatry* 37:8, 1974.

17. Bell J, Carmichael EA: On hereditary ataxia and spastic paraplegia. In Fisher RA (eds): *The Treasury of Human Inheritance.* London, Cambridge University Press, 1939, vol 4. part 3.

18. Biemond A: Clinisch-anatomische demonstratie over een bijzondere vorm van hereditaire ataxie. *Ned T Geneesk* 1014, 1946.

19. Biemond A: Les dégénérations spino-cérébelleuse. *Folia Psychiatr Neerl* 54:216, 1951.

20. Biemond A: Hereditary posterior column ataxia. In: Vinken PJ, Bruyn GW (eds): *System Disorders and Atrophies. Handbook of Clinical Neurology.* Amsterdam, North-Holland, 1975, part 1.

21. Bird ED, Spokes EG: Huntington's chorea. In: Crow JG (eds): *Disorders of Neurohumoural Transmission.* New York, Academic Press, 1982.

22. Blass JP: Spinocerebellar degenerations (hereditary ataxias). In Davison AN, Thompson RHS (eds): *The Molecular Basis of Neuropathology.* Tokyo, Igaku-Shoin, 1981.

23. Boller F, Segarra JM: Spino-pontine degeneration. *Eur Neurol* 2:356, 1969.

24. Boller F, Segarra JM: Spino-pontine degeneration. In Vinken PJ, Bruyn GW (eds): *System Disorders and Atrophies. Handbook of Clinical Neurology.* Amsterdam, North-Holland, 1975, part 1.

25. Boller F, et al: Parkinson disease, dementia, and Alzheimer disease: clinicopathological correlations. *Ann. Neurol.* 7:329, 1980.

26. Bonduelle M: The myoclonias. In: *Handbook of Clinical Neurology.* Amsterdam, North-Holland, 1968, vol 6.

27. Bonduelle M: Amyotrophic lateral sclerosis. In Vinken PJ, Bruyn GW (eds): *System Disorders and Atrophies. Handbook of Clinical Neurology.* Amsterdam, North-Holland, 1975, part 2.

28. Bradley WG: Morphometric and biochemical studies of peripheral nerves in amyotrophic lateral sclerosis. *Ann. Neurol.* 14:267, 1983.

29. Brodal A: *Neurological Anatomy in Relation to Clinical Medicine.* Oxford, Oxford University Press.

30. Bronson RT, Schoene WC: Spontaneous pallido-nigral accumulation of iron pigment and spheroid-like structures in Macaque monkeys. *J Neuropathol Exp Neurol* 39:181, 1980.

31. Brown S: On hereditary ataxia, with a series of twenty-one cases. *Brain* 15:250, 1892.

32. Brownell B, et al: The central nervous system in motor neurone disease. *J Neurol Neurosurg Psychiatry* 33:338, 1970.

33. Buchthal F, Olsen PZ: Electromyography and muscle biopsy in infantile spinal muscular atrophy. *Brain* 93:15, 1970.

34. Brunt PW, McKusick VA: Familial dysautonomias. *Medicine* 49:343, 1970.

35. Burns RS, et al: A primate model of parkinsonism: Selective destruction of dopaminergic neurons in the pars compacta of the substantia nigra by N-methyl-4-phenyl-1,2,3,6-tetrahydropyridine. *Proc Natl Acad Sci USA* 80:4546, 1983.

36. Calne DB, Langston JW: Aetiology of Parkinson's disease. *Lancet* 24(31): 1457, 1983.

37. Candy JM, et al: Pathological changes in the nucleus of Meynert in Alzheimer's and Parkinson's disease. *J Neurol Sci* 54(59):277, 1983.

38. Carlo J, et al: Examination of dental pulp to diagnose infantile neuroaxonal dystrophy. *Arch Neurol* 39:422, 1982.

39. Carpenter S: Proximal axonal enlargement in motor neuron disease. *Neurology (Minneap)* 18:842, 1968.

40. Carpenter S, et al: Lafora's disease: peroxisomal storage in skeletal muscle. *Neurology (Minneap)* 24:531, 1974.

41. Charcot JM, Joffroy A: Deux cas d'atrophie musculaire progressive avec lésions de la substance grise et des faisceaux antéro-latéraux de la moelle épinière. *Arch Physiol* (Paris) 2:354, 629, 744, 1869.

42. Charcot JM: De la sclérose latérale amyotrophique. *Prog Médicale* 2:325, 341, 453, 1874.

43. Chou SM, et al: Axonal balloons in subacute motor neuron disease. *J Neuropathol Exp Neurol* 29:141, 1970.

44. Chou SM: Pathognomy of intraneuronal inclusions in ALS. In Tsubaki T, Toyokura Y (eds): *Amyotrophic Lateral Sclerosis.* Tokyo, University of Tokyo Press, 1979.

45. Collins GH, et al: Myoclonus epilepsy with Lafora bodies on ultrastructural and cytochemical study. *Arch Pathol* 86:239, 1968.

46. Cooper JA, et al: Autosomal dominant motor system degeneration in a black family. *Ann. Neurol.* 14:585, 1983.

47. Cork LC, et al: Hereditary canine muscular atrophy. *J Neuropathol Exp Neurol* 38:209, 1979.

48. Corsellis JAN: Aging and the dementias. In Blackwood W, Corsellis JAN (eds): *Greenfield's Neuropathology.* London, Edward Arnold, 1976.

49. Coutinho P, Andrade C: Autosomal dominant system. Degeneration in Portuguese families of the Azores Islands. *Neurology* 28:703, 1978.

50. Cowen D, Olmstead EV: Infantile neuroaxonal dystrophy. *J Neuropathol Exp Neurol* 22:175, 1963.

51. Dancis J: Familial dysautonomia (Riley-Day syndrome). In Bannister R (ed): *Autonomic Failure: A Textbook of Clinical Disorders of the Autonomic Nervous System.* Oxford, Oxford University Press, 1983.

52. Davis GC, et al: Chronic Parkinsonism secondary to intravenous injection of meperidine analogues. *Psychiatr Res* 1:249, 1979.

53. Déjerine J, Thomas A: L'atrophie olivo-ponto-cérébel-leuse. *Nouv Iconogr Salpêt* 13:330, 1900.

54. Dooling EC, et al: Hallervorden-Spatz syndrome. *Arch Neurol* 30:70, 1974.

55. Dooling EC, et al: Computed tomography in Hallervor-den-Spatz disease. *Neurology* 30:1128, 1980.

56. Dubowitz V: Infantile spinal muscular atrophy. In Vin-ken PJ, Bruyn GW (eds): *System Disorders and Atro-phies. Handbook of Clinical Neurology.* Amsterdam, North-Holland, 1975, part 3.

57. Duchenne GBA: Étude comparie des lésions anato-miques dans l'atrophie musculaire progressive et dans la paralysie générale. *Union Médicale* 7:246, 1853.

58. Duffy PE, Tennyson VM: Phase and electron micro-scopic observations of Lewy bodies and melanin granules in the substantia nigra and locus ceruleus in Parkinson's disease. *J Neuropathol Exp Neurol* 24:398, 1965.

59. Duncan C, et al: Peripheral nerve biopsy as an aid to diagnosis in infantile neuroaxonal dystrophy. *Neurology* 20:1024, 1970.

60. Dunlap CB: Pathologic changes in Huntington's chorea with special reference to corpus striatum. *Arch Neurol Psychiatry* 18:867, 1927.

61. Dyck PJ, et al: Frequency of nerve fiber degeneration of peripheral motor and sensory neurons in amyotrophic lateral sclerosis. Morphometry of deep and superficial peroneal nerves. *Neurology* 25:781, 1975.

62. Eadie MJ: Hereditary spastic ataxia. In Vinken PJ, Bruyn GW (eds): *System Disorders and Atrophies. Hand-book of Clinical Neurology.* Amsterdam, North-Holland, 1975, part 1.

63. Eadie MJ: Olivo-ponto-cerebellar atrophy (variants). In Vinken PJ, Bruyn GW (eds): *System Disorders and Atrophies. Handbook of Clinical Neurology.* Amsterdam, North-Holland, 1975, part 1.

64. Eadie MJ: Olivo-ponto-cerebellar atrophy (Déjerine-Thomas type). In Vinken PJ, Bruyn GW (eds): *Systems Disorders and Atrophies. Handbook of Clinical Neurology.* Amsterdam, North-Holland, 1975, part 1.

65. Eadie MJ: Cerebello-olivary atrophy (Holmes type). In Vinken PJ, Bruyn GW (eds): *System Disorders and Atrophies. Handbook of Clinical Neurology.* Amsterdam, North-Holland, 1975, part 1.

66. Eadie MJ: Olivo-ponto-cerebellar atrophy (Menzel type). In Vinken PJ, Bruyn GW (eds): *System Disorders and Atrophies. Handbook of Clinical Neurology.* Amsterdam, North-Holland, 1975, part 1.

67. Fisher CM: Pure spastic paralysis of cortico-spinal ori-gin. *Can J Neurol Sci* 4:251, 1977.

68. Fraser D: Defect of the cerebellum occurring in a brother and sister. *Glasgow Med J* 13:199, 1880.

69. Friedreich N: Ueber degenerative Atrophie der spinalen Hinterstränge. Versammlung deutsche Naturforsch. *U Arzte,* 1861.

70. Friedreich N: Ueber degenerative Atrophie der spinalen Hinterstränge. *Virchows Arch Pathol Anat* 26:391, 433; 27:1, 1863.

71. Gambetti P, et al: Neurofibrillary change in human brain. An immunocytochemical study with a neurofila-ment antiserum. *J Neuropathol Exp Neurol* 42:69, 1983.

72. Gilbert GJ: Dyssynergia cerebellaris myoclonica. In Vin-ken PJ, Bruyn GW (eds): *System Disorders and Atro-phies. Handbook of Clinical Neurology.* Amsterdam, North-Holland, 1975.

73. Goldman JE, et al: Lewy bodies of Parkinson's disease contain neurofilament antigens. *Science* 221:1082, 1983.

74. Graham JG, Oppenheimer DR: Orthostatic hypotention and nicotine sensitivity in a case of multiple system atrophy. *J Neurol Neurosurg Psychiatry* 32:28, 1969.

75. Greenfield JG: *The Spinocerebellar Degenerations,* Blackwell (ed). Oxford, Vincent-Baxter Press, 1954.

76. Grufferman S: Alzheimer's disease and senile dementia: one disease or two? In Katzman R, Terry RD, Bick KL (eds): *Alzheimer's Disease: Senile Dementia and Related Disorders.* New York, Raven Press, 1978, vol 7.

77. Gusella JF, et al: A polymorphic DNA marker genetically linked to Huntington's disease. *Nature* 306:234, 1983.

78. Hakim AM, Mathieson G: Dementia in Parkinson dis-ease: a neuropathologic study. *Neurology* 29:1209, 1979.

79. Hallervorden J, Spatz H: Eigenartige Erkrankung im extrapyramidalen System mit besonderer Beteiligung des Globus pallidus und der Substantia Nigra. *Z ges Neurol* 79:254, 1922.

80. Harriman DGF, Millar JHD: Progressive familial my-oclonic epilepsy in three families: its clinical features and pathological basis. *Brain* 78:343, 1955.

81. Hausmanowa-Petrusewicz I: *Spinal Muscular Atrophy: Infantile and Juvenile Type.* Warsaw, Poland, Foreign Scientific Publications Department of the National Cen-ter for Scientific, Technical and Economic Information, 1978.

82. Healton EB, et al: Presumably Azorean disease in a presumably non-Portuguese family. *Neurology* 30:1084, 1980.

83. Hirano A, et al: Parkinsonism-dementia complex: an epidemic disease on the island of Guam. I. Clinical features. *Brain* 84:642, 1961.

84. Hirano A, et al: Parkinsonism-dementia complex, an epidemic disease on the island of Guam. II. Pathological features. *Brain* 84:662, 1961.

85. Hirano A: Pathology of amyotrophic lateral sclerosis. In Gajdusek DC, Gibbs CJ, Alpers M (eds): *Slow, Latent, and Temperate Virus Infections.* Washington, DC, NINDB Monograph, National Institutes of Health, 1965, vol 2, p 23.

86. Hirano A, et al: Amyotrophic lateral sclerosis and Par-kinsonism-dementia complex on Guam. Further patho-logic studies. *Arch Neurol* 15:35, 1966.

87. Hirano A, et al: Familial amyotrophic lateral sclerosis. *Arch Neurol* 16:232, 1967.

88. Hirano A, et al: The fine structures of some intragan-glionic alterations. Neurofibrillary tangles, granulovac-uolar bodies and "rod-like" structures as seen in Guam. Amyotrophic lateral sclerosis and Parkinsonism-demen-tia complex. *J Neuropathol Exp Neurol* 27:167, 1968.

89. Hirano A: Aspects of the ultrastructure of amyotrophic lateral sclerosis. In Rowland LP (ed): *Human Motor Neuron Diseases. Advances in Neurology.* New York, Raven Press, 1982, vol 36.

90. Holmes G: A form of familial degeneration. *Brain* 30:466, 1907.

91. Holmes G: An attempt to classify cerebellar disease, with a note on Marie's hereditary cerebellar ataxia. *Brain* 30:545, 1907.

92. Hudson AJ: Amyotrophic lateral sclerosis and its asso-ciation with dementia, Parkinsonism and other neuro-logical disorders: a review. *Brain* 104:217, 1981.

93. Hughes JT: Pathology of amyotrophic lateral sclerosis. In Rowland LP (ed): *Human Motor Neuron Diseases. Advances in Neurology.* New York, Raven Press, 1982, vol 36.

94. Hughes RC, et al: Primary neurogenic orthostatic hypo-tention. *J Neurol Neurosurg Psychiatry* 33:363, 1970.

95. Hunt JR: Dyssynergia cerebellaris myoclonica: primary atrophy of the dentate system. A contribution to the pathology and symptomatology of the cerebellum. *Brain* 44:490, 1921.

96. Ishii T, Nakamura Y: Distribution and ultrastructure of Alzheimer's neurofibrillary tangles in postencephalitic Parkinsonism of economo type. *Acta Neuropathol.* (Berl) 62:55, 1981.

97. Ishino H, et al: An autopsy case of Marie's hereditary ataxia. *Psychiatr Neurol Jpn* 73:747, 1971.

98. Iwata M, Hirano A: Current problems in the pathology of amyotrophic lateral sclerosis. In: Zimmerman HM (ed): *Progress in Neuropathology.* New York, Raven Press, 1979, vol 4.

99. Jackson JF, et al: Genetic linkage and spinocerebellar ataxia. In Kark RAP, Rosenberg RN, Schut LJ (eds): *Advances in Neurology.* New York, Raven Press, 1978.

100. Jellinger K: Neuroaxonal dystrophy: its natural history and related disorders. In Zimmerman HM (ed): *Progress in Neuropathology.* New York, Grune & Stratton, 1973, vol 2.

101. Kark RAP, et al: Evidence for a primary defect of li-poamide dehydrogenase in Friedreich's ataxia. In Kark RAP, Rosenberg RN, Schut LJ (eds): *Advances in Neurology.* New York, Raven Press, 1978, vol 21.

102. Kark RAP, et al: The inherited ataxias: biochemical, viral and pathological studies. In *Advances in Neurology.* New York, Raven Press, 1978, vol 21.

103. Kessler II: Parkinson's disease in epidemiologic perspective. *Acta Neurol* 19:358, 1978.

104. Klippel M, Durante G: Contribution à l'étude des affections nerveuse familiales et héréditaires. *Rev Méd* (Paris) 12:745, 1892.

105. Kugelberg E: Chronic proximal (pseudomyopathic) spinal muscular atrophy. In Vinken PJ, Bruyn GW (eds): *System Disorders and Atrophies. Handbook of Clinical Neurology.* Amsterdam, North-Holland, 1975.

106. Lafora GR: Uber das Vorkommen amylioder Korperchen im Innern der Ganglienzellen. Zugleich ein Beitrug zum Studium der amyloiden Substanz im Nervensystem. *Virchows Arch* 205:295, 1911.

107. Lafora GR, Glück B: Beitrag zur Histopathologie der myoklonischen Epilepsie. *Z ges Neurol Psychiatr* 6:1, 1911.

108. Lafora GR, Glück B: Beitrag zur Kenntnis der Alzheimerschen Krankheit oder Präsenilen Demenz mit Herdsymptomen. *Z ges Neurol Psychiatr* 6:1, 1911.

109. Lafora GR: Myoclonus: physiological and pathological considerations. In *Proceedings of the Second International Congress of Neuropathology.* Amsterdam, Excerpta Medica, 1955, part 1.

110. Lampert PW: A comparative electron microscopic study of reactive, degenerating, regenerating, and dystrophic axons. *J Neuropathol Exp Neurol* 26:345, 1967.

111. Langston JW, Ballard, PA Jr: Parkinson's disease in a chemist working with 1-methyl-4-phenyl-1,2,5,6-tetra-hydropyridine. *N Engl J Med* 309:310, 1983.

112. Langston JW, et al: Chronic parkinsonism in humans due to a product of meperidine-analog synthesis. *Science* 219:979, 1983.

113. Lapresle J: The spinocerebellar degenerations: spinal forms. In: *Proceedings of the International Symposium on Spinocerebellar Degenerations,* October 12–14, Tokyo. Baltimore, University Park Press, 1978.

114. Lundborg H: Die Progressive Myoklonus-Epilepsie (Unverrichts Myoklonie). Uppsala, Sweden, Almquist & Wiksells, 1903.

115. Malmström-Groth AG, Kristensson K: Neuroaxonal dystrophy in childhood. *Acta Pediatr Scand* 71:1045, 1982.

116. Mannen T, et al: Neuropathological study of the Onufrowicz nucleus and the anal sphincter muscles in amyotrophic lateral sclerosis and the Shy-Drager syndrome. *Clin Neurol (Tokyo)* 19:125, 1979.

117. Mannen T, et al: The Onuf's nucleus and the external anal sphincter muscles in amyotrophic lateral sclerosis and Shy-Drager syndrome. *Acta Neuropathol* 58:255, 1982.

118. Mansvelt J van: *Pick's Disease. A Syndrome of Lobar Cerebral Atrophy.* The Netherlands, Enschede, 1954.

119. Marie P: Clinique des maladie nerveuses. Sur l'hérédo-ataxie cérébelleuse. *Semin Méd* (Paris) 13:444, 1893.

120. Marie P, et al: De l'atrophie cérébelleuse tardive a pre-dominance corticale. *Rev Neurol* 38:849, 1082, 1922.

121. Marsden CD: Extrapyramidal diseases. In Davison AN, Thompson RHS (eds): *The Molecular Basis of Neuropathology.* London, Edward Arnold, 1981.

122. Marsden CD: Basal ganglia. *Lancet* 2:1141, 1982.

123. Matheson JK, et al: Abnormalities of somatosensory, visual, and brainstem auditory evoked potentials in amyotrophic lateral sclerosis (abstr.). *Muscle Nerve* 6:529, 1983.

124. McMenemey WH: The dementias and progressive diseases of the basal ganglia. In Blackwood W, et al (eds): *Greenfield's Neuropathology.* London, Edward Arnold, 1963.

125. McMenemey WH: System degenerations of the cerebellum, brainstem, and spinal cord. In Blackwood W, et al (eds): *Greenfield's Neuropathology.* London, Edward Arnold, 1963.

126. Meier C, Sollmann H: Glial outgrowth and central-type myelination of regenerating axons in spinal nerve roots following transection and suture. Light and electron microscopic study in the pig. *Neuropathol Appl Neurobiol* 4:21, 1978.

127. Menzel P: Beitrag zur Kenntnis der hereditären ataxie und Kleinhirnatrophie. *Arch Psychiatr Nervenkr* 22:160, 1891.

128. Meyer A: The morbid anatomy of a case of hereditary ataxia. *Brain* 20:276, 1897.

129. Mindham RHS, et al: A controlled study of dementia in Parkinson's disease. *J Neurol Neurosurg Psychiatry* 45:969, 1982.

130. Mulder DW, et al: Motor neuron disease (ALS): Evaluation of detection thresholds of cutaneous sensation. *Neurology* 33:1625, 1983.

131. Nakano KK, et al: Machado disease: a hereditary ataxia in Portuguese immigrants to Massachusetts. *Neurology* 22:49, 1972.

132. Nakano I, Hirano A: Neuron loss in the nucleus basalis of Meynert in Parkinsonism-dementia complex of Guam. *Ann Neurol* 13:87, 1983.

133. Nielson SL: Striatonigral degeneration in familial disorders. *Neurology (Minneap)* 27:306, 1977.

134. Nishimura RN, et al: Lafora disease: diagnosis by liver biopsy. *Ann Neurol* 8:409, 1980.

135. Nonne M: Ueber eine eigenthüm liche familiäre Erkrankungs form des Zentral nervensystems. *Arch Psychiatr Nervenkr* 22:283, 1891.

136. Oppenheimer DR: Diseases of the basal ganglia, cerebellum and motor neurons. In Blackwood W, Corsellis JAN: *Greenfield's Neuropathology.* London, Edward Arnold, 1976.

137. Oppenheimer DR: Neuropathology of progressive autonomic failure. In Bannister R (ed): *Autonomic Failure: A Textbook of Clinical Disorders of the Autonomic Nervous System.* Oxford, Oxford University Press, 1983.

138. Parkinson J: An essay on the shaking palsy, London, 1817. Reproduced in Critchley M (ed): *James Parkinson.* London, MacMillan, 1955.

139. Pearce GW: *The neuropathology of parkinsonism.* In Smith WI, Cavanagh JB (eds): *Recent Advances in Neuropathology.* London, Churchill-Livingstone, 1979.

140. Pearson J, et al: Current concepts of dysautonomia: neuropathological defects. *Ann NY Acad Sci* 228:288, 1974.

141. Pearson J, et al: The sural nerve in familial dysautonomia. *J Neuropathol Exp Neurol* 34:413, 1975.

142. Pearson J, Pytel BA: Quantitative studies of sympathetic ganglia and spinal cord intermedio-lateral gray columns in familial dysautonomia. *J Neurol Sci* 39:47, 1978.

143. Pentland B, Fox K: The heart in Friedreich's ataxia. *J Neurol Neurosurg Psychiatry* 46:1138, 1983.

144. Perry TL, et al: Abnormalities in neurotransmitter aminoacids in dominantly inherited cerebellar disorders. In Kark RAP, Rosenberg RN, Schut LJ (eds): *Advances in Neurology.* New York, Raven Press, 1978, vol 21.

145. Pilleri G: The Klüver-Bucy syndrome in man. *Psychiatr Neurol* (Basel) 152:65, 1966.

146. Postkanser DC, Schwab RS: Cohort analysis of Parkinson's syndrome. Evidence for a single etiology related to subclinical infection about 1920. *J Chron Dis* 16:961, 1963.

147. Rewcastle NB, Ball MJ: Electron microscopic structures of the "inclusion bodies" in Pick's disease. *Neurology* 18:1205, 1968.

148. Richardson JC, et al: Supranuclear ophthalmoplegia, pseudobulbar palsy, nuchal dystonia and dementia. *Trans Am Neurol Assoc* 88:25, 1963.

149. Riley CM, et al: Central autonomic dysfunction with defective lacrimation. I. Report of 5 cases. *Pediatrics*

3:468, 1949.

150. Roessmann U: Primary orthostatic hypotention. In Vinken PJ, Bruyn GW (eds): System Disorders and Atrophies. *Handbook of Clinical Neurology.* Amsterdam, North-Holland, 1975.

151. Roizin L, et al: Neuropathologic observations in Huntington's chorea. In Zimmerman HM (ed): *Progress in Neuropathology.* New York, Grune & Stratton, 1977.

152. Romanul FGA, et al: Azorean disease of the nervous system. *N Engl J Med* 296:505, 1977.

153. Rosenberg RN, et al: Autosomal dominant striato-nigral degeneration. A clinical, pathologic and biochemical study of a new genetic disorder. *Neurology* 26:703, 1976.

154. Rosenberg RN: Dominant ataxias. In Kety SS, et al (eds): *Genetics of Neurological and Psychiatric Disorders.* New York, Raven Press, 1983.

155. Rowland LP: Human motor neuron diseases. In Rowland LP (ed): *Advances in Neurology.* New York, Raven Press, 1982.

156. Roy S, Wolman L: Ultrastructural observations in Parkinsonism. *J Pathol* 99:39, 1969.

157. Russell DS: Myocarditis in Friedreich's ataxia. *J Pathol Bacteriol* 58:739, 1946.

158. Sachdev HS, et al: Joseph disease: a multisystem degenerative disorder of the nervous system. *Neurology* 32:192, 1982.

159. Sakai T, et al: Joseph disease in a non-Portuguese family. *Neurology* 33:74, 1983.

160. Schaumburg HH, et al: *Disorders of Peripheral Nerves.* Philadelphia, F. A. Davis, 1983.

161. Schochet SS Jr, et al: Fine structure of the Pick and Hirano bodies in a case of Pick's disease. *Acta Neuropathol* 11:330, 1968.

162. Schochet SS Jr, McCormick WF: Ultrastructure of Hirano bodies. *Acta Neuropathol* 21:56, 1972.

163. Schwab RS, England AC Jr: Parkinson syndromes due to various specific causes. In Vinken PJ, Bruyn GW (eds): *Diseases of the Basal Ganglia. Handbook of Clinical Neurology.* Amsterdam, North-Holland, 1968.

164. Schwartz GA: Dysautonomic syndromes in adults. In Vinken PJ, Bruyn GW (eds): *System Disorders and Atrophies. Handbook of Clinical Neurology.* Amsterdam, North-Holland, 1975, part 2.

165. Seitelberger F: Eine unbekannte form von infantiler Lipoid-Speicher-Krankheit des Gehirns. In *Proceedings of the First International Congress of Neuropathology.* Rome, 1952, vol 3, p 323.

166. Seitelberger F: Pigmentary disorders. In Minkler JH (ed): *Pathology of the Nervous System.* New York, McGraw-Hill, 1971, vol 2, p 1324.

167. Selby G: Parkinson's disease. In Vinken PJ, Bruyn GW (eds): *Diseases of the Basal Ganglia. Handbook of Clinical Neurology,* Amsterdam, North-Holland, 1968, vol 6.

168. Shy GM, Drager GA: A neurological syndrome associated with orthostatic hypotension. *Arch Neurol* 2:511, 1960.

169. Smith AA, et al: Ocular responses to autonomic drugs in familial dysautonomia. *Invest Ophthalmol* 4:358, 1965.

170. Smith MC: Nerve fibre degeneration in the brain in amyotrophic lateral sclerosis. *J Neurol Neurosurg Psychiatry* 23:269, 1960.

171. Sobue I: Spinocerebellar degenerations. In Sobue I (ed): *Proceedings of the International Symposium on Spinocerebellar Degenerations,* October 12–14, Tokyo. Baltimore, University Park Press, 1978.

172. Staal A, Bots GThAM: A case of hereditary juvenile amyotrophic lateral sclerosis complicated with dementia. *Psychiatr Neurol Neurochir* 72:129, 1969.

173. Steele JC, et al: Progressive supranuclear palsy. *Arch Neurol* 10:333, 1964.

174. Steele JC: Progressive supranuclear palsy. In Vinken PJ, Bruyn GW (eds): *System Disorders and Atrophies. Handbook of Clinical Neurology.* Amsterdam, North-Holland 1975, part 2.

175. Stover ML, et al: Skin ultrastructural changes in Haller-

vorden-Spatz syndrome. Abstract 67, vol 31, 33rd American Academy Meeting, 1981, p 93.

176. Strümpell A: Beiträge zur Pathologie des Rückenmarks. *Arch Psychiatr Nervenkr* 10:676, 1880.

177. Strümpell A: Ueber eine bestimmte form der primären kombinierten Systemerkrankung des Rückenmarks. *Arch Psychiatr Nervenkr* 17:227, 1886.

178. Strümpell A: Die primäre Seitenstrangs-klerose (spasticsche Spinalparalyse). *Dtsch Z Nervenheilk* 27:291, 1904.

179. Swaiman KF, et al: Sea-blue histiocytes, lymphocytic cytosomes, movement disorder and ^{59}Fe-uptake in basal ganglia: Hallervorden-Spatz disease or ceroid storage disease with abnormal isotope scan? *Neurology* 33:301, 1983.

180. Takahashi K, et al: Hereditary amyotrophic lateral sclerosis. Histochemical and electron microscopic study of hyaline inclusions in motor neurons. *Arch Neurol* 27:292, 1972.

181. Taniguchi R, Konigsmark BW: Dominant spino-pontine atrophy. Report of a family through three generations. *Brain* 94:349, 1971.

182. Terry RD: Aging, senile dementia, and Alzheimer's disease. In Katzman R, Terry RD, Blick KL (eds): *Alzheimer's Disease: Senile Dementia and Related Disorders.* New York, Raven Press, 1978, vol 7.

183. Terry RD, Katzman R: Senile dementia of the Alzheimer type. *Ann Neurol* 14:497, 1983.

184. Towfighi J: Early Pick's disease: a light and ultrastructural study. *Acta Neuropathol* 21:224, 1972.

185. Tyler JH: Friedreich's ataxia. In Vinken PJ, Bruyn GW (eds): *Systemic Disorders and Atrophies. Handbook of Clinical Neurology.* Amsterdam, North-Holland, 1975, part 1.

186. Uhl GR, et al.: Pick's disease (lobar sclerosis). Depletion of neurons in the nucleus basalis of Meynert. *Neurology* 33:1470, 1983.

187. Unverricht H: *Die myoklonie.* Leipzig and Vienna, Deuticke. 1891.

188. Vonsattle J-P, et al: Neuropathologic classification of Huntington's disease, in preparation.

189. Ward CD, et al: Parkinson's disease in sixty-five pairs of twins and in a set of quadruplets. *Neurology* 33:815, 1983.

190. Wechsler AF, et al: Pick's disease: a clinical computed tomographic and histological study with Golgi impregnation observations. *Arch Neurol* 39:287, 1982.

191. White P, et al: Neocortical cholinergic neurons in elderly people. *Lancet* 1:668, 1977.

192. Whitehouse PJ, et al: Alzheimer's disease and senile dementia. Loss of neurons in the basal forebrain. *Science* 215:1237, 1982.

193. Whitehouse PJ, et al: Basal forebrain neurons in the dementia of Parkinson disease. *Ann Neurol* 13:243, 1983.

194. Williams HW: The peculiar cells of Pick's disease. *Arch Neurol Psychiatry* 34:508, 1935.

195. Wisniewski HM, et al: Pick's disease. *Arch Neurol* 26:97, 1972.

196. Woods BT, Schaumburg HH: Nigro-spino-dentatal degeneration with nuclear ophthalmoplegia: a unique and partially treatable clinicopathological entity. *J Neurol Sci* 17:149, 1972.

197. Woods BT, Schaumburg HH: Nigrospinodentatal degeneration with nuclear ophthalmoplegia. In Vinken PJ, Bruyn GW (eds): *System Disorders and Atrophies Handbook of Clinical Neurology.* Amsterdam, North-Holland 1975, part 2.

198. Yen S-H, et al: Immunocytochemical comparison of neurofibrillary tangles in senile dementia of Alzheimer type, progressive supranuclear palsy, and postencephalitic Parkinsonism. *Ann Neurol* 13:172, 1983.

199. Yoshimura M: Cortical changes in Parkinsonian brain: a contribution to the delineation of "diffuse Lewy body disease." *J Neurol* 229:17, 1983.

CHAPTER 16

Alzheimer's Disease

ROBERT D. TERRY, M.D.

CLINICAL ASPECTS, FUNCTION, AND FREQUENCY

In the industrialized nations of the west, Alzheimer's disease is the most common cause of dementia, a condition perhaps best defined as a progressive loss of intellectual abilities of such severity as to interfere with social and/or occupational functioning in an otherwise alert patient (2). The disease, with certain relatively minor clinical differences, is found in both senium and presenium, which only arbitrarily have been divided at the age of 65 as to time of onset. Most characteristic of the clinical findings are a loss of memory, beginning with that concerning recent events, and a loss of initiative. Difficulty in word finding and in performing calculations and disorientation in time and place are also common early in the course. Apraxias, dysphasia, and agnosias are also to be found. Personality change including reactive depression may be early, but myoclonus is rarely evident until later. The advanced patient becomes incontinent and is often ultimately confined to bed where joint contractures and decubitus ulcers may develop. The course of the disease is rarely less than 6 months, and may last 10 or even 15 yr. Life expectancy is, on average, shortened to about one-third that of the age-matched normal (62). While the clinical course is usually steadily progressive, occasional plateaus are reported, and momentary improvements may be noted. Death is most often the result of pneumonia or some other extraneural infection, although there is also an increased rate of accidents and of other systemic disease. Inanition is often a factor contributory to the demise.

In Alzheimer's disease, the cerebral blood flow is reduced parallel to the loss of brain parenchyma and especially of grey matter (56). Positron emission tomography has revealed that the metabolism of oxygen and glucose in the cerebum is also lessened, but the oxygen extraction ratio is normal, and this indicates that cerebral ischemia is not a pathogenetic factor (32). The intracranial vessels are usually strikingly normal. The basic background electrical rhythmicity of the brain is slowed to five or 6 Hz (63).

It is important, both conceptually and practically, to note that normal aging does not include any degree of dementia; that dementia connotes disease; and that, therefore, Alzheimer's disease, the major cause of dementia, is not accelerated normal aging but is, rather, abnormal, and is a disease sui generis. Although it is most commonly found in the aged population, that is among those who are senile, it, or something very similar in most ways, is also found among those younger than 65 and even very rarely as young as 30. In the younger cohort it is to be thought of as presenile dementia not in the sense of accelerated senescence, but simply as a disease which has occurred in a younger person comparable to a myocardial infarction found in a 30-yr-old, rather than one who is 60.

This relationship between age and Alzheimer's disease is particularly evident in the older population, where it is found that at age 65 the prevalence rate is less than 1 or 2%, while in a group aged 85 the prevalence is at least 10% (39). For the physician concerned with patients at nursing homes, the frequency of senile dementia of the Alzheimer type (SDAT) will be extraordinarily high, reaching 25–30% of those con-

824

fined to such institutions. Data are still inadequate concerning prevalence in the tenth or later decades. One study would have it that the rate beyond age 90 is lower than in the preceding decade (71). This would represent a survivorship pattern similar to that of diabetes mellitus. That is, beyond a certain age most of those who are going to get the disease have already done so and have died with it or even because of it, leaving behind smaller numbers of people with the disease, that is, a lower prevalence rate in the older cohort.

It is, as a matter of fact, not yet certain whether the prevalence rate of Alzheimer's disease rises steadily with age or whether there are two peaks, the first in the sixth decade and the second in the eighth to early ninth. If there are two peaks, it would be significant further evidence that classical presenile Alzheimer's disease as described by Alzheimer (1) is fundamentally different from SDAT.

To put this matter of prevalence in some perspective, it may be pointed out that in the total population of the United States, SDAT is five to ten times as common as multiple sclerosis, and 50 to 100 times as frequent as amyotrophic lateral sclerosis or Huntington's disease. Of patients with dementia coming to autopsy, Alzheimer's disease accounts for at least half, multiple cerebral infarcts about 20%, and both Alzheimer's and infarcts another 15 to 20%. Multiple other causes account for the rest (101).

GENETICS

There are three general patterns of inheritance of this disorder. The least common but most dramatic is one in which the disease appears clearly as a simple Mendelian dominant, and this is more often found among the presenile patients (15). The second form, amounting to about 30 or 40% of cases, is where at least one relative had a similar disease process, but in which there is neither a recessive nor a dominant pattern. The third type is one with no evidence of any relatives with similar disease, and is, therefore, truly sporadic. In sum, the risk to first order relatives of those with Alzheimer's disease is about four-fold the expected rate (43).

Concordance of Alzheimer's disease in identical twin pairs was originally found to be unexpectedly low (52), but this conclusion was probably based on studies of inadequate duration. It has recently been reported that a difference of nearly 15 yr existed between the age of onset of proven Alzheimer's disease in one set of twins (16). This long interval might suggest an environmental etiologic factor in addition to the genetic one.

Several HLA haplotypes have been cited as being significantly increased in frequency in patients with Alzheimer's disease, but none has been confirmed in more than a single laboratory (70, 103).

Patients with Down's syndrome, or trisomy 21, who survive beyond age 40 essentially invariably have histologic changes identical to those of Alzheimer's disease (13). Reports vary as to the frequency with which these histologic changes are reflected in an altered clinical state, but progressive dementia is a very common if not universal finding in adult Down's syndrome (109). Nevertheless, chromosome 21 is, at least to that extent, implicated in Alzheimer's disease. Among the many proteins coded by genes on this chromosome are superoxide dismutase and interferon, which have both been implicated in other aspects of cellular aging (102). On the other hand, chromosomal abnormality, except for hypodiploidy (51) in some cases, has not been reliably demonstrated (11).

GROSS EXAMINATION

The weight and volume of the brain declines to a small but significant extent in normal aging, especially after age 65 (27). The normal wide variation of brain weight is such as to make simple regression analysis of brain weight as a function of age appear to be weak, but when the volume of the individual brain is compared with that of its own cranial cavity, it becomes quite clear that there is very real shrinkage. Through the sixth decade the brain fills about 92% of the cavity, but this ratio falls to 83% in the ninth decade, and 81% in the tenth (25). It is also to be noted that this gross atrophy is not uniform throughout the brain, or even throughout the cerebral hemisphere. The brain stem and cerebellum do not participate significantly, while the temporal lobe, especially after age 80, is more affected than the other cerebral areas (46). White matter atrophy is said to parallel that of grey in one report (46), while another has it that the ratio between cerebral grey and white matter falls during the first 50 yr of life, and then rises (17).

The averages of brain weights and volumes in Alzheimer's disease are significantly decreased below those normal for the age. Very severe, general cerebral atrophy with brain weight less than 900 g is somewhat more common in the presenile group, where the patient has survived a decade or more (Fig. 16.1). In the senile age group, the most common weight range for patients even with quite severe clinical Alzheimer's disease is 950–1050 g, and many cases will overlap with the normal weight range. The gyri are usually at least mildly atrophic, with a corresponding widening of the sulci. This alteration is quite symmet-

rical and diffuse over the hemispheres, but is usually less severe than elsewhere in the occipital lobe and the paracentral region. Generally, the most severely affected area is the hippocampal gyrus, which not infrequently shrinks to less than 1 cm in coronal width. In occasional cases the atrophy may be strikingly asymmetric or focal, giving the examiner the strong false impression that it is an example of Pick's disease (89). In other individuals the gross changes are so mild as to be inapparent. Very severe gyral atrophy, in fact, is quite unusual in senile dementia of the Alzheimer type (SDAT).

The cortical ribbon in disease is usually just below normal thickness, but some gyri may display an obviously thinner cortex (Fig. 16.2). The cerebral grey to white matter ratio is similar to that in the normal (17, 46), with obvious shrinkage of white matter. The basal ganglia, substantia nigra, and cerebellum are not atrophic, but the

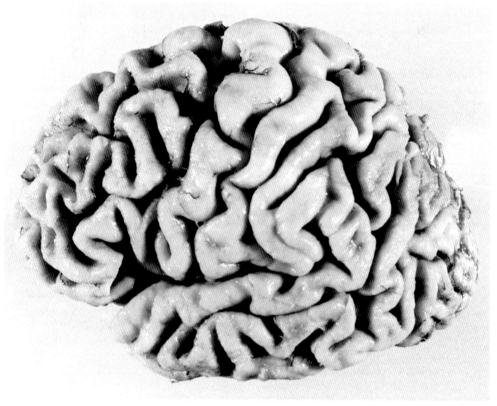

Figure 16.1. Lateral view of the cerebrum from a patient with clinically and microscopically proven Alzheimer's disease. It displays moderately severe diffuse cortical atrophy with widened sulci. In this instance the parietal lobe is less involved than frontal or temporal.

locus ceruleus is often pale, especially in advanced cases. The size of the lateral ventricles is quite variable, but they are usually at least rounded at the lateral angles adjacent to the head of the caudate nucleus. Sometimes the hydrocephalus ex vacuo is more extensive (Fig. 16.2), with sizeable enlargement of frontal and temporal horns of the lateral ventricles and some enlargement of the third ventricle with stretching of the massa intermedia. Many cases in the senile age group, however, will fall well within normal limits of ventricular size (50). This is far less often the situation with younger patients.

NEURONAL SHAPE AND SIZE

Golgi impregnations of long fixed neocortical or hippocampal tissue from patients with Alzheimer's disease display some pyramidal cells with a significant loss of dendrites, especially the horizontal ones (80). These basilar dendrites, particularly susceptible in Alzheimer's disease according to some investigators, normally synapse primarily with granule cells in layers 2 and 4 (34) to form the local circuitry thought to be involved in higher mental functions. In

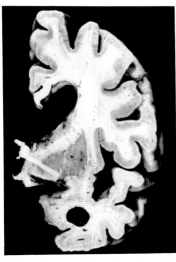

Figure 16.2. A coronal section through the anterior commissure displays widening of the lateral ventricle, including its temporal horn, as well as of several sulci especially in the insula. The white matter is shrunken. The cortical ribbon is narrowed in some areas, most obviously in the insular region. The substantia innominata is to be seen ventral to the anterior commissure.

addition, there are fewer dendritic spines per unit length of dendrite in Alzheimer's disease (61). Both these changes may be present to a lesser degree in normal aging (81). It should be noted, however, that artifactitious changes in tissue fixed for a long time are sometimes prominent in Golgi impregnations and may give a false impression of dendritic breakage and loss (106). Also reported in normal aging, moreover, are pyramidal cells with a significant *increase* in the extent and complexity of the dendritic arbor (12). Apparently, remodeling and growth of the dendritic tree continue throughout normal life, even into old age. This synaptogenesis is cut off, and a dying-back phenomenon is noteworthy in Alzheimer's disease.

It has been stated that biopsies of temporal lobe cortex in Alzheimer's disease revealed a 40% shrinkage of normal neuronal nucleoli. Later, at autopsy, the nucleoli of neurons with tangles were even more shrunken. The inference was drawn that there was both early and additional late reduction of the capacity of neurons to synthesize proteins (58).

CELL COUNTS

The classical morphometric work of Brody (10) on normal aging of the human neocortex would have it that there is a major loss of neurons, involving especially the small neurons in layers 2 and 4. The neuronal loss approached 50% in the superior temporal area and, although somewhat less elsewhere in the neocortex, was of significant numbers. Another report stated that there was also much loss of large cells (42). Still other studies, however, have not been able to confirm this decrement or its emphasis on small neurons, even though overall atrophy of the cerebrum indicates some loss of cells (41). One analysis has shown that there is a major decrement in the category of large neurons, which may correspond to a real cellular loss or to a general shrinkage of the neurons so that there are actually increased numbers of small ones (R. D. Terry and R. DeTeresa, manuscript in preparation, 1983). All agree that there is a mild to moderate increase in the number of astrocytes, especially obvious in the molecular layer.

In neocortical tissue from Alzheimer

cases, there is a marked increase in the number of fibrous astrocytes in layers 2 through 6 without a change in the total number of glia (79). As to neurons, there is a 35–45% drop out of large pyramids (98), but it is not known whether these large neurons represent a single transmitter group. Their loss does not seem to be simply a matter of shrinkage, since there is also a decrease in the number of small neurons, although this is statistically insignificant. The disappearance of the large neurons is very subtle, in that one rarely sees karyorrhexis or neuronophagia. The cytoarchitecture of the cortex is made irregular in the most severely affected cases, in that the area of each plaque is devoid of neuronal perikarya and of most myelin. Axon stains in these severe cases reveal a somewhat disrupted and irregular pattern in the neuropil.

Aside from the neocortex, major cell loss has been enumerated in the area of the basal nucleus of Meynert within the substantia innominata (105) (Fig. 16.3). These neurons, as discussed below, are the major source of choline acetyltransferase and thus of acetylcholine to the neocortex. Furthermore, pyramidal neurons of the hippocampus may also be significantly decreased in Alzheimer's disease. In some severe cases, the locus ceruleus is similarly affected (8, 66), but the substantia nigra, basal ganglia and thalamus are not apparently involved in this disease-related decrement. In advanced stages of the disorder, where nutrition may be a major factor, one often finds a deficiency of granule cells in the rostral cerebellar vermis, but this is a secondary and separate process.

HISTOLOGIC LESIONS

There are four major histologic lesions found in Alzheimer's disease: Alzheimer's

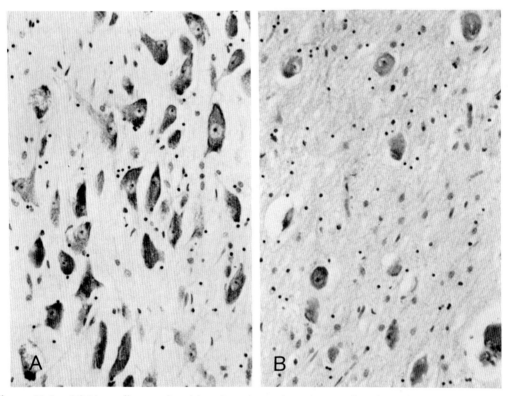

Figure 16.3. (A) Normally populated basal nucleus of Meynert within the substantia innominata from a normal control specimen. Paraffin, H&E. (Original magnification ×120.) (B) A comparable area of the basal nucleus of Meynert from a patient with Alzheimer's disease is impoverished of neurons and has a loosened neuropil. The remaining neurons are somewhat shrunken. Paraffin, H&E. (Original magnification ×120.)

neurofibrillary tangle (1), the neuritic or senile plaque (7), the granulovacuolar body of Simchowicz (85), and the Hirano body (45). None is altogether specific, since each can be found in normal aged brain tissue as well as in a variety of disease conditions. Despite this nonspecificity, the distribution and frequency of these lesions in Alzheimer's disease is highly characteristic, and not to be confused with other conditions where they are either alone, or sparse, or overwhelmed by gross and histologic changes indicative of another disorder.

Neurofibrillary *tangles* (NFT) may be found in small to moderate numbers in the pyramidal cells of the entorhinal cortex and hippocampus in most people in the course of normal cerebral aging. The prevalence of NFT in this area is quite high by the tenth decade (26, 60, 100). They are, however, extremely sparse in the neocortex in the normal elderly at any age. Because of their normal presence in the aged hippocampal area, a section of this region must never be used alone for diagnostic purposes.

In Alzheimer's disease, on the other hand, the tangles are present in great profusion in the neocortex as well as the paleocortex (Fig. 16.4). They are widespread in frontal, parietal, and temporal regions in approximately equivalent concentrations even in early cases. The occipital pole and paracentral gyri have fewer tangles than elsewhere. Their greatest concentration is in the subiculum, entorhinal cortex, and the amygdala, the limbic system being particularly involved (Fig. 16.5). Among the deep grey areas, the basal nucleus of Meynert (4), hypothalamus (48), and rostral brain stem tegmental nuclei are those most often found to contain tangles, but rarely as concentrated as in the other indicated regions.

Up to age 75, NFT are always present in significant numbers in the neocortex in Alzheimer's disease. Beyond that age, however, many cases of clinically typical dementia come to autopsy without neocortical NFT, but with many plaques. Some pathologists do not regard these as examples of Alzheimer's disease, but this writer does on four counts: (a) Alzheimer himself ap-

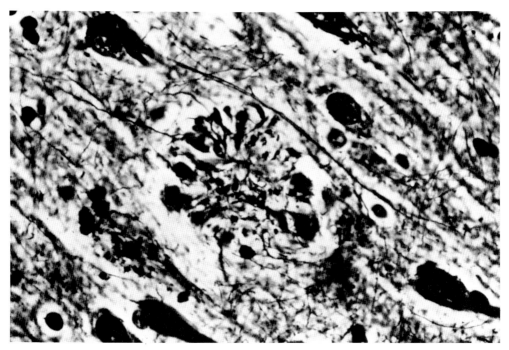

Figure 16.4. A neuritic plaque occupies the center of the field. Hazy material within the plaque represents amyloid, but the core is not well developed here. The very dense irregular shapes at the periphery of the plaque represent abnormal neurites. Surrounding the plaque are several neurons containing dense neurofibrillary tangles. Paraffin, Bodian. (Original magnification ×300.)

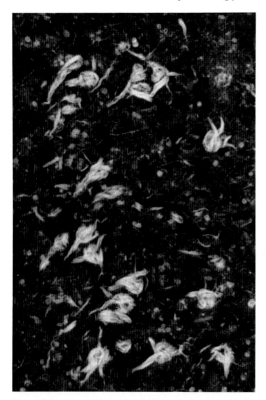

Figure 16.5. Numerous tangles mark the entorhinal cortex in this specimen from a patient with SDAT. Paraffin, thioflavine S. (Original magnification ×200.)

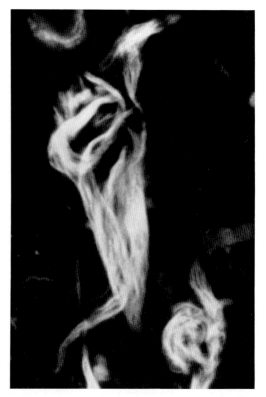

Figure 16.6. A neurofibrillary tangle in a cortical neuron displays abnormal fibers twisting through the cytoplasm and extending into the proximal neurites. A smaller tangle lies in the lower right corner. Paraffin, thioflavine S. (Original magnification ×1000.)

parently did (H. M. Zimmerman, personal communication, 1982); (b) the neuronal losses are identical to those of the similarly aged cases with both tangles and plaques (91); (c) typical plaques are present in numbers similar to those cases with both lesions (91) and, furthermore, those plaques contain paired helical filaments; and (d) evidence of other pathology relevant to dementia is lacking.

The neurofibrillary tangle occupies part or even most of the cytoplasm of pyramidal cells of medium and large size. The argentophilic, congophilic fibers making up the NFT are arranged in bundles which course erratically through the cytoplasm and extend into proximal neurites (Fig. 16.6). They sometimes seem to form knots and curves which are quite unlike the nearly straight configuration of the more delicate normal neurofibers, which are also argentophilic but not congophilic. These lesions are most often demonstrated by silver impregnations, of which there are many types including Bodian, Bielschowski, King, etc. The proteins making up the abnormal fibers also have the capacity to bind amyloid stains. The Congo red stain, especially when examined with crossed polarizing filters is very sensitive, but thioflavine stains (82) are even more so and, furthermore, are easier to prepare, although they require microscopic examination with fluorescent illumination (Figs. 16.5 and 16.6). Although NFT are sometimes apparent as bluish bundles in hematoxylin-eosin (H&E) preparations, a negative H&E is never acceptable as indicating the absence of these lesions. Occasionally one finds, especially in Sommer's sector, a tangle without a nucleus. This probably represents a dead neuron which has left the PHF behind to be phagocytosed by astrocytic activity (53).

At electron microscope magnifications it

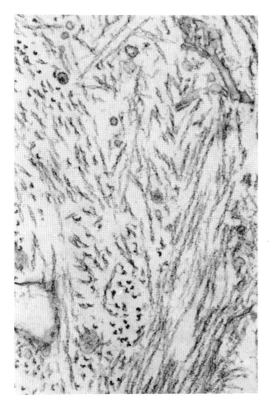

Figure 16.7. An electron micrograph of the paired helical filaments which make up the neurofibrillary tangle. The regularly spaced twists at 80 nm are readily apparent. Poorly seen in this image are the irregular side arms on these abnormal fibers. (Original magnification ×70,000.) (From R. D. Terry et al. (97).)

width and frequent short side arms (Fig. 16.8). In occasional cases, another sort of structure has been found to comprise at least some of the tangles. These are 15-nm untwisted, tubule-like structures (112) (Fig. 16.9). In these cases, most if not all tangles are made up of one or the other fiber, but not both. It is interesting to note that antisera which react with the neurofibrillary tangles made up of PHF have been found to react with these smaller straight tubules which also occur in progressive supranuclear palsy (90), as well as with the neurofibrillary tangles in the substantia nigra of postencephalitic Parkinson's disease (113).

The PHF are not specific to Alzheimer's disease, having been reported in large quantities in dementia pugilistica, in Guam Parkinson-dementia complex, in postencephalitic Parkinsonism, and in rare examples of a variety of other disorders, including adult lipofuscinosis, subacute sclerosing panencephalitis, and others (110).

The PHF are remarkably resistant to autolysis, and they are very stable in the common fixatives. It has recently been found that they are insoluble in reagents at concentrations generally used to prepare proteins for electrophoresis (83), and this insolubility has delayed their analysis and understanding. This insolubility has implied that there is a covalent linkage be-

is found that the tangle is made up of close-packed, paired helical filaments (PHF) (55) (Fig. 16.7). Each filament in the pair is about 10 nm in width and twists over or under its twin at approximately 80-nm intervals. The maximum distance between the elements of the pair is about 4 nm, so that its greatest width is 24 nm, although this is usually 20–22 nm. Where the pair is crossing, the width narrows to that of a single filament, since the two lie in coincidence. Short, indistinct side arms are occasionally seen, but these are less frequent, less regular, and less prominent than the side arms on either microtubules or normal neurofilaments (Y. Kress and R. D. Terry, unpublished data, 1983).

The PHF in situ are sometimes mixed with significant numbers of normal neurofilaments, displaying the usual 10-nm

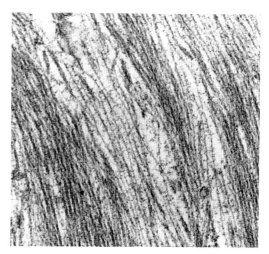

Figure 16.8. An electron micrograph of a tangle which contains not only the usual paired helical filaments, but an admixture of normal neurofilaments. (Original magnification ×12,000.) (Courtesy of Ms. Yvonne Kress.)

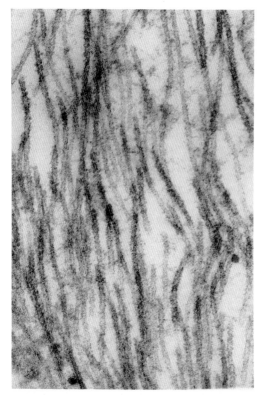

Figure 16.9. This electron micrograph displays the straight 15-nm fibers which are occasionally found to make up the neurofibrillary tangle. Side arms are to some extent visible. (Original magnification ×85,000.) (Courtesy of Ms. Yvonne Kress.)

of the neocortex as well as the hippocampus. Only occasionally, however, in the normal situation do they exceed five or even ten plaques per microscope field as visualized in 10-μm section with the 10× objective. The histologic picture of more than 15 plaques per field is almost always accompanied by a history of clinical dementia. There is a good correlation between the concentration of cortical plaques and the severity of the clinical symptoms of Alzheimer's disease, at least until the disease is very severe. The plaques are to be found in Alzheimer's disease not only in the neocortex and hippocampus, but also in the innominata, hypothalamus, claustrum, and tegmentum of mesencephalon and rostral pons. They are occasionally reported in the cerebellar cortex, and this most often in familial cases. They are unusual in the basal ganglia. Plaques are found throughout the thickness of the cortical neuropil, and sometimes even in the subcortical white matter. They are approximately spherical, with a diameter up to about 200 μm. A capillary often, but not always, lies adjacent to or within the plaque.

At light microscopic magnifications, the core of the plaque is globular or sometimes stellate, staining as does amyloid (28) (Fig. 16.10). Surrounding this core there is often a relatively clear halo and then a ring of

tween the filaments of each pair. It has proven difficult to isolate PHF by physical means, but enriched fractions are being studied extensively by chemical and immunocytochemical techniques. It is apparent that they are in some way related to the proteins of normal neurofibers (3, 33, 40), but the nature of this relationship or whether the cross-reaction is due simply to an admixture in the tangles of PHF with normal neurofilaments has not been finally determined (47).

Since senile *plaques* are found prior to as well as during the senium, and since they are made up primarily of neurites, it was suggested some years ago that they be called neuritic plaques rather than senile plaques (96), and this terminology will be utilized here. These lesions are present in small numbers in the great majority of normally aged brains by age 70, and this is true

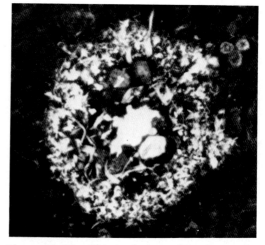

Figure 16.10. This typical neuritic plaque displays a dense central core surrounded by an empty halo and a ring of abnormal neurites and further wisps of amyloid. Paraffin, thioflavine S. (Original magnification ×400.)

granules, and wisps and irregular rods which are argentophilic and often also stain in part as amyloid. Microglial and astrocytic nuclei are commonly nearby, or even within the periphery of the plaque. Immunocytochemical stains for glial fibrous acidic protein demonstrate an intense participation within the plaque by processes of reactive fibrous astrocytes.

Some of these lesions do not have a solid core of amyloid, which is, instead, distributed only as wisps among the other elements of the plaque (Fig. 16.11). Such lesions are thought to be immature plaques, although this may simply represent a tangential section. Other lesions have a very solid, dense core, but lack the surrounding ring of argentophilia, having only astrocytic processes around the amyloid mass. These plaques are considered to be hypermature or burned out (94) (Fig. 16.12).

The nature of the amyloid in the plaque is not yet agreed upon. γ-Globulin (49), APUDamyloid (68), and prealbumin (84) have all been suggested on the basis of histochemical studies.

Electron microscopic studies of the cor-

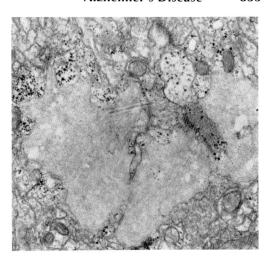

Figure 16.12. This hypermature or burned out plaque is made up of dense masses of amyloid surrounded by astrocytic processes marked by their granular, dense glycogen. Abnormal neurites have been almost entirely lost from this region. (Original magnification ×17,000.) (From R. D. Terry and H. M. Wisniewski (94).)

tex in Alzheimer's disease resolved the composition of the plaque after decades of uncertainty (97). It became clear that the central core was indeed extracellular amyloid (Fig. 16.13), that the halo around this center was, in large measure, an artefact of preparation for light microscopy, and that the wide external ring was made up of abnormal unmyelinated neuronal processes ultimately shown to be mostly presynaptic boutons (36). These abnormal neurites are massively enlarged and contain paired helical filaments identical to those in the neurofibrillary tangle, granular degenerating mitochondria, and many lysosomes (88), most of which appear to be concentrically laminated (Fig. 16.14). Occasionally one finds a dendritic bouton containing numerous PHF in its matrix (94). Astrocytic fibers pass between the other cellular elements of the plaque. Microglia-like cells contain lipofuscin and occasionally are seen to have bundles of amyloid fibers within their cytoplasm, without a bounding membrane (94).

It has been shown that at least some of the presynaptic boutons in the plaque contain acetyl cholinesterase (67, 87), and this is presumptive evidence of their being cholinergic terminals. These plaque compo-

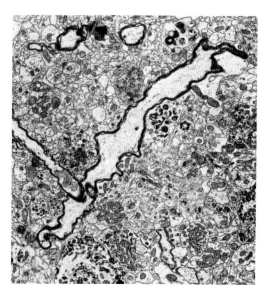

Figure 16.11. An electron micrograph of an immature plaque displays, at low magnification, abnormal neurites containing numerous degenerating mitochondria and lysosomes. Among them are a few wisps of amyloid. The myelin sheaths have not been displaced from this early lesion. (Original magnification ×2,700.) (From R. D. Terry and H. M. Wisniewski (94).)

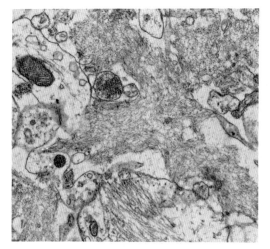

Figure 16.13. Amyloid filaments 9–10 nm in width are clustered in the extracellular space to form the core of the mature plaque. (Original magnification ×19,000.) (From R. D. Terry (97).)

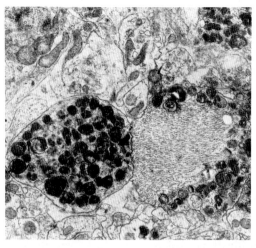

Figure 16.14. This electron micrograph displays two enlarged abnormal neurites found in the periphery of a typical plaque. The unmyelinated terminal on the left is filled with partially laminated lysosomes, while the one to the right displays numerous paired helical filaments as well as lysosomes. Cut in another plane both might have displayed the markings of presynaptic terminals. (Original magnification ×18,000.)

nents, therefore, probably come from cell bodies in the basal nucleus of Meynert (87). Other axonal terminals of the plaque contain 5-HT (serotonin), somatostatin, or substance P. Some dendritic components

come from nearby cortical neurons as seen in Golgi preparations (69).

Scrapie-induced plaques in mice (107) closely resemble those of the human disorder, except that they lack PHF. At this time there is no other evidence that Alzheimer's disease is related to an infectious agent, although there are occasional reports of virion-like structures seen in the tissue (38).

The *granulovacuolar degeneration* (GVD) of Simchowicz (85) is found in the pyramidal cell bodies of the hippocampus, and occasionally in the innominata and amygdaloid. Their frequency in the former area is very greatly increased in Alzheimer's disease, but a few can be found in normal aging. These lesions are best seen with a light microscope in hematoxylin and eosin or Bodian type silver preparations (Fig. 16.15). The cytoplasm of the affected neurons contains one or more circular clear zones, contained in which is a small, basophilic, argentophilic body. There may be great numbers of these in a single, somewhat ballooned cell, most granules having their own vacuoles. In such instances the nucleus may not be apparent. One finds with the electron microscope that the vacuole is bounded by a unit membrane, while the granule is made up of very finely divided, uniform, electron-dense material (95) (Fig. 16.16). Because of the exclusive location of these lesions, they have not been obtained fresh enough for investigation by histochemical techniques, and literally nothing is known about them beyond their morphology. Woodard (111) first quantified their diagnostic significance in 1962, stating that an incidence of GVD greater than 9% among hippocampal neurons was diagnostic of Alzheimer's disease. That is not to say that all cases of the disorder have so many GVD. Subsequently, Ball (5) showed a strong correlation between the frequency of hippocampal tangles and that of neurons with granulovacuolar degeneration.

The eosinophilic rod or *Hirano body* was originally found in patients with Guam Parkinson-dementia (44), and only later in Alzheimer's disease. Like the granulovacuolar bodies, they are almost exclusive to the hippocampal pyramidal layer, where the Hirano body is found generally adjacent to

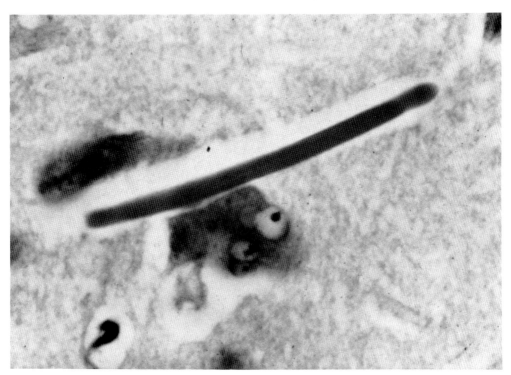

Figure 16.15. A Hirano body runs diagonally through this light micrograph and is seen as a rod which was bright red in the H&E preparation. It lies immediately adjacent to a hippocampal pyramidal cell containing at least three granulovacuolar bodies. Paraffin, H&E. (Original magnification ×800.)

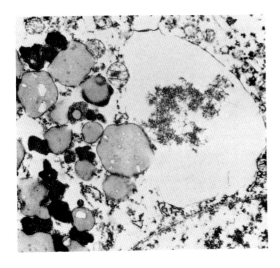

Figure 16.16. An electron micrograph of a postmortem granulovacuolar body displays the remnants of the boundary membrane and the finely divided granular body. Adjacent to the vacuole are several lipofuscin bodies. (Original magnification ×7,300.) (From R. D. Terry and H. M. Wisniewski (95).)

the neuronal cell bodies, and occasionally within them. They resemble a close-packed column of red cells in the H&E stain, but the diameter is usually somewhat greater, often 10–15 μm, and sometimes their fibrillar composition is apparent (Fig. 16.15). Their electron microscopic appearance is quite striking as a body of alternating rows of filaments, each 5–6 nm in thickness, first in longitudinal section and then in cross-section, lying within the neuronal perikaryon or in a neurite (45). The rows are quite close packed in most instances, giving a paracrystalline appearance (Fig. 16.17). These bodies react with antiactin sera, indicating that they may be made up of this important contractile protein (35). It is doubtful that the abnormal aggregation of actin filaments could explain the atrophy of the dendritic tree in Alzheimer's disease, since this change is so diffuse while the Hirano body is focal, but normal contractile apparatus is undoubtedly essential to normal remodeling.

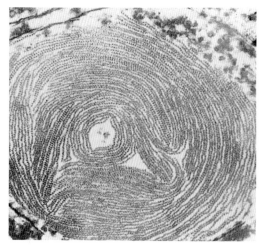

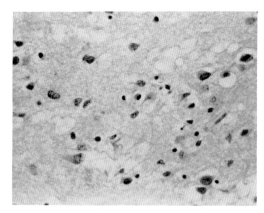

Figure 16.18. This is an image of the spongy encephalopathy found in the superficial cortical layers of some cases of Alzheimer's disease. The neuropil is vacuolated, and some of the neurons are shrunken and surrounded by an artifactitious space, adding to the impression of sponginess. Paraffin, H&E. (Original magnification ×250.)

Figure 16.17. This electron micrograph reveals the cross-sectioned appearance of a typical Hirano body. Note the concentrically arranged filaments and the adjacent cross-sectioned filaments placed at regular intervals, giving a paracrystalline appearance. (Original magnification ×19,000.) (From H. M. Wisniewski and R. D. Terry: *Progress in Brain Research* 40:167, 1973.)

In addition to these four consistent histologic lesions are two which are not always present. One is to be seen in some of the most severe cases of Alzheimer disease. This is a fine, delicate spongy change in the upper cortical layers (Fig. 16.18) and is similar to that found in a more widespread and more intense form in Creutzfeldt-Jakob disease and the other spongy encephalopathies (31). The differential diagnosis should not be difficult because of this difference in distribution of sponginess, the florid astrocytosis, and absence of tangles in Creutzfeldt-Jakob disease (57).

The final histologic change, as seen in about half the cases, is a greater or lesser degree of amyloid infiltration in the walls of cortical and leptomeningeal vessels. This is segmental in linear distribution, but often involves the full thickness of the arterial muscular coat (Fig. 16.19). The amyloid sometimes extends out into the neural parenchyma, but is usually confined to the wall of the vessel. Occasionally, numerous capillaries are involved, seeming to have furry coats representing amyloid fibers pointing out into the parenchyma. Although *amyloid angiopathy*, as this whole range of abnormality might best be called,

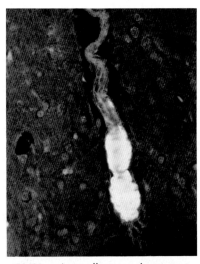

Figure 16.19. A small parenchymatous vessel affected segmentally by amyloid which, here, has infiltrated the full thickness of the wall. Paraffin, thioflavine S. (Original magnification ×250.)

is usually quite diffuse, it is often most prominent in the occipital pole.

NEUROTRANSMITTERS

The major functional biochemical abnormality in Alzheimer's disease is a severe deficiency of acetylcholine in neocortex, hippocampus (23, 65, 100), and innominata (77). This very unstable transmitter itself is measured directly in biopsies, while choline acetyltransferase (the enzyme which synthesizes acetylcholine and is far more stable than the transmitter) is readily measurable in frozen or fresh autopsy material. It has been found that the enzyme is present in normal concentrations in spinal cord and putamen, and only mildly reduced in the caudate (76). The deficiency is thus quite specifically located parallel to the structural changes. Biopsy fragments metabolize glucose to carbon dioxide at a normal or even increased rate, but utilize glucose to produce acetylcholine at a much reduced rate, even in the presence of high concentrations of substrate (86). The deficiencies of synthetic enzyme and transmitter range from 70–90% in the neocortex and hippocampus. Cholinergic activity in the disease has been found to correlate negatively with the concentration of plaques and positively with the mental ability of the patients. Muscarinic receptor concentrations remain normal (23).

About 70% of the cholinergic input to the neocortex is reported to come from the basal nucleus of Meynert in the substantia innominata, ventral to the anterior commissure and the lentiform nucleus (54). These large cholinergic neurons are significantly reduced in number in Alzheimer's disease (105), although, according to some investigators (14), to a lesser extent than is the reduction of transmitter in the cortex. This disparity indicates the possibility that the basal nucleus neurons are turning off production of the cholinergic enzyme or that their axons degenerate before the cell bodies disappear. Other cortical cholinergic input is thought to come from cell bodies in the tegmentum of mesencephalon and rostral pons (78), but although some histologic lesions are to be found in these areas, their relevance to Alzheimer's disease is not certain. Cholinergic neurons intrinsic to the cortex are very sparse.

Further confirmation of the clinical significance of the cholinergic deficiency has come from at least two other directions. First, memory loss, difficulty in word finding, and some disorientation can be induced in normal volunteers by using an anticholinergic drug such as scopolamine (29). Second, Alzheimer patients treated with the antiesterase, physostigmine, are found to improve in regard to memory tests (30, 99).

Norepinephrine, coming to the cortex essentially exclusively from neurons in the locus ceruleus, is reduced in some cases of Alzheimer's disease, most often in the very severely affected patients. Gross pallor and microscopic cell loss (8, 66) are also to be found in some cases, although this structural change does not correlate well with the biochemical assays, indicating the possibility of sprouting of axons from residual neurons in some cases and loss of terminals before loss of cell bodies in others.

Among neuropeptides, somatostatin has repeatedly been found to be significantly depressed in the cortex of Alzheimer's disease (24, 72). Substance P has also been reported as deficient in the disorder, but not so uniformly as somatostatin or acetylcholine (22). On the other hand, vasoactive intestinal polypeptide (73), cholecystokinin octapeptide (75), thyroid-releasing hormone (6), and vasopressin (74) are all normal.

Although dopamine has been reported as diminished in Alzheimer's disease (37), it is probable that this is based on the inclusion of cases where Parkinson's disease was present, either coincident with or without Alzheimer's. The dopamine metabolite, homovanillic acid or HVA, is normal in spinal fluid of patients with biopsy-proven Alzheimer's disease, implying normality of the dopaminergic system in these cases (9).

γ-aminobutyric acid (GABA) is an inhibitory transmitter widespread in the central nervous system, and it is relatively spared in Alzheimer's disease, although again, the neocortex in some cases may have diminished concentrations (76).

OTHER CHEMICAL ABNORMALITIES

Aluminum, in either the metallic form or as a salt, inoculated into the cerebrospinal fluid of susceptible animals such as rabbits, induces the formation of neurofilamentous masses within neurons in several parts of the central nervous system (93). Although this model is not identical to that of the human tangle, it led to the finding that in certain specimens of Alzheimer's disease the aluminum concentration is increased to three or four times normal (19). The level of cerebral aluminum is even greater in dialysis dementia which, however, lacks plaques and tangles (21). These quantitative findings have been amplified with electron probe studies which located the aluminum in neurons with neurofibrillary tangles, but not in adjacent normal neurons in histologic sections (64). More recent, however, and coming from a part of the country where alum is not used to purify water, is a report to the effect that aluminum concentrations are normal in Alzheimer brain tissue (59). The issue of the causal significance of aluminum has not yet been settled, but it seems possible that aluminum is not the cause of Alzheimer's disease, but rather might be aggregated on degenerating neurons when the metal is particularly common in the environment.

Chromatin alterations have also been reported in Alzheimer's disease (20). Although there have been no confirmations of these findings, it was stated that euchromatin falls by about one-quarter in neuron-enriched fractions and by nearly 40% in glia-enriched fractions. The rise in heterochromatin is statistically significant. Nevertheless, those authors have pointed out that the euchromatin incorporated labeled nucleotides at normal rates and that the elongation of ribonucleic acid in vitro was normal in the Alzheimer material. mRNA has been found to be deficient in the diseased cortex, and this has been reported (114) as due to increased activity of alkaline ribonuclease, which in turn is due to the reduced inhibitor bound to the latter enzyme.

A final note in regard to the biochemical abnormalities in SDAT is in order. Recent data from numerous laboratories indicate that in older patients the transmitter concentrations are closer to those of age-matched controls (76), while the differences are great in regard to younger patients. That is, in old people factors other than currently recognized deficiencies of neurotransmitters become more important in producing dementia. These other factors obviously include the formation of plaques and tangles in the demented patients.

PATHOLOGIC DIAGNOSIS OF ALZHEIMER'S DISEASE AND SDAT

The situation is usually simple when a demented patient younger than 60 yr comes to brain biopsy. Most often there will be numerous plaques and tangles in the specially stained (thioflavine, Bodian, etc.) sections. If both lesions are indeed identified, the diagnosis of Alzheimer's disease is obviously justified. If only plaques are present, this diagnosis can be made if they are very numerous, and the patient is at least 75 yr old. Tangles alone might indicate dementia pugilistica (18) or Guam Parkinson-dementia (44). Absence of both plaques and tangles must call for a search for other local or remote causes of dementia.

Autopsy situations are often more difficult, since the clinical impression of dementia may have been much less certain. Without a strong clinical history of progressive loss of intellect, the pathologist must insist on the presence of large numbers of plaques (more than 15 per 10× field) in widespread areas of the neocortex. Frequent neurofibrillary tangles as well as neocortical plaques assure the diagnosis.

Finally, what should one call the situation in which a few plaques are found in neocortex and a few tangles in hippocampus without a clinical history of dementia? This writer simply says "Alzheimer changes," not Alzheimer's disease, although some observers would call this subclinical Alzheimer's disease.

ACKNOWLEDGMENTS

The author is grateful to a series of coworkers, but especially to Dr. Peter Davies and Richard DeTeresa. Finally, a number of grants from the National Institutes of Health, AG-02478, NS-02255, NS-03356, AG-01066, and from the Kresge and the McKnight Foundations have been essential.

References

1. Alzheimer A: Uber eine eigenartige Erkrankung der Hirnrinde. *Algemeine Zeitschrift Psychiatric* 64:146, 1907.
2. American Psychiatric Association, Task Force on Nomenclature and Statistics: *Diagnostic and Statistical Manual of Mental Disorders*, ed 3. Washington DC, 1980, p 111.
3. Anderton BH, et al: Monoclonal antibodies show that neurofibrillary tangles and neurofilaments share antigenic determinants. *Nature* 298:84, 1982.
4. Averback P: Lesions of the nucleus ansa peduncularis in neuropsychiatric disease. *Arch Neurol* 38:230, 1981.
5. Ball MJ: Neuronal loss, neurofibrillary tangles and granulovacuolar degeneration in the hippocampus with ageing and dementia. A quantitative study. *Acta Neuropathol (Berl)* 37:111, 1977.
6. Beggins JA, et al: Postmortem levels of thyrotropin-releasing hormone and neurotensin in the amygdala in

Alzheimer's disease, schizophrenia and depression. *J Neurol Sci* 58:117, 1983.

7. Blocq P, Marinescu G: Sur les lesions et la pathogenie de l'epilepsie dite essentielle. *Sem Med Paris* 12:445, 1892.

8. Bondareff W, et al: Loss of neurons of origin of the adrenergic projection to cerebral cortex (nucleus locus ceruleus) in senile dementia. *Neurology* 32:164, 1982.

9. Bowen DM, et al: Treatment of Alzheimer's disease: a cautionary note. *N Engl J Med* 305:1016, 1981.

10. Brody H: Organization of the cerebral cortex. III. A study of aging in the human cerebral cortex. *J Comp Neurol* 102:511, 1955.

11. Brun A, et al: Normal chromosome banding pattern in Alzheimer's disease. *Gerontology (Basel)* 24:369, 1978.

12. Buell SJ, Coleman PD: Dendritic growth in the aged human brain and failure of growth in senile dementia. *Science* 206:854, 1979.

13. Burger PC, Vogel FS: The development of the pathologic changes of Alzheimer's disease and senile dementia in patients with Down's syndrome. *Am J Pathol* 73:457, 1973.

14. Candy JM, et al: Pathological changes in the nucleus of Meynert in Alzheimer's and Parkinson's diseases. *J Neurol Sci* 54:277, 1983.

15. Cook RH, et al: Studies in aging of the brain. IV. Familial Alzheimer disease: relation to transmissible dementia, aneuploidy, and microtubular defects. *Neurology* 29:1402, 1979.

16. Cook RH, et al: Twins with Alzheimer's disease. *Arch Neurol* 38:300, 1981.

17. Corsellis JAN: Discussion. In Katzman R, Terry RD, Bick KL (eds): *Alzheimer's Disease: Senile Dementia and Related Disorders.* New York, Raven Press, 1978, p 397. *Aging,* vol 7.

18. Corsellis JAN, et al: The aftermath of boxing. *Psychol Med* 3:270, 1973.

19. Crapper DR, et al: Brain aluminum distribution in Alzheimer's disease and experimental neurofibrillary degeneration. *Science* 180:511, 1973.

20. Crapper DR, et al: Altered chromatin conformation in Alzheimer's disease. *Brain* 102:483, 1979.

21. Crapper DR, et al: Intranuclear aluminum content in Alzheimer's disease, dialysis encephalopathy and experimental aluminum encephalopathy. *Acta Neuropathol (Berl)* 50:19, 1980.

22. Crystal HA, Davies P: Cortical substance P-like immunoreactivity in cases of Alzheimer's disease and senile dementia of the Alzheimer type. *J Neurochem* 38:1781, 1982.

23. Davies P, Maloney AJR: Selective loss of central cholinergic neurons in Alzheimer's disease. *Lancet* 2:1403, 1976.

24. Davies P, et al: Reduced somatostatin-like immunoreactivity in cerebral cortex from cases of Alzheimer disease and Alzheimer senile dementia. *Nature* 288:279, 1980.

25. Davis PJM, Wright EA: A new method for measuring cranial cavity volume and its application to the assessment of cerebral atrophy at autopsy. *Neuropathol Appl Neurobiol* 3:341, 1977.

26. Dayan AD: Quantitative histologic studies on the aged human brain. *Acta Neuropathol (Berl)* 16:95, 1970.

27. Dekaban AS, Sadowsky D: Changes in brain weights during the span of human life: relation of brain weights to body heights and body weights. *Ann Neurol* 4:345, 1978.

28. Divry P: Etude histo-chimique des plaques seniles. *J Belge Neurol Psychiatry* 27:643, 1927.

29. Drachman DA, Leavitt J: Human memory and the cholinergic system. *Arch Neurol* 30:113, 1974.

30. Drachman DA, Zaks MS: The "memory cliff" beyond span in immediate recall. *Psychol Rep* 21:105, 1967.

31. Flament-Durand J, Couck AM: Spongiform alterations in brain biopsies of presenile dementia. *Acta Neuropathol (Berl)* 46:159, 1979.

32. Frackowiak RSJ, et al: Regional cerebral oxygen supply and utilization in dementia. A clinical and physiological study with oxygen ^{15}O and positron tomography. *Brain* 104: 753, 1981.

33. Gambetti P, et al: Alzheimer neurofibrillary tangles: an immunohistochemical study. In Amaducci L, Davison AN, Antuono P (eds): *Aging of the Brain and Dementia.* New York, Raven Press, 1980, pp 55–63. *Aging,* vol 13.

34. Globus A, Scheibel AB: Pattern and field in cortical structure of the rabbit. *J Comp Neurol* 131:155, 1967.

35. Goldman JE: The association of actin with Hirano bodies. *J Neuropathol Exp Neurol* 42:146, 1983.

36. Gonatas NK, et al: The contribution of altered synapses in the senile plaque: an electronmicroscopic study in Alzheimer's dementia. *J Neuropathol Exp Neurol* 26:25, 1967.

37. Gottfries CG, et al: Homovanillic acid and 5-hydroxyindoleacetic acid in the cerebrospinal fluid of patients with senile dementia, presenile dementia and Parkinsonism. *J Neurochem* 16:1341, 1969.

38. Goudsmit J, et al: Evidence for and against the transmissibility of Alzheimer disease. *Neurology* 30:945, 1980.

39. Gruenberg EM: A mental health survey of older people. III. *Psychiatr Q Suppl* 34–35:34–75, 1960–1961.

40. Grundke-Iqbal I, et al: Alzheimer neurofibrillary tangles: antiserum and immunohistological staining. *Ann Neurol* 6:532, 1979.

41. Haug H: Quantitative investigations of the human cerebral cortex. *Gerontology* 27:105, 1981.

42. Henderson G, et al: Cell counts in human cerebral cortex in normal adults throughout life using an image analysing computer. *J Neurol Sci* 46:113, 1980.

43. Heston LL, et al: Dementia of the Alzheimer type. Clinical genetics, natural history and associated conditions. *Arch Gen Psychiatry* 38:1085, 1981.

44. Hirano A, et al: Parkinsonism-dementia complex, an endemic disease on the island of Guam.—II. Pathological features. *Brain* 84:662, 1961.

45. Hirano A, et al: The fine structure of some intraganglionic alterations. Neurofibrillary tangles, granulo-vacuolar bodies and "rod-like" structures as seen in Guam amyotrophic lateral sclerosis and parkinsonism-dementia complex. *J Neuropathol Exp Neurol* 27:167, 1968.

46. Hubbard BM, Anderson JM: A quantitative study of cerebral atrophy in old age and senile dementia. *J Neurol Sci* 50:135, 1981.

47. Ihara Y, et al: Antibodies to paired helical filaments in Alzheimer's disease do not recognize normal brain protein. *Nature* 304:727, 1983.

48. Ishii T: Distribution of Alzheimer's neurofibrillary changes in the brain stem and hypothalamus of senile dementia. *Acta Neuropathol (Berl)* 6:181, 1966.

49. Ishii T, Haga S: Immuno-electron microscopic localization of immunoglobulins in amyloid fibrils of senile plaques. *Acta Neuropathol. (Berl)* 36:243, 1976.

50. Jacobs L, et al: Computerized tomography in dementia with special reference to changes in size of normal ventricles during aging and normal pressure hydrocephalus. Alzheimer's disease: senile dementia and related disorders. *Aging NY,* vol 7, 1978.

51. Jarvik LF, et al: Organic brain syndrome and chromosome loss in aged twins. *Dis Nerv Syst* 32:159, 1971.

52. Jarvik LF, et al: Organic brain syndrome and aging. A six year follow-up of surviving twins. *Arch Gen Psychiatry* 37:280, 1980.

53. Johnson AB, Blum NR: Nucleoside phosphatase activities associated with the tangles and plaques of Alzheimer's disease: a histochemical study of natural and experimental neurofibrillary tangles. *J Neuropathol Exp Neurol* 29:463, 1970.

54. Johnston MV, et al: Evidence for a cholinergic projection to neocortex from neurons in basal forebrain. *Proc Natl Acad Sci (USA)* 76:5392, 1979.

55. Kidd M: Paired helical filaments in electron microscopy in Alzheimer's disease. *Nature* 197:192, 1963.

56. Lassen NA, Ingvar DH: Blood flow studies in the aging normal brain and in senile dementia. In Amaducci L, Davison AN, Antuono P (eds): *Aging of the Brain and Dementia.* New York, Raven Press, 1980, pp 91–98. *Aging,* vol 13.

57. Mancardi GL, et al: Ultrastructural study of spongiform-like abnormalities in Alzheimer's disease. *J Neuropathol Exp Neurol* 40:360, 1981.

58. Mann DMA, Yates PO: Ageing, nucleic acids and pigments. In Smith, WT, Cavanagh JB (eds): *Recent Advances in Neuropathology,* Number Two. Edinburgh, Churchill Livingstone, 1982.

59. Markesbery WR, et al: Brain trace element levels in Alzheimer's disease by instrumental neutron activation analysis. *J Neuropathol Exp Neurol* 40:359, 1981.

60. Matsuyama H, et al: Senile changes in the brain in the Japanese. Incidence of Alzheimer's neurofibrillary change and senile plaques. In Luthy F, Bischoff A (eds): *Proceedings of the Fifth International Congress of Neuropathology.* Amsterdam, Excerpta Medica Series 100, 1966.

61. Mehraein P, et al: Quantitative study on dendrites and dendritic spines in Alzheimer's disease and senile dementia. In Kreutzberg GW (ed): *Physiology and Pathology of Dendrites. Advances in Neurobiology.* New York, Raven Press, 1975, vol 12.

62. Nielsen J, et al: Followup 15 years after a gerontopsychiatric prevalence study. *J Gerontol* 32:554, 1977.

63. Obrist WD: Electroencephalographic changes in normal aging and dementia. In Hoffmeister F, Muller C (eds): *Brain Function in Old Age.* Berlin, Springer-Verlag, 1979.

64. Perl DP, Brody AR: Alzheimer's disease: x-ray spectrometric evidence of aluminum accumulation in neurofibrillary tangle-bearing neurons. *Science* 208:207, 1980.

65. Perry EK, et al: Necropsy evidence of central cholinergic deficits in senile dementia. *Lancet* 1:189, 1977.

66. Perry EK, et al: Neuropathological and biochemical observations on the noradrenergic system in Alzheimer's disease. *J Neurol Sci* 51:279, 1981.

67. Perry RH, et al: Histochemical observations on cholinesterase activities in the brains of elderly normal and demented (Alzheimer type) patients. *Age Ageing* 9:9, 1980.

68. Powers JM, Spicer SS: Histochemical similarity of senile plaque amyloid to APUDamyloid. *Virchows Arch (Pathol Anat)* 376:107, 1978.

69. Probst A, et al: Neuritic plaques in senile dementia of Alzheimer type: a Golgi analysis in the hippocampal region. *Brain Res* 268:249, 1983.

70. Renvoise EB, et al: Possible association of Alzheimer's disease with HLA-BW 15 and cytomegalovirus infection. *Lancet* 1:1238, 1979.

71. Rosenwaike I, et al: The recent decline in mortality of the extreme aged: an analysis of statistical data. *Am J Public Health* 70:1074, 1980.

72. Rossor MN, et al: Reduced amounts of immunoreactive somatostatin in the temporal cortex in senile dementia of Alzheimer type. *Neurosci Lett* 20:373, 1980.

73. Rossor MN, et al: Reduced cortical choline acetyltransferase activity in senile dementia of Alzheimer type is not accompanied by changes in vasoactive intestinal polypeptide. *Brain Res* 201:249, 1980.

74. Rossor MN, et al: Arginine vasopressin and choline acetyltransferase in brains of patients with Alzheimer type senile dementia. *Lancet* 2:1367, 1980.

75. Rossor MN, et al: Normal cortical concentration of cholecystokinin-like immunoreactivity with reduced choline acetyltransferase activity in senile dementia of the Alzheimer type. *Life Sci* 29:405, 1981.

76. Rossor MN, et al: A post-mortem study of the cholinergic and GABA systems in senile dementia. *Brain* 105:313, 1982.

77. Rossor MN, et al: The substantia innominata in Alzheimer's disease: an histochemical and biochemical study of cholinergic marker enzymes. *Neurosci Lett* 28:217, 1982.

78. Saper CB, Loewy AD: Projections of the pedunculopontine tegmental nucleus in the rat: evidence for additional extrapyramidal circuitry. *Brain Res* 252:367, 1982.

79. Schechter R, et al: Fibrous astrocytes in senile dementia of the Alzheimer type. *J Neuropathol Exp Neurol* 40:95, 1981.

80. Scheibel AB: Structural aspects of the aging brain: spine systems and the dendritic arbor. In Katzman R, Terry RD, Bick KL (eds): *Alzheimer's Disease: Senile Dementia and Related Disorders.* New York, Raven Press, 1978, pp 353–373. *Aging,* vol 7.

81. Scheibel ME, Scheibel AB: Structural changes in the aging brain. In Brody H, Harman D, Ordy JM (eds): *Clinical, Morphologic, and Neurochemical Aspects in the Aging Central Nervous System.* New York, Raven Press, 1975, pp 11–37. *Aging,* vol 1.

82. Schwarz P: Amyloid degeneration and tuberculosis in the aged. *Gerontologia* 18:321, 1972.

83. Selkoe DJ, et al: Alzheimer's disease: insolubility of partially purified paired helical filaments in sodium dodecyl sulfate and urea. *Science* 215:1243, 1982.

84. Shirahama T, et al: Senile cerebral amyloid. Prealbumin as a common constituent in the neuritic plaque, in the neurofibrillary tangle, and in the microangiopathic lesion. *Am J Pathol* 107:41, 1982.

85. Simchowicz T: Histopathologische studien über die senile demenz. In Nissl F, Alzheimer A (eds): *Histologie und Histopathologische Arbeiten über die Grosshirnrinde.* Jena, Germany, Fisher, 1911, vol 4.

86. Sims NR, et al: (^{14}C)Acetylcholine synthesis and (^{14}C)carbon dioxide production from (U-^{14}C)glucose by tissue prisms from human neocortex. *Biochem J* 196:867, 1981.

87. Struble RG, et al: Cholinergic innervation in neuritic plaques. *Science* 216:413, 1982.

88. Suzuki K, Terry RD: Fine structural localization of acid phosphatase in senile plaques in Alzheimer's presenile dementia. *Acta Neuropathol (Berl)* 8:276, 1967.

89. Tariska I: Circumscribed cerebral atrophy in Alzheimer's disease: a pathological study. In Wolstenholme GEW, O'Connor M (eds): *CIBA Foundation Symposium on Alzheimer's Disease and Related Conditions.* London, J&A Churchill, 1970.

90. Tellez-Nagel I, Wisniewski HM: Ultrastructure of neurofibrillary tangles in Steele-Richardson-Olszewski syndrome. *Arch Neurol* 29:324, 1973.

91. Terry RD, Davies P: Some morphologic and biochemical aspects of Alzheimer's disease. In Samuel D, Algeri S, Gershon S, et al (eds): *The Aging of the Brain.* New York, Raven Press, 1983, pp 47–59. *Aging,* vol 22.

92. Terry RD, DeTeresa R: The importance of video editing in automated image analysis in studies of the cerebral cortex. *J Neurol Sci* 53:413, 1982.

93. Terry RD, Pena C: Experimental production of neurofibrillary degeneration. 2. Electron microscopy, phosphatase histochemistry and electron probe analysis. *J Neuropathol Exp Neurol* 24:200, 1965.

94. Terry RD, Wisniewski HM: The ultrastructure of the neurofibrillary tangle and the senile plaque. In Wolstenholme GEW, O'Connor M (eds): *CIBA Foundation Symposium on Alzheimer's disease and Related Conditions.* London, J&A Churchill, 1970.

95. Terry RD, Wisniewski HM: Ultrastructure of senile dementia and of experimental analogs. In Gaitz CM (ed): *Aging and the Brain. The Proceedings of the Fifth Annual Symposium Held at the Texas Research Institute of Mental Sciences in Houston, October, 1971.* New York, Plenum Press, 1972, pp 89–116. *Adv Behav Biol,* vol 3.

96. Terry RD, Wisniewski HM: Structural and chemical changes of the aged human brain. In Gershon S, Raskin A (eds): *Genesis and Treatment of Psychologic Disorders in the Elderly.* New York, Raven Press, 1975, pp 13–15. *Aging,* vol 2.

97. Terry RD, et al: Ultrastructural studies in Alzheimer's presenile dementia. *Am J Pathol* 44:269, 1964.

98. Terry RD, et al: Some morphometric aspects of the brain in senile dementia of the Alzheimer type. *Ann Neurol* 10:184, 1981.

99. Thal LJ, et al: Oral physostigmine and lecithin improve memory in Alzheimer's disease. *Ann Neurol* 13:491, 1983.

100. Tomlinson BE, et al: Observations on the brains of non-demented old people. *J Neurol Sci* 7:331, 1968.

101. Tomlinson BE, et al: Observations on the brains of demented old people. *J Neurol Sci* 11:205, 1970.

102. Van Keuren ML, et al: Protein variations associated with Down's syndrome, chromosome 21, and Alzheimer's disease. Alzheimer's disease, Down's syndrome, and aging. *Ann NY Acad Sci* 396:55–67, 1982.

103. Walford RL, Hodge S: HLA distribution in Alzheimer's disease. In Terasaki PI (ed): *Histocompatibility Testing.* Los Angeles, University of California Press, 1980.

104. White P, et al: Neocortical cholinergic neurons in elderly people. *Lancet* 1:668, 1977.

105. Whitehouse PJ, et al: Alzheimer's disease: evidence for selective loss of cholinergic neurons in the nucleus basalis. *Ann Neurol* 10:122, 1981.

106. Williams RS, et al: The Golgi rapid method in clinical neuropathology: the morphologic consequences of suboptimal fixation. *J Neuropathol Exp Neurol* 37:13, 1978.

107. Wisniewski HM, et al: Infectious etiology of neuritic (senile) plaques in mice. *Science* 190:1108, 1975.

108. Wisniewski HM, et al: Ultrastructural studies of the neuropil and neurofibrillary tangle in Alzheimer's disease and post-traumatic dementia. *J Neuropathol Exp Neurol* 35:367, 1976.

109. Wisniewski K, et al: Precocious aging and dementia in patients with Down's syndrome. *Biol Psychiatry* 13:616, 1978.

110. Wisniewski K, et al: Alzheimer neurofibrillary tangles in diseases other than senile and presenile dementia. *Ann Neurol* 5:288, 1979.

111. Woodard JS: Clinicopathologic significance of granulovacuolar degeneration in Alzheimer's disease. *J Neuropathol Exp Neurol* 21:85, 1962.

112. Yagashita S, et al: The fine structure of neurofibrillary tangles in a case of atypical presenile dementia. *J Neurol Sci* 48:325, 1980.

113. Yen S-H, et al: Immunocytochemical comparison of neurofibrillary tangles in senile dementia of Alzheimer type, progressive supranuclear palsy, and postencephalitic Parkinsonism. *Ann Neurol* 13:172, 1983.

114. Sajdel-Sulkowska EM, Marotta CA: Alzheimer's disease brain: alterations in RNA levels and in a ribonuclease-inhibitor complex. *Science* 225-947, 1984.

CHAPTER 17

Cerebrospinal Trauma

JOHN M. HARDMAN, M.D.

INTRODUCTION

Accidents have become one of the most important causes of injury, disability, and death in industrialized society. Vehicle accidents are by far the most important cause of head and spinal injuries of adults and older children, but falls still cause more head injuries among small children than vehicles do (46, 250). In the United States accidents at home, work, and play all cause serious head injuries. Likewise, serious head injuries commonly occur in victims of assault, suicide, or homicide.

For many years pathologists have recognized the characteristic focal lesions that are found in fatal head injuries. However, these abnormalities often failed to explain the dramatic neurophysiologic abnormalities that were evident clinically. Recently pathologic features which may explain these changes have been identified which are attributable to diffuse brain injury. The experimental production of injury patterns in primates comparable to injuries of man has underscored the significance of these abnormalities. Gennarelli *et al.* have demonstrated that coma can be produced in monkeys by rapid acceleration of the head without striking the head (83). In this model widespread axonal injury and subdural hematomas are produced which appear to be identical to such lesions found in humans.

In this chapter a survey of the essential clinicopathologic features of the various lesions encountered in head and spinal injuries are presented. Finally several unique trauma-associated syndromes are discussed. Hopefully this survey will provide useful information concerning the essential clinicopathologic features of the injuries of the head and brain found in humans.

EPIDEMIOLOGY

Epidemiologic studies of head-injured patients admitted to medical treatment centers or accident victims from defined populations have remarkably similar characteristics (6, 12, 79, 128, 131, 139, 140, 179, 250). Head injuries occur in young adults ages 15–24 yr most frequently, and they occur in men twice as often as in women (12, 131). Accidents produce higher case fatality ratios among older adults (140) and occur in over half of all moving vehicle accidents (46, 139). Accidents occur more frequently in individuals who have been drinking alcoholic beverages than persons who have not (79, 127, 128), and they occur in individuals who have one or more of the following conditions: alcoholism, prior head injury, prior meningitis, seizure disorder, mental retardation, or significant psychiatric disorder (6, 45, 46, 127). Finally, accidents cause death in more than half of fatally injured patients before they reach a medical treatment facility (46, 79). The National Center for Health Statistics surveys indicate that there is a 1% annual rate of nonfatal head injuries among all individuals living in the United States (251). Two epidemiologic studies of head injuries occurring in populations living in San Diego and Rochester areas document annual incidence rates of 0.3% for serious head injuries (12, 139). By comparison the mortality rate for all accident victims was reported to be 48/100,000 persons in the United

States, whereas the rate for motor vehicle accident victims was 23/100,000 (251). In other industrialized countries of the world the annual mortality rates have ranged from a low of 12/100,000 in England and Wales to a high of 27/100,000 in Australia (263). In the United States accidents are now the fourth most common cause of death for persons of all ages and are the leading cause of death for individuals below 40 yr of age (251).

Injuries in vehicular crashes are related primarily to the second collision within the vehicle and ejection (88). Deaths from fire, immersion, or intrusion of objects from the environment are less frequent. Epidemiologic studies indicate that the drivers, vehicles, and highways are the principal factors which contribute to crashes but that the vehicle itself produces the injuries. Since the 1950s improvement in the crashworthiness of vehicles has resulted from crash investigations. Two principles have been identified which reduce the likelihood of injury. First, design changes have allowed distribution of the impact forces over as large an anatomic area as possible, and second, modifications to eliminate sharp interior objects have been made. Such changes distribute the force of impact over a greater area, thus reducing the potential for injury. Crash helmets also are designed to reduce forces this way. Vehicle crashes occur in four ways: frontal, side, rear, and rollover. Studies by Stapp with human volunteers indicate that deceleration forces of 40 g or less are survivable (231). The use of shoulder and lap belts and rollover bars have all improved crash survivability.

In the investigation of fatalities from car crashes, the pathologist should inspect the vehicle or at least view pictures of the exterior and interior of the vehicle to help establish the pathogenesis of injuries sustained in a specific collision. Unfortunately this approach is all too often neglected. Even so the civil and criminal litigation that often results makes such study an important and essential aspect of the investigation.

Head injuries account for nearly three-fourths of accidental deaths. The relative importance of head injury and death is quite apparent when such percentages are compared to injuries of other body areas

(see Table 17.1) (187). Even though many excellent clinical and pathologic studies regarding head injuries have been reported in the last 20 yr (6, 42, 100, 161), gaps still exist in assessing the incidence, severity, etiology, and the specific types of injuries. Gennarelli and his coworkers (7, 86, 256) have elucidated some of the fundamental pathophysiologic and neuropathologic features of experimentally induced injuries of primates which closely mimic rotation-induced injuries of humans. Likewise, the comprehensive neuropathologic studies of victims of fatal head injuries induced by blunt nonmissile trauma have also advanced our understanding of the pathophysiologic and morphologic features of brain injuries in humans. In Table 17.2 a summary of the pathologic features of 151 such cases reported by Adams et al. (6) is listed. The correlative studies presented by these two groups have significantly advanced our basic understanding of traumatic brain injury.

TYPES OF INJURY

Concussion

Cerebral concussion is defined as a temporary, reversible neurological deficiency caused by trauma which results in immediate, temporary loss of consciousness (85, 255). Historically the term *commotio cerebri* has been used to describe this posttraumatic state. Recognition of this neurologic dysfunction dates to ancient times. However, our basic understanding of the pathophysiologic events encountered in this disorder have only recently been clarified by Gennarelli and his coworkers (7, 85–87).

Table 17.1
Traumatic Injury: Roles of Injury and Death

Body area	% Injured[a]	% Fatal
Head	70	5
Neck and cervical spine	9	16
Thorax and thoracic spine	39	6
Abdomen, pelvis, lumbar spine	16	4
Upper extremities	35	<0.5
Lower extremities	48	<0.5

[a] Total percentage adds up to greater than 100% because many patients sustained injury to two or more parts of their body.

	%
Sex distribution:	
Male	81
Female	19
Primary complications:	
Skull fracture	79
Contusions/lacerations	93
Diffuse axonal injury	13
Primary complications:	
Intracranial hemorrhage	64
Brain swelling	17
Secondary complications:	
Raised intracranial pressure	83
Ischemic damage	91
Meningitis	2.6
Fat embolism	1.3

This traumatic condition is always accompanied by both retrograde and posttraumatic amnesia. The length of amnesia is indicative of the severity of concussion, but unconsciousness should be completely reversed within 24 h; otherwise, diffuse brain injury of greater severity will be found. Experimental studies of concussion have shown minimal nonspecific neuronal changes but nothing else (7, 96). As would be expected neuropathologic studies of classical cerebral concussion in humans have rarely been available to study. Other types of brain injury were encountered in 64% of patients with classical concussion evaluated by Gennarelli (85). Focal injuries like cortical contusions and skull fractures were seen in 28% of injured patients, and multiple brain injuries were identified in 36% of them. Focal lesions like cortical contusions do not as a rule cause loss of consciousness. Head-injured patients may have a "lucid interval" after an initial concussion and become unconscious again after transtentorial herniation and irreparable damage of the brain stem has occurred. Typically a "mass lesion" like an epidural hematoma can follow such a clinical course. Consequently the morbidity and mortality of cerebral concussion is dependent upon the severity of the associated brain injuries. The relationship of concussion to diffuse axonal injury and to the posttraumatic encephalopathy (pugilistic

dementia) encountered in boxers is discussed in more detail below.

Skull Fractures

The presence of a skull fracture signifies that traumatic cranial injury has occurred, and skull fractures are reported in up to 80% of fatal head injuries (3). Concomitant brain injuries also occur frequently, but they are by no means an invariable consequence of skull fractures. Likewise, fatal brain injuries do occur in the absence of skull fractures. In children skull fractures rarely result from falls out of a bed or crib, and when fractures are produced they are seldom associated with significant brain injury (102, 107). This observation has prompted authorities on child abuse to suspect such maltreatment whenever a child is alleged to have fallen from a bed or crib and found to have both skull fractures and significant brain injury (133, 189). The neuropathologic findings in child abuse are discussed in more detail below.

A skull fracture is generally classified by the configuration or pattern it displays (26, 61, 150, 253). When a straight crack or break is produced by a blow to the skull, the resultant fracture is the most frequent type found and is termed a *linear* fracture. If the fracture is depressed by a distance equal to the thickness of the skull or more it is called a *depressed* skull fracture, and occasionally such a fracture is referred to as a *bending* fracture. If the fracture shows bending outward distal to the impact site it is termed a *bursting* fracture. When fractures separate the cranial sutures they are referred to as *diastatic* fractures. Fractures are further divided into closed or open (compound) fractures, depending upon the nature of injuries of the overlying soft tissues and scalp.

Hinge fractures are produced when the head is fixed on the ground, run over by a heavy object like the wheel of a truck, and crushed (218). Typically in such cases, diastatic fractures are found between the petrous portion of each temporal bone, the greater wing of each sphenoid bone, and the petrosquamous fissures. In turn these diastatic fractures are connected by a fracture across the dorsum sella. Such extensive fractures allow the base of the skull to be moved like a hinge. Even so, bilateral petrous bone fractures may be produced in other ways such as blow to the chin (101).

The pattern of a skull fracture may indicate the direction, the location, and force of the impact producing the injury (26, 61, 150, 253). Fracture lines usually radiate from the impact point and will often extend into the base of the skull and connect with cranial nerve foramina. Depressed skull fractures commonly result from low velocity impacts to a limited area of the calvarium. Such fractures are most frequently located in the frontal and parietal regions. When interlacing fracture lines are found, multiple impact sites must be suspected. The appearance and the location of the impact site may identify the cause of the injury and determine the pattern of fractures. Linear fractures frequently result from falls and commonly occur in children. Ring fractures circumscribing the foramen magnum may result from sudden deceleration after impacts to the base of the spine, i.e., in falls impacting on the buttocks.

Fractures of the orbital roofs and ethmoid plates remote from the site of cranial impact may be produced by crushing injuries, in falls, and in gunshot wounds (112, 221). Orbital roof fractures should always be suspected whenever "black eyes" (periorbital ecchymoses) are seen.

Missiles, particularly low-velocity bullets, produce characteristic fracture patterns at the points of entrance and exit through the skull (66). At the point of entrance the outer table defect is smaller than is the inner table defect, whereas the converse is true at the point of exit of the bullet from the skull. High-velocity missiles frequently explode the skull (8). Even low-velocity bullets may occasionally be as devastating if the gun is fired with the muzzle in direct contact with the scalp.

Fractures of the base of the skull are not reliably depicted by x-ray examination (61, 64). In fact they are much better demonstrated at autopsy, providing the dura mater is stripped from the base of the skull to ensure good visualization of the bones and suture lines. In the autopsy examination of trauma victims, careful removal of the dura mater from the skull should be done routinely to identify fractures.

Traumatic cerebrospinal fluid fistulas are produced by compound and basal skull fractures. When the fractures traverse the paranasal sinuses rhinorrhea results, and fractures of the petrous portion of the temporal bone may cause otorrhea. Rhinorrhea was found in 2.3% and otorrhea in 1.8% of 1187 skull fractures among children (102). Pneumocephalus may also occur and is demonstrable by plain skull films and/or computed tomography (270). As little as 0.5 cm^3 of air can be seen by computed tomography (195). The presence of cerebrospinal fluid fistulas predisposes the patient to central nervous system infection, and in one recent report meningitis occurred in 27% of 164 patients with rhinorrhea and in 9% of 33 patients with otorrhea (149).

Another unique lesion is the *growing* fracture which is produced by an enlarging traumatically induced leptomeningeal cyst (136, 152, 175, 241). The cyst protrudes through a tear in the underlying dura mater and arachnoid meninges, enlarges a linear fracture, and erodes the bone along the fracture margin. The enlargement and erosion of bone are believed to be caused by pulsation of the brain (241). Such fractures nearly always occur in young children less than 3 yr of age and are usually not associated with significant injury of the brain.

Accurate assessment of each case depends on careful reconstruction of the fractures and evaluation of the soft tissue and scalp wounds. Such study helps make accurate localization of impact sites and may determine the cause of the skull fractures.

Contusion

A cortical contusion is defined as a bruise of the brain's surface and is covered by intact dura mater. A cerebral contusion is distinctive if not pathognomonic of mechanical injury. Such injuries were first accurately described by Spatz in 1930 (230). Later Lindenberg and Freytag (155, 156) identified different types and considered each one to be caused by different biomechanical forces. Contusions formed at the site of cranial impact are called coup contusions, opposite the cranial impact—contrecoup contusions, and in the margins of brain hernias—herniation contusions. The latter lesions are most frequently located along the margin of the falx cerebri, tentorium, or foramen magnum.

Contusions found adjacent to the skull

fractures are called fracture contusions. The so-called gliding contusions as described by Lindenberg are injuries which may or may not be comparable to surface contusions.

Cortical contusions (Fig. 17.1):

1. Involve the crowns of gyri.
2. Are wedge-shaped.
3. Cause full-thickness necrosis of the cortex and leptomeninges.
4. Are regularly associated with perivascular hemorrhages of the cortical vessels. Hemorrhage regularly extends to the cortical surface and spreads in the cerebrospinal fluid.

Contusions are more likely to be found at certain anatomic sites. These patterns of injury have been observed at autopsy and reflect the position and motion of the body at the time of impact in victims of accidents. Recent experimental studies using the monkey as a model have helped elucidate the underlying pathophysiologic events in the formation of cortical contusions (83, 86). Such studies have confirmed that the injury patterns differ whether the victim's head is stationary or in motion at the moment of impact. When the free mobile head is motionless at the moment of impact, cortical contusions, so-called coup contusions, appear most prominently beneath the point of cranial impact. When the free mobile head is accelerating as in a fall and impacts against a firm or unyielding surface, contusions form in cortical surfaces opposite the cranial impact site and are called contrecoup contusions (60). The inferior frontal lobes and the temporal poles sustain the brunt of such blows (Fig. 17.2). Some lateralization of the contusions will be evident, although such injuries rarely involve the superior and posterior aspects of the cerebral hemispheres. However, lateral cranial impacts will cause prominent contralateral contusions of the frontotemporal regions (Fig. 17.3). The localization of contusions to the inferior temporal and frontal regions may be explained by movement of the brain surface over the irregular bony prominences regularly found in the anterior and middle fossae of the skull.

Laceration

A laceration is a tear or rent in normal tissues which is produced by mechanical forces. Such injuries are commonly found in the same anatomic sites that contusions are observed and likely reflect more severe effects of trauma. Lacerations are most frequently found along fracture lines and are

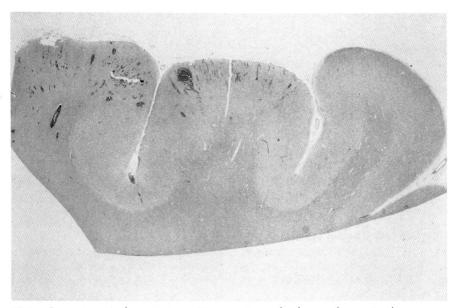

Figure 17.1.   Recent cortical contusions. Note perivascular hemorrhages in the crowns of two adjacent gyri of the inferior frontal lobe. H&E. (Original magnification ×2.)

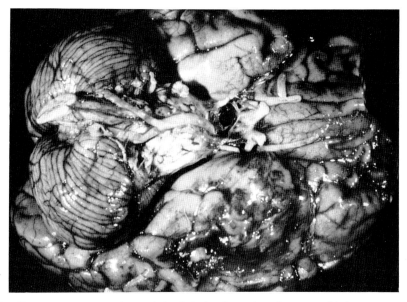

Figure 17.2. Contrecoup contusions of the inferior frontal and temporal lobes sustained in a fall with impact to the right occipital region.

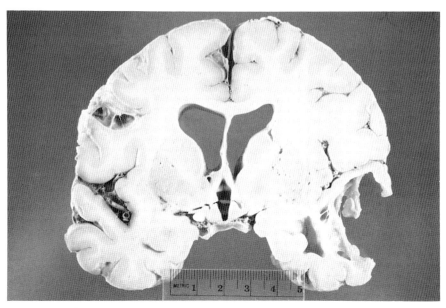

Figure 17.3. Healed small coup and large contrecoup contusions of the left frontal and right temporal lobes, respectively.

invariably found about penetrating or perforating wounds. Lacerations produced by blunt nonmissile head trauma may be found with or without associated skull fractures. Such injuries may be accompanied by microhemorrhages or large hematomas. Cerebral lacerations are found preferen-

tially in the inferior frontal lobes and temporal tips in so-called contrecoup injuries (Fig. 17.4). They commonly accompany diffuse axonal injury, and the lacerations are regularly located in the corpus callosum and the rostral brain stem. Rents of the pontomedullary junction (Fig. 17.5) and

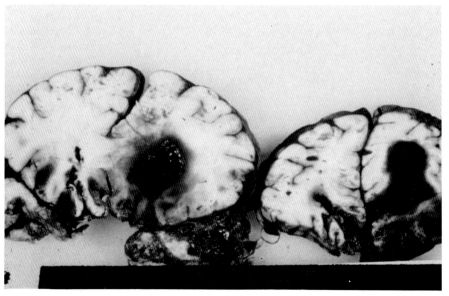

Figure 17.4. Contrecoup contusions, lacerations, and intracerebral hematomas of inferior frontal and anterior temporal lobes in automobile accident victim.

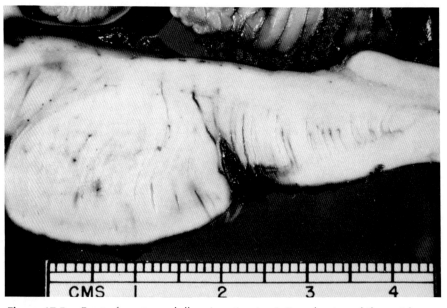

Figure 17.5. Rent of pontomedullary junction in victim of automobile accident.

cerebral peduncles are usually seen in vehicular accidents and are presumably caused by sufficient hyperextension to stretch and snap the axons at these sites. Except for fracture contusions such sudden fatal injuries have been remarkably free of other traumatic lesions. In Table 17.3, the findings in 13 cases I have studied are presented. One of these also had an asymmetric tegmental injury of the midbrain comparable to the damage seen in patients with diffuse axonal injuries. Such findings would suggest that these apparently unique lacerations may in fact be variants of the axonal damage produced in other sites by angular acceleration of the head in man or

Table 17.3
Pontomedullary Rents: Pathologic Findings (13 Cases)[a]

Rent of pyramids	
Partial	10
Complete	2
Subarachnoid hemorrhage	11
Basilar artery laceration	2
Transverse basal skull fractures	9
Atlanto-occipital dislocation without odontoid fracture	5
Other primary CNS traumatic lesions	
Contusion, cerebral cortex	3
Contusion/laceration, spinal cord	2
Contusion/laceration, midbrain	3
Major extracranial skeletal and visceral injuries	8
Impact site	
Face	9
Upper thorax	1
Undetermined	2
Accident type	
Automobile	6
Motorcycle	2
Pedestrian	2
Airplane	1
Fight	1
Child abuse	1

[a] Three cases had concomitant basal skull fractures.

experimental animals. Rents of the pontomedullary junction were first recognized by Patscheider (199); then studies by others further characterized this distinctive mechanical tear (5, 28, 42, 89, 100, 141, 160, 264). Circumferential fractures through the petrous bones and over the cranium, ring fractures about the foramen magnum, and fracture dislocations of the first and second cervical vertebrae have accompanied these tears. These patterns of fractures allow the brain to be displaced or stretched with hyperextension, and the pontomedullary junction or cerebral peduncles are disrupted.

Diffuse Axonal Injury

Diffuse axonal injury (DAI) was first recognized as an essential component of posttraumatic dementia by Strich in 1956 (237). Her studies and the reports of others confirmed that axonal injury was a key feature of the posttraumatic encephalopathies which developed as a consequence of blunt nonmissile injuries of the brain (125, 161, 194, 201, 236, 238). Most frequently these injuries occur in vehicle accidents, and less often after falls. The characteristic features of this entity include diffuse axonal injury of the brain and focal lesions of the corpus callosum and dorsolateral rostral brain stem.

Clinically these patients become unconscious immediately after injury and either remain comatose or develop a persistent vegetative state and die after a protracted time. About one-half of severely injured victims present in a comatose state and do not have "mass lesions" as viewed by computed tomography, but do have focal eccentric hemorrhages in the corpus callosum, near the third ventricle, and the cerebral white matter. Zimmerman et al. (270) first recognized this CT pattern in 3% of acute head injuries. This injury pattern may also be seen in association with contusions, increased intracranial pressure, brain swelling, intracranial hematomas, and hypoxic/ischemic brain damage.

In these cases the brain may appear surprisingly normal when viewed with the naked eye, yet show strikingly microscopic abnormalities. Widely distributed lesions containing reactive axonal swellings (retraction balls) are found in the cerebral white matter, corpus callosum, and upper brain stem (Fig. 17.6). Axonal swelling becomes apparent within hours after injury and may persist for years. Microglial stars (clusters of microglial cells) develop in these damaged sites and eventually may replace the swollen axons as they disappear. In time long tract degeneration will evolve, and ventricular dilation will follow. Foci of hemorrhage and necrosis may accompany the sites of axonal damage and will evoke the usual cellular reactions to injury. The callosal injury may be focal (Fig. 17.7), segmental, or extend from the genu to the splenium. Such lesions are often hemorrhagic and may disrupt or tear the corpus callosum (Fig. 17.8). The lesions in the rostral dorsolateral brain stem (Fig. 17.9) exhibit similar histologic changes to those found in the corpus callosum. Often these lesions involve the brachium conjunctivum and lead to central tegmental tract degeneration with hypertrophy, neuronal swelling and vacuolation, and gliosis of the

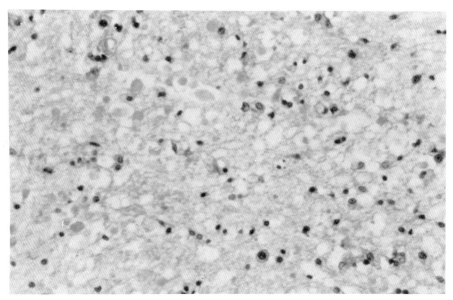

Figure 17.6.   Diffuse axonal injury. Reactive axonal swelling in margin of necrotic lesion of corpus callosum 2 days after injury.

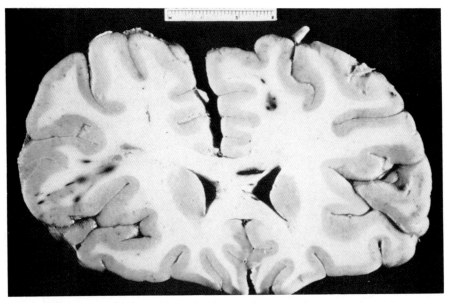

Figure 17.7.   Diffuse axonal injury. Note tiny hemorrhages and necrotic foci of corpus callosum and bifrontal white matter.

corresponding inferior olivary nucleus. Similar hemorrhagic and necrotic lesions are found in the periaqueductal tissue. Such lesions may be important in producing lasting coma or the persistent vegetative state that accompanies these injuries. Evoked potentials are abnormal in such cases. The periaqueductal lesions are almost always accompanied by hemispheric injury. The reports of Adams et al. (5) and Rosenblum et al. (215) suggest that the incidence of this kind of primary brain stem injury varies considerably and likely reflects the bias of the cases available for study.

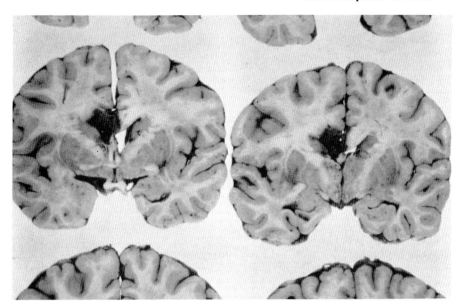

Figure 17.8 Laceration of corpus callosum in diffuse axonal injury 5 days after automobile accident. Victim never regained consciousness after the accident.

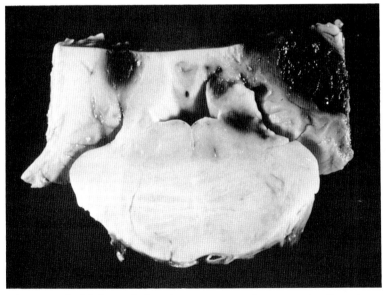

Figure 17.9. Asymmetrical injury of dorsal tegmentum of pons and adjacent cerebellar white matter. Victim was considered to have "brain death" when first seen but was maintained on a respirator for 72 hours before somatic death occurred.

Theoretical, experimental, and morphologic studies indicate that the diffuse axonal injury of the cerebral white matter, brain stem, and corpus callosum is produced by sudden angular rotation of the head (41, 161, 194, 201, 245, 270). Strich believed that shear forces caused the damage and cited the theoretical work of Holbourn (114) and the experimental studies of Pudenz and Shelden (207) in support of this thesis. Holbourn, a physicist, using gelatin models of the brain predicted that the brain would be more vulnerable to shear stains than to compressibility and argued that this type of mechanical deformation would cause the brain damage with rotation of the head. Later Pudenz and Shelden replaced the monkey's calvarium with clear lucite plastic and could see swirling motion of the brain after cranial impacts. Clark noted that microglial clusters were located in the corpus callosum ipsilateral to the external applied force and the internal capsule and brain stem contralateral to the applied force in 90% of patients with head injuries severe enough to cause loss of consciousness (41). However, Adams et al. (5) found this distribution pattern in only 16% of comparable cases. Even so this pattern of injury closely matched Holbourn's earlier predictions of likely sites to be injured by shear forces. Other favored hypotheses based on the effects of direct cranial impacts seem to be invalidated by the experimental studies recently reported by Genarelli et al. (86). Using the monkey as an experimental model, he produced injury patterns identical to that seen in human cases with diffuse axonal injury by using angular acceleration alone. The injuries are believed to be produced by shear and/or tensile strains causing axonal injury of the cerebral white matter, corpus callosum, and brain stem. These same experiments also demonstrated that angular acceleration of the head causes axonal injury of the brain proportional to the degree of coronal motion. These findings confirm that minute injuries sometimes found after concussion may be directly related to angular acceleration. Such observations suggest that concussion is not the completely reversible physiologic disorder that it has always been considered. In fact boxers who are known to suffer permanent brain damage after repeated concussive insults may also be injured this way.

Brain Swelling

After head injury, brain swelling may or may not develop in conjunction with other injuries of the brain. The term brain swelling is used here to include both edema and severe cerebrovascular congestion (hyperemia).

Since computed tomography has been so widely used in evaluation of patients with head injuries, two closely related clinicopathologic syndromes of *diffuse brain swell-*

ing have been identified (31, 32). These syndromes occur almost exclusively in children. In one the diffuse brain swelling is attributed to brain edema, whereas in the other the swelling is believed to be caused by severe hyperemia and increased blood flow (30, 31, 191). In the first type patients often followed a relentless course to death, whereas in the second type the patients nearly all recover without sequelae if properly treated. In children diffuse brain swelling may evolve without other apparent injury. In these patients rapid neurological deterioration may begin within minutes to hours following head injury. Cerebral blood flow and computed tomographic density studies suggest that this swelling is due to cerebral hyperemia and increased blood volume but not edema. Children in this category with Glasgow coma scales of greater than 8 make a complete recovery and have normal CT on follow-up studies; however, children with coma scales of 8 or less usually do well, although some die (less than 10%) from the effects of the severe brain swelling. Autopsy studies confirm these findings, but to date only a few deaths have been carefully studied pathologically (229). By comparison adults who show similar clinical neurological deterioration usually develop a mass lesion, often an expanding hematoma.

Children rendered unconscious immediately after an injury often have diffuse brain swelling caused by edema and other injuries comparable to those found in adults (2). Such patients have remained comatose for weeks to months. In follow-up of CT examinations of these patients, a high incidence of other injuries are seen. In one study 17 of 34 children developed increased intracranial hypertension, and 5 of 34 patients died (31). In the 29 survivors follow-up CT exams demonstrated extracerebral collections of presumed cerebrospinal fluid in 27% of the patients and ventricular dilation associated with cortical atrophy in 35%. Such changes suggest that these patients suffered severe diffuse injury of the white matter.

Diffuse swelling is readily appreciated when flattening of gyri, narrowing of sulci, and symmetrical collapse of the ventricular system are evident. With localized swelling distortion and herniation may be evident.

However, subtler or minimal swelling is not so easily recognized. The histologic criteria of cerebral edema include pallor of the myelin, distention of the perivascular and pericellular spaces, rarefaction of subpial spaces, a vacuolar appearance of the neuropil, and pools of protein-rich fluid in the spongy-appearing areas (18, 67, 68, 170). However, such criteria are hard to standardize and are always subject to challenge. A more reliable way to assess the presence of cerebral edema is to measure the water content of tissues (267). Here, too, such studies need to be widely used to establish their feasibility and practicality. Ultrastructural studies have been invaluable in elucidating the features of cerebral edema experimentally, but again such studies cannot be easily or reliably applied to the study of routine autopsies (111).

Hemorrhage

Following traumatic injuries of the head, hemorrhages have a predilection to develop in the epidural, subdural, and subarachnoidal spaces and in the brain. When such bleeds form mass lesions, they often produce devastating neurophysiologic effects and may cause death of the victim. Studies by Jamieson and Yelland (119–121) of approximately 11,000 head injury victims admitted to hospitals in Brisbane, Australia documented 1.5% extradural, 5% subdural, and 0.6% intracerebral hematomas among these patients. In Table 17.4 a summary of the mortality rates and the levels of con-

sciousness recorded for these hematomas are listed. These findings are typical and provide an overview of the essential features of these traumatically induced intracranial hemorrhages. Even so considerable variation is reported for the outcome of such injuries and is very likely related to many difficult to control factors including the acuteness and severity of injury, associated cranial, skeletal, and visceral injuries, the treatment given and follow-up time after injury (48, 108, 167, 168, 172, 183, 202, 209, 260). With the advent of computed tomography, rapid and accurate assessment of these lesions has become commonplace.

The various types of hemorrhage are discussed separately in the following sections.

EPIDURAL HEMATOMA

Epidural hematomas form when bleeding occurs between the calvarium and the dura mater (endosteum) (Fig. 17.10). Such hematomas are typically caused by blows to the head, with fracture of the temporal bone and laceration of branches of the middle meningeal artery (48, 108, 113, 116, 119–122, 167, 168, 172, 174, 183, 197, 202, 209, 260). Bleeding may be minimal or massive and be localized or diffusely layered between the calvarium and separated dura. The clots are most frequently found in the temporoparietal region, less commonly in the frontal and occipital regions, and rarely in the posterior fossa. Although epidural hematomas are said to be uncommonly associated with other significant intracranial

Table 17.4
Intracranial Hematomas (84–86)

	Extradural	Subdural	Intra-cerebral
Mortality rate	15.6%	35.1%	25.4%
Course of consciousness			
Unconscious to lucid to unconscious	12.0	14.0	19.0
Unconscious to lucid	19.8	25.0	17.5
Lucid to unconscious	21.0	16.3	15.9
Unconscious throughout course	22.8	29.0	14.3
Lucid throughout course	24.6	29.0	33.3
Associated intradural lesions	47.3	55.0	—[a]

[a] Does not include hematomas found beneath compound or simple depressed fractures, nor hematomas found in relation to cerebral lacerations. However, there were associated subdural hematomas in 10 cases, extradural hematomas in 6 cases, and extradural and subdural hematomas combined in 4 cases.

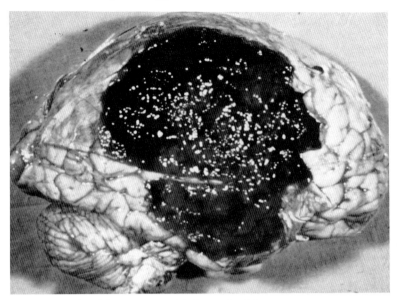

Figure 17.10.   Acute epidural hematoma of left cerebral hemisphere. Note that clotted blood overlays dura mater.

injuries (48, 122, 197), recent reports show that nearly one-third of patients do have other significant injuries, such as contusions and subdural hematomas (113, 119, 120, 121, 174). Clotted blood forming in an epidural hematoma seldom liquifies but in every other respect is removed by the inflammatory and reparative responses in a manner comparable to that observed in subdural hematomas (113, 174, 183). Within a few days a thin layer of granulation tissue will form on the surface of the dura adjacent to the blood clot (169, 182). Ossification will also be noted infrequently at interface between the granulation tissue and the dura. A well formed neomembrane of vascular fibrous tissue will encapsulate the loculated blood after a month or more has lapsed from the time of injury. Rarely false aneurysms of the middle meningeal artery develop.

Epidural hematomas are usually characterized by an acute rapidly progressing clinical course. Such lesions are now usually quickly identified and treated surgically. If not they continue to enlarge and may rapidly progress to cause coma and death of the victim. Epidural hematomas may become symptomatic after a protracted period following injury. Chronic variants comprised 28% surgical cases in one report (116).

Arterial lacerations were identified as the source of bleeding in 61% of acute epidural hemorrhages in one report (174). Bleeding from torn veins, dural sinuses, and bone accounted for the remainder. By comparison arterial bleeding accounted for only 24% of chronic epidural hematomas in another study (13).

The intense heat produced in fires may lead to the diffuse accumulation of coagulated blood in the epidural space of burn victims (Fig. 17.11). This lesion is believed to be caused by heat and should not be confused with traumatical epidural hematomas as described above.

In Table 17.5 the distinctive features of epidural and acute subdural hematomas are compared (10, 13, 23, 38, 39, 40, 48, 59, 76, 91, 108, 113, 116, 119–122, 135, 167–169, 172, 174, 182, 183, 197, 202, 226, 243, 260, 266).

SUBDURAL HEMATOMA

Subdural hematomas develop when blood accumulates in the subdural space from bleeding of torn bridging veins (Fig. 17.12). Traumatic subdural hematomas may be caused by either open (penetrating) or closed head injuries. Subdural hematomas remain one of the most important causes of death of severely injured patients. Such hemorrhages occur commonly after

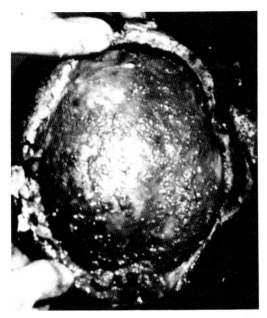

Figure 17.11. Diffuse epidural hemorrhage believed to be artifactually produced by the heat of the fire. Victim incinerated in airplane accident.

falls and assaults, in vehicular accidents, in victims of child abuse, and in sporting accidents. Older age and alcoholism have been important predisposing factors for their development. Rarely ventricular decompression for hydrocephalus and pneumoencephalography have been implicated (182, 232, 260, 266). However, in one recent report 23.6% of 212 surgically diagnosed subdural hematomas were not preceded by significant injury (260). Traditionally the distinction between acute, subacute, and chronic subdural hematomas has been arbitrary and based on the time interval between injury and the onset of symptoms. Hematomas becoming symptomatic within 3 d were regarded as acute, those with symptoms between 3 and 21 d were classified subacute, and those becoming symptomatic after 21 d were considered chronic (122). Even so in 154 traumatic subdural hematomas reported by Wintzen (260) such a crisp distinction was not found (260).

With sudden angular (rotational) acceleration of the movable head, the inert brain lags behind the accelerated skull stretching and snapping veins which connect the brain and the dural sinuses. Blood accumulation then may form a mass lesion and cause compression, edema, and herniation of the brain. Recent experimental studies have demonstrated that sudden angular acceleration of the head of the monkey will produce subdural hematomas independently from direct blows to the head (84). Such experiments closely simulate the way traumatic subdural hematomas appear to develop in man and indicate that this mechanism is the principal way such hematomas are produced.

Bleeding may be minimal or massive. In Stehben's review the prevalence of bilateral subdural hematomas was 18.5% in adults and 76.7% in children (232). Although the correlation of the size of the hematoma and the severity of the clinical manifestations is imperfect, such lack of agreement is likely related to how quickly the hematoma forms and how severe the associated injuries are. Studies by Aronson and Okazaki (13) indicated that a hematoma of 50 ml or more was invariably associated with neurologic and psychiatric disturbances, and clots measuring 100 ml or more are likely to cause death (13). One or more blows to the head may precipitate subdural hematomas, and blows to the occipital region are most frequently documented. However, indirect injury such as a fall on the buttocks, blast, and whiplash injuries have produced subdural hematomas (1, 177, 193, 254). These latter reports tend to validate the importance of angular acceleration in the production of these lesions. Subdural hematomas form characteristically over the frontoparietal regions of the cerebral hemispheres (Fig. 17.12). Extensive bleeds may cover the entire hemisphere and even extend into the middle and frontal fossae. Supra- and infratentorial hematomas may be found concurrently. Posterior fossa subdural hematomas may be found rarely at any age, but the neonate is thought to be the most vulnerable. Either acute or chronic spinal subdural hematomas are equally rare, and when found they usually do not cause spinal cord compression (27, 63). Other significant injuries like skull fractures, extradural and intracerebral hematomas, cortical contusions and lacerations, and diffuse injuries may occur concomitantly. The relative frequency of these associated injuries depends upon the nature of the cases examined. For example, skull

Table 17.5
Comparison of Acute Subdural and Epidural Hematomas

Subdural hematoma	Epidural hematoma
Etiology	
1. Trauma in >75% of cases	1. Trauma in 95% of cases
2. Blood dyscrasias	2. Blood dyscrasias
3. Hemodialysis	3. Other: rare
4. Ruptured aneurysms, etc.	
Associated clinical conditions	
1. Alcoholism	1. Ventricular decompression for
2. Pneumoencephalography	hydrocephalus
3. Ventricular decompression for	2. Battered child syndrome
hydrocephalus	
4. Battered child syndrome	
5. Boxing	
Sex: Males predominate	Males predominate
Bleeding source: Bridging cortical veins	Middle meningeal artery, vein,
	or venous sinuses
Location	
Frontoparietal most common	Temporal, 80%; do not respect cranial
Bilateral: 20% adults, 80%	suture line
children	Unilateral, 97%
Posterior fossa neonate: rare	Spinal canal, uncommon
Spinal canal: rare	
Size	
Significant: >50 ml blood	Significant: 25–50 ml blood
Lethal: >100 ml blood	Lethal: 75–100 ml blood
Maximum: approx 300 ml blood	Maximum: approx 300 ml blood
Associated neuropathologic conditions	
Skull fracture: 67% adults; approx.	Skull fracture: in approximately
10% children	90% of all cases
Hematoma: intracerebral and sub-	Hematoma: subdural, subarachnoid,
arachnoid common; extradural	and or intracerebral in 33%; epi-
infrequent	cranial, uncommon
Edema: ipsilateral cerebral hemi-	Herniation: brainstem in most un-
sphere	treated patients
Herniation: brainstem in 33%	
Infarcts: posterior cerebral artery	
distribution	
Sequelae	
Secondary hemorrhage common	None
Hydrocephalus untreated infants	
Spontaneous resorption	
Secondary infection rare	
Mortality	
Untreated acute: dependent on size	Untreated: dependent on size
and rapidity of onset (up to 100%)	and rapidity of onset
Treated subacute, 24%	Treated: average approx 30%;
Treated chronic, 6%	range: 8–76%

fractures were found in 69.7% of 861 forensic autopsies (76), but in only 8.1% of 136 patients surgically treated for subdural hematomas (108). The clinicopathologic features of acute subdural hematoma and epidural hematomas are listed in Table 17.5, modified from the review by Hardman (100).

The gross and microscopic appearance of subdural hematomas has long been the subject of interest to pathologists and neurosurgeons alike. The typical histologic features of these lesions are listed in Table 17.6 also modified from the review by Hardman (100). A note of caution is in order for anyone trying to assess the age on subdural

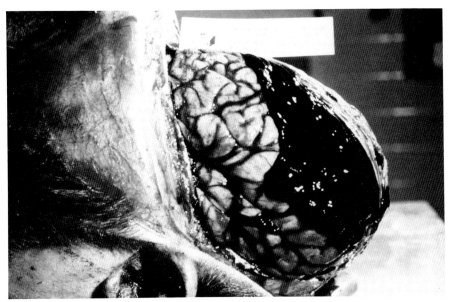

Figure 17.12. Acute subdural hematoma over left cerebral hemisphere. Note that clotted blood looks like "currant jelly" and is not organized.

Table 17.6
Histologic Features of Subdural Hematomas[a]

Time after injury	Clot	Dural side	Arachnoid side
To 24 h	Fresh erythrocytes	Fibrin	Fibrin
36–48 h	Fresh erythrocytes	Few fibroblasts at dural junction	Fibrin
4–5 d	Erythrocytes loose; some lysis; pigment-laden macrophages	Fibroblastic layer 2–5 cells thick	Fibrin
1 wk	Erythrocytes laking; angiofibroblastic invasion of clot	Fibroblastic layer approx 12 cells thick	May be a single layer of flat, epithelioid-like cells
2 wk	Clot breaks up; vascular sinusoids ("giant capillaries") apparent	Fibroblastic layers are one-half thickness of the dura	Fibroblastic membrane. Very few capillaries
3 wk	Vascular sinusoids are well developed		
4 wk	Liquefied clot	Fibroblastic membrane equal to the dura in thickness; pigment-laden macrophages	Well-formed fibrous fibrous membrane; relatively avascular
1–3 mo	There is hyalinization of the membranes of both the dural and the arachnoid side. There are large (giant) capillaries early, and there are often secondary hemorrhages.		
3–12 mo	The nonmembranes usually fuse, consist of more mature fibrous tissue, and contain scattered pigment-laden macrophages. Beyond 3 months, it is not possible to give a very accurate approximation of the age of the hematoma.		
Beyond 1 yr	The neomembrane forms a distinct fibrous connective tissue layer which closely resembles the adjacent dura mater. Occasionally calcification and/or ossification will appear after approximately 3 years.		

[a] Modified from JM Hardman (100).

hematomas, as it is particularly difficult to get adequate tissue samples on surgical biopsies for histologic study. The history may be the only reliable indicator of the age of a given hematoma. Nevertheless, I believe that this table does provide useful guidelines to assess the age of most lesions. At autopsy reliable histologic evaluations are easier to obtain. Multiple segments of the hematoma and the neomembranes must be examined microscopically. Sections must include the neomembranes at the junction of the dural and arachnoidal meninges, as early fibroblastic proliferation begins at this point and is easiest to assess (Fig. 17.13A and B). Most acute subdural hematomas resolve leaving a yellow-brown (xanthochromic) stain and a layer of dense

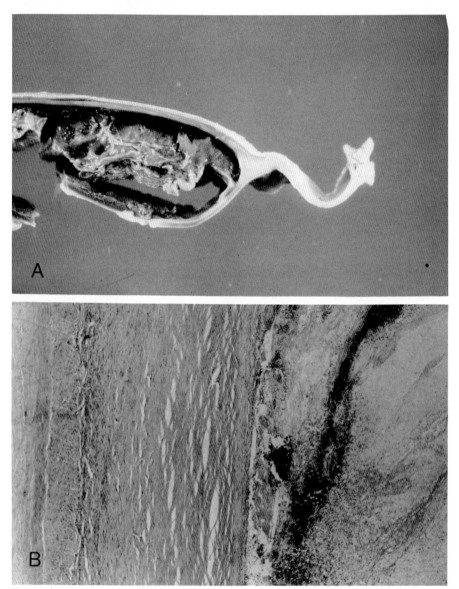

Figure 17.13. Chronic subdural hematoma in elderly alcoholic patient. (A) A thick subdural neomembrane surrounds a large hematoma over one cerebral hemisphere (note outer layer of fibrous tissue, the dura mater). (B) Enlargement of circled area of A showing the normal dura mater (arrows) and the attached dense fibrous neomembrane surrounding the blood clot. (H&E, original magnification - 2×).

fibrous tissue fused with the normal dura mater. The underlying brain may be atrophic with dilated ventricles and contain scars of old injuries, or appear normal.

The origin of the neomembranes that form about hematomas in the subdural space have been shown by Friede and Schachenmayr (78) to be the result of proliferation and thickening of the normal dural border cells. The proliferating cells form layers and clusters with interspersed

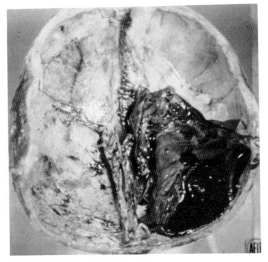

Figure 17.14. Subdural hematoma encapsulated by neomembranes attached to calvarium 1 month after injury.

collagen fibrils and elastic fibers. New capillaries originate from the inner dural face and penetrate the dural cell proliferations. These investigators have also shown that the fine structure of the normal dura-arachnoid interface in humans contains a distinct layer of nonadherent cells devoid of collagen (223). These unique structural features make cleavage of these cells an innate characteristic and may explain why until now the dura and arachnoid have always been considered anatomically separate membranes. Presumably the inherent lack of adhesion exhibited by proliferated dural border cells (the neomembrane) also explains why the neomembrane does not fuse with the arachnoid (Fig. 17.15). Based on such unique structural features, these investigators believe that any pathologic condition separating the dura and arachnoid meninges in the dural border cell layer will produce a neomembrane. If so the long held postulate that proliferation of the inner dural border cells always results from traumatic hemorrhage is no longer valid and might explain the long-recognized clinical observation that a history of significant traumatic injury is lacking more often than one would expect, especially in patients with chronic subdural hematomas (17.14). For example, in the report by Wintzen (260) a history of significant head trauma was absent in only 5% of acute subdural

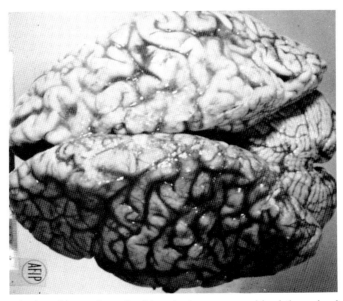

Figure 17.15. Marked molding of cerebral hemispheres caused by bilateral subdural hematomas which were not adherent to the leptomeninges and were easily removed.

hematomas but in 85% of chronic subdural hematomas.

SUBARACHNOID HEMORRHAGE

Subarachnoid hemorrhage is most frequently caused by trauma and is usually associated with injuries like contusions or lacerations. Blood entering the subarachnoid space is circulated widely in the cerebrospinal fluid and provokes an aseptic meningitis (118). Within a few hours fever, meningismus (stiff neck) and an acute inflammatory response in the cerebrospinal fluid becomes apparent. Polymorphonuclear leukocytes appear first, and they are replaced by lymphocytes and macrophages within a few days. The macrophages consume the red blood cells within a few days or weeks and are identified by the presence of lipid vacuoles and iron-pigment granules in the cell cytoplasm (246). Such cells may persist for months to years in the arachnoid meninges and Virchow-Robin spaces; however, in children these cells seem to disappear faster and more completely (235). Finally massive or repeated subarachnoid hemorrhages can produce hydrocephalus (5, 91, 161).

INTRACEREBRAL HEMATOMA

Hematomas may develop in the brain after closed or open head injury. Traumatic intracerebral hematomas measuring 0.5 cm or more in diameter are reported in 0.4–9% of all intracranial hematomas treated neurosurgically (209). They are found in nearly 20% of acute subdural hematomas and are found with epidural hematomas alone or in combination with a subdural hematoma. Such hemorrhages are more likely to be solitary in clinical studies, whereas at autopsy the relative frequency of multiple intraparenchymal hematomas is much greater and may approach 40% of parenchymal hematomas (42).

Hematomas of the brain are found most frequently in the temporal and frontal lobes associated with cortical contusions and lacerations (Fig. 17.4). Rarely other sites may contain them. For example, a hematoma originating in the lateral ventricles may form following traumatic laceration of the septum pellucidum and fornices. Recently Adams et al. (6) have used the term "burst lobe" to describe an injury pattern characterized by intraparenchymal hematoma and either laceration or contusion in continuity with a subdural hematoma. Whether this combination of injuries needs to be distinguished from parenchymal hematomas remains to be seen.

Hematomas confined to the parasagittal white matter of the frontal lobes were originally termed "gliding contusions" by Lindenberg (156) (Fig. 17.16). The formation

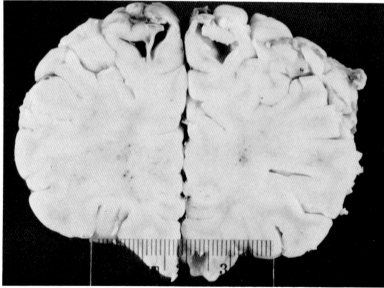

Figure 17.16.   Bilateral intracerebral hematomas of the subcortical regions of each frontal lobe in an infant who was an alleged victim of child abuse.

of these lesions in decelerative head injuries has been recognized for a long time; however, their pathogenesis has not been well established. The mechanism by which subdural hematomas are produced may be equally applicable to the genesis of these lesions and would suggest that tears of cortical veins in the brain itself rather than in the overlying parasagittal subdural space bleed to produce these lesions. Such tears could be produced by angular acceleration.

In the past, intracerebral hematomas that become symptomatic after a delay of a week or more were classified as *delayed posttraumatic hematomas* (of Bollinger) (29). These hematomas may become symptomatic within 24 hours of injury, and the development of delayed intracerebral hemorrhages can be identified by serial CT scans (268). How frequently these hemorrhages develop is not known; however, a small percentage of patients scanned for acute head injuries will develop them.

Recent studies indicate that alcohol intoxication may enhance the development of hematomas by disturbing the function of platelets, coagulation, and membrane-bound enzymes (51, 69). Disseminated intravascular coagulation may be initiated by either open or closed head injuries, and bleeding seems to be most pronounced in those injured patients with thrombocytopenia (16, 17). Since alcohol remains a primal factor in vehicle accidents, cognizance of its effects becomes even more important in the assessment and treatment of accident victims.

Subdural Hygroma

The accumulation of watery (serous) fluid resembling cerebrospinal fluid in the subdural space has been termed either "subdural hydroma" or "hygroma" (97). Following head injury, such collections may develop immediately or after a delay and may occur unilaterally or bilaterally over the cerebral hemispheres. Hygromas may be found alone or concomitantly with other head and brain injuries (219, 234, 270). The associated intracranial injuries that have been reported most often include chronic subdural hematoma, epidural hematoma, skull fractures, and/or ventricular enlargement. Symptoms vary, depending on the size of and rapidity with which the fluid

collections form. Some patients remain asymptomatic and, in others, the fluid accumulation forms a progressively expanding "mass lesion" that may lead to coma and death. Subdural hygromas are found in males and females of all ages, and they are caused by motor vehicle accidents, domestic accidents, fights, and child abuse (219, 234, 270).

Hygromas may be produced by tears of the arachnoid or by impaired cerebrospinal fluid absorption (56, 57, 184). With the passage of cerebrospinal fluid into the subdural space, absorption is impaired or blocked. The delayed onset of this condition suggests that hygromas may also evolve from subdural hematomas.

Traumatic subdural hygromas comprise 13% of operated subdural lesions (234), but recognition of them preoperatively has only become feasible with the advent of computed tomography (74, 219, 234, 270). Clinical reports indicate that hygromas can be distinguished from hypodense subdural hematomas by their lower attenuation coefficients on computed tomography (74, 219, 234, 270). Such low values correspond to the markedly reduced protein content of cerebrospinal fluid as compared to blood (188). Nevertheless, some authors contend that differentiation of a hypodense subdural hematoma from a subdural hygroma is not possible (183, 225).

OPEN (MISSILE) WOUNDS

Gunshot Wounds

Low velocity bullets fired from handguns cause most civilian deaths, whereas high velocity bullets fired from military firearms usually account for military deaths. Death by suicide ranked as the 9th leading cause of death of Americans in 1978, and homicide ranked 12th (186). Firearms were used in the majority of these deaths, and they were even the cause of 1.9% of all accidental deaths in the United States in 1979 (250). In studies from large neurosurgical treatment facilities, mortality rates of 93% were observed in unconscious victims and 22% in conscious patients with gunshot wounds of the brain admitted for treatment (109).

Gunshot wounds of the head cause penetrating and perforating wounds. If the bullet traverses the head, the resultant injury is classified as a perforating head wound (Fig. 17.17). If not, the injuries are characterized as penetrating. Lacerations and contusions are readily appreciated about bullet tracks, whether the bullet follows a penetrating or perforating course (137). Single tracks are found in 80% of fatal gunshot wounds to the head, and up to three tracts may be found in the remainder (75). Intracranial richochet and tangential courses beneath the calvarium account for most cases with more than one track. Bone chips that frequently impact into the brain virtually always originate from the entrance wound. The paths these bone fragments take define the course that the bullet has taken. Typically, tracks of low velocity missiles are not related to the caliber of the firearm, and they show considerable variation in their size. The amount of tissue damage about the track varies and is largely dependent upon the speed and weight of the bullet. The faster the bullet travels, the greater the damage is and the less important the weight becomes in causing damage. The damaging effects of missiles are largely related to the cavity that is formed transiently in the wake of the bullet as it releases its energy. For the interested reader, the comprehensive report by Belkin (22) regarding wound ballistics should be consulted for more information about this complex subject.

Careful inspection of the wounds of entrance and exit through the scalp and skull are invaluable in determining the course of a bullet. The patterns of entrance and exit bullet wounds of the skull are identified by the characteristic beveling of the skull's inner and outer tables. The larger bevel invariably occurs on the side opposite the entry point of the bullet in the bone (see Fig. 17.18). Linear fractures of the vault and base of the skull regularly radiate from points of entry and exit from the skull.

Other injuries are found at a distance from the course of the bullet. Herniation contusions are typically found on the unci along the margins of the tentorium and in the medulla and the cerebellar tonsils along the rim of the foramen magnum. Such damage was reported in 85% of deaths from civilian gunshot wounds of the brain (137). Based on these observations death is believed to be caused by acute pressure on the brain stem from passage of the bullet through the brain. Contusions along the margin of the falx occur not infrequently, and contusions of the inferior frontal lobes were found in 24% of fatal civilian gunshot wounds of the brain (137). Unilateral or bilateral orbital plate fractures are also frequently encountered.

If the patient survives the initial head injury, residual neurologic deficits, cerebrospinal fistulas and secondary infections be-

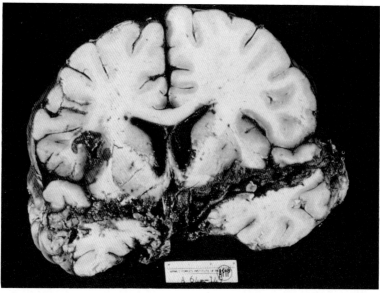

Figure 17.17.   Perforating gunshot wound of head. Note a single track traverses the brain.

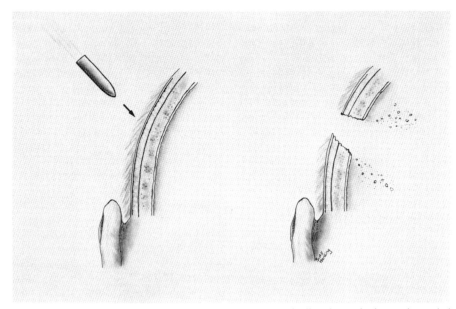

Figure 17.18.   Diagram depicting the entrance path of a bullet through the scalp and skull.

come problems. Infections may develop as complications of cerebrospinal fistulas, surgical intervention, displaced bone chips, or retained missile fragments (208). Meningitis or abscesses can occur months to years after injury.

Other Missile Wounds

Although gunshots cause the overwhelming majority of open craniocerebral wounds, such injuries can be produced in many other ways. Potentially, any sharp instrument can penetrate the skull, particularly through the thin orbital roof or squamous portion of the temporal bone. Periorbital punctures may appear superficial and may be considered trivial until a delayed complication like meningitis or brain abscess appears (35). Intracranial penetration of the orbital plate by an ordinary lead pencil is notorious for producing such injuries in a young child who accidentally falls on a pencil. Likewise, in falls or in vehicle accidents any protruding sharp object can be driven through the skull into the brain and create an open wound. Crushing blows of the cranium may also produce extensive bursting fractures and open craniocerebral wounds. Such devastating injuries are practically always fatal. Finally, severe scalp injuries and compound depressed skull fractures have been reported,

rarely, in young infants and children who have suffered severe dog bites of the head (259).

Emboli

Nonthrombotic embolic injuries of the brain and spinal cord may develop after blunt trauma, such as complications from cardiovascular and neurosurgical procedures, central and peripheral venous catheterization, mechanical ventilation of neonates, and dysbarism. Fat, air, and other particulate material form the emboli.

FAT

Fat emboli to the lungs occur regularly after severe injuries to soft tissues and bones of accident victims (24). With such damage, and particularly with long bone fractures, the fat embolism syndrome develops in a small percentage (<10%) of casualties (24). Such patients typically have fever, dyspnea, and tachypnea; restlessness and confusion; petechiae in the skin and conjunctiva; bilateral diffuse alveolar infiltrates on chest roentgenograms; hypoxemia and hypocalcemia; and lipuria (15, 34, 62, 242). The patients become confused and restless 2–3 days after injury, and some progress to stupor, coma, and death.

In the fat embolism syndrome, the brain may appear normal or contains widely distributed petechial hemorrhages of the white matter (Fig. 17.19). Fat emboli will be demonstrable in both pulmonary and cerebral vessels by staining them with fat-soluble dyes like oil red 0 or sudan IV. Earlier studies indicate that both depot fat released from the injured tissues and plasma fat coalesced by injury from free fatty acids make up the emboli (152). The delayed onset of injury of the lungs and brain is attributed to chemical injury produced by the embolized lipids and fatty acids. The respiratory distress syndrome evolves and is believed to be the principle cause of death in the fat embolism syndrome (258).

Fat globules most likely reach the systemic circulation through the alveolar capillaries (62); yet, there are reports that the fat may be shunted through a patent foramen ovale (192) and through bronchopulmonary or pulmonary arteriovenous shunts (171, 206). When fat emboli are not demonstrable in the brain, the patients have either not had cerebral symptoms or they have lived sufficient time for the body's normal healing responses to remove them. Even so, clinicopathologic correlations remain imperfect and need further clarification.

AIR

Air embolism has been recognized as a serious complication of open cardiovascular and neurosurgical procedures for many years, but the frequency with which they occur had not been accurately determined until recently (90). Air embolism was reported in 80% of 100 consecutive neurosurgical procedures evaluated (21) and in 0.2% of 3620 cardiopulmonary bypass operations examined (180). In addition air embolism has been reported as a serious, if not fatal, complication of coronary bypass surgery (25), positive pressure ventilation in neonates (178), central venous catheterization (205), and peritoneoscopy (173). Air embolism is an important feature in the pathogenesis of the pathologic changes in dysbarism and is discussed separately below.

The amount of air necessary to cause serious injury has not been established with certainty, although the studies of Bedford et al. (21) suggest that more than 20 ml of air are needed to cause paradoxical air embolism. When the right atrial pressure exceeds the pulmonary capillary wedge pressure, air can readily pass through a probe patent foramen ovale and cause damaging systemic air emboli. Even so, Bedford et al. observed only one such case among 29 patients who had such pressure reversal. Finally, it should be noted that shunting of air from the venous to the arterial circulations is not always dependent upon the presence of a septal defect (65).

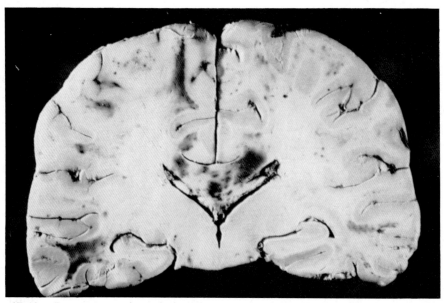

Figure 17.19. Posttraumatic fat embolism. Note multiple tiny hemorrhages in the corpus callosum and cerebral white matter.

Experimentally, cerebral air embolism causes severe cardiac arrhythmias and acute hypertension (81). That arrhythmias are mediated by the autonomic nervous system presumably would explain sudden death. With delayed death, multifocal discrete infarcts are found in the gray and white matter (92). Such injuries are believed to be a consequence of either decreased blood flow or arterial air embolism (81). Now, with the use of hyperbaric oxygen therapy, such damage may be minimized or averted (25).

OTHER

Patients undergoing open heart surgery may embolize calcified fragments from diseased valves (92). Other materials such as silicone have also caused damage (92).

Finally, brain tissue itself may be dislodged, enter a torn cerebral vein or lacerated venous sinus, and embolize to the pulmonary arteries (151). Brain emboli have been found in the pulmonary arteries of a hydrocephalic infant delivered vaginally after cranioclasty (72) and in an apparently normal infant following a breech delivery (72). They have also been reported in fatal gunshot wounds which traverse the venous sinuses (100).

SITES OF INJURY

Brain Stem Injuries

Direct injury of the brain stem has been recognized with increasing frequency in recent years. Such damage is found in combination with diffuse axonal injury, with fractures of the clivus, and fractures or fracture-dislocation of the cervical spine (3, 42, 47, 62, 89, 100, 141, 157, 181). Whether direct injury of the brain stem can occur alone is challenged by some (11). If such injuries occur they must be quite rare.

Contusions and lacerations of the pons occur with transverse fractures of the clivus. Lacerations of the cervicomedullary and pontomedullary junctions and cerebral peduncles result from hyperextension and basilar skull fractures or cervical fracture-dislocations (Fig. 17.5). Hemorrhages and necrosis of the rostral dorsal brain stem may involve the brachium conjunctivum and adjacent cerebellum (Fig. 17.9). In the past, such asymmetrical injuries have been

attributed to impacts of the incisura of the tentorium (125, 141); however, recently these lesions have been considered a component of diffuse axonal injury (6). In fact, such lesions have been found constantly with other components of diffuse axonal injury, namely, corpus callosal and diffuse white matter lesions.

Secondary injury of the brain stem occurs regularly with transtentorial herniation. These hernias not infrequently complicate supratentorial mass lesions like epidural and subdural hematomas. Rarely, entrapment of the posterior inferior cerebellar artery producing a medullary infarct is found after head injury (62). Finally, transneuronal degeneration with olivary hypertrophy may occur after injury of the central tegmental tract or dentate nucleus (62, 166).

Hypothalamus and Pituitary

Injuries of the hypothalamus and pituitary are found quite frequently in head-injured victims. The clinicopathologic syndromes of diabetes insipidus and inappropriate antidiuretic hormone (ADH) secretion may develop in surviving patients, particularly individuals with fractures of the sphenoid bone (53). Although these distinctive metabolic disturbances develop infrequently, injuries of the hypothalamus and pituitary are quite common and are reported in more than one-half of deaths caused by closed head trauma (62). In the comprehensive review by Crompton (54) ischemic or hemorrhagic lesions of the anterior hypothalamus were found in 42.5% of patients dying of acute closed (blunt) head injuries. Such lesions were often found in combination with skull fractures and contusions and/or lacerations at remote cortical sites. Likewise, damage of the pituitary was also frequently associated. In McCormick's comprehensive review, pituitary lesions were identified at autopsy in more than 60% of closed head injury victims (62). Among the lesions found, capsular hemorrhages, focal hemorrhages of the posterior lobe, and infarcts of variable size of the anterior lobe were encountered most often, while stalk lacerations and anterior hypophyseal hemorrhages were found in less than 10 per cent of such casualties.

Cranial Nerve Injury

Cranial nerve injuries are produced by both open and closed head trauma and are most frequently complications of basal skull fractures (2, 100, 106, 126, 161, 162, 166, 217). While missile wounds may produce damage to any cranial nerve, blunt trauma is more likely to damage the rostral cranial nerves (I to VIII). In closed (blunt) head injuries, the most frequently injured cranial nerve is reported to be the acoustic (VIII) nerve (126, 244). However, at autopsy the olfactory (I) and optic nerves (II) may be as frequently traumatized (93). The relative frequency with which each cranial nerve is injured is not well established, as such injuries are usually not well documented in autopsy reports. In the routine autopsy examination, the cranial nerves are *not* usually dissected beyond the point of their penetration of the dura and passage through the skull foramina. The inherent difficulties encountered in the removal and accurate dissection of the cranial nerves as they course through bone precludes doing such studies routinely.

OLFACTORY NERVE

Contusion or laceration of the olfactory bulbs (Fig. 17.2) is found frequently in closed head injuries associated with inferior frontal contusions, and fractures of the orbital plates may or may not be associated (126, 162).

OPTIC NERVE (II)

Direct and posttraumatic ischemic injury of the optic nerves and tracts occur in closed head injuries (52, 93, 100, 126, 162, 166, 222). Skull fractures may cause direct injury of the nerve segments in the optic foramen or optic chiasm (222). Diffuse axonal (shearing) injury with edema and ischemic necrosis of the optic nerve in the optic foramen and/or its intracranial segment are frequently encountered at autopsy in deaths caused by traumatic head injuries (52). Rarely, posttraumatic brain swelling with compression of the anterior choroidal artery will cause an infarct of an optic tract (166).

OCULOMOTOR NERVES (III, IV, AND VI)

Direct injuries of the oculomotor nerves may be produced by either penetrating or closed head injuries (126, 217). Penetrating injuries are usually produced by gunshots, the most frequent cause of direct injury of the third nerve. Basilar skull fractures produced by blunt trauma may also damage one or more of the oculomotor nerves. Damage may occur in the roots or intraosseus segments of the third, fourth, and sixth nerves; yet, avulsions are more apt to be seen with injuries of the fourth and sixth nerves (33, 217, 239). An oblique cranial blow may cause injury of one trochlear nerve, whereas frontal cranial blows have caused injury of both trochlear nerves. Such contusions are postulated to be caused by impaction of the nerves against the incisura of the tentorium. With occipitosphenoid synchondrosis separation or a clivus fracture, the sixth nerve may be directly injured (211).

Indirect injuries of the oculomotor nerves (III, IV, and VI) occur much more frequently than direct injuries and are nearly always the consequence of transtentorial herniation (100, 257). With herniation the hemorrhagic necrotic segment of the third nerve opposes the pulsating posterior cerebral artery (100, 211).

TRIGEMINAL NERVE (V)

Direct injury of this nerve rarely occurs, but when it does it is caused by basilar skull fractures involving the roots or intraorbital branches of the nerve (239).

FACIAL AND AUDITORY NERVES (VII AND VIII)

Fractures of the petrous portion of the temporal bone frequently cause direct injury of the facial and auditory nerves (190, 244). Transverse fractures are more likely to cause nerve injury than are longitudinal ones. Frontal or occipital impacts usually cause transverse fractures of the petrous bones, whereas lateral impacts will produce longitudinal fractures (244, 249). Delayed transient facial palsy may occur after closed head injuries and presumably is caused by swelling of the intraosseus segment of the nerve (126).

Traumatic Arterial Injuries

Severe closed or open head injuries may occasionally cause lacerations, avulsions, thromboses, and arteriovenous fistulas of intracranial arteries (166). The concomitant head and brain injuries may be slight or quite severe. The common or internal carotid arteries are thrombosed most frequently, with the vertebral arteries being involved less often and other arteries being thrombosed quite rarely. By comparison thromboses of the dural sinuses or cortical veins occur even less frequently following head injury (44, 164). Posttraumatic arteriovenous fistulas are found almost exclusively in the cavernous sinus. The cogent features of these posttraumatic vascular lesions are discussed in succeeding paragraphs.

A carotid artery occlusion is most often found several centimeters above the carotid bifurcation or in the carotid canal. The occlusion may develop in hours, days, or a few weeks after injury. Blunt trauma to the neck, hyperextension, and lateral flexion of the neck; paratonsillar trauma; or skull fractures involving the petrous bone may stretch the carotid arteries sufficiently to tear the intima and lead to secondary thrombosis (37, 71, 73, 129, 164, 203, 214, 248, 265). The resultant thrombotic occlusions may produce cerebral infarcts, and when they do, they usually cause significant neurologic impairment which may even result in death. Thromboses of the supraclinoid portion of the carotid arteries and the middle cerebral arteries have also been reported (153, 213). The vertebral arteries are most often damaged at the C5-6 interspace, the atlantoaxial joint, or the allanto-occipital joint (228, 233).

Carotid-cavernous fistulas most frequently develop following head trauma, particularly following blows to the frontal-temporal regions of the head. They are estimated to occur in approximately 2% of patients sustaining severe head injuries (220). Basal skull fractures or penetrating wounds cause tears of the tightly encased vessel in the carotid canal or contuse the vessel wall, leading to its later dehiscence. With development of a carotid-cavernous sinus fistula, marked venous engorgement occurs. Then chemosis and proptosis appear, and papilledema and optic atrophy with loss of vision may follow (14). When such fistulas are bilateral, the maintenance of cerebral perfusion may be sufficiently compromised to cause ischemic brain damage (14).

Traumatic aneurysms of the intracranial arteries have been described in superficial branches of the middle cerebral and anterior cerebral arteries most frequently (70, 117). However, they may also rarely develop in the anterior choroidal, posterior cerebral, superior cerebellar, vertebral, and posterior inferior cerebellar arteries (115, 165, 198, 200, 224). Most traumatic aneurysms are false aneurysms because the disrupted vessel wall is incorporated into the organized surrounding hematoma. When the vessel wall is partially disrupted, true aneurysmal dilation of the weakened vessel wall results. To distinguish traumatic aneurysms from congenital (saccular) aneurysms, the following criteria need to be satisfied. First, the aneurysm should be located peripherally at a nonbranching point of the artery; second, there should be delayed emptying and filling of the aneurysmal sac; third, a demonstrable neck of the aneurysm should be missing; and, fourth, the aneurysmal sac should have an irregular contour (198). Finally, multifocal injuries of the arterial wall adjacent to but not contiguous with the weakened vessel wall forming the aneurysm should be demonstrable (200). Whether closed head injury can cause rupture of a preexisting saccular congenital aneurysm remains debatable, even though such a relationship is alleged in litigation and workmen's compensation cases. Again, certain criteria should be met to satisfy such a relationship. The criteria listed by McCormick (165) include: (a) there should be clear and unequivocal evidence of significant head trauma; (b) the time relationships between trauma and the rupture of the aneurysm should be such that the likelihood of an association is present; (c) the location of the aneurysm relative to the objective evidence of trauma should be such that forces generated by trauma would impact the aneurysm. Even so, blunt trauma seems to have a very weak causal relationship for rupturing a preexisting saccular intracranial aneurysm (165).

Spinal Cord Injuries

Traumatic injuries of the spinal cord and the surrounding vertebral column cause significant morbidity but are less likely to cause death than brain wounds. Such injuries are produced by both blunt trauma and missiles. With vertebral fractures, subluxation, and/or dislocation, the spinal cord may be contused over an extended area that is often well above and below the point of bruising (Fig. 17.20). Hemorrhagic necrosis ensues, and cylindrical areas of necrosis may extend a considerable distance above and below the initial point of injury. The spinal cord can be traumatized at multiple levels, and such injuries are reported in approximately 15% of patients who have sustained traumatic spinal cord injuries (166). Injuries to the cervical spinal cord are particularly devastating and frequently cause death. Cervical spinal cord injuries

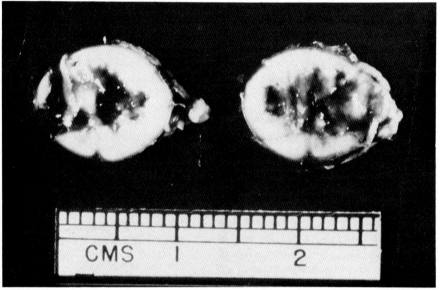

Figure 17.20. Hemorrhagic contusion of spinal cord caused by vertebral fracture dislocation.

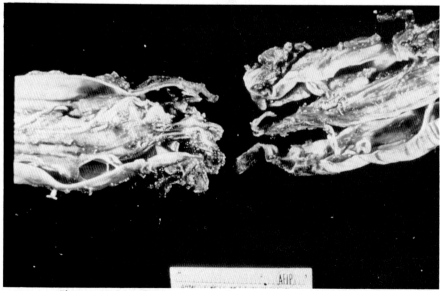

Figure 17.21. Remote traumatic transsection of spinal cord.

are also likely to coexist with brain injuries. Likewise, infarcts of the cervical cord can develop as a consequence of vertebral artery injury caused by hyperextension (224).

Standard autopsy techniques are often inadequate for good visualization of the cervical spine, spinal cord, and cervicomedullary junction. Hooper (115) has shown that excellent visualization can be obtained by changing the standard techniques for removal of the brain and spinal cord (115). He makes a midline incision from the top of the head of the sacrum. The skull is sawed in a circle from one side of the foramen magnum around the top of the skull to the other side of the foramen magnum. The lamina of the neural arches are sectioned. With removal of the posterior half of the skull and the posterior portions of the neural arches, the posterior cerebral hemispheres, cerebellum, cervical medullary junction, and spinal cord can be well visualized in situ. Then the brain and spinal cord can be removed intact, examined, and fixed for further study.

With recovery gliosis, cavitation and

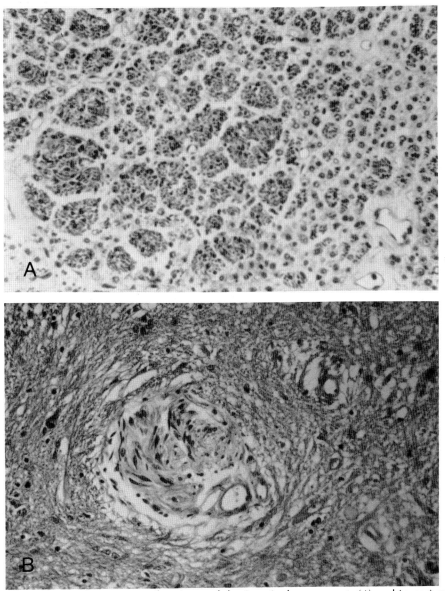

Figure 17.22. Traumatic neuromas forming nodules in spinal nerve roots (A) and in perivascular space of the spinal cord (B) years after injury of cauda equina. H&E. (Original magnification ×160).

complete transsection (Fig. 17.21) of the damaged cord may be seen. Ascending and descending Wallerian degeneration of injured fiber tracts evolve with atrophy of the affected tracts becoming readily apparent. In addition, two unique lesions, traumatic neuromas and posttraumatic syringomyelia, develop. The traumatic neuromas commonly form nodular masses in the region of the injured nerve roots and spinal cord and with time probably form in nearly all cases with significant spinal nerve injury (262) (Fig. 17.22). In the follow-up studies of Barnett and Jousse (19) posttraumatic syringomyelia was found in 2.3% of 934 paraplegics and 0.3% of 580 tetraplegics they have studied.

For more comprehensive information about the pathology of spinal cord and vertebral injuries, reviews by Jellinger (124) and Kakulas and Bedbrook (130) should be consulted.

BIRTH INJURY

Injuries of the brain and meninges may occur during the process of birth. The application of the forceps and compression of the skull against the pelvis during uterine contractions are believed to be the most significant factors causing these injuries (77). Birth injuries may involve the skull, meninges, brain, and spinal cord.

Linear and depressed skull fractures are seen rarely, and most do not have other associated injuries. So-called ping-pong fractures occur fairly frequently and are believed to be the result of pressure on the scalp from the mother's bony pelvis and are not related to forceps application (32). The ping-pong fracture is identified by a small or large depression in the skull and resembles such depressions formed on damaged ping-pong balls. These fractures are usually not associated with injury of the scalp or a subgaleal hematoma. Neurosurgeons usually recommend surgical treatment for ping-pong fractures if they do not resolve spontaneously in a few days.

Intradural hemorrhages are commonly found in infants of all ages, either as isolated or multiple lesions confined to the loose connective tissue of the dura mater (77). Such lesions have a predilection to occur in the falx cerebri or tentorium cerebelli and are usually not considered to cause or contribute to death.

Subdural hemorrhages resulting from tears of the free edge of the tentorium at its junction with the falx have been recognized for many years, and their frequency of occurrence increases with gestational age or birth weight (147). Lacerations of the falx cerebri are also reported in a small percentage of dural lacerations (94). The true frequency of occurrence of these lesions is not known; however, the continued improvements in obstetrical care have made their occurrence a rarity.

Subarachnoid hemorrhages occur with surprising frequency and have been reported in approximately 10% of all newborns (212). Such hemorrhages also seem to resolve with little or no adverse effect.

Epidural hemorrhages are distinctly rare in the neonate, and when they are found they are frequently associated with a fracture, often a depressed one (240). Subdural hematomas happen more often and tend to follow an acute progressive clinical course (9). Such bleeds may be resolved without need of surgical removal. Intraventricular and intracerebral hemorrhages that are now seen so frequently in the premature infant are not related to trauma but presumably to other factors like hypoxia.

Finally, spinal cord injuries, although quite rare, still occur (185, 227). The cervical or upper thoracic spinal cord is particularly susceptible to damage with the application of excessive traction during breech delivery. Now, such risks are minimized or avoided by delivering these infants by caesarean section. Extreme congestion and interstitial hemorrhage of the epidural adipose tissue of newborns has been observed frequently (247); however, its clinocopathologic relevance remains to be established.

CHILD ABUSE

Head injuries all too often disable or kill physically abused children (80, 133, 148, 189). In 1962 Kempe and coworkers (132) introduced the term "battered child syndrome" to characterize the uniqueness of these injuries. Subsequently, Dr. Kempe has been particularly successful in establishing the importance of this condition in the United States, as well as in other nations. Now laws exist in every state of the United States mandating reports on all cases of suspected child abuse (189). Nevertheless, cases of child abuse are still missed. Physicians, including knowledgeable pathologists, are often reticent to take the necessary action to ensure that such cases are handled appropriately. How often such injuries occur is still difficult to determine exactly, but in one recent study 13% of acute head injuries in children under 18 years of age were attributed to child abuse (270). Violence toward children is a leading cause of mortality. In children less than 3 years old, deaths are usually attributed to intrafamilial child abuse, whereas in children over 12 years of age, deaths are related to extrafamilial criminal acts or arguments (123). Young children, usually less than 2 years of age, and infants are particularly vulnerable to abuse, with beating or shaking being the ways most injuries are produced. With child abuse significant risks of mental retardation, psychological impairment, neurological impairment, or death caused by intracranial injuries are observed (133, 189, 270). In Table 17.7 the distribution of injuries demonstrated by computed tomography in 26 battered children is listed (270). Note that injuries attributed to shaking were identified in 10 of 15 patients with interhemispheric hematomas and 80% of the cases with retinal hemorrhages.

Bruises and fractures of different ages commonly accompany the craniocerebral injuries produced by beatings. Bruises of different ages distributed in an "assaultive" pattern are considered pathognomonic for child abuse (189). Bruises of the chest, back, buttocks, thighs, upper arms, or face are considered "assaultive" and are only rarely the consequence of accidental injury at play. When such injuries are symmetrical and bilateral, the concern for child abuse is even more compelling (145). "Pat-

17.7
Initial Findings in Child Abuse (26 Cases)

Findings	%
Hematomas, subdural and intracerebral	69
Hygromas, subdural	12
Brain swelling	50
Cerebral contusions	4
Cerebral infarcts	12
Skull fractures	23
Cutaneous bruises	31
Retinal hemorrhages	65

terned" bruises may provide a clue as to how a given injury was produced. For example, gripping or pinching of the cheeks or arms produces circular bruises, whereas blows with belts, straps, or sticks typically cause parallel bruises. The resultant patterned bruises (circular or parallel) make the suspicion of child abuse very great. The epiphyseal-metaphyseal junctions of long bones are particularly vulnerable to injury by pulling, jerking, or shaking. By comparison, external signs of head injury are apt to be missing in victims with shaking injuries, even though severe or lethal injury of the brain may be present (270). Metaphyseal avulsions and subperiosteal hemorrhages are produced by grabbing the infants by the extremities and shaking them. Shaking in turn causes the intracranial injuries and retinal hemorrhages that are frequently associated with such assaults (36).

Although direct cranial blows often produce bruises of the scalp, they do not always do so. Such blows may cause skull fractures with or without severe injury of brain and meninges. In young children, falls from heights of 3 ft or less rarely produce significant brain injury, and even falls from heights up to 10 ft seldom cause serious head injury (55, 107). Hence, serious brain injury in children attributed to falls, particularly out of bed, must always be suspect for child abuse. The morbidity and mortality caused by child abuse are most frequently due to injuries of the brain. Subdural hematomas are the most serious of the injuries found, but any of the primary types of injury and even an infarct may result (176). Depressed skull fractures frequently tear the dura and cause cerebral contusions, and in one report such injuries were found in 20% of 323 cases (102).

Interhemispheric hemorrhage in the parieto-occipital region is a typical feature of injuries caused by violent shaking (Fig. 17.23) (269, 271). Intracerebral hematomas, particularly of the parasagittal frontal white matter, are also demonstrated occasionally (Fig. 17.16). In the reports by Lindenberg and Freytag (156, 159), such lesions were believed to be induced by blunt trauma, but whether shaking injury in child abuse was an underlying cause is not addressed. The studies of Voight et al. (256) would support the thesis that such intra-

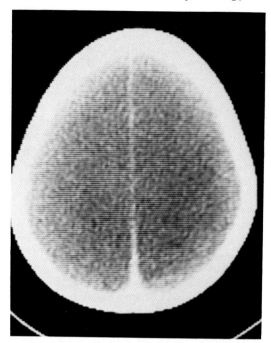

Figure 17.23. Interhemispheric hemorrhage and brain swelling seen by means of computed tomography in young victim of child abuse.

cerebral hematomas could be produced by rotational acceleration of the head, as such movements occur with shaking or whiplash injuries (256). The recent experience of Zimmerman et al. (270) documented permanent neurologic sequelae in a high percentage (53%) of child abuse cases. These observations suggest that diffuse axonal injury may be a significant feature of shaking injuries (271). Although retinal hemorrhages commonly result from violent shaking (36), they may also occur in response to increased intracranial pressure not related to traumatic injury (20).

DYSBARISM

The general term "dysbarism" is applied to any group of symptoms produced by rapid pressure changes encountered among sport (SCUBA) divers, military and commerical divers, high altitude personnel exposed to hypobaric decompression, and compressed air workers (98). Decompression sickness and air embolism identify the common forms of dysbarism.

Decompression sickness is characterized by joint pains, respiratory manifestations, skin lesions, and neurologic signs (43). The severe joint and bone pains cause writhing and are referred to as the "bends" by the afflicted victims. If the illness is limited and nonparalyzing, it is categorized as Type I decompression sickness. If paralysis or other neurologic abnormalities appear, the illness is then classified as Type II decompression sickness. Any part of the nervous system may be affected, and paralysis, particularly paraplegia, may result. In severe cases the damage is permanent and often disabling. For example from 1976 to 1979, 59% of 210 civilian and military patients treated for dysbarism in Hawaii had Type II decompression sickness (138).

Decompression illness particularly affects the lower thoracic and lumbar spinal cord, and damage of the spinal cord occurs in two-thirds of serious (Type II) cases of decompression sickness (138). Experimental studies have demonstrated that the white matter of the spinal cord in the watershed regions of the thoracic and lumbar areas of the spinal cord are especially likely to be damaged (110). Nevertheless, only a few reports have demonstrated these injury patterns in humans (99, 103–105, 196). In my personal experience, tiny spots of softening may be grossly visible, and necrotic foci with disruption of the myelin sheaths and axons are found microscopically. With inflammation and repair, inflammatory cells remove cellular debris, and glial scars form. With recovery, axonal injury is appreciated by the presence of reactive axonal swellings (Fig. 17.24A and B) and Wallerian degeneration.

Recent studies of decompression sickness suggest that gas bubbles form extravascularly in tissue interfaces, since the pia arachnoid meninges form a rigid outer casing against which a cord enlarged by internal gas formation can no longer expand without greatly elevating the pressure within the cord itself. The gas bubbles then compress the tissues and cut off the blood supply by producing pressure which equals or exceeds the perfusion pressure (110). In the spinal cord this injury pattern occurs most frequently in the watershed zones (T_4 and L_1) and would account for the clinical findings and readily explain the unique localization of injury to these regions (99, 196). Such a thesis would explain why spinal symptoms exceed cerebral symptoms

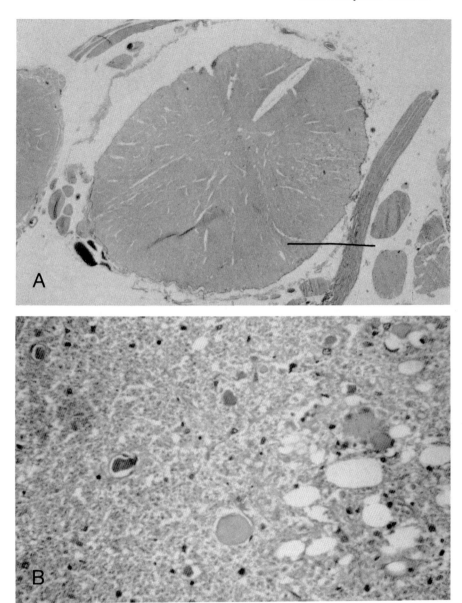

Figure 17.24. Decompression sickness, 28 days after SCUBA diving accident. (*A*) Focal necrosis of lower thoracic spinal cord. H&E. (Original magnification ×2). (*B*) Reactive axonal swelling in spongiotic area of *A*. H&E. (Original magnification ×160).

of neurological decompression sickness by about 3:1, even though the brain receives 75–85 times as much blood as the spinal cord. Therefore, the cerebral hemispheres should suffer embolic injury more severely if damage were strictly related to intravascular air emboli.

Air embolism is a feature of dysbarism in approximately 10% of patients requiring recompressive treatment (138). In this dis-

order involvement of the cerebrum is much more likely and may even be the cause of sudden death. Pathologically, the infarcts may vary from tiny foci of necrosis to large infarcts, depending on the size of an obstructed artery (Fig. 17.25*A* and *B*). Such infarcts are said to be located most frequently in the distribution of the middle cerebral artery or one of its branches and are indistinguishable grossly and micro-

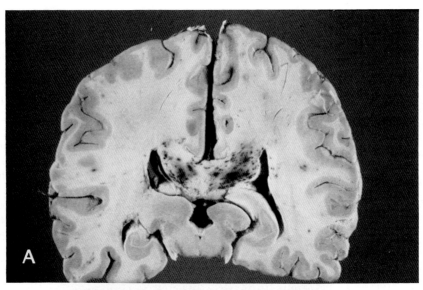

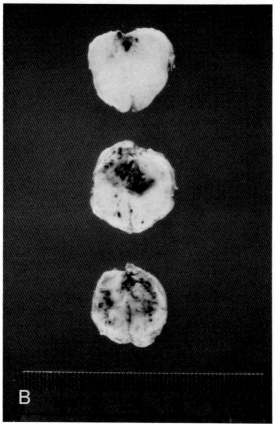

Figure 17.25.   Air embolism with hemorrhagic infarcts of corpus callosum (*A*) and caudal medulla oblongata (*B*), 5 days after SCUBA diving accident.

scopically from other infarcts, like those caused by arteriosclerosis. Infarcts caused by air emboli evoke the same inflammatory and repair responses seen with other destructive processes of the central nervous system.

BOXING INJURIES

Although pleas to ban or rigidly control boxing abound, wide public support for the sport continues (50). Unlike other sports the primary aim of the boxer is to inflict injury to his opponent. Both acute and chronic brain damage are produced, with death resulting occasionally (146). Blows to the head produce sudden rotational or angular acceleration of the movable head. These movements appear to be the most likely way serious injuries are caused (252). The bridging veins are torn between the brain and the superior sagittal sinus, and blood accumulates in the subdural space, causing compression, edema, and herniation of the brain. The resultant subdural hematomas are the most frequent cause of death among fighters (261). Hemorrhages can also be expected to occur in the deep cerebral white matter, corpus callosum, and cerebellar peduncles. After a knockout (cerebral concussion), the boxer may hit the ropes or mat and sustain contrecoup cortical contusions of the inferior frontal and temporal lobes.

Finally, chronic brain damage emerges as the cause of the punch-drunk syndrome (dementia pugilistica) and develops in up to 20% of professional boxers (49, 210). Recent studies indicate that the number of bouts, rather than the number of knockouts, correlates best with the development of this disorder (40, 216). The victims have speech difficulties, clumsiness, disequilibrium or ataxia, spasticity, and extrapyramidal disturbances. Ventricular dilation, with fenestration of the septum pellucidum and cerebral atrophy, are noted. Widespread neuronal degeneration with neurofibrillary tangles is found in the brains of demented ex-boxers (Fig. 17.26). The medial temporal cortex, the amygdaloid nucleus, and the hippocampal gyrus are preferentially involved. Unlike Alzheimer's disease, neuritic (senile) plaques are either absent or barely discernible. Depigmentation of the substantia nigra correlates with the extrapyramidal signs of parkinsonism (49). Loss of Purkinje cells in the cerebellar tonsils has also been described.

SECONDARY BRAIN LESIONS

Once brain injury has occurred, a series of more or less predictable pathophysiologic events ensue. Among them, brain swelling, hemorrhage, and neuronal damage with or without increased intracranial pressure and herniations is most significant.

Although most lethal injuries involve the central nervous system, visceral, soft-tissue, and skeletal injuries commonly accom-

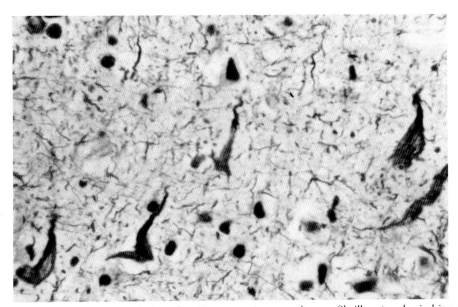

Figure 17.26.   Pugilistic encephalopathy. Note prominence of neurofibrillary tangles in hippocampal neurons and absence of neuritic (senile) plaques. Bodian silver. (Original magnification ×160).

pany them. Blood loss with hypotension and hypoxia contribute to cerebral edema and hypoxic encephalopathy. Hypoxia produces variable damage but gray matter, particularly in the anastomotic border zones between the major cerebral and cerebellar arteries, hippocampi, and basal ganglia, is especially vulnerable (82). Such ischemic damage was identified in 91% of 151 consecutive cases of deaths from nonmissile head injury examined (95).

Following closed head injuries with significantly increased intraventricular pressure (>40 mm Hg), pressure necrosis in one or both parahippocampal gyri is found in more than 90% of cases (4) (Fig. 17.27). There is also a concomitant high incidence of calcarine infarcts and pressure necrosis in the cingulate gyrus. In addition reports have documented that with increased intracranial pressure, regardless of its origin, any major artery of the circle of Willis can be obstructed and can produce an infarct (154, 158, 161).

Primary injuries of the central nervous system are frequently localized and produce swelling and bleeding. The mass effect of such lesions predisposes the injured brain to herniate from one cranial compartment to another. Subfalcial hernias usually shift the anterior cerebral arteries, but they do not produce specific neurologic deficits. On the other hand, transtentorial and foraminal herniations are life threatening. Most frequently, transtentorial herniation displaces the rostral brain stem caudally, tethers the oculomotor nerves against the posterior cerebral arteries, and dislocates the midline penetrating arterial branches supplying the tegmental gray matter of the midbrain and rostral pons. The resultant hemorrhages and focal necroses often lead to coma and death. In fact, any structure that traverses the incisura of the tentorium cerebelli can be damaged (114, 141–144, 161). Likewise, increased intracranial pressure may be sufficiently great so as to interfere with the blood supply to the pituitary and cause necrosis, usually of the anterior lobe (58). This reaction is also frequently found in those injured patients maintained on mechanical respirators (163).

Finally, with injury of the neuron and its

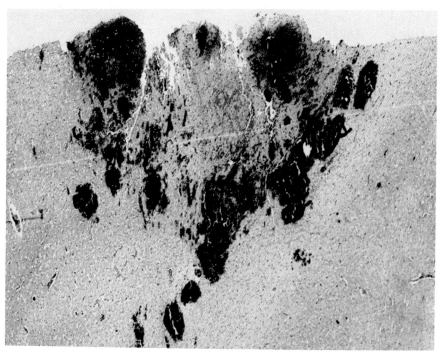

Figure 17.27. Herniation contusion of uncus against the margin of the tentorium cerebelli in a patient with prolonged increased intracranial pressure caused by large subdural hematoma. H&E. (Original magnification ×25).

processes, Wallerian, retrograde, and transneuronal degeneration occur. The morphologic details of how the neuron responds to injury is discussed in more detail in an earlier chapter. In the future I believe that ways in which transneuronal degeneration can be better studied will likely provide a clearer understanding of the pathophysiologic effects of traumatic brain injuries.

UNSPECIFIC CHANGES

Many unspecific changes may be found which can be easily misinterpreted by the unwary observer. Recognition of alterations related to postmortem trauma is particularly important. Lacerations of the spinal cord, cerebral peduncles, cranial nerves, and corpus callosum are easily produced during removal of the brain. The corpus callosum is often cut to facilitate fixation, but since this area is selectively injured in diffuse axonal injury, we strongly discourage this practice to minimize confusing gross and microscopic artifacts. Finally, intravital hemorrhage is considered to be one of the earliest signs of injury; yet, small petechial hemorrhages, particularly of the hypothalamus and pontine tegmentum, are noted occasionally in patients dying from disorders not related to trauma and are believed to be more common in patients with short agonal periods associated with severe hypoxemia (20).

ACKNOWLEDGMENT

"Mahalo" to Haruko Hazama for typing this manuscript.

References

1. Abbott WD, Due FO, Nosik WA: Subdural hematoma and effusion as a result of blast injuries. *Bull Amer Coll Surg* 28:123, 1948.
2. Adams H, Graham DI: Pathology of blunt head injuries. In *Scientific Foundations of Neurology.* Philadelphia, FA Davis, 1972, pp 478–491.
3. Adams JH: The neuropathology of head injuries. In Vinken PJ, Bruyn GW (eds): *Handbook of Clinical Neurology.* Amsterdam, North-Holland, 1975, vol 23, p 35.
4. Adams JH, Graham DI: The relationship between ventricular fluid pressure and the neuropathology of raised intracranial pressure. *Neuropathol Appl Neurobiol* 2:323, 1976.
5. Adams JH, Mitchell DE, Graham DI, Doyle D: Diffuse brain damage of immediate impact type. *Brain* 100:489, 1977.
6. Adams JH, Graham DI, Scott G, Parker LS, Doyle D: Brain damage in fatal non-missile head injury. *J Clin Pathol* 33:1132, 1980.
7. Adams JH, Graham DI, Gennarelli TA: Acceleration induced head injury in the monkey. *Acta Neuropathol* (Suppl) 7:26, 1981.
8. Allen IV, Scott, R, Tanner JA: Experimental high-velocity missile head injury. *Injury* 14:183, 1982.
9. Alvarez-Garijo JA, Gomila DT, Aytes AP, Mengual MV, Martin AA: Subdural hematomas in neonates. Surgical treatment. *Child's Brain* 8:31, 1981.
10. Anderson FM: Subdural hematoma, a complication of operation for hydrocephalus. *Pediatrics* 10:11, 1952.
11. Anderson JR, Treip CS: Hypertrophic olivary degeneration and Purkinje cell degeneration in a case of long-standing head injury. *J Neurol Neurosurg Psychiatry* 34:826, 1973.
12. Annegers JF, Grabow JD, Kurland LT, Laws ER Jr: The incidence, causes and secular trends of head trauma in Olmstead County, Minnesota 1935–1974. *Neurology* 30:912, 1980.
13. Aronson SA, Okazaki H: A study of some factors modifying response of cerebral tissue to subdural hematomata. *J Neurosurg* 20:89, 1963.
14. Asari S, Nakamura S, Yamada O, Beck H, Sugatani H, Higashi T: Traumatic aneurysms of peripheral cerebral arteries. *J Neurosurg* 46:795, 1977.
15. Ashbaugh DG, Petty TL: The use of corticosteroids in the treatment of respiratory failure associated with massive fat embolism. *Surg Gynecol Obstet* 123:493, 1966.
16. Auer L: Disturbances of the coagulatory system in patients with severe cerebral trauma. I. *Acta Neurochir* 43:51, 1978.
17. Auer L: Disturbances of the coagulatory system in patients with severe cerebral trauma. II. *Acta Neurochir* 49:219, 1979.
18. Bakay L, Lee JC: *Cerebral Edema.* Springfield, IL, Charles C Thomas, 1965.
19. Barnett HJM, Jousse AT: Posttraumatic syringomyelia (cystic myelopathy). In Vinken PJ, Bruyn GW (eds): *Handbook of Clnical Neurology.* Amsterdam, North-Holland, 1976, vol 26, p 113.
20. Barsewisch B: *Perinatal Retinal Haemorrhages.* Berlin, Springer-Verlag, 1979, p 113.
21. Bedford RF, Marshall WK, Butler A, Welsh JE: Cardiac catheters for diagnosis and treatment of venous air embolism: a prospective study in man. *J Neurosurg* 55:610, 1981.
22. Belkin M: Wound ballistics. *Prog Surg* 16:7, 1978.
23. Bell WE, McCormick WF: *Major Problems in Clinical Pediatrics. Increased Intracranial Pressure in Children,* Schafer AJ (ed). Philadelphia, WB Saunders, 1971, vol 8, pp 123–146.
24. Benatar SR, Ferguson AD, Goldschmidt RB: Fat embolism—some clinical observations and a review of controversial aspects. *Q J Med* 41:85, 1972.
25. Bove AA, Clark JM, Simon AJ, Lambertsen CJ: Successful therapy of cerebral air embolism with hyperbaric oxygen at 2.8 ATA. *Undersea Biomed Res* 9:75, 1982.
26. Braakaman R, Jennett B: Depressed skull fracture (non-missile). In Vinken PJ, Bruyn GW (eds): *Handbook of Neurology.* Amsterdam, North-Holland, 1975, vol 23, p 403.
27. Brandt RA: Chronic spinal subdural haematoma. *Surg Neurol* 13:121, 1980.
28. Britt RH, Herrick MK, Mason RT, Dorfman LJ: Traumatic lesions of the ponto-medullary junction. *Neurosurgery* 6:623, 1980.
29. Brown FD, Mullan S, Duda EE: Delayed traumatic intracerebral hematomas. *J Neurosurg* 48:1019, 1978.
30. Bruce D, Obrist W, Zimmerman R, Bilaniuk L, Dolinskas C, Kuhl D, Schut L: The pathophysiology of acute severe brain swelling following pediatric head trauma. Cerebral blood flow and metabolism. *Acta Neurol Scand* 60(Suppl 72):372, 1979.
31. Bruce DA, Alavi A, Bilaniuk L, Dolinskas C, Obrist W, Uzzell B: Diffuse cerebral swelling following head injuries in children: the syndrome of "malignant brain edema." *J Neurosurg* 54:170, 1981.
32. Bruce DA: Special considerations of the pediatric age group. In Cooper PR (ed): *Head Injury.* Baltimore, William & Wilkins, 1982, p 315.

33. Burger LJ, Kalvin NH, Smith JL: Acquired leisons of the fourth cranial nerve. *Brain* 93:567, 1970.
34. Burgher LW, Dines DE, Linscheid RL, Didier EP: Fat embolism and the adult respiratory distress syndrome. *Mayo Clin Proc* 49:107, 1974.
35. Bursick DM, Selker RG: Intracranial pencil injuries. *Surg Neurol* 16:427, 1981.
36. Caffey J: The whiplash shaken infant syndrome: manuel shaking by the extremities with whiplash-induced intracranial and intraocular bleedings, linked with residual permanent brain damage and mental retardation. *Pediatrics* 54:396, 1974.
37. Calhoun CL: Cerebral infarction due to internal carotid hypoplasia precipitated by head injury. *South Med J* 65:114, 1972.
38. Calkins RA, Van Allen MW, Sahs AL: Subdural hematoma following pneumoencephalography. *J Neurosurg* 27:56, 1967.
39. Carter LP, Pitman HW: Posterior fossa subdural hematoma of the newborn. *J Neurosurg* 34:423, 1971.
40. Casson IR, Sham R, Campbell EA, Tarlau M, Didmenico A: Neurological and CT evaluation of knocked-out boxers. *J Neurol Neurosurg Psychiatry* 45:170, 1982.
41. Clark JM: Distribution of microglial clusters in the brain after head injury. *J Neurol Neurosurg Psychiatry* 37:463, 1974.
42. Clifton GL: McCormick WF, Grossman RG: Neuropathology of early and late deaths after head injury. *Neurosurgery* 8:309, 1981.
43. Cockett ATK, Pauley SM, Zehl DN, Pilmanis AA, Cockett WS: Pathophysiology of bends and decompression sickness. An overview with emphasis on treatment. *Arch Surg* 114:296, 1979.
44. Cohn D, Streifler M: Post-traumatic thrombosis of cerebral and neck blood vessels. *Bull Los Angeles Neurol Soc* 39:60, 1974.
45. College of American Pathologists News Release: Pathologists say alcohol factor far greater than suspected in motor vehicle accidents. Skokie, IL, December 26, 1983.
46. Cooper PR: Epidemiology of head injury. In Cooper PR (ed): *Head Injury.* Baltimore, Williams & Wilkins, 1982, p 1.
47. Cooper PR, Maravilla K, Kirkpatrick J, Moody SF, Sklar FH, Diehl J, Clark WK: Traumatically induced brain stem hemorrhage and the computed tomographic scan: clinical, pathological and experimental observations. *Neurosurgery* 4:115, 1979.
48. Cordobes F, Lobato RD, Rivas JJ, Munoz MJ, Chillon D, Portillo JM, Lamas E: Observations on 82 patients with extradural hematoma. *J Neurosurg* 54:179, 1981.
49. Corsellis JAN, Bruton CJ, Freeman-Browne D: The aftermath of boxing. *Psychol Med* 3:270, 1973.
50. Council on Scientific Affairs: Brain injury in boxing. Council report. *JAMA* 249:254, 1983.
51. Cowan DH: The platelet defect in alcoholism. *Ann NY Acad Sci* 252:328, 1975.
52. Crompton MR: Visual lesions in closed head injury. *Brain* 93:785, 1970.
53. Crompton MR: Hypothalamic lesions following closed head injury. *Brain* 94:165, 1971.
54. Crompton MR: Hypothalamic and pituitary lesions. In Vinken PJ, Bruyn GW (eds): *Handbook of Clinical Neurology.* Amsterdam, North-Holland, 1975, vol 23, p 465.
55. Cummins D, Potter J: Head injury due to falls from heights. *Injury* 2:61, 1970.
56. Da Costa DG, Adson AW: Subdural hygroma. *Arch Surg* 43:559, 1941.
57. Dandy WE: Chronic subdural hygroma and serious meningitis (pachymeningitis serosa; localized external hydrocephalus). In Lewis D (ed): Hagerstown, MD, WF Prior Co, 1955, vol 12, p 291.
58. Daniel PM, Spicer EJF, Treip CS: Pituitary necrosis in patients maintained on mechanical respirators. *J Pathol* 111:135, 1973.
59. Davidoff IM, Feiring EH: Subdural hematoma occurring in surgically treated hydrocephalic children. With a note on a method of handling persistent accumulations. *J Neurosurg* 10:557, 1953.
60. Dawson SL, Hirsch CS, Lucas FV, Sebek BA: The contrecoup phenomenon. *Human Pathol* 11:155–165, 1980.
61. De Grood MPAM: Skull fractures. In Vinken PJ, Bruyn GW (eds): *Handbook of Neurology.* Amsterdam, North-Holland, 1975, vol 23, p 387.
62. Dines DE, Burgher LW, Okasaki H: The clinical and pathologic correlation of fat embolism syndrome. *Mayo Clin Proc* 75:407, 1975.
63. Edelson RN: Spinal subdural hematomas. In Vinken PJ, Bruyn GW (eds): *Handbook of Clinical Neurology.* Amsterdam, North-Holland Publishing Co, 1976, vol 26, p 31.
64. Ehler E, Ivankievicz D, Schomacher GH: Diagnosis of skull fractures by autopsy and radiology. *Acta Morphol* 28:291, 1980.
65. Evans DE, Kobrine AI, Weatherby PK, Bradley ME: Cardiovascular effects of cerebral air embolism. *Stroke* 12:338, 1981.
66. Fatteh A: *Medicolegal Investigation of Gunshot Wounds.* Philadelphia, JB Lippincott, 1976, p 101.
67. Feigin I, Popoff N: Neuropathological observations on cerebral edema. *Arch Neurol* 6:151, 1962.
68. Feigin I: Sequence of pathological changes in brain edema. In Klatzo I, Seitelberger F (eds): *Brain Edema.* New York, Springer-Verlag, 1967, pp 129–151.
69. Flamm ES, Demopoulous HB, Seligman MI, Tomasula JJ, DeCrescito V, Ransohoff J: Ethanol potentiation of central nervous system trauma. *J Neurosurg* 46:328, 1977.
70. Fleischer AS, Patton JM, Tindall GT: Cerebral aneurysms of trauma origin. *Surg Neurol* 4:233, 1975.
71. Fleming JFR, Petrie D: Traumatic thrombosis of the internal carotid artery with delayed hemiplegia. *Can J Surg* 11:166, 1968.
72. Fobes CD, Hirst AE: Brain embolism to the lung, a complication of breech delivery. *JAMA* 218:735, 1971.
73. Frantzen E, Jacobson HH, Therkelsen J: Cerebral artery occlusions in children due to trauma to the head and neck. *Neurology* 11:695, 1961.
74. French BN, Dublin AB: The value of computerized tomography in the management of 1000 consecutive head injuries. *Surg Neurol* 7:171, 1977.
75. Freytag E: Autopsy findings in head injuries from firearms. Statistical evaluation of 254 cases. *Arch Pathol* 76:215, 1963.
76. Freytag E: Autopsy findings in head injuries from blunt forces. Statistical evaluation of 1367 cases. *Arch Pathol* 75:402, 1963.
77. Friede RL: Cerebral lesions from physical trauma. In Friede RL (ed): *Developmental Neuropathology.* New York, Springer-Verlag, 1975, p 37.
78. Friede RL, Schachenmayr W: The origin of subdural neomembranes. *Am J Pathol* 92:69, 1978.
79. Gale JL, Dikmen S, Wyler A, Temkin N, McLean A: Head injury in the Pacific Northwest. *Neurosurgery* 12:487, 1983.
80. Galleno H, Oppenheim WL: The battered child syndrome revisited. *Clin Orthop* 162:11, 1982.
81. Garcia JH, Klatzo I, Archer T, Lassinsky AS: Arterial air embolism: structural effects on the gerbil brain. *Stroke* 12:414, 1981.
82. Garcia JH: Ischemic injuries of the brain. *Arch Pathol Lab Med* 107:157, 1983.
83. Gennarelli TA, Adams JH, Graham DI: Acceleration induced head injury in the monkey: the model, its mechanical and physiologic correlates. *Acta Neuropathol (Berl)* (Suppl) 7:23, 1981.
84. Gennarelli TA, Thibault LE: Biomechanics of acute subdural hematoma. *J Trauma* 22:680, 1982.
85. Gennarelli TA: Cerebral concussion and diffuse brain injuries. In Cooper PR (ed): *Head Injury.* Baltimore, William & Wilkins, 1982, p 83.

86. Gennarelli TA, Thibault LE, Adams JH, Graham DI, Thompson CJ, Marcincin RP: Diffuse axonal injury and traumatic coma in the primate. *Ann Neurol* 12:564, 1982.

87. Gennarelli TA, Spielman GM, Langfit TW: Influence of the type of intracranial lesion on outcome from severe head injury: a multicenter study using a new classification system. *J Neurosurg* 56:26, 1982.

88. Gikas P: Forensic aspects of the highway crash. In: *Pathology Annual*: 1983, part 2, Appleton-Century Crofts, Norwalk, p 147.

89. Gilbert JJ, Thierry D: Unusual brainstem findings following closed head injury. *J Pediatr* 81:343, 1972.

90. Gillen HW: Air embolism. In Vinken PJ, Bruyn GW (eds): *Handbook of Clinical Neurology. Injuries of the Brain and Skull Part I*. Amsterdam, North-Holland, 1975, vol 23, p 609.

91. Gilles FH, Shillito J Jr: Infantile hydrocephalus. Retrocerebellar subdural hematoma. *J Pediatr* 76:529, 1970.

92. Gilman S: Cerebral disorders after open-heart operations. *N Engl J Med* 272:489, 1965.

93. Gjerris F: Traumatic lesions of the visual pathways. In Vinken PJ, Bruyn GW (eds): *Handbook of Clnical Neurology*. Amsterdam, North-Holland, 1976, vol 24, p 27.

94. Goerttler K, Draisbach FJ: On the genesis of tentorium ruptures and intracranial hemorrhages. Formal basis and patho-anatomical findings. *Biol Neonate* 5:59, 1963.

95. Graham DI, Adams JH, Doyle D: Ischaemic brain damage in fatal non-missile head injuries. *J Neurol Sci* 39:213, 1978.

96. Groat RA, Windle WF, Magoun HW: Functional and structural changes in the monkey's brain during and after concussion. *J Neurosurg* 2:26, 1945.

97. Gurdjian ES, Brihaye J, Christenson JC, Frowein RA, Lindgren S, Luyendij KW, Norlen G, Ommaya AK, Oprescu I, de Vasconcellas Marques A, Vigouroux RP: Glossary of neurotraumatology. *Acta Neurochir (Wein)* (Suppl) 25:36, 1978.

98. Hallenbeck JM, Bove AA, Elliott DH: Mechanisms underlying spinal cord damage in decompression sickness. *Neurology* 25:308, 1975.

99. Halpern P, Greenstein A, Melamed Y, Margulies JY, Robin GC: Spinal decompression sickness with delayed onset, delayed treatment, and full recovery. *Br Med J* 284:1014, 1982.

100. Hardman JM: The pathology of traumatic brain injuries. *Adv Neurol* 22:15, 1979.

101. Harvey FH, Jones AM: "Typical" basilar skull fractures of both petrous bones: an unreliable indicator of head impact site. *J Forensic Sci* 25:280, 1980.

102. Harwood-Nash D, Hendrick EB, Hudson AP: The significance of skull fractures in children: a study of 1,187 patients. *Radiology* 101:151, 1975.

103. Haymaker W: Decompression sickness. In Scholz W (ed): *Handbuch Des Speziellen Pathologischen Anatomie und Histologie*. 1957, Pt 1, vol 13, p 1600.

104. Haymaker W, Davison C: Fatalities resulting from exposure to simulated high altitudes in decompression chambers. *J Neuropathol Exp Neurol* 98:29, 1950.

105. Haymaker W, Johnston AD: Pathology of decompression sickness. A comparison of the lesions in airmen with those in caisson workers and divers. *Milit Med* 117:285, 1955.

106. Heinze J: Cranial nerve avulsion and other neural injuries in road accidents. *Med J Aust* 2:1246, 1969.

107. Helfer RE, Slovis TL, Black M: Injuries resulting when small children fall out of bed. *Pediatrics* 60:533, 1977.

108. Hernesniemi J: Outcome following acute subdural haematoma. *Acta Neurochir* 49:191, 1979.

109. Hernesniemi J: Penetrating craniocerebral gunshot wounds in civilians. *Acta Neurochir (Wien)* 49:199, 1979.

110. Hills BA, James PB: Spinal decompression sickness: mechanical studies and a model. *Undersea Biomed Res* 9:185, 1982.

111. Hirano A: The fine structure of the brain in edema. In Bourne GH (ed): *The Structure and Function of Nervous Tissue*. New York, Academic Press, 1969, vol 2, pp 69–135.

112. Hirsch CS, Kaufman B: Contrecoup skull fractures. *J Neurosurg* 42:530, 1975.

113. Hirsh LF: Chronic epidural hematomas. *Neurosurg* 6:508, 1980.

114. Holbourn AHS: Mechanics of head injuries. *Lancet* 2:438, 1943.

115. Hooper AD: A new approach to upper cervical injuries. *J Forensic Sci* 24:39, 1979.

116. Iwakuma T, Brunngraber CV: Chronic extradural hematomas. A study of 21 cases. *J Neurosurg* 38:488, 1973.

117. Jackson FE, Gleave JRW, Janon E: The traumatic cranial and intracranial aneurysms. In Vinken PJ, Bruyn GW (eds): *Handbook of Clinical Neurology*. Amsterdam, North-Holland, 1976, vol 24, p 381.

118. Jackson IJ: Aseptic hemogenic meningitis. *Arch Neurol Psychiatry* 62:572, 1949.

119. Jamieson KG, Yelland JDN: Extradural hematoma: report of 167 cases. *J Neurosurg* 29:13, 1968.

120. Jamieson KG, Yelland JDN: Surgically treated traumatic subdural hematoma. *J Neurosurg* 37:137, 1972.

121. Jamieson, KG, Yelland JDN: Traumatic intracerebral hematoma. Report of 63 surgically treated cases. *J Neurosurg* 3:528, 1972.

122. Jamieson KG: Epidural haematoma. In Vinken PJ, Bruyn GW (eds): *Handbook of Clinical Neurology*. Amsterdam, North-Holland, 1976, vol 24, pp 261–274.

123. Jason J: Child homicide spectrum. *Am J Dis Child* 137:578, 1983.

124. Jellinger K: Neuropathology of cord injuries. In Vinken PJ, Bruyn GW (eds): *Handbook of Clinical Neurology*. Amsterdam, North-Holland, 1976, vol 25, p 43.

125. Jellinger K, Seitelberger F: Protracted post-traumatic encephalopathy, pathology, pathogenesis and clinical implications. *J Neurol Sci* 10:51, 1970.

126. Jennett WB: Injury to cranial nerves and optic chiasm. In Feiring EH (ed): *Brock's Injuries of the Brain and Spinal Cord and Their Coverings*, ed 5. New York, Springer, 1974, p 162.

127. Jennett B, Teasdale G, Galbraith S, Pickard J, Grant H, Braakman R, Avezaat C, Mass A, Minerhoud J, Vecht CJ, Heiden L, Small R, Catin W, Kurze T: Severe head injuries in three countries. *J Neurol Neurosurg Psychiatry* 40:291, 1977.

128. Jennett B, Teasdale G: *Management of Head Injuries*. Philadelphia, FA Davis, 1981, p 1.

129. Jernigan WR, Gardner WC: Carotid artery injuries due to closed cervical trauma. *J Trauma* 11:429, 1971.

130. Kakulas BA, Bedbrook GM: Pathology of injuries of the vertebral column. In Vinken PJ, Bruyn GW (eds): *Handbook of Clinical Neurology*. Amsterdam, North-Holland, 1976, vol 25, p 27.

131. Kalsbeek WD, McLaurin RL, Harris BSH III, Miller JD: The national head and spinal cord injury survey: major findings. *J Neurosurg* 53:519, 1980.

132. Kempe CH, Silverman FN, Steele BF, Droegemueller W, Silver NK: The battered child syndrome. *JAMA* 181:17, 1962.

133. Kempe CH, Helfer RE: *Helping the Battered Child and His Family*. Philadelphia, JB Lippincott, 1972.

134. Kernohan JW, Woltman HW: Incisura of the crus due to contralateral brain tumor. *Arch Neurol Psychiatry* 21:274, 1929.

135. Khalifeh RR, Van Allen MW, Sahs AL: Subdural hematoma following pneumoencephalography in an adult. *Neurology* 14:77, 1964.

136. Kingsley D, Till K, Hoare R: Growing fractures of the skull. *J Neurol Neurosurg Psychiatry* 41:312, 1978.

137. Kirkpatrick JB, Di Maio V: Civilian gunshot wounds of the brain. *J Neurosurg* 49:185, 1978.

138. Kizer KW: Dysbarism in paradise. *Hawaii Med J* 39:109, 1980.

139. Klauber MR, Barrett-Conner E, Marshall LF, Bowers SA: The epidemiology of head injury: a prospective study of an entire community—San Diego County, California, 1978. *Am J Epidemiol* 113:500, 1981.

140. Klauber MR, Marshall LF, Barrett-Conner E, Bowers SA: Prospective study of patients hospitalized with head

injury in San Diego County, 1978. *Neurosurgery* 9:236, 1981.

141. Klingle TG, Schulz R, Murphy MG: Pointine gaze paresis due to traumatic craniocerebral hyperextension. *J Neurosurg* 53:249, 1980.

142. Klintworth GK: Grooving of the uncus in the absence of intracranial disease. *J Forensic Med* 9:137, 1962.

143. Klintworth GK: Paratentorial grooving of human brains with particular reference to transtentorial herniation and the pathogenesis of secondary brainstem hemorrhages. *Am J Pathol* 53:391, 1968.

144. Klintworth GK: The pathogenesis of secondary brainstem hemorrhages as studied in an experimental model. *J Neurosurg* 17:368, 1968.

145. Laing S, Buchan A: Bilateral injuries in childhood: an alerting sign? *Br Med J* 2:940, 1976.

146. Lampert PW, Hardman JM: Morphologic changes in brains of boxers. *JAMA* 251:2676, 1984.

147. Larroche JC: Hemorrhagie cerebrales intraventriculaires chez le premature. *Biol Neonate* 7:26, 1964.

148. Lauer B, Broeck ET, Grossman M: Battered child syndrome: review of 130 patients with controls. *Pediatrics* 54:57, 1974.

149. Laun A: Traumatic cerebrospinal fluid fistulas in the anterior and middle cranial fossae. *Acta Neurochir (Wien)* 60:215, 1982.

150. LeCount ER, Apfelbach CW: Pathologic anatomy of traumatic fractures of cranial bones and concomitant brain injuries. *JAMA* 74:501, 1920.

151. Legier J, Rinaldi I: Gross pulmonary embolization with cerebral tissue following head trauma. Case report. *J Neurosurg* 39:109, 1972.

152. Lende RA, Erickson TC: Growing fractures of childhood. *J Neurosurg* 18:479, 1961.

153. Levy RL, Dugan TM, Bernat JL, Keating J: Lateral medullary syndrome after neck injury. *Neurology (Minneap)* 30:788, 1980.

154. Lindenberg R: Compression of brain arteries as pathogenetic factor for tissue necroses and their areas of predilection. *J Neuropathol Exp Neurol* 14:223, 1955.

155. Lindenberg R, Freytag E: Morphology of cortical contusions. *Arch Pathol* 63:23, 1957.

156. Lindenberg R, Freytag E: A mechanism of cerebral contusions. A pathologic-anatomic study. *Arch Pathol* 69:440, 1960.

157. Lindenberg R: Significance of the tentorium in head injuries from blunt forces. *Clin Neurosurg* 12:129, 1966.

158. Lindenberg R, Walsh FB: Vascular compression involving intracranial visual pathways. *Trans Am Acad Ophthalmol Otolarngol* 64:677, 1968.

159. Lindenberg R, Freytag E: Morphology of brain lesions from blunt trauma in early infancy. *Arch Pathol* 87:298, 1969.

160. Lindenberg R, Freytag E: Brainstem lesions characteristic of traumatic hyperextension of the head. *Arch Pathol* 90:509, 1970.

161. Lindenberg R: Trauma of meninges and brain. In Minckler J (ed): *Pathology of the Nervous System.* New York, McGraw-Hill, 1971, vol 2, p 1705.

162. Lindenberg R, Walsh FB, Sacks JG: *Neuropathology of Vision. An Atlas.* Philadelphia, Lea & Febiger, 1973.

163. McCormick WF, Halmi NS: The hypophysis in patients with *coma depasse* ("respirator brain"). *Am J Clin Pathol* 54:374, 1970.

164. McCormick WF, Schochet SS Jr: Brain herniation. In: *Atlas of Cerebrovascular Disease.* Philadelphia, WB Saunders, 1976, p 380.

165. McCormick WF: The relationship of closed-head trauma to rupture of saccular intracranial aneurysms. *Am J Forensic Med Pathol* 1:223, 1980.

166. McCormick WF: Trauma. In Rosenberg RN, Schochet SS Jr (eds): *The Clinical Neurosciences. Neuropathology.* New York, Churchill Livingstone, 1983, vol 3, p III:241.

167. McKissock W, Taylor JC, Bloom WH, Til K: Extradural hematoma-observation on 125 cases. *Lancet* 2:167, 1960.

168. McLaurin RL, Tutor FT: Acute subdural hematoma, review of ninety cases. *J Neurosurg* 18:61, 1961.

169. McLaurin RL, McLaurin KS: Clacified subdural hematomas in childhood. *J Neurosurg* 24:648, 1966.

170. Manz HJ: The pathology of cerebral edema. *Hum Pathol* 5:291, 1974.

171. Marchand P, Gilroy JC, Wilson VH: An anatomical study of the bronchial vascular system and its variations in disease. *Thorax* 5:207, 1950.

172. Markwalder T-M: Chronic subdural hematomas: a review. *J Neurosurg* 54:637, 1981.

173. Marquez J, Sladen A, Gendell H, Boehnke M, Mendelow H: Paradoxical cerebral air embolism without an intracardiac septal defect. Case report. *J Neurosurg* 55:997, 1981.

174. Mathur PPS, Dharker SR, Agarwall SK, Sharma M: Fluid chronic extradural haematoma. *Surg Neurol* 14:81, 1980.

175. Matson DD: Leptomeningeal cyst. In *Neurosurgery of Infancy and Childhood.* Springfield, IL, Charles C Thomas, 1969, p 304.

176. Ment LR, Duncan CC, Rowe DS: Central nervous system manifestations of child abuse. *Conn Med* 46:315, 1982.

177. Meredith JM: Chronic or subacute subdural hematoma. *J Neurosurg* 8:444, 1951.

178. Mikhael MA, Paise ML, Port RB: Detection of pneumocephaly secondary to mechanical ventilation in neonates. *CT* 5:328, 1981.

179. Miller JD, Sweet RC, Narayan R, Becker DP: Early insults to the injured brain. *JAMA* 240:439, 1978.

180. Mills NL, Ochsner JL: Massive air embolism during cardiopulmonary bypass. Causes, prevention, and management. *J Thorac Cardiovasc Surg* 80:708, 1980.

181. Mitchell DE, Adams JH: Primary focal impact damage to the brainstem in blunt head injuries. Does it exist? *Lancet* 2:215, 1973.

182. Munro D, Merritt HH: Surgical pathology of subdural hematoma. Based on a study of one hundred and five cases. *Arch Neurol Psychiatry* 35:64, 1936.

183. Munro D: Cerebral subdural hematoma: a study of three hundred and ten verified cases. *N Engl J Med* 227:87, 1942.

184. Naffziger HC: Subdural fluid accumulations following head injury. *JAMA* 82:1751, 1924.

185. Natelson and Sayers MP: The fate of children sustaining severe head trauma during birth. *Pediatrics* 51:169, 1973.

186. National Center of Health Statistics: *Vital Statistics of the United States, 1978,* Vol II, Part A, DHHS Pub No (PHS) 83-101. Washington, DC, Public Health Service, US Government Printing Office, 1982.

187. National Safety Council: *Body Area of Motor Vehicle Occupant Injured in Motor Vehicle Accident.* Chicago, National Safety Council, 1966.

188. Norman D, Price D, Boyd D, Fishman R, Newton TH: Quantitative aspects of computed tomography of blood and cerebrospinal fluid. *Radiology* 123:335, 1977.

189. Norton LE: Child abuse. *Clin Lab Med* 3:321, 1983.

190. Noseworthy JH, Miller J, Murray TJ: Auditory brainstem responses in postconcussion syndromes. *Arch Neurol* 38:275, 1981.

191. Obrist WD, Thompson HK Jr, Wang HS, Wilkinson WE: Regional cerebral blood flow estimated by 133^{Xenon} inhalation. *Stroke* 6:245, 1975.

192. O'Farrell PT: The clinical diagnosis of congenital heart disease. *Ir J Med Sci* 11:597, 1938.

193. Ommaya AK, Yarnell P: Subdural haematoma after whiplash injury. *Lancet* 2:237, 1969.

194. Oppenheimer DR: Microscopic lesions in the brain following head injury. *J Neurol Neurosurg Psychiatry* 31:299, 1968.

195. Osborn AG, Daines JH, Wing SD, Anderson RE: Intracranial air on computerized tomography. *J Neurosurg* 48:355, 1978.

196. Palmer AC, Calder IM, McCallum RI, Mastaglia FL: Spinal cord degeneration in a case of "recovered" spinal decompression sickness. *Br Med J* 283:888, 1981.

197. Parkinson D, Reddy V, Taylor J: Ossified epidural hematoma: case report. *Neurosurgery* 7: 171, 1980.

198. Parkinson D, West M: Traumatic intracranial aneu-

rysms. *J Neurosurg* 52:11, 1980.

199. Patscheider H: Zur Entstehung von Ringbruchen des Schadelgrundes. *Deutsch Z Ges Gerichtl Med* 52:13, 1962.

200. Paul GA, Shaw C-M, Wray IM: True traumatic aneurysm of the vertebral artery. *J Neurosurg* 53:101, 1980.

201. Peerless SJ, Rewcastle NB: Shear injuries of the brain. *Can Med Assoc J* 96:577, 1967.

202. Phonprasert C, Suwanwela C, Hongsaprabhas C, Prichayudh P, O'chavoen S: Extradural hematoma: analysis of 138 cases. *J Trauma* 20:679, 1980.

203. Pitner SE: Carotid thrombosis due to intraoral trauma. *N Engl J Med* 274:767, 1966.

204. Pitts LH: Medical complications of head injury. In Cooper PR (ed): *Head Injury.* Baltimore, William & Wilkins, 1982, p 327.

205. Ponsky JL, Pories WJ: Paradoxical cerebral air embolism. *N Engl J Med* 284:985, 1971.

206. Prinzmetal M, Ornitz EM Jr, Simkin B, Bergman HC: Arterio-venous anastomoses in liver, spleen and lungs. *Am J Physiol* 152:48, 1948.

207. Pudenz RH, Shelden CH: The leucite clavarium—a method for direct observation of the brain. II. Cranial trauma and brain movement. *J Neurosurg* 3:487, 1946.

208. Rish BL, Caveness WF, Dillon JD Jr, Kistler JP, Mohr JP, Weiss GH: Analysis of brain abscess after penetrating craniocerebral injuries in Vietnam. *Neurosurgery* 9:535, 1981.

209. Rivano C, Borzone M, Carta F, Michelozzi G: Traumatic intracerebral hematomas. Seventy-two cases surgically treated. *J Neurosurg Sci* 24:77, 1980.

210. Roberts AH: *Brain Damage in Boxers.* A study of the prevalence of traumatic encephalopathy among exprofessional boxers. London, Pitman Medical & Scientific Publishing Co, 1969.

211. Roberts M: Lesions of the ocular motor nerves (III, IV, and VI). In Vinken PJ, Bruyn GW (eds): *Handbook of Clinical Neurology.* Amsterdam, North-Holland, 1976, vol 24, p 59.

212. Roberts MH: The spinal fluid in the newborn with special reference to intracranial hemorrhage. *JAMA* 85:500, 1925.

213. Roessmann U, Miller RT: Thrombosis of the middle cerebral artery associated with birth trauma. *Neurology (Minneap)* 30:889, 1980.

214. Rose EF, O'Connor ML: Traumatic carotid artery occlusion. ASCP Check Sample-Forensic Pathology No. FP-78.

215. Rosenblum WI, Greenberg RP, Seelig JM, Becker DP: Midbrain lesions: frequent and significant prognostic feature in closed head injury. *Neurosurgery* 9:613, 1981.

216. Ross RJ, Cole M, Thompson JS, Kim KH: Boxers—computed tomography, EEG, and neurological evaluation. *JAMA* 249:211, 1983.

217. Rucker CW: The causes of paralysis of the third, fourth and sixth cranial nerves. *Am J Ophthalmol* 61:1293, 1966.

218. Russell R, Schiller F: Crushing injury of the skull: clinical and experimental observations. *J Neurol Neurosurg Psychiatry* 12:52, 1949.

219. St John JN, Dila C: Traumatic subdural hygroma in adults. *Neurosurgery* 9:621, 1981.

220. Sanders MD, Hoyt WF: Hypoxic ocular sequelae of carotid-cavernous fistulae. *Br J Ophthalmol* 53:82, 1969.

221. Sato O, Kamitani H, Kamitani T: Blow-in fractures of both orbital roofs caused by shear strain of the skull. *J Neurosurg* 49:734, 1978.

222. Savino PH, Glaser JS, Schatz NJ: Traumatic chiasmal syndrome. *Neurology (Minneap)* 30:963, 1980.

223. Schachenmayr W, Friede RL: The origin of subdural neomembranes. I. Fine structure of the dura-arachnoid interface in man. *Am J Pathol* 92:53, 1978.

224. Schneider RC, Schemm GW: Vertebral arterial insufficiency in acute and chronic spinal trauma. *J Neurosurg* 18:348, 1961.

225. Scotti G, Terbrugge K, Melancon D, Belanger G: Evaluation of the age of subdural hematomas by computerized tomography. *J Neurosurg* 47:311, 1977.

226. Sherwood D: Chronic subdural hematoma in infants. *Am J Dis Child* 39:980, 1930.

227. Shulman ST, Madden JD, Shankin DR, Esterly JR: Transection of the spinal cord. A rare obstetrical complication of cephalic delivery. *Arch Dis Child* 46:291, 1971.

228. Six EG, Stringer WL, Cowley AR, Davis CH Jr: Posttraumatic bilateral vertebral artery occlusion. *J Neurosurg* 54:814, 1981.

229. Snoek J, Jennett B, Adams JH, Graham DI, Doyle D: Computerized tomography after recent severe head injury in patients without acute intracranial haematoma. *J Neurol Neurosurg Psychiatry* 42:215, 1979.

230. Spatz H: Kann man alte Rindendefekte traumatischer und arteriosklerotischer Genese voneinauder unterscheiden? Die Bedeutung des Etat vermoulu. *Arch Psychiatry* 90:885, 1930.

231. Stapp JP: Trauma caused by impact and blast. *Clin Neurosurg* 11:324, 1966.

232. Stehbens WE: *Pathology of the Cerebral Blood Vessels.* St Louis, CV Mosby, 1972, pp 207–283.

233. Stern WE: Carotid-cavernous fistula. In Vinken PJ, Bruyn GW (eds): *Handbook of Clinical Neurology.* Amsterdam, North-Holland, 1976, vol 24, p 399.

234. Stone JL, Lang RGR, Sugar O, Moody RA: Traumatic subdural hygroma. *Neurosurgery* 8:542, 1981.

235. Strassman G: Formation of hemosiderin and hematoidin after traumatic and spontaneous cerebral hemorrhages. *Arch Pathol* 47:205, 1949.

236. Strich SJ: Cerebral trauma. In Blackwood W, Corsellis JAN (eds): *Greenfield's Neuropathology.* London, Edward Arnold, 1976.

237. Strich SJ: Diffuse degeneration of the cerebral white matter in severe dementia following head injury. *J Neurol Neurosurg Psychiatry* 19:163, 1956.

238. Strich SJ: Shearing of nerve fibers as a cause of brain damage due to head injury, a pathological study of twenty cases. *Lancet* 2:443, 1961.

239. Summers CG, Wirtschafter JD: Bilateral trigeminal and abducens neuropathies following low-velocity crushing head injury. *J Neurosurg* 50:508, 1979.

240. Takagi T, Nagai R, Wakabayashi S, Mizawa I, Hayashi K: Extradural hemorrhage in the newborn as the result of birth trauma. *Child's Brain* 4:306, 1978.

241. Taveras J, Ransokoff J: Leptomeningeal cysts of the brain following trauma with erosion of the skull: a study of seven cases treated by surgery. *J Neurosurg* 10:233, 1953.

242. Thomford NR, Sirinek KR: Fat embolism. In Vinken PJ, Bruyn GW (eds): *Injuries of the Brain and Skull. Part I. Handbook of Clinical Neurology.* Amsterdam, North-Holland, 1975, vol 23, p 631.

243. Till K: Subdural hematoma and effusion in infancy. *Br Med J* 3:400, 1968.

244. Toglia JU, Katinsky S: Neuro-otological aspects of closed head injury. In Vinken PJ, Bruyn GW (eds): *Handbook of Clinical Neurology.* Amsterdam, North-Holland, 1976, vol 24, p 119.

245. Tomlinson BE: Brain stem lesions after head injury. *J Clin Pathol* 23:(Suppl 4):154, 1970.

246. Tourtellote WW, Metz LN, Bryan ER, DeJong RN: Spontaneous subarachnoid hemorrhage. Factors affecting the rate of clearing the cerebrospinal fluid. *Neurology* 14:301, 1964.

247. Towbin A: Latent spinal cord and brain stem injury in newborn infants. *Dev Med Child Neurol* 11:54, 1969.

248. Towne NE, Neis DD, Smith JW: Thrombosis of the internal carotid artery following blunt cervical trauma. *Arch Surg* 104:565, 1972.

249. Travis LW, Stalnaker RL, Melvin JW: Impact of the human temporal bone. *J Trauma* 17:761, 1977.

250. US Bureau of the Census: *Statistical Abstract of the United States: 1982–83* (103rd edition). Washington, DC, 1982, p 76.

251. US Department of Health, Education, Welfare: *National Center for Health Statistics.* Hyattsville, MD, Vital Sta-

tistics of the United States 1975, 1979.

252. Unterharnscheidt F, Sellier K: Vom boxen mechanik, pathomophologie und klinik der traumatischn schaden des ZNS bei boxern. *Fortschr Neurol Psychiatr* 39:109, 1971.

253. Vance BM: Fractures of the skull. Complications and causes of death: a review of 512 necropsies and 61 cases studied clinically. *Arch Surg (Chicago)* 14:1023, 1927.

254. Van Gijn J, Wintzen AR: Whiplash injury and subdural haematoma. *Lancet* 2:592, 1969.

255. Verjaal A, van T Hooft F: Commotio and contusion cerebri (cerebral concussion). In Vinken PJ, Bruyn GW (eds): *Injuries of the Brain and Skull. Part I. Handbook of Clinical Neurology.* Amsterdam, North-Holland, 1975, vol 23, p 417.

256. Voight GE, Lowenhielm CGP, Ljung CBA: Rotational cerebral injuries near the superior margin of the brain. *Acta Neuropathol (Berl)* 39:201, 1977.

257. Weintraub CM: Bruising of the third cranial nerve and the pathogenesis of mid brain hemorrhage. *Br J Surg* 48:62, 1960.

258. Weisz GM, Steiner E: The cause of death in fat embolism. *Chest* 59:511, 1971.

259. Wilberger JE Jr, Pang D: Craniocerebral injuries from dog bites. *JAMA* 249:2685, 1983.

260. Wintzen AR: The clinical cause of subdural haematoma. *Brain* 103:855, 1980.

261. Wolff K: Boxsport und boxverletzungen. Eine kritische studie unter mitteilung eigener beobachtungen. *Dtsch Z Chir* 208:397, 1928.

262. Wolman L: Axon regeneration after spinal cord injury. *Paraplegia* 4:175, 1966.

263. World Health Organization: *World Health Statsitics Annual (1973–1976)* Geneva, World Health Organization, 1976.

264. Wuermeling von HB, Struck G: Brainstem ruptures in traffic accidents. *Beitr Gerichtl Med* 23:297, 1965.

265. Yamada S, Kindt GW, Youmans JR: Carotid artery occlusion due to non-penetrating injury. *J Trauma* 7:333, 1967.

266. Yashon D, Jane JA, White RJ, Sugar O: Traumatic subdural hematoma in infancy. *Arch Neurol* 18:370, 1968.

267. Yates AJ, Thelmo W, Pappins HM: Postmortem changes in the chemistry and histology of normal and edematous brains. *Am J Pathol* 79:555, 1975.

268. Young HA, Gleave JRW, Schmidek HH, Gregory S: Delayed traumatic intracerebral hematoma: report of 15 cases operatively treated. *Neurosurgery* 14:22, 1984.

269. Zimmerman RA, Bilaniuk LT, Bruce D, Schut L, Uzzell B, Goldberg HI: Interhemispheric acute subdural hematoma: a computed tomographic manifestation of child abuse by shaking. *Neuroradiology* 16:39, 1978.

270. Zimmerman RA, Bilaniuk LT, Brice D, Schut L, Uzzell B, Goldberg HI: Computed tomography of craniocerebral injury in the abused child. *Radiology* 130:6807, 1979.

271. Zimmerman RA, Bilaniuk LT: Head trauma. The clinical neurosciences. *Neuroradiology* 4:483, 1984.

Index

Page numbers in italics denote figures; those followed by "*t*" or "*f*" denotes tables or footnotes, respectively